ILLUSTRATED
Orthopedic Physical Assessment

ILLUSTRATED
Orthopedic Physical Assessment

Third Edition

RONALD C. EVANS, D.C., F.A.C.O., F.I.C.C.

Fellow, Academy of Chiropractic Orthopedists
Fellow, International College of Chiropractic
Diplomate, American Board of Chiropractic Orthopedists
Past-Chairman of the Iowa Board of Chiropractic Examiners of the Department of
Professional Licensure, State of Iowa, Des Moines, Iowa (Ret)
Examiner Emeritus, American Board of Chiropractic Orthopedists
Examiner Emeritus, Academy of Chiropractic Orthopedists
Member, Chiropractic Healthcare Benefits Advisory Committee, Department of
Defense, United States of America
Chief Executive Officer, Iowa Chiropractic Physicians Clinic, Des Moines, Iowa
Chairman, Department of Defense Committee, Foundation for Chiropractic
Education and Research
Chiropractic Orthopedist, Private Practice
Trustee and Vice President, Foundation for Chiropractic Education
and Research
Chair, Evidence-Based Resource Center, Foundation for Chiropractic
Education and Research

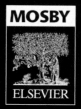

MOSBY

ELSEVIER

11830 Westline Industrial Drive
St. Louis, Missouri 63146

ILLUSTRATED ORTHOPEDIC PHYSICAL ASSESSMENT, Third Edition   ISBN: 978-0-323-04532-2
Copyright © 2009, 2001 by Mosby, Inc., an affiliate of Elsevier Inc.

ISBN: 978-0-323-04532-2

Vice President and Publisher: Linda Duncan
Senior Acquisitions Editor: Kellie F. White
Senior Developmental Editor: Jennifer Watrous
Associate Developmental Editor: Kelly Milford
Publishing Services Manager: Julie Eddy
Senior Project Manager: Andrea Campbell
Designers: Renee Duenow, Jessica Williams

Printed in Canada

Last digit is the print number: 9 8 7 6 5 4 3 2 1

DEDICATION

For Linda,

Inspiration Everlasting

For

PJS, VR, JG, KB, MAB, CG, LA, CH, KH, DH, RM, RS, JC, PS, MLP, DRG, NJR,

JS, MF, RH, MHN, SAA, EJW, MAN, LLS, FLVW, RMS, MHA, SMR, JD, CMC, MC, ADS . . .

and all other patients, past and present, participating in my continued search for their wellness . . .

For JRB

. . . because many scientific premises first illuminate in eddies of single malts, plumes of Cuban smoke, and at the end of tight lines . . . a consummate physician/scientist . . .

And finally,

For my mother:

An Irish woman who bore a Welsh son. I am blessed by her endless creativity and, compassion, and gift of gab. Were it not for her, I would have less to say . . . how very dull.

Dr. Ronald C. Evans is a Doctor of Chiropractic and a 1976 graduate of Northwestern Health Sciences Univeristy, and Chaired its Chiropractic Orthopedics Residency Program from 1980 to 1984. He is a Diplomate of the American Board of Chiropractic Orthopedists (DABCO) and Examiner Emeritus of that Board. He is a Fellow of the Academy of Chiropractic Orthopedists (FACO) and Examiner Emeritus of that Board. Dr. Evans is a Fellow of the International College of Chiropractors (FICC), and has lectured in orthopedics and neurology for 35 years, speaking extensively throughout the United States, Canada, New Zealand and Australia, and Scotland. Dr. Evans has lectured on the campuses of Northwestern Health Sciences, Drake University, Texas College of Chiropractic, Logan University/College of Chiropractic, Southern California University of Health Sciences, and Palmer College of Chiropractic, Western States Chiropractic College, as well as at the Center for Alternative Medicine Research, Harvard Medical School. Dr. Evans has addressed diverse audiences that include the Association of Trial Lawyers of Iowa, the American Bar Association, the Australian Chiropractor's Association, the Defense Research Institute of the American Bar Association, the American Public Health Association, and the Royal Academy of Physicians and Surgeons.

Dr. Evans is retired from an 11-year term of office on the Iowa Board of Chiropractic Examiners, serving as chairperson of the Board for nearly half that term. He maintains a private practice in Des Moines, and is the senior chiropractic orthopedic staff of a multi-provider, multi-disciplinary health care facility specializing in the non-surgical management of orthopedic and neurological disorders. He is a Trustee of the Foundation for Chiropractic Education and Research, and served as Editorial Advisor for its publication "*Staying Well*" for many years. Dr. Evans is the Vice President of FCER and continues to serve the FCER as the Chairman of its Department of Defense Committee. Dr. Evans is the Chair of the Evidence-Based Resource Center of FCER. He was an appointee to the RAND Consensus Panel for the study of the Appropriateness of Manipulative Care for the Cervical Spine. He is an appointee, by the Secretary of Defense of the United States, to the Oversight Advisory Committee for Chiropractic Health Care, Department of Defense, now serving as a Senior Member of that Committee, as well as its successor committee, the Chiropractic Healthcare Benefits Advisory Committee. Dr. Evans has served as an Editorial Advisor for DC TRACTS, and is a Prepublication Book Reviewer for Lippincott Williams & Wilkins Publishers; Elsevier, and Aspen Publishing. He is an Associate Editor for the *Journal of Neuromusculoskeletal*

System of the ACA and a Forum Acquisitions Editor for the ACA Press.

Dr. Evans was an appointee by Iowa Governor Terry E. Branstad to the Iowa Health Reform Council, the Iowa Health Regulation Review Task Force, and the Iowa Community Health Management Information System (CHMIS). He is the CEO of the Iowa Chiropractic Physicians Clinic, (ICPC) a single-specialty independent provider network for Iowa and surrounding Midwestern states.

Dr. Evans is the recipient of the Chiropractic Orthopedist of the Year Award (1984) and the Distinguished Service Award (1994) from the American College of Chiropractic Orthopedists, receiving the ACCO Distinguished Service Award again for 2001-2002. The Council on Chiropractic Orthopedics recognized Dr. Evans for Lifetime Achievement in 1992 and he received the President's Citation for Distinguished Service by the American Board of Chiropractic Orthopedists in 1991. Dr. Evans received the Award of Excellence in 1993-1994, the Presidential Award in 1994, and the Outstanding ICS Member in 1996-1997, all from the Iowa Chiropractic Society. Most recently, he received the Iowa Board of Chiropractic Examiners Service Award: Iowa Chiropractic Society 1990-2001. Dr. Evans received the Distinguished Service Award from the Academy of Chiropractic Orthopedists in March 2003.

Dr. Evans' writings include *Orthopedic Test and Signs, A Compendium*, NWUHS, 1979, third edition, 1984, 1985; *Differential Diagnosis of Conditions Presenting Neck and Arm Pain*, NWCC, 1980, second edition, 1984, 1985; *Orthopedic Considerations of the Low Back and Lower Extremity*, NWUHS, 1980, second edition, 1984, 1985; *The Impairment Rating*, NWCC, 1981, second edition, 1984; "The Injured Worker: Role of the Chiropractor," *Journal of the Australian Chiropractor's Association*; 1985;15(2); "Malingering and Symptom Embellishment," Chapter 15, *Chiropractic Family Practice*, Williams & Wilkins, 1990; *Thoracic Spinal Examination Procedures*; audio lecture for DC TRACTS bimonthly publications, 1989, 1990; "Truncal Pain," Chapter 5, as a contribution to *Scoliosis*, by D. Aspergren, Williams & Wilkins, 1991; "*Back School; a statistical correlation to demonstrate efficacy of a Back School Education Program in the therapeutic regimen: a one year study,*" completed 12/31/82; "*CPT/ICD-9 coding and reference glossary*" for Iowa Chiropractic Society; *The Role of The Doctor of Chiropractic In Health Care Reform in The State of Iowa Within the Context of the Principles of Reform Of the Iowa Health Reform Council*; Notice of Intended Action Insurance Division [191], New Chapter 75, "*Iowa Individual Health Benefits Plans*"; *Managed Care In The United*

States Perspectives on Chiropractic Health Care Delivery in Total Managed Care Systems, 1995; Noticed Rules, Chapter 110, *"Center for Rural Health and Primary Care,"* New Section. 514c.11 *Patient Access to Types of Physicians Under Managed Care Health Plan or Indemnity Plan With Limited Provider Network*; *Analysis of the Final Report on the Physician Utilization Study as authorized by Iowa State Senate*, Senate File 2470(1996) and completed by Donald G. Hamm, Jr., FSA William M. Mercer, Incorporated, as the *Clinical and Cost Effectiveness of Various Types of Physicians* for the Iowa Division of Insurance January 6, 1997 by Ronald C. Evans, DC, FACO, FICC, and Anthony I. Rosner, Ph.D. February 10, 1997; *Fibromyalgia: A Conservative Perspective on Definition, Diagnosis and Management*, a video presentation for FCER 5/95; *Identifying and Understanding Lateral Elbow Pain with Emphasis on Lateral Epicondylitis*; *Alternative Medicine: Implications for Clinical Practice Chiropractic Health Care*; *Basic Chiropractic Testing and Evaluation Techniques PAIN: "Is it real, or is it Memorex,"* Iowa Trial Lawyers Association Medical Damages Seminar June 9, 1995; *Testing Methodology and Protocol of the American Board of Chiropractic Orthopedists*, Evans RC, Brandt JR; Evans RC, Rosner AL. "Alternatives in Cancer Pain Treatment: The Application of Chiropractic Care," *Seminars in Oncology Nursing* 2005;21(3):184-189. His textbooks include *The Illustrated Essentials in Orthopedic Physical Assessment*, 1993; *Illustrated Orthopedic Physical Assessment*, 2001; and *Instant Access to Orthopedic Physical Assessment*, 2002; and Iatrogenic Tendinopathy Associated with Levaquin (Levofloxacin); case report, 2008.

Dr. Evans holds the copyright and trademark for the Greenfield Babinski Neurological Reflex Hammer; IMPSTAT (a computer program for the Evaluation and Rating of Physical Impairments (coauthored with Logic Unlimited, Inc.); and he is the co-developer of EXAM-MAKER, a computerized exam-making program, based on multi-statistical permutations, with Logic Unlimited, Inc.

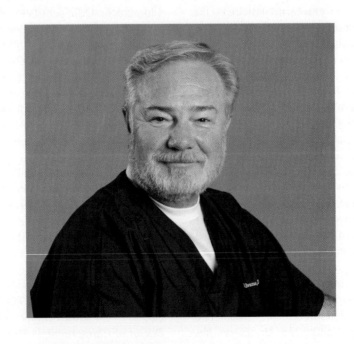

PREFACE

The basic observation of a patient's painful stance and aggravating movements usually allows the formulation of the presenting signs and symptoms into a recognizable constellation of a disease syndrome. The essence of orthopedic diagnosis is the clinically demonstrable or reproducible signs of disease or injury.

Many physicians associate an aura of mysticism with the ease and speed with which the orthopedic specialist arrives at a diagnosis. In fact, the specialist's development of interviewing, observation, and physical testing skills allows proceeding directly to the heart of the patient's problem.

I have been privileged in clinical practice to be challenged by the myriad orthopedic health problems presented by my patients. I believe that my early and fumbling years were well tolerated by these gracious people. They became well in spite of my efforts. They have remained loyal indeed.

In these latter years of practice, many of the early patients return with new diseases. These maladies are often much more difficult to diagnose and treat. My skills as an orthopedic specialist have been honed to a fine edge out of necessity. Some of these patients will not outlive me to give me yet another chance to get it right.

The perspective of the role of the physician in modern medicine has changed. Physicians are no longer viewed as the omnipotent beings they were formerly thought to be. The physician is expected to recognize personal skill limitations and make appropriate consultations and referrals. Patients expect the correct diagnosis the first time around. At the least, they deserve that.

This book is created to alleviate the frustration and discomfort for two parties in their respective quests for health and wellness. First are the physicians and orthopedic specialists, who labor mightily in pushing, pulling, poking, bending, and twisting patients' body parts in the sometimes less than compassionate search for the cause of the suffering. Second are the patients who have been not-so-gently pushed, pulled, poked, bent, and twisted into inhuman configurations as they wait furtively for the discovery of the cause of their anguish. I salute both parties for their endurance in seeking the origin of disease and discomfort.

Although the first edition of *Instant Access to Orthopedic Physical Assessment* was an unqualified success—voted into the 1994-1995 Top 250 Books of the Year by *Doody's Health Sciences Book Review Journal*—it could be made to be better. Much of what made the first edition so successful succeeded into a second edition, and now a third edition. There are many major changes to the contents: increasing the information on disease assessment, including more illustrations, and creating many more Orthopedic Gamuts.

Readers will enjoy the "At the View Box," contributions of Dr. Timothy Mick, DC, DACBR, as well as the expanded critical thinking elements. *Illustrated Orthopedic Physical Assessment, Third Edition*, remains clinically relevant and useful for both the student and the practicing clinician.

The scope and organization of *Illustrated Orthopedic Physical Assessment, Third Edition*, makes it a suitable companion for the clinician at all levels of sophistication, progressing from the initial procedures of orthopedic diagnosis to the requirements of the advanced student and the experienced practitioner. Included in the thirteen chapters are diagnostic facts in orthopedics, organized in a manner most likely to be useful during the examination of patients. The book's compact physical dimensions invite constant use as a reference volume on the physician's office desk, in the instrument bag, and in the clinical setting; its functional internal design, with liberal use of **Orthopedic Gamuts**, offers a convenient vehicle for refreshing one's memory about seldom encountered and easily forgotten clinical orthopedic phenomena.

Only the unusual reader and clinician could master the contents of *Illustrated Orthopedic Physical Assessment* by studying it in sequence from beginning to end. Rather, the student or clinician should digest the principles and procedures in segments as general diagnostic knowledge progresses. First, the reader should become familiar with Chapters 1 and 2 and the descriptions of the "**Cardinal Signs and Symptoms**". From these chapters, the clinician should explore the regional chapters. As contact with patients increases and specific questions arise, the reader should become familiar with the "Comments" for each diagnostic procedure. The "Comments" section of each test or sign amplifies the knowledge of an underlying pathology that is often discovered with the pertinent test or procedure.

Chapter 13 presents rationale and procedures for investigating malingering or non-organically–based complaints. Included with Chapter 13 are numerous medical record forms, outcomes assessment forms, and pain scale analogs.

Each chapter of *Illustrated Orthopedic Physical Assessment, Third Edition*, has a specific format. The format lends to the quick referencing of tests and maneuvers and cross-referencing of associated procedures.

Each chapter begins with **indexing of the tests found** therein. Each chapter also begins with **cross-reference tables** for the syndrome assessed and by the syndrome suspected. Further, each chapter presents the separate protocols for the regional joint assessment procedures and for assessment of pain in the particular joint or region. These are presented as testing procedural flow charts. These charts identify the test procedure(s) used to objectify the symptoms of pain, paralysis, weakness, and loss of sensation. The chart provides a plan of examination and selections of tests for the joint.

Each chapter begins with a set of axioms. **Axioms** are self-evident or universally recognized truths. Axioms are also established rules, principles, or laws. An axiom used in this text is also a principle accepted as true, without proof as the basis for argument.

Each **chapter introduction** addresses the various unique considerations or pathologies of the focal joint. The introductory section contains the index of the tests presented and illustrated in the chapter.

Laced throughout a chapter are **Orthopedic Gamuts**. The various gamuts present a range or spectrum of facts or concepts in assessing orthopedic disease. The gamuts in each chapter may represent universal orthopedic precepts as well as specific regional principles and maxims. The gamuts serve as diagnostic rubric in examining a patient.

Essential anatomy is presented in each chapter. The essential anatomy section is not all-encompassing, but rather discusses only the typical tissues that can be examined in orthopedic physical procedures.

Essential motion assessment for the joint is included. These illustrations depict the expected full ranges of movement for the joint. The discussion further identifies the amount of lost motion that can affect the activities of daily living.

Essential muscle function for each joint is also included. This section identifies the musculature that is the prime mover of the joint, the innervation, and the action of the muscle, and limited discussion of the muscular anatomy.

Essential imaging elements are addressed in each chapter, specific for the region or joint discussed. Again, not all imaging techniques or modalities are discussed, only those procedures germane to the physical orthopedic testing of a patient.

Each test, maneuver, sign, law, or phenomenon is presented separately. The common usage name for the test, as identified in *Stedman's*, *Taber's*, *Mosby's*, *Dorland's*, or *Churchill's* medical dictionaries, is the heading for the test. Equally, common synonyms and eponyms follow this name.

Eponyms for certain examinations vary from locale to locale or among institutions within the same area. Such observations are a reflection of the training center's influence. This is especially true where the names of prominent local physicians or clinicians or researchers are frequently used for these examinations. On occasion, the same test is given two or more names, or the name can apply to more than one test or sign. In a problem-oriented situation, eponyms are routinely used in the physical evaluation process. Familiarity with the terms and techniques used in determining regional problems enables the physician and assistant to record and clarify an orthopedic examination. Following the name of the test, maneuver, or sign is identification of the specific pathology the test is suited to elicit.

A **test** is part of the physical examination in which direct contact with the patient is made. It also may be a chemical test, x-ray, or other study. All tests described in his book will relate to the physical examination.

A **sign** is elicited by a test or a particular maneuver. A sign can be simply a visual observation (e.g., antalgia), and it is an indication of the existence of a problem perceived by the examiner.

A **maneuver** is a complex motion or series of movements, used either as a test or treatment. A maneuver is also a method or technique.

A **phenomenon** is any sign or objective symptom or any observable occurrence or fact.

A **law** is a description of a phenomenon that is so thoroughly tested and accepted that it is regarded as a principle governing like phenomena.

For each testing procedure in the book, a **general comment** is presented about the pathologic condition targeted by the test. Numerous citations from current research literature annotate the discussions of underlying pathologies. Following the comment section is a bulleted delineation of how the test is conducted. Each procedure is supported by photo illustrations and legends.

Each test is cross-referenced with other supportive tests and procedures as "**Next Steps/Procedures**". Where pertinent, a "**Clinical Pearl**" identifies the subtle nuances or finesse of the tests that the author has gleaned from empirical practice.

For selected tests or procedures, **At the Viewbox** case studies are presented. The case studies exemplify the typical and salient diagnostic image findings for the disease pathology discussed. The case studies have been graciously supplied from the teaching library of Dr. Timothy Mick, DC, DACBR.

At the close of each chapter, a "**critical thinking**" section is included. The critical thinking section is a range of questions germane to the specific region or joint of the chapter. The questions pertain largely to information contained in this text, but may occasionally require the reader to cross-reference with other pieces of literature or current scientific journals. The answers for each question are contained in this reference as well.

The **references** are listed for each chapter. The bibliographic listing is new, updated, and extensive. In some instances, the bibliography reflects older volumes or works than are commonly found in scientific literature today. These older references are the original work of the creators of various tests or procedures in this book. Preserving the books in these reference lists is an attempt to preserve a continuum in the development of orthopedic investigation.

In an effort to accurately depict tissues and pathology involved in orthopedic disease and injury, **numerous new illustrations** are included in *Illustrated Orthopedic Physical Assessment, Third Edition*. Largely the new illustrations are from the outstanding and benchmark works of selected authors. Their works are exemplary in great scientific writing, strongly contributing to the fund of knowledge of modern physicians. The artwork and line drawings used in these works are unsurpassed.

Although the various tests and procedures in this book are presented in an anatomical or regional format, the application of the tests is accomplished in a more natural flow of examination procedures. The natural flow of the examination usually moves the patient from the standing position, through sitting, supine, and side-lying positions to the prone position. **Appendix A** is a Listing of Tests, Alphabetically and Anatomically; **Appendix B** is a Listing of Tests According to the Position of the Patient. A **Glossary of Abbreviations** is also included.

ACKNOWLEDGMENTS

Many individuals come to mind for their contributions to the continuum of this reference work, and they are indeed too numerous to list. They are, especially, the physicians who attend my lectures and symposia and take the time to tell me about or demonstrate for me various orthopedic tests and signs. I am sure that in many instances the uninformed or casual onlookers thought that grown men were wrestling in public, when, in fact, we were exchanging the latest testing procedures. I will always be grateful to these keepers of the empirical body of medicine and science. Without their thirst for knowledge and scientific evidence and support, this book could not be written or continue in its evolution.

More specifically, I must acknowledge three great mentors in chiropractic orthopedics: **Dr. Joseph J. Sweere, Dr. Russell G. Hass (dec.),** and **Dr. Robert N. Solheim (dec.).** It was my fortune to be their student in orthopedic health science. Their challenges kept me advancing in my fundamental knowledge in orthopedic medicine, and their educational excellence caused me to grow. This book is a product of that growth. Their guidance and vitality have been the breath of life for the entity of orthopedic specialization within the scope of chiropractic practice. Perhaps more especially, I acknowledge **Dr. John F. Allenberg,** former President, Northwestern University of Health Sciences, as the individual responsible for my completion of the arduous, if not overwhelming, residency program at Northwestern. Although I may have had the talent and intellect for the task, he provided the necessary stimulus at the right times to help me see the endeavor to completion. Without that, I would not be a chiropractic orthopedist.

It is hard to define the driving force that propels one to aspire to excellence. **Samuel C. Evans, DC,** my father, and partner in practice, in his life and love of quietly but efficiently caring for people, embodied the greatest attributes in health science and art. His dedication to truth in science and compassion in ministering to the sick and injured inspired me to greater heights as a physician and as a person. This book, the editions before it, and those that will come after, is penned with eternal respect, admiration, and humility for his lifetime work and contribution to the human condition. The greatest man I ever knew.

My contemporary, **Dr. James R. Brandt,** continued to serve in the development of the third edition of this text, as well as for its companion, *Instant Access to Orthopedic Physical Assessment, Second Edition.* Dr. Brandt remained steadfast in critical assessment of the work and dedicated to making me strive for excellence in my writing.

Dr. Kim A. Skibsted contributed to the third edition with astute clinical photography. Dr. Skibsted's keen eye and sense of photographic composition are unparalleled and add to the advancement of the images used in various chapters. In many instances, the clinical photography of Dr. Skibsted is unsurpassed in depicting important positions and postures. Dr. Skibsted not only grasped the concept and framing issues of the illustrations, he worked tirelessly to perfect the quality of this book. I am ever indebted.

For the third edition, **Mrs. Linda K. Evans** saw to it that manuscripts for both *Illustrated Orthopedic Physical Assessment, Third Edition,* and *Instant Access to Orthopedic Physical Assessment, Second Edition,* were ready, accurate, and finished ahead of time. Her zeal to make these editions as successful as the previous ones is unparalleled. She made the task of revision more interesting and less heavy. I will seek her guidance for future works.

For the third edition—and to quote, "It takes a village" —to produce the stunning new color images for the various tests and maneuvers. At the outset, **Logan University/ College of Chiropractic president Dr. George Goodman,** and **Dr. Elizabeth Goodman, Ms. Ann Carter,** Assistant to **Drs. Goodman,** and **Ms. Kim Sullivan,** Graduation & Event Planner at the Purser Center, are commended for their generosity in providing a magnificent location for the author, crew, editorial photographer, and models, in the production of the art. The Purser Center is unparalleled in its beauty and functionality. Certainly, the college administration and staff saw to every need for this project, ensuring its success. I am grateful to the **ITC** company for providing the set backdrop and carpet, without which, the art would be less charming.

Mr. Jim Visser, primary still photographer, and **Mr. Chuck Leroi,** and his videographic assistants **Matt Aiskenen,** and **Ryan Cannon,** could not have worked harder to achieve any higher degree of excellence with the color photos and illustrations and video footage. They both pushed the models to exceed their known abilities, squeezing out every detail of movement or position. Their collective work embodies the constant search for perfection, serving as a guide for me to create prose equal to the illustrations. I look forward to working with both in future endeavors.

The primary photographic models include **Ms. Kim Alvis, Mr. Sean Brasfield, Ms. Candyse Burns, Mr. Ryan Collart, Mr. Ochuko Ekpere, Ms. Angela Fain, Dr. LT Faison, Ms. Sheena Gordon, Mr. John Knott, Mr. Patrick Milford, Ms. Julie Mowczuo, Mr. Gary Taylor,** and **Ms. Annie Walters.** Both Mr. Brasfield and Dr. Faison rose far above the call of duty in providing either specialized and critical equipment for the photos, or in helping recruit suitable models for the shoot. Each of the models demonstrated interminable patience in achieving just the right position or look of a test or procedure. I am grateful for their stamina and physical pliability. It is worthwhile noting that some of these able models subsequently entered successful practice as chiropractic physicians.

Ms. Bailey Schechinger is a superb model for the clinical illustrations. She was tireless, well-poised, and eager to learn the meanings and usefulness of the procedures. Because of this, she helped make this book better.

The Mosby/Elsevier staff for this edition included: **Ms. Jennifer Watrous**, Senior Developmental Editor, Health Professions I department of Editorial. I am pleased that Ms. Watrous elected to engage in the work on my new editions. She worked diligently on the second edition of *Illustrated Orthopedic Physical Assessment,* and it has been exciting to have her working on the third. Her attention to detail previously made the book into a definitive reference. That same perseverance with editing my writing this time pushes the book yet one notch higher. It is always a pleasure to work with people who truly want to see a project succeed. Ms. Watrous exemplifies this trait. **Ms. April Falast**, Editorial Assistant, Health Professions I department of Editorial. We could not have completed the work on time or in an organized fashion without Ms. Falast's creative work in making the photographic masters from the second edition. The enlarged illustrations were the perfect tool for both the stills and videos. I am sure this was hard work, but the resulting photo catalog is unsurpassed. I am also grateful for her attention to the needs of the models. Without Ms. Falast's leadership, I am certain the freezing models would simply have left the building, along with Elvis. **Ms. Kelly Milford**, Associate Developmental Editor, Health Professions I department of Editorial, is exceptional in her work. Her attention to detail and dedication to completion of the project kept the manuscripts, models, photographers, and the author moving forward. I am ever indebted to her patience in waiting for the final draft(s). Her professionalism is unsurpassed, especially tested in frequent e-mail and tele-conference contact from the beginning until the first bound copy. One could not ask for more of an editor. Her activities in compiling the manuscript schedules, arranging the photo shoot, arranging for the models and organizing the video and audio studios, as well as keeping everyone on the same page were invaluable. I could not have done any of the work without her at the "director's table." **Ms. Andrea Campbell**, Senior Project Manager, juggled communication with numerous staff constantly. She was the last stop before the "work" becomes a book. She is *the* sous chef for my manuscripts: I gave her the ingredients and she turned them into something everyone will like to look at and want to read. Ms. Campbell helped to sort out the art problems and keep track of what needed to be redrawn and what needed replacing (according to my seemingly interminable corrections). Quite a task. I am ever grateful for her skills. **Ms. Kellie White,** Senior Acquisitions Editor, Health Professions I department of Editorial. Worked with me from the earliest stages of *Illustrated Essentials in Orthopedic Physical Assessment*, through to *Illustrated Orthopedic Physical Assessment, Second Edition*, and *Instant Access to Orthopedic Physical Assessment*, and now for *Illustrated Orthopedic Physical Assessment, Third Edition*, and *Instant Access to Orthopedic Physical Assessment, Second Edition*. Ms. White continues to provide the necessary latitude and unwavering encouragement for the development of both books to evolve them into nationally recognized, definitive works. She embodies the attributes of a senior editor for which every author hopes. She and her excellent staff brought professionalism, interest, and dedication to the project. I have now written two editions under her guidance, with great result. The current revisions will surpass both our expectations, which I attribute to her skills at marshaling all the creative elements, models, photographers, and the author, to their best. Developing a book with her and for her is a joy. Elsevier is both astute and fortunate to have Ms. White in its Editorial leadership, and I am fortunate to enjoy her friendship and creative counsel. I will continue to strive to give her the best manuscripts. I look forward to future collaborations.

INTRODUCTION

Solving a patient's health problem can be a demanding exercise of orthopedic medical detection and logical deduction. Each health problem is a new diagnostic jigsaw puzzle for which the pieces must be found and fitted together in a carefully organized manner.

Each examination or investigation should have a plan for including or excluding a specific member of a "short list" of suspected conditions. It is always the failure to have such an organized plan or approach that makes the diagnosis of orthopedic health problems so artificially difficult. Certainly, common or customary steps must be followed, but not blind routine or blunderbuss investigations.

ORTHOPEDIC GAMUT

Success requires an organized thought process in approaching the patient's problem. There must be a clear plan to follow and a particular aim in each stage of the investigation.

- **First**, it must be determined whether a lesion of the musculoskeletal system is present. This determination is accomplished by analysis of the history and physical examination.
- **Second**, the location of the lesion must be determined. Is it possible to locate the lesion at one site, or are multiple sites involved? A system must be developed by the examiner to relate the signs and symptoms to a basic knowledge of musculoskeletal anatomy.
- **Third**, what pathologic conditions are capable of producing the lesions?
- **Fourth**, from careful analysis of the history and examination and by intelligent use of ancillary tests, which of these suspected conditions is most likely to be present?

Diagnosis purely by comparison with previous cases is reserved for the physician or orthopedic specialist who is very experienced and very accurately remembers the cases, but this combination is not the norm. The entry level physician or orthopedic specialist will come nearer to diagnostic accuracy by progressing logically through the medical investigation paradigm.

Despite all this, however, the right approach will never be achieved until one misconception is laid to rest. This misconception is that the exact solution of an orthopedic problem does not matter very much and that such a solution will be of academic interest only, with no useful nonsurgical treatment. Such a view is nonsense. It is true that health science is frustrated in treating motor neuron disease; no cure exists for hereditary ataxia, and no reliable method exists to prevent relapses in disseminated sclerosis. Contrary to many beliefs, these diseases occupy only a small part of the orthopedist's time.

Think for a moment of the transformation in the last 30 years in the treatment of cervical spine trauma, intervertebral disc prolapse, carpal tunnel syndrome, and deficiency neuropathies. Think of the influence of physiologic therapeutics in hypersensitivity states and in acute episodes of soft-tissue disease, of the continuing progress of manipulative therapy in certain facets of the migraine headache process, mechanical lower-back disorders, and in trigeminal neuralgia. Consider the advances of chiropractic orthopedics in treating various forms of benign spinal compression.

Finally, the solution of an orthopedic problem takes time. A solution cannot be rushed, and the examiner must never allow the approach to be influenced by the exhortations of optimistic colleagues to "just glance at this case while passing" or to "just run over the musculoskeletal system, it won't take 5 minutes." It will, it always does, and so it should.

CONTENTS

CHAPTER ONE
PRINCIPLES IN ASSESSING MUSCULOSKELETAL DISORDERS

INTRODUCTION

Health care providers assess patients every day in clinical practice. Commonly, clinical practice is impossible without structured assessments and tests. Examination procedures appear to be straightforward; results are either positive or negative. However, all assessment and testing in clinical practice is based on the assumption of uncertainty: Does the patient have a disease? The probability of a particular disease can be established only by performing a test or a chain of tests.

The accuracy of a test for detecting a disease or a condition is determined by sensitivity and specificity. A high sensitivity (or a high specificity) does not suffice to make a test useful in clinical practice; a test should be as sensitive as possible. The sensitivity and specificity of examination procedures and tests can often be found in the literature. Sensitivity and specificity are important characteristics of evidence-based physical assessment procedures but only in the context of a specific disease or condition.

The probability of a disease or condition after having performed a test (Bayes theorem) is dependent on two things: (1) the specificity and sensitivity of the procedure (test characteristics) and (2) the probability of the disease or condition before conducting the procedure. Interpretation of Bayes' theorem is that the probability of having a disease is not only dependent on the test or examination procedure result and the characteristics of the procedure, but is also

ORTHOPEDIC GAMUT 1-1

ORTHOPEDIC EVALUATION PROCESS

The orthopedic evaluation process has three phases:
1. History taking
2. Examination
3. Diagnosis

ORTHOPEDIC GAMUT 1-2

CLINICAL ASSESSMENTS

In clinical practice, assessments occur all day, every day, including:
1. Elucidating complaints
2. Establishing impact of the complaints
3. Checking the complaint consistency with specific diagnoses
4. Performing a general physical examination
5. Performing special physical examinations
6. Performing laboratory and imaging tests
7. Interpreting test results
8. Formulating a diagnosis
9. Commencing treatment
10. Evaluating treatment efficacy
11. Referring to a specialist, as needed

dependent on how likely the existence of the disease is before the procedure is actually conducted. This likelihood is dependent on the prevalence of the disease.

The decision on whether to perform a new test depends on the result of the previous test. Procedures with the lowest burden, risk, and costs for the patient are performed first, and those with the highest burden, risk, or costs are reserved for specific patients in which the prior probability is highest. Examination procedures in the context of a low prior probability of disease is rarely, if ever, informative. The yield of diagnostic testing will increase the prior probability in the range of approximately 50%. Very experienced clinicians intuitively apply these rules and arrange *their* diagnostic process in such a way that the highest possible yield (a

---

ORTHOPEDIC GAMUT 1-3

BAYES THEOREM

Rules of Thumb **rationale for use in clinical situations:**

1. Highly sensitive and specific tests will not perform very well in the clinical context if the *a priori* probability is very low.
2. No single diagnostic test exists that turns an *a priori* risk of disease of less than 10% into a probability that makes a clinician sufficiently convinced to establish a diagnosis.
3. Testing is most valuable if the *a priori* probability of the disease is somewhere in the range of 40% to 60%.
4. Diagnostic tests can turn such a probability into a sufficiently high posttest probability onto which to base further action.

ORTHOPEDIC GAMUT 1-4

PRÉCIS OF PHYSICAL EXAMINATION

- Sensitivity and specificity do not exclusively make a diagnostic test as appropriate for clinical use.
- Test results that are considered *normal* or *abnormal* should always be interpreted in the context of the individual patient.
- The probability of having a disease is not totally dependent on the test result and the characteristics of the test.
- The probability of having a disease is also dependent on how prevalent the disease is before the test is actually conducted.
- Testing in the context of a low probability of disease is rarely, if ever, informative.
- Highly sophisticated and costly diagnostic techniques may fail as easily as simple, cheap, diagnostic maneuvers.

---

highly probable diagnosis) will be obtained at the lowest possible burden, risk, and costs for the patient. Less experienced clinicians may learn from experienced colleagues by recalling Bayes theorem and implementing its principles in everyday clinical practice.

Health care providers cannot function adequately without physical examination procedures. In the real world, examiners accomplish clinical practice appropriately *without* a detailed knowledge of the principles of tests. However, the benefits from physical testing can be easily increased by recognizing that these tests do nothing more than increase the probability of a certain condition or diagnosis. Test results are never infallible.

BOX 1-1

PRÉCIS IN ORTHOPEDIC DIAGNOSIS

1. History
2. Examination
3. Determination of disability (PILS):
   Preventable causes of disability
   Independent living
   Lifestyle
   Social support

From the moment of the first encounter with a patient, the examiner is simultaneously observing and examining the movements and mannerisms of the patient, as well as listening to what is being said. The diagnostic process is complex; the examiner needs to establish the physical issues that are of greatest importance to the patient (those most disrupting to the activities of daily living) and try to differentiate the anatomic and pathologic aspects of any disease or injury that might be present.

The **history** provides much information about what difficulties the patient is experiencing and the impact of these difficulties on the patient. Orthopedic **examination** is essential to define the structures involved; together, these processes allow differentiation of orthopedic disorders into various **diagnostic categories** (Box 1-1).

HISTORY TAKING

A carefully elicited history is a most crucial element in orthopedic assessment. An experienced examiner can form an idea of the extent and magnitude simply from the patient's history. In the modern era of electronic patient medical record keeping, the examiner has new tools and methods for not only capturing patient information, but also tracking clinically significant changes.

Health care providers are increasingly under pressure to deliver efficient and high-quality care. Important reasons for this pressure are the ageing population, increasing demands and expectations by patients, rising medical costs, and a decrease of full-time employed specialists. Various innovations in information technology have been proposed to enhance the efficiency and quality of health care. Consequences of these innovations are altered health care processes, as well as a redefinition of responsibilities and a change in workload for caregivers and patients involved in these processes. A health care innovation that is increasingly applied in many medical specialties is telemedicine (TM). TM can be defined as "the use of telecommunications technology for medical diagnostic, monitoring and therapeutic purposes when distance and/or time separates the participants" (Berghout et al, 2006).

A recent Institute of Medicine (IOM) report characterized increased utilization of advances in health care informa-

---

ORTHOPEDIC GAMUT 1-5

- An integrated electronic patient record (EPR) is essential for the future of health care services.
- The EPR assists in the sharing of patient information and helps promote efficiency.
- The most important resource for the development of the EPR is the patient.
- Computer systems can take appropriate directed medical histories from patients based on chief complaint.

ORTHOPEDIC GAMUT 1-6
WORKING DIAGNOSIS

Essential steps in formulating a working diagnosis include:
1. History taking
2. Observation
3. Palpation
4. Orthopedic testing
5. Clinical laboratory and imaging procedures

ORTHOPEDIC GAMUT 1-7
OBSERVATION AND INSPECTION

Observation and inspection of the patient occur anytime during the examination or history interview, especially when the patient is not aware of the observation. In this way, the examiner notes:
1. Antalgia or deformities of posture
2. Gait disturbances, especially if the patient needs assistance
3. Spinal symmetry, including prominences or elevations, flattening or depressions, scoliosis, or abnormalities of the anteroposterior curvature
4. Surface scars and wounds

---

tion technology (IT) (e.g., automation of clinical, financial, and administrative transactions) as essential to improving quality and efficiency, preventing errors, and enhancing consumer confidence in the health care system. Research shows that IT tools, such as computerized clinical decision support systems and computerized physician order entry, can improve physician performance and patient outcomes (Nowinski et al, 2007).

Clearly, IT has had an extraordinary impact on the provision of health services. Over 40 years has passed since the vision of a comprehensive electronic patient record (EPR) system was first established. Integration of the EPR has been less than successful partly because it relies heavily on physicians and other highly skilled professionals for data acquisition. Some EPR systems have attempted to improve physician use and acceptance by standardizing medical prose or creating templates; acceptance is still suboptimal (Benaroia, Elinson, Zarnke, 2007).

Burt and Hing found that although 73% of physician offices used computers for billing, only 17% used them for maintaining medical records and 8% for ordering prescriptions. The proportion of U.S. physicians who have adopted electronic health records is estimated to be between 20% and 25% (Schleyer, Spallek, Hernandez, 2007).

The complaint history of a musculoskeletal condition covers certain essential points. History of trauma helps differentiate between acquired ligamentous (soft-tissue) insufficiency, inherent laxity, and past instability. If trauma or overuse caused the problem, the examiner must determine whether the patient stopped the injurious activity immediately and self-treated the resulting condition. Finding traumatized joints and adjacent structures neglected, deconditioned, weakened, or atrophied caused by prolonged periods of protection is common.

An accurate description of the traumatic event, including the exact position of the part at the moment of injury, is essential.

The exact site of the pain is also important. Patients often identify pain in one location, such as the hip, but point somewhere else, such as the sacroiliac joint. The more distal the pain is, the more accurately patients define its location.

CHIEF COMPLAINT

Patients who have more than one complaint, such as those with pain of spinal origin coupled with other body region symptoms or extremity problems, must be guided in ranking the complaints in priority. Although patients occasionally seek attention for stiffness or some other joint-related complaint, most patients with musculoskeletal conditions do so for reasons related to pain, especially when it compromises the activities of daily living.

The basic elements of examining the patient include observation and inspection, palpation, neurologic evaluation, vital signs, range-of-motion studies, clinical laboratory studies, orthopedic tests, and diagnostic imaging.

Most examiners perform routine comprehensive examinations on patients with even minimal initial chief complaints (Phelps, Rodriguez, 2005).

OBSERVATION AND INSPECTION

The first impressions—observations made while taking the patient's history—are often the most revealing.

Reasoning within these (pain-based clinical) categories appears to be useful in helping providers and patients understand and account for clinical presentations of pain. Such reasoning influences planning of physical assessments and treatment (Smart, Doody, 2007).

A useful approach in the clinical examination of the neuromusculoskeletal system is to seek answers to the *Critical*

5 questions for an orthopedic specialist. Once all five questions are answered, a differential diagnosis can usually be established (Box 1-2).

A rapid general screening examination suffices initially. Abnormal joints are subjected to a more focused regional orthopedic examination procedure.

The examiner must determine the presence of active or current inflammation, the presence of irreversible joint damage from past injury or inflammation, and existing mechanical defects. These findings are not mutually exclusive.

The distribution of joint involvement is important in reaching a diagnosis. Certain patterns characterize specific disorders. The number of involved joints may also be of diagnostic significance.

Learning what exacerbates or relieves the symptom pattern is important. Equally important is how long the complaints have existed (Table 1-1).

Several other features may be of diagnostic importance. Some of these features produce skin signs or nodules. Examples include rheumatoid nodules (Fig. 1-1), gouty tophi (Fig. 1-2), dermatomyositis (Fig. 1-3), and psoriatic arthritis (Fig. 1-4).

ORTHOPEDIC GAMUT 1-8
PAIN-BASED CLINICAL REASONING

Five main categories of pain-based clinical reasoning are:
- Biomedical (structural-functional source)
- Psychosocial (perception-interpretation of pain)
- Pain mechanisms (underlying pathophysiologic factors)
- Chronicity (temporal aspects of pain)
- Irritability or severity (degree of pain)

ORTHOPEDIC GAMUT 1-9
DETERMINING EXTENT OF INJURY

Other characteristic features of diagnostic importance in determining the extent of the disease or injury:
1. Is involvement symmetric or asymmetric?
2. Are large or small joints affected?
3. Is the distribution of the condition peripheral or axial?
4. Does the condition affect upper versus lower limbs, or vice versa?

BOX 1-2
CRITICAL QUESTIONS IN ORTHOPEDIC PHYSICAL EXAMINATION

1. Are any joints abnormal?
2. What is the nature of the abnormality?
3. What is the extent of the involvement?
4. Are other features of diagnostic importance present?
5. Do the answers to questions 1 through 4 provide sufficient data?

TABLE 1-1
JOINT PATTERNS IN ORTHOPEDIC/RHEUMATIC DISORDERS

Diagnosis	Symmetry	Number of Joints Involved*	Large/Small Joints	Peripheral/Central Distribution	Upper/Lower Limb	Predilection
Rheumatoid arthritis	Symmetric	Mono-, oligo-, polyarthritis	Large/small	Peripheral	Upper/lower	MCPs, PIPs, MTPs, DIPs
Ankylosing spondylitis	—	—	—	Central	—	Sacroiliac joints, hip, shoulder
Psoriatic arthritis	Asymmetric	Polyarthritis	Large/small	Peripheral	Upper/lower	DIPs, sacroiliac joints
Reactive arthritis	Asymmetric	Oligoarthritis/Polyarthritis	Large	Peripheral	Lower	Sacroiliac joints, DIPs (toes)
Gout	Asymmetric	Monoarthritis/Oligoarthritis	Large/small	Peripheral	Lower more than upper	First MTP, Knee, Hip

DIPs, Distal interphalangeal joints; *MCPs,* metacarpophalangeal joints; *MTPs,* metatarsophalangeals; *PIPs,* proximal interphalangeal joints.
***Monoarthritis** denotes inflammation in a single joint, **oligoarthritis** denotes two to four joints, and **polyarthritis** denotes five or more joints.

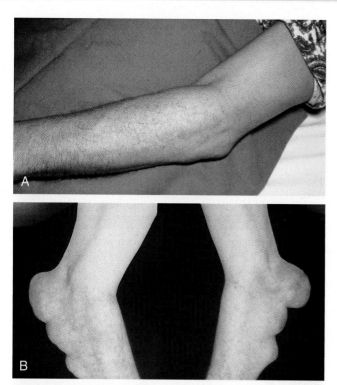

FIG. 1-1 **A,** Rheumatoid nodules. **B,** Large nodules may develop in the olecranon bursa as well as in the subcutaneous tissue. (From Klippel JH, Dieppe PA: *Rheumatology,* vol 1-2, ed 2, London, 1998, Mosby.)

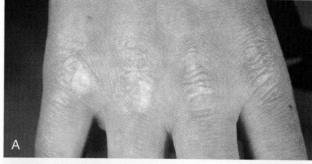

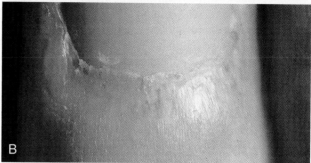

FIG. 1-3 Skin and nail fold lesions seen in dermatomyositis. Patches (**A**) and periungual edema and nail fold (**B**). (From Klippel JH, Dieppe PA: *Rheumatology,* vol 1-2, ed 2, London, 1998, Mosby.)

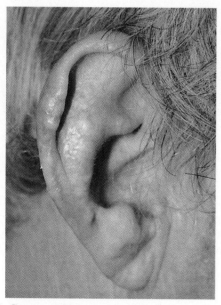

FIG. 1-2 Gouty tophi represent deposits of urate crystals. (From Klippel JH, Dieppe PA: *Rheumatology,* vol 1-2, ed 2, London, 1998, Mosby.)

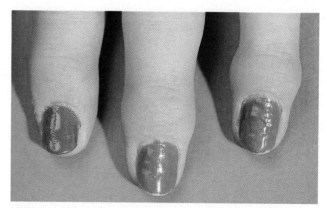

FIG. 1-4 Psoriatic arthritis, with swelling of the distal interphalangeal joint and pitting in the adjacent fingernails. (From Klippel JH, Dieppe PA: *Rheumatology,* vol 1-2, ed 2, London, 1998, Mosby.)

The answers to the *Critical 5* questions usually provide sufficient information to establish a differential diagnosis. They must. If not, the examiner will need to retrace each examination step until a logical and credible diagnosis can be reached.

PALPATION

Palpation is the process of assessing the physical characteristics of joints and contiguous structures by touching or feeling the patient's body. The purpose of palpation is to locate and substantiate areas of tenderness, swelling, and abnormal muscle tone. Palpation allows the examiner to identify a localized increase or decrease in surface temperature and the presence of induration and mass. Palpation is classically performed with the fingertips or with the blunt end of a cotton-tip applicator. However, instruments can be used in percussion (gently tapping with a reflex hammer), with vibration (using a C-128 tuning fork).

ORTHOPEDIC GAMUT 1-10

SPINAL PALPATION

Effective spinal palpation can be accomplished with the patient in the sitting or kneeling variants of Adam's position:

- In palpating various structures, the examiner assesses the skin and subcutaneous tissue. Rolling of the skin (Kibler's test) can be performed. The examiner observes for surface temperature, hypesthesia, hyperhidrosis, and muscle splinting.
- Tenderness of muscles and tendons and their attachments is assessed, in both the anatomic resting position and through various ranges of motion.

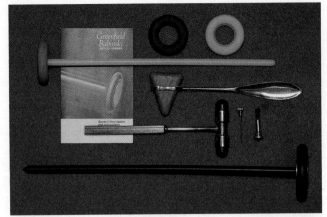

FIG. 1-5 From top to bottom, the Greenfield Babinski reflex hammer, Taylor reflex hammer, Buck's neurologic hammer, and Babinski reflex hammer.

Tendon sheaths and bursae are palpated for thickness, crepitus (especially silken versus snowball crepitus), and tenderness. The joints are palpated for all anatomic components to include bones, capsule, ligaments, any specialized structures, swelling, a change of shape or deformity, positional deficits, and tenderness. Palpation also aids in establishing the integrity of local circulation.

Using a stethoscope or similar instrument improves crepitation grading by enhancing the auditory component in conjunction with palpation and is especially useful with patients who display mild or moderate crepitation grade subclassifications.

NEUROLOGIC EVALUATION

The neurologic evaluation involves locating the lesion; testing deep tendon, superficial, and pathologic reflexes (Fig. 1-5); testing cranial nerve and brainstem function; measuring body parts (mensuration); grading muscular strength; and testing the gross sensory modalities (Fig. 1-6).

Cerebral dysfunction is determined during the consultation by noting the patient's mannerisms and orientation to time, space, and body parts (usually noted in the chart as oriented *×3*). Further evaluations of lesions in the cerebrum require advanced imaging procedures and electroneurodiagnostic testing.

Cerebellar lesions are characterized by repeated cogwheel-type muscle actions while the patient's eyes are open. The posterior columns of the spinal cord are the source of the dysfunction when repeated muscle actions are smooth and occur while the patient's eyes are open. However, these same muscular actions cannot be repeated as smoothly with the eyes closed. Brainstem dysfunction is discerned through testing of the cranial nerves. The type and quality of paralysis, reflexes, muscle tone, clonus, atrophy, fasciculation, and reactions of degeneration can differentiate spinal cord lesions from lower motor neuron disorders.

Moritz Heinrich Romberg (1795–1873), the founder of clinical neurology in Germany, described his now famous

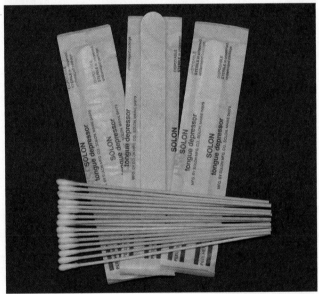

FIG. 1-6 Single-tipped cotton applicators are both economical and versatile and can be used in the following settings: in emergency rooms, examining rooms, outpatient clinics, and laboratories and on dressing carts. Sterile tongue depressors are usually made from white Birchwood that is $\frac{1}{16}$-inch thick. These tongue depressors are evenly cut and highly polished for smooth and clean edges, ends, and surfaces.

sign in the second edition of his *Lehrbuch der Nervenkrankheiten des Menschen* (1851). After discussing a reduction of the motor power in the lower extremities, Romberg states, "The individual keeps his eyes on his feet to prevent his movements from becoming still more unsteady. If he is ordered to close his eyes while in the erect posture, he at once commences to totter. The insecurity of his gait also exhibits itself more in the dark" (Romberg, 1853). Romberg thought the sign was pathognomonic of tabes dorsalis (Cole, Michael, Robert, 2003).

ORTHOPEDIC GAMUT 1-11
DEEP-TENDON REFLEXES

1. Scapulohumeral C5–C6
2. Biceps C5–C6
3. Radial C5–C6
4. Triceps C7–C8
5. Wrist C7–C8
6. Ulnar C8–T1
7. Patellar L2–L4
8. Hamstring L4–S1
9. Achilles S1–S2

ORTHOPEDIC GAMUT 1-12
SUPERFICIAL REFLEXES

1. Corneal III, V
2. Upper abdominal T7–T9
3. Lower abdominal T10–T12
4. Cremasteric
5. Gluteal
6. Plantar
7. T12–L2
8. L4–L5
9. S1–S2

ORTHOPEDIC GAMUT 1-13
PATHOLOGIC REFLEXES

1. Hoffmann
2. Babinski
3. Chaddock
4. Oppenheim
5. Bechterew-Mendel
6. Rossolimo
7. Gordon
8. Schaeffer

ORTHOPEDIC GAMUT 1-14
CRANIAL NERVES AND BASIC FUNCTION

I:	Smell
II:	Vision
III:	Light accommodation
III, IV, VI:	Eye movement
V:	Sensation (wink)
VII:	Facial muscle (taste)
VIII:	Auditory (balance)
IX:	Taste (gag)
X:	Voice (swallow)
XI:	Shoulder (shrug)
XII:	Tongue (motor)

ORTHOPEDIC GAMUT 1-15
COMMONLY ACCEPTED DEEP-TENDON REFLEX GRADING SCHEME

0 = Absent
1 = Diminished or hyporeactive
2 = Average
2+ = Slightly exaggerated (hyperreactive)
3 = Exaggerated (hyperreactive)
4 = Associated with myoclonus

Deep-tendon reflexes help the examiner locate the lower motor neuron lesion and differentiate it from an upper motor neuron lesion.

Superficial reflexes differentiate lower motor neuron lesions from upper motor neuron lesions.

Pathologic reflexes determine the presence of upper motor neuron lesions.

Cranial nerve function is determined by testing brainstem activity.

On occasion, eliciting a particular reflex is difficult; distraction techniques are helpful in such situations. If less-than-normal reactivity is encountered in the upper or lower extremities, the patient is directed to perform an isometric contraction in the opposite upper or lower extremities (Jendrassik maneuver).

Jendrassik facilitation is different between age groups and weight bearing versus non–weight bearing. Young patients often demonstrate a significant Jendrassik facilitation effect in the standing position, whereas, very often, no difference is seen in the elderly patients.

Mensuration of body parts is used to determine atrophy and functional and anatomic abnormalities (Fig. 1-7).

Grip strength testing examines the function of the ulnar nerve and can help differentiate myoneural dysfunction from malingering activity (Fig. 1-8). The examiner can use three methods of grip strength evaluation (one trial, the mean of three trials, and the best of three trials) when using the Jamar dynamometer. Two different static grip tests are the five-rung test and the maximal static grip test.

The five-rung test involves performing one repetition (trial) with the handle of the Jamar dynamometer on each of the five handle settings, whereas the maximal static grip test involves performing three repetitions with the handle on either the second or third setting (Fess, 1992; Joughin et al, 1993).

The main difference between the static grip test and the rapid exchange grip (REG) maneuver is the duration of the muscular contraction during gripping.

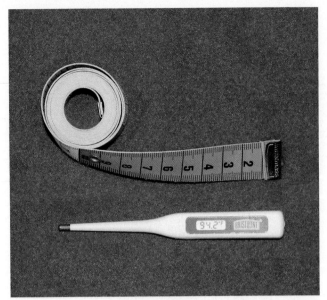

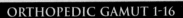

FIG. 1-7 Soft linen tape is marked in inches on one side and centimeters on the other. The fast-reading clinical thermometer.

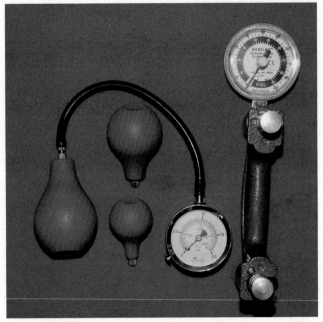

FIG. 1-8 Martin Vigorimeter aneroid dynamometer *(left)* and Jamar hand grasp mechanical five-position dynamometer *(right)*.

ORTHOPEDIC GAMUT 1-16

COMMON AREAS OF MENSURATION

1. Excursion of the chest during inspiration and expiration
2. Upper-extremity circumference (brachium and antebrachium); measured in the noncontracted and contracted state
3. Lower-extremity circumferences (thigh and calf); measured in the noncontracted and contracted states
4. Leg length (measured standing versus supine or prone); differentiates a functional short leg from an anatomic short leg

---

ORTHOPEDIC GAMUT 1-17

CERVICAL SPINE EXTRINSIC MUSCULATURE WITH SPECIFIC NERVE ROOTS NOTED

1. Deltoid (C5)
2. Biceps (C6)
3. Wrist extensors (C6)
4. Triceps (C7)
5. Wrist flexors (C7)
6. Finger extensors (C7)
7. Finger flexors (C8)
8. Finger abductors (T1)

During the static grip test, the duration of muscular contraction of each hand grip is 3 to 5 seconds, whereas during the REG maneuver, the hands alternate rapidly, resulting in a shorter duration of each grip (less than 1.5 seconds per grip) (Taylor et al, 2000).

A *positive* REG test is obtained when REG scores are greater than static grip scores, which indicates a submaximal or a feigned effort. A *negative* REG test is obtained when static grip scores are greater than REG scores, indicating a maximal or a sincere effort (Shechtman, Taylor, 2002).

Cervical intrinsic muscle testing relates to the cervical spine functions of flexion, extension, lateral flexion, and rotation.

Thoracolumbar intrinsic muscle function is associated with trunk flexion, extension, lateral flexion, and rotation.

ORTHOPEDIC GAMUT 1-18

THORACOLUMBAR EXTRINSIC MUSCULATURE AND SPECIFIC ASSOCIATED NERVE ROOT LEVELS

1. Hip flexors (L2–L3)
2. Knee extensors (L3–L4)
3. Ankle extensors (L4–L5)
4. Hip extensors (L4–L5)
5. Knee flexors (L5–S1)
6. Ankle flexors (S1–S2)

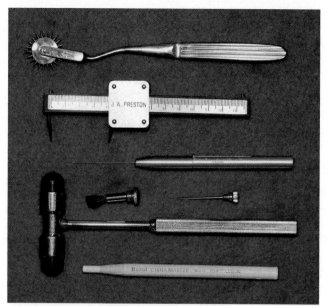

FIG. 1-9 From top to bottom, the Wartenberg pinwheel; Boley two-point discrimination gauge; von Frey anesthesimeter; Buck camel hair brush, pin, and neurologic hammer; and a Berol China marker.

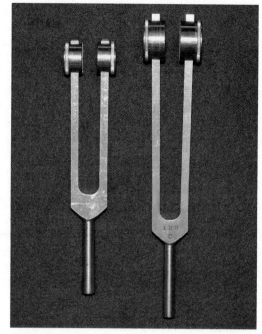

FIG. 1-10 Aluminum alloy tuning forks, available in C-64, C-128, C-256, C-512, C-1024, C-2048, and C-4096 vibrations. The lower-frequency tuning forks are the usual choices for bone vibration conduction studies.

Testing of the gross sensory modalities allows for evaluation of the dermatomes involved in superficial and deep sensations and proprioception (Fig. 1-9).

The superficial sensations include light touch, pain, and temperature. Light touch is mediated by the dorsal columns and easily examined with a cotton ball. Pain receptors are mediated by the lateral spinothalamic tracts and are tested by a pinprick and hot and cold temperatures. Temperature, or thermal sensation, mediated by the dorsal columns is tested with warm (not hot) and cool (not cold) temperatures.

The deep sensations are vibration and deep pressure perception. The dorsal columns of the spinal cord (Fig. 1-10) mediate vibration, tested with a C-128 or lower-frequency tuning fork. Deep pressure is tested by squeezing any muscular part of the body and is mediated in the dorsal columns.

Proprioception, or joint position sense, is mediated by the dorsal columns and can be tested by having the patient point to a particular part of the body while keeping the eyes closed.

PAIN AND PATTERNS OF PAIN

Pain that arises with activity and decreases with rest is likely to have mechanical causes. The pain may be position dependent; most cases of mechanical spinal pain have both a provocative and palliative arc of motion.

Spinal pain is the most difficult to differentially diagnose. The three primary patterns are dermatogenous, myogenous, and scleratogenous (Fig. 1-11).

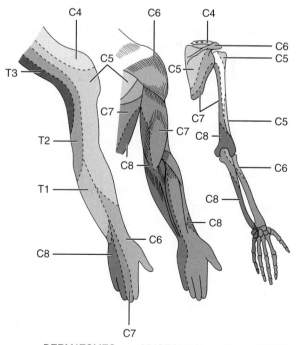

DERMATOMES   MYOTOMES   SCLEROTOMES

FIG. 1-11 Primary patterns of pain originating in the spine: dermatomes, myotomes, and sclerotomes. Demonstrated for the right upper extremity. (From Saidoff DC, McDonough A: *Critical pathways in therapeutic interventions: upper extremities,* St Louis, 1997, Mosby.)

A dermatome is the area of sensation attributed to a particular nerve root level. Dermatomal pain is often described as sharp, stabbing, and well demarcated. It may result from herniated discs, stretch injuries, or tumors.

Pain referral within muscular or fascial tissue is myogenous pain. Areas known as *trigger points* refer pain to distant sites. Trigger points are evident in patients with myofascial pain syndromes. Specific sites of tenderness that do not result from referred pain are termed *tender points*. Tender points develop in patients with varied soft-tissue, rheumatic, and collagen-vascular disorders, such as systemic lupus erythematosus and fibromyalgia.

Pain referred from somatic structures such as cartilage, ligament, joint capsule, or bone often does not follow dermatome patterns, as does nerve root pain. This pain is known as *scleratogenous pain*. Patients may describe this type of pain as dull, achy, diffuse, and difficult to pinpoint. Scleratogenous pain is one of the more common spinal pain patterns.

Local Versus Referred Pain

Patients with referred pain often point to large generalized areas, whereas patients with localized lesions can be more specific. A patient complaining of unrelenting spinal pain, demonstrating full, pain-free range of motion presents a problem. The patient likely has either viscerosomatic pain, which mandates further diagnostic testing, or pain resulting from a psychosocial cause. If referred pain from a diseased organ system is mimicking a local orthopedic problem, the examiner should not hesitate to order appropriate tests.

Every effort should be made to objectify the patient's report of pain and discomfort. Measurement instruments such as the **visual analog scale** (Fig. 1-12) are reliable and valid for examining a patient's pain. The **McGill Short Form Questionnaire** (Fig. 1-13) is helpful for pain measurement in a clinical setting.

Pain is associated with a very high disability rate, significantly affecting the three domains evaluated by the **Sheehan Disability Scale,** which assesses patient functional impairment in three domains: work impairment, social impairment, and impairment of family life or home responsibilities. Two further items gather data on patient-perceived stress and social support.

| No pain | On the line below, place a mark indicating your pain level | Worst pain |

0   10

FIG. 1-12 Visual analog scale for objective pain measurement. (From Malone TR, McPoil TG, Nitz AJ: *Orthopedic and sports physical therapy,* ed 3, St Louis, 1997, Mosby.)

VITAL SIGNS

Vital signs include the brachial blood pressure, peripheral pulse rate, respiration rate, height, weight, and vital capacity. The instrumentation for these measurements includes stethoscopes, spirometers, scales, tape measures, and blood pressure cuffs (Fig. 1-14).

RANGE OF MOTION

Of all the orthopedic tests that an examiner can perform on a patient, none is more crucial than range-of-motion (ROM) testing of the affected articulation. Range of motion testing often reveals the origin of the patient's discomfort, because movement may reproduce the pain. The patient is examined symmetrically for *active* ROM of all the joints that may be involved in the dysfunction or injury (Fig. 1-15). The examiner then takes the patient through *passive* ROM, evaluating the *end-feel* (i.e., springiness) of the affected joint.

Any movable joint in the body, including the spine, can be tested for ROM. ROM is assessed bilaterally by comparing findings with a given set of normal values. Normal values can vary dramatically, depending on the reference source used. An examiner must exercise careful professional judgment to ensure objectivity. Any ROM that is less than normal may indicate or be the result of muscle spasm, sprain, strain, joint subluxation, general arthritic degeneration, postsurgical condition, or obesity.

Recently, Childs and colleagues found in a clinical trial that spinal stiffness was one of five predictors of which patients with low back pain would respond favorably to a particular physical therapy manipulation. In their study, they used a manual assessment to grade the relative stiffness of the L4-L5 and L5-S1 joints. A palpable difference in the stiffness at these joints helped predict which patients were more likely to respond favorably to manipulative therapy. Manual palpation methods have been notoriously difficult to quantify and suffer from a lack of objectivity. Interexaminer

---

ORTHOPEDIC GAMUT 1-19

JOINT END-FEEL CATEGORIES

In passive joint motion assessment, the end-feel is important. The accepted end-feel categories are:

- Bone-to-bone: an abrupt halt to movement when two hard surfaces meet
- Capsular end-feel: a *leathery* resistance to movement with a slight amount of give at the very end of the range
- Springy block: a usually pathologic end-feel, generally representing an intraarticular displacement
- Tissue approximation: no further joint movement available
- Empty feel: usually pathologic

Check only one item for each category to describe your pain today.

1	2	3	4
1 Flickering 2 Quivering 3 Pulsing 4 Throbbing 5 Beating 6 Pounding	1 Jumping 2 Flashing 3 Shooting	1 Pricking 2 Boring 3 Drilling 4 Stabbing 5 Lancinating	1 Sharp 2 Cutting 3 Lacerating

5	6	7	8
1 Pinching 2 Pressing 3 Gnawing 4 Cramping 5 Crushing	1 Tugging 2 Pulling 3 Wrenching	1 Hot 2 Burning 3 Scalding 4 Searing	1 Tingling 2 Itchy 3 Smarting 4 Stinging

9	10	11	12
1 Dull 2 Sore 3 Hurting 4 Aching 5 Heavy	1 Tender 2 Taut 3 Rasping 4 Splitting	1 Tiring 2 Exhausting	1 Sickening 2 Suffocating

13	14	15	16
1 Fearful 2 Frightful 3 Terrifying	1 Punishing 2 Grueling 3 Cruel 4 Vicious 5 Killing	1 Wretched 2 Blinding	1 Annoying 2 Troublesome 3 Miserable 4 Intense 5 Unbearable

17	18	19	20
1 Spreading 2 Radiating 3 Penetrating 4 Piercing	1 Tight 2 Numb 3 Drawing 4 Squeezing 5 Tearing	1 Cool 2 Cold 3 Freezing	1 Nagging 2 Nauseating 3 Agonizing 4 Dreadful 5 Torturing

FIG. 1-13 McGill Short Form Pain Questionnaire. (From Malone TR, McPoil TG, Nitz AJ: *Orthopedic and sports physical therapy*, ed 3, St Louis, 1997, Mosby; from Melzacker R: The McGill Pain Questionnaire: major properties and scoring methods, *Pain* 1:277, 1975.)

reliability of chiropractic palpation of segmental fixation is typically poor to slight. Intraexaminer reliability is usually rated somewhat better, in the moderate to substantial range, depending on the experience of the examiner. Similarly, stiffness measures commonly used by physical therapists show little interexaminer agreement. Childs and colleagues were able to achieve acceptable reliability in the lumbar mobility test they used by reducing the assessment to three levels: (1) hypomobile, (2) normal, and (3) hypermobile (Owens et al, 2007).

STABILITY TESTING

Because clinical examination reveals the degree of ligamentous or joint sprain, the examiner must be able to test accurately for joint instability (Table 1-2). Stability testing moves joint and periarticular structures through their respective arcs and end-range motions. Stability testing involves stressing ligamentous tissues and joint capsules (Fig. 1-16).

MUSCULAR ASSESSMENT

Movement restrictions in a joint's passive ROM are not exclusively articular. Muscular hypertonicity limits passive movement and often occurs in association with articular lesions (joint dysfunction). Chronic joint problems are also commonly associated with myofascitis.

CLINICAL LABORATORY

For the examiner concerned with musculoskeletal disorders, differential diagnosis becomes a challenge. Complete blood

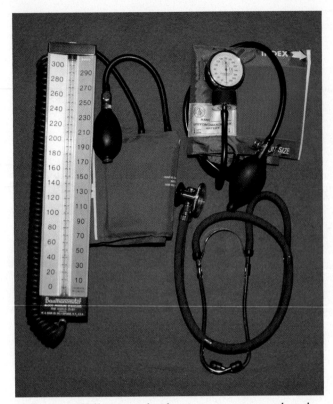

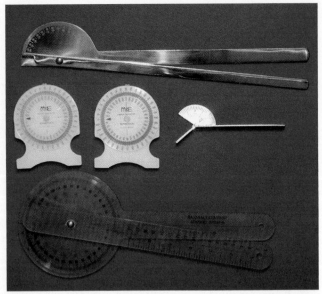

FIG. 1-15 From top to bottom, stainless steel goniometer measures movement of joints from 0 to 180 degrees. Bubble inclinometers measure the angular motion from 0 to 360 degrees. Finger or small joint goniometer measures the movement of interphalangeal joints of fingers and toes. Plastic radiographic goniometer provides standard orthopedic measurements of joint motion and neutral position.

FIG. 1-14 Wall-mounted sphygmomanometer and stethoscope *(left)*. Portable blood pressure cuff *(top right)*. Most significant heart sounds occur in the frequency range of 200 to 500 Hz, but human auditory sensitivity is limited to those sounds below 1000 Hz. Stethoscopes amplify the lower frequencies *(bottom right)*.

TABLE 1-2

INJURED LIGAMENT RESIDUAL FUNCTION

Extent of Failure	Sprain	Damage*	Joint Motion, Subluxation	Residual Strength	Residual Functional Length	Residual Functional Capacity
Minimal	First degree	Less than one third of fibers failed; includes most sprains with few to some fibers failed. Microtears also exist.	None	Retained or slightly decreased	Normal	Retained
Partial	Second degree	One-third to two-thirds ligament damage; significant damage, but parts of the ligament are still functional. Microtears may exist.	In general, minimal or no increased motion. Remaining fibers in ligament resist opening.	Marked decrease. At risk for complete failure	Increased, still within functional range but may later act as a check rein rather than subtle control of joint motions	Marked compromise; requires healing to regain function
Complete	Third degree	More than two-thirds to complete failure; continuity remains in part. Continuity lost and gross separation between fibers	Depends on secondary restraints Depends on secondary restraints	Little to none None	Lost Lost	Severely compromised or lost Lost

*Estimate of damage is often difficult; however, the different types listed can usually be differentiated. Note: Anterior and posterior cruciate tears commonly exist with little to no abnormal laxity. The examination for medial and lateral ligamentous injury is usually more accurate.
From Feagin JA, editor: *The crucial ligaments*, New York, 1988, Churchill Livingstone.

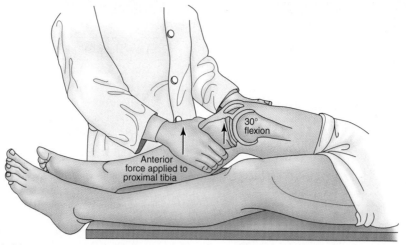

FIG. 1-16 Lachman test of the anterior cruciate ligament. (From Scuderi GR, McCann PD, Bruno PJ: *Sports medicine: principles of primary care,* St Louis, 1997, Mosby.)

ORTHOPEDIC GAMUT 1-20
RESISTED MUSCLE MOVEMENT

In assessing muscle tissue, resisted movements are the most revealing. Standard interpretations of resisted muscle testing movements include:

- Painful and strong is equated with a minor lesion of muscle or tendon.
- Painful and weak equates with a major lesion of the muscle or tendon.
- Painless and weak equates with neurologic injury or complete rupture of the muscular attachment.
- Painless and strong is normal.

ORTHOPEDIC GAMUT 1-21
LABORATORY RESULTS INTERPRETATIONS

For laboratory testing in orthopedic evaluations, results interpretation errors usually involve one of four areas:

- False-positive results
- False-negative results
- Measurement error
- Differences in groups of patients compared with individual patients

---

and urine tests can help determine a diagnosis. Diseases of the heart, liver, kidney, pancreas, and prostate can mimic back pain of spinal origin.

Most laboratory testing has limited utility for orthopedic diagnosis (Table 1-3). As an example, in **rheumatoid arthritis,** the diagnosis is often established from the history and physical examination; for **systemic lupus erythematosus,** from the laboratory test antinuclear antibody (ANA); for **gout,** from a synovial fluid examination; and for **ankylosing spondylitis,** from a radiograph. In common disorders such as osteoarthritis, fibromyalgia, or muscular strains and sprains, essentially no diagnostic role exists for laboratory tests except to exclude other diagnostic possibilities.

The simplest orthopedic screen includes rheumatoid arthritis factor, ANA, and uric acid, although more elaborate screens are available, which may include erythrocyte sedimentation rate, C-reactive protein, antistreptolysin-O titer, protein electrophoresis, quantitative immunoglobulins, and ANA subsets such as anti-Ro and anti-LA, anti-Sm, and anticentromere antibodies.

INDIVIDUAL BLOOD AND URINE TESTS

Acid Phosphates

Dietary deficiencies in phosphorus are rare but may be seen with alcoholism and malnutrition. Low levels of phosphorus (hypophosphatemia) may also be caused by or associated with:

- Hypercalcemia (high levels of calcium), especially as a result of hyperparathyroidism
- Overuse of diuretics (drugs that encourage urination)
- Severe burns
- Diabetic ketoacidosis (after treatment)
- Hypothyroidism
- Hypokalemia (low levels of potassium)
- Chronic antacid use
- Rickets and osteomalacia (caused by vitamin-D deficiencies)

Higher-than-normal levels of phosphorus (hyperphosphatemia) may be caused by or associated with:

TABLE 1-3

LABORATORY STUDIES USEFUL IN DIAGNOSING LOW BACK SYNDROMES

Test	Measurement	Low Back Implication
Complete blood count Hematocrit hemoglobin	A measure of volume of circulating red blood cells	May be diminished in systemic diseases (e.g., neoplasm) and in chronic spinal infections.
White blood count and differential	Amount and type of circulating white blood cells	Total white blood cell and shifts in differential may be present in spinal infections or occasionally in spondyloarthropathies.
Sedimentation rate	Nonspecific test of inflammation	Increased in spinal infections, may be increased in neoplasms and spondyloarthropathies.
Chemistry Calcium Phosphorus	A measure of circulating calcium and phosphorus	Calcium is elevated in hyperparathyroidism, may be elevated with primary and secondary osseous tumors, alterations in the distribution of calcium and phosphorus accompany many metabolic disorders but are normal in osteoporosis.
Alkaline phosphatase	Enzyme associated with bone formation; therefore; elevation implies increased bone formation.	May be elevated in primary or secondary osseous neoplasms.
Acid phosphatase	An enzyme associated with tumors metastatic to bone	Increased in prostatic tumors.
Serum proteins (albumin globulin protein electrophoresis) protein	Measurement of amount and type circulating	Elevations of one fraction of globulin are associated with multiple myeloma.
HLA-B27 antigen	A circulating antigen	Usually individuals with spondyloarthropathies are HLA-B27 positive. Note 6-8% of men have this antigen and therefore its presence is not confirmatory of a spondyloarthropathy.

HLA, Human leukocyte antigen.
Adapted from Pope ML: *Occupational low back pain, assessment, treatment and prevention,* St Louis, 1991, Mosby.

- Kidney failure
- Hypoparathyroidism (underactive parathyroid gland)
- Diabetic ketoacidosis (when first seen)
- Phosphate supplementation

Alkaline Phosphatase

Increased serum alkaline phosphatase is seen in states of increased osteoblastic activity (hyperparathyroidism, osteomalacia, primary and metastatic neoplasms), hepatobiliary diseases characterized by some degree of intra- or extrahepatic cholestasis, and in sepsis, chronic inflammatory bowel disease, and thyrotoxicosis. Isoenzyme determination may help determine the organ or tissue responsible for an alkaline phosphatase elevation.

Decreased serum alkaline phosphatase may not be clinically significant. However, decreased serum levels have been observed in hypothyroidism, scurvy, kwashiorkor, achondroplastic dwarfism, deposition of radioactive materials in bone, and in the rare genetic condition hypophosphatasia.

Amylase

In acute pancreatitis, amylase in the blood increases (often to four to six times higher than the highest reference value, sometimes called the *upper limit of normal*). The increase occurs within 12 hours of injury to the pancreas and generally remains elevated until the cause is successfully treated.

Then the amylase values will return to normal in a few days. In chronic pancreatitis, amylase levels will initially be moderately elevated but often decrease over time with progressive pancreas damage.

Amylase levels may also be significantly increased in patients with pancreatic duct obstruction, cancer of the pancreas, and gallbladder attacks. Urine and blood amylase levels may also be elevated with a variety of other conditions, such as ovarian cancer, lung cancer, tubal pregnancy, mumps, intestinal obstruction, or perforated ulcer, but amylase tests are not generally used to diagnose or monitor these disorders. Decreased blood and urine amylase levels may indicate permanent damage to the amylase-producing cells in the pancreas. Increased blood amylase levels with normal to low urine amylase levels may indicate decreased kidney function or the presence of a macroamylase, a benign complex of amylase and other proteins that accumulates in the blood.

Given that reference values for amylase vary from laboratory to laboratory, depending on the test method used, no universally accepted number exists that can be called normal or high.

Anti-Nuclear Antibody

Anti-nuclear antibody (ANA) tests are performed using different assays (indirect immunofluorescence microscopy or by enzyme linked immunoabsorbent assay), and results are reported as a titer with a particular type of immunofluorescence pattern (when positive). Low-level titers are considered negative, whereas increased titers, such as 1:320, are positive and indicate an elevated concentration of ANAs.

ANA shows up on indirect immunofluorescence as fluorescent patterns in cells that are fixed to a slide that is evaluated under a microscope. Different patterns are associated with a variety of autoimmune disorders. Some of the more common patterns include:

- Homogenous (diffuse)—associated with systemic lupus erythematosus (SLE) and mixed connective tissue disease
- Speckled—associated with SLE, Sjögren syndrome, scleroderma, polymyositis, rheumatoid arthritis, and mixed connective tissue disease
- Nucleolar—associated with scleroderma and polymyositis
- Outline pattern (peripheral)—associated with SLE

An example of a positive result might be *positive at 1:320 dilution with a homogenous pattern.*

A positive ANA test result may suggest an autoimmune disease, but further specific testing is required to assist in making a final diagnosis. ANA test results can be positive in people without any known autoimmune disease. Although this finding is not common, the frequency of a false positive ANA result increases as people get older.

Approximately 95% of patients with SLE have a positive ANA test result. If a patient also has symptoms of SLE, such as arthritis, a rash, and autoimmune thrombocytopenia, then the patient probably has SLE. In cases such as these, a positive ANA result can be useful to support the SLE diagnosis. Two subset tests for specific types of autoantibodies, such as anti-dsDNA and anti-Sm, may be ordered to help confirm that the condition is SLE.

A positive ANA can also mean that the patient has drug-induced lupus. This condition is associated with the development of autoantibodies to histones, which are water-soluble proteins rich in the amino acids lysine and arginine. An antihistone test may be ordered to support the diagnosis of drug-induced lupus.

Other conditions in which a positive ANA test result may be seen include:

- Sjögren syndrome: Between 40% and 70% of patients with this condition have a positive ANA test result. Even though this finding supports the diagnosis, a negative result does not rule it out. The examiner may want to test for two subsets of ANA: anti-SS-A (Ro) and anti-SS-B (La). The frequency of autoantibodies to SSA in patients with Sjögren syndrome can be 90% or greater.
- Scleroderma: Approximately 60% to 90% of patients with scleroderma have a positive ANA finding. In patients who may have this condition, ANA subset tests can help distinguish two forms of the disease, limited versus diffuse. The diffuse form is more severe. Limited disease is most closely associated with the anticentromere pattern of ANA staining (and the anticentromere test), whereas

the diffuse form is associated with autoantibodies to the anti–Scl-70.

- A positive result on the ANA may also show up in patients with Raynaud disease, rheumatoid arthritis, dermatomyositis, mixed connective tissue disease, and other autoimmune conditions.

Because symptoms may come and go, months or years may be required to show a pattern that might suggest SLE or any of the other autoimmune diseases.

A negative ANA result makes SLE an unlikely diagnosis. Immediately repeating a negative ANA test is not usually necessary; however, because of the episodic nature of autoimmune diseases, repeating the ANA test at a future date may be worthwhile.

Aside from rare cases, further autoantibody (subset) testing is not necessary if a patient has a negative ANA result.

Antistreptolysin-O Titer

Antistreptolysin-O (ASO) titer test results can be reported in several different ways; however, the interpretation is generally the same: The higher the result is, the more antibody that is present in the blood (unless a titer is performed, which is a ratio and therefore is interpreted differently).

The ASO antibody is either absent or present in very low concentrations in patients who have not had a recent streptococcal (strep) infection. Antibodies are produced approximately a week to a month after the initial strep infection. ASO levels peak at approximately 4 to 6 weeks after the illness and then taper off but may remain at detectable levels for several months after the strep infection has resolved.

If the test is negative, or if ASO is present in very low concentrations, then the patient most likely has not had a recent strep infection, especially if a sample taken 10 to 14 days later is also negative or minimal.

If the ASO level is high or is rising, then a recent strep infection has likely occurred. ASO levels that are initially high and then decline suggest that an infection has occurred and may be resolving.

The ASO test does not predict whether complications will occur after a strep infection, nor do they predict the severity of the disease. If symptoms of rheumatic fever or glomerulonephritis are present, an elevated ASO level may be used to confirm the diagnosis.

Bence-Jones Protein

A Bence-Jones protein is a monoclonal globulin protein found in the blood or urine. The isolated finding of a Bence-Jones protein is known as monoclonal gammopathy of uncertain significance. Finding this protein in the context of end-organ manifestations such as renal failure, lytic bone disease, or anemia, or large numbers of plasma cells in the bone marrow of patients can be diagnostic of multiple myeloma.

The proteins are antibody immunoglobulin–free light chains (paraproteins) and are produced by neoplastic plasma cells. The light chains can be detected by heating or electrophoresis of concentrated urine. Light chains precipitate when heated to 50° to 60° C and re-dissolve at 90° to 100° C. These tests are essential in patients who may bave Bence-Jones proteins in their urine because these proteins do not react with the reagents normally used in urinalysis dipsticks. This circumstance leads to false-negative results in people with Bence-Jones proteins in their urine undergoing standard urinalysis. Various rarer conditions can produce Bence-Jones proteins, such as Waldenström macroglobulinemia and other malignancies.

Bilirubin

Newborns

Excessive bilirubin kills developing brain cells in infants and may cause mental retardation, physical abnormalities, or blindness. Bilirubin in newborns must not become too high. When the level of bilirubin is above a critical threshold, special treatments are initiated to lower it. An excessive bilirubin level may result from the breakdown of red blood cells (RBCs) caused by Rh blood typing incompatibility. (The mother is Rh negative [Rh–], the father is Rh positive [Rh+], and the fetus is Rh+; the mother develops antibodies against the newborn's RBCs, which are destroyed.)

Adults and Children

Bilirubin levels can be used to identify liver damage or disease or to monitor the progression of jaundice. A conjugated bilirubin that is elevated may indicate some kind of blockage of the liver or bile duct, hepatitis, trauma to the liver, a drug reaction, or long-term alcohol abuse. Inherited disorders caused by abnormal bilirubin metabolism (Gilbert, Rotor, Dubin-Johnson, or Crigler-Najjar syndromes) may also cause increased levels.

Blood Urea Nitrogen

Increased blood urea nitrogen (BUN) levels suggest impaired kidney function. This elevation may be caused by acute or chronic kidney disease, damage, or failure; it may also be caused by a condition that results in decreased blood flow to the kidneys, such as congestive heart failure, shock, stress, recent heart attack, or severe burns; to conditions that cause obstruction of urine flow; or to dehydration.

BUN concentrations may be elevated in the setting of excessive protein catabolism (breakdown), significantly increased protein in the diet, or gastrointestinal bleeding (because of the proteins present in the blood).

Low BUN levels are not common and are not usually a cause for concern. They may be seen in severe liver disease, malnutrition, and sometimes when a patient is overhydrated (excessive fluid volume); but the BUN test is not normally used to diagnose or monitor these conditions.

Both decreased and increased BUN concentrations may be seen during a normal pregnancy.

If one kidney is fully functional, BUN concentrations may be normal even when significant dysfunction is present in the other kidney.

Calcium

A normal calcium result with other normal laboratory results means that the patient has no problems with calcium metabolism (use by the body).

Because approximately one half of the calcium in the blood is bound by albumin (a protein), these two tests are usually ordered together. Calcium values must be interpreted in combination with albumin to determine if the calcium concentration of serum is appropriate. As albumin levels rise, calcium rises as well, and vice versa.

A high calcium level is called *hypercalcemia*, requiring treatment for the underlying condition. Hypercalcemia is usually caused by:

- Hyperparathyroidism (increase in parathyroid gland function): This condition is usually caused by a benign tumor on the parathyroid gland. This form of hypercalcemia is usually mild and can be present for many years before being noticed.
- Cancer: Cancer can cause hypercalcemia when it spreads to the bones, which releases calcium into the blood, or when cancer causes a hormone similar to parathyroid hormone to increase calcium levels.

Other causes of hypercalcemia include:

- Hyperthyroidism
- Sarcoidosis
- Tuberculosis
- Bone breaks combined with bed rest or not moving for a long periods
- Excess vitamin D intake
- Kidney transplantation
- High protein levels (e.g., if a tourniquet is used for too long while blood is collected)

In this case, free or ionized calcium remains normal. High levels of ionized calcium occur with all the conditions previously mentioned, except high protein levels.

Low calcium levels, called *hypocalcemia*, mean that the patient has insufficient calcium in the blood or that the patient has insufficient protein in the blood. The most common cause of low total calcium is low protein levels, especially low albumin. When low protein is the problem, the ionized calcium level remains normal.

Low calcium, known as *hypocalcemia*, is caused by many conditions:

- Low protein levels
- Underactive parathyroid gland (hypoparathyroidism)
- Decreased dietary intake of calcium
- Decreased levels of vitamin D
- Magnesium deficiency
- Excessive phosphorus
- Acute inflammation of the pancreas
- Chronic renal failure
- Calcium ions becoming bound to protein (alkalosis)
- Bone disease
- Malnutrition
- Alcoholism

Causes of low ionized calcium levels include all of these condition except low protein levels.

Chloride

Increased levels of chloride *(hyperchloremia)* usually indicate dehydration, but high levels can also occur with any other problem that causes high blood sodium. Hyperchloremia also occurs when excessive base is lost from the body (producing metabolic acidosis) or when a person hyperventilates (causing respiratory alkalosis).

Decreased levels of chloride *(hypochloremia)* occur with any disorder that causes low blood sodium. Hypochloremia also occurs with prolonged vomiting or gastric suction, chronic diarrhea, emphysema or other chronic lung disease (causing respiratory acidosis), and with loss of acid from the body (causing metabolic alkalosis).

Cholesterol

In a routine setting in which testing is performed to screen for risk factors, the test results are grouped in three categories of risk:

- Desirable: A cholesterol level below 200 mg/dL (5.18 mmol/L) is considered desirable and reflects a low risk of heart disease.
- Borderline high: A cholesterol level of 200 to 240 mg/dL (5.18-6.22 mmol/L) is considered to reflect moderate risk.
- High risk: A cholesterol level above 240 mg/dL (6.22 mmol/L) is considered high risk.

Creatinine

Increased creatinine levels in the blood suggest diseases or conditions that affect kidney function, including the following:

- Damage to or swelling of blood vessels in the kidneys (glomerulonephritis) caused by, for example, infection or autoimmune diseases
- Bacterial infection of the kidneys (pyelonephritis)
- Death of cells in the kidneys' small tubes (acute tubular necrosis) caused, for example, by drugs or toxins
- Prostate disease, kidney stone, or other causes of urinary tract obstruction
- Reduced blood flow to the kidney caused by shock, dehydration, congestive heart failure, atherosclerosis, or complications of diabetes

Creatinine can also increase temporarily as a result of muscle injury. Low levels of creatinine are not common and are not usually a cause for concern and can be seen with conditions that result in decreased muscle mass. Creatinine levels are generally slightly lower during pregnancy.

Creatinine Phosphokinase

A high creatinine phosphokinase (CK) level, or one that goes up from the first to the second or later samples, generally indicates some damage to the heart or other muscles; it can also indicate that the patient's muscles have experienced heavy use. If the patient has experienced a heart attack and the CK is high, a more specific test (troponin or CK-MB) should be ordered to determine if the patient's heart is damaged.

Glucose

High levels of glucose most frequently indicate diabetes, but many other diseases and conditions can also cause elevated glucose. The following information summarizes the meaning of the test results. These points are based on the clinical practice recommendations of the American Diabetes Association (Table 1-4).

Some of the other diseases and conditions that can result in elevated glucose levels include:

- Acromegaly
- Acute stress (response to trauma, heart attack, and stroke for instance)
- Chronic renal failure
- Cushing syndrome
- Drugs (e.g., corticosteroids, tricyclic antidepressants, diuretics, epinephrine, estrogens [birth control pills and hormone replacement medications], lithium, phenytoin [Dilantin®], salicylates)
- Excessive food intake
- Hyperthyroidism
- Pancreatic cancer
- Pancreatitis

Low to nondetectible urine glucose results are considered normal. Anything that raises blood glucose levels also has the potential to elevate urine glucose levels. Increased urine glucose levels may be seen with medications such as estrogens and chloral hydrate and with some forms of renal disease.

Moderately increased levels may be seen with prediabetes. This condition, if left untreated, often leads to type 2 diabetes.

Low glucose levels (hypoglycemia) are also seen with:

- Adrenal insufficiency
- Drinking alcohol
- Drugs (e.g., acetaminophen, anabolic steroids)
- Extensive liver disease
- Hypopituitarism
- Hypothyroidism
- Insulin overdose
- Insulinomas (insulin-producing pancreatic tumors)
- Starvation

Heavy Metal Screens

Heavy metals are increasingly responsible for the production of free radicals, as well as undermining the *internal environment* and body chemistry. The main concern is not so much the type of metal that may be detected but rather if metals in their ionic form are present. Chemical analyses can establish the exposure to excessive amounts of toxic substances. Many analytical procedures can be performed if the problem warrants the investment of time and the client is willing to pay for the procedure. Although screening samples for certain groups of chemicals is possible, *analyzing for everything* or *checking for poisons* is not feasible. Heavy metals include arsenic, cadmium, calcium, cobalt, copper,

TABLE 1-4	
SUMMARY OF GLUCOSE TOLERANCE TESTS AND INTERPRETATIONS	
Fasting Blood Glucose	
From 70 to 99 mg/dL (3.9 to 5.5 mmol/L)	Normal glucose tolerance
From 100 to 125 mg/dL (5.6 to 6.9 mmol/L)	Impaired fasting glucose (prediabetes)
126 mg/dL (7.0 mmol/L) and above on more than one testing occasion	Diabetes
Oral Glucose Tolerance Test (OGTT) [except pregnancy] (2 hours after a 75-gram glucose drink)	
Less than 140 mg/dL (7.8 mmol/L)	Normal glucose tolerance
From 140 to 200 mg/dL (7.8 to 11.1 mmol/L)	Impaired glucose tolerance (pre-diabetes)
Over 200 mg/dL (11.1 mmol/L) on more than one testing occasion	Diabetes
Gestational Diabetes Screening: Glucose Challenge Test (1 hour after a 50-gram glucose drink)	
Less than 140* mg/dL (7.8 mmol/L)	Normal glucose tolerance
140* mg/dL (7.8 mmol/L) and over	Abnormal, needs OGTT (see below)
Gestational Diabetes Diagnostic: OGTT (100-gram glucose drink)	
Fasting†	95 mg/dL (5.3 mmol/L)
1 hour after glucose load†	180 mg/dL (10.0 mmol/L)
2 hours after glucose load†	155 mg/dL (8.6 mmol/L)
3 hours after glucose load†‡	140 mg/dL (7.8 mmol/L)

*Some use a cutoff of >130 mg/dL (7.2 mmol/L) because that identifies 90% of women with gestational diabetes, compared to 80% identified using the threshold of >140 mg/dL (7.8 mmol/L).

†If two or more values are above the criteria, gestational diabetes is diagnosed.

‡A 75-gram glucose load may be used, although this method is not as well validated as the 100-gram OGTT; the 3-hour sample is not drawn if 75 grams is used.

cyanide, fluoride, iron, lead, magnesium, manganese, mercury, molybdenum, phosphorus, potassium, selenium, sodium, and zinc.

Hematocrit

Decreased hematocrit indicates anemia, such as that caused by iron deficiency or other deficiencies. Further testing may be necessary to determine the exact cause of the anemia.

Other conditions that can result in a low hematocrit include vitamin or mineral deficiencies, recent bleeding, cirrhosis of the liver, and malignancies.

The most common cause of increased hematocrit is dehydration, and with adequate fluid intake, the hematocrit returns to normal. However, increased levels may reflect a condition called *polycythemia vera*—that is, when a person has more than the normal number of RBCs. Increased hematocrit can be caused by a problem with the bone marrow or, more commonly, as compensation for inadequate lung function (the bone marrow manufactures more RBCs to carry enough oxygen throughout the body).

Hemoglobin

Normal values in an adult are 12 to 18 g/dL (100 mm/dL) of blood. Above-normal hemoglobin levels may be the result of:

- Dehydration
- Excessive production of RBCs in the bone marrow
- Severe lung disease
- Several other conditions

Below-normal hemoglobin levels may lead to anemia that can be the result of:

- Iron deficiency or deficiencies in essential vitamins of other elements such as vitamin B12, folate, vitamin B6
- Inherited hemoglobin defects, such as sickle cell anemia or thalassemias
- Other inherited defects affecting the RBCs
- Cirrhosis of the liver (during which the liver becomes scarred)
- Excessive bleeding
- Excessive destruction of RBCs
- Kidney disease
- Other chronic illnesses
- Bone marrow failure or aplastic anemia
- Cancers that affect the bone marrow

Human Leukocyte Antigen-B27

Human leukocyte antigen (HLA)-B27 will be present or absent. If it is present, then the HLA-B27 antigen (protein structure) exists on the surface of the body's white blood cells (WBCs) and nucleated cells. If a patient has HLA-B27 and has symptoms such as chronic pain, inflammation, and degenerative changes to his bones (as seen on X-ray examination), then it supports a diagnosis of ankylosing spondylitis (AS), Reiter syndrome, or another autoimmune disorder that is associated with the presence of HLA-B27. This circumstance is especially true if the patient is young, male gender, and if the patient experienced the first symptoms before the age of 40.

The presence of HLA-B27 may also seen with other autoimmune conditions such as:

- Isolated acute anterior uveitis
- Undifferentiated spondyloarthropathies
- Enteropathic synovitis

If HLA-B27 is not present, then the symptoms are likely the result of an HLA-B27–associated autoimmune disorder. (Exceptions to this rule, however, are approximately 10% of patients with AS and 40% to 50% of those with Reiter syndrome will be negative for HLA-B27.)

At this time, identifying the presence of HLA-B27 does not predict the likelihood of developing an autoimmune disease. If a patient does have an associated disorder, the presence of HLA-B27 cannot be used to tell which disease is present, how quickly it will progress, its severity, prognosis, or the degree of organ involvement.

Lactic Dehydrogenase Compression Test II

Elevated levels of lactic dehydrogenase (LDH) and changes in the ratio of the LDH isoenzymes usually indicate some type of tissue damage. LDH levels will usually rise as the cellular destruction begins, peak after some time period, and then begin to fall. For instance, when someone has a heart attack, blood levels of total LDH will rise within 24 to 48 hours, peak in 2 to 3 days, and return to normal in 10 to 14 days.

Elevated levels of LDH may be seen with:

- Cerebrovascular accident (CVA, stroke)
- Drugs (e.g., anesthetics, aspirin, narcotics, procainamide, alcohol)
- Hemolytic anemia
- Pernicious anemias (megaloblastic anemias)
- Infectious mononucleosis
- Intestinal and pulmonary infarction (tissue death)
- Kidney disease
- Liver disease
- Muscular dystrophy
- Pancreatitis
- Some cancers

With some chronic and progressive conditions, and some drugs, moderately elevated LDH levels may persist.

Low and normal levels of LDH do not usually indicate a problem. Low levels are sometimes seen when a patient ingests large amounts of ascorbic acid (vitamin C).

Latex Agglutination

Various rapid tests identifying bacterial antigen from body fluids are becoming increasingly available. One of these techniques, latex agglutination, is frequently used to test cerebrospinal fluid in children being evaluated for possible meningitis. Early diagnosis of meningitis can lead to prompt treatment.

Leucine Aminopeptidase

Serum leucine aminopeptidase determination is a useful screening procedure for hepatobiliary disease in jaundiced and unjaundiced patients. Values under 1000 units are of no help in the differential diagnosis of jaundice, but values above 1000 units are highly indicative of biliary obstruction. The differentiation of intra- from extrahepatic obstruction, as well as of malignant from benign jaundice, cannot generally be established by this single test.

Lipase

In acute pancreatitis, lipase levels are frequently very high, often 5 to 10 times higher than the highest reference value (often called the *upper limit of normal*). In acute pancreatitis, lipase concentrations rise within 24 to 48 hours of an acute pancreatic attack and may remain elevated for approximately 5 to 7 days. Concentrations may also be increased with pancreatic duct obstruction, pancreatic cancer, and other pancreatic diseases.

Moderately increased lipase values may occur in other conditions such as kidney disease (caused by decreased clearance from the blood), salivary gland inflammation, a bowel obstruction, or peptic ulcer disease, although the lipase test is not normally used to monitor these conditions. Decreased lipase levels may indicate permanent damage to the lipase-producing cells in the pancreas.

Lipids

The lipid profile includes total cholesterol, high-density lipoprotein (HDL) cholesterol (often called *good* cholesterol), low-density lipoprotein (LDL) cholesterol (often called *bad* cholesterol), and triglycerides. The report will sometimes include additional calculated values such as HDL/LDL ratio or a risk score based on lipid profile results, age, sex, and other risk factors.

A normal level for fasting triglycerides is less than 150 mg/dL (1.70 mmol/L). Having high triglycerides without also having high cholesterol is unusual. Most treatments for heart disease risk will be aimed at lowering LDL cholesterol. However, the type of treatment used to lower LDL cholesterol may differ depending on whether triglycerides are high or normal.

Triglycerides that are very high (greater than 1000 mg/dl [11.30 mmol/L]) increases the risk of developing pancreatitis. Treatment to lower triglycerides should be started as soon as possible.

Lupus Erythematosus Cell Prep

The lupus erythematosus (LE) cell prep was the primary diagnosis of SLE for nearly 50 years, having a sensitivity of nearly 50%. This test has been replaced by a more sensitive test, ANA, which measures the binding of a patient's serum antibodies to HEp-2 cell nuclei.

The results of each of the lupus anticoagulant tests lead either toward or away from the likelihood of having a lupus anticoagulant. Although the tests performed may vary, they usually begin with a prolonged partial thromboplastin time (PTT).

- If the PTT or lupus anticoagulant (LA)-PTT is prolonged, and mixing it with normal pooled plasma does not *correct* the result, then an inhibitor is likely present. If the pro-longed test corrects when phospholipid is added, then a lupus anticoagulant is likely present. (After heparin con-tamination, a lupus anticoagulant is the most common reason for a prolonged PTT.)

- If the PTT is not prolonged, a lupus anticoagulant may not be present, the test reagents may contain too much phospholipid, or the test may not be sufficiently sensitive to pick up the lupus anticoagulant. The LA–sensitive PTT may need to be performed.
- If a dilute Russell viper venom time or modified Russell viper venom time test is prolonged and does not correct when mixed with normal pooled plasma but does correct with the addition of phospholipids, then a phospholipid antibody is likely present.
- If a thrombin time test is normal, then heparin contamina-tion is excluded.
- If a fibrinogen test is normal, then fibrinogen is likely sufficient for normal clot formation.

Other tests that may be performed to help confirm the diagnosis of a lupus anticoagulant include:

- Platelet neutralization (This test uses platelets as a source of phospholipids.)
- Hexagonal (II) phase phospholipid assay (Staclot-LA test)
- Kaolin clotting time
- Tissue thromboplastin inhibition test
- Venereal Disease Research Laboratory (VDRL) or rapid plasma reagin (RPR) (These tests are used to detect syphilis. Their reagents are made of cardiolipin and they may give a false positive result for both anticardiolipin antibodies and for lupus anticoagu-lant.)
- Coagulation factors (These tests may be ordered to rule out factor deficiencies that may cause a prolonged PTT and bleeding episodes.)
- Prothrombin time

Other tests that may be performed in addition to lupus anticoagulant testing include:

- Anticardiolipin and anti-beta2-glycoprotein I antibod-ies to check for antiphospholipid syndrome
- Platelet count (Mild to moderate thrombocytopenia is often seen along with the lupus anticoagulant and may be caused by anticoagulant [heparin] therapy.)

Phosphorus

Dietary deficiencies in phosphorus are rare but may be seen with alcoholism and malnutrition. Low levels of phosphorus (hypophosphatemia) may also be caused by or associated with:

- Hypercalcemia (high levels of calcium) especially as a result of hyperparathyroidism
- Overuse of diuretics (drugs that encourage urination)
- Severe burns
- Diabetic ketoacidosis (after treatment)
- Hypothyroidism
- Hypokalemia (low levels of potassium)

- Chronic antacid use
- Rickets and osteomalacia (caused by vitamin-D deficiencies)

Higher-than-normal levels of phosphorus (hyperphos-phatemia) may be caused by or associated with:

- Kidney failure
- Hypoparathyroidism (underactive parathyroid gland)
- Diabetic ketoacidosis (when first seen)
- Phosphate supplementation

Potassium

Increased potassium levels indicate hyperkalemia. Increased levels may also indicate the following health conditions:

- Excessive dietary potassium intake (Fruits are par-ticularly high in potassium; therefore, excessive intake of fruits or juices may contribute to high potassium.)
- Excessive intravenous potassium intake
- Acute or chronic kidney failure
- Addison disease
- Hypoaldosteronism
- Injury to tissue
- Infection
- Diabetes
- Dehydration

Certain drugs can also cause hyperkalemia in a small percentage of patients. Among these drugs are nonsteroidal antiinflammatory drugs (e.g., Advil®, Motrin®, Nuprin®), beta-blockers (e.g., propranolol atenolol), angiotensin-converting enzyme inhibitors (e.g., captopril, enalapril, lisinopril), and potassium-sparing diuretics (e.g., triam-terene, amiloride, spironolactone).

Decreased levels of potassium indicate hypokalemia. Decreased levels may occur in several conditions, particu-larly:

- Dehydration
- Vomiting
- Diarrhea
- Deficient potassium intake (rare)

Protein-Bound Iodine

Iodine binds to protein, mainly thyroxin, in the plasma. The thyroid hormone is precipitated by protein-denaturing agents, and the amount of iodine in a protein precipitate generally indicates the amount of thyroid hormone present and is thus an index of thyroid activity. Various values are given for thyroid function: hypothyroidism, 0 to 3.5 mcg/mL of protein-bound iodine; euthyroidism, 3.5 to 8.0 g/mL; hyperthyroidism, values higher than 8 mcg/mL.

Red Blood Cell Count

A high RBC count may indicate congenital heart disease, dehydration, obstructive lung disease, or bone marrow overproduction. A high RBC count is also seen in beta-thalassemia trait, a benign condition with little or no anemia. A low RBC count may indicate anemia, bleeding, kidney disease, bone marrow failure (for instance, from radiation or a tumor), malnutrition, or other causes. A low count may also indicate nutritional deficiencies of iron, folate, vitamin B12, and vitamin B6.

Rheumatoid Arthritis Factor (RA Latex) Test

A rapid latex slide agglutination test for the qualitative and semi-quantitative determination of rheumatoid arthritis factor in human serum. The presence of these autoantibodies to human immunoglobulin G (IgG) is a useful diagnostic tool for active rheumatoid arthritis (RA) because high titres indicate severe disease.

Serum Glutamate Oxaloacetate Transaminase

Very high levels of aspartate aminotransferase (AST) (more than 10 times the highest normal level) are usually the result of acute hepatitis, often caused by a virus infection. In acute hepatitis, AST levels usually stay high for approximately 1 to 2 months but can take as long as 3 to 6 months to return to normal. In chronic hepatitis, AST levels are usually not as high as they are in acute hepatitis, often less than four times the highest normal level. In chronic hepatitis, AST often varies between normal and slightly increased; therefore, examiners will typically order the test frequently to determine the pattern.

In some diseases of the liver, especially when the bile ducts are blocked, or with cirrhosis and certain cancers of the liver, AST may be close to normal, but it increases more often than alanine aminotransferase (ALT). When liver damage is the result of alcohol, AST often increases much more than ALT. (This pattern is seen with a few other liver diseases.) AST is also increased after heart attacks and with muscle injury, usually to a much greater degree than is ALT.

Serum Ionized Calcium

Blood calcium is tested to screen for, diagnose, and monitor a range of conditions relating to the bones, heart, nerves, kidneys, and teeth. Blood calcium levels do not directly tell how much calcium is in the bones, but rather, how much calcium is circulating in the blood.

A total calcium level is often measured as part of health screening. It is included in the comprehensive metabolic panel (CMP) and the basic metabolic panel (BMP)—groups of tests that are performed together to diagnose or monitor a variety of conditions. When an abnormal total calcium result is obtained, it is viewed as an indicator or some kind of underlying problem. To help diagnose the underlying problem, additional tests are often done to measure ionized calcium, urine calcium, phosphorous, magnesium, vitamin D, and parathyroid hormone (PTH). Parathyroid hormone and vitamin D are responsible for maintaining calcium concentrations in the blood within a narrow range of values.

Measuring calcium and PTH together can help determine whether the parathyroid gland is functioning normally. Measuring urine calcium can help determine whether the kidneys are excreting the proper amount of calcium, and testing for vitamin D, phosphorus, and/or magnesium can help deter-

mine whether other deficiencies or excesses exist. Frequently the balance among these different substances, and the changes in them, are just as important as the concentrations. Calcium can be used as a diagnostic test if the patient presents with symptoms that suggest:

- Kidney stones
- Bone disease
- Neurologic disorders

The total calcium test is the test most frequently ordered to evaluate calcium status. In most cases, it is a good reflection of the amount of free calcium involved in metabolism since the balance between free and bound is usually stable and predictable. However, in some patients, the balance between bound and free calcium is disturbed and total calcium is not a good reflection of calcium status. In those circumstances, measurement of ionized calcium is necessary. Some conditions where ionized calcium should be the test of choice include: critically ill patients who are receiving transfusions or IV fluids, patients undergoing major surgery, and patients with blood protein abnormalities like low albumin. Large fluctuations in ionized calcium can cause the heart to slow down or to beat too rapidly, can cause muscles to go into spasm (tetany), and can cause confusion or even coma. In critically ill patients, it is extremely important to know the ionized calcium level to be able to intervene and prevent serious complications. These include the following:

1. Kidney disease, because low calcium is especially common in those with kidney failure;
2. Symptoms of too much calcium, such as fatigue, weakness, loss of appetite, nausea, vomiting, constipation, abdominal pain, urinary frequency, and increased thirst;
3. Symptoms of low calcium, such as cramps in your abdomen, muscle cramps, or tingling fingers; or
4. Other diseases that have been associated with abnormal blood calcium, such as thyroid disease, intestinal disease, cancer, or poor nutrition.

An ionized calcium test is ordered when the patient has numbness around the mouth and in the hands and feet and muscle spasms in the same areas. These can be symptoms of low levels of ionized calcium. However, when calcium levels fall slowly, many people have no symptoms at all. The patient may need calcium monitoring when they have certain kinds of cancer (particularly breast, lung, head and neck, kidney, and multiple myeloma), have kidney disease, or have had a kidney transplant. Monitoring may also be necessary when the patient is being treated for abnormal calcium levels to evaluate the effectiveness of treatments such as calcium or vitamin D supplements.

Calcium absorption, use, and excretion are regulated and stabilized by a feedback loop involving PTH and vitamin D. Conditions and diseases that disrupt calcium regulation can cause inappropriate acute or chronic elevations or decreases in calcium and lead to symptoms of hypercalcemia or hypocalcemia. In most cases, total calcium is measured because the test is more easily performed than the ionized calcium test and requires no special handling of the blood sample. Total calcium is usually a good reflection of free calcium since the free and bound forms are typically each about half of the total. However, because about half the calcium in blood is bound to protein, total calcium test results can be affected by high or low levels of protein. In such cases, it is more useful to measure free calcium directly using an ionized calcium test.

Normal Calcium

A normal total or ionized calcium result together with other normal lab results generally means that calcium metabolism is normal and blood levels are being appropriately regulated.

High Total Calcium—Hypercalcemia

Two of the more common causes of hypercalcemia are:

1. Hyperparathyroidism, an increase in parathyroid gland function: This condition is usually caused by a benign tumor of the parathyroid gland. This form of hypercalcemia is usually mild and can be present for many years before being noticed.
2. Cancer: Cancer can cause hypercalcemia when it spreads to the bones, which releases calcium into the blood, or when a cancer produces a hormone similar to PTH, resulting in increased calcium levels.

Some other causes of hypercalcemia include:

1. Hyperthyroidism
2. Sarcoidosis
3. Tuberculosis
4. Prolonged immobilization
5. Excess Vitamin D intake
6. Kidney transplant

Low Total Calcium—Hypocalcemia

The most common cause of low total calcium is:

1. Low blood protein levels, especially a low level of albumin. In this condition, only the bound calcium is low. Ionized calcium remains normal and calcium metabolism is being regulated appropriately.

Some other causes of hypocalcemia include:

1. Underactive parathyroid gland (hypoparathyroidism)
2. Inherited resistance to the effects of parathyroid hormone
3. Extreme deficiency in dietary calcium
4. Decreased levels of vitamin D
5. Magnesium deficiency
6. Increased levels of phosphorus
7. Acute inflammation of the pancreas (pancreatitis)
8. Renal failure
9. Malnutrition
10. Alcoholism

Serum Protein Electrophoresis

Protein and immunofixation electrophoresis tests give the examiner a rough estimate of how much of each protein is present. The value of protein electrophoresis lies in the proportions of proteins and in the patterns they create on the electrophoresis graph. The value of immunofixation electrophoresis is in identifying the presence of a particular type of immunoglobulin. For example, certain conditions or diseases may be associated with decreases or increases in various serum proteins, as reflected as follows:

- Albumin
  - *Decreased:* with malnutrition and malabsorption, pregnancy, kidney disease (especially nephrotic syndrome), liver disease, inflammatory conditions, and protein-losing syndromes
  - *Increased:* with dehydration
- Alpha$_1$ globulin
  - *Decreased:* in congenital emphysema (α_1-antitrypsin deficiency, a rare genetic disease) or severe liver disease
  - *Increased:* in acute or chronic inflammatory diseases
- Alpha$_2$ globulin
  - *Decreased:* with hyperthyroidism or severe liver disease, hemolysis (RBC breakage)
  - *Increased:* with kidney disease (nephrotic syndrome), acute or chronic inflammatory disease
- Beta globulin
  - *Decreased:* with malnutrition, cirrhosis
  - *Increased:* with hypercholesterolemia, iron deficiency anemia, some cases of multiple myeloma, or monoclonal gammopathies of undetermined significance (MGUS)
- Gamma globulin
  - *Decreased:* variety of genetic immune disorders, and in secondary immune deficiency
  - *Increased:* polyclonal—chronic inflammatory disease, RA, SLE, cirrhosis, chronic liver disease, acute and chronic infection, recent immunization.
  - *Increased:* monoclonal—Waldenström macroglobulinemia, multiple myeloma, MGUS
- Total protein

Low total protein levels can suggest a liver disorder, a kidney disorder, or a disorder in which protein is not digested or absorbed properly. Some laboratories also report the calculated ratio of albumin to globulins (A/G ratio). Normally, albumin slightly exceeds globulins, giving a normal A/G ratio of slightly over 1. Because disease states affect the relative changes in albumin and globulins in different ways, this ratio may provide a clue to the physician as to the cause of the change in protein levels. A low A/G ratio may reflect overproduction of globulins, such as seen in multiple myeloma or autoimmune diseases, or underproduction of albumin, such as occurs with cirrhosis, or selective loss of albumin from the circulation, as occurs with nephrotic syndrome. A high A/G ratio suggests underproduction of immunoglobulins, as may be seen in some genetic deficiencies and in some leukemias. More specific tests, such as albumin, liver enzyme tests, and serum protein electrophoresis, must be performed to make an accurate diagnosis.

Sodium

Hyponatremia is rarely caused by decreased sodium intake (deficient dietary intake or deficient sodium in intravenous fluids). Most commonly, hyponatremia is caused by sodium loss (Addison disease, diarrhea, excessive sweating, diuretic administration, or kidney disease). In some cases, hyponatremia is caused by increased water (drinking too much water, heart failure, cirrhosis, kidney diseases that cause protein loss [nephrotic syndrome]). In a large number of diseases (particularly those involving the brain and the lungs, many kinds of cancer, and with some drugs), the body makes too much antidiuretic hormone, causing the patient to keep too much water in the body.

A high blood sodium level means the patient has hypernatremia, almost always caused by excessive loss of water (dehydration) without enough water intake. Symptoms include dry mucous membranes, thirst, agitation, restlessness, acting irrationally, and coma or convulsions if levels rise extremely high. In rare cases, hypernatremia may be caused by increased salt intake without enough water, Cushing syndrome, or insufficient antidiuretic hormone (*diabetes insipidus*).

Sodium urine concentrations must be evaluated in association with blood levels. Concentrations may mirror blood levels or be the opposite. The body normally excretes excess sodium; thus the concentration in the urine may be elevated because it is elevated in the blood. It may also be elevated in the urine when the body is losing excessive sodium. In this case, the blood level would be normal to low. If blood sodium levels are low as a result of insufficient intake, then urine concentrations will also be low.

Uric Acid

Higher-than-normal uric acid levels mean that the body is not handling the breakdown of purines well. Increased concentrations of uric acid can cause crystals to form in the joints, which leads to the joint inflammation and pain characteristics of gout. Uric acid can also form crystals or kidney stones that can damage the kidneys.

Low levels of uric acid in the blood are seen much less commonly than high levels and are seldom considered cause for concern. Although low values can be associated with some kinds of liver or kidney diseases, exposure to toxic compounds, and rarely as the result of an inherited metabolic defect, these conditions are typically identified by other tests and symptoms and not by an isolated low uric acid result.

Urinalysis

pH
Acidity of urine is measured by the pH.

Specific Gravity
Specific gravity (SG) measures how dilute the urine is. Water has a SG of 1.000. Most urine is approximately 1.010, but it can vary greatly depending on when the patient drank fluids last or if the patient is dehydrated.

Glucose
Normally, urine contains no glucose. A positive glucose occurs in diabetes. The number of people who have glucose in their urine with normal blood glucose levels is small; however, any glucose in the urine would raise the possibility of diabetes or glucose intolerance.

Protein
Normally no protein is detectable on a urinalysis strip. Protein can indicate kidney damage, blood in the urine, or an infection. Up to 10% of children can have protein in their urine. Certain diseases require the use of a special, more sensitive (and more expensive) test for protein called a microalbumin test. A microalbumin test is useful in screening for early damage to the kidneys from diabetes, for instance.

Blood
Normally, urine contains no blood. Blood can indicate an infection, kidney stones, trauma, or bleeding from a bladder or kidney tumor and may be hemolyzed (dissolved blood) or nonhemolyzed (intact RBCs). Rarely, muscle injury can cause myoglobin to appear in the urine, which also causes the reagent pad to indicate blood falsely.

Bilirubin
Normally, urine contains no bilirubin or urobilinogen. These substances are pigments that are cleared by the liver. In liver or gallbladder disease, they may appear in the urine as well.

Nitrate
Normally negative, nitrate in the urine usually indicates a urinary tract infection.

Leukocyte Esterase
Leukocyte esterase is normally negative. Leukocytes are the WBCs (or pus cells). WBCs in the urine suggest a urinary tract infection.

Sediment
Items such as mucous cells and squamous cells are commonly seen. Abnormal findings would include >15 RBCs/hpf (hematuria)—additional investigation must be done to determine the source of the hematuria (renal or postrenal); or >10 WBCs/hpf (pyuria)—additional investigation must be done to determine the source of the pyuria (renal or postrenal); or the presence of crystals, casts, renal tubular cells, or bacteria (bacteria can be present if contamination was present at the time of collection).

White Blood Cell Count

An elevated number of white blood cells (WBCs) is called *leukocytosis,* which can result from bacterial infections, inflammation, leukemia, trauma, or stress.

A decreased WBC count is called *leukopenia,* which can result from many different situations, such as chemotherapy, radiation therapy, or diseases of the immune system.

Blood and serum panels that are useful in the differential diagnosis include:

- Bone panel
- Alkaline phosphatase
- Calcium
- Complete blood count (CBC)

Table 1-5 explains what increases or decreases in each of the components of the CBC may mean.

SPECITIC PROFILES
Arthritis Panel

- ANA screen
- C-reactive protein (CRP)

A high or increasing amount of CRP in the blood suggests an acute infection or inflammation. In a healthy person, CRP is usually less than 10 mg/L. Most infections and inflammations result in CRP levels above 100 mg/L. If the CRP level drops, it means inflammation is being reduced. When results fall below 10 mg/L, clinically active inflammation is no longer present.

- RA latex

Liver Function Tests

- Alkaline phosphatase
- Bilirubin-total and direct
- Cholesterol
- Gamma-glutamyl transpeptidase (GGT) or peptidase

Elevated GGT levels indicate that something is going on with the liver but not specifically what. In general, the higher the level is, the greater the *insult* will be to a liver. Elevated levels may be caused by liver disease, but they may also be caused by congestive heart failure, alcohol consumption, and use of many prescription and nonprescription drugs, including nonsteroidal antiinflammatory drugs, lipid-lowering drugs, antibiotics, histamine blockers (used to treat excess stomach acid production), antifungal agents, seizure control medications, antidepressants, and hormones such as testosterone. Oral contraceptives (birth control pills) and clofibrate can decrease GGT levels.

TABLE 1-5		
SUMMARY OF CBC COMPONENTS AND INTERPRETATIONS		
Test	**Name**	**Increased/Decreased**
WBC	White blood cell	May be increased with infections, inflammation, cancer, leukemia; decreased with some medications (such as methotrexate), some autoimmune conditions, some severe infections, bone marrow failure, and congenital marrow aplasia (marrow doesn't develop normally)
% Neutrophil	Neutrophil/Band/Seg	This is a dynamic population that varies somewhat from day to day depending on what is going on in the body. Significant increases in particular types are associated with different temporary/acute and/or chronic conditions. An example of this is the increased number of lymphocytes seen with lymphocytic leukemia. For more information, see Blood Smear and WBC.
% Lymphs	Lymphocyte	
% Mono	Monocyte	
% Eos	Eosinophil	
% Baso	Basophil	
Neutrophil	Neutrophil/Band/Seg	
Lymphs	Lymphocyte	
Mono	Monocyte	
Eos	Eosinophil	
Baso	Basophil	
RBC	Red blood cell	Decreased with anemia; increased when too many made and with fluid loss due to diarrhea, dehydration, burns
Hgb	Hemoglobin	Mirrors RBC results
Hct	Hematocrit	Mirrors RBC results
MCV	Mean corpuscular volume	Increased with B_{12} and Folate deficiency; decreased with iron deficiency and thalassemia
MCH	Mean corpuscular hemoglobin	Mirrors MCV results
MCHC	Mean corpuscular hemoglobin concentration	May be decreased when MCV is decreased; increases limited to amount of Hgb that will fit inside a RBC
RDW	Red blood cell distribution width	Increased RDW indicates mixed population of RBCs; immature RBCs tend to be larger
Platelet	Platelet	Decreased or increased with conditions that affect platelet production; decreased when greater numbers used, as with bleeding; decreased with some inherited disorders (such as Wiskott-Aldrich, Bernard-Soulier), with Systemic lupus erythematosus, pernicious anemia, hypersplenism (spleen takes too many out of circulation), leukemia, and chemotherapy
MPV	Mean platelet volume	Vary with platelet production; younger platelets are larger than older ones

- LDH (See previous discussion.)
- Serum glutamate pyruvate transaminase (SGPT) (See previous discussion.)
- Serum glutamate oxaloacetate transaminase (SGOT)
- Total protein—albumin and globulin

Parathyroid Function and Calcium Metabolism

- Alkaline phosphatase
- Serum calcium
- Serum phosphorus
- Total protein
- Urine calcium
- Pancreas function tests
- Amylase
- CBC
- Glucose tolerance
- Lipase

Joint Pain or Swelling Tests

- ANA screen
- CBC
- Heavy metal screen
- RA latex
- Sedimentation rate

Although it is frequently ordered, the erythrocyte sedimentation rate (ESR) is not a useful screening test; it is useful only for diagnosing three diseases: (1) myeloma, (2) temporal arteritis, and (3) polymyalgia rheumatica (in which it may exceed 100 mm/hour).

ESR is commonly used for a differential diagnosis for Kawasaki disease, and it may be increased in some chronic infective conditions such as tuberculosis and infective endocarditis. The ESR is a component of the Pediatric Crohn Disease Activity Index (PDCAI), an index for assessment of severity of inflammatory bowel disease in children.

The clinical usefulness of ESR is limited to monitoring the response to therapy in certain inflammatory diseases such as temporal arteritis, polymyalgia rheumatica, and rheumatoid arthritis; it can also be used as a crude measure of response in Hodgkin disease.

The use of ESR as a screening test in asymptomatic persons is limited by its low sensitivity and specificity. When a moderate suspicion of disease exists, the ESR may have some value as a *sickness index*.

An elevated ESR in the absence of other findings should *not* trigger an extensive laboratory or radiographic evaluation.

- Uric acid
- Synovial fluid analysis, including culture

Synovial fluid analysis is inexpensive and may be diagnostic in patients with bacterial infections or crystal-induced synovitis. According to the American College of Rheumatology (ACR) clinical guidelines committee, this analysis should be performed in the febrile patient with an acute flare of established arthritis to rule out superimposed septic arthritis. In other situations, its main value is to permit classification into an inflammatory or noninflammatory category. Thus, synovial fluid analysis should be performed if it is readily obtainable and the diagnosis is uncertain after history interview, physical examination, and standard laboratory tests (Table 1-6).

The WBC count, differential count, cultures, Gram stain, and polarized light microscopy are the most valuable studies. Noninflammatory fluids generally have fewer than 2000 WBCs/mm^3, with fewer than 75% polymorphonuclear leukocytes. The ACR committee suggests that unexplained inflammatory fluid, particularly in a febrile patient, is assumed to be infected until proven otherwise by appropriate culture.

Normal joints contain a small amount of synovial fluid with the following characteristics:

- Highly viscous
- Clear
- Essentially acellular

TABLE 1-6

CATEGORIES OF SYNOVIAL FLUID BASED UPON CLINICAL AND LABORATORY FINDINGS

Measure	Normal	Noninflammatory	Inflammatory	Septic	Hemorrhagic
Volume, mL (knee)	<3.5	Often >3.5	Often >3.5	Often >3.5	Usually >3.5
Clarity	Transparent	Transparent	Translucent-opaque	Opaque	Bloody
Color	Clear	Yellow	Yellow to opalescent	Yellow to green	Red
Viscosity	High	High	Low	Variable	Variable
WBC, per mm3	<200	200-2,000	2000-10,000	>100,000*	200-2,000
PMNs, percent	<25	<25	≥50	≥75	50-75
Culture	Negative	Negative	Negative	Often positive	Negative
Total protein, g/dl	1-2	1-3	3-5	3-5	4-6
LDH (compared to levels in blood)	Very low	Very low	High	Variable	Similar
Glucose, mg/dl	Nearly equal to blood	Nearly equal to blood	>25, lower than blood	<25, much lower than blood	Nearly equal to blood

LDH, Lactic dehydrogenase; *PMN,* polymorphonuclear cell; *WBC,* white blood cell.
*Lower with infections caused by partially treated or low virulence organisms

- Protein concentration approximately one-third that of plasma
- Glucose concentration similar to that in plasma

If a synovial effusion is present and arthrocentesis is indicated, joint fluid should be routinely analyzed for volume, clarity, color, viscosity, crystals cell count, differential, Gram stain, and culture. In certain circumstances, the presence and type of crystals should also be assessed. Synovial fluid is subsequently categorized as either normal, noninflammatory, inflammatory, septic, or hemorrhagic based on the clinical and laboratory analysis. The differential diagnosis of each of these specific categories is broad and not necessarily exclusive:

- *Noninflammatory* effusions may be caused by degenerative joint disease (osteoarthritis), trauma, osteochondritis dissecans, neuropathic arthropathy, subsiding or early inflammation, hypertrophic osteoarthropathy, and pigmented villonodular synovitis.
- *Inflammatory* effusions may be caused by RA, acute crystal-induced synovitis, reactive arthritis (formerly Reiter syndrome), ankylosing spondylitis, psoriatic arthritis, arthritis associated with inflammatory bowel disease, rheumatic fever, SLE, hypertrophic osteoarthropathy, and scleroderma. Rheumatic fever, SLE, and scleroderma can also cause a noninflammatory effusion.
- *Septic* effusions may be caused by bacteria, mycobacteria, or fungus.
- *Hemorrhagic* effusions may be caused by hemophilia or other hemorrhagic diathesis, scurvy, trauma with or without fracture, neuropathic arthropathy, pigmented villonodular synovitis, synovioma, hemangioma, and other benign neoplasms.

Thyroid Profile

Free Thyroxine Index

The free thyroxine index (FTI or T7) is a mathematical computation that allows the laboratory to estimate the free thyroxine index from the thyroxine (T4) and triiodothyronine (T3) uptake tests. The results tell how much thyroid hormone is free in the blood stream to work on the body. Unlike the T4 alone, FTI is not affected by estrogen levels.

Thyroid-Stimulating Hormone

A high thyroid-stimulating hormone (TSH) result often means an underactive thyroid gland that is not responding adequately to the stimulation of TSH because of some type of acute or chronic thyroid dysfunction. In rare instances, a high TSH result can indicate a problem with the pituitary gland, such as a tumor that produces unregulated levels of TSH, in what is known as *secondary hyperthyroidism*. A high TSH value can also occur when patients with a known thyroid disorder (or those who have had their thyroid gland removed) are receiving inadequate thyroid hormone medication.

A low TSH result can indicate an overactive thyroid gland (hyperthyroidism) or excessive amounts of thyroid

TABLE 1-7			
SUMMARY OF THYROID-STIMULATING HORMONE TEST RESULTS AND INTERPRETATIONS			
TSH	**T4**	**T3**	**Interpretation**
High	Normal	Normal	Mild (subclinical) hypothyroidism
High	Low	Low or normal	Hypothyroidism
Low	Normal	Normal	Mild (subclinical) hyperthyroidism
Low	High or normal	High or normal	Hyperthyroidism
Low	Low or normal	Low or normal	Rare pituitary (secondary) hypothyroidism

T3, Triiodothyronine; *T4,* thyroxine; *TSH,* thyroid-stimulating hormone.

hormone medication in patients who are being treated for an underactive (or removed) thyroid gland. In rare cases, a low TSH result may indicate damage to the pituitary gland that prevents it from producing adequate amounts of TSH.

Whether high or low, an abnormal TSH indicates an excess or deficiency in the amount of thyroid hormone available to the body, but it does not indicate the reason why. An abnormal TSH test result is usually followed by additional testing to investigate the cause of the increase or decrease.

Table 1-7 summarizes test results and their potential meaning.

Thyroxine

In general, high free or total T4 results may indicate an overactive thyroid gland (hyperthyroidism), and low free or total T4 results may indicate an underactive thyroid gland (hypothyroidism). The test results alone are not diagnostic but will prompt the examiner to perform additional testing to investigate the cause of the excess or deficiency. Both decreased and increased T4 results are associated with a variety of temporary and chronic thyroid conditions. Low T4 results in conjunction with a low TSH level, or high T4 results along with a high TSH, may indicate a pituitary gland condition.

Table 1-8 summarizes test results and their potential meaning.

Triiodothyronine

Increased or decreased thyroid hormone results indicate an imbalance between the body's requirements and supply, but they do not tell the examiner specifically what is causing the excess or deficiency.

Table 1-9 summarizes test results and their potential meaning.

If a patient is being treated with antithyroid medication for hyperthyroidism and the T3 (or, more frequently, the T4 or TSH) is normal, then the medication is likely controlling the condition. If the T3 (or T4) is elevated, then the medication is not sufficient to control the condition, and the patient

TABLE 1-8

SUMMARY OF THYROXINE (T4) TEST RESULTS AND INTERPRETATIONS

T4	TSH	T3	Interpretation
Normal	High	Normal	Mild (subclinical) hypothyroidism
Low	High	Low or normal	Hypothyroidism
Normal	Low	Normal	Mild (subclinical) hyperthyroidism
High or normal	Low	High or normal	Hyperthyroidism
Low or normal	Low	Low or normal	Rare pituitary (secondary) hypothyroidism

T3, Triiodothyronine; *T4,* thyroxine; *TSH,* thyroid-stimulating hormone.

TABLE 1-9

SUMMARY OF TRIIODOTHYRONINE (T3) TEST RESULTS AND INTERPRETATIONS

T3	T4	TSH	Interpretation
Normal	Normal	High	Mild (subclinical) hypothyroidism
Low or normal	Low	High	Hypothyroidism
Normal	Normal	Low	Mild (subclinical) hyperthyroidism
High or normal	High or normal	Low	Hyperthyroidism
Low or normal	Low or normal	Low	Rare pituitary (secondary) hypothyroidism

T3, Triiodothyronine; *T4,* thyroxine; *TSH,* thyroid-stimulating hormone.

may be experiencing symptoms associated with hyperthyroidism.

Prostate Profile

Prostate-Specific Antigen

The normal value for total prostate-specific antigen (PSA) has been set at less than 4.0 ng/mL blood. Some experts believe that this level should be lowered to 2.5 ng/mL to detect more cases of prostate cancer. Others argue that this change would exacerbate overdiagnosing and overtreating cancers that are not clinically significant.

Most experts agree that patients with a total PSA level greater than 10.0 ng/mL are at an increased risk for prostate cancer (more than a 67% chance, according to the American Cancer Society). Levels between 4.0 and 10.0 ng/mL may indicate prostate cancer (approximately a 25% chance, according to the American Cancer Society), benign prostate hyperplasia, or prostatitis. These conditions are more common in older adult males, as is a general increase in PSA levels. Concentrations of total PSA between 4.0 and 10.0 ng/mL are often called the *gray zone*. The free PSA is

the most useful in this range. When patients in the gray zone have decreased levels of free PSA, they have a higher probability of prostate cancer; when they have elevated levels of free PSA, the risk is diminished. The ratio of free to total PSA can help the examiner decide whether a prostate biopsy should be performed.

When the complexed PSA (cPSA) test is used as a screening tool, increased levels may indicate an increased risk of prostate cancer, whereas lower levels indicate a decreased risk.

In addition to the introduction of the free PSA and cPSA tests, efforts have been made to increase the usefulness of the total PSA as a screening tool. Although none of these efforts have been widely accepted yet, researchers are studying them, and some examiners are using them. These factors include:

- PSA velocity. This test measures the change in PSA concentrations over time. If the PSA continues to rise significantly over time, such as 3 or more years, then prostate cancer is more likely present. If it climbs rapidly, then the patient may have a more aggressive form of cancer.
- PSA doubling time. This test is another version of the PSA velocity. It measures how rapidly the PSA concentration doubles.
- PSA density. This test is a comparison of the PSA concentration and the volume of the prostate (as measured by ultrasound). Patients with larger prostates tend to produce more PSA; thus, this factor is an adjustment to compensate for the size.
- Age-specific PSA ranges. Given that PSA levels naturally increase as a man ages, experts have proposed that normal ranges be tailored to a man's age.

During treatment for prostate cancer, the PSA level should begin to fall. At the end of treatment, it should be at very low or undetectable levels in the blood. If concentrations do not fall to very low levels, then the treatment has not been fully effective. After treatment, the PSA test is performed at regular intervals to monitor the patient for recurrence. Because even tiny increases can be significant, patients may want to have their monitoring PSA tests performed by the same laboratory each time so that testing variation is kept to a minimum.

Prostatic Acid Phosphatase

Prostatic acid phosphatase (PAP) is an enzyme produced by the prostate. It may be found in increased amounts in men who have prostate cancer or other diseases. This same enzyme is also found in significant amounts in female ejaculate.

The highest levels of PAP are found in metastasized prostate cancer. Diseases of the bone (e.g., Paget disease, hyperparathyroidism), diseases of blood cells (e.g., sickle-cell disease, multiple myeloma), or lysosomal storage diseases (e.g., Gaucher disease) will show moderately increased levels.

Certain medications can cause temporary increases or decreases in PAP levels. Manipulation of the prostate gland through massage, biopsy, or rectal examination before a test can increase the level.

Hypertension (Coronary Risk Profile)

- Cholesterol
- Coronary risk indicator

This is a group of tests and health factors have been proven to indicate a patient's chance of having a coronary event. They have been refined to indicate the degree of risk: slight, moderate, or high.

Perhaps the most important indicators for cardiac risk are those of the personal health history. Age, hereditary factors, weight, smoking, blood pressure, exercise history, and diabetes are all important in determining risk. The lipid profile is the most important blood test for risk assessment. Other tests, both invasive and noninvasive, may be used in cardiac risk assessment. Noninvasive tests may include an electrocardiographic stress test, thallium stress test, electrocardiogram, computed tomographic scan, and echocardiogram. Invasive tests include an arteriogram and cardiac catheterization.

The lipid profile measures cholesterol, triglycerides, HDL (*good* cholesterol), and LDL (*bad* cholesterol). Triglycerides are the major form of fat found in the body, and their function is to provide energy for the cells. The desirable ranges for the components of the lipid profile include the following:

- Cholesterol <200 mg/dL (5.18 mmol/L)
- HDL cholesterol >40 mg/dL (1.04 mmol/L)
- LDL cholesterol <100 mg/dL* (2.59 mmol/L)
- Triglycerides <150 mg/dL (1.70 mmol/L)

If any or all of the results are significantly outside these ranges, the risk of a cardiac event is increased. If they are only slightly outside the desirable level, diet, exercise, medication, or any combination of these treatments may be sufficient to reduce the abnormal levels, thereby reducing risk.

Another test gaining importance is serum homocysteine. Homocysteine is an amino acid that comes from the normal breakdown of proteins in the body and appears to be a better test than cholesterol testing for predicting heart disease, stroke, and reduced blood flow to the hands and feet. Lipoprotein A (Lp[a]) is a lipoprotein consisting of an LDL molecule with another protein (apolipoprotein A) attached to it. Lp(a) is similar to LDL but does not respond to typical strategies to lower LDL such as diet, exercise, or most lipid-lowering drugs. Given that the level of Lp(a) appears to be genetically determined and not easily altered, the presence of a high level of Lp(a) may be used to identify individuals who might benefit from more aggressive treatment of other risk factors. A fairly new test, high-sensitivity (hsCRP), may be measured on apparently healthy patients to determine if they are at risk for a coronary event, even if their lipid levels are normal or borderline elevated.

---

*Optimal levels will depend on the number and type of risk factors present and whether testing is being used in primary or secondary intervention

High-Density Lipoprotein Cholesterol
- LDL cholesterol
- Triglycerides

Health Screen

- Albumin

Low albumin levels can suggest liver disease. Other liver enzyme tests are ordered to determine exactly which type of liver disease. Low albumin levels can also reflect diseases in which the kidneys cannot prevent albumin from leaking from the blood into the urine and being lost. In this case, the amount of albumin (or protein) in the urine also may be measured. Low albumin levels can also be seen in inflammation, shock, and malnutrition. Low albumin levels may also suggest conditions in which the body does not properly absorb and digest protein (e.g., Crohn disease, sprue) or in which large volumes of protein are lost from the intestines.

High albumin levels usually reflect dehydration.
- A/G ratio (See previous discussion.)
- Alkaline phosphatase
- Anion gap

Anion gap can be classified as high, normal, or, in rare cases, low. A high anion gap indicates a loss of bicarbonate without a subsequent increase in chloride. Electroneutrality is maintained by the increased production of anions such as ketones, lactate, phosphate, and sulfate; these anions are not part of the anion-gap calculation, and therefore a high anion gap results. In patients with a normal anion gap, the drop in bicarbonate is compensated for by an increase in chloride and hence is also known as hyperchloremic acidosis.

High Anion Gap
The bicarbonate lost is replaced by an unmeasured anion, and thus a high anion gap will be present in the following disorders:

Lactic acidosis
Ketoacidosis
    Diabetic ketoacidosis
    Alcohol abuse
Toxins:
    Ethanol
    Ethylene glycol
    Lactic acid
    Methanol
    Paraldehyde
    Aspirin
    Cyanide, coupled with elevated venous oxygenation
    Iron
    Isoniazid

The mnemonic MUDPILES is used to remember the causes of a high anion gap.
    Methanol/metformin
    Uremia
    Diabetic ketoacidosis

Paraldehyde/propylene glycol
Infection/ischemia/isoniazid
Lactate
Ethylene glycol/ethanol
Salicylates/starvation

Some people, especially those not in the emergency room, find the mnemonic KILU easier to remember and also more useful clinically:

Ketones
Ingestion
Lactic acid
Uremia

All of the components of MUDPILES are also covered with the KILU device, with the added imperative that these things can kill a patient.

Ketones: more straightforward than remembering diabetic ketosis, starvation ketosis, and so forth.

Ingestion: methanol, metformin, paraldehyde, propylene glycol, isoniazid, ethylene glycol, ethanol, and salicylates are covered by ingestion. These substances can be considered as a single group—*ingestions*—during the initial consideration, especially when not triaging a patient in the emergency room.

Lactic Acid: including that caused by infection and shock (Usually the bicarbonate lost is replaced by a chloride anion, and thus the anion gap is normal.)
Gastrointestinal loss of bicarbonate (e.g., diarrhea) (Note: Vomiting causes hypochloremic alkalosis.)
Renal loss of bicarbonate (e.g., proximal renal tubular acidosis)

Uremia: Renal dysfunction (e.g., renal failure, hypoaldosteronism, distal renal tubular acidosis)

A low anion gap is relatively rare but may occur from the presence of abnormal positively charged proteins, as in multiple myeloma, or in the setting of a low serum albumin level.

- Bilirubin (total)
- BUN (See earlier discussion.)
- BUN-creatinine ratio

The BUN/creatinine ratio is a ratio of two laboratory test values: the BUN and serum creatinine. It is used in the United States. Elsewhere (Canada, Europe), urea is used instead of BUN; thus, it is the urea-to-creatinine ratio, also urea-creatinine ratio, and urea/creatinine ratio.

The BUN/creatinine ratio is predictive of prerenal failure, if the BUN-to-creatinine ratio is greater than 20 or the urea-to-creatinine ratio of more than 0.10 and urea of more than 10. In prerenal failure, urea rises out of proportion to the creatinine because of enhanced proximal tubular reabsorption.

The BUN/creatinine ratio is useful for the diagnosis of upper gastrointestinal (GI) bleeding in patients who do not exhibit overt vomiting of blood. In children, a BUN/creatinine ratio of 30 or above has a sensitivity of 68.8% for upper GI bleeding and a specificity of 98%.

The reason the urea concentration increases in upper GI bleeds is as follows:

- Blood, which consists largely of the protein hemoglobin, is broken down by digestive enzymes of the upper GI tract into amino acids.
- The amino acids, which originate from the hemoglobin, are reabsorbed by the lower GI tract.
- Urea is a break-down product of amino acid catabolism; therefore, the *protein meal* from an upper GI bleed shows up in the blood as urea.

Because of decreased muscle mass, elderly patients may have an elevated BUN/creatinine ratio at baseline.

- Calcium
- Calculated LDL
- CBC
- Chloride
- Cholesterol
- Cholesterol-HDL ratio
- Creatinine
- GGT (See earlier discussion.)
- Globulin

Globulins are roughly divided into alpha, beta, and gamma globulins. These values can be separated and measured in the laboratory by techniques called electrophoresis and densitometry. The gamma fraction includes the various types of antibodies (immunoglobulins M, G, and A).

Normal values are:

- Serum globulin: 2.0 to 3.5 g/dL
- IgM component: 75 to 300 mg/dL
- IgG component: 650 to 1850 mg/dL
- IgA component: 90 to 350 mg/dL

Increased gamma globulin proteins may indicate:

- Multiple myeloma
- Chronic inflammatory disease (e.g., RA, SLE)
- Hyperimmunization
- Acute infection
- Waldenström macroglobulinemia
- Glucose
- HDL
- Ionized calcium
- LDH
- Phosphorus
- Potassium
- Serum glutamate oxaloacetate transaminase
- Serum glutamate pyruvate transaminase
- Sodium
- T4 radioimmunoassay (RIA)

T4 by RIA is the most widely used thyroid test of all. It is frequently called a T7, which means that a resin T3 uptake (RT3u) has been accomplished to correct for certain medications such as birth control pills, other hormones, seizure medication, cardiac drugs, or even aspirin that may alter the routine T4 test. The T4 reflects the amount of T4 in the blood. If the patient does not take any type of thyroid medication, this test is usually a good measure of thyroid function.

- Total carbon dioxide

Carbon dioxide levels that are higher or lower than normal suggest that the body is having trouble maintaining

---

ORTHOPEDIC GAMUT 1-22

SYNOVIAL FLUID

For three significant aspects, analysis of synovial fluid differs from other body fluids:

1. Neoplastic processes rarely affect synovial joints.
2. Recognition of noncellular particulate material, such as microorganisms and crystals and cartilage fragments, is essential for defining the disease process affecting the joint.
3. Diagnostic information comes not only from recognition of cell types but also from their quantification.

---

its acid-base balance or that the electrolyte balance is upset, perhaps by losing or retaining fluid. Both of these imbalances may be the result of a wide range of dysfunctions.

- Total protein
- Triglycerides
- Uric acid
- Synovial fluid

BOX 1-3

NORMAL SYNOVIAL FLUID

Osmolarity	296 mOsm/L
pH	7.44
Carbon dioxide pressure	6.0 kPa (range 4.7–7.3)
Oxygen pressure	<4.0 kPa
Potassium	4.0 mmol/L
Sodium	136 mmol/L
Calcium	1.8 mmol/L
Urea	2.5 mmol/L
Uric acid	0.23 mmol/L
Glucose	100 mmol/L
Chondroitin sulfate	40 mg/L
Hyaluronate	2.14 g/L
Cholesterol	Small amounts
Total protein	~25 g/L
Albumin	~8 g/L
α_1-antitrypsin	0.78 mcg/L
Ceruloplasmin	~43 mg/L
Haptoglobin	~90 mg/L
α_2-macroglobin	0.31 g/L
Lactoferrin	0.44 mg/L
IgG	2.62 g/L
IgA	0.85 g/L
IgM	0.14 g/L
IL-1β	20 pg/mL
IL-2	15.1 U/mL
TNF-α	1.38 hg/mL
INF-α	350 U/mL
INF-δ	13.7 U/mL

IgA, *Immunoglobulin A;* IgG, *immunoglobulin G;* IgM, *immunoglobulin M;* IL, *interleukin;* INF, *interferon;* TNF, *tumor-necrosis factor.*
Adapted from Klippel JH, Dieppe PA: *Rheumatology, vol 1-2,* ed 2, London, 1998, Mosby.

Normal synovial fluid is a hypocellular, avascular connective tissue. In disease, the synovial fluid increases in volume and can be aspirated. Synovial fluid is a transudate of plasma supplemented with high molecular weight, saccharide-rich molecules. The most notable of these is hyaluronan (hyaluronic acid), which is produced by fibroblast-derived type B synoviocyte (Box 1-3). Variation in the volume and composition of synovial fluid reflects pathologic processes within the joint.

ORTHOPEDIC TESTS

In the orthopedic physical examination, a test is positive or a sign is present when the procedure duplicates the patient's complaint or symptom. Tests are based on joint, muscle, or nerve function. If testing causes different pain or symptoms, it may indeed be significant, but the result is not positive for the findings that the test was designed to elicit.

During an examination, the examiner must use techniques that defeat the human tendency of exaggeration. The examiner must conduct several tests and multiples of similar tests so that the patient is not aware of which specific tissue function is being examined. With time and exposure to a myriad of orthopedic disorders, examiners develop the skill and accuracy necessary to reach diagnoses efficiently. However, interpreting the results of examination processes in a clinically meaningful way requires the examiner to consider the reliability of the clinical measurements and tests.

Interpretation and analysis of examination procedures depend not only on the reliability and validity of such measures, but also on the sensitivity and specificity of the *signs* elicited by the test procedures.

DIAGNOSTIC IMAGING MODALITIES IN ORTHOPEDICS

Imaging procedures are important to the diagnosis and management of an orthopedic condition. The decision to use any diagnostic imaging procedure, especially ionizing imaging procedures, should be based on a demonstrated need and should be used only after an adequate medical history is obtained and a physical examination is conducted. The decision to use any imaging procedure must also be based on the assumption that the results of the examination, even if negative, will significantly affect the treatment of the patient. The value of the information gained from the imaging examination must be worth the possible detrimental effects of the procedure. In imaging modalities that use ionizing radiation (plain-film radiography, fluoroscopy, and CT), the possible effect of radiation on the patient or future offspring must be considered (Fig. 1-17).

Plain-Film Radiography (Conventional Radiography)

Plain-film radiography, or conventional radiography, provides a wide and diverse array of diagnostic data about musculoskeletal problems, such as soft-tissue injury, bony malalignment, loss of integrity of the osseous structures, and joint space abnormality.

Plain-film X-ray examination is an efficient way to discover dislocations, fractures, the static component of anatomic subluxations, certain types of stress injuries, metastatic disease, some types of primary tumors, metabolic disease, degenerative arthropathic diseases (Table 1-10), and abnormalities in the growth plate.

Soft-tissue structures require careful scrutiny on film because they may offer subtle clues to serious or underlying pathologic abnormalities.

A radiologic evaluation of the traumatized sites should include films of the adjacent joints. If a need exists for special projections, other radiologic investigation may be necessary (Table 1-11).

Care must be taken to investigate the possibility of associated injuries in trauma victims (Table 1-12). Patients may not realize that such injuries have occurred.

The patient's history and clinical evaluation are guides that help determine which portion or portions of the body requires plain-film imaging and how many different views should be produced (Fig. 1-18).

Radiography is a useful tool in the initial assessment of rheumatologic disorders because it may provide specific information that contributes to establishing a diagnosis. Various rheumatologic disorders have unique features that can be easily detected with plain-film radiographs. Abnormalities on plain-film radiographs can be detected with a high degree of sensitivity. Serial radiography is useful in measuring structural damage, and features such as erosions, joint space narrowing, and disease-specific findings can help gauge response to therapy (Ory, 2003).

Tomography

Conventional tomography is also known as *thin-section radiography, planigraphy*, and *linear tomography*. Conventional tomography is largely replaced by CT. However, some circumstances, such as evaluating subtle alterations of bone density and ruling out fracture, necessitate conventional tomography. CT scans are used for more detailed appreciation of skeletal pathologic processes, which can help evaluate suspected intervertebral disc protrusions or herniations, facet disease, or central canal and lateral recess stenosis. If spinal disease is suspected and is not well identified on plain films and the patient is not responding to care, a CT scan is indicated. A CT scan is especially useful for the appreciation of bone and calcifications and surpasses magnetic resonance imaging (MRI) in this regard.

CT has been useful in a wide variety of musculoskeletal disorders, including those related to trauma (Fig. 1-19), back pain (e.g., herniated nucleus pulposus) (Fig. 1-20), and metabolic bone disease (e.g., osteoporosis, tumor and soft-tissue masses).

Two thirds of patients with multiple injuries suffer from blunt chest trauma, and severe thoracic trauma is associated with multiple injuries in 70% to 90% of cases (LoCicero J 3rd, Mattox, 1989; Pinilla, 1982).

TABLE 1-10	
PLAIN-FILM EVALUATION IN DEGENERATIVE ARTHROPATHIC DISORDERS	
Diagnosis	**Site of Plain-Film Findings**
Psoriatic arthritis	Hand, sacroiliac joints (common); pubis symphysis, hip, knee (less common)
Rheumatoid arthritis	Wrist and hand, shoulder, knee, cervical spine, hip
Spondyloarthropathy	Sacroiliac joints, thoracolumbar spine
Osteoarthritis	Lumbosacral spine, hip, knee, foot and ankle, hand

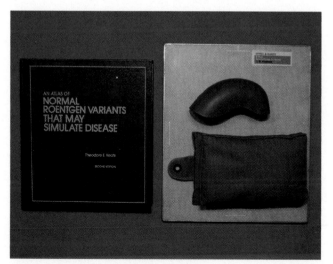

FIG. 1-17 From left to right and top to bottom, *An atlas of normal roentgen variants that may simulate disease* (by Theodore E. Keats), gonadal shielding, sandbag, DuPont Quanta Detail Rare Earth X-ray cassette screens, and compatible film.

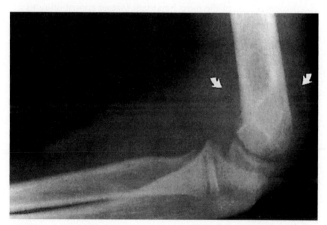

FIG. 1-18 Displacement of fat pads in the elbow by joint effusion. (From Klippel JH, Dieppe PA: *Rheumatology,* vol 1-2, ed 2, London, 1998, Mosby.)

ORTHOPEDIC GAMUT 1-23

ARTHRITIDES: DIAGNOSIS AND CLINICAL PROGRESSION ASSESSMENT STEPS IN RHEUMATOID ARTHRITIS, PSORIATIC ARTHRITIS, ANKYLOSIS SPONDYLITIS, AND OSTEOARTHRITIS

Rheumatoid arthritis
- Serial radiographs (posteroanterior [PA] view) of hands, wrists, and feet at baseline and at 6-month intervals for a minimum of 2 years after onset
- Monitoring frequency decreased after 2 years in patients without erosions at 2 years
- Distinguishing radiographic features: bilateral symmetrical involvement of the small joints (hands, wrists, and feet), juxtaarticular osteopenia, lack of proliferative bone response, marginal erosions, joint space narrowing.

Psoriatic arthritis
- Serial radiographs (PA view) of hands, wrists, and feet (and spine and other joints if symptoms are present) at baseline and at 6-month intervals for a minimum of 2 years after onset
- Distinguishing radiographic features: asymmetric and possibly oligoarticular joint involvement, initially marginal erosions that become irregular and ill defined, distal interphalangeal joint involvement, abnormalities in phalangeal tufts and at sites of attachments of tendons and ligaments to the bone, possible spondylitis, paramarginal syndesmophytes in nonconsecutive vertebrae, *sausage digits,* proliferative bone changes, and ankylosis

Ankylosing spondylitis
- Serial radiographs (anteroposterior [AP] view) of pelvis, sacroiliac joints, and axial spine
- If early ankylosing spondylitis is suspected, repeat pelvic radiographs 6 months from baseline; otherwise, serial

radiographs of pelvis, sacroiliac joints, and axial spine annually or every other year
- Serial radiographs (lateral and AP views) of cervical, thoracic, and lumbar spine annually or every other year
- Radiographs (PA view) of hands and feet at baseline; follow-up radiographs based on clinical features
- Distinguishing radiographic features: cervical lesions not typically associated with instability and subluxations of the lower five vertebrae as in rheumatoid arthritis, less-severe hip lesions than in rheumatoid arthritis without protrusions, osteophytes along the margin of articular cartilage of the femoral head, marginal syndesmophytes in consecutive vertebrae, sacroiliitis, 'bamboo spine,' smaller and more localized erosions, and less frequent joint space narrowing and osteopenia compared with rheumatoid arthritis

Osteoarthritis
- Radiographs (PA view) of the hands and feet annually
- Radiographs of the hips (AP pelvic in supine position) and knees (standing, weight-bearing AP with full knee extension) annually
- Distinguishing radiographic features of osteoarthritis: osteophytes, subchondral sclerosis
- Distinguishing radiographic features of erosive osteoarthritis: distribution in distal joints of fingers similar to that of psoriatic arthritis; centrally located erosions; erosions typically absent in metacarpophalangeal joints

Adapted from Ory PA: Radiography in the assessment of musculoskeletal conditions, *Best Pract Res Clin Rheum* 17(3):495-512, 2003.

Among blunt injuries to the chest, lung contusion is considered one of the most important factors contributing to the increased morbidity and mortality of patients with multiple injuries (Johnson, Cogbill, Winga, 1986; Schild et al, 1986).

The usual diagnostic work-up in the emergency department for blunt injuries to the chest includes a routine chest x-ray taken in the supine position and an ultrasound. Despite this approach, significant injuries such as pneumothoraces, hemothoraces, and lung contusions can be missed during the initial trauma assessment (Wagner, Jamieson, 1989).

CT scanning is accurate in visualizing intrathoracic injuries. In addition, the availability, reliability, and low complication rate of CT scans has led to its widespread use in the evaluation of blunt trauma.

Clinicians often use the noninvasive technique of quantitative CT to measure bone mineral density.

Discography

Although effective, discography has been a controversial imaging modality for spinal disc disease. Clinicians use discography for specific cases of spinal pain that are recalcitrant to conventional therapy.

Discography is an important diagnostic procedure in which disc pressure controlled by needle injection is correlated with degree of lumbar pain reported by the patient. Although imaging studies, such MRI, can be used to document pathologic changes in the disc, some studies have shown a poor correlation between MRI findings and clinical symptoms because disc degeneration and herniation increase with normal aging (Boden et al, 1990).

The high incidence of asymptomatic findings on MRI makes interpretation of patient studies more difficult because each imaging finding must be closely correlated to symptoms that can be relatively nonspecific in many patients. MRI alone is not able to differentiate symptomatic from

TABLE 1-11

PREFERRED RADIOGRAPHIC VIEWS IN SKELETAL TRAUMA

Area	Specific Views	Area	Specific Views
Skull	Posteroanterior or anteroposterior Caldwell Townes Lateral (one lateral should be upright)	Sternum, sternoclavicular joints	Posteroanterior Right and left anterior obliques with cephalad angle of tube Lateral
Facial bones	Waters Modified Waters Caldwell Lateral	Elbow	Anteroposterior Lateral Capitellum
Cervical spine	Anteroposterior Coned odontoid or orthopantogram Odontoid Lateral (cross-table or upright) Swimmer lateral (cross-table) Both obliques, when possible	Radioulnar joints (forearm)	Anteroposterior or posteroanterior Lateral
Thoracic spine	Anteroposterior Lateral (cross-table or routine) Swimmer (coned to upper thoracic spine)	Wrist and hand	Posteroanterior Oblique internal, external, or both Lateral Navicular views, if needed
Lumbar spine	Anteroposterior Lateral (cross-table or upright) Lateral (coned to L5–S1)	Pelvis, acetabulum	Anteroposterior Obliques (Judet)
Sacrum	Anteroposterior (tube-angled cephalad) Lateral	Hip, proximal part of femur	Anteroposterior pelvis Frog-leg or cross-table lateral Obliques
Chest	Posteroanterior or anteroposterior Left lateral (may not be possible in trauma) Lateral decubitus (pneumothorax, pleural fluid)	Femur	Anteroposterior (to include hip and knee) Lateral (to include hip and knee)
Ribs	Anteroposterior or posteroanterior Oblique	Distal part of femur and knee	Anteroposterior Lateral Tunnel Internal oblique
Shoulder	Anteroposterior (internal rotation) Anteroposterior (neutral) Transscapular lateral (Neer) Axillary	Tibia, fibula	Anteroposterior (to include ankle and knee) Lateral (to include both joints)
Humerus	Anteroposterior (to include elbow and shoulder) Lateral (to include both joints)	Ankle	Anteroposterior Oblique (mortise) Lateral
Clavicle	Anteroposterior or posteroanterior (to include both joints with and without weight bearing)	Calcaneus	Tangential Lateral
		Foot	Lateral Anteroposterior Oblique Lateral

From Gustilo RB, Kyle RF, Templeman DC: *Fractures and dislocations, vol 1*, St Louis, 1993, Mosby.

asymptomatic degenerative disc changes (Scuderi et al, in press).

Magnetic Resonance Imaging

MRI is a computerized, thin-section imaging procedure that uses a magnetic field and radio-frequency waves rather than ionizing radiation. MRI can produce thin-section images in the sagittal, coronal, or axial planes, as well as any other oblique plane desired. The MRI can image neurologic structures and other soft tissues and can reveal disc degeneration before any other imaging method. Indications for MRI are similar to those for CT. MRI is superior to CT for the evaluation of suspected spinal cord tumors or damage, intracranial disease, and various types of central nervous system

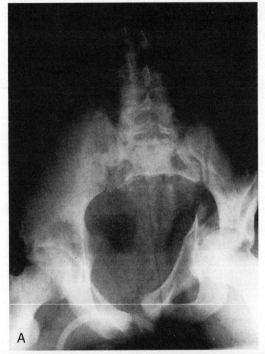

ORTHOPEDIC GAMUT 1-24

ASSESSMENT ABILITIES AND LIMITATIONS OF PLAIN-FILM RADIOGRAPHY

1. Plain-film radiography is the least expensive and most widely available imaging technique.
2. Radiography offers higher spatial resolution than any other modality, providing extremely high contrast for cortical and trabecular bone.
3. Radiography affords only a projectional viewing perspective.
4. Projection of three-dimensional anatomy onto a two-dimensional film results in morphologic distortion and superimposition of overlapping structures.
5. The sensitivity for trabecular bone loss is relatively poor.
6. As much as 30% to 50% of trabecular bone must be removed before the change becomes perceptible on conventional radiographs.
7. The contrast for soft tissues that are not calcified or fatty is relatively poor.
8. Radiography cannot directly visualize the articular cartilage, inflamed synovial tissue, joint effusion, bone marrow edema, or intraarticular fat pads.

ORTHOPEDIC GAMUT 1-25

ASSESSMENT ABILITIES AND LIMITATIONS OF COMPUTED TOMOGRAPHY

1. The greatest advantage of CT over conventional radiography is its tomographic nature.
2. CT provides high contrast between bone and adjacent tissues and is excellent for evaluating osseous structures.
3. CT offers slightly greater soft-tissue contrast than radiography.
4. Image contrast is insufficient to visualize the articular cartilage or synovial tissue or to discriminate between tendonitis and tendon rupture.
5. CT reveals only the surfaces of these structures; it does not disclose intra substance changes that may precede gross morphologic disruption.

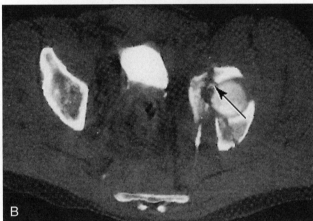

FIG. 1-19 Complex acetabular fracture. **A,** Anteroposterior plain film. **B,** Axial computed tomography scan. (From Gustilo RB, Kyle RF, Templeman DC: *Fractures and dislocations,* vol 1, St Louis, 1993, Mosby.)

disease (e.g., multiple sclerosis). MRI is especially useful in identifying small differences among similar soft tissues and surpasses CT in this regard.

The evaluation of a child with a suspected soft tissue mass in the hand is a challenge. Imaging evaluation should begin with radiographs that may reveal the diagnosis. Further imaging with ultrasound, CT, or MRI is often required for either diagnosis or operative planning. A soft-tissue mass in the hand may be a manifestation of neoplasm, congenital malformation, infection, other inflammatory process, or trauma. Infectious and traumatic causes are more prevalent in pediatric patients than neoplasia or congenital malformation. The evaluation of these masses should include an assessment of the extent of the soft-tissue, osseous, and neurovascular involvement. Of all the imaging modalities, MRI is best suited for this role (Jimenez, Jaramillo, Connolly, 2005).

In the management of low back pain and lumbar degenerative kyphosis disorders, paraspinal muscles are subjected to many studies using ultrasound, CT, needle electromyography (EMG), and histopathologic analysis. MRI can evalu-

TABLE 1-12

INJURIES ASSOCIATED WITH SKELETAL TRAUMA

Fracture	Associated Injury
Bone and bone	Remote additional spinal fracture
Spine	Scapula fracture
Chest wall	Sacrum fracture or dislocated
Anterior pelvic arch	sacroiliac joint
Femoral shaft	Fracture or fracture-dislocation of
Tibia (severe)	hip
Calcaneus	Dislocated hip
	Fractured thoracolumbar spine
Bone and viscera	Ruptured mesentery or small bowel
Chance fracture of spine	Laceration of liver, spleen, kidney,
Lower ribs	or diaphragm
Pelvis	Ruptured bladder or urethra
Pelvis	Ruptured diaphragm
Bone and vascular	Ruptured aorta
Ribs 1, 2, or 3	Myocardial contusion
Sternum	Laceration of pelvic arterial tree
Pelvis	Laceration of femoral artery
Distal third femur	Popliteal artery laceration
Knee dislocation	

Adapted from Rogers LF, Hendrix RW: Evaluating the multiple injured patient radiographically, *Orthop Clin North Am* 21(3):444, 1990.

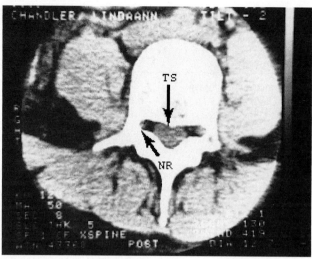

FIG. 1-20 Axial image showing a right paracentral herniation of the nucleus pulposus. (From Brier SR: *Primary care orthopedics*, St Louis, 1999, Mosby.)

ORTHOPEDIC GAMUT 1-26

USES OF DISCOGRAPHY

- To rule out disc involvement, especially as a cause of postoperative pain
- To determine the appropriate level for spinal fusion
- To test the potential effectiveness of chemonucleolysis
- To visualize internal disc anatomy

ORTHOPEDIC GAMUT 1-27

FOR CERTAIN PATHOLOGIC CONDITIONS, MAGNETIC RESONANCE IMAGING IS THE DIAGNOSTIC PROCEDURE OF CHOICE

1. Spinal disc disease
2. Medullary tumor
3. Multiple sclerosis
4. Cerebral edema
5. Spinal stenosis
6. Metastatic disease
7. Herniated disc
8. Discitis (or infection)
9. Meniscal tear (fibrocartilage abnormalities)
10. Central nervous system tumor
11. Soft-tissue tumor

ate fatty infiltration in the muscles and the fascia status overlying the muscles. The MRI enables the examiner to distinguish between muscle and fibrous tissue.

The fatigue of the lumbar muscles is probably one of the most important causes of pain in lumbar degenerative kyphosis deformity because the lumbar extensors overwork to maintain secure balance (Takemitsu et al, 1988).

Experts also suggest that weakness is a consequence, rather than a cause, of low back pain, whereby pain limits movement and muscle atrophy occurs (Stokes, Young, 1984).

For patients who have sustained head trauma with skull fractures, MRI is an efficient way to identify the early signs of cerebral edema. The test procedure of choice for diagnosing metastatic disease is an MRI scan (Table 1-13).

ORTHOPEDIC GAMUT 1-28

ASSESSMENT ABILITIES ND LIMITATIONS OF MAGNETIC RESONANCE IMAGING

1. Diarthrodial joints are particularly suitable for MRI.
2. MRI is unparalleled in its ability to depict soft-tissue detail.
3. MRI is the only modality that can examine all components of the joint simultaneously.

TABLE 1-13

MAGNETIC RESONANCE IMAGING VERSUS COMPUTED TOMOGRAPHY

Anatomic Area	Indications	Recommended Procedure
Brain (including brainstem)	Initial evaluation (e.g., demyelination disease seizures)	MRI
	Previous normal CT	MRI
	Previous abnormal CT	CT or MRI*
	Unchanged abnormal CT with increase in symptoms	MRI
	Contrast allergy	MRI
	Acute trauma	CT
	Pituitary tumors	MRI
Ear, nose, throat, and eye	Neurosensory hearing loss (e.g., to rule out acoustic neuroma)	CT
	Conductive hearing loss	CT
	Cancer staging (including laryngeal cancer)	CT or MRI*
	Cholesteatoma of temporal bone	CT
	Fractures of facial bones	CT
	Thyroid or parathyroid dysfunction (after US)	MRI
	Sinus conditions	CT or MRI*
	Orbital disease	MRI or CT*
	Disease of optic tracts and chiasm	MRI
	Internal derangement of temporomandibular joint	MRI
Musculoskeletal spine	Lower back or radicular pain in younger person	MRI
	Lower back or radicular pain in older person	MRI or CT*
	Cervical disk disease	MRI
	Spinal stenosis	MRI
	Cervical	CT or MRI*
	Lumbar	MRI
	Tumors	MRI
	Metastatic disease	
Hips	Early detection of aseptic necrosis	MRI
	Congenital hip dislocation or reduction	US
Extremities	Tumors, disease, or injury to muscle, ligaments, or cartilage	MRI
	Confirmation of calcification or fracture	CT
Chest	Diseases of the hila	MRI
	Diseases of the mediastinum	MRI or CT*
	Lung disease	CT
Abdomen and pelvis	General survey (e.g., to rule out tumor)	CT
	Liver disease	CT or MRI*
	Renal cell cancer staging	MRI
	Prostate disease	MRI, CT, or US
	Bladder disease	MRI or CT
	Abdominal aortic aneurysm	MRI*
	Other	

CT, Computed tomography; *MRI*, magnetic resonance imaging; *US*, ultrasonography.
*Consult radiologist for imaging options.
From Brier SR: *Primary care orthopedics,* St Louis, 1999, Mosby; originally courtesy of Robert Goodman, MD, South Suffolk MRI, PC, Bayshore, New York.

The guideline for using the imaging modalities to best advantage can be summarized as follows: Using *state of the art* MR techniques with high resolution, at least two planes, fast sequences, phased-array coils, and established technical parameters, MRI can answer all clinical questions. This guideline applies to conditions treated conservatively or surgically, as well as to all manifestations of degenerative spine disease. In particular, only MRI can identify abnormalities within the spinal cord as syringomyelia or myelopathy (Kretzschmar, 1998).

Contrast Arthrography

The conventional use of arthrography in musculoskeletal disease involves the use of air to distend a synovial joint and a radiopaque contrast agent to outline anatomic structures. The injection of contrast material into the joint space results in a radiographic outline of the cartilage, menisci, ligaments, or synovium. Conventional arthrography is used in diagnosing the scope and magnitude of orthopedic trauma to the shoulder, wrist, knee, and ankle (Table 1-14).

TABLE 1-14

JOINTS TYPICALLY STUDIED WITH COMPUTED TOMOGRAPHIC ARTHROGRAPHY FOLLOWING TRAUMA

Joint	To Observe
Knee	Meniscus, cruciate and collateral ligaments, hyaline cartilage tears, osteochondral defects
Shoulder	Rotator cuff, glenoid labrum disruption
Hip	Hyaline cartilage integrity and tears, prosthetic joint loosening
Wrist	Triangular fibrocartilage, intercarpal ligament integrity
Elbow	Hyaline cartilage integrity, osteochondral defects
Ankle	Ligamentous tears, osteochondral defects
Temporomandibular	Disc and condylar integrity

Adapted from Gustilo RB, Kyle RF, Templeman DC: *Fractures and dislocations, vol 1,* St Louis, 1993, Mosby.

ORTHOPEDIC GAMUT 1-29

ASSESSMENT ABILITIES AND LIMITATIONS OF RADIONUCLIDE SCANNING

1. The principal advantage of scintigraphy over other imaging modalities is its ability to help in identifying tissues or organs with abnormal physiologic or biochemical properties.
2. Increased skeletal uptake can be seen at sites of elevated blood flow or increased bone metabolism.
3. Scintigraphy is a convenient way of surveying the entire skeleton for multifocal processes.

Contrast-enhanced cartilage imaging can visualize early degenerative cartilage lesions before substantial morphologic changes occur. The application of contrast agent can be performed as either direct or indirect MR arthrography. Despite the advantages of indirect MR arthrography using intravenous contrast material, direct MR arthrography has gained increasing popularity as a safe diagnostic tool in assessing subtle intraarticular derangements, including the evaluation of articular cartilage especially in the shoulder, the hip, the ankle, and the postoperative knee (Guntern et al, 2003; Kassarjian et al, 2005; McCauley, 2005; Schmid et al, 2003).

Radionuclide Scanning

Examinations conducted with the use of nuclear medicine techniques, including bone scans, positron emission tomography (PET) scans, and single-photon emission computed

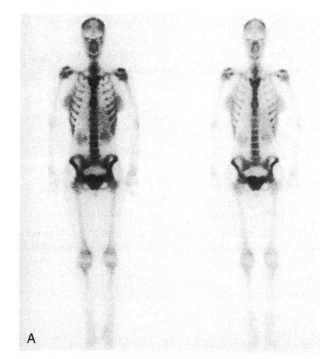

A

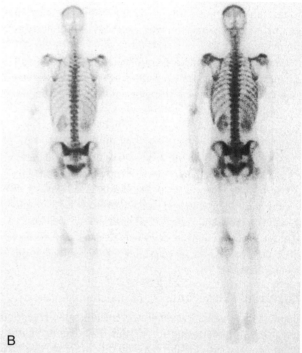

B

FIG. 1-21 Normal bone scans. (From Early PJ, Sodel DB: *Principles and practice of nuclear medicine,* St Louis, 1995, Mosby.)

tomography (SPECT) scans, are valuable in diagnostic imaging because of their highly sensitive and noninvasive nature. Whole-body scanning for metastatic and infectious diseases, as well as inflammatory and ischemic processes, is possible with scintigraphy (Fig. 1-21).

Highly active individuals (e.g., competitive athletes) are prime candidates for bone scanning when the diagnosis is uncertain. A bone scan may show increased uptake of the radioactive isotope consistent with a stress fracture (Fig. 1-22).

Because of the high incidence of false-negative radiographs early in the course of stress fractures, additional diagnostic imaging is often indicted. Radionuclide bone scanning has traditionally been the test of choice in this situation but is being supplanted by MRI. An increased uptake observed on a bone scan correlates with increased bone activity caused by fatigue failure and confirms the diagnosis of stress fracture (Schils et al, 1992).

Despite being sensitive, bone scanning is not specific and can yield false-positive rates between 13% and 24%. Additionally, localizing the precise anatomic location of injury can be difficult (Steinbronn, Bennett, Kay, 1994).

Bone scanning has become common in the evaluation of child abuse. Very young children typically do not develop stress fractures of multiple fracture sites in normal living situations (Fig. 1-23).

Video Fluoroscopy

Video fluoroscopy is used when a function study of the joint is warranted. Video fluoroscopy should be used when a biomechanical abnormality is present but is not adequately demonstrated by plain-film stress surveys or other examination methods.

Three-dimensional motion visualization in the context of clinical and biomechanical analyses of the musculoskeletal system is becoming a key instrument for investigating its complex mechanisms and the awkward characteristics (Leardini et al, 2006).

Conventional instrumented gait analysis with skin-mounted markers has the disadvantage of measuring artefacts because of skin movement relative to the underlying bones. Video fluoroscopy is a well-established method of more accurately measuring knee joint kinematics by avoiding the use of skin markers. The small field of view of the image intensifier and the ability only to gain kinematic data are the two main disadvantages of this system (Zihlmann et al, 2006).

Diagnostic Ultrasound

Diagnostic ultrasound, a sound wave echo study, is particularly useful for evaluating soft tissues. The diagnostic ultrasound does not provide the same quality of image as CT or MRI.

Diagnostic ultrasound requires high-resolution equipment, including a high-frequency transducer. Diagnostic ultrasound performs well in the detection of rotator cuff tears and other tendon abnormalities, as well as in identifying some metabolic disease. In cases of suspected pediatric hip disease, diagnostic ultrasound is the recommended primary imaging technique.

Preoperative ultrasound-guided marking of calcium deposits significantly enhances the clinical results of arthroscopic removal of calcium deposits. The success of this type of surgery is largely dependent on the exact localization and removal of calcium deposits. Complete removal of calcium

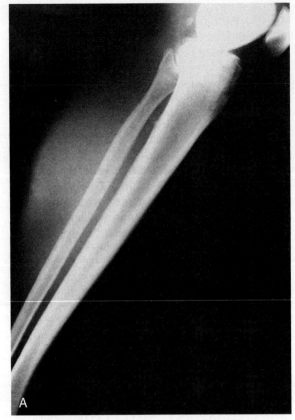

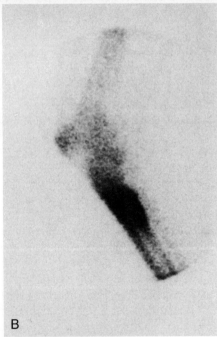

FIG. 1-22 Radiographic film (**A**) and bone scan (**B**) demonstrating stress fracture. (From Nicholas JA, Hershman EB: *The lower extremity and spine in sports medicine*, ed 4, St Louis, 1995, Mosby.)

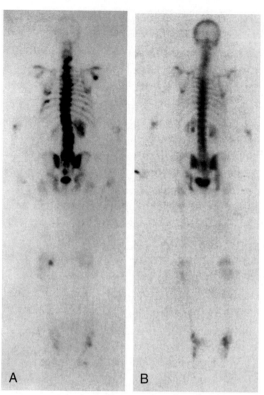

FIG. 1-23 **A,** Whole-body scintigraphy. **B,** Normal bone scan is shown for comparison. (From Klippel JH, Dieppe PA: *Rheumatology,* vol 1-2, ed 2, London, 1998, Mosby.)

BOX 1-4

STRENGTHS AND LIMITATIONS OF MYELOGRAPHIC STUDIES

Strengths

Studies of the subarachnoid space are possible.
Intraarachnoid lesions are shown.
Demarcation of multi-disc levels is shown.
Information on surgical scars is provided.
Assessment of flexion and extension dynamic are possible.

Limitations

Lesions removed from outside of the thecal sac can be missed.
Study variations are problematic.
Detail shown in the dorsal spine is poor.
Postoperative studies are impossible to read with accuracy.
Testing procedure is invasive.

From Brier SR: *Primary care orthopedics,* St Louis, 1999, Mosby.

ORTHOPEDIC GAMUT 1-30

ASSESSMENT ABILITIES AND LIMITATIONS OF ULTRASONOGRAPHY

1. Ultrasonography offers direct multiplanar tomography without any need for image reformatting.
2. Ultrasonography can also provide images in real time, without any exposure to ionizing radiation.
3. The modality is inexpensive and widely available.
4. Ultrasonography offers relatively good soft-tissue contrast and is particularly effective at helping to identify fluid collections such as bursitis and abscesses.
5. Ultrasound waves cannot penetrate bone.

---

deposits correlates with good or excellent clinical results (Porcellini et al, 2004; Rupp, Seil, Kohn, 2000).

Identifying the course of the calcium deposit is therefore extremely important. The presence of a calcium deposit with an atypical course and location more proximal to the joint complicates the operation even further. Failure to locate the calcium deposit can make the surgical process extremely frustrating and may result in a very long operative time (Kayser et al, 2007).

Myelography

Traditional myelographic techniques involve the introduction of small amounts of water-soluble contrast medium into the subarachnoid space, either through a lumbar approach below the level of the conus medullaris or at the level of C1–C2 through a posterolateral approach. Standard films of the spinal canal are made to determine the presence or absence of a filling defect. In cases of acute spinal trauma, myelography may be used in conjunction with CT (Fig. 1-24).

Myelography remains valuable in evaluating intrinsic spinal cord lesions, nerve root lesions, and dural tears associated with severe trauma (Box 1-4).

Depending on patient selection and therapeutic strategy, the role of plain CT and MRI, as well as myelography combined with myelo-CT, in the diagnostic evaluation of degenerative changes of the spine is judged differently (Kretzschmar, 1998).

In patients with disk disease, plain-film CT for initial diagnostic examination is recommended, if the complaints are nonspecific (Thornbury et al, 1991, 1993).

If the clinical findings suggest a herniated disk, MRI should be given preference over myelography combined with myelo-CT. The use of nonionic contrast media without meningeal irritation or neurotoxicity has reduced the morbidity of myelography (Kretzschmar, 1998).

Thermography

Using temperature differentials of the body, thermography illustrates neurovascular changes in injury or disease. Thermograms do not provide specific information regarding the cause of nerve fiber irritation (e.g., herniated disc, scar tissue, myospasm).

Reflex sympathetic dystrophy is part of a spectrum of sympathetically mediated pain syndromes that usually occur

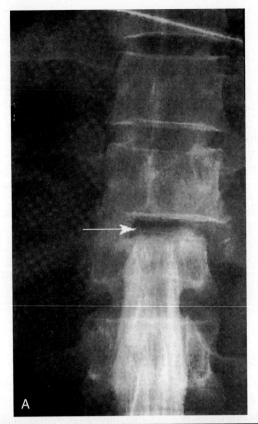

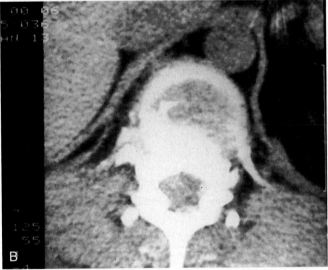

FIG. 1-24 Lumbar myelogram (**A**), with computed tomography axial image (**B**) through the T12 body. (From Gustilo RB, Kyle RF: *Fractures and dislocations,* vol 1, St Louis, 1993, Mosby.)

Motor and trophic symptoms, however, characterize complex regional pain syndromes but are not found after acute trauma. These latter symptoms obviously need time to develop, and the duration of disease clearly separates complex regional pain syndromes (weeks) and trauma (days) (Birklein et al, 2000).

Electrodiagnostic Testing

Although electrodiagnostic testing provides valuable information, it does not stand alone as a diagnostic entity (Table 1-15). The data obtained must be correlated with the physical examination findings and case history.

Electrodiagnostic testing can potentially differentiate asymptomatic disk herniations from symptomatic ones. A minimal amount of denervation can occur in asymptomatic spines.

With surface measurement of motor nerve conduction, velocity provides a valuable ancillary procedure in the diagnosis of various peripheral nerve lesions in both the upper and lower extremities. This form of testing involves stimulating a peripheral nerve at two separate positions along its course and recording the action potentials observed on an oscilloscopic screen. Slow conduction times indicate nerve entrapment syndromes across the point at which the impulses are delayed.

The electrical responses of nervous system sensory tracks are *somatosensory-evoked potentials* (SSEPs). SSEPs evaluate various pathologic variations from the peripheral nerve through the spinal cord to the somatosensory region of the brain. SSEPs assess diseases of the spinal cord, trauma to the spine, neuromuscular disease, and demyelinating disorders.

Using needle electrodes, needle EMG is widely used to diagnose nerve root lesions at the level of the spine. EMG

in an extremity after a seemingly minor injury or surgical procedure.

Even though certain similarities exist between acute complex regional pain syndromes (reflex sympathetic dystrophy) and patients with acute trauma, detailed investigation of these signs reveals striking differences. The clinical similarity comprises pain, hyperalgesia, and some presumably autonomic disturbances (edema and skin temperature changes).

TABLE 1-15

STRENGTHS AND LIMITATIONS OF ELECTRODIAGNOSTIC TESTING

Testing Modality	Strengths	Limitations
Nerve conduction velocity	Helpful in ruling out peripheral entrapment neuropathic conditions (e.g., prolonged latencies exhibited in carpal tunnel syndrome, tarsal tunnel syndrome) and ulnar neuropathic variations	Provides imperfect sensitivity; limited localization and determination of injury severity; timing of study an important factor
F waves	Provides screening for late motor response with distal sweeps starting at the foot	Evaluates motor reflex only; possibly evaluates abnormal findings only in the presence of multiple-level injury
H reflex	Equivalent of ankle joint reflex; evaluates monosynaptic reflex with sensory and motor S1 function	Provides assessment of S1 nerve root only
SSEPs	Helpful in documenting sensory pathway disturbances in proximal neural injury and central conduction delays, as in myopathies and multiple sclerosis	Offers imperfect localization; findings are rarely abnormal if results of other electrodiagnostic tests within normal limits
Needle EMG	Useful in assessing conductivity of neural tissues; helpful in determining site and severity of lesion; may be helpful in early assessment of recovery, screening for fibrillation potentials, and signs of denervation from nerve root compression disorders	Unable to detect denervation potentials for 14 to 28 days after injury; provides imperfect sensitivity; study timing an important factor; proximal lesions sometimes inaccessible anatomically; effectiveness reduced after surgery

EMG, Electromyography; *SSEPs,* somatosensory-evoked potentials.
Adapted from Brier SR: *Primary care orthopedics,* St Louis, 1999, Mosby.

ORTHOPEDIC GAMUT 1-32

ASSESSMENT ABILITIES AND LIMITATIONS OF NERVE CONDUCTION VELOCITY

1. Studies of nerve conduction velocity (NCV) can rule out peripheral neuropathic conditions.
2. Routine NCV tests are not specific for conditions such as radiculopathy, but they may be helpful in cases of chronic pain that have a questionable spinal origin.

ORTHOPEDIC GAMUT 1-33

ASSESSMENT ABILITIES AND LIMITATIONS OF ELECTROMYOGRAPHY

1. Electromyography (EMG) shows fibrillation potentials and possible motor unit changes in denervated muscles.
2. Denervation of paraspinal muscle, indicates that the patient has a lesion at the nerve root level.
3. The usual finding of needle EMG in a patient who has dorsal root disease is normal.
4. It does not provide any information with respect to the locus of injury (e.g., root, nerve, muscle) and, in fact, often reflects associated tissue injury rather than neurovascular dysfunction.

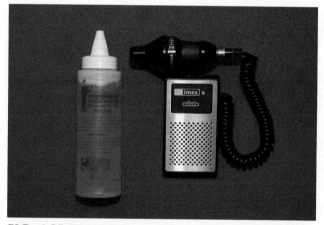

FIG. 1-25 The IMEX portable Doppler *(right),* audibly monitors pulses in noisy environments when palpation is questionable or not possible or when the pulse is especially weak or rapid. The Doppler also aids in the assessment of circulation distal to fractures, burns, and other injuries to quickly determine the extent of injury. Transmission gel *(left)* is used to couple the Doppler head to the skin surface and eliminate air gaps that can degrade sound transmission.

differentiates a central spinal lesion from a peripheral neuropathic condition. Results of the procedure are accurate in differentiating disease of a neuromuscular origin.

Doppler Ultrasonic Vascular Testing

Doppler vascular testing allows the assessment of pulses in noisy environments or when pulses are weak. This test is efficient when palpation of a pulse is questionable or not possible. The Doppler instrument aids in the assessment of circulation distal to fracture sites, burns, and other injuries that potentially compromise vascular tissue, quickly determining the extent of injury (Fig. 1-25).

Laser Doppler flowmetry is a valuable noninvasive method for investigation of the very early skin venoarteriolar dysfunctions, for evaluation of focal autonomic dysregulation and skin vasomotor abnormalities in patients with Raynaud phenomenon. Laser Doppler-recorded venoarteriolar reflex testing is a simple procedure and an adequate additional diagnostic tool, which contributes to diagnose Raynaud phenomenon and differentiate primary from secondary Raynaud phenomenon (Stoyneva, 2004).

CRITICAL THINKING

1. In the complaint history of a musculoskeletal condition, what essential points should be included for proper history taking by an experienced examiner?
2. Name the five essential steps in drawing a working diagnosis for your patient.
3. Name the *Critical 5* questions in orthopedics.
4. Describe Jendrassik maneuver.
5. You have a patient who is complaining of unrelenting spinal pain who demonstrates full and pain-free range of motion. What two problems should you consider with this presentation?
6. Describe the difference and what information can be obtained from the five rung test and the *maximal static grip* when using a Jamar dynamometer.
7. What are the significances of the clinical findings of the static grip test and the REG test?
8. How are the two tests performed?
9. How would you describe the presentation of a patient with scleratogenous pain?
10. Why is serial radiography useful in a patient with rheumatoid arthritis?
11. What area or areas would you monitor?
12. How frequent should radiography be used?
13. You have just diagnosed a case of AS. How frequent should you perform serial studies of this patient?
14. What areas should be monitored?
15. A question of causation arises in a child with multiple complaints. What imaging procedure would you recommend for this child?
16. SSEPs are useful in the evaluation of various pathologic conditions. What part of the nervous system is evaluated with this process?

BIBLIOGRAPHY

American Medical Association: *Guides to the evaluation of permanent impairment,* ed 4, Chicago, 1993, American Medical Association.

Anderson KN, Anderson LE: *Mosby's pocket dictionary of medicine, nursing, & allied health,* ed 2, St Louis, 1994, Mosby.

Arabi A et al: Discriminative ability of dual-energy X-ray absorptiometry site selection in identifying patients with osteoporotic fractures, *Bone* 40(4):1060, 2007.

Ashford RF, Nagelburg S, Adkins R: Sensitivity of the Jamar dynamometer in detecting submaximal grip effort, *J Hand Surg* 21(3):402, 1996.

Atkinson G, Nevill A, Hopkins WG: Typical error versus limits of agreement, *Sports Med* 30 (5):375, 2000.

Atkinson G, Nevill AM: Statistical methods for assessing measurement error (reliability) in variables relevant to sports medicine, *Sports Med* 26(4):217, 1998.

Ballou SP, Kushner I: C-reactive protein and the acute phase response, *Adv Intern Med* 37:313, 1992.

Barboi AC, Barkhaus PE: Electrodiagnostic testing in neuromuscular disorders. *Neurologic Clin* 22(3):619, 2004.

Barkauskas VH et al: *Health & physical assessment,* ed. 2, St Louis, 1998, Mosby.

Barker S et al: Guidance for pre-manipulative testing of the cervical spine, *Physiotherapy* 87(6):318, 2001.

Beaton DE, O'Driscoll SW, Richards RR: Grip strength testing using the BTE work simulator and the Jamar dynamometer: a comparative study, *J Hand Surg* 20(2):293, 1995.

Bechman H et al: Getting the most from a 20-minute visit, *Am J Gastroenterol* 89:662, 1994.

Birklein F, Kunzel W, Sieweke N: Despite clinical similarities there are significant differences between acute limb trauma and complex regional pain syndrome I (CRPS I). *Pain* 93(2):165, 2001.

Bland JM, Altman DG: Measurement error and correlation coefficients. *BMJ* 313(7048):41, 1996.

Bogduk N, Aprill C, Derby R: Discography. In White AH, Schofferman JA, editors: *Spine care,* vol 1, St Louis, 1995, Mosby.

Botwin KP, Gruber RD, Savarese R: Lumbar discography, *Tech Reg Anesth Pain Manag* 9(1):3, 2005.

Bowlus B: *Mosby's regional atlas of human anatomy,* St Louis, 1997, Mosby.

Brannan SR, Jerrard DA: Synovial fluid analysis, *J Emerg Med* 30(3):331, 2006.

Brier SR: *Primary care orthopedics,* St Louis, 1999, Mosby.

Bushong SC: *Radiologic science for technologist: physics, biology, and protection,* ed. 5, St Louis, 1993, Mosby.

Canale T: *Campbell's operative orthopaedics,* vol 1-4, ed 9, St Louis, 1998, Mosby.

Cardinal E, Lafortune M, Burns P: Power Doppler US in synovitis: reality or artifact? *Radiology* 200:868, 1996.

Chance PF: Survey of inherited peripheral nerve diseases. *Electroencephalogr Clin Neurophysiol* 103(1):12, 1997.

Chandnani VP, et al: Knee hyaline cartilage evaluated with MR imaging: a cadaveric study involving multiple imaging sequences and intraarticular injection of gadolinium and saline solution, *Radiology* 178:557, 1991.

Chiodo A et al: Needle EMG has a lower false positive rate than MRI in asymptomatic older adults being evaluated for lumbar spinal stenosis, *Clin Neurophysiol* 118(4):751, 2007.

Cipriano JJ: *Photographic manual of regional orthopaedic and neurological test,* ed 3, Baltimore, 1997, Williams & Wilkins.

Coldham F, Lewis J, Lee H: The reliability of one vs. three grip trials in symptomatic and asymptomatic subjects, *J Hand Ther* 19(3):318, 2006.

Conwell TD: *Documenting patient progress "daily office charting seminar" thorough accurate quick procedures,* ed 11, Lakewood, CO, 1990, Clinical Advancement Plus Seminars.

Dambro MR, Griffith JA: *Griffith's 5 minute clinical consult,* Baltimore, 1997, Williams & Wilkins.

Datz FL: *Handbook of nuclear medicine,* ed 2, St Louis, 1993, Mosby.

Delitto A, Snyder-Mackler L: The diagnostic process: examples in orthopedic physical therapy, *Phys Ther* 75:203, 1995.

Derby R et al: P153. The influence of pain tolerance and psychological factors on discography in chronic axial LBP patients, *Spine J* 5(4, suppl 1):S184, 2005.

Dickenson AH: Spinal cord pharmacology of pain, *Br J Anaesth* 75:193, 1995.

Disler DG, et al: Fat-suppressed three-dimensional spoiled gradient-echo MR imaging of hyaline cartilage defects in the knee: comparison with standard MR imaging and arthroscopy, *AJR* 167:127, 1996.

Doherty M: *Color atlas and text of osteoarthritis,* London, 1994, Wolfe.

Doherty M, Doherty J: *Clinical examination in rheumatology,* London, 1992, Wolfe.

Doherty M, George E: *Self-assessment picture tests in rheumatology,* London, 1995, Mosby-Wolfe.

Doody C, McAteer M: Clinical reasoning of expert and novice physiotherapists in an outpatient orthopaedic setting, *Physiotherapy* 88(5):258, 2002.

Dray A: Inflammatory mediators of pain, *Br J Anaesth* 75:125, 1995.

Early PJ, Sodee DB: *Principles and practice of nuclear medicine,* St Louis, 1995, Mosby.

Epstein O et al: *Clinical examination,* ed 2, London, 1997, Mosby.

Feagin JA. *The crucial ligaments: diagnosis and treatment of ligamentous injuries about the knee,* New York, 1988, Churchill Livingstone.

Feldmann E: *Current diagnosis in neurology,* St Louis, 1994, Mosby.

Freemont AJ, Denton J: *Atlas of synovial fluid cytopathology,* vol 18, Dordrecht, Netherlands, 1991, Kluwer Academic.

Freemont FJ et al: The diagnostic value of synovial fluid cytoanalysis: a reassessment, *Ann Rheum Dis* 50:101, 1991.

Galvez R et al: Cross-sectional evaluation of patient functioning and health-related quality of life in patients with neuropathic pain under standard care conditions, *Eur J Pain* 11(3):244, 2007.

Ge H-Y et al: Hypoalgesia to pressure pain in referred pain areas triggered by spatial summation of experimental muscle pain from unilateral or bilateral trapezius muscles, *Eur J Pain* 7(6):531, 2003.

Gemmell H, Miller P: Should chiropractors recommend provocative discography for diagnostic purposes in patients with chronic low back pain? *Clin Chiropr* 8(1):20, 2005.

Ghanem N et al: MRI and discography in traumatic intervertebral disc lesions, *Clin Imaging* 31(2):147, 2007.

Goker B et al: The effects of minor hip flexion, abduction or adduction and x-ray beam angle on the radiographic joint space width of the hip, *Osteoarthr Cartil* 13(5):379, 2005.

Goldie BS: *Orthopaedic diagnosis and management a guide to the care of orthopaedic patients,* ed 2, Oxford, UK, 1998, ISIS Medical Media.

Greenstein G: *Clinical assessment of neuromusculoskeletal disorders,* St Louis, 1997, Mosby.

Guckel C, Nidecker A: Diagnosis of tears in rotator-cuff-injuries, *Eur J Radiol* 25(3):168, 1997.

Gustilo RB, Kyle RF, Templeman DC: *Fractures and dislocations,* St Louis, 1993, Mosby.

Haack E, Tkach J: Fast MR imaging: techniques and clinical applications, *AJR* 155:951, 1990.

Hall LD, Tyler JA: Can quantitative magnetic resonance imaging detect and monitor the progression of early osteoarthritis? In Kuetner KE, Goldberg VM, editors: *Osteoarthritic disorders,* Rosemont, Ill, 1995, American Academy of Orthopaedic Surgeons.

Hamilton J, Manrique L, Scarborough N: Development of an intervertebral disc model for testing a new discography system, *J Pain* 7(4, suppl 1):S26, 2006.

Hartley A: *Practical joint assessment lower quadrant,* ed 2, St Louis, 1995, Mosby.

1

Hawkins RJ: *An organized approach to musculoskeletal examination and history taking,* St Louis, 1995, Mosby.

Hayes KW, Petersen C, Falconer J: An examination of Cyriax's passive motion tests with patients having osteoarthritis of the knee, *Phys Ther* 74:697, 1994.

Herndon WA: Acute and chronic injury: its effect on growth in the young athlete. In Frana WA, et al, editors: *Advances in sports medicine fitness,* vol 3, Chicago, 1990, Year-Book Medical.

Hillman TE et al: A practical posture for hand grip dynamometry in the clinical setting, *Clin Nutr* 24(2):224, 2005.

Hinkle CZ: *Fundamentals of anatomy and movement: a workbook and guide,* St Louis, 1997, Mosby.

Huckell CB, Simmons ED, Zheng Y: The significance of annular tear of cervical disc for positive discography by age in discogenic pain, *Spine J* 5(4, suppl 1):S48, 2005.

Ido K et al: The validity of upright myelography for diagnosing lumbar disc herniation, *Clin Neurol Neurosurg* 104(1):30, 2002.

Jablonski S: *Dictionary of medical acronyms & abbreviations,* ed 3, Philadelphia, 1998, Hanley & Belfus.

Jones MA: Clinical reasoning in manual therapy, *Phys Ther* 72:875, 1992.

Kang CH et al: MRI of paraspinal muscles in lumbar degenerative kyphosis patients and control patients with chronic low back pain, *Clin Radiol* 62(5):479, 2007.

Katirji B: *Electromyography in clinical practice a case study approach,* St Louis, 1998, Mosby.

Keats TE: *Atlas of normal roentgen variants that may simulate disease,* ed 6, St Louis, 1996, Mosby.

Kessler RM, Herling D: Assessment of musculoskeletal disorders. In Kessler RM, Herling D, editors: *Management of common musculoskeletal disorders,* ed. 2, Philadelphia, 1990, JB Lippincott.

Kettenbach G: *Writing s.o.a.p. notes,* Philadelphia, 1990, FA Davis.

Khurana R, Berney SM: Clinical aspects of rheumatoid arthritis, *Pathophysiology* 12(3):153-165, 2005.

Kim H-S et al: Comparison of the predictive value of computed tomography with myelography versus MRI using exercise treadmill exam in lumbar spinal stenosis, *Spine J* 3(5, suppl 1):84-95, 2003.

Kleinrensink GJ et al: Upper limb tension tests as tools in the diagnosis of nerve and plexus lesions: anatomical and biomechanical aspects, *Clin Biomech* 15(1):9-14, 2000.

Klippel JH, Dieppe PA: *Rheumatology,* vol 1-2, ed. 2, London, 1998, Mosby.

Konowitz KB: Reflex sympathy dystrophy syndrome sometimes misdiagnosed, often misunderstood, *J Am Chiro Assoc* 35:58, 1998.

Lancaster AR, Nyland J, Roberts CS: The validity of the motion palpation test for determining patellofemoral joint articular cartilage damage. *Phys Ther Sport* 8(2):59-65, 2007.

Lander PH: Lumbar discography: current concepts and controversies, *Semin Ultrasound CT MRI* 26(2):81-88, 2005.

Landewe RBM, van der Heijde DMFM: Principles of assessment from a clinical perspective, *Best Pract Res Clin Rheumatol* 17(3):365-379, 2003.

Lassere M et al: Smallest detectable difference in radiological progression, *J Rheumatol* 1 26(3):731-739, 999.

Lewis CB, Knortz KA: *Orthopedic assessment and treatment of the geriatric patient,* St Louis, 1993, Mosby.

Licht PB, Christensen HW, Hoilund-Carlsen PF: Is there a role for premanipulative testing before cervical manipulation? *J Manipulative Physiol Ther* 23(3):175-179, 2000.

Long L, Huntley A, Ernst E: Which complementary and alternative therapies benefit which conditions? A survey of the opinions of 223 professional organizations, *Complement Ther Med* 9(3):178-185, 2001.

Mader TJ, Ames A, Letourneau P: Pain management in paediatric trauma patients with long bone fracture, *Injury* 37(1):61-65, 2006.

Magee DJ: *Orthopedic physical assessment,* ed 3, Philadelphia, 1997, WB Saunders.

Maher C, Adams R: Reliability of pain and stiffness assessments in clinical manual lumbar spine examination, *Phys Ther* 74:801, 1994.

Malanga GA et al: Physical examination of the knee: a review of the original test description and scientific validity of common orthopedic tests, *Arch Phys Med Rehabil* 84(4):592-603, 2003.

Malone TR, McPoil TG, Nitz AJ: *Orthopedic and sports physical therapy,* ed 3, St Louis, 1997, Mosby.

Mathers LH: *Clinical anatomy principles,* St Louis, 1996, Mosby.

Matsuo T et al: Application of thermography for evaluation of mechanical load on the muscles of upper limb during wheelchair driving, *J Biomech* 39(suppl 1):S537, 2006.

Maurissen JPJ et al: Factors affecting grip strength testing, *Neurotoxicol Teratol* 25(5):543-553, 2003.

McDonnell MN et al: Impairments in precision grip correlate with functional measures in adult hemiplegia, *Clin Neurophysiol* 117(7):1474-1480, 2006.

McKinnis LN: Fundamentals of radiology for physical therapists. In Richardson JK, Iglarsh ZA, editors: *Clinical orthopedic physical therapy,* Philadelphia, 1994, WB Saunders.

McRae R: *Clinical orthopaedic examination,* ed 3, Edinburgh, 1990, Churchill Livingstone.

Mengel MB, Schwiebert LP: *Ambulatory medicine the primary care of families,* ed 2, Stamford, Conn, 1996, Appleton & Lange.

Mennell JM: *The musculoskeletal system differential diagnosis from symptoms and physical signs,* Gaithersburg, Md, 1992, Aspen.

Mercier LR, Pettid FJ: *Practical orthopedics,* ed 5, St Louis, 2000, Mosby.

Micheli LJ: Reflex sympathetic dystrophy may stem from sports (news brief), *Phys Sports Med* 18:35, 1990.

Middleton GD, McFarlin JE, Lipsky PE: Prevalence and clinical impact of fibromyalgia in systemic lupus erythematous, *Arthritis Rheum* 8:1181, 1994.

Moreau JF. Re: "Ultrasound: is there a future in diagnostic imaging?" *J Am Coll Radiol* 4(1):78-79, 2007.

Morse JL et al: Maximal dynamic grip force and wrist torque: the effects of gender, exertion direction, angular velocity, and wrist angle, *Appl Ergon* 37(6):737-742, 2006.

Mosby-Year Book, Inc: *Expert 10-minute physical examination,* St Louis, 1997, Mosby.

Mower WR et al: Use of plain radiography to screen for cervical spine injuries, *Ann Emerg Med* 38(1):1-7, 2001.

Nardone DA et al: A model for the diagnostic medical interview: nonverbal, verbal and cognitive assessments, *J Gen Intern Med* 7:437, 1992.

Nettina SM: *The Lippincott manual of nursing practice,* ed 6, Philadelphia, 1996, JB Lippincott.

Newman JS et al: Power Doppler sonography of synovitis: assessment of therapeutic response—preliminary observations, *Radiology* 198:582, 1996.

Ng GYF, Fan ACC: Does elbow position affect strength and reproducibility of power grip measurements? *Physiotherapy* 87(2):68-72, 2001.

Nicholas JA, Hershman EB: *The lower extremity & spine in sports medicine,* ed 2, St Louis, 1995, Mosby.

Niere KR, Torney SKSK: Clinicians' perceptions of minor cervical instability, *Man Ther* 9(3):144-150, 2004.

Pagana KD, Pagana TJ: *Mosby's manual of diagnostic and laboratory tests,* St Louis, 1998, Mosby.

Palmgren PJ et al: Improvement after chiropractic care in cervicocephalic kinesthetic sensibility and subjective pain intensity in patients with nontraumatic chronic neck pain, *J Manipulative Physiol Ther* 29(2):100-106, 2006.

Paoloni JA, Appleyard RC, Murrell GAC: The Orthopaedic Research Institute—Tennis Elbow Testing System: a modified chair pick-up test—interrater and intrarater reliability testing and validity for monitoring lateral epicondylosis, *J Shoulder Elbow Surg* 13(1):72-77, 2004.

Papacharalampous X et al: The effect of contrast media on the synovial membrane, *Eur J Radiol* 55(3):426-430, 2005.

Pascual E, Jovani V: Synovial fluid analysis, *Best Pract Res Clin Rheum* 19(3):371-386, 2005.

Patton K: *Student survival guide for anatomy and physiology,* St Louis, 1999, Mosby.

Peterfy CG et al: MR imaging of the arthritic knee: improved discrimination of cartilage, synovium and effusion with pulsed saturation transfer and fat-suppressed T1-weighted sequences, *Radiology* 191:413, 1994.

Pincus T et al: Persistent back pain—why do physical therapy clinicians continue treatment? A mixed methods study of chiropractors, osteopaths and physiotherapists, *Eur J Pain* 10(1):67-76, 2006.

Pope MH: *Occupational low back pain: assessment, treatment, and prevention,* St Louis, 1991, Mosby Year Book.

Raspe HH: Back pain. In Silman AJ, Hochberg M, editors: *Epidemiology of the rheumatic diseases,* Oxford, UK, 1993, Oxford University Press.

Ravaud P et al: Assessing smallest detectable change over time in continuous structural outcome measures: application to radiological change in knee osteoarthritis, *J Clin Epidemiol* 52(12):1225-1230, 1999.

Ravel R: *Clinical laboratory medicine clinical application of laboratory data,* ed. 6, St Louis, 1995, Mosby.

Rogers LF, Hendrix RW: Evaluating the multiple injured patients radiographically, *Orthop Clin North Am* 21:437, 1990.

Ross JS: *Diagnostic imaging. Spine.* Salt Lake City, 2004, Amirsys.

Sahin G, Demirtas M: An overview of MR arthrography with emphasis on the current technique and applicational hints and tips, *Eur J Radiol* 58(3):416-430, 2006.

Saidoff DC, McDonough AL: *Critical pathways in therapeutic intervention: lower extremity,* St Louis, 1997, Mosby.

Sasaki H et al: Grip strength predicts cause-specific mortality in middle-aged and elderly persons, *Am J Med* 120(4):337-342, 2007.

Schreuders TAR et al: Strength measurements of the intrinsic hand muscles: a review of the development and evaluation of the Rotterdam intrinsic hand myometer, *J Hand Ther* 19(4):393-402, 2006.

Schueller G: MRI atlas of orthopedics and traumatology of the knee, *Eur J Radiol* 51(3):293-238, 2004; from Teller P et al. *Eur J Radiol* 51(3):293-298.

Schumacher HR, Klippel JH, Koopman WJ: *Primer on the rheumatic diseases,* ed 10, Atlanta, 1993, Arthritis Foundation.

Schwartz ML, Al-Zahrani S: Diagnostic imaging of elbow injuries in the throwing athlete, *Oper Tech Sports Med* 4(2):84-90, 1996.

Scuderi GR, McCann PD, Bruno PJ: *Sports medicine: principles of primary care,* St Louis, 1997, Mosby.

Scutellari PN, Orzincolo C: Rheumatoid arthritis: sequences, *Eur J Radiol* 27(suppl 1):S31-S38, 1998.

Seo K-S et al: In vitro measurement of pressure differences using manometry at various injection speeds during discography, *Spine J* 7(1):68-73, 2007.

Shankman GA: *Fundamental orthopedic management for the physical therapist assistant,* St Louis, 1997, Mosby.

Shechtman O, Taylor C: How do therapists administer the rapid exchange grip test? A survey. *J Hand Ther* 15(1):53-61, 2002.

Sheehan DV H-SK, Raj BA: The measurement of disability, *Int Clin Psychopharmacol* 11:S89-S95, 1996.

Sherbondy PS, Sebastianelli WJ: Stress fractures of the medial malleolus and distal fibula, *Clin Sports Med* 25(1):129-137, 2006.

Sieper J et al: Diagnosing reactive arthritis: role of clinical setting in the value of serologic and microbiologic assays, *Arthritis Rheum* 46(2):319-327, 2002.

Slipman CW et al: Provocative cervical discography symptom mapping, *Spine J* 5(4):381-388, 2005.

Smart K, Doody C: The clinical reasoning of pain by experienced musculoskeletal physiotherapists, *Man Ther* 12(1):40-49, 2007.

Smith RC, Hoppe RB: The patient's story: integrating the patient and physician centered approaches to interviewing, *Ann Intern Med* 115:470, 1991.

St. Claire SM: Diagnosis and treatment of fibromyalgia syndrome, *J Neuromusc Syst* 2:3, 1994.

Stamford JA: Descending control of pain, *Br J Anaesth* 75:217, 1995.

Stevenson J: When the trauma patient is elderly, *J Perianesth Nurs* 19(6):392-400, 2004.

Stojilovic N et al: Analysis of prosthetic knee wear debris extracted from synovial fluid, *Appl Surface Sci* 252(10):3760-3766, 2006.

Stone JA: MR myelography of the spine and MR peripheral nerve imaging, *Magn Reson Imaging Clin N Am* 11(4):543-558, 2003.

Storm S et al: Compliance with electrodiagnostic guidelines for patients undergoing carpal tunnel release, *Arch Phys Med Rehabil* 86(1):8-11, 2005.

Sugimoto H et al: Early-stage rheumatoid arthritis: diagnostic accuracy of MR imaging, *Radiology* 198:185, 1996.

Tamai K et al: Dynamic magnetic resonance imaging for the evaluation of synovitis in patients with rheumatoid arthritis, *Arthritis Rheum* 37:1151, 1994.

Thibodeau G, Patton K: *Pocket reference to accompany anatomy & physiology,* ed 3, St Louis, 1996, Mosby.

Thibodeau GA, Patton KT: *Anatomy & physiology,* ed 3, St Louis, 1996, Mosby.

Thibodeau GA, Patton KT: *Anatomy & physiology,* ed 4, St Louis, 1999, Mosby.

Thompson JM: *Clinical outlines for health assessment,* St Louis, 1997, Mosby.

Toghill PJ: *Examining patients an introduction to clinical medicine,* London, 1990, Edward Arnold.

Torg JS, Shepard RJ: *Current therapy in sports medicine,* ed 3, St Louis, 1995, Mosby.

Traub M et al: The use of chest computed tomography versus chest x-ray in patients with major blunt trauma, *Injury* 38(1):43-47, 2007.

Tredgett MW, Davis TRC: Rapid repeat testing of grip strength for detection of faked hand weakness, *J Hand Surg* 25(4):372-375, 2000.

Tsuruike M et al: Age comparison of H-reflex modulation with the Jendrassik maneuver and postural complexity, *Clin Neurophysiol* 114(5):945-953, 2003.

Turnbull TJ, Dymowski JJ: Emergency department use of hand-held Doppler ultrasonography, *Am J Emerg Med* 7(2):209-215, 1989.

Van De Kar THJ et al: Clinical value of electrodiagnostic testing following repair of peripheral nerve lesions: a prospective study, *J Hand Surg* 27(4):345-349, 2002.

Weinstein SL, Buckwalter JA: *Turek's orthopaedics principles and their application,* ed 5, Philadelphia, 1994, JB Lippincott.

White KP et al: Fibromyalgia in rheumatology practice: a survey of Canadian rheumatologists, *J Rheumatol* 22:722, 1995.

Whitmore I, Willan P: *Multiple choice questions in human anatomy,* London, 1995, Mosby.

Wiener E et al: Contrast enhanced cartilage imaging: comparison of ionic and non-ionic contrast agents, *Eur J Radiol* (in press, corrected proof).

Wolfe F et al: The prevalence and characteristics of fibromyalgia in the general population, *Arthritis Rheum* 38:19, 1995.

Woolf CJ: Somatic pain-pathogenesis and prevention, *Br J Anaesth* 75:169, 1995.

Zatouroff M: *Diagnosis in color physical signs in general medicine,* ed 2, London, 1996, Mosby-Wolfe.

Zeitz K, McCutcheon H: Observations and vital signs: ritual or vital for the monitoring of postoperative patients? *Appl Nurs Res* 19(4):204-211, 2006.

Zembsch A et al: Positioning device for optimal active kinematic real-time magnetic resonance imaging of the knee joint: a technical note, *Clin Biomech* 13(4-5):308-313, 1998.

Zitelli BJ, Davis HW: *Atlas of pediatric physical diagnosis,* ed 2, London, 1992, Wolfe.

CITATIONS

Benaroia M, Elinson R, Zarnke K: Patient-directed intelligent and interactive computer medical history-gathering systems: a utility and feasibility study in the emergency department, *Int J Med Inform* 76(4):283-238, 2007.

Berghout RM et al: Evaluation of general practitioner's time investment during a store-and-forward teledermatology consultation, *Int J Med Inform* 76 (supplement): S384–S391.

Birklein F et al: Neurological findings in complex regional pain syndromes—analysis of 145 cases, *Acta Neurol Scand* 101(4):262-269, 2000.

Boden SD et al: Abnormal magnetic-resonance scans of the lumbar spine in asymptomatic subjects. A prospective investigation, *J Bone Joint Surg* 72(3):403-408, 1990.

Cole M, Michael JA, Robert BD: Romberg's sign. In *Encyclopedia of the neurological sciences*, New York, 2003, Academic Press.

Fess EE: Grip strength. In Casanova JS, editor: *Clinical assessment recommendations* ed 2, Chicago, 1992, American Society of Hand Therapists.

Guntern DV et al: Articular cartilage lesions of the glenohumeral joint: diagnostic effectiveness of MR arthrography and prevalence in patients with subacromial impingement syndrome, *Radiology* 226(1):165-170, 2003.

Jimenez RM, Jaramillo D, Connolly SA: Imaging of the pediatric hand: soft tissue abnormalities, *Eur J Radiol* 56(3):344-357, 2005.

Johnson JA, Cogbill TH, Winga ER: Determinants of outcome after pulmonary contusion, *J Trauma* 26(8):695-697, 1986.

Joughin K et al: An evaluation of rapid exchange and simultaneous grip tests, *J Hand Surg* 18(2):245-252, 1993.

Kassarjian A et al: Triad of MR arthrographic findings in patients with cam-type femoroacetabular impingement, *Radiology* 236(2):588-592, 2005.

Kayser R et al: Value of preoperative ultrasound marking of calcium deposits in patients who require surgical treatment of calcific tendinitis of the shoulder, *Arthroscopy* 23(1):43-50, 2007.

Kretzschmar K: Degenerative diseases of the spine. The role of myelography and myelo-CT. *Eur J Radiol* 27(3):229-234, 1998.

Leardini A et al: A new software tool for 3D motion analyses of the musculo-skeletal system, *Clin Biomech* 21(8):870-879, 2006.

LoCicero J 3rd, Mattox KL: Epidemiology of chest trauma, *Surg Clin North Am* 69(1):15-19, 1989.

McCauley TR: MR imaging evaluation of the postoperative knee, *Radiology* 234(1):53-61, 2005.

Nowinski CJ et al: The impact of converting to an electronic health record on organizational culture and quality improvement. *Int J Med Inform* 76(suppl 1):S174-S183, 2007.

Ory PA: Radiography in the assessment of musculoskeletal conditions, *Best Pract Res Clin Rheum* 17(3):495-512, 2003.

Owens JEF et al: The reliability of a posterior-to-anterior spinal stiffness measuring system in a population of patients with low back pain, *J Manipulative Physiol Ther* 30(2):116-123, 2007.

Phelps MA, Rodriguez RM: The comprehensive physical exam: when and why do emergency medicine residents perform them on patients with minor chief complaints? *Ann Emerg Med* 46(3, suppl 1):28-29, 2005.

Pinilla JC: Acute respiratory failure in severe blunt chest trauma, *J Trauma* 22(3):221-226, 1982.

Porcellini G et al: Arthroscopic treatment of calcifying tendinitis of the shoulder: clinical and ultrasonographic follow-up findings at two to five years, *J Shoulder Elbow Surg* 13(5):503-508, 2004.

Rupp S, Seil R, Kohn D: [Tendinosis calcarea of the rotator cuff], *Orthopade* 29(10):852-867, 2000.

Schild H et al: [Computed tomography of lung contusion. An experimental study], *Fortschr Geb Rontgenstr Nuklearmed* 145(5):519-526, 1986.

Schils JP et al: Medial malleolar stress fractures in seven patients: review of the clinical and imaging features, *Radiology* 185(1):219-221, 1992.

Schleyer T, Spallek H, Hernandez P: A qualitative investigation of the content of dental paper-based and computer-based patient record formats, *J Am Med Inform Assoc* 14(4):515-526, 2007.

Schmid MR et al: Cartilage lesions in the hip: diagnostic effectiveness of MR arthrography, *Radiology* 226(2):382-386, 2003.

Scuderi GJ et al: Towards a more scientific understanding of lumbar discography in patients with lumbar intervertebral disc disease, *Spine J* (in press, corrected proof).

Shechtman O, Taylor C: How do therapists administer the rapid exchange grip test? A survey, *J Hand Ther* 15(1):53-61, 2002.

Smart K, Doody C: The clinical reasoning of pain by experienced musculoskeletal physiotherapists, *Man Ther* 12(1):40-49, 2007.

Steinbronn DJ, Bennett GL, Kay DB: The use of magnetic resonance imaging in the diagnosis of stress fractures of the foot and ankle: four case reports, *Foot Ankle Int* 15(2):80-83, 1994.

Stokes M, Young A: The contribution of reflex inhibition to arthrogenous muscle weakness, *Clin Sci* 67(1):7-14, 1984.

Stoyneva Z: Laser Doppler-recorded venoarteriolar reflex in Raynaud's phenomenon, *Auton Neurosci* 116(1-2):62-68, 2004.

Takemitsu Y et al: Lumbar degenerative kyphosis. Clinical, radiological and epidemiological studies, *Spine* 13(11):1317-1326, 1988.

Taylor C, Shechtman O: The use of the rapid exchange grip test in detecting sincerity of effort, part I: administration of the test, *J Hand Ther* 13(3):195-202, 2000.

Thornbury JR et al: Disk-caused nerve compression in patients with acute low-back pain: diagnosis with MR, CT myelography, and plain CT, *Radiology* 186(3):731-738, 1993.

Thornbury JR et al: Increasing the scientific quality of clinical efficacy studies of magnetic resonance imaging, *Invest Radiol* 26(9):829-835, 1991.

Wagner RB, Jamieson PM: Pulmonary contusion. Evaluation and classification by computed tomography, *Surg Clin North Am* 69(1):31-40, 1989.

Zihlmann MS et al: Three-dimensional kinematics and kinetics of total knee arthroplasty during level walking using single plane video-fluoroscopy and force plates: a pilot study, *Gait Posture* 24(4):475-481, 2006.

CHAPTER TWO

ASSESSING CARDINAL MUSCULOSKELETAL SYMPTOMS AND SIGNS

INTRODUCTION

The actual technique of examination varies according to individual preference. Nevertheless, developing and adhering to a particular routine is useful. Familiarity with such a routine ensures that an examiner does not overlook any step in the examination.

The part or region under evaluation must be adequately exposed and in good lighting. Many mistakes are made simply because the examiner does not insist on removing enough of the patient's clothing to allow proper evaluation

---

ORTHOPEDIC GAMUT 2-1
VISUAL INSPECTION

Systematically, visual inspection focuses on four areas:
1. Bones: Observe the general alignment and position of the parts to detect any deformity, shortening, or unusual posture.
2. Soft tissues: Observe the soft-tissue contours, comparing bilaterally and noting any visible evidence of general or local swelling or muscle wasting.
3. Color and texture of the skin: Look for rubor, cyanosis, pigmentation, shininess, loss of hair, or other changes.
4. Scars or tissue sinuses: If a scar is present, determine from its appearance whether it was caused by operation (linear scar with suture marks), injury (irregular scar), or suppuration (broad, adherent, puckered scar).

ORTHOPEDIC GAMUT 2-2
PALPATION

Four elements are the focus of palpation:
1. Skin temperature: By careful bilateral comparison, determine whether an area of increased warmth or unusual coolness exists. An increase in local temperature denotes increased blood flow, the usual cause is an inflammatory reaction. A rapidly growing tumor also may cause marked local hyperemia.
2. Bones: Investigate the general shape and outline of the bone. Palpate in particular for thickening, abnormal prominence, or disturbed relationship of the normal landmarks. Spinal palpation accuracy is clinically acceptable for noninvasive therapeutic intervention, given that any given vertebra obviously articulates with vertebra above and below.
3. Soft tissue: Direct attention is given to the muscle (spasm, atrophy), joint tissue (synovial membrane, joint distension), and the detection of any local or general swelling of the part.
4. Local tenderness: The exact borders of any local tenderness should be delineated. An attempt is made to relate this tenderness to a particular structure.

ORTHOPEDIC GAMUT 2-3
PRESENTING MUSCULOSKELETAL SYMPTOMS AND SIGNS

Presenting symptoms and signs will differentiate musculoskeletal complaints into five main types:
- Inflammatory disease
- Mechanical articular or periarticular disorder
- Systemic disease presenting with musculoskeletal symptoms or signs
- Idiopathic
- Functional disorder

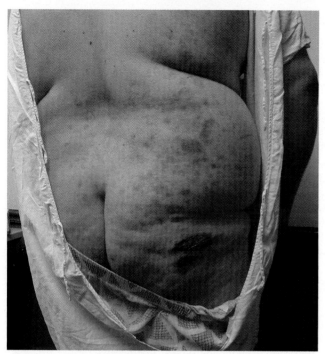

FIG. 2-1 Male patient with chronic piriformis syndrome and sciatica. Examination revealed healed third-degree burns and scarring over the right lower lumbar spine and the right gluteal region secondary to splash injury with molten brass in a foundry. Customary hyperalgesia associated with burn recovery complicated the examination.

and inspection (Fig. 2-1). When examining the involved extremity, the uninvolved extremity is always be used for comparison.

CARDINAL SYMPTOMS

Pain and Sensibility

Among presenting symptoms, pain is usually most important for the patient. Among presenting signs, swelling of a joint or periarticular tissue is important. With regard to pain, the examiner must be certain of the site of origin and distribution. The patient's verbal description may be misleading. The patient should be able to point to or define the site of maximal intensity and map out the area over which pain is experienced.

The deep muscles of the vertebral column, predominantly those of the upper cervical complex, are arranged in a diversity of orientations. Deep muscles of the cervical spine have higher concentrations of mechanoreceptors in areas flanking the articulations than in the more superficial areas. Signals from muscle receptors in individual neck muscles or muscle subsections may have a substantial potential to provide a detailed representation of head position and head movement (Palmgren et al, 2006).

Articular or periarticular pain may radiate widely and may be felt in a spot distant from the originating tissues. Such referred pain is a perceptual error occurring at the

sensory cortex and reflects shared innervation by structures derived from the same embryonic segment. Cortical cells most commonly receive stimuli from the skin. When the same cells receive an initial painful stimulus from a deeply situated myotomal or sclerotomal structure, they interpret the signal based on experience. The patient feels pain in the area of the skin (dermatome) that shares the connection. An important distinction for dermatomal pain is that referred pain is felt deeply, rather than in the skin itself, and its boundaries are indistinct. Referred pain radiates segmentally without crossing the midline.

Differences in pain sensitivity are reported over different parts of the body. Interpretation of both spatial interactions and spatial radiation of pain are significantly complicated by systematic site-to-site differences. Radiation of pain is a common phenomenon seen in clinical pain states. However, instead of radiation to proximal areas, higher inhibition on distal areas produces an illusion that pain radiates to the proximal stimulus location. A possible explanation for this phenomenon is that in the presence of multiple noxious stimuli, the proximal stimulus is more important for driving the withdrawal responses because it optimizes the defensive behaviors (Quevedo, Coghill, 2007).

Because the dermatome often extends more distally than the myotome, the pain is mainly referred distally. The more distal the originating structure from the spinal cord is, the more accurate the pain localization is likely to be. In addition to pain referral, tenderness may also be experienced at a distant site. Dermatomes are variable between individuals. For example, the precise area of pain referral may differ between patients with the same musculoskeletal problem. The more superficial a soft-tissue structure is, the more precise its pain localization will be. Massage over the area of referred pain may improve rather than worsen the pain, and pressure over the originating tissue may reproduce the pain.

The quality of musculoskeletal pain sometimes provides important diagnostic clues. For example, nerve entrapment may produce pain that is described as being similar to an electric shock and of a shooting type. In contrast, vascular pain may be throbbing, and joint pains are severe aching sensations.

The patient's description of the quality of the pain is often not helpful in diagnosis. Pain descriptions are based on the patient's frame of reference and shaded by their emotional state.

In particular, pain detection in older adults with dementia and communication disorders is particularly challenging. The relationship between pain and cognitive impairment is not well explained. Theories suggest that the neuropathologic processes involved in dementia seem to influence pain experience. Unfortunately, no objective biologic markers of pain exist (Costardi et al, 2007).

Helpful descriptions include sharp, shooting pain that travels a distance and is characteristic of root entrapment or extreme pain, typical of crystal deposition synovitis. Although topographic localization occurs at the sensory cortex level, pain appreciation and severity are determined by cells in the supraorbital region of the frontal lobe, which is why the patient's emotional state has such an influence over the severity of the pain. The memory of pain resides in the temporal lobe.

Factors that exacerbate or ameliorate the pain are important. Pain during activity suggests a mechanical problem, particularly if it worsens during the activity and quickly improves when resting. Pain while at rest and pain that is worse at the beginning rather than at the end of use implies a marked inflammatory component. Night pain is a distressing symptom that reflects intraosseous hypertension and accompanies serious problems, such as avascular necrosis, bone neoplastic activity, or bone collapse adjacent to a severely arthritic joint. Persistent bony pain is characteristic of neoplastic invasion. The activities that create a mechanical pain may provide clues as to the appropriate diagnosis. Periarticular problems are often induced by a specific type of activity but are also divided by region (Table 2-1).

Testing sensibility to both light touch and pinprick throughout the affected area is appropriate. In unilateral afflictions, the opposite side should be similarly tested. From knowledge of the cutaneous distribution of the peripheral nerves, the particular nerve is identified.

The sense of pain is served by free nerve endings located in the skin and certain visceral tissues. Pain can be caused by stimuli of different natures. Strong mechanical stimuli (intense pressure) and very hot and very cold stimuli (thermal and certain chemical stimuli, such as acidic substances) can both cause pain. Pain receptors have a high threshold of stimulation. These receptors are usually activated when stimulus strength is very high. Because such strong stimuli are usually noxious, the evoked sensation is also called *nociception* (pain sense). The pain receptors activated by noxious stimuli are the *nociceptors*.

Tissue damage results in the local release of certain internal nociceptive substances such as serotonin, pressor substance (substance P), histamine, and kinin peptides (bradykinin) in the injured area. These substances then act on the free nerve endings, activating pain signals. Sharp pain is conveyed by thin, myelinated, fast, type-A delta fibers. Dull, aching, and hurting pain travels through the unmyelinated, slow, conducting type-C fibers.

Peripheral Nociceptors

The skin, joint structures, arterial walls, and periosteum are richly supplied with nociceptors that are activated by a variety of mechanical (stretching), thermal (heat and cold), and chemical stimuli (Fig. 2-2). The main neurotransmitters involved in pain inhibitory pathways are serotonin, norepinephrine, and the endogenous opioids (Fig. 2-3).

TABLE 2-1	
REGIONAL PERIARTICULAR SYNDROMES	
Region	**Periarticular Syndrome**
Jaw	Temporomandibular joint dysfunction (myofascial pain syndrome)
Shoulder	Subacromial bursitis
	Long-head bicipital tendinopathy
	Rotator cuff tear
Elbow	Olecranon bursitis
	Epicondylitis
Wrist	Extensor tendinopathy (including de Quervain tenosynovitis)
	Gonococcal tenosynovitis
Hand	Palmar fasciitis (Dupuytren contracture)
	Ligamentous or capsular injury
Hip	Greater trochanteric bursitis
	Adductor syndrome
	Ischial bursitis
	Fascia lata syndrome
Knee	Anserine bursitis
	Prepatellar bursitis
	Meniscal injury
	Ligamentous tear-laxity
	Baker cyst
Ankle	Peroneal tendinopathy
	Achilles tendinopathy
	Retrocalcaneal bursitis
	Calcaneal fasciitis
	Sprain
	Erythema nodosum
Foot	Plantar fasciitis
	Pes planus *(fallen arches)*

Adapted from Kelley WN, et al: *Textbook of rheumatology,* ed 5, Philadelphia, 1997, WB Saunders.

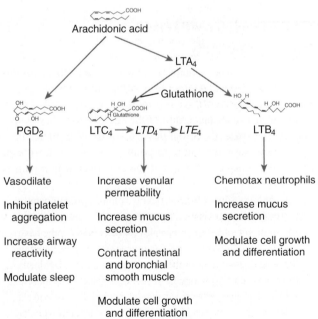

FIG. 2-2 Major leukotriene and prostaglandin products of mast cells and basophils. *LT,* Leukotriene; *PG,* prostaglandin. (From Kelley WN, et al: *Textbook of rheumatology,* ed 5, Philadelphia, 1997, WB Saunders.)

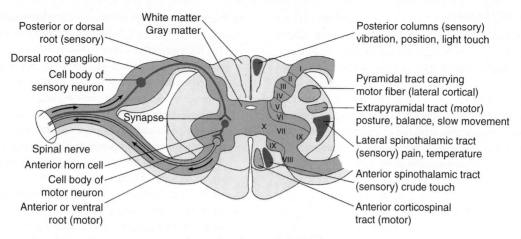

FIG. 2-3 Cross-section of the spinal cord. Spinal nerve roots and their neurons appear on the left side. Spinal nerve tracts appear in white matter on right side. All tracts and nerves are bilateral. (From Barkauskas VH et al: *Health and physical assessment,* ed 2, St Louis, 1998, Mosby.)

Weakness

Weakness of limbs or of the whole body can be an important clue. The pattern of asymmetric or symmetric muscle weakness and its central or peripheral distribution may give vital clues to the diagnosis. *Weakness* may describe the difficulty that the patient has with movement because of joint disease or the feeling of insecurity associated with a loss of proprioception that accompanies many forms of joint disease. Patients may also use the term *weakness* to describe general fatigue rather than loss of muscle power. True generalized muscular weakness often affects gait and stance. Ankle, knee, and hip movements and strength need to be assessed.

After midstance, the ankle plantar flexor movement normally provides upright support and forward progression while accelerating the hip into extension. When the hip flexors are too weak to control this hip extension, individuals can alter lower-extremity joint positions and movements to produce forward progression while minimizing hip extension acceleration. These compensatory strategies permit independent ambulation although at a reduced speed as compared with normal gait (Siegel, Kepple, Stanhope, 2007).

Stiffness

Stiffness is a subjective sensation of resistance to movement that probably reflects fluid distension of the limiting boundary of the inflamed tissue. Stiffness resulting from this phenomenon is most noticeable when arising from bed and after inactivity or rest. As normal use resumes, fluid clears from the inflamed structures, and stiffness wears off. The duration and severity of early-morning stiffness and inactivity stiffness reflect the degree of local inflammation.

Falls are the leading cause of accidental death in older adults and lead to approximately 185,000 hip fractures each year. Fallers tend to have a slower self-selected walking speed compared with nonfallers and are more susceptible to falling laterally, which increases their potential for hip fractures.

Compared with young adults, older adults exhibit a slower preferred walking speed, smaller step length, shorter swing phase time, and decreased range of motion in their lower-extremity joints. The underlying mechanisms causing these gait adaptations, however, are not well understood, with various musculoskeletal parameters being put forth as contributing factors, including increased joint stiffness and decreased isometric strength (Goldberg, Neptune, 2007).

Spontaneous locking of a joint, a limb, or the spine is less common in the absence of injury, such as sustained in falls. In the nontraumatic instance, *locking* may be used to describe very severe stiffness. However, more commonly, it is used to describe a specific mechanical event in which some internal derangement of a joint actually causes it to lock in one position. In the knee, for example, the mechanical locking continues until the patient initiates a *trick* movement or gets help from someone else who frees it up. However, the singular event of a knee (or other joint) locking does not make a diagnosis; the event is only a finding until other tests and procedures support the clinical suspicion.

Regarding the knee, composite examination can improve the examiner's ability to diagnose meniscal tears accurately, as shown by the high positive predictive value of composite tests. As the number of positive composite findings increases, the probability of accurately diagnosing a meniscal tear increases. Improved diagnostic ability allows the physician to counsel the patient better regarding surgery and other management decisions. However, when anterior cruciate ligament injuries and degenerative joint disease are suspected along with a tear of the meniscus, the physician should be cautious about relying solely on the history and physical findings (Lowery et al, 2006).

Such mechanical locking experienced in spinal elements is typical in many patients with ankylosing spondylitis (Fig. 2-4). Mechanical locking is also seen in advanced kyphoscoliosis (Fig. 2-5).

Disability and Handicap

Disability is present when a tissue, organ, or system cannot function adequately. A handicap exists when disability interferes with a patient's daily activities or social or occupational performance. A marked disability does not necessarily cause a handicap. Conversely, minor disability may produce a major handicap. Both states of disability and handicap require separate assessment, with the evaluation of disability purely a medical activity, whereas handicap assessment is often a medicolegal function. Patients' perception of their problems is a product of their adaptation to the depreciated tissue, as well as aspirations for recovery (Box 2-1).

Low back pain affects approximately 60% of the population in Western industrialized countries. Chronic low back pain has become a major medical, social, and economic problem. Chronic low back pain costs are comparable to those incurred by coronary heart disease, diabetes, or depression, and reducing these costs is a major public health issue. One approach to achieving this goal is to determine subgroups of patients at high risk for chronic disabling pain. Working-age adults with subacute low back pain (i.e., pain duration of more than 4 weeks and less than 12 weeks) are thought to be at risk for chronic pain, and therapeutic strategies are needed to decrease the rate at which patients experience chronic disabling low back pain. Among factors related to

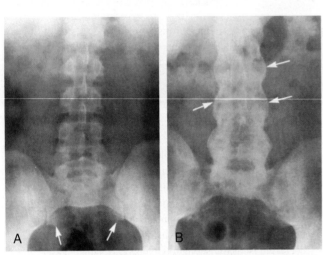

FIG. 2-4 Ankylosing spondylitis with bilateral symmetric sacroiliitis (**A**) *(arrows)*. Ten years later, sacroiliac joint appears similar to previous film (**B**), but the spine exhibits advanced syndesmophytes not noted on previous film *(arrows)*. (From Marchiori DM: *Clinical imaging,* St Louis, 1998, Mosby.)

BOX 2-1

ABILITY DEPRECIATION ASSESSMENT

Question
Ability to perform key task
Loss of work capacity
Adequacy for job
Adequacy for occupation
Maximal dependable ability

Compared with:
Preinjury ability
Normal values
Specific job demands
General occupational demands
General employment standards

Adapted from Demeter SL: *Disability evaluation,* St Louis, 1996, Mosby.

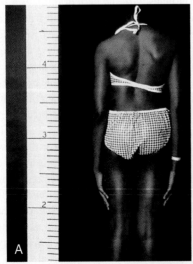
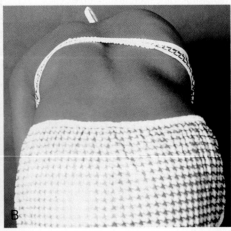

FIG. 2-5 Scoliosis lateral curvature of the spine, with increased convexity to the right. **A,** Scapular asymmetry is easily discernible in the upright position. **B,** Forward flexion reveals a mild rib hump deformity. (From Seidel HM, et al: *Mosby's guide to physical examination,* ed 4, St Louis, 1998, Mosby.)

ORTHOPEDIC GAMUT 2-4

ASSESSING DISABILITY

An aide in assessing the more important aspects of disability is the *PILS mnemonic,* which considers four issues:

1. **P**reventable causes of disability (e.g., falls, direct trauma)
2. **I**ndependence (e.g., self-care)
3. **L**ifestyle (e.g., roles, goals)
4. **S**ocial factors (e.g., family, friends, shelter)

---

the onset and persistence of chronic low back pain, psychosocial factors may play a pivotal role in the development of disability, and especially cognitive behaviors may be more important than sociodemographic features. Several authors have supported the theory that fear-avoidance beliefs may be the most important cognitive factors in the development of chronic disability in patients with low back pain (Poiraudeau et al, 2006).

Assessing a disorder affecting the locomotor system, local or generalized, is not complete without evaluating the patient's functional status and quality of life. This process includes assessing the impact of the condition or injury on the patient's ability to perform activities of daily living and

---

ORTHOPEDIC GAMUT 2-5

SPECIFIC ELEMENTS TO CONSIDER IN ACTIVITIES OF DAILY LIVING ASSESSMENT

Feeding:
- Utensil, cup, plate management, and napkin use
- Tidiness and organization
- Awareness of swallowing, chewing, or pocketing problems
- Ability to handle different food consistencies (e.g., finger foods versus soups)
- Mouth care after eating

Bathing:
- Assembling of items and appropriate equipment
- Management of caps, lids, sprays, etc.
- Facial cleansers and cosmetic applications
- Shaving foam or soap application versus electric razor
- Shaving face, underarms, or legs
- Hair care
- Deodorant application
- Tooth/denture care
- Nail care
- Replacement of care items
- Location of bath facilities in hospital or home
- Transfer ability to bathtub or shower

Dressing:
- Selection of clothing
- Assembling of clothing
- Application of underwear
- Management of fasteners
- Application of trousers/slacks, belts, or suspenders
- Management of pullover tops
- Application of shirt, jacket, dress (front opening) or tie
- Management of buttons
- Application of socks or stockings
- Application of shoes or tying laces
- Location of dressing activities: bed, sitting, or standing
- Ability to care for and apply eyeglasses, contact lenses, or hearing aid

Toileting and elimination management:
- Transfer ability
- Clothing management
- Cognitive function
- Bowel and bladder control
- External devices—assembly, application, removal and care of equipment
- Suppository insertion (including preparation of suppository and cleaning of insertion device if used)
- Post toileting hygiene
- Timing of bowel program (morning or evening)
- Employment/school/home/environment considerations
- Colostomy or ileal conduit care
- Performance of bladder management programs
- Accident management

Sleep:
- Lying still
- Turning over at night in bed
- Getting up and walking in the morning

Movement and transfer:
- Standing upright
- Sitting
- Walking on a flat surface
- Walking on uneven ground
- Ascending stairs
- Descending stairs

Grasp and lifting:
- Performing overhead work
- Scratching own back
- Lifting light objects
- Carrying out chores at home or at work
- Lifting heavy objects
- Throwing objects

Miscellaneous:
- Having sexual intercourse
- Participating in athletics

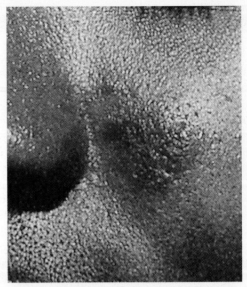

FIG. 2-6 Discoid lupus erythematosus. (From Barkauskas VH, et al: *Health and physical assessment,* ed 2, St Louis, 1998, Mosby.)

FUNCTIONAL ASSESSMENT

A complete functional assessment includes evaluation of the following:
1. Self-care: ability to wash, bathe, attend to toilet needs, dress, cook, and feed oneself
2. Mobility: ability to stand, transfer, walk, negotiate stairs, drive, and use public transportation
3. Lifestyle: nature of occupation, work capacity, and Social Security benefits

---

on the patient's capacity to carry out a normal daily routine, including work, leisure, and other social activities.

Systemic Illness

Inflammatory musculoskeletal disease may trigger a marked acute-phase response and cause nonspecific symptoms of systemic upset. Symptoms may include fever, reduced appetite, weight loss, fatigue, lethargy, and irritability. The patient might not volunteer specific complaints but might report feeling ill. Florid, acute inflammation may cause confusion, especially in older adults.

> Acute pancreatitis is an example of an acute inflammatory disease with a clinical course that may vary from mild to severe. Although in the majority of patients the inflammation resolves with conservative medical management, a minority develop life-threatening complications (Siva, Pereira, 2007).

Chronic cutaneous lesions may occur in the absence of any systemic manifestations, particularly in discoid lupus or systemic lupus erythematosus. Lesions associated with these systemic diseases often begin as erythematous papules or plaques, with scaling that may become thick and adherent with a hypopigmented central area (Fig. 2-6).

Sleep Disturbance

Several factors may interfere with normal sleep patterns and cause anxiety and depression. These factors include chronic pain, triggering of the acute-phase response, unreasonable anxiety concerning deformity and morbidity, central nervous system (CNS) side effects from pain-relieving drugs, and severe arthropathy. Features of masked or overt depression should be sought, particularly in patients with severe musculoskeletal disease. A poor sleep pattern is also a feature of fibromyalgia.

> Disrupted circadian rhythmicity, such as with shift work, affects reproductive function in women. Working shifts increases menstrual cycle irregularities and painful menstruation; 53% of premenopausal women working shifts experience changes in menstrual function compared with approximately 20% of women in the general population. Sleep disturbances have been reported in female shift workers. Based on surveys of female nurses, flight attendants, and industrial workers who work rotating or night shifts, women experience more menstrual irregularities and health problems than those working other shifts (Baker, Driver, in press).

Fatigue

Fatigue is sometimes functional or the result of overexertion. It can be prominent in noninflammatory conditions such as fibromyalgia. Fatigue can be a good indicator of the systemic activity of the disease. In fibromyalgia, most patients report profound fatigue. Seemingly, minor activities aggravate the pain and fatigue, although prolonged inactivity also heightens fibromyalgic symptoms.

> The findings on sleep quality, depression, and negative affect are only partially consistent with individual differences in fatigue. Patients with greater fatigue on average also experience more depression, more sleep problems, and higher levels of negative affect than patients with less fatigue (Zautra et al, 2007).

Emotional Lability

Patients are usually anxious that they may have some severe disease or injury that will cause permanent disfigurement or disability. Pain is a potent cause of anxiety. Much of the important information regarding the patient's perception of pain and accommodation is gleaned during the clinical evaluation from the history, either during the examination, or from a health assessment questionnaire.

> Theorists have argued that the inability to regulate, monitor, and adjust to psychologic pain and pleasure is the essence of psychopathology (Widiger, Sankis, 2000).

> Affective and self-esteem instability are core symptoms of borderline personality disorder, and self-esteem instability has been examined as a factor in the etiology and maintenance of depression (Koenigsberg et al, 2002).

> If these variables are relevant to depression, then the shared features between depression and posttraumatic stress

disorder (PTSD) and high levels of comorbidity between these conditions suggest potential relevance to PTSD (Kashdan et al, 2006).

Referred Symptoms

When the source of the symptom is still in doubt after a thorough examination of the part, attention must be directed to possible extrinsic disorders. Determination of extrinsic disorders requires examination of other regions of the body that might be responsible. For instance, in a case of pain in the shoulder, examining the neck for evidence of a lesion interfering with the brachial plexus might be necessary. For pain in the thigh, the examination often includes a study of the spine, abdomen, pelvis, and genitourinary system, as well as the local examination of the hip and thigh.

The afferent pain fibers originating from the same area demonstrate extensive convergence onto the dorsal horn relay cells. In certain cases, the convergence may take place by fibers from different areas, causing relay cell activation by pain originating in different body parts. This mechanism underlies the phenomenon of referred pain (e.g., pain originating in the heart is often felt at the inner aspects of the left arm). Referred pain is either caused by convergence of pain fibers from both zones onto the same spinal relay cell or caused by facilitation of somatic signals during excessive pain traffic from a visceral source. Classic examples of this circumstance include the referral of neck or shoulder pain to the upper arm (Table 2-2).

Phantom pains, may be a maladaptive failure of the neuromatrix to maintain global bodily constructs. Phantom pains can originate from an amputated limb. Irritation of

severed endings of pain fibers at the site of the amputation signals pain to the same areas of the cortex. These signals are projected to their original source in the limb or body, creating a phantom sensation.

The body schema most likely provides the template for phantom limb perception, particularly considering the complexity of phantom limb sensations (notably, proprioception, kinesthesia, and kinetics), the nature of the triggers of phantom sensations and pain (e.g., referred sensations, vestibular stimulation, visual capture through the mirror box paradigm), and the likely role of phantom limb perception in prosthesis use and embodiment (Giummarra et al, 2007).

CARDINAL SIGNS

Posture

The way the patient positions an affected region or joint is important. A joint with synovitis has **intraarticular hypertension** and is most comfortable in the position that minimizes any pressure increases. Usually the part is adducted and held in internal rotation or flexion. The opposite movements, abduction and external rotation or extension, are the earliest movements affected and the most uncomfortable because they maximize intraarticular hypertension. The attitude of the body part and pattern of restricted movement may suggest the underlying problem.

In spinal conditions, the direction of limitation of spinal motion does not clearly indicate the area of the lesion, however. Spinal muscular strain more likely produces limitation in either the anterior or the posterior direction; arthritic spinal changes more likely produce universal limitation of motion.

Changes in Dimension of the Part

Measurement of the circumference of an extremity provides an index of muscle atrophy, soft-tissue swelling, or bony thickening. Signs of active current inflammation and abnormal tissue responses are crucial in distinguishing arthritides from arthralgia of noninflammatory origin (e.g., mechanical defects, hypermobility).

In addition to physiologic repair mechanisms, an abnormal tissue response may contribute to disease progression and loss of joint function. Cartilage metaplasia, cartilage calcification, synovial hypertrophy and fibrosis, and ectopic and heterotopic bone formation with ankylosis are all consequences of disturbed tissue responses, and an understanding of their cellular and molecular basis is required to control these inappropriate events (Luyten et al, 2006).

Decreased Circulation

Symptoms in a region or joint may be associated with impairment of the arterial circulation. Time should be spent in assessing the state of the circulation by examining the color, temperature, and texture of the skin and the nails and by measuring the arterial pulses. This examination is

TABLE 2-2

CERVICAL SPINE SYNDROMES REFERRING PAIN TO THE UPPER EXTREMITY

Lesions Producing Neck and Shoulder Pain	Lesions Producing Predominantly Shoulder Pain
Postural disorders	Rotator cuff tears and tendinopathy
Rheumatoid arthritis	Calcareous tendinopathy
Fibrositis syndromes	Subacromial bursitis
Musculoligamentous injuries to neck and shoulder	Bicipital tendonitis
Osteoarthritis (apophyseal and Luschka)	Adhesive capsulitis
	Reflex sympathetic dystrophy
	Frozen shoulder syndromes
Cervical spondylosis	Acromioclavicular secondary osteoarthritis
Intervertebral osteoarthritis	Glenohumeral arthritis
Thoracic outlet syndrome	Septic arthritis
Nerve injuries (serratus anterior, C3–C4 nerve root, long thoracic nerve)	Tumors of the shoulder

Modified from Kelley WN, et al: *Textbook of rheumatology,* ed 5, Philadelphia, 1997, WB Saunders.

particularly important in the extremities and extremely important in the lower extremities. An important point to remember is that position, exertion, and endogenous blood pressures all play a role in tissue health.

Hampering of blood flow and reduction in muscle tissue oxygenation during sustained repetitive work can contribute to the development of upper-extremity muscle disorders (Carayon, Smith, Haims, 1999).

A more widely supported explanation for the lack of blood supply is an increased intramuscular pressure, which impedes microcirculation. The intramuscular pressure is related to the produced force, the shape, and location of the muscle with high pressure at high forces in cylindrical and deep muscles (Jensen et al, 1995).

Circulation becomes completely blocked when intramuscular pressure exceeds blood pressure (Visser, van Dieen, 2006).

Diffuse Joint Swelling

Soft-tissue swelling is pathognomonic of inflammation (Table 2-3). Joint, bursal, or tenosynovial inflammation is almost invariably accompanied by the presence of an inflammatory exudate (Figs. 2-7 and 2-8). An important step in confirming inflammation is detecting effusion. In small joints, cross-fluctuation is applied with the examiner's index finger pressing dorsally while the joint is gently squeezed from the sides between the examiner's index finger and thumb (Fig. 2-9).

Swelling is variable, depending on its cause. Various signs are used in the knee (Fig. 2-10), elbow (Fig. 2-11), wrist, ankle, small finger, and toe joints to establish the presence of a joint effusion (by fluctuation using the index finger against the contralateral thumb or index finger in combination).

Bone thickening is detected by deep palpation through the soft tissues. The bone outlines are compared bilaterally. A fluid effusion gives a clear sense of fluctuation in the examiner's hands. Synovial thickening gives a characteristic spongy sensation, as if a layer of soft sponge or rubber had been placed between the skin and the body. Synovial thickening is always accompanied by a well-marked increase in local tissue warmth.

Swelling may be caused by the presence of fluid, soft tissue, or bone. Fluid within a joint collects initially and maximally at the site of least resistance within the capsular confines, producing characteristic swelling (Fig. 2-12).

TABLE 2-3

JOINT AND SOFT-TISSUE EDEMA

Tissue	Indicative of:
Joint synovium/effusion	Inflammatory joint disease
Subcutaneous tissue	Inflammatory joint disease
Bursa/tendon sheath	Inflammation of structure
Articular ends of bone	Osteoarthritis

ORTHOPEDIC GAMUT 2-7

DIFFUSE JOINT SWELLING

Diffuse swelling of a joint as a whole can have only three causes:
1. Thickening of the bone end
2. Fluid within the joint
3. Thickening of the synovial membrane

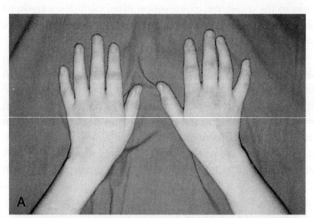

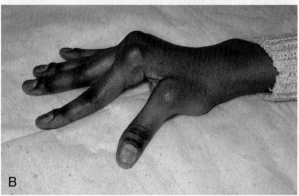

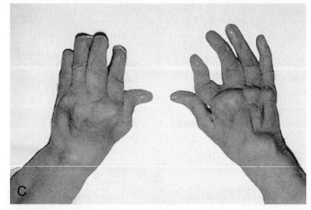

FIG. 2-7 Subcutaneous nodules, called arthritic nodules, are usually found at pressure points such as in the hands or elbows. **A,** Rheumatoid arthritis, early stage. **B,** Rheumatoid arthritis, intermediate stage. **C,** Rheumatoid arthritis, advanced stage. (From *Mosby's dictionary of medicine, nursing, and health professions,* St Louis, 2006, Mosby.)

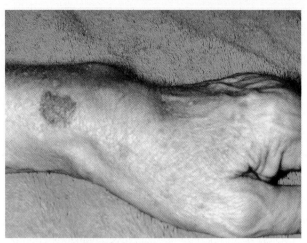

FIG. 2-8 Dorsal sheath effusion in rheumatoid arthritis.

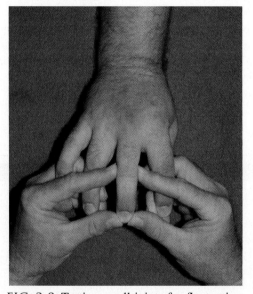

FIG. 2-9 Testing small joints for fluctuation.

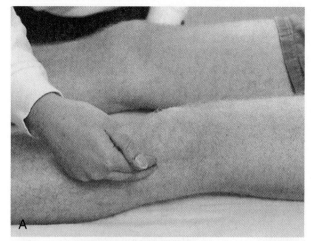

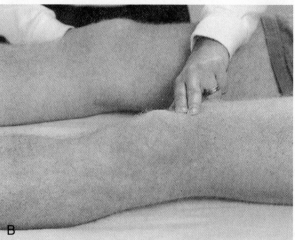

FIG. 2-10 Testing for the bulge sign in examination of the knee. **A,** Milk the medial aspect of the knee two or three times. **B,** Then tap the lateral side of the patella. (From Seidel et al, *Mosby's guide to physical examination*, ed 4, St Louis, 1999, Mosby.)

For small fluid volumes in a confined cavity, a bulge sign may be produced. Larger volumes produce a balloon sign (fluctuance) in which pressure over one point causes ballooning at other parts of the swelling. This ballooning is the most specific sign of fluid. Capsular swelling is the most specific sign of synovitis. The swelling is delineated by the capsular confines and becomes firmer toward the extremes of movement (e.g., swelling associated with pigmented villonodular synovitis).

Pigmented villonodular synovitis is a locally aggressive synovial proliferative tumor disorder of unknown etiology affecting the linings of joints, tendon sheaths, and bursae. The most commonly occurring sites are the knee, flexor tendon sheaths of the hand, and hip joints followed by the ankle and shoulder.

Benign and malignant soft-tissue tumors may resemble each other in terms of clinical presentation; therefore, a high index of suspicion must be observed for appropriate man-

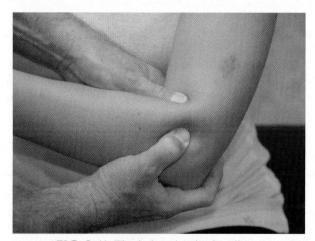

FIG. 2-11 The bulge sign in the elbow.

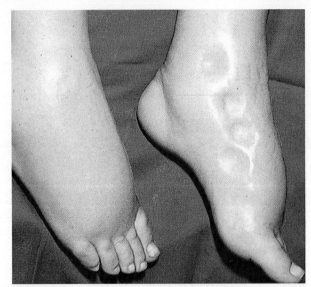

FIG. 2-12 Pitting edema. (From *Mosby's medical, nursing, & allied health dictionary,* St Louis, 2006, Mosby.)

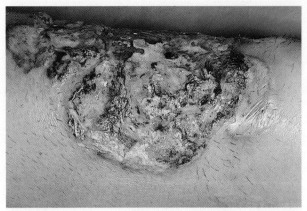

FIG. 2-13 Pyoderma gangrenosum. Pyoderma gangrenosum (PG) is an uncommon ulcerative cutaneous condition of uncertain etiology. PG was first described in 1930. It is associated with systemic diseases in at least 50% of patients who are affected. The diagnosis is made by excluding other causes of similar-appearing cutaneous ulcerations, including infection, malignancy, vasculitis, collagen vascular diseases, diabetes, and trauma. Ulcerations of PG may occur after trauma or injury to the skin in 30% of patients; this process is termed *pathergy.* (From *Mosby's medical, nursing, & allied health dictionary*, St Louis, 1998, Mosby.)

agement. Among the digits and on the dorsum of the foot, localized pigmented villonodular synovitis and giant-cell tumor of the tendon sheath are two of the most common tumors. A combination of clinical, radiologic, and histologic correlation is necessary to make the diagnosis with certainty (Sharma, Jane, Reid, 2006).

Skin Changes

Overlying scars or skin disease may be important clues to causation of deeper rheumatic symptoms. Erythema, commonly followed by desquamation, is an important sign, reflecting periarticular inflammation. Although erythema may occur in several conditions, a red joint or bursa should always raise the suspicion of sepsis or crystals.

Ulcerations secondary to ischemia may result from vasospasm in Raynaud phenomenon, vascular thrombosis, and vascular necrosis. Vascular, infectious, and tumor-associated causes must be considered in the patient with cutaneous ulceration and musculoskeletal symptoms (Fig. 2-13).

Ulcers occur over bony prominences associated with undue pressure. They can become quite deep and are often infected in patients with moderate or severe peripheral neuropathies (Fig. 2-14).

Pressure ulcers remain a frequently occurring problem for hospitalized patients. They are caused by pressure and shearing forces. These two forces can inhibit blood circulation to underlying tissues (Panel for the Prediction and Prevention of Pressure Ulcers in Adults, 1992).

Continuous focal pressure on tissue, especially overlying bony prominences, coupled with shearing of tissue layers from each other as maceration begins causes insufficient blood supply to soft tissues and muscles, resulting in non-blanchable erythema, seen as discoloration of the skin (Fig. 2-15).

ORTHOPEDIC GAMUT 2-8

CAUSES OF ERYTHEMA OVERLYING A JOINT

Sepsis
- Crystals (gout, pseudogout, calcific periarthritis)
- Rheumatoid arthritis
- Acute Reiter or reactive arthropathy
- Early Heberden or Bouchard nodes
- Inflammatory (erosive) osteoarthritis of the hands
- Rheumatic fever

Warmth, edema, induration, or hardness may also be used as an indicator, particularly on individuals with dark skin (European Pressure Ulcer Advisory Panel, 1999).

Nonblanchable erythema is the most important symptom of grade 1 pressure ulcer. Two methods are commonly used to observe nonblanchable erythema, namely, the finger method and the transparent disk method. In the first method, a finger is used to press on the erythema. Erythema that does not blanch when the finger is removed is considered as nonblanchable erythema. In the transparent disk method, a transparent plastic disk is used to press on the erythema. If the skin under the transparent disk does not blanch, the type is also regarded as nonblanchable erythema (Vanderwee et al, 2006).

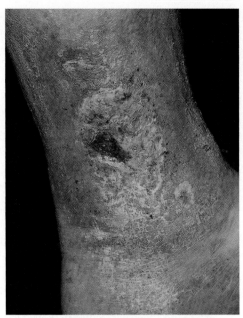

FIG. 2-14 Stasis ulcer. (From Habif TP: *Clinical dermatology,* ed 3, St Louis, 1996, Mosby.)

Erythema

Redness is uncommon but is encountered in gout, especially around the big toe or fingers (see Fig. 2-16), and sepsis in any joint (Fig. 2-17). The primary lesion of erythema migrans, which is nearly pathognomonic of acute Lyme disease, is usually found at the site of the tick bite (Fig. 2-18).

Discoid lupus has a virtually diagnostic appearance and distribution (Table 2-4) but may require histopathologic and immunofluorescence studies.

Misdiagnosis of acute lupus can occur in patients expressing other photosensitive eruptions and in patients with conditions that produce vascular dilation (Table 2-5). A clinical history and examination are usually sufficient to discriminate acute lupus from other photosensitive eruptions.

Features of dermatomyositis rash (Figs. 2-19 and 2-20) allow discrimination from lupus. These features include occasional nasolabial fold involvement, prominent heliotrope and extrafacial involvement (Figs. 2-21 and 2-22), erythema following the course of extensor tendons, and scaling and fissuring of lateral aspects of the fingers (mechanic's hands). A heliotrope rash and Gottron papules are

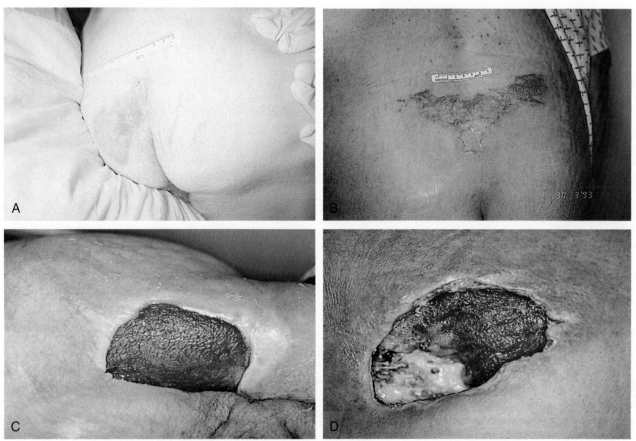

FIG. 2-15 **A,** Stage I pressure ulcer. **B,** Stage II pressure ulcer. **C,** Stage III pressure ulcer. **D,** Stage IV pressure ulcer resulting from ischemic hypoxia of the tissues caused by prolonged pressure on them. Pressure ulcers are most often seen in aged, debilitated, immobilized, or cachectic patients.

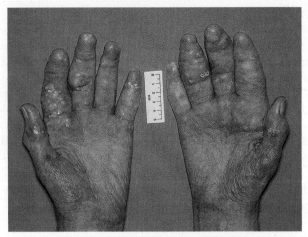

FIG. 2-16 Chronic tophaceous gouty arthritis. (From Nuki G: Gout. *Medicine* 34(10): 417-423, 2006.)

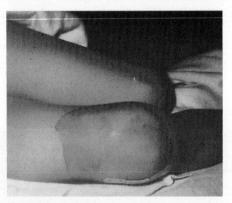

FIG. 2-17 Septic arthritis. (From *Mosby's medical, nursing, & allied health dictionary,* St Louis, 1998, Mosby.)

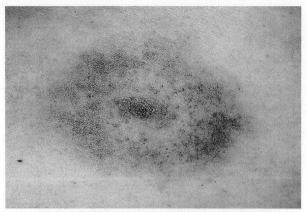

FIG. 2-18 Erythema migrans. (From *Mosby's medical, nursing, & allied health dictionary,* St Louis, 1998, Mosby.)

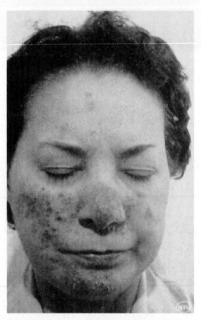

FIG. 2-19 Acne rosacea. (From Barkauskas VH et al: *Health and physical assessment,* ed 2, St Louis, 1998, Mosby.)

TABLE 2-4

FACIAL DISEASES CONFUSED WITH LUPUS

Polymorphous light eruption (occasional)
Benign lymphocytic infiltration of Jessner (rare)
Seborrheic dermatitis (common)
Acne rosacea (common)
Tinea faciei (occasional)
Lupus vulgaris tuberculous (rare)
Lupus pernio sarcoid (rare)

characteristic and possibly pathognomonic cutaneous features of dermatomyositis (Fig. 2.23). The heliotrope rash consists of a violaceous to dusky erythematous rash, with or without edema, in a symmetrical distribution involving periorbital skin.

Sometimes this sign (heliotrope rash) is quite subtle and may involve only a mild discoloration along the eyelid margin (Callen, 2000).

Gottron papules are found covering bony prominences, particularly the metacarpophalangeal joints, proximal interphalangeal joints, and distal interphalangeal joints; they may also be found overlying the elbows, knees, feet, or a combination of these. The lesions consist of slightly raised violaceous papules and plaques.

Tenderness

Precise localization of tenderness is the most useful sign in determining the cause of the problem. Joint line or capsular tenderness signifies arthropathy or capsular disease around the whole margin. Localized joint line tenderness suggests intracapsular pathologic processes. Periarticular point tenderness, away from the joint line, usually indicates bursitis or enthesopathy.

The only reliable finding on examination in fibromyalgia is the presence of multiple tender points. The diagnostic

TABLE 2-5

REVISED CRITERIA FOR THE CLASSIFICATION OF SYSTEMIC LUPUS ERYTHEMATOSUS (1982)

Criterion	Definition
1. Malar rash	Fixed erythema, flat or raised, over the eminences, tending to spare the nasolabial folds
2. Discoid rash	Erythematous raised patches with adherent keratotic scaling and follicular plugging; atrophic scarring may occur in older lesions
3. Photosensitivity	Skin rash as a result of unusual reaction to sunlight, by patient history or physician observation
4. Oral ulcers	Oral or nasopharyngeal ulceration, usually painless, observed by a physician
5. Arthritis	Nonerosive arthritis involving two or more peripheral joints, characterized by tenderness, swelling, or effusion
6. Serositis	(a) Pleuritis—convincing history of pleuritic pain or rub heard by a physician or evidence of pleural effusion *or*
	(b) Pericarditis—documented by electrocardiogram or rub or evidence of pericardial effusion
7. Renal disorder	(a) Persistent proteinuria greater than 0.5 g/day *or* greater than 3+ if quantification not performed *or*
	(b) Cellular casts—may be red cell, hemoglobin, granular, tubular, or mixed
8. Neurologic disorder	(a) Seizures—in the absence of offending drugs or known metabolic derangements, for example, uremia, ketoacidosis, or electrolyte imbalance *or*
	(b) Psychosis—in the absence of offending drugs or known metabolic derangements, for example, uremia, ketoacidosis, or electrolyte imbalance
9. Hematologic disorders	(a) Hemolytic anemia—with reticulocytosis *or*
	(b) Leukopenia—less than 4000/mm^3 total on two or more occasions *or*
	(c) Lymphopenia—less than 1500 cells/mm^3 on two or more occasions *or*
	(d) Thrombocytopenia—less than 100,000 cells/mm^3 in the absence of offending drugs
10. Immunologic disorder	(a) Positive lupus erythematosus cell preparation *or*
	(b) Anti-DNA; antibody to native DNA in abnormal titer *or*
	(c) Anti-Smith antibody: presence of antibody to Smith nuclear antigen *or*
	(d) False-positive serologic test for syphilis known to be positive for at least 6 months and confirmed by *Treponema pallidum* immobilization or fluorescent treponemal antibody absorption test
11. Antinuclear antibody	An abnormal titer of antinuclear antibody by immunofluorescence or an equivalent assay at any point in time and in the absence of drugs known to be associated with *drug-induced lupus* syndrome

From Tan EM, et al: The 1982 revised criteria for the classification of SLE, *Arthritis Rheum* 25:1271, 1982.

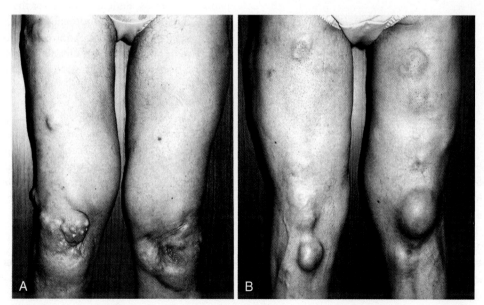

FIG. 2-20 **A** and **B,** A 46-year-old woman with juvenile dermatomyositis (JDM) and extensive cutaneous calcinosis. The first calcific lesions appeared at 18 months and they progressed in size and number along the following 44 years, while muscle involvement subsided. (From Iannuccelli C, et al: Juvenile dermatomyositis with extensive calcinosis: Clinical and radiologic life-long follow-up, *Eur J Radiol Extra* 60(1):33-35, 2006.)

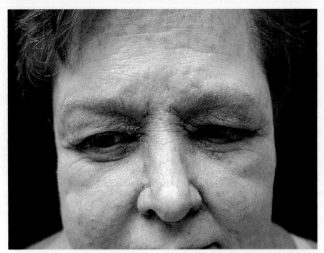

FIG. 2-21 Heliotrope eruption. The periorbital changes represent the heliotrope eruption. (From Callen JP: *Dermatomyositis, Lancet* 355(9197):53-57, 2000.)

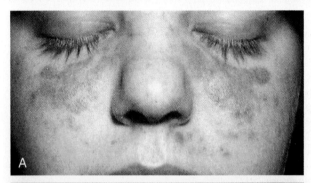

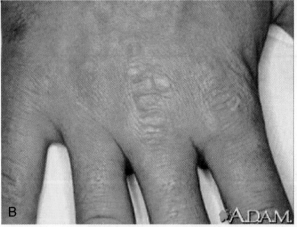

FIG. 2-22 **A,** Classic butterfly rash of systemic lupus erythematosus. (From *Mosby's medical, nursing, and health professions dictionary*, ed 7, St Louis, 2006, Mosby.) **B,** This violet-colored inflammation (erythema) over the knuckles is caused by dermatomyositis. Other skin conditions produce more redness, while the color of this lesion is violet. There may also be inflammation in the muscle tissue. (From Michael Lehrer, MD, Department of Dermatology, University of Pennsylvania Medical Center, Philadelphia, PA. Review provided by VeriMed Healthcare Network, A.D.A.M., Inc., 1600 River Edge Parkway, Suite 100, Atlanta, GA 30328. Tel: 770-980-0888; fax: 770-955-3088; available online at: *http://apps. uwhealth.org/healthy/adam/hie/1/000839.htm.*)

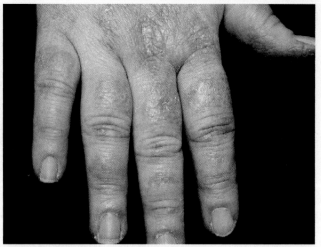

FIG. 2-23 Gottron papules. Erythematous scaly plaques are present on the dorsal hands, particularly over the bony prominences (metacarpal phalangeal [MCP]; proximal interphalangeal [PIP]; distal interphalangeal [DIP] joints). This patient also has some disease between the MCP and PIP joints and demonstrates early changes of *mechanics hands* on the lateral thumb. (From Callen JP: *Dermatomyositis, Lancet* 355(9197):53-57, 2000.)

utility of a tender-point evaluation has been objectively documented with the use of a dolorimeter or algometer, with pressure-loaded gauges that accurately measure force per area, and with manual palpation. The criteria of at least 11 of 18 tender points are recommended for classification purposes but should not be considered essential in individual patient diagnoses. Patients with fewer than 11 tender points can be diagnosed with fibromyalgia provided other symptoms and signs are present. An investigation must be made to determine whether the fibromyalgia is primary or secondary. The Leeds Assessment of Neuropathic Symptoms and Signs helps differentiate neuropathic pain and fibromyalgic pain (Box 2-2).

Patients with chronic widespread pain have symptoms similar to fibromyalgia though less severe. The most important factor that affects the criteria for fulfilling the number of tender points in patients with chronic widespread pain is the neuropathic pain score, which suggests that fibromyalgia is primarily a neuropathic pain syndrome (Pamuk, Yeil, Cakir, 2006).

Warmth

Warmth is one of the cardinal signs of inflammation. The back of the examiner's hand is a sensitive area for comparing skin temperature above, over, and below an inflamed structure (Fig. 2-24).

Painful Arc of Movement

Ligament injuries are detected by eliciting tenderness over the damaged portion of the affected tendon. Injuries are also

BOX 2-2

LEEDS ASSESSMENT OF NEUROPATHIC SYMPTOMS AND SIGNS (THE LANSS PAIN SCALE)

A. Pain questionnaire
- Think about how your pain has felt over the last week.
- Please say whether any of the descriptions match your pain precisely.
  1. Does your pain feel like strange, unpleasant sensations in your skin? Words such as *pricking, tingling,* and *pins and needles* might describe these sensations.
     - a. NO ☐ (0)
     - b. YES ☐ (5)
  2. Does your pain make the skin in the painful areas look different from normal? Words such as *mottled* or *looking more red or pink* might describe the appearance.
     - a. NO ☐ (0)
     - b. YES ☐ (5)
  3. Does your pain make the affected skin abnormally sensitive to touch? Getting unpleasant sensations when lightly stroking the skin or getting pain when wearing tight clothes might describe the abnormal sensitivity.
     - a. NO ☐ (0)
     - b. YES ☐ (5)
  4. Does your pain come on suddenly and in bursts for no apparent reason when you are still? Words such as *electric shocks, jumping,* and *bursting* describe these sensations.
     - a. NO ☐ (0)
     - b. YES ☐ (5)

  5. Does your pain feel as if the skin temperature in the painful area has changed abnormally? Words such as *hot* and *burning* describe these sensations.
     - a. NO ☐ (0)
     - b. YES ☐ (5)

B. Sensory testing
   Skin sensitivity can be examined by comparing the painful area with a contralateral or adjacent nonpainful area for the presence of allodynia and an altered pinprick threshold (PPT).
  1. Allodynia
     Examine the response to lightly stroking cotton wool across the nonpainful area and then the painful area. If normal sensations are experienced in the painful site, but pain or unpleasant sensations (tingling, nausea) are experienced in the painful area when stroking, then allodynia is present.
     - a. NO, normal sensation in both areas ☐ (0)
     - b. YES, allodynia in painful areas only ☐ (5)
  2. Altered pin-prick threshold
     If a sharp pinprick is felt in the nonpainful area, but a different sensation is experienced in the painful area, for example none or blunt only (raised PPT) or a very painful sensation (lowered PPT), altered PPT is present.
     - a. NO, equal sensation in both areas ☐ (0)
     - b. YES, altered PPT in painful area ☐ (5)

Scoring:
Add values in parentheses for sensory description and examination findings to obtain overall score.
Total score (maximum 20) _____
Score <12: Neuropathic mechanisms are ***unlikely*** to be contribution to the patient's pain.
Score ≥12: Neuropathic mechanisms are ***likely*** to be contribution to the patient's pain.
This pain scale can help determine whether the nerves that are carrying the patient's pain signals are working normally. The examiner should know this information in case different treatments are needed to control the patient's pain.
Adapted from Kaki AM, El-Yaski AZ, Youseif E: Identifying neuropathic pain among patients with chronic low-back pain: use of the Leeds Assessment of Neuropathic Symptoms and Signs Pain Scale. *Reg Anesth Pain Med* 30(5):422.e1-422.e9, 2005.

ORTHOPEDIC GAMUT 2-9

COMMON TERMS TO DESCRIBE PERIPHERAL JOINT DEFORMITIES

Dislocation: **articulating surfaces are displaced to the degree that they are no longer in contact with each other**
1. Fixed flexion: loss of joint extension, resulting in permanent flexion
2. Valgus: the distal part of the joint is directed laterally from the midline
3. Varus: the distal part of the joint is directed medially toward the midline

detected by eliciting a *painful arc* of active movement in the plane of action of the affected tendon. Passive movement in the same plane is almost pain free (Table 2-6).

Fixed Deformity

Although articular deformity may be observed at rest, most become more apparent when the limb is bearing weight or being used. The examiner should determine whether the deformity is correctable or noncorrectable. Many conditions are associated with characteristic deformities, but no deformity is pathognomonic of any single disease (Table 2-7). Shorthand terms are used for combined deformities, such as **swan-neck finger deformity** for hyperextension at the proximal and fixed flexion at the distal interphalangeal joints.

Fixed deformity exists when a joint cannot be placed in the neutral (anatomic) position. The degree of fixed deformity at a joint is determined by moving the joint, as near as it will come, to the neutral position and then measuring the remaining angle. In valgus deformity the distal part of the

detected in attempting to distract the bony structures held together by the ligament of interest.

When the tendon is subject to disease or excessive load, it may rupture. In tendon disease or injury less than rupture, tendon inflammation usually results. Tendinopathy is extremity is deviated laterally (outward) in relation to the proximal part. In hallux valgus, the first metatarsal is deviated outward in relation to the foot. In genu valgum, the lower leg is deviated outward in relation to the thigh. Varus deformity is the opposite. The distal part of an extremity is deviated medially (inward) in relation to the proximal part (Fig. 2-25).

Children with Morquio syndrome have skeletal manifestations that result from a unique spondyloepiphyseal dysplasia with ligament laxity. Growth and development are normal in the first 1 or 2 years of life, and the diagnosis is usually made between 2 and 4 years of age, although the severity of the features varies and milder forms of the syndrome may go undiagnosed. They can be distinguished from other mucopolysaccharidosis syndromes at an early age, given that they have normal mental function and do not have coarse facial features. Severe growth retardation is observed, usually with disproportionate short stature (short trunk), a large head and short neck, a prominent maxilla with wide-spaced teeth, thoracolumbar kyphosis with other spine and rib abnormalities, hip dysplasia, genu valgum, and marked joint and skin laxity. The combined abnormalities result in a *duck-waddling* gait (Fig. 2-25) (Lankester, Whitehouse, Gargan, 2006).

Movement

Every joint has a normal range of motion. The ranges of motion for any joint vary with age, gender, and ethnic origin. A range of movement that is beyond the upper limit represents hypermobility. Ranges below the lower limit represent hypomobility. The normal joint range of motion is diminished by joint inflammation or by irreversible damage to the joint structures. In trauma or disease, movement is first lost from the extreme end ranges. Increasing joint damage results in more profound loss of range of motion. The complete loss of movement of a joint is known as *fixation ankylosis* or *joint ankylosis,* depending on soft-tissue versus bony involvement. Fixation or joint ankylosis is further compli-

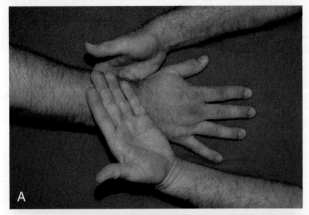
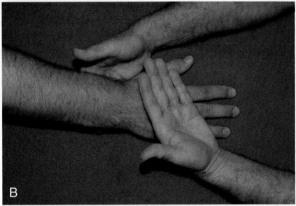

FIG. 2-24 Testing for warmth.

TABLE 2-6			
DIAGNOSTICALLY USEFUL CLINICAL FEATURES IN THE INITIAL EVALUATION OF THE PATIENT WITH ACUTE MUSCULOSKELETAL SYMPTOMS			
	Tendinopathy/Bursitis	**Noninflammatory Joint Problems***	**Systemic Rheumatic Disease**
Symptoms			
Morning stiffness	Focal, brief	Focal, brief	Significant, prolonged
Constitutional symptoms	Absent	Absent	Present
Peak period of discomfort	With use	After prolonged use	After prolonged inactivity
Locking or instability	Unusual, except rotator cuff tear, trigger finger	Implies loose body, internal derangement, or weakness	Uncommon
Symmetry	Uncommon	Occasional	Common
Signs			
Tenderness	Focal, periarticular, or tender points (fibromyalgia)	Unusual	Over entire exposed joint spaces
Inflammation (fluid, pain, warmth, erythema)	Over tendon or bursa	Unusual	Common
Instability	Uncommon	Occasional	Uncommon
Multisystem disease	No	No	Often

*For example, osteoarthritis or internal derangement.
From Kelley WN et al: *Textbook of rheumatology,* ed 5, Philadelphia, 1997, WB Saunders.

TABLE 2-7

SPECIFIC MUSCULOSKELETAL DEFORMITIES

Lower Limb
Hallux abductovalgus
Genu varum
Genu valgum
Dislocation of the patella
Valgus deformity of the heel
Coxa vara
Pes planovalgus
Fixed flexion of the knee
Fixed flexion of the hip

Upper Limb
Fixed flexion of DIPs/PIPs/MCPs (*benediction prayer* sign)
Ulnar deviation
Swan neck deformity of finger
Boutonni Agere deformity
Z-shaped thumb
Volar subluxation of wrist
Dorsal subluxation of inferior radioulnar joint
Fixed flexion of elbow
Cubitus valgus
Upward subluxation of shoulder
Anterior dislocation of shoulder
Posterior dislocation of shoulder

DIPs, Distal interphalangeal joints; *IP,* interphalangeal; *MCPs,* metacarpo-phalangeal joints; *PIP,* proximal interphalangeal joints.

TABLE 2-8

JOINT PLANE MOTION CHARACTERISTICS

Type	Planes	Joints
Hinge	1	Elbow, knee, ankle, MCP, PIP, DIP, MTP
Two-way hinge	2 (circumduction)	Wrist, trapeziometacarpal
Ball and socket	All planes	Shoulder, hip

DIP, Distal interphalangeal; *MCP,* metacarpophalangeal; *MTP,* metatarso-phalangeal; *PIP,* proximal interphalangeal.

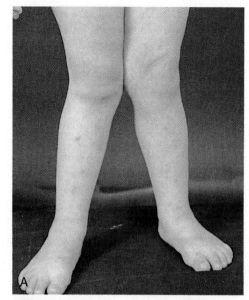

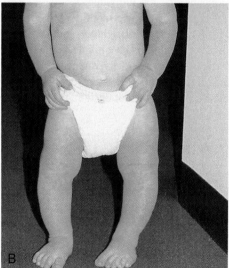

FIG. 2-25 Valgus **(A)** and Varus **(B)** deformities. (From *Mosby's medical, nursing, & allied health dictionary,* St Louis, 1998, Mosby.)

cated by the involvement or loss of multiple planes of motion (Table 2-8).

Synovitis reduces most or all joint movements, but tenosynovitis and periarticular lesions affect movement in only one plane. Synovitis and arthropathy cause a similar reduction of active and passive movement. The pattern of pain during movement is of diagnostic significance. Pain that is absent or minimal in the midrange but increases toward the extremes of restricted movement is capsular stress pain. Universal capsular stress pain is the most sensitive sign of synovitis. Selective stress pain, occurring in one plane of movement only, is characteristic of a localized intraarticular or periarticular lesion. Pain uniformly present throughout a range of movement reflects mechanical rather than inflammatory problems.

A useful method for demonstrating periarticular problems is the use of resisted, active (isometric) movement. This method requires the patient to push against the examiner's restraining hand to contract the muscle of interest without moving the adjacent joints. If the patient's pain is reproduced and no joint has moved, the pain probably arises from muscle, tendon, or tendon insertion. Conversely, passive stress tests produce pain by stretching the responsible ligament or tendon.

Enthesis is defined as the site of insertion of a tendon, ligament, fascia, or articular capsule into bone. Pain originating in the free nerve endings–enriched entheses (enthesalgia) may represent a potential cause of chronic musculoskeletal pain in some individuals. Enthesis involvement in the disease process is well appreciated in spondyloarthropathies and in rheumatoid arthritis, though overshadowed by **synovitis** in the latter. Calcium deposition diseases may constitute the most significant articular cause of enthesopathies in the general population (Slobodin et al, in press).

The normal range of motion varies from patient to patient. Limitation of movement in all directions suggests an arthritic process. Selective limitation of movement in specific directions with free movement in others suggests an articular mechanical derangement.

Passive movement range is usually equal to the active range. The passive range will exceed the active range only when the muscles responsible for movement are paralyzed or when the muscles or their tendons are torn, severed, or unduly slack.

Hypermobility is recognized by a series of passive maneuvers collectively known as the **9-point scale of Beighton** (Box 2-3). The Beighton modification of the Carter and Wilkinson scoring system has been used for many years as an indicator of widespread hypermobility. A high Beighton score by itself does not mean that an individual has HMS. It simply means that the individual has widespread hypermobility. Diagnosis of Hypermobility Syndrome or HMS should be made using the Brighton Criteria. The Beighton score is an easy to administer 9-point scale where points are given for the performance of five maneuvers. It is generally considered that hypermobility is present if 4 out of 9 points are scored. The scale was not designed for clinical use and has been criticized because it only samples a few joints and gives no indication of the degree of hypermobility.

Joint hypermobility is defined as a condition in which most of an individaul's synovial joints move beyond the normal limits taking into consideration the age, gender and ethnic background of the individual. Hypermobility may be inherited, or acquired through years of training and stretching, as seen in ballet dancers and gymnasts. Furthermore, hypermobility may also develop as a result of changes in connective tissue in a number of other diseases. Hypermobility may pose no problems, but in some individuals it predisposes to a wide variety of soft tissue injuries and internal joint derangements, arthritis, arthralgias or myalgias, which lead sufferers to seek medical attention (Grahame, 1990).

Joint hypermobility, when associated with symptoms is termed the joint hypermobility syndrome or hypermobility syndrome (JHS) (Simmonds and Keer 2007).

ORTHOPEDIC GAMUT 2-10

RANGE OF MOTION

Range of motion is assessed as follows:
1. Range of active movement
2. Passive versus active movement
3. Pain during movement
4. Movement crepitation

BOX 2-3

MODIFIED BEIGHTON JOINT LAXITY INDEX

1. Hyperextension of the elbows
2. Hyperextension of the knees
3. Apposition of the thumb to the flexor aspect of the forearm
4. Passive dorsiflexion of the metacarpophalangeal joints to 90 degrees
5. Passive dorsiflexion of the ankle past 90 degrees
6. Dorsolumbar flexion, placing hands flat on floor with knees fully extended

1 point is awarded for each side of the body for each extremity clinically involved.

1 point is awarded for dorsolumbar flexion hypermobility.

ORTHOPEDIC GAMUT 2-11

BRIGHTON CRITERIA (DIAGNOSTIC CRITERIA FOR HYPERMOBILITY SYNDROME)

Major criteria
1. A Beighton score of 4/9 or greater (either currently or historically)
2. Arthralgias for longer than 3 months in four or more joints.

Minor criteria
- 1. A Beighton score of 1, 2, or 3/9 (0,1,2,or 3 if aged 50+).
- 2. Arthralgias (for 3 months or longer) in one to three joints or back pain for (for 3 months or longer), spondylosis, spondylolysis/spondylolisthesis.
- 3. Dislocation/subluxation in more than one joint, or in one joint on more than one occasion.
- 4. Soft tissue rheumatism: three or more lesions (e.g., epicondylitis, tenosynovitis, bursitis).
- 5. Marfanoid habitus (tall, slim, span/height ration >1.03 upper: lower segment ration <0.89, arachnodactyly (positive Steinberg/wrist signs).
- 6. Abnormal skin striae, hyperextensibility, thin skin, papyraceous scarring.
- 7. Eye signs: drooping eyelids or myopia or antimongoloid slant.
- 8. Varicose veins or hernia or uterine/rectal prolapse.

BJHS is diagnosed in the presence of **two major criteria** or **one major** and **two minor criteria**, or four minor criteria. Two minor criteria will suffice where there is an unequivocally affected first-degree relative. BJHS is excluded by the presence of Marfan or Ehlers—Danlos syndromes other than the EDS hypermobility type (formerly EDS III). Criteria Major 1 and Minor 1 are mutually exclusive, as are Major 2 and Minor 2. From Grahame R: Pain distress and joint hyperlaxity, *Joint Bone Spine* 67:157-163, 2000.

The recognition of joint hypermobility rests on the ability of the patient to perform a series of passive joint maneuvers (Figs. 2-26 and 2-27).

Stability

Localized ligamentous or capsular instability may result from traumatic or inflammatory lesions. Arthropathy, particularly inflammatory, may produce instability via cartilage loss and capsular inflammation, as well as by ligamentous rupture. Instability is determined by demonstration of excessive movement on stressing the joint. Comparison with the unaffected side is helpful.

The stability of a joint depends partly on the integrity of its articulating surfaces and partly on its intact ligaments. When a joint is unstable, mobility is abnormal. When testing for abnormal mobility, the examiner must ensure that the muscles controlling the joint are relaxed. A muscle in

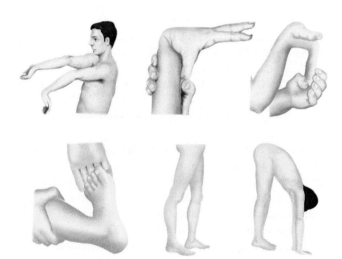

FIG. 2-26 Maneuvers that may be used to establish the presence of clinically significant joint laxity. Finding extreme laxity of the small joints and less laxity in large joints in not unusual. Laxity decreases with age. (Redrawn and modified from Wynne-Davies R: Acetabular dysplasia and familial joint laxity: two etiological factors in congenital dislocation of the hip. A review of 589 patients and their families, *J Bone Joint Surg* 52B:704, 1970.)

strong contraction can often conceal ligamentous instability (Table 2-9).

Crepitation

Crepitation is palpable crunching sensation present throughout the movement of the involved joint or enthesis structure. Fine crepitation may be audible only by stethoscope and is not transmitted through the adjacent bone. Fine crepitation may accompany inflammation of the tendon sheath, bursa, or synovium. Coarse crepitation may be audible at a distance and is palpable through the bone. Coarse crepitation usually reflects cartilage or bone damage (Table 2-10).

Muscular Atrophy

Muscle atrophy is a common sign but can be difficult to detect, particularly in older adults. Synovitis quickly produces local spinal reflex inhibition of muscles acting across the joint. Atrophy can be rapid (within several days) in septic arthritis. Severe arthropathy produces widespread periarticular wasting. Localized atrophy is more characteristic of a mechanical tendon or muscle problem or nerve entrapment. Disuse atrophy is a complex and highly regulated biochemical process (Table 2-11).

> Almost certainly, some signaling pathways involved in muscle atrophy are interacted or interdependent with each other. Activation or inhibition of a single pathway may have

TABLE 2-9
JOINT INSTABILITY
Finding
Passive side-to-side movement of the tibia on the femur (collateral knee ligaments)
Passive anteroposterior movement of the tibia on the femur (cruciate ligaments)
Gross genu recurvatum
Positive Trendelenburg sign
Arthritis mutilans—flail interphalangeal joints
Spontaneous dislocation of the shoulder or patella
Pes planus (collapse of the longitudinal arch)

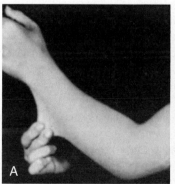
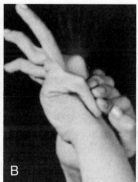
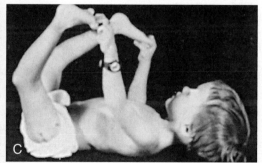

FIG. 2-27 Joint hypermobility. Recurrent dislocations may require surgical repair. (From Kelley WN, et al: *Textbook of rheumatology,* ed 5, Philadelphia, 1997, WB Saunders.)

TABLE 2-10

CREPITATION GRADING SCALE

	None	Mild	Moderate	Severe
Palpable	Smooth silky motion	Fine-grade sandpaper	Medium-grade sandpaper	Bone-on-bone grinding
Audible	Quiet	Barely audible	Consistent squeak	Popping-cracking-crunching

Adapted from Lancaster AR, Nyland J, Roberts CS: The validity of the motion palpation test for determining patellofemoral joint articular cartilage damage, *Phys Ther Sport* 8(2):59-65, 2007.

TABLE 2-11

SIGNALS INVOLVED IN DISUSE-INDUCED MUSCLE ATROPHY

Signals	Finding	Function
PI3K, Akt	Decreased	Promotes protein degradation Inhibits protein synthesis
FOXO1, FOXO3	Increased	Promotes protein degradation Down-regulates type I fiber genes?
mTOR, p70S6K, eIF4B	Decreased	Inhibits protein synthesis
PHAS-I	Increased	Inhibits protein synthesis
p50, c-Rel, Bcl-3	Increased	Promotes protein degradation
Myostatin, ActIIB	Increased	Inhibits protein synthesis?
p38	Increased	Promotes protein degradation
Erk	Increased	Promotes glucose uptake?
JNK	Increased	Increases insulin resistance
Calcineurin	Increased	Compensatory mechanism?
ROS	Increased	Promotes protein degradation
MAFbx, MuRF1	Increased	Promotes protein degradation

Signal Abbreviations: *ACTIIB*, Myostatin receptor; *AKT*, serine/threonine kinase; *Bcl-*, transcriptional coactivtor; *Calcineurin*, serine/threonine phosphatase; *c-REL*, NF-kB family transcription factor; *E1F4B*, eukaryotic translation initiation factor 4B (homo sapiens); *ERK*, extracellular signal-regulated kinase; *FOXO*, Forkhead family of transcription factor; *JNK*, c-JUN N-terminal kinase; *MAFbx*, muscle atrophy f-box ubiquitin ligase; *mTOR*, mammalian target of rapamycin; *MuRF1*, muscle ring finger 1 ubiquitin ligase; *Myostatin*, inhibitor of skeletal muscle mass; *p38*, p38 isoform mitogen activated protein; *p50*, NF-kB family transcription factor; *p70S6K*, 70-kDa ribosomal protein S6 kinase; *PHAS-I*, eukaryotic initiation factor 4E-binding protein; *PI3K*, Phosphatidylinositol 3-OH kinase; *ROS*, reactive oxygen species.
Adapted from Zhang P, Chen X, Fan M: Signaling mechanisms involved in disuse muscle atrophy, *Med Hypotheses* (in press, corrected proof).

ORTHOPEDIC GAMUT 2-12

CREPITUS NOISES (OTHER THAN FINE OR COARSE)

Ligamentous snaps—usually single, loud, and painless—that are common around the upper femur as a clicking hip
1. Cracking by joint distraction, which is common at the finger joints and is caused by production of an intraarticular gas bubble (such cracking cannot be repeated until the bubble has reformed)
2. Reproducible clunking noises that occur at irregular surfaces, such as when the scapula moves on the ribs

als and in muscle of normal strength and size. Fascicular twitches noted during rest, with exaggerated muscular weakness and atrophy, are characteristic of peripheral motor neuron disorders. Acute denervation of skeletal muscles results in spontaneous contractions of muscle fibers.

The fine contractions of muscle fibers are best observed at the tongue because of its special and unique anatomic structure: the architecture of the intrinsic musculature is composed of a three-dimensional network of highly interwoven muscle fibers inserting directly in the lingual aponeurosis, which is tightly connected with the tongue dorsum (Gilbert, Napadow, 2005).

Since the late 1800s, quivering or flickering of muscle fibers is called *fibrillation*. The term *fibrillation* is derived from fibril, the diminutive form of fiber.

If involuntary tongue movement is visible in infants with spinal muscular atrophy (SMA) and can be distinguished from normal movement of the tremulous tongue during crying, this phenomenon is termed *fasciculation*. However, this term is incorrect from an electromyographer's viewpoint because fasciculation potentials are rarely seen in childhood SMA (Hausmanowa-Petrusewicz, 1988).

The correct term of individual muscle fiber activity would seem to be *fibration*. The same rule applies for electromyographic findings of acute denervation because the observed patterns derive from membrane potential changes of muscle fibers and not of fibrils. Therefore, instead of *fibrillation* potentials, the correct term would seem to be *fibration* potentials (Baalen, Stephani, in press).

cascade effects on muscle protein balance, but no evidence has been found to prove that the pathway is the sole regulator of the process (Zhang, Chen, Fan, in press).

Fasciculations

Fasciculations are visible, spontaneous contractions of muscle fibers supplied by a single motor nerve filament. Visible dimpling or twitching may occur. Fasciculations occurring during muscular contraction (twitching) are associated with conditions of irritability, resulting in poorly coordinated contraction of small and large motor units (spasmophilia). Benign fasciculation occurs in normal individu-

TABLE 2-12

TREMOR CLASSIFICATION

Cause	Type and Rate of Movement	Description
Anxiety	Fine, rapid, 10 to 12/sec	Irregular, variable
		Increased by attempts to move part; decreased by relaxation of part
Parkinsonism	Fine, regular, or coarse, 2 to 5/sec	Occurs at rest
		May be inhibited by movement
		Involves flexion of finger and thumb *pill rolling*
		Accompanied by rigidity, *cogwheel* phenomena, bradykinesia
Cerebellar tremor	Variable rate	Evident only on movement (most prominent on finger-to-nose test)
		Dysmetria (seen when patient is asked to pat rapidly; pats are of unequal force and do not all arrive at same point)
Essential or senile	Coarse, 3 to 7/sec	Involves the jaw, sometimes the tongue, and sometimes the entire head
Metabolic		Disappears on complete relaxation or in response to alcohol
		Variable
		Patient is obviously ill; if illness is a result of hepatic failure, patient will have other signs, such as palpable liver, spider nevi

From Barkauskas VH et al: *Health & physical assessment,* ed 2, St Louis, 1998, Mosby.

Cramps and Spasm

Muscular spasm, or tremor (Table 2-12), may occur at rest or with movement. Spasms and tremors occur in the normal individual with metabolic and electrolyte alterations. Cramping is a common complaint after excessive sweating and subsequent **hyponatremia, hypocalcemia, hypomagnesemia,** or **hyperuricemia.**

Exercise-associated muscle cramping is a painful, involuntary contraction of skeletal muscle that occurs immediately after exercise. Any athlete who exhibits repeated episodes of muscle spasms should undergo a comprehensive history and physical examination and, in most cases, laboratory studies to evaluate electrolytes. Athletes should also have a urinalysis to check for blood or myoglobin. The initial history should include questions pertaining to hydration status, frequency of stretching, and the use of ergogenic supplements such as steroids or creatine. Questions to define the athlete's medical history should inquire about how the muscle cramping relates to temperature, diet, family history, urine color changes (myoglobinuria), and how long the symptoms last (Nadler et al, 2004).

Tetany

Hypocalcemia and hypomagnesemia often cause the involuntary spasms of skeletal muscle, which resemble cramping. Tetanic cramps can be elicited by repeatedly percussing the motor nerve, which leads to a muscle group contraction-cramp-spasm at frequencies of 15 to 20 per second. Chvostek sign is the spasm of facial muscles produced by tapping over the facial nerve near its foraminal exit. Chvostek sign may also occur with normocalcemia, as well as with hypocalcemia.

Patients with hypocalcemic seizures demonstrate marked Chvostek sign, positive Trousseau sign, sweaty hands, and hyperreflexia (Ahmed et al, 2004).

ORTHOPEDIC GAMUT 2-13

GAIT

Gait impairments of predominant neurologic origin include the following (in descending order of frequency):
1. Disorders of the corticospinal pathways (spasticity)
2. Basal ganglia (parkinsonism)
3. Cerebellum and connections (ataxia)
4. Cerebral cortex (gait apraxia)
5. Neuromuscular system (weakness)
6. Sensation (ataxia)

Trousseau sign is demonstrated by inflating a sphygmomanometer around the wrist area of the left hand to above systolic blood pressure for 3 minutes while observing the hand. Typical carpal spasm, which relaxes approximately 5 seconds after the cuff is released, is considered a positive Trousseau sign.

Tetany is most commonly caused by hypocalcemia. Low levels of free or ionized extracellular calcium reduce the normal transmembrane potential of the nerve by increasing sodium conductance, thus reducing the threshold required to cause depolarization. Normal serum ionized calcium levels range from 5.9 to 6.5 mg/dl. Levels falling below 4.3 mg/dl can cause tetany. Hypocalcemia is observed in hypoparathyroidism, vitamin-D deficiency, malabsorption syndromes, acute pancreatitis, malignancy, sepsis, and drug effect. Hyperventilation leading to respiratory alkalosis and secondary reduction of ionized calcium may precipitate tetany (Freeman, Michael, Robert, 2003).

Impairment of Gait

Finding a spinal or lower extremity orthopedic or neurologic disorder that does not produce abnormalities of gait at some time during its course is difficult.

> Gait disturbances after a stroke are multifaceted and hence must be studied from multiple perspectives. Biomechanical measurements such as temporal distance parameters, kinematics, kinetics, mechanical energy, and energy costs, as well as electromyography, can evaluate the behavioral profile of gait and reflect CNS adaptation with respect to internal and external demands. Electrophysiologic measurements such as stretch reflex, H-reflex, and cutaneous reflexes can evaluate the integrity of spinal cord functions during gait and indirectly assess the integrity of the descending control system (Lamontagne, Stephenson, Fung, 2007).

Bladder Control

Incontinence and other disturbances of urinary bladder function are occasionally the first manifestation of disease of the spinal cord, as well as the rest of the nervous system. The physiologic mechanism of micturition is complex. The terms *atonic bladder* and *spastic bladder* are no longer useful in describing different levels of neurologic involvement because they are related mainly to local factors in the bladder wall.

> Compressive lesions to the cauda equina or conus medullaris are a common cause of neurogenic lower urinary tract dysfunction, although more peripheral lesions may also cause sacral disease. In patients with suspected focal sacral disease,

---

ORTHOPEDIC GAMUT 2-14

IMPAIRED MICTURITION

Localization of impaired micturition depends on the following:

1. Loss of bladder sensation
2. Perineal sensory loss
3. Patulous anal sphincter
4. Absence of the bulbocavernous and anocutaneous reflexes
5. Sensory, motor, and reflex changes in the lower extremities

---

bilateral-needle electromyographic examination of the external anal sphincter and sometimes of the bulbocavernosus muscle needs to be considered first. Detection of spontaneous denervation activity, most appropriately in the bulbocavernosus muscle, is common in the interval from 3 weeks to several months after a lower motor neuron injury (Podnar, in press).

An associated history of erectile dysfunction or rectal incontinence should clearly suggest the presence of a common neurogenic cause for urinary incontinence. The additional presence of sacral pain should suggest tumor in the sacral region.

CRITICAL THINKING

1. What are the five groups of signs and symptoms differentiating musculoskeletal complaints?
2. Why can articular or periarticular pain radiate widely and be felt in a spot distant from its originating tissue?
3. What typical sensations differentiate pain with nerve entrapment, vascular compromise, and articular or joint involvement?
4. In listening to a patient's description of pain, i.e., when present, what relieves it, what makes it worse, and what improves it, pain at rest, night, or with use suggests what kinds of problems?
5. What is the leading cause of accidental death in older adults?
6. What subgroup of patients is at high risk of developing chronic lower back pain?
7. What four issues are important in assessing a patient's disability?
8. After thoroughly examining the patient's painful part, you have doubt of the source of the symptoms. What would your next step be?
9. What are the two most common tumors of the digits of the hand and on the dorsum of the foot?
10. A heliotropic rash and Gottron papules are characteristic and possibly pathognomonic cutaneous features of what condition?
11. Where can Gottron papules most commonly be found?
12. The Leeds Assessment of Neuropathic Symptoms and Signs is used in the assessment of what type of conditions?
13. You have a very athletic patient with reoccurring episodes of muscle cramping with exercise. What would be your immediate action steps for this case presentation?
14. Gait impairments from disorders of the corticospinal pathways are manifested by what?
15. Gait impairments from the cerebellum and its connections are characterized by what?

BIBLIOGRAPHY

Abrams WB, Berkow R: *The Merck manual of geriatrics,* Rahway, NJ, 1990, Merck Sharp & Dohme Research Laboratories.

Adams JC, Hamblen DL: *Outline of orthopaedics,* ed 11, Edinburgh, 1990, Churchill Livingstone.

Ahwee Leftwich S et al: High incidence disabilities: placement determinants and implications for instruction and service delivery. In Scruggs TE, Mastropieri MA, editors: *Advances in learning and behavioral disabilities,* vol 18, Greenwich, Conn, 2005, JAI Press.

Alario AJ: *Practical guide to the care of the pediatric patient,* St Louis, 1997, Mosby.

Alberti A: Headache and sleep, *Sleep Med Rev* 10(6):431-437, 2006.

Anderson KN, Anderson LE: *Mosby's pocket dictionary of medicine, nursing, & allied health,* ed 2, St Louis, 1994, Mosby.

Atkinson G, Davenne D: Relationships between sleep, physical activity and human health, *Physiol Behav* 90(2-3):229-235, 2007.

Barkauskas VH et al: *Health & physical assessment,* ed 2, St Louis, 1998, Mosby.

Bechman H et al: Getting the most from a 20 minute visit, *Am J Gastroenterol* 89:662, 1994.

Beighton L et al: Articular mobility in an African population, *Annu Rheum Dis* 32:413-417, 1973.

Boukhris S et al: Pain as the presenting symptom of chronic inflammatory demyelinating polyradiculoneuropathy (CIDP), *J Neurol Sci* 254(1-2):33-38, 2007.

Brotzman SB: *Clinical orthopaedic rehabilitation,* St Louis, 1996, Mosby.

Brown DE, Neumann RD: *Orthopedic secrets,* Philadelphia, 1995, Hanley & Belfus.

Brucini M et al: Pain thresholds and electromyographic features of periarticular muscles in patients with osteoarthritis of the knee, *Pain* 10(1):57-66, 1981.

Bucholz RW: *Orthopaedic decision making,* ed 2, St Louis, 1996, Mosby.

Bunker TD, Schranz PJ: *Clinical challenges in orthopaedics: the shoulder,* Oxford, UK, 1998, ISIS Medical Media.

Calvino B, Grilo RM: Central pain control, *Joint Bone Spine* 73(1):10-16, 2006.

Campbell JB, Campbell JM: *Mosby's survival guide to medical abbreviations & acronyms prefixes & suffixes symbols Greek alphabet,* St Louis, 1995, Mosby.

Campbell JN, Meyer RA: Mechanisms of neuropathic pain, *Neuron* 52(1):77-92, 2006.

Canale ST: *Campbell's operative orthopaedics,* vol 1-4, ed 9, St Louis, 1998, Mosby.

Cardinal E, Lafortune M, Burns P: Power Doppler US in synovitis: reality or artifact? *Radiology* 200:868, 1996.

Chard MD et al: Shoulder disorders in the elderly: a community survey, *Arthritis Rheum* 34:766, 1991.

Cipriano JJ: *Photographic manual of regional orthopaedic and neurological test,* ed 3, Baltimore, 1997, Williams & Wilkins.

Cleeman E, Auerbach JD, Springfield DS: Tumors of the shoulder girdle: a review of 194 cases, *J Shoulder Elbow Surg* 14(5):460-465, 2005.

Cohn RE: *Impairment rating examination and disability evaluation,* ed 3, Wilkesboro, NC, 1994, R Ernest Cohn.

Colloca CJ, Keller TS: Stiffness and neuromuscular reflex response of the human spine to posteroanterior manipulative thrusts in patients with low back pain, *J Manipulative Physiol Ther* 24(8):489-500, 2001.

Colvin LA, Power I: Neurobiology of chronic pain states, *Anaesth Intensive Care Med* 6(1):10-13, 2005.

Conwell TD: *Documenting patient progress "daily office charting seminar" thorough accurate quick procedures,* ed 11, Lakewood, Colo, 1990, Clinical Advancement Plus Seminars.

Copeland SA et al: *Joint stiffness of the upper limb,* St Louis, 1997, Mosby.

Coutaux A et al: Hyperalgesia and allodynia: peripheral mechanisms, *Joint Bone Spine* 72(5):359-371, 2005.

Craik RL, Oatis CA: *Gait analysis theory and application,* St Louis, 1995, Mosby.

Dambro MR, Griffith JA: *Griffith's 5 minute clinical consult,* Baltimore, 1997, Williams & Wilkins.

Daruwalla P, Darcy S: Personal and societal attitudes to disability, *Ann Tourism Res* 32(3):549-570, 2005.

Demeter SL, Andersson GBJ, Smith GM: *Disability evaluation,* St Louis, 1996, Mosby.

Dickenson AH: Spinal cord pharmacology of pain, *Br J Anaesth* 75:193, 1995.

Dionysian E et al: Proximal interphalangeal joint stiffness: measurement and analysis, *J Hand Surg* 30(3):573-579, 2005.

Doherty M: *Color atlas and text of osteoarthritis,* London, 1994, Wolfe.

Doherty M et al: The "GALS" locomotor screen, *Ann Rheum Dis* 51:1165, 1992.

Doherty M, Doherty J: *Clinical examination in rheumatology,* London, 1992, Wolfe.

Doherty M, George E: *Self-assessment picture tests in rheumatology,* London, 1995, Mosby-Wolfe.

Dray A: Inflammatory mediators of pain, *Br J Anaesth* 75:125, 1995.

Epstein O et al: *Clinical examination,* ed 2, London, 1997, Mosby.

Farasyn A: Referred muscle pain is primarily peripheral in origin: the "barrier-dam" theory, *Med Hypotheses* 68(1):144-150, 2007.

Feldmann E: *Current diagnosis in neurology,* St Louis, 1994, Mosby.

Ferezy JS: *The chiropractic neurological examination,* Gaithersburg, Md, 1992, Aspen.

Field T et al: Lower back pain and sleep disturbance are reduced following massage therapy, *J Bodywork Move Ther* 11(2):141-145, 2007.

Fitzpatrick TB et al: *Color atlas and synopsis of clinical dermatology common and serious diseases,* ed 2, New York, 1992, McGraw-Hill.

Gatts SK, Woollacott MH: How Tai Chi improves balance: biomechanics of recovery to a walking slip in impaired seniors, *Gait Posture* 25(2):205-214, 2007.

Goldie BS: *Orthopaedic diagnosis and management a guide to the care of orthopaedic patients,* ed 2, Oxford, UK, 1998, ISIS Medical Media.

Gracely RH, Undem BJ, Banzett RB: Cough, pain and dyspnoea: similarities and differences, *Pulm Pharmacol Ther* 20(4):433-437, 2007.

Gramaglia L et al: Worsening of chronic pain: the treatment, *Arch Gerontol Geriatr* 44(suppl 1):207-211, 2007.

Greenstein GM: *Clinical assessment of neuromusculoskeletal disorders,* St Louis, 1997, Mosby.

Gunther M, Blickhan R: Joint stiffness of the ankle and the knee in running, *J Biomech* 35(11):1459-1474, 2002.

Gurwood AS, Drake J: Guillain-Barré syndrome. *J Am Optom Assoc* 77(11):540-546, 2006.

Haack E, Tkach J: Fast MR imaging: techniques and clinical applications, *AJR* 155:951, 1990.

Hanley MA et al: Self-reported treatments used for lower-limb phantom pain: descriptive findings, *Arch Phys Med Rehabil* 87(2):270-277, 2006.

Hanley MA et al: Preamputation pain and acute pain predict chronic pain after lower extremity amputation, *J Pain* 8(2):102-109, 2007.

Hartley A: *Practical joint assessment lower quadrant,* ed 2, St Louis, 1995, Mosby.

Hassell AB et al: The relationship between serial measures of disease activity and outcome in rheumatoid arthritis, *Q J Med* 86:601, 1995.

Hawkins RJ: *An organized approach to musculoskeletal examination and history taking,* St Louis, 1995, Mosby.

Hinkle CZ: *Fundamentals of anatomy & movement a workbook and guide,* St Louis, 1997, Mosby.

Hofer M, Mahlaoui N, Prieur A-M: A child with a systemic febrile illness—differential diagnosis and management, *Best Pract Res Clin Rheumatol* 20(4):627-640, 2006.

Jagoda A, Riggio S: Mild traumatic brain injury and the postconcussive syndrome, *Emerg Med Clin North Am* 18(2):355-363, 2000.

Karkin-Tais A et al: 367 13-year study of pain in phantom limbs of amputees—victims of war in Sarajevo (period 1992-2005), *Eur J Pain* 10(suppl 1):S98-S211, 2006.

Katirji B: *Electromyography in clinical practice a case study approach,* St Louis, 1998, Mosby.

Kline CR, Martin DP, Deyo RA: Health consequences of pregnancy and childbirth as perceived by women and clinicians, *Obstet Gynecol* 92(5):842-848, 1998.

Klippel JH, Dieppe PA: *Rheumatology,* vol 1-2, ed 2, London, 1998, Mosby.

Kuruganti U et al: Strength and muscle coactivation in older adults after lower limb strength training, *Int J Ind Ergon* 36(9):761-766, 2006.

Lautenbacher S, Kundermann B, Krieg J-C: Sleep deprivation and pain perception, *Sleep Med Rev* 10(5):357-369, 2006.

Lewis CB, Knortz KA: *Orthopedic assessment and treatment of the geriatric patient,* St Louis, 1993, Mosby.

Lovejoy CO: The natural history of human gait and posture: Part 3. The knee, *Gait Posture* 25(3):325-341, 2007.

Lynch GS, Schertzer JD, Ryall JG: Therapeutic approaches for muscle wasting disorders, *Pharmacol Ther* 113(3):461-487, 2007.

Magee DJ: *Orthopedic physical assessment,* ed 3, Philadelphia, 1997, WB Saunders.

Makhsous M, Lin F, Zhang L-Q: Multi-axis passive and active stiffness of the glenohumeral joint, *Clin Biomech* 19(2):107-115, 2004.

Malone TR, McPoil TG, Nitz AJ: *Orthopedic and sports physical therapy,* ed 3, St Louis, 1997, Mosby.

Mathews DA, Suchman AL, Branch WT: Making "connexions": enhancing the therapeutic potential of patient-clinician relationships, *Ann Intern Med* 118:973, 1993.

McRae R: *Clinical orthopaedic examination,* ed 3, Edinburgh, 1990, Churchill Livingstone.

Mengel MB, Schwiebert LP: *Ambulatory medicine the primary care of families,* ed 2, Stamford, Conn, 1996, Appleton & Lange.

Mennell JM: *The musculoskeletal system differential diagnosis from symptoms and physical signs,* Gaithersburg, Md, 1992, Aspen.

Mercier LR, Pettid FJ: *Practical orthopedics,* ed 5, St Louis, 2000, Mosby.

Moriwaki K et al: Neuropathic pain and prolonged regional inflammation as two distinct symptomatological components in complex regional pain syndrome with patchy osteoporosis—a pilot study, *Pain* 72(1-2):277-282, 1997.

Mosby-Year Book, Inc: *Mosby's expert 10-minute physical examination,* St Louis, 1997, Mosby.

Murphy AJ et al: Reliability of a test of musculotendinous stiffness for the triceps-surae, *Phys The Sport* 4(4):175-181, 2003.

Nardone DA et al: A model for the diagnostic medical interview: nonverbal, verbal and cognitive assessments, *J Gen Intern Med* 7:437, 1992.

Nettina SM: *The Lippincott manual of nursing practice,* ed 6, Philadelphia, 1996, Lippincott.

Newton RW: *Color atlas of pediatric neurology,* St Louis, 1995, Mosby-Wolfe.

Ogilvie-Harris DJ, Saleh K: Generalized synovial chondromatosis of the knee: a comparison of removal of the loose bodies alone with arthroscopic synovectomy, *Arthroscopy* 10:166, 1994.

Oleson M, Adler D, Goldsmith P: A comparison of forefoot stiffness in running and running shoe bending stiffness, *J Biomech* 38(9):1886-1894, 2005.

Olson WH et al: *Handbook of symptom-oriented neurology,* ed 2, St Louis, 1994, Mosby.

Patin JR, Hamot HB, Singer JM: Replicated evidence on the construct validity of the SCAG (Sandoz Clinical Assessment-Geriatric) scale, *Prog Neuropsychopharmacol Biol Psychiatry* 8(2):293-306, 1984.

Perhala RS et al: Local infectious complications following large joint replacement in rheumatoid arthritis patients treated with methotrexate versus those not treated with methotrexate, *Arthritis Rheum* 34:146, 1991.

Peterfy CG et al: MR imaging of the arthritic knee: improved discrimination of cartilage, synovium and effusion with pulsed saturation transfer and fat-suppressed T1-weighted sequences, *Radiology* 191:413, 1994.

Peterfy CG, Genant HK: Emerging applications of magnetic resonance imaging for evaluating the articular cartilage, *Radiol Clin North Am* 34:195, 1996.

Rachlin ES: *Myofascial pain and fibromyalgia trigger point management,* St Louis, 1994, Mosby.

Raspe HH: Back pain. In Silman AJ, Hochberg M, editors: *Epidemiology of the rheumatic diseases,* Oxford, UK, 1993, Oxford University Press.

Robertson CM, Coopersmith CM: The systemic inflammatory response syndrome, *Microbes Infect* 8(5):1382-1389, 2006.

Rubens DJ et al: Rheumatoid arthritis: evaluation of wrist extensor tendons with clinical examination versus MR imaging—a preliminary report, *Radiology* 187:831, 1993.

Schumacher HR, Klippel JH, Koopman WJ: *Primer on the rheumatic diseases,* ed 10, Atlanta, 1993, Arthritis Foundation.

Smith RC, Hoppe RB: The patient's story: integrating the patient and physician centered approaches to interviewing, *Ann Intern Med* 115:470, 1991.

Spacek E et al: Disability induced by hand osteoarthritis: are patients with more symptoms at digits 2-5 interphalangeal joints different from those with more symptoms at the base of the thumb? *Osteoarthr Cartil* 12(5):366-373, 2004.

Stamford JA: Descending control of pain, *Br J Anaesth* 75:217, 1995.

Stein C: The control of pain in peripheral tissue by opioids, *N Engl J Med* 332:1685, 1995.

Stevens JC et al: Conditions associated with carpal tunnel syndrome, *Mayo Clin Proc* 67:541, 1992.

Stochkendahl MJ et al: Manual examination of the spine: a systematic critical literature review of reproducibility, *J Manipulative Physiol Ther* 29(6):475-462, 2006.

Sugimoto H et al: Early-stage rheumatoid arthritis: diagnostic accuracy of MR imaging, *Radiology* 198:185, 1996.

Tan JC, Horn SE: *Practical manual of physical medicine and rehabilitation,* St Louis, 1998, Mosby.

Thibodeau GA, Patton KT: *Anatomy & physiology,* ed 3, St Louis, 1996, Mosby.

Thibodeau GA, Patton KT: *Pocket reference to accompany anatomy & physiology,* ed 3, St Louis, 1996, Mosby.

Thompson JM: *Clinical outlines for health assessment,* St Louis, 1997, Mosby.

Toghill PJ: *Examining patients an introduction to clinical medicine,* London, 1990, Edward Arnold.

Wakefield TS, Frank RG: *The clinician's guide to neuromusculoskeletal practice,* Abbotsford, Wisc, 1995, Allied Health of Wisconsin, S.C.

Weinstein SL, Buckwalter JA: *Turek's orthopaedics principles and their application,* ed 5, Philadelphia, 1994, JB Lippincott.

White G: *Levene's color atlas of dermatology,* ed 2, London, 1997, Mosby-Wolfe.

White G: *Regional dermatology,* London, 1994, Mosby-Wolfe.

White KP et al: Fibromyalgia in rheumatology practice: a survey of Canadian rheumatologists, *J Rheumatol* 22:722, 1995.

Windsor RE, Lox DM: *Soft tissue injuries: diagnosis and treatment,* Philadelphia, 1998, Hanley & Belfus.

Wolfe F et al: The prevalence and characteristics of fibromyalgia in the general population, *Arthritis Rheum* 38:19, 1995.

Woolf CJ: Somatic pain-pathogenesis and prevention, *Br J Anaesth* 75:169, 1995.

Yeamans DC et al: Pain, management of. In *International encyclopedia of the social & behavioral sciences,* Oxford, UK, 2001, Pergamon.

Zatouroff M: *Diagnosis in color physical signs in general medicine,* ed 2, London, 1996, Mosby-Wolfe.

Zitelli BJ, Davis HW: *Atlas of pediatric physical diagnosis,* ed 2, London, 1992, Wolfe.

CITATIONS

Ahmed MAS et al: Chvostek's sign and hypocalcaemia in children with seizures. *Seizure* 13(4):217-222, 2004.

Baalen AV, Stephani U: Fibration, fibrillation, and fasciculation: say what you see, *Clin Neurophysiol* (in press, corrected proof).

Baker FC, Driver HS: Circadian rhythms, sleep, and the menstrual cycle, *Sleep Med* (in press, corrected proof).

Callen JP. Dermatomyositis, *Lancet* 355(9197):53-57, 2000.

Carayon P, Smith MJ, Haims MC: Work organization, job stress, and work-related musculoskeletal disorders, *Human Factors* 41(4):644-663, 1999.

Costardi D et al: The Italian version of the pain assessment in advanced dementia (PAINAD) scale, *Arch Gerontol Geriatr* 44(2):175-180, 2007.

European Pressure Ulcer Advisory Panel (EPUAP): Gotopu, *EPUAP Rev* 1:31-33, 1999.

Freeman MC, Michael JA, Robert BD: Tetany. In *Encyclopedia of the neurological sciences,* New York, 2003, Academic Press.

Gilbert RJ, Napadow VJ. Three-dimensional muscular architecture of the human tongue determined in vivo with diffusion tensor magnetic resonance imaging. *Dysphagia* 20(1):1-7, 2005.

Giummarra MJ et al: Central mechanisms in phantom limb perception: the past, present and future, *Brain Res Rev* 54(1):219-232, 2007.

Goldberg EJ, Neptune RR: Compensatory strategies during normal walking in response to muscle weakness and increased hip joint stiffness, *Gait Posture* 25(3):360-367, 2007.

Grahame R: The hypermobility syndrome, *Ann Rheumatol Dis* 49:199-200, 1990.

Grahame R: Pain, distress and joint hyperlaxity. *Joint Bone Spine* 67(3):157-163, 2000.

Hausmanowa-Petrusewicz I: Electrophysiological findings in childhood spinal muscular atrophies, *Revue Neurologique* 144(11):716-720, 1988.

Jensen BR et al: Soft tissue architecture and intramuscular pressure in the shoulder region, *Eur J Morphol* 33(3):205-220, 1995.

Kashdan TB et al: Fragile self-esteem and affective instability in posttraumatic stress disorder, *Behav Res Ther* 44(11):1609-1619, 2006.

Koenigsberg HW et al: Characterizing affective instability in borderline personality disorder, *Am J Psychiatry* 159(5):784-788, 2002.

Lamontagne A, Stephenson JL, Fung J: Physiological evaluation of gait disturbances post stroke, *Clin Neurophysiol* 118(4):717-729, 2007.

Lankester BJA, Whitehouse M, Gargan MF: Morquio syndrome, *Curr Orthopaed* 20(2):128-131, 2006.

Lowery DJ et al: A clinical composite score accurately detects meniscal pathology, *Arthroscopy* 22(11):1174-1179, 2006.

Luyten FP et al: Contemporary concepts of inflammation, damage and repair in rheumatic diseases, *Best Pract Res Clin Rheumatol* 20(5):829-848, 2006.

Nadler SF et al: Sports and performing arts medicine. 1. General considerations for sports and performing arts medicine, *Arch Phys Med Rehabil* 85(suppl 1):48-51, 2004.

Palmgren PJ et al: Improvement after chiropractic care in cervicocephalic kinesthetic sensibility and subjective pain intensity in patients with nontraumatic chronic neck pain, *J Manipulative Physiol Ther* 29(2):100-106, 2006.

Pamuk ON, Yeil Y, Cakir N: Factors that affect the number of tender points in fibromyalgia and chronic widespread pain patients who did not meet the ACR 1990 criteria for fibromyalgia: are tender points a reflection of neuropathic pain? *Semin Arthritis Rheum* 36(2):130-134, 2006.

Panel for the Prediction and Prevention of Pressure Ulcers in Adults: *Pressure ulcers in adults: prediction and prevention. Clinical practice guideline number 3,* Rockville, Md, 1992, Agency for Health Care Policy and Research, Public Health Service, U.S. Department of Health and Human Services.

Podnar S: Neurophysiology of the neurogenic lower urinary tract disorders, *Clin Neurophysiol* (in press, corrected proof).

Poiraudeau S et al: Fear-avoidance beliefs about back pain in patients with subacute low back pain. *Pain* 124(3):305-311, 2006.

Quevedo AS, Coghill RC: An illusion of proximal radiation of pain due to distally directed inhibition, *J Pain* 8(3):280-286, 2007.

Sharma H, Jane MJ, Reid R: Pigmented villonodular synovitis of the foot and ankle: forty years of experience from the Scottish bone tumor registry, *J Foot Ankle Surg* 45(5):329-336, 2006.

Siegel KL, Kepple TM, Stanhope SJ: A case study of gait compensations for hip muscle weakness in idiopathic inflammatory myopathy, *Clin Biomech* 22(3):319-326, 2007.

Simmonds JV, Keer RJ: Hypermobility and the hypermobility syndrome. *Manual Ther* 12(4):298-309, 2007.

Siva S, Pereira SP: Acute pancreatitis, *Medicine* 35(3):171-177, 2007.

Slobodin G et al: Varied presentations of enthesopathy, *Semin Arthritis Rheum* (in press, corrected proof).

Vanderwee K et al: The reliability of two observation methods of non-blanchable erythema, grade 1 pressure ulcer, *Appl Nurs Res* 19(3):156-162, 2006.

Visser B, van Dieen JH: Pathophysiology of upper extremity muscle disorders, *J Electromyogr Kinesiol* 16(1):1-16, 2006.

Widiger TA, Sankis LM: Adult psychopathology: issues and controversies, *Ann Rev Psychol* 51:377-404, 2000.

Zautra AJ et al: Daily fatigue in women with osteoarthritis, rheumatoid arthritis, and fibromyalgia, *Pain* 128(1-2):128-135, 2007.

Zhang P, Chen X, Fan M: Signaling mechanisms involved in disuse muscle atrophy, *Med Hypotheses* (in press, corrected proof).

CHAPTER THREE

CERVICAL SPINE

INTRODUCTION

Neck discomfort commonly appears after sudden and unusual motion of the neck because the cervical spine is the most mobile segment of the spine. Many delicate and vital structures pass through the cervical spinal column, including the carotid and vertebral arteries, the spinal cord, and the spinal nerves, all of which require great protection.

Normal function of the cervical spine requires that all movements be accomplished without injury to the spinal cord and the millions of nerve fibers that pass through it. The spinal cord has the capacity to adapt itself to marked alteration in the length of the cervical spinal canal. Flexion of the neck lengthens the spinal canal, and extension shortens it. The thickness of the cervical spinal cord and the diameter of the spinal canal vary considerably from person to person.

The nerve roots in the neck are particularly vulnerable to injury because of their relatively horizontal position in comparison with those of the lumbar spine (Fig. 3-2). Stretching of the spinal cord itself is greatest at the cervical

---

AXIOMS IN ASSESSING THE CERVICAL SPINE

- Cervical spine syndromes are extremely common and are probably the fourth most common cause of musculoskeletal pain.
- At any given time, 9% of men and 12% of women have neck pain with or without arm and hand pain, and 35% of the population can remember having had neck pain at some time.
- The cervical spine is the origin of a large proportion of shoulder, elbow, hand, and wrist disorders.
- Most people who develop pain in the neck do not seek medical attention because they regard such pain as a part of life, and they simply wait for it to disappear.

ORTHOPEDIC GAMUT 3-1

CERVICAL SPINE PAIN

Differential diagnostic possibilities of cervical spine pain:

- Cardiovascular disease
- Myocardial infarction
- Aortic dissection
- Meningitis
- Cervical osteoarthritis
- Hypertension
- Temporal arteritis
- Polymyalgia rheumatica
- A spectrum of neurologic diseases and syndromes
- Various metabolic bone diseases
- Primary and metastatic cancer
- Infection
- Lymphoma
- Myeloma

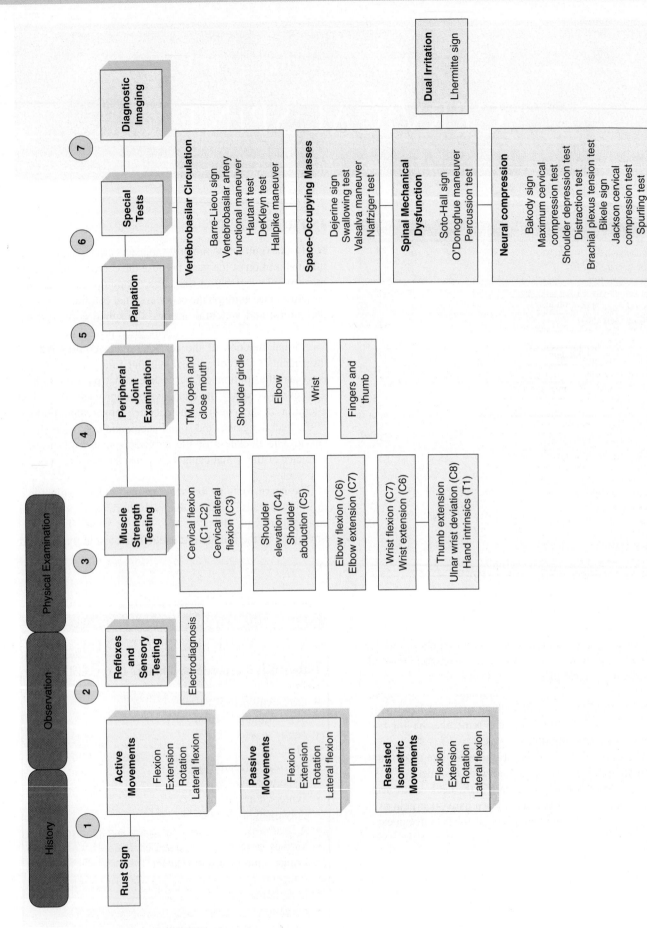

FIG. 3-1 Cervical spine assessment chart. *TMJ*, Temporomandibular joint.

TABLE 3-1

CERVICAL SPINE CROSS-REFERENCE TABLE BY SYNDROME OR TISSUE DISEASE ASSESSED

Cervical Spine Test/Sign	Nerve Root	VBA Syndrome	Brachial Plexus	Meningitis	IVD Syndrome	Tumor	Fracture	Dural Irritation	Sprain	Facet	Myospasm	Subluxation	Arthritis
Bakody sign	•												
Barré-Liéou sign		•											
Bikele sign			•	•									
Brachial plexus tension test		•		•		•	•	•					
Dejerine sign	•												
DeKleyn test			•										
Distraction test	•									•	•		
Foraminal compression test	•												
Hallpike maneuver		•											
Hautant test		•											
Jackson compression test					•	•				•		•	•
Lhermitte sign								•					
Maximum cervical compression test	•									•	•		
Naffziger test	•					•					•		
O'Donoghue maneuver									•		•		
Rust sign							•		•			•	•
Shoulder depression test	•							•		•			
Soto-Hall sign				•	•		•		•			•	•
Spinal percussion test					•		•				•		
Spurling test	•												
Swallowing test					•	•							•
Underburg test		•											
Valsalva maneuver					•	•							
Vertebrobasilar artery functional maneuver		•											

IVD, Intervertebral disc; *VBA*, vertebrobasilar artery.

ORTHOPEDIC GAMUT 3-2

ORTHOPEDIC EXAMINATION

An orthopedic examination of the cervical spine includes the following:
1. History
2. Vital signs
3. Inspection
4. Palpation of superficial and deep tissues and joint play
5. Percussion
6. Instrumentation (other physical measurement)
7. Range-of-motion evaluation
8. Orthopedic maneuvers
9. Neurologic examination
10. Imaging
11. Laboratory evaluation

ORTHOPEDIC GAMUT 3-3

CATEGORIES OF INTRACTABLE SPINAL CORD INJURY PAIN:

1. **Above-level pain,**
   a. At dermatomes rostral to the injury site in areas where normal sensation persists following injury
2. **At-level pain,**
   a. In dermatomes near the spinal injury, develops shortly after spinal cord injury, and is often characterized as either stabbing pain or a stimulus-independent type that is accompanied by allodynia (nonnoxious stimuli become noxious)
3. **Below-level pain,**
   a. Localized to dermatomes distal to the injury site, develops more gradually than does at-level pain, and is often classified as a stimulus-independent continuous, burning pain

TABLE 3-2

CERVICAL SPINE CROSS-REFERENCE TABLE BY SYNDROME OR TISSUE

Arthritis	Jackson cervical compression test Rust sign Soto-Hall sign Swallowing test	Nerve root	Bakody sign Brachial plexus tension test Dejerine sign Distraction test Maximum cervical compression test Naffziger test Shoulder depression test Spurling test
Brachial plexus	Bikele sign Brachial plexus tension test	Sprain	Naffziger test O'Donoghue maneuver Rust sign Soto-Hall sign
Dural irritation	Lhermitte sign Shoulder depression test	Subluxation	Jackson cervical compression test Rust sign Soto-Hall sign
Facet	Distraction test Jackson cervical compression test Maximum cervical compression test Shoulder depression test	Tumor	Brachial plexus tension test Jackson cervical compression test Swallowing test Valsalva maneuver
Fracture	Brachial plexus tension test Rust sign Soto-Hall sign Spinal percussion test	Vertebrobasilar artery syndrome	Barré-Liéou sign DeKleyn test Hallpike maneuver Hautant test Underburg test Vertebrobasilar artery functional maneuver
Intervertebral disc syndrome	Brachial plexus tension test Jackson cervical compression test Naffziger test Soto-Hall sign Spinal percussion test Swallowing test Valsalva maneuver		
Meningitis	Brachial plexus tension test Soto-Hall sign		
Myospasm	Distraction test Maximum cervical compression test Naffziger test O'Donoghue maneuver Soto-Hall sign Spinal percussion test		

spine, which also predisposes the cord and nerve roots to trauma (Tables 3-1 and 3-2).

Many provocative tests have been developed for the cervical spine. The anatomic structures commonly tested are dural tension, foraminal and vertebral canal patency, and muscle, tendon, or ligamentous injuries (Table 3-3). During investigation of the upper extremity, the examiner must differentiate between canal or nerve root lesions by physical examination and, if necessary, electrodiagnostic studies. Cervical spine canal stenosis, whether of bony or soft-tissue origins, can cause lower extremity signs and symptoms. Most notable is long tract pain, or rhizalgia, appearing in an ipsilateral leg with a cervical nerve root lesion (Table 3-4).

ORTHOPEDIC GAMUT 3-4

NEURAL RESPONSES

Pathologic neural responses to cervical injury can be grouped into four categories (Fig. 3-3):

1. Transient neurologic deficit (lasting less than 8 weeks) involving the nerve roots, trunk or the brachial plexus, or motor unit
2. Longstanding, consistent neurologic deficit (lasting more than 8 weeks)
3. Cervical myelopathy (clonus, lower or upper limb findings)
4. Gross spinal cord impairment (quadriplegia)

TABLE 3-3

COMMON PROVOCATIVE TESTS TO EVALUATE THE SPINE

Provocative Test	Anatomic Structures Being Tested	Positive Finding(s)
Cervical spine		
Jackson compression test	Dural sheath, nerve root, spinal nerve	Radicular pain
Spurling compression test	Dural sheath, nerve root, spinal nerve	Radicular pain
Maximal foraminal compression test	Dural sheath, nerve root, spinal nerve	Radicular pain
Distraction test	Dural sheath, nerve root, spinal nerve	Relief of radicular pain
Shoulder depression test	Dural sheath, nerve root, spinal nerve, brachial plexus	Radicular pain to one or more dermatomes
E.A.S.T. test	Subclavian artery	Vascular compromise
Eden test	Scalene musculature	Radiculopathy to multiple dermatomes or vascular compromise
Thoracic spine		
Wright hyperabduction test	Pectoralis minor	Vascular compromise, subclavian artery, TOS
Tests for anterior thoracic wall	Peripheral nerve, muscles	Radicular pain, dull ache
Lumbar spine		
Straight leg raise (SLR)	Dural sheath, nerve root, spinal nerve	Radiculopathy to one dermatome usually
Bragard test	Dural sheath, nerve root, spinal nerve	Radiculopathy to one dermatome usually
Bekhterev test (Bechterew)	Dural sheath, nerve root, spinal nerve	Radiculopathy to one dermatome usually
Neri bow string test	Dural sheath, nerve root, spinal nerve	Radiculopathy to one dermatome usually

E.A.S.T., Elevated arm stress test; *TOS*, thoracic outlet syndrome.
(From Greenstein GM: *Clinical assessment of neuromusculoskeletal disorders*, St Louis, 1997, Mosby.)

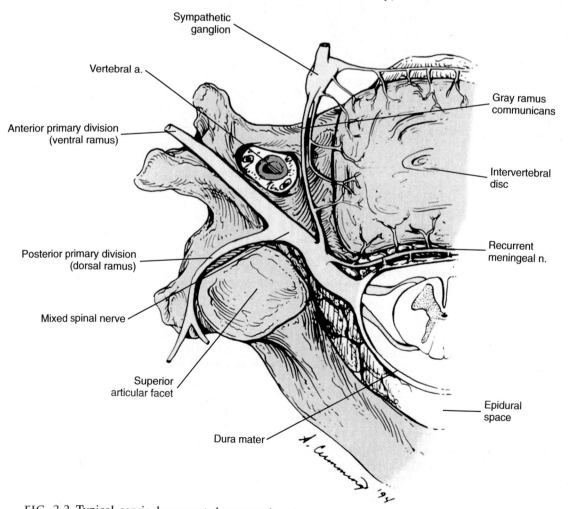

FIG. 3-2 Typical cervical segment demonstrating the neural elements. (From Cramer GD, Darby SA: *Basic and clinical anatomy of the spine, spinal cord, and ANS*, St Louis, 1995, Mosby.)

TABLE 3-4

CLASSIFICATION OF POST–SPINAL CORD INJURY PAIN STATES

Acute Phase Pain	Chronic Phase Pains
Acute nociceptive (spinal injury site)	Nociceptive (musculoskeletal, spasm)
Early neurogenic	Neurogenic
Early burning	Peripheral
Transitional zone pain	Transitional zone pain
	Double lesion syndrome pain
	Visceral pain (?)
	Central
	Central dysesthesia syndrome pain
	Syringomyelia pain
	Visceral pain (?)
	Psychogenic

(Adapted from Beric A: Post-spinal cord injury pain states, *Anesthesiol Clin North Am* 15(2):445-463, 1997.)

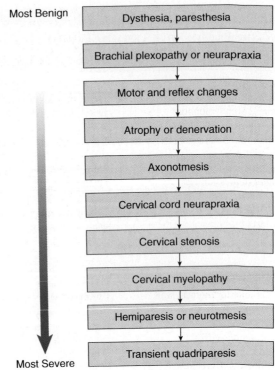

FIG. 3-3 Pathologic neurologic responses in cervical trauma. (From Brier SR: *Primary care orthopedics*, St Louis, 1999, Mosby.)

Multiple studies indicate that the incidence of people with some form of chronic pain after spinal cord injury is up to 90%, with most studies reporting moderate to severe pain in the majority of cases (Crown et al, 2005).

The early pain that is neurogenic in origin includes transitional zone pain in thoracic injuries and cauda equina pain in lumbosacral spine injuries. In these cases, an overlap exists between the acute traumatic pain and early development of these neurogenic pains (Beric, 1997).

ESSENTIAL CLINICAL ANATOMY

The atlas consists of a pair of strong lateral masses that are linked by the anterior arch and the posterior arch (Fig. 3-4). The posterior arch of the atlas is attached to the posterior rim of the foramen magnum by the atlantooccipital membrane (Fig. 3-5).

Children often have lax ligaments, which increases spinal motion. This condition most commonly occurs in the cervical region. Increased motion seen during physical or x-ray examination should be differentiated from pathologic subluxation. On imaging of the cervical spine, the predental space should not exceed 3 mm. A predental space greater than 3 mm has been found in 20% of normal patients younger than 8 years and can be followed on patients into early adulthood.

Pathologic subluxation of the atlas on the axis that compromises the spinal cord (compressive myelopathy) is associated with rheumatoid arthritis and ankylosing spondylitis. The common characteristic of these disorders is the destructive weakening of the atlantooccipital ligament system, with resultant translation of the structures.

The costal element in C7 is one of the most common from which accessory ribs may form (e.g., a *cervical rib*). Abnormal positioning of a cervical rib heightens the risk of compression of the nerves and vessels (Fig. 3-6).

The articulations of the vertebral column are of great importance. The vertebral column supports much weight; serves as an axis for movement of the limbs, trunk, head, and neck; and protects the spinal cord from trauma (Fig. 3-7).

The intervertebral discs are fibrocartilaginous flattened structures interposed between adjacent vertebral bodies (Fig. 3-8). Each disc consists of a gelatinous inner region (i.e., the nucleus pulposus), surrounded by a solid ring of stiffer material (i.e., the annulus fibrosus) (Fig. 3-9).

The vertebral artery (VA) is closely related to the cervical spine and is the first branch of the subclavian artery. It enters the foramen of the transverse process of C6 and ascends through the remaining foramina of the tops of the cervical vertebrae (Fig. 3-10). The vertebral artery passes beneath the posterior atlantooccipital membrane (Fig. 3-11). The union of the two VAs forms the basilar artery.

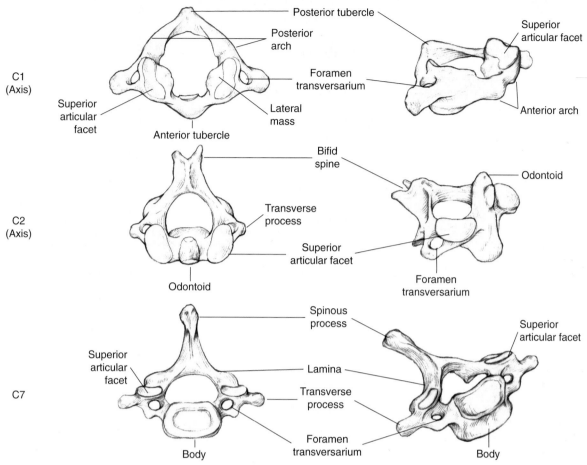

C1
(Axis)

Posterior tubercle

Posterior arch

Superior articular facet

Foramen transversarium

Superior articular facet

Lateral mass

Anterior arch

Anterior tubercle

C2
(Axis)

Bifid spine

Transverse process

Superior articular facet

Odontoid

Odontoid

Foramen transversarium

C7

Spinous process

Superior articular facet

Superior articular facet

Lamina

Transverse process

Transverse process

Foramen transversarium

Body

Foramen transversarium

Body

FIG. 3-4 Cervical vertebrae C1, C2, and C7. (From Mathers LH, et al: *Clinical anatomy principles,* St Louis, 1996, Mosby.)

ESSENTIAL MOTION ASSESSMENT

During a cervical spine range-of-motion assessment, active then passive movements should be examined. For flexion, the patient brings the chin onto the chest; for extension, the patient bends the head backward as far as possible (Fig. 3-12). For lateral flexion, the patient brings an ear toward the shoulder, first on one side and then on the other. For rotation, the patient looks over one shoulder and then the other. Repeating the movements while applying gentle pressure over the vertex of the skull may trigger pain or paresthesia in the arm if a critical degree of narrowing exists at an intervertebral foramen (Fig. 3-13). In evaluating cervical spine range of motion, the examiner observes not only the total range of movement, but also the smoothness and comfort with which the patient accomplishes the motions (Figs. 3-14 to 3-21).

ESSENTIAL MUSCLE FUNCTION ASSESSMENT

The muscles of the vertebral column are often in an increased state of contraction, which stiffens the vertebral column to serve as a platform for movement of the head or limbs (Fig. 3-22).

The intrinsic longitudinal vertebral muscles, placed more superficially, are collectively called the *erector spinae* (Fig. 3-23). The cervical region contains elongated muscles

Text continued on p. 90

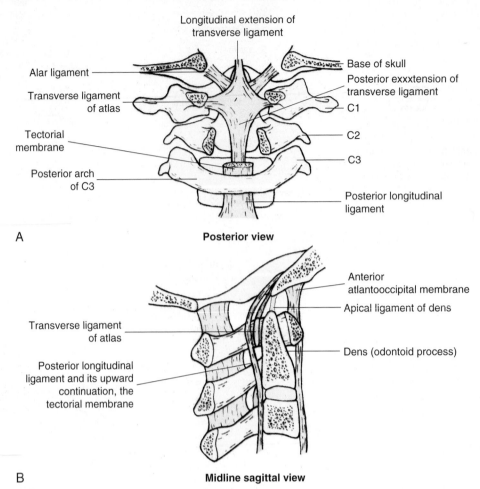

FIG. 3-5 Ligaments connecting the skull and vertebral column. (From Mathers LH, et al: *Clinical anatomy principles,* St Louis, 1996, Mosby.)

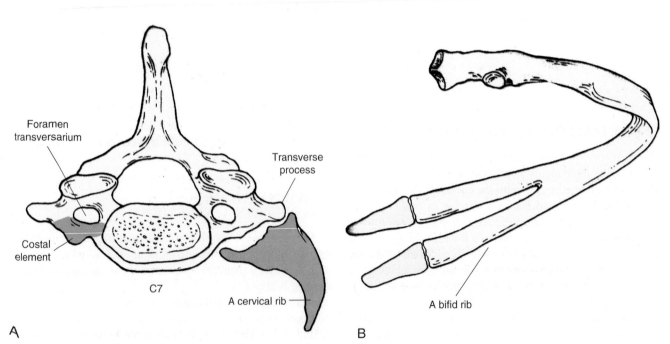

FIG. 3-6 Variations in rib structures. **A,** Cervical rib. **B,** Bifid rib with two costal cartilages. (From Mathers LH, et al: *Clinical anatomy principles,* St Louis, 1996, Mosby.)

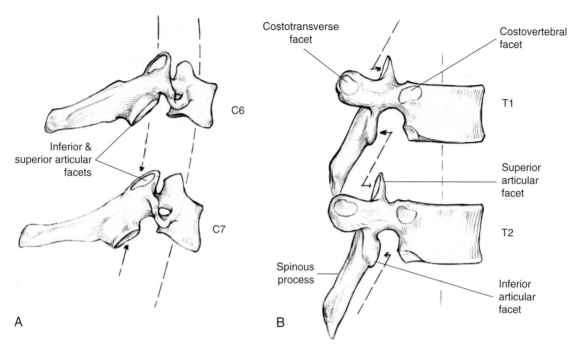

FIG. 3-7 Vertebral articulations. **A,** Cervical vertebrae. **B,** Thoracic vertebrae. (From Mathers LH, et al: *Clinical anatomy principles,* St Louis, 1996, Mosby.)

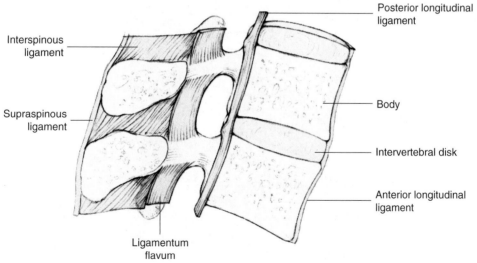

FIG. 3-8 Midsagittal section through a typical vertebra. (From Mathers LH, et al: *Clinical anatomy principles,* St Louis, 1996, Mosby.)

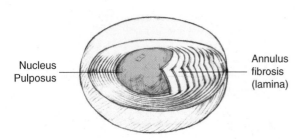

FIG. 3-9 Intervertebral disc. (From Mathers LH, et al: *Clinical anatomy principles,* St Louis, 1996, Mosby.)

Nucleus Pulposus

Annulus fibrosis (lamina)

ORTHOPEDIC GAMUT 3-5

VERTEBRAL MUSCLES

The vertebral muscles are divided into two large groups:

1. Extrinsic muscles, which are important in the attachment of limbs and limb girdles to the vertebrae and contribute to motions of the trunk
2. Intrinsic muscles, which stabilize and carry out motions of the vertebral column itself

---

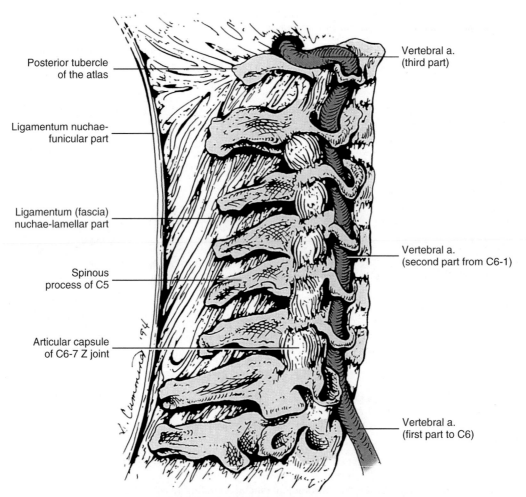

Posterior tubercle of the atlas

Ligamentum nuchae-funicular part

Ligamentum (fascia) nuchae-lamellar part

Spinous process of C5

Articular capsule of C6-7 Z joint

Vertebral a. (third part)

Vertebral a. (second part from C6-1)

Vertebral a. (first part to C6)

FIG. 3-10 Lateral view of the cervical portion of the vertebral column. (From Cramer GD, Darby SA: *Basic and clinical anatomy of the spine, spinal cord, and ANS,* St Louis, 1995, Mosby.)

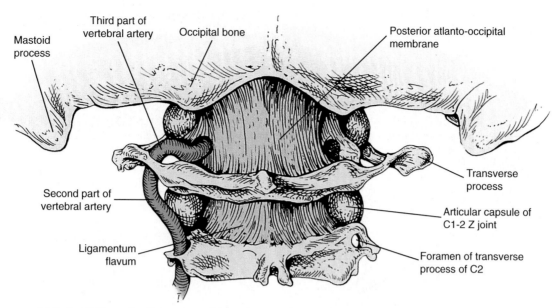

FIG. 3-11 Posterior ligaments of the upper cervical region. (From Cramer GD, Darby SA: *Basic and clinical anatomy of the spine, spinal cord, and ANS,* St Louis, 1995, Mosby.)

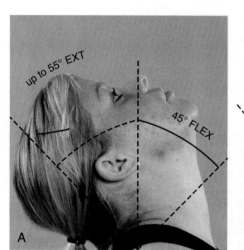
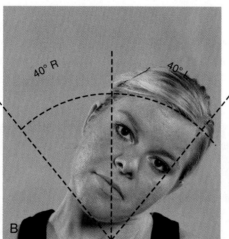
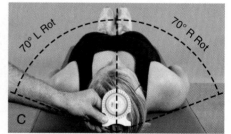

FIG. 3-12 Range of motion of the cervical spine.

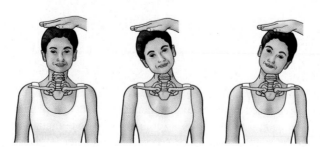

FIG. 3-13 Compression of the vertex of the skull to reproduce cervical root pain. (From Epstein O et al: *Clinical examination, ed 2,* London, 1997, Mosby.)

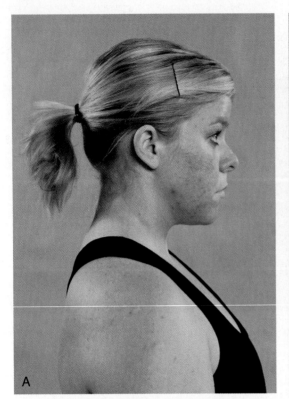
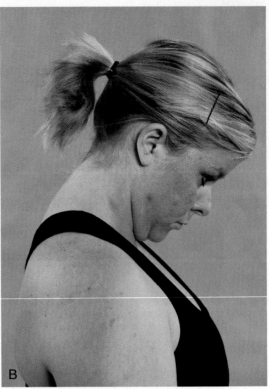

FIG. 3-14 Flexion. **A,** To assess cervical range of motion, the examiner has the patient sit with the head upright. **B,** The examiner then instructs the patient to tuck the chin in toward the chest. The expected range of motion is 80 to 90 degrees. Excessive range is when the chin can reach the chest while the patient's mouth is closed. Two finger widths' distance between the chin and the chest can be considered normal. Forty degrees or less of retained cervical flexion is an impairment of neck function in the activities of daily living.

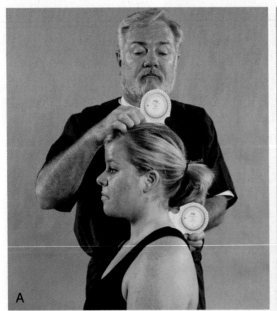
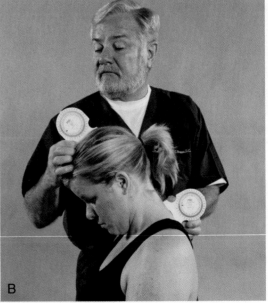

FIG. 3-15 Flexion assessed with an inclinometer. **A,** With the patient seated and the cervical spine in the neutral position, the examiner places one inclinometer over the T1 spinous process in the sagittal plane. The second inclinometer is placed at the superior aspect of the occiput, or on top of the head, also in the sagittal plane. Both inclinometers are zeroed in these positions. **B,** The patient flexes the head and neck forward. The examiner records both angles. The T1 inclination is subtracted from the cranial inclination to determine the cervical flexion angle. The expected range of motion is 60 degrees or greater from the neutral position.

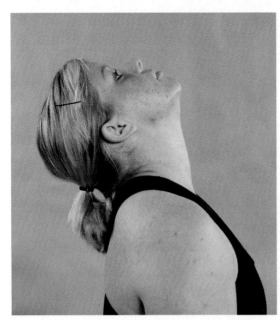

FIG. 3-16 Extension. Extension range of motion is 70 degrees. In extension the plane of the nose and forehead should be nearly horizontal. Fifty degrees or less of retained cervical extension is an impairment of neck function in the activities of daily living.

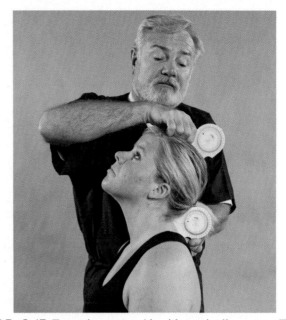

FIG. 3-17 Extension assessed with an inclinometer. The patient is seated with the cervical spine in the neutral position. The examiner places one inclinometer slightly lateral to the T1 spinous process in the sagittal plane. The second inclinometer is placed at the superior aspect of the occiput, or on top of the head, in the sagittal plane. Both inclinometers are zeroed in these positions. The patient extends the head and neck, and the examiner records the angle of both inclinometers. The T1 inclination is subtracted from the occipital inclination to determine the cervical extension angle. The expected range of motion is 75 degrees or greater from the neutral position.

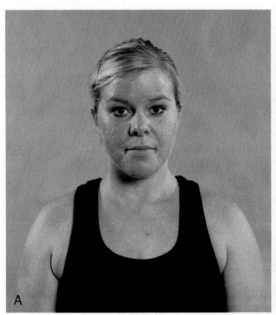
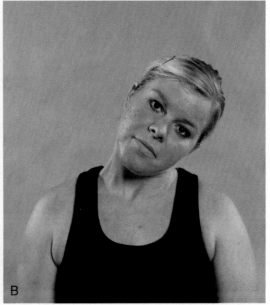

FIG. 3-18 Lateral flexion. **A,** The patient begins with the cervical spine in the neutral position. **B,** Lateral flexion of the cervical spine is normally about 20 to 45 degrees to the right and left. Most lateral flexion occurs between the occiput and C1 and between C1 and C2. Thirty degrees or less of retained lateral flexion is an impairment of neck function in the activities of daily living.

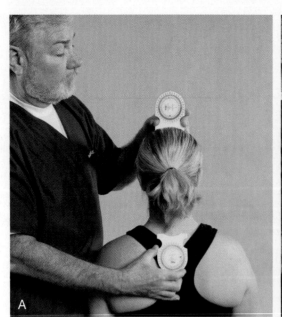
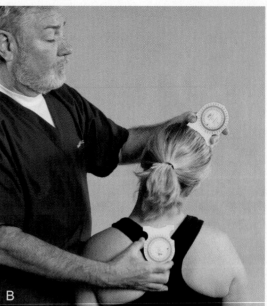

FIG. 3-19 Lateral flexion assessed with an inclinometer. **A,** With the patient seated and the cervical spine in a neutral position, the examiner places one inclinometer on the T1 spinous process in the coronal plane. The examiner places the second inclinometer at the superior aspect of the occiput, or on top of the head, also in the coronal plane. Both instruments are then zeroed. **B,** The patient laterally flexes the head and neck to one side. The examiner records the angles of both instruments. The T1 inclination is subtracted from the occipital inclination to determine the cervical lateral flexion angle. The expected range of motion is 45 degrees or greater from the neutral position. The procedure should be repeated for the opposite side.

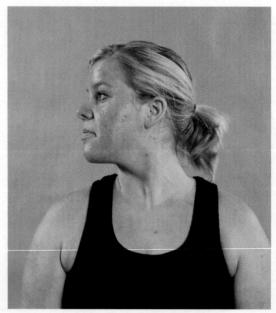

FIG. 3-20 Rotation. Normal rotation of the cervical spine is 70 to 90 degrees. In many instances, the patient's chin does not reach the plane of the shoulder. Sixty degrees or less of retained cervical rotation is an impairment of the cervical spine in the activities of daily living.

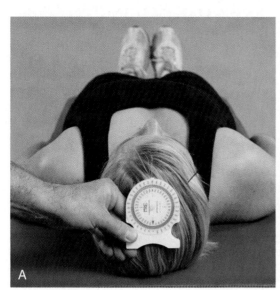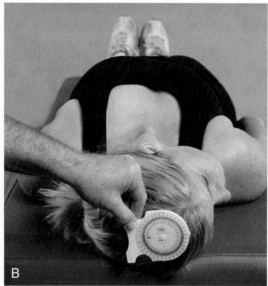

FIG. 3-21 Rotation assessed with an inclinometer. **A,** With the patient in a supine position, the examiner places the inclinometer at the crown of the head in the coronal plane. The instrument is zeroed. **B,** The patient rotates the head to one side, and the examiner records the angle indicated on the instrument. This angle is the cervical spine rotation angle. The procedure is repeated for the opposite side. The expected range of motion is 80 degrees or greater from the neutral position.

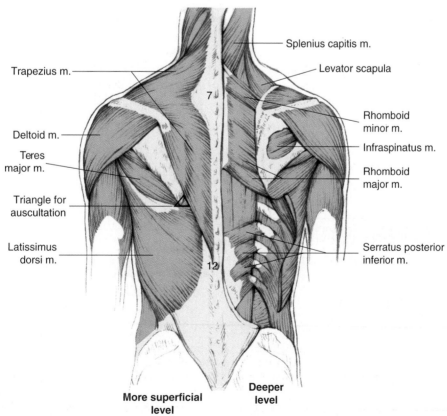

FIG. 3-22 Superficial back muscles. (From Mathers LH, et al: *Clinical anatomy principles,* St Louis, 1996, Mosby.)

originating from the spinous process (the splenius muscles) and others from the transverse processes (the semispinalis muscles). The suboccipital muscles are a special group of muscles linking the atlas, the axis, and the base of the skull (Fig. 3-24).

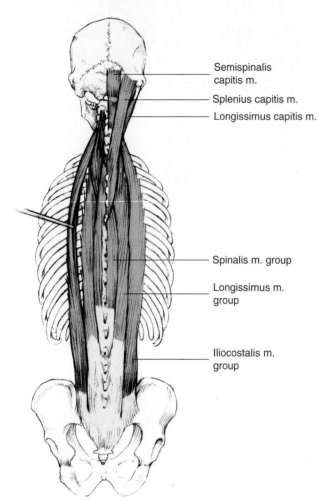

FIG. 3-23 Erector spinae muscles. (From Mathers LH, et al: *Clinical anatomy principles,* St Louis, 1996, Mosby.)

Semispinalis capitis m.

Splenius capitis m.

Longissimus capitis m.

Spinalis m. group

Longissimus m. group

Iliocostalis m. group

ESSENTIAL IMAGING
Plain-Film Imaging

The minimal set of films for the cervical spine includes the anteroposterior (AP), lateral, open-mouth, and odontoid views. The vertebra C7 must be visualized on the lateral projection when the cervical spine is being examined because many fracture-dislocations occur in the lower cervical spine or at the cervicothoracic junction (see Fig. 3-29).

The open-mouth view is essential in assessing the normal articulation of the lateral masses of the atlas (C1) with those of the axis (C2), especially when assessing a possible Jefferson burst fracture with disruption of the normal neural ring of C1, causing lateral displacement of its lateral masses.

Of equal importance is the articulation between the anterior arch of C1 and the odontoid process of C2 on the lateral projection. Laxity or disruption of the transverse ligament may result in an unstable atlantoaxial joint (Fig. 3-30). In the lower cervical spine, the translation of a single vertebra over the inferior vertebral segment, greater than 3 or 3.5 mm signifies instability.

Oblique views of the cervical spine aid in evaluating the neural foramina and the posterior elements (Fig. 3-31).

Text continued on p. 95

ORTHOPEDIC GAMUT 3-7

CERVICAL SPINE INSTABILITY

Plain-film lateral, flexion, or extension views reveal evidence of cervical spine instability, which includes the following:
1. Anterolisthesis (sagittal displacement of vertebral body more than 3.5 mm)
2. Increased spinous spacing
3. Subluxation of facet joints
4. Acute angular deformity at level of injury (11-degree angulation of adjacent vertebral bodies)
5. Sagittal diameter of spinal canal less than 13 mm
6. Fracture or dislocation
7. Atlantodental interval greater than 3 mm in adults and 4 mm in children

---

ORTHOPEDIC GAMUT 3-8

CERVICAL SPINE PLAIN FILM SERIES

The typical cervical spine plain-film series consists of the following:
1. AP open-mouth (APOM) view (Figs. 3-33 to 3-35)
2. AP lower cervical (APLC) view (Figs. 3-36 to 3-38)
3. Lateral cervical view (Figs. 3-39 and 3-40)
4. Oblique views (Figs. 3-41 to 3-43)

ORTHOPEDIC GAMUT 3-6

CERVICAL SPINE MUSCLE STRENGTH

To evaluate cervical spine muscle strength, the patient does the following:
1. Pushes a cheek against the examiner's hand (This maneuver also tests the motor function of cranial nerve XI [sternocleidomastoid muscle]) (Fig. 3-25)
2. Pushes the back of the head against the examiner's hand (Fig. 3-26)
3. Pushes the forehead against the examiner's hand (Figs. 3-27 and 3-28)

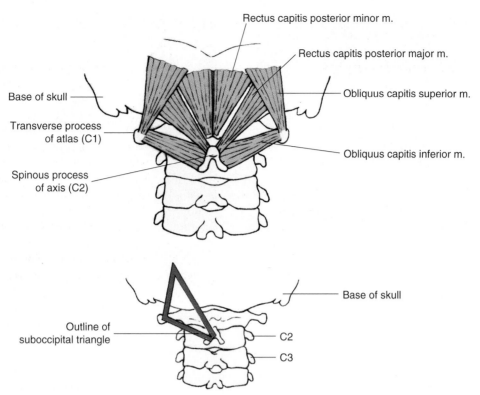

FIG. 3-24 Suboccipital triangle. (From Mathers LH, et al: *Clinical anatomy principles,* St Louis, 1996, Mosby.)

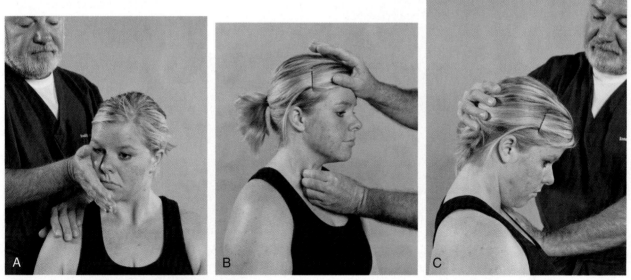

FIG. 3-25 Examining the strength of the sternocleidomastoid and trapezius muscles. **A,** Rotation against resistance. **B,** Flexion with palpation of the sternocleidomastoid muscle. **C,** Extension against resistance.

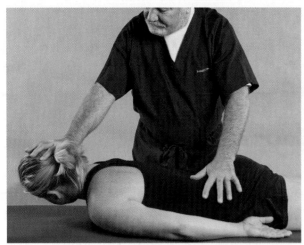

FIG. 3-26 Posterolateral head and neck extensors. The muscles included in this test are chiefly the splenius capitis and cervicis, semispinalis capitis and cervicis, and cervical erector spinae. The patient is prone on the examining table. Slight fixation is necessary. The patient tries a posterolateral extension with the face turned toward the side tested. The upper trapezius, also a posterolateral neck extensor, is tested in a similar manner with the face turned away from the side examined. The examiner applies pressure in an anterior direction against the posterolateral aspect of the head.

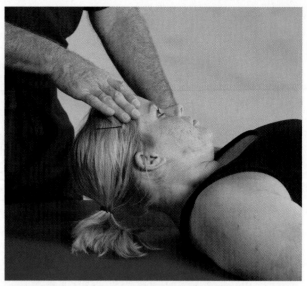

FIG. 3-27 Anterolateral head and neck flexors. The muscles acting in this test are chiefly the sternocleidomastoid and scaleni. The patient is supine on the examination table. If the patient's anterior abdominal muscles are weak, the examiner can give fixation by firm downward pressure on the thorax. The patient attempts anterolateral neck flexion. The examiner applies pressure to the temporal region of the head in an obliquely posterior direction. If the neck muscles are strong enough to hold the head but not strong enough to flex completely, the patient may try to lift the head from the table by raising the shoulders. This movement occurs especially in the tests for right and left neck flexors because the patient attempts to aid the maneuver by taking some weight on the elbow or hand, allowing the shoulder to rise from the table. To prevent this movement, the examiner holds the patient's shoulder flat on the table.

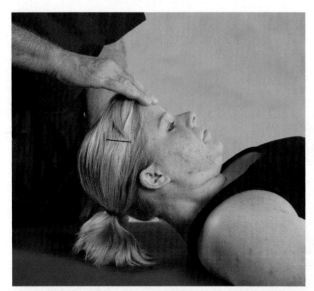

FIG. 3-28 Anterior head and neck flexors. The patient is resting on the examination table in the supine position with elbows bent and hands over the head. The anterior abdominal muscles must be strong enough to give anterior fixation of the thorax to the pelvis. This strength allows the head to be raised by the neck flexors. If the abdominal muscles are weak, the examiner can provide fixation by applying firm, downward pressure on the thorax. Children 5 years or younger should always have fixation of the thorax provided by the examiner. The patient tries to flex the cervical spine by lifting the head from the table toward the sternum while keeping the mouth closed and the chin depressed. The examiner applies pressure to the forehead in a posterior direction.

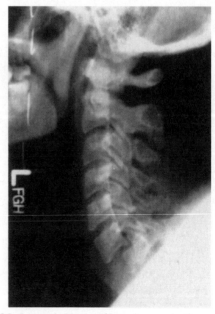

FIG. 3-29 Lateral X-ray film demonstrating significant anterior subluxation (translation) of C6 on C7 with depression of the shoulders. (From Watkins RG: *The spine in sports,* St Louis, 1996, Mosby.)

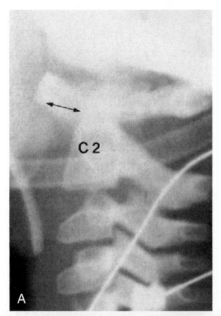

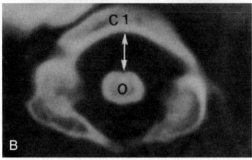

FIG. 3-30 Lateral X-ray film (**A**) and axial computed tomography scan (**B**) demonstrating widening between the anterior arch of C1 and the odontoid process of C2. (From Watkins RG: *The spine in sports,* St Louis, 1996, Mosby.)

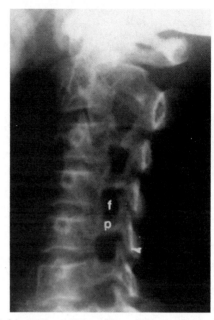

FIG. 3-31 Oblique X-ray film of the cervical spine demonstrating patent normal foramina. (From Watkins RG: *The spine in sports,* St Louis, 1996, Mosby.)

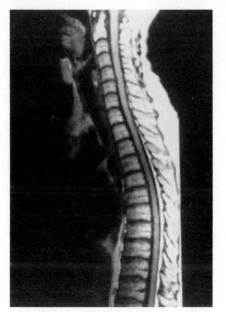

FIG. 3-32 Sagittal T1-weighted image of the entire cervical and thoracic spine. (From Watkins RG: *The spine in sports,* St Louis, 1996, Mosby.)

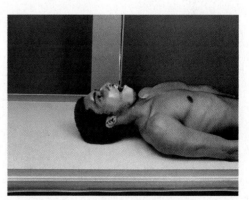

FIG. 3-33 AP atlas and axis. (From Frank ED, et al: *Merrill's atlas of radiographic positioning and procedures,* vol 1-3, ed 11, St Louis, 2007, Mosby.)

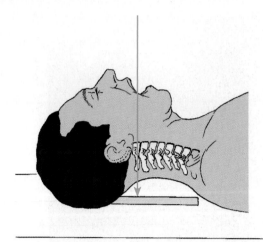

FIG. 3-34 Open-mouth spine alignment. (From Frank ED, et al: *Merrill's atlas of radiographic positioning and procedures,* vol 1-3, ed 11, St Louis, 2007, Mosby.)

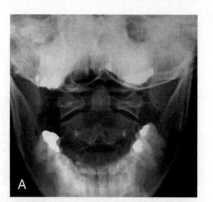

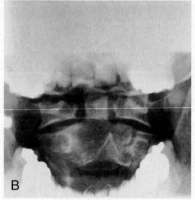

FIG. 3-35 **A** and **B,** Open-mouth atlas and axis. (From Frank ED, et al: *Merrill's atlas of radiographic positioning and procedures,* vol 1-3, ed 11, St Louis, 2007, Mosby.)

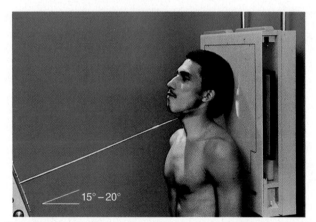

FIG. 3-36 AP axial cervical vertebrae, upright. (From Frank ED, et al: *Merrill's atlas of radiographic positioning and procedures,* vol 1-3, ed 11, St Louis, 2007, Mosby.)

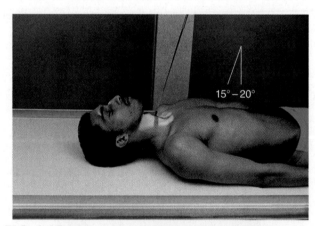

FIG. 3-37 AP axial cervical vertebrae, recumbent. (From Frank ED, et al: *Merrill's atlas of radiographic positioning and procedures,* vol 1-3, ed 11, St Louis, 2007, Mosby.)

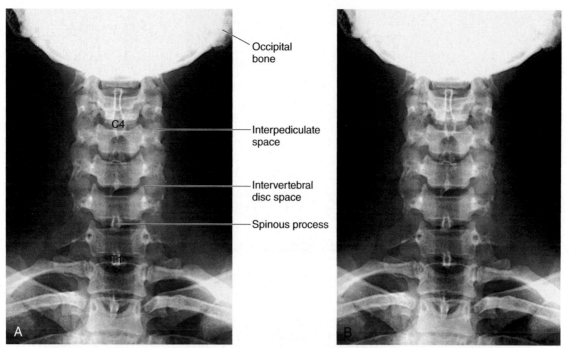

Occipital bone

Interpediculate space

Intervertebral disc space

Spinous process

FIG. 3-38 **A** and **B,** AP axial cervical vertebrae. (From Frank ED, et al: *Merrill's atlas of radiographic positioning and procedures,* vol 1-3, ed 11, St Louis, 2007, Mosby.)

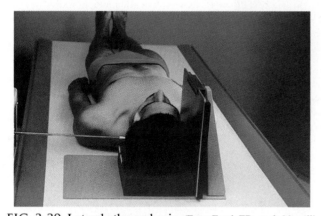

FIG. 3-39 Lateral atlas and axis. (From Frank ED, et al: *Merrill's atlas of radiographic positioning and procedures,* vol 1-3, ed 11, St Louis, 2007, Mosby.)

BOX 3-1

ACCEPTED CERVICAL SPINE PLAIN FILM IMAGING

- Anteroposterior lower cervical view (APLC)
- Anteroposterior open-mouth view (APOM)
- Lateral view
- Anterior oblique views (right and left)
- Additional views:
  - Flexion and extension lateral view
  - Fuch's view
  - Pillar or Boyleston view

Data from Greenstein GM, *Clinical assessment of neuromusculoskeletal disorders*, St Louis, 1997, Mosby.

The pillar view is another special-view plain film. Using 20 to 30 degrees of caudal angulation of the x-ray beam enables a more precise inspection of the lateral masses when pillar fractures and facet dislocations are suspected in hyperextension and rotational injuries.

Magnetic Resonance Imaging

Magnetic resonance imaging (MRI) has gained recognition based on its high soft-tissue contrast, lack of ionizing radiation, and direct multiplanar acquisition. In many institutions, MRI has become the most widely used screening method for evaluating the spine. A wide variety of specialized surface coils have been produced. With each of these coils,

the entire cervical, lumbar, or most of the thoracic spine may be imaged in one acquisition. Improvements in coil technology consisting of phased-array coils have allowed imaging of most of the spinal column in one acquisition with no additional scanning time (Fig. 3-32).

Specific views are used to evaluate complex regions of anatomy or spinal placement at extremes of motion (Box 3-1).

In assessing the sagittal diameter of the spinal canal, on a lateral view, the shortest distance from the posterior aspect of the vertebral body to the spinolaminar line is measured. The distance between the posterior aspect of the dens and the posterior cervical line is measured at C1. The ranges for diameter by level are listed in Table 3-5.

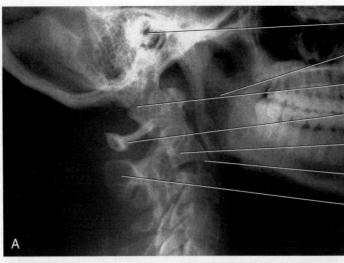

External acoustic meatus

Superimposed mandibular rami

Atlantooccipital articulation

Posterior arch, atlas

Transverse process, axis

Body of axis

Spinous process, axis

A

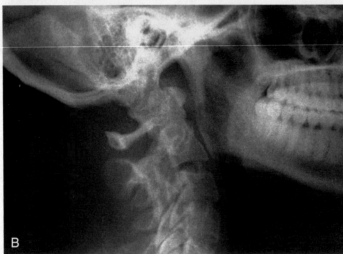

B

FIG. 3-40 Lateral atlas and axis. (From Frank ED, et al: *Merrill's atlas of radiographic positioning and procedures,* vol 1-3, ed 11, St Louis, 2007, Mosby.)

TABLE 3-5		
ACCEPTED SAGITTAL CANAL DIAMETER OF THE CERVICAL SPINE		
	Diameter (mm)	
Level	Minimum	Maximum
C1	16	31
C2	14	27
C3	13	23
C4 to C7	12	22

Adapted from Greenstein GM: *Clinical assessment of neuromusculo-skeletal disorders*, St Louis, 1997, Mosby.

McGregor line is used to evaluate for basilar invagination. The measurement can be affected by changes in the shape of the occiput unrelated to basilar invagination. On a lateral view, a line is drawn from the posterior aspect of the hard palate to the most inferior surface of the occiput. The tip of the odontoid process should not project above this line more than 8 mm in men and 10 mm in women.

Atlantodental interspace is the measurement made on a lateral view in assessing the distance between the posterior surface of the anterior arch of C1 and the anterior surface of the dens.

The maximal measurement (in any position) in adults is 3 mm and in children is 5 mm. An increase in this

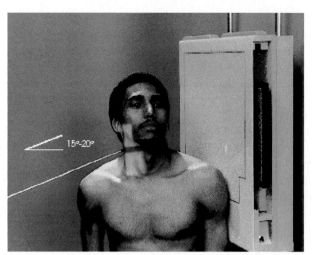

FIG. 3-41 Upright AP axial oblique intervertebral foramina, left posterior oblique. (From Frank ED, et al: *Merrill's atlas of radiographic positioning and procedures,* vol 1-3, ed 11, St Louis, 2007, Mosby.)

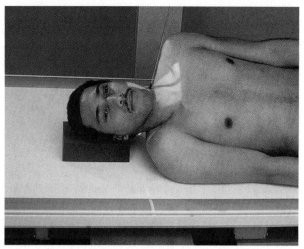

FIG. 3-42 Recumbent AP axial oblique left intervertebral foramina, right posterior oblique. (From Frank ED, et al: *Merrill's atlas of radiographic positioning and procedures,* vol 1-3, ed 11, St Louis, 2007, Mosby.)

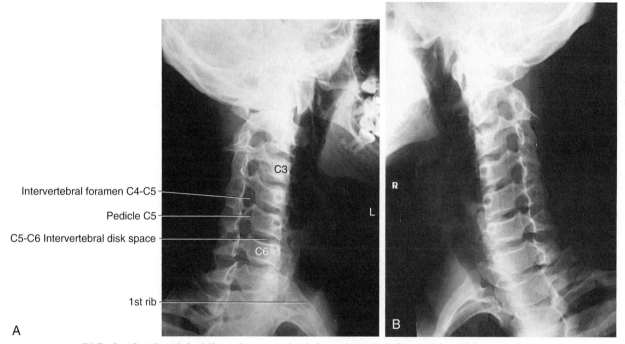

FIG. 3-43 AP axial oblique intervertebral foramina. **A,** left posterior oblique position. **B,** right posterior oblique position. (From Frank ED, et al: *Merrill's atlas of radiographic positioning and procedures,* vol 1-3, ed 11, St Louis, 2007, Mosby.)

measurement indicates loss of integrity of the transverse ligament, which is seen in such conditions as rheumatoid arthritis and pharyngeal infections, as well as in traumatic rupture of the ligament.

George line, made on a lateral view, is a line drawn along the posterior aspect of all the vertebral bodies. These lines should be in relatively good alignment, thus forming a smooth, continuous line. A break in the continuity of this line suggests listhesis of a vertebra on the one below. The

amount of slippage should be measured. Two millimeters or less of displacement or translation is considered to be within physiologic limits.

Posterior cervical line, made on a lateral view, is a line drawn connecting the spinolaminar (posterior cervical) lines from C1 to T1 (if visible). Similar to George line, the posterior cervical line should form a relatively smooth, continuous line, and it should be drawn in conjunction with George line.

The cervical gravity line is assessed on the neutral lateral view. The cervical gravity line is a vertical line drawn down from the apex of the odontoid process. This line should intersect the C7 vertebral body. If the line falls anterior to C7, anterior carriage of the head is indicated, which is commonly seen in patients with whiplash in association with loss of the lordosis. If the line falls posterior to C7, posterior carriage of the head is indicated (an uncommon finding).

To measure the lordotic angle, a line is drawn through the anterior and posterior tubercles of C1. Another line is drawn along the inferior end-plate of C7. Perpendicular lines are constructed from these lines. At the point of intersection of these lines, the superior angle is measured. The normal range is 35 to 45 degrees. An angle smaller than 35 degrees indicates hypolordosis, and an angle greater than 45 degrees indicates hyperlordosis.

Retropharyngeal and retrotracheal spaces are assessed in making two measurements on a neutral lateral view: (1) the distance from the anteroinferior corner of the C2 vertebral body to the posterior border of the pharyngeal air shadow (retropharyngeal) and (2) the distance from the anteroinferior corner of the C6 vertebral body to the posterior border of the tracheal air shadow (retrotracheal). The maximal measurement for the retropharyngeal space is 7 mm and for the retrotracheal space is 10 to 21 mm. An increase in either of these measurements indicates the presence of a space-occupying lesion, including hematoma, infection, or tumor.

Shoulder Abduction Relief Sign/Test
Cervical Foraminal Compression Test

Assessment for Cervical Nerve Root Compression

Comment

Annular fissures, or rents, develop in a degenerating disc and may coalesce, ultimately allowing nuclear material to extrude into the neural canals. When the extruded nucleus pulposus forms a broad-based extension of the disc beyond the peripheral confines of the vertebral end-plate, it is bulging. When focal asymmetric nuclear material extends beyond the end-plate but is still contained by the posterior longitudinal ligament, the nucleus is protruding. With further expulsion of nuclear material, disc extrusion occurs. With disc extrusion, free or sequestered disc fragments may migrate away from the parent disc level (Fig. 3-44).

Intervertebral discs provide a strong yet flexible bond between adjacent vertebrae. As a consequence of this flexibility, intervertebral discs are subject to a variety of disruptions that include peripheral, circumferential, radial and transverse tears of the annulus, bulging discs, protruding discs (i.e., focal bulges), and frank herniation. When her-niation is absent, this constellation of pathologies is known as internal disc disruption (IDD) (Oliphant, Frayne, Kawchuk, 2006).

Cervical radiculopathy is more common than cervical myelopathy. Cervical radiculopathy consists of pain and neurologic dysfunction produced by irritation or injury to a spinal nerve. The injury may be caused by a herniated cervical disc, cervical foraminal stenosis, tumors, fractures, or dislocations. The pathognomic characteristic of cervical radiculopathy is pain in the distribution of nerve (Table 3-6).

Although cervical nerve root compression is a part of the syndrome of cervical osteoarthritis, particularly with zygapophyseal joint (Z joint) and Luschka joint involvement, faulty posture of the cervical spine may contribute to the cervical nerve root compression, or it may be the primary cause of compression.

Hyperextension of the cervical spine, performed with the chin in a forward position, compresses the Z joints and Luschka joints on the posterior surfaces of the cervical vertebrae. Hyperextension is the cause and pathogenesis of the compression.

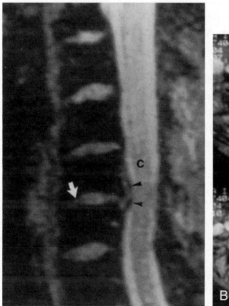 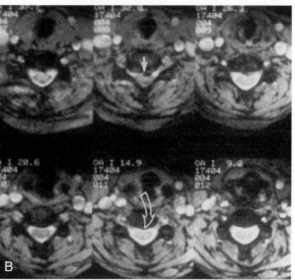

FIG. 3-44 Sagittal (**A**) and axial gradient-recalled (**B**) magnetic resonance imaging scans of the cervical spine showing central disc extrusion effacing ventral subarachnoid space in contrast to normal subarachnoid space. (From Watkins RG: *The spine in sports,* St Louis, 1996, Mosby.)

TABLE 3-6

CLINICAL FINDINGS ASSOCIATED WITH THE CERVICAL NERVE ROOTS

Root	Disc	Muscle	Reflex	Sensation	Myelogram/CT/MR Deficit
C5	C4–C5	Deltoid Biceps	Biceps	Lateral arm Deltoid area Axillary nerve	C4–C5
C6	C5–C6	Biceps Wrist extensors	Brachioradialis	Thumb, index, ring fingers Lateral forearm Musculocutaneous nerve	C5–C6
C7	C6–C7	Triceps Wrist flexors Finger extensors	Triceps	Middle finger, ring finger, or both	C6–C7
C8	C7–T1	Hand intrinsics Finger flexors		Ring and fifth fingers Medial forearm Medial anterior brachial cutaneous nerve	C7–T1
T1	T1–T2	Hand intrinsics		Medial arm Medial brachial cutaneous nerve	

CT, Computed tomography; *MR*, magnetic resonance.
Adapted from Watkins RG: *The spine in sports*, St Louis, 1996, Mosby.

ORTHOPEDIC GAMUT 3-9

CERVICAL NERVE ROOT COMPRESSION SYMPTOMS

The symptoms of nerve root compression include:
- Proximal (root) pain and neck pain
- Distal paresthesia in dermatome patterns
- Muscle weakness in one or several muscles supplied by a single root
- Loss of deep-tendon reflexes
- Muscle fasciculation
- Radiating pains that are further aggravated by movements of the neck

---

Neither specific genetic and environmental factors nor specific epidemiologic factors exist for cervical compression. In cervical hyperextension syndromes, radiographic characteristics may include those typical of cervical osteoarthritis in addition to other postural factors.

A cervical nerve root compression syndrome may result from direct trauma to the nerve roots from the pincer-like action of the foraminal architecture during an acute hyperextension trauma, from chronic irritation from hypertrophic spurring, or from disc disease. This last source may be a traumatic aggravation of chronic disc disease or an acute herniation or prolapse of disc material. Symptoms of nerve root compression are distinctly different from those of neurovascular compression syndromes or reflex sympathetic dystrophy.

Irritation of the cervical nerve roots may cause pain, sensory changes, muscle atrophy, or spasm and alteration of the tendon reflexes anywhere along the segmental distribution. Any condition causing a narrowing of the intervertebral canals may cause compression of the nerve roots and the spinal branches of the VAs, venous congestion and irritation, and compression of the recurrent meningeal nerves.

Encroachment, or narrowing, of the intervertebral canals may be the result of some involvement of the proximate soft-tissue structures or bony structures. Any condition that causes inflammation and swelling of the dural sleeves of the nerve roots may also cause neural compression (Figs. 3-45 and 3-46).

Intervertebral disk calcification in children is a rare but well-recognized clinical entity. It was first reported in 1924, and since then, more than 400 cases have been reported in patients 20 years of age or younger. This disorder peaks between 6 and 10 years. The cervical spine is the area mostly commonly involved, especially at the C6-C7 vertebral level. In children, such a calcification may be an incidental finding or may cause spinal symptoms. The most common symptom is spinal pain, regardless of the spinal level affected. Other symptoms include local tenderness, limited motion in the affected region of the spine, and occasionally torticollis (Park, Kim, Sung, 2005).

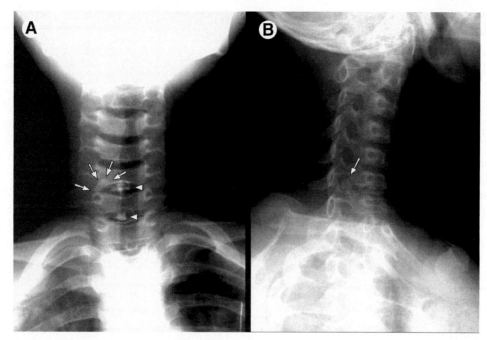

FIG. 3-45 Anteroposterior plain radiograph showing the calcification material *(white arrows without stalk)* occupying the nucleus pulposus in the center of the intervertebral disk space at the C6–C7 and the C7–T1 level. (From Park SM, Kim E-S, Sung DH: Cervical radiculopathy caused by neural foraminal migration of a herniated calcified intervertebral disk in childhood: a case report, *Arch Phys Med Rehabil* 86[11]:2214-2217, 2005.)

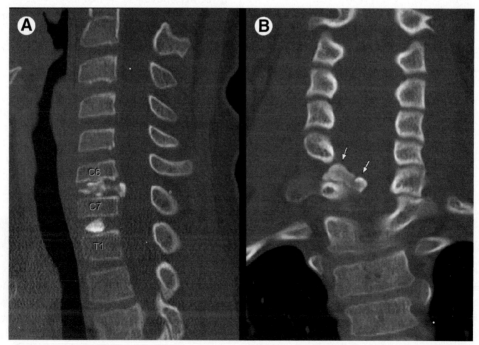

FIG. 3-46 Sagittal reformatted CT scan of the cervical spine shows the herniated calcification material from the C6–C7 intervertebral disk. (From Park SM, Kim E-S, Sung DH: Cervical radiculopathy caused by neural foraminal migration of a herniated calcified intervertebral disk in childhood: a case report, *Arch Phys Med Rehabil* 86[11]:2214-2217, 2005.)

PROCEDURE

- While in the seated position, the patient actively places the palm of the affected extremity on top of the head, raising the elbow to a height approximately level with the head (Fig. 3-47).
- By elevating the suprascapular nerve, traction of the lower trunk of the brachial plexus is relieved (Fig. 3-48).
- Overall, this maneuver decreases stretching of the compressed nerve root.
- The sign is present when the radiating pain is lessened or disappears with this maneuver.
- The test is as reliable as Spurling test and is less painful for the patient to endure.
- A cervical nerve root compression is suggested by a positive Bakody sign.

Next Steps/Procedures

Dejerine sign, Valsalva maneuver, Naffziger test, reflexes, maximum foraminal compression test, distraction test, brachial plexus tension test, Bikele sign, Jackson cervical compression test, Spurling test, electrodiagnosis, and diagnostic imaging

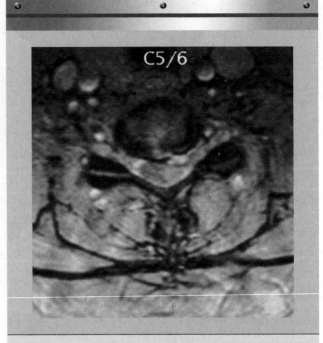

C5/6

AT THE VIEWBOX

Patient with left C6 upper extremity radicular symptoms. The extruded (noncontained) left posterolateral to foraminal disc herniation at C5–6, with underlying full thickness annular tear, impinges upon the left C6 axillary sleeve and nerve root and accounts for the radiculopathy. Note the increased signal within the left hemi cord, compatible with cord edema, hematoma, or myelomalacia, which may be associated with nondermatomal signs and symptoms. (From the teaching file of Timothy Mick, DC, DACBR)

CLINICAL PEARL

Patients with moderate to severe radicular symptoms usually do not have to be directed into the Bakody sign position because it also is an antalgic pain–relieving posture. The more difficult it is for the patient to lower the arm, the more difficult the condition will be to treat conservatively. If the patient cannot lower the arm without severe exacerbation of pain, surgery is probably indicated. Patients with moderate to severe cervical nerve root compression find the most comfortable sleeping positions to be those that involve abduction and elevation of the arm. Again, this position relieves the traction of the neural elements and is an antalgic position for someone experiencing cervical nerve root compression. A patient often voluntarily assumes the Bakody sign position while in the examination room.

3

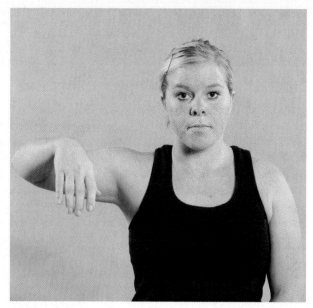

FIG. 3-47 The patient abducts and externally rotates the ipsilateral shoulder by moving the hand toward the head.

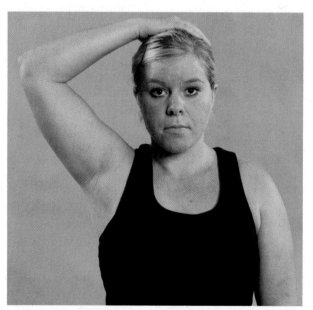

FIG. 3-48 The hand is placed on top of the head. If this position relieves radicular pain, this is a positive sign that suggests a nerve root syndrome.

BARRÉ-LIÉOU SIGN

Assessment for Vertebral Artery Syndrome

Comment

Rotation of the neck to one side usually decreases circulatory flow in the atlantoaxial portion of the **contralateral VA.** When kinking of the artery, atheromata, or encroaching osteoarthritis occurs, such movement reduces the circulation even more. Other mechanisms that can alter the blood supply to the brainstem are carotid sinus compression, use of a cervical collar, fighting (boxing, wrestling, contact sports, etc.), manipulation of the neck that causes the release of emboli from atheromatous plaques in the great vessels, and thrombosis with infarction of the cerebellum or brainstem.

Lamberty and Zivanovic identify the ponticulus posticus (PP) as the causative factor in headaches, vertigo, Barré-Liéou syndrome, *eye* pain, and photophobia. The mechanism is unclear, although some authorities believe it to be the result of compression of the VA by the PP, leading to ischemia of the vertebrobasilar circulation. In 1957, Tatlow and Bammer were among the first researchers who reported several cases of Barré-Liéou syndrome to be caused by VA compression by the PP—a view that has gained considerable support in more recent years because the logical progression of such a scenario was that surgical excision of the PP should decompress the VA and therefore alleviate the symptoms. Sun in 1990 and Li and colleagues in 1995 reported the alleviation of vertigo, headaches, and nausea with such a surgical procedure (Wight, Osborne, Breen, 1999).

Vertebral artery insufficiency, whether permanent or transitory, has been identified as the explanation for some of the symptoms seen with hyperextension or hyperflexion injuries. The course of the VA in the cervical spine is tortuous, and the artery passes through, over, and around structures that may become malaligned after trauma (Fig. 3-49). Abnormal pressures or tractional stresses may impede circulation through these arteries. The VAs may also be compressed as a result of chronic degenerative disease of the cervical spine. This compression may occur at any point along its usual course from C6 to C2 and may become symptomatic after cervical spine trauma (Fig. 3-50).

Vertebrobasilar insufficiency may produce symptoms ranging from dizziness, syncope, and nausea to motor and sensory deficits.

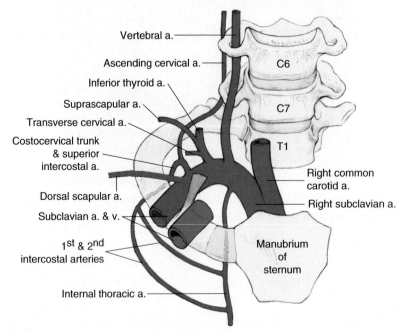

FIG. 3-49 VA and cervical vertebrae. (From Mathers LH, et al: *Clinical anatomy principles,* St Louis, 1996, Mosby.)

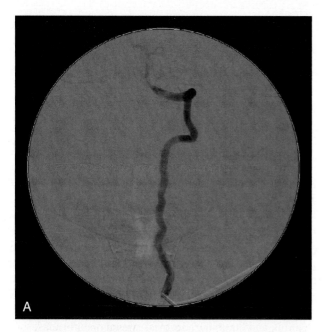

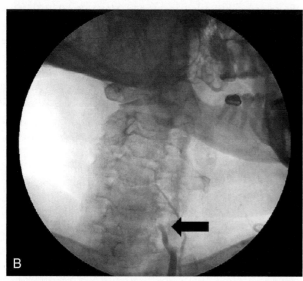

FIG. 3-50 Cervical angiography in the neutral position. **A,** Showing no compromise of the VA and with the patient's head turned to the left. **B,** Demonstrating complete occlusion of the VA at the level of the C6 vertebral body *(arrow)*. (From Velat GJ et al: Intraoperative dynamic angiography to detect resolution of bow hunter's syndrome: technical case report, *Surg Neurol* 66[4]:420-423, 2006.)

Bow hunter syndrome is a rare form of vertebrobasilar insufficiency caused by occlusion or stenosis of the VA during head rotation along the craniocervical axis. In most cases, occlusion of the dominant VA occurs with contralateral head rotation, causing mechanical stretching or compression of the ipsilateral C1 through C2 VA segment. This phenomenon may also be reproduced along subaxial segments of the VA in the setting of occlusive fibrous tissue bands or osteophyte formation. Transient rotational compression of the VA does not usually fall into the category of bow hunter's syndrome

---

ORTHOPEDIC GAMUT 3-10

VERTEBRAL ARTERY COMPRESSION

Three mechanisms of vertebral artery compression include:
1. Osteophytes from the lateral disc margin
2. Anteriorly extending osteophytes from the facet joint
3. Compression from the inferior facet as a result of posterior subluxation and a scissoring effect by the adjacent superior facet

---

ORTHOPEDIC GAMUT 3-11

TRAUMA TO THE VERTEBRAL ARTERY

Three areas in which the vertebral artery is most susceptible to trauma include:
1. The posterior atlantooccipital membrane, which is dense and inelastic and may become calcified (firmly attached to the artery)
2. The space between the occiput and posterior arch of the atlas, especially during extension
3. The area between the lateral mass of the atlas and the transverse process of the axis, especially during extension and rotation

---

because of compensatory blood flow from the vertebrobasilar system (Velat et al, 2006).

Increased tissue pressures from myospasm, edema, or hemorrhage may also compromise the blood flow through the VA, especially when patency is already compromised because of atherosclerosis or a congenital anomaly. Arterial spasm may also occur.

Older patients with preexisting atherosclerotic disease are at a greater risk of injury that results in VA syndrome or vertebrobasilar artery insufficiency.

The history is important in patients with carotid artery stenosis or occlusion. The symptoms may range from a minor problem, such as blurring of vision in one eye, to profound obtundation, aphasia, and hemiparesis.

In mid-basilar artery occlusion, the effect is profound *(locked-in* syndrome). Locked-in syndrome is a condition of total consciousness, with or without impaired sensation, and no voluntary movement except vertical eye movement and convergence. The syndrome results from interference of basilar artery blood flow in the region of the mid-pons, producing bilateral ventral pontine infarction; this serves as a transection of the brainstem at the mid-pons region.

The **locked-in syndrome** (pseudocoma) describes patients who are awake and conscious but selectively de-efferented

ORTHOPEDIC GAMUT 3-12

CLASSIFICATION OF LOCKED-IN SYNDROME

Locked-in syndrome (LIS) is subdivided based on the extent of motor impairment:

A. Classical LIS is characterized by total immobility except for vertical eye movements or blinking
B. Incomplete LIS permits remnants of voluntary motion
C. Total LIS consists of complete immobility including all eye movements combined with preserved consciousness

ORTHOPEDIC GAMUT 3-13

THE AMERICAN CONGRESS OF REHABILITATION MEDICINE (1995) DEFINITION OF LOCKED-IN SYNDROME

1. The presence of sustained eye opening (bilateral ptosis should be ruled out as a complicating factor)
2. Preserved basic cognitive abilities
3. Aphonia or severe hypophonia
4. Quadriplegia or quadriparesis
5. A primary mode of communication that uses vertical or lateral eye movement or blinking of the upper eyelid

ORTHOPEDIC GAMUT 3-14

LOCKED-IN SYNDROME

Locked-in syndrome characteristics:
1. Retained consciousness
2. No volitional movement of the body
3. Nuclei of cranial nerves V to XII destroyed, resulting in their paralysis
4. Loss of sensations carried in the medial lemniscus
5. Normal hearing
6. Sparing of cranial nerve IV nucleus and the superior colliculus of the quadrigeminal plate

(i.e., those who have no means of producing speech or limb or facial movements). Acute ventral pontine lesions are its most common cause. People with such brainstem lesions often remain comatose for some days or weeks, needing artificial respiration, and then gradually wake up but remaining paralyzed and voiceless, superficially resembling patients in a vegetative state or akinetic mutism (Laureys et al, 2005).

In 1926, Barré studied and established a syndrome that was further described in 1928 by his student Liéou. So diverse and widespread is the combination of symptoms and signs that some people no longer regard the syndrome as a disorder associated with the cervical spine; rather, they view the syndrome as one caused by VA insufficiency and its multivariate characteristics. The symptoms of this syndrome include pain in the head, neck, eyes, ears, face, sinuses, and throat; sensory disturbances in the pharynx and larynx; paroxysmal hoarseness and aphonia; tinnitus that is synchronous with the pulse; various auditory hallucinations, such as whistling and humming; deafness; visual disturbances, such as blurring, scintillating scotomata, photophobia, blepharospasm, squinting sensations, and a peculiar pulling at the back of the eyes; flushing; sweating; salivation; lacrimation; nausea; vomiting; and rhinorrhea.

PROCEDURE

- The examiner instructs the patient to rotate the head slowly from side to side while in a seated position (Fig. 3-51).
- Rotating the head causes compression of the VAs (Fig. 3-52).
- Vertigo, dizziness, visual disturbances, nausea, syncope, and nystagmus are signs of a positive test (Fig. 3-53).
- A positive finding strongly suggests a buckling of the ipsilateral VA, constituting vertebrobasilar insufficiency.

Next Steps/Procedures

Vertebrobasilar artery functional maneuver, Hautant test, DeKleyn test, Hallpike maneuver, Underburg test, Doppler vascular investigation, carotid auscultation, and diagnostic imaging

CLINICAL PEARL

The patient with a positive Barré-Liéou sign is a poor risk for aggressive cervical spine manipulation. Such manipulation should not be undertaken until all vascular causes have been investigated. Aggravation of the *sympathetic ganglia* of the cervical spine can produce many, if not all, of these symptoms (vertigo, dizziness, visual disturbances, nausea, syncope, and nystagmus), in which case cervical spinal manipulation is not contraindicated. The examiner *must* be able to distinguish between vascular and neural origins before manipulation is performed.

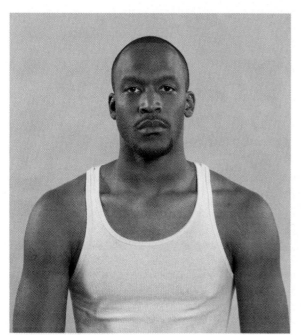

FIG. 3-51 The patient is seated as comfortably and as erect as possible. Blood pressure and pulse are examined and recorded before starting the test.

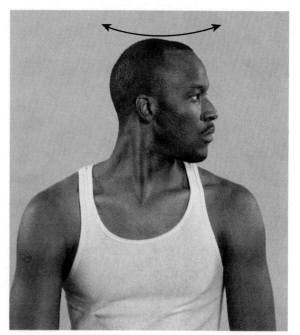

FIG. 3-52 The patient rotates the head maximally from side to side. This movement is performed slowly at first and then accelerated until the patient's tolerance is reached.

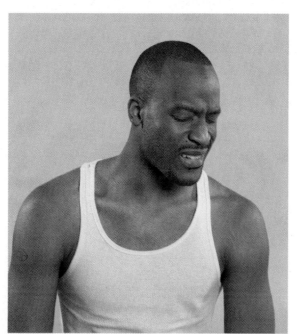

FIG. 3-53 A VA syndrome is suggested by vertigo, blurred vision, nausea, syncope, or nystagmus. These symptoms may occur singly or in combination.

3

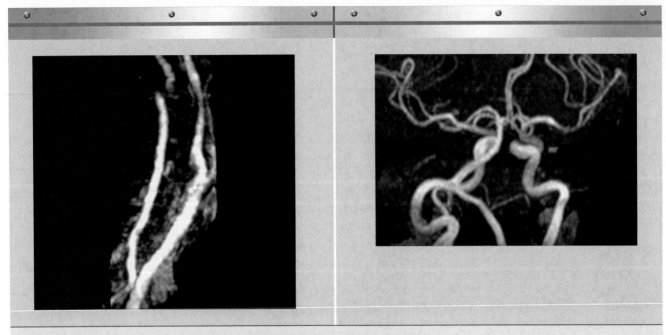

AT THE VIEWBOX

A, 3-D time-of-flight magnetic resonance angiogram (MRA) of the neck vessels in a 73-year-old female with dizziness and positive tests for vertebrobasilar insufficiency. There were regions of stenosis bilaterally. MRA, CT, and ultrasound represent noninvasive options for vascular imaging. Magnetic resonance angiography and conventional angiography require injection of contrast media. **B,** A second patient, a 44-year-old male with recent onset of dizziness, had a normal MRA of the circle of Willis and neck vessels (not shown). His dizziness resolved spontaneously and the etiology was never determined.

(From the teaching file of Timothy Mick, DC, DACBR)

BIKELE SIGN

Assessment for Brachial Plexus Neuritis and Meningitis

Comment

The most common and least understood cervical neural injury is neurapraxia of the nerve roots and brachial plexus. Brachial plexus lesions result in motor and sensory syndromes of muscles of the upper extremities. The brachial plexus is made up of the anterior primary rami of the four lower cervical nerves, C5 through C8, and the greater part of T1. The C5 and C6 rami form the upper trunk, the C7 ramus forms the middle trunk, and the C8 and T1 rami form the lower trunk. The brachial plexus lies in the supraclavicular fossa distal to the anterior scalene muscle. Each trunk splits into an anterior and posterior division, with derivation of three cords from them.

The lateral cord is formed by the anterior division of the upper and middle trunks, the medial cord by the anterior division of the lower trunk (C8 and T1), and the posterior cord by the posterior divisions of all three trunks and nerves. The upper trunk branches to the supraclavicular nerve, innervating the supraspinatus and infraspinatus muscles, as well as the subclavius muscles. The lateral cord branches to the lateral anterior thoracic nerve, innervating the greater pectoral muscle. The medial cord becomes the medial anterior thoracic cord, which goes to the pectoral muscles and the medial antebrachial and brachio cutaneous nerves.

The posterior cord branches to the subscapular nerve, which innervates the subscapular and teres major muscle, and the thoracodorsal nerve, which innervates the latissimus dorsi muscles. Terminal branches of the posterior cord are the axillary and radial nerves, and the terminal branches of the lateral cord are the musculocutaneous (biceps) component and the lateral component of the median nerve. The terminal branches of the medial cord are the ulnar nerve and the medial component of the median nerve.

Brachial plexopathy (sometimes called a *stinger*, *burner*, or *dead arm*) is also a possible result of a lateral flexion traction injury. The neurologic deficit may last for only a few seconds, or it may occur intermittently for several days. Swelling at the nerve root or distal to the spine can combine with traction to the nerve sleeves, making the deficit more severe (Fig. 3-54).

Idiopathic brachial plexitis was first reported by Feinberg in 1897. Various terms have been ascribed to it, such as brachial plexus neuropathy, acute brachial plexitis, acute shoulder neuritis, and Parsonage-Turner syndrome. The pathophysiologic mechanism of disease is unknown; however, the condition is generally thought to be an immune-mediated inflammatory reaction. Various events or factors can pre-

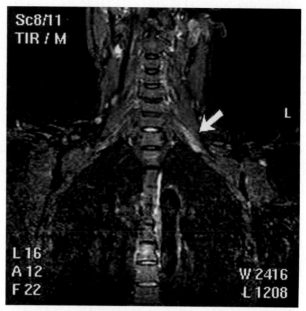

FIG. 3-54 Coronal short T1 inversion recovery (STIR) image showing increased signal intensity in the posterior cord of the left brachial plexus *(arrow)*. (Sarikaya S et al: Magnetic resonance neurography diagnosed brachial plexitis: a case report, *Arch Phys Med Rehabil* 86[5]:1058-1059, 2005.)

cipitate the condition, such as trauma, infection, viral disease, heavy exercise, surgery, immunization, and autoimmune mechanism. The most common symptom is an acute-onset severe pain in the shoulder girdle. The pain generally radiates from the shoulder to the upper arm or neck. Patients usually have weakness after the pain subsides. Weakness commonly occurs in the deltoid, supraspinatus, infraspinatus, and biceps muscles (Sarikaya et al, 2005).

PROCEDURE

- With the arm held upward and backward and the elbow fully flexed, the patient extends the elbow (Fig. 3-55).
- If this movement meets with resistance and increases radicular pain from the cervicodorsal region, the test is positive (Fig. 3-56).
- This finding suggests brachial plexus neuritis or meningitis because this maneuver stretches the brachial plexus nerve roots or their coverings.

Next Steps/Procedures

Reflexes, sensory testing, Bakody sign, Dejerine sign, Valsalva maneuver, maximum foraminal encroachment testing, shoulder depression test, distraction test, brachial

When reflex sympathetic symptoms are present, additional tests may be indicated. These tests include matchstick testing, pilomotor response testing, and thermography.

CLINICAL PEARL

Injury to the C8 and T1 roots, the lower trunk, or the medial cord of the brachial plexus may be caused by tumors, disease of the pulmonary apex, or a fractured clavicle or cervical rib. Aneurysm of the arch of the aorta, fracture or dislocation of the humeral head, or unusually abrupt and severe upward traction of the arm may also injure the nerves.

Although Bikele sign does not usually produce a profound finding in minor cervical nerve root compression syndromes, the maneuver often produces startling results in lower brachial plexopathy in the thoracic outlet. Reflex sympathetic changes may be present with the plexopathy and should be correlated with other physiologic findings.

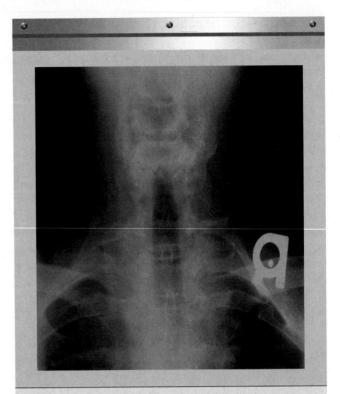

AT THE VIEWBOX

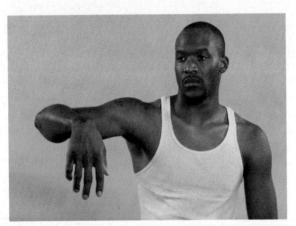

FIG. 3-55 The patient is seated and abducts the shoulder to 90 degrees. The internally is internally rotated.

A 59-year-old female with a long history of rheumatoid arthritis. Prior cervical spine surgical fusion and multiple peripheral joint arthroplasties. Manipulation of the cervicothoracic spine resulted in sudden, severe right axillary pain, gradually subsiding over the next two weeks (evidence of neuropraxia). Note large cervical ribs, more prominent on the right, with accessory articulation between the left C7 rib and the first thoracic rib, a variant of Srb's anomaly. This is nearly obscured by the right side marker. Cervical and upper thoracic rib anomalies may cause neurovascular compression syndromes of the brachial plexus. Other causes include tumor, trauma, and vascular lesions, which may be further assessed with MRI. When intrinsic abnormality of the brachial plexus is suspected, dedicated MRI of the brachial plexus is appropriate, but lesions of the brachial plexus may be occult on radiographs and on both cervical spine and brachial plexus MRI. Signs or symptoms of vascular compression would warrant angiography, which could include magnetic resonance angiography (MRA), a noninvasive option. These disorders are most often diagnosed based on clinical findings. (From the teaching file of Timothy Mick, DC, DACBR)

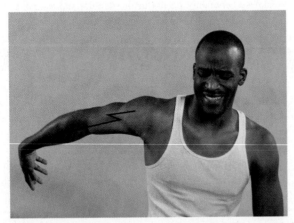

FIG. 3-56 The arm is fully extended at the elbow, and the patient attempts to reach behind. In the presence of radiculopathy or plexopathy, this maneuver produces the radicular pain.

Assessment for Cervical Nerve Root Syndrome or Compression (C5)

Comment

A direct traumatic insult to the nerve roots causes inflammation in the dural sleeves and perineural tissues, which may result in fibrosis. Adhesions may occur between the dural sleeves and the adjacent capsular tissues. Normally, the nerve roots are free in the intervertebral canals and can move $1/4$ to $1/2$ of an inch. Nerve roots that are injured or compressed by capsular thickening or bony encroachments cannot move within the intervertebral canals. Nerve roots subjected to compressive forces by osteophytic encroachments have varying amounts of distortion and perineural fibrosis.

In many instances, at least one fiber of a nerve root fails to continue in that particular nerve root. The aberrant fiber descends to join the adjacent distal nerve root. For instance, one of the fourth cervical nerve root fibers that leaves the cord at that level may actually leave the spinal canal with fibers of the fifth cervical nerve root. If the fourth cervical nerve root is irritated within the foramen of the fifth cervical nerve root, the examiner may find that the fourth cervical nerve is also involved.

The fifth cervical nerve root is irritated most often, and the sixth, fourth, third, second, and seventh roots become irritated in that order of frequency. Irritation or compression of a nerve root may cause pain-sensory changes anywhere along its distribution. Localized areas of tenderness and muscle spasm will be found at the site of the pain. The examiner often finds some areas of segmental tenderness of which the patient is not aware. These myalgic areas are found only by deep palpation because hyperalgesia, or superficial tenderness, is not present.

In cases affecting the fifth cervical root, the pain extends from the scapular area to the front of the arm and forearm and can extend as far as the radial side of the hand. However, the pain does not reach the thumb, and the pins-and-needles sensation is absent. The weak muscles are the supraspinatus, the infraspinatus, the deltoid, and the biceps. The biceps reflex may be sluggish or absent, and the brachioradialis reflex is sluggish, absent, or inverted.

From its position at the thoracic outlet, the brachial plexus is the neurologic switchboard responsible for transferring the sensory and motor impulses from the cervical nerve roots to the peripheral nerves of the first thoracic nerve root contributing to the plexus.

The examination of a person with a brachial plexopathy should begin with observation for round shoulders, forward neck, or obvious swelling. The examiner should palpate the

---

ORTHOPEDIC GAMUT 3-15

SLEEP PALSY OF THE BRACHIAL PLEXUS

- Positive neurologic examination
  - Winging of the scapula is usually caused by weakness of either serratus anterior (long thoracic nerve; C5–C7) or rhomboids (dorsal scapular nerve; C4–C5)
- Positive MRI
  - Increased T2-weighted signal on the MRI in supraspinatus, infraspinatus (suprascapular nerve; C5–C6), and teres minor (axillary nerve; C5–C6)
- Positive nerve-conduction study or electromyographic findings
  - More severe in the upper trunk as exhibited by prominent proximal arm weakness and electromyographic evidence of denervation in the shoulder muscles

---

paraspinal region for spasm or hypertonicity in the musculature. Similarly, the examiner should palpate the supraclavicular area for swelling, spasm, or masses that can adversely affect the brachial plexus.

The individual with brachial plexopathy usually has transient paresis of the upper limb because of an excessive lateral flexion injury of the cervical spine, with or without shoulder depression. Paresthesia generally emanates from the middle or lower cord of the plexus, reproducing the usual distribution of the dysesthetic response seen in contact sports injuries called *burners* or *stingers*. Sometimes the entire hand goes numb and weak, and the individual tries to shake the limb to reduce the pain.

> Sleep palsy, or so-called *Saturday night palsy*, has been reported in patients who sleep on their arm at night after an alcohol binge, and typically affects the radial nerve. Similarly, sciatic, peroneal and tibial nerve injuries related to prolonged compression from poor positioning have also been reported (Sathornsumetee, Morgenlander, 2006).

Brachial neurapraxia involves demyelination of the axon sheath without disruption. In some neuronal injuries, the axon is interrupted, but the surrounding tissues remain intact. Degeneration of the affected muscles (axonotmesis) appears on electrodiagnostic studies 2 to 3 weeks after sustaining the neural injury. Patterns of reinnervation often develop. In contrast, recovery from neurotmesis, a severe injury that destroys the axon and supporting structures, is unlikely.

The **brachial plexus tension test** is used clinically to *test the dynamics of the neural tissues of the upper quadrant. The* upper trapezius muscle and the nerves of the **brachial plexus** share common anatomic locations and are jointly affected by brachial plexus tension test movements (Balster, Jull, 1997).

PROCEDURE

- The examiner passively elevates the patient's shoulders through abduction (Figs. 3-57 and 3-58).
- The elbows are extended to a point just short of the onset of pain and are maintained in that position.
- The shoulders are externally rotated to the point just short of the onset of pain and maintained (Fig. 3-59).
- The examiner supports the shoulders and forearms in this position as the patient flexes the elbows (Fig. 3-60).
- Reproduction of symptoms suggests cervical spine disorders, most likely the C5 nerve root.
- In addition, from this challenge position, symptoms increase when the cervical spine is flexed.

Next Steps/Procedures

Dejerine sign, Valsalva maneuver, reflex testing, Bakody sign, maximum foraminal encroachment test, shoulder depression test, distraction test, Bikele sign, Jackson cervical compression test, Spurling test, and diagnostic imaging

CLINICAL PEARL

Although the brachial plexus tension test involves shoulder joint movement, it also provides maximal stretch on the brachial plexus, which affects the lower branches of the cervical spine (C5) the most. If this test is positive, the early stages of a C5 nerve root disorder may be present along with the subtle signs of a positive *doorbell sign* (pain that occurs at the superior scapulo-vertebral border and radiates with deep palpation to the C5 segment) and pain in the deltoid area. The deltoid pain is often misconstrued as an articular problem of the shoulder.

3

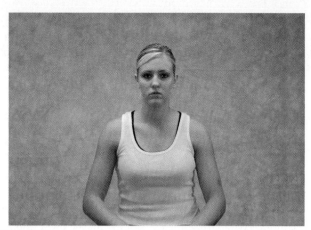

FIG. 3-57 The patient is sitting erect. *An alternative is to have the patient assume the supine position on the examination table.*

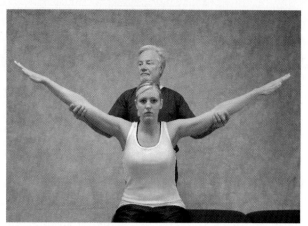

FIG. 3-58 The examiner fully elevates the patient's shoulders through abduction to the end-point of joint play. The elbows are fully extended. The examiner supports the patient's arms in this position.

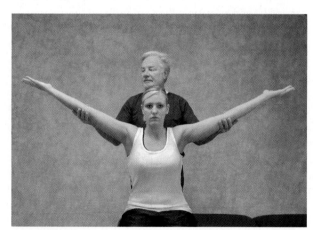

FIG. 3-59 The patient externally rotates the shoulders to the end-point of joint play or to the onset of discomfort. The examiner continues to support the patient's arms in this position.

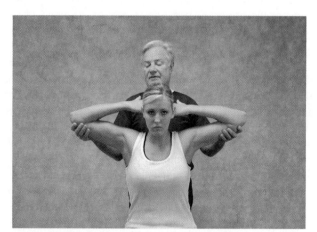

FIG. 3-60 As the shoulders are supported in this position, the patient flexes the elbows, maintaining ***full external rotation of the shoulders*** (the backs of the hands should contact the back of the patient's head or neck). In more severe nerve root compression syndromes, external rotation of the shoulders and full flexion of the elbows may not be possible to complete. Reproduction of the radicular symptoms suggests a nerve root syndrome that probably involves C5. If symptoms do not appear, a final maneuver is flexion of the cervical spine.

DEJERINE TRIAD
TRIAD OF DEJERINE

Assessment for Herniated or Protruding Intervertebral Disc and Spinal Cord Tumor or Spinal Compression Fracture

Comments

The symptoms of a cervical disc injury vary according to the status and site of the injury. Acute disc protrusions typically have radicular symptoms down one arm; the pain can be bilateral if the spinal canal is compromised and the protrusion is central or large. Motor, reflex, or sensory changes are a distinct possibility, and the examiner should examine the patient regularly for such changes during the first 2 weeks of care. The presence of Dejerine sign (pain on coughing, sneezing, or straining) suggests a space-occupying lesion. Compression tests with the patient in various positions are elucidating. The position of the disc bulge or the site of the canal-nerve root compromise of the cervical spine causes pain in patients with disc and nerve root lesions; distraction maneuvers are usually palliative.

Referred pain to the arm, hand, and scapula is common. Injury to the C5 nerve root level often causes scapular pain. During the acute phase the patient experiences muscle spasm and guarding, local or referred pain from annular nerve fiber stimulation or posterior joint dysfunction. A distinct loss of range of motion is observed, and some swelling may be present. Patients often complain of instability, such as difficulty rising from the recumbent position.

Infections and tumors, benign or malignant, are rare occurrences in the cervical spine. The cervical spine is unique, anatomically and physiologically, with its concentration of crowded, critical structures. Rapid clinical catastrophe is a constant threat unless early diagnosis of tumor and infection is instituted. Neurologic structures have little tolerance to mechanical compression. The possibilities of quadriplegia, spinal cord stroke, and death are always in the background. The close anatomic and physiologic relationships among the spinal cord, nerve roots, and peripheral nervous system and the structurally confining implications of the skeletal and soft tissues make early diagnosis mandatory in these cervical spinal disorders.

Space-occupying lesions that are in or around the spinal canal cause a broad spectrum of clinical syndromes ranging from neck pain, radiculitis, and paresthesia to quadriparesis and death. Cervical cord compression can be caused by the gross space occupation of an expanding abscess; a rapidly growing vertebral, medullary, or extramedullary tumor; or the fracture, collapse, and dislocation of the supporting structures. These structures include the bones, discs, joints, ligaments, and tendons.

Critical structures that are at risk when tumors and infections of the cervical spine are present include the lower brainstem, cervical spinal cord, nerve roots and rootlets, ganglia and common spinal nerves, VAs, carotid artery, trachea, and esophagus.

Radiating pain in the cervical spine, shoulder, and arm that is accompanied by tenderness, muscle spasms, and decreased cervical spine movements may be the only clinical manifestations of a benign, space-occupying mass. Torticollis is more common in masses involving the upper cervical spine. Mass enlargement or bony displacement may cause clinical symptoms and signs of radiculitis or spinal cord compression. Spinal stroke occurs when the radicular arteries, the end arteries in the cord itself, or the anterior and posterior spinal arteries are constricted. Myelopathy caused by disc herniation in the cervical and thoracic spine without symptoms or abnormal neurologic signs in the upper extremities, is a rare condition.

Clinical manifestations of cervical disc disease are highly variable. Patients may have many complaints and physical findings. Generally, signs and symptoms can be categorized as neurogenic or discogenic.

Neurogenic symptoms result from pressure on the cervical nerve roots or the spinal cord by disc material or by posterior or posterolateral osteophytes. Patients may have radicular symptoms alone, or they may have signs and symptoms of nerve root and spinal cord compression simultaneously.

Patients with *discogenic* symptoms have no objective dermatomal neurologic findings. Patients complain of intermittent, chronic pain in the posterior cervical region and the shoulder, chest wall, and scapular region. Occipital headaches are common. The pain experienced by patients with discogenic symptoms results from the stimulation of the sensory receptors of the sinuvertebral nerve. The sinuvertebral nerve is located in the fibrous ring of the intervertebral disc and in the posterior and anterior longitudinal ligament.

Root pain is often produced or aggravated by coughing, sneezing, or straining, such as during defecation or any other measures that suddenly increase intrathoracic and intra-abdominal pressure. Because the intervertebral veins do not contain valves, such pressure increases block the venous flow from the epidural space through the intervertebral veins or permit a retrograde flow of blood. This pressure increase causes distension of the veins in the epidural space, which in turn forces the dura, which envelops the nerve roots, toward the spinal cord. Because the nerve roots are fixed to the spinal cord proximally and peripherally at the intervertebral foramen, the displacement of the dura results in a stretching of the involved nerve root, which may result in pain. In addition, distension of the intervertebral vein may result in direct compression of the nerve root.

Reports show that 52% to 69% of cervical disc herniation causing radiculopathy occur at the C6-C7 level, whereas only 4% to 6% of such herniation causing myelopathy occur at this level. Matsumoto and colleagues retrospectively analyzed the neurologic signs of 106 patients with cervical myelopathy caused by single-level soft disc herniation. According to this report, only 6 patients (6%) had disc herniation at C6-C7, and their neurologic signs included normal deep-tendon reflexes in the upper extremities in all patients, sensory disturbances below the C8 level and numbness on the ulnar side of the hands in three patients, no sensory deficits in the upper extremities in the other three patients, and positive Hoffmann's reflex in only one patient (Sasai et al, 2006).

PROCEDURE

- Coughing, sneezing, and straining during defecation may aggravate radiculitis symptoms (Fig. 3-61).
- This aggravation results from the mechanical obstruction of spinal fluid flow.
- Dejerine sign is present when one of the following exists: herniated or protruding intervertebral disc, spinal cord tumor, or spinal compression fracture.
- The course of the radiculitis helps identify the location of the lesion.

Next Steps/Procedures
Swallowing test, Valsalva maneuver, Naffziger test, vascular assessment, and diagnostic imaging (e.g., MRI)

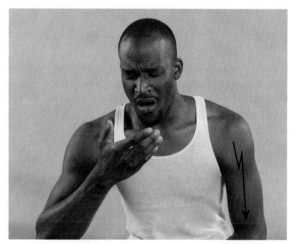

FIG. 3-61 Coughing, sneezing, or straining during defecation causes a reproduction of radicular symptoms, which suggests a space-occupying mass that is creating neurologic compression.

CLINICAL PEARL

Patients with radicular symptoms and pronounced Dejerine sign, especially if it is in the lumbar spine, should be told to bend the knees and lean into a wall during a cough or sneeze. This maneuver reduces intradiscal pressure and minimizes the effect of the cough or sneeze on the nerve root. A more worrisome situation is the sudden, unexpected absence of Dejerine sign when all other clinical findings indicate an active nerve root compression. The loss of the sign indicates fragmentation of the disc with momentary decompression of the nerve.

DEKLEYN TEST

Assessment for Vertebral Artery Syndrome

Comment

The VA is often the first and largest branch of the subclavian artery. It passes upward to enter the foramen in the sixth cervical transverse process. It continues to course upward, encased by the bony rings formed by the transverse foramina. After emerging from the transverse foramen of the atlas, the VA proceeds to wind posteriorly and medially around the lateral mass of the atlas. The VA then passes through the foramen magnum and at the lower border of the pons unites with the VA of the opposite side to form the basilar artery. The posterior inferior cerebellar arteries leave the VAs just before they join each other (Fig. 3-62).

VA syndrome (also called *VA compression syndrome* or *vertebrobasilar artery insufficiency*) is characterized by recurring transient episodes of cerebral symptoms (Fig. 3-63). The notable cerebral symptoms include vertigo, nystagmus, and sudden postural collapse without unconsciousness. These symptoms are precipitated by rotation and hyperextension of the neck and are caused by temporary occlusion of the VA. This mechanical action produces ischemia at the base of the brain. A combination of cerebrovascular arteriosclerosis and cervical spondylosis is fundamental in this syndrome.

Vertebral basilar arterial dissection frequently causes headache and cervical pain. However, the reported interval between dissection and the appearance of neurologic symptoms has varied among previous studies. Most patients

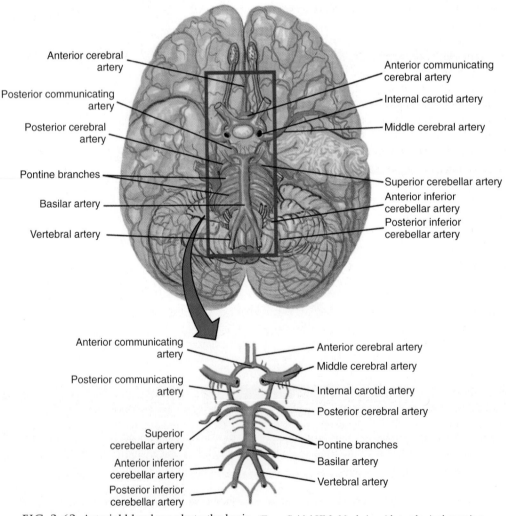

FIG. 3-62 Arterial blood supply to the brain. (From Seidel HM: *Mosby's guide to physical examination,* ed 4, St Louis, 1999, Mosby.)

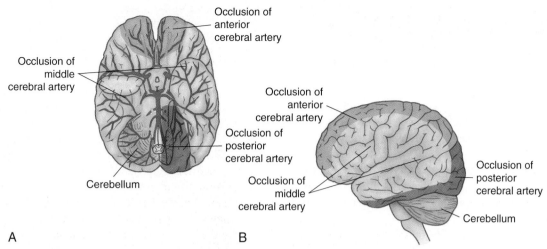

FIG. 3-63 Areas of the brain affected by occlusion of the anterior, middle, and posterior cerebral artery branches. **A,** Inferior view. **B,** Lateral view. (From Seidel HM: *Mosby's guide to physical examination,* ed 4, St Louis, 1999, Mosby.)

develop neurologic symptoms immediately or within 24 hours after onset. However, some patients develop these symptoms a few weeks after onset. Noninvasive MRI may be useful for definitively diagnosing cerebral arterial dissection. Some authors have reported that an intramural thrombus suggesting vertebral basilar arterial dissection on T1-weighted images and an intimal flap or double lumen on T2-weighted images are more frequently detected by MRI than by cerebral angiography (Nomura et al, 2004).

The main tributaries to the basilar artery at the base of the brain are the internal carotid and VAs. Occlusive arterial disease gradually reduces blood flow to a certain critical point. Any further reduction in the caliber of the vessel, unless an adequate collateral supply has developed, will result in ischemia and cerebral symptoms.

Normally, hyperextension and rotation of the neck compresses and may occlude the VA on the contralateral side at the level of the atlas and axis. However, symptoms do not develop because collateral circulation is adequate. When vessels are occluded by atheromatous plaques and compressed by osteophytes, collateral blood flow may be insufficient, and symptoms may develop as the VA becomes blocked momentarily during the rotation and hyperextension movement of the cervical spine.

Various causes of dizziness must first be ruled out, particularly those caused by labyrinthine or cerebellar disease. The drop attack must be differentiated from epilepsy, syncope, and Stokes-Adams syndrome. Carotid sinus sensitivity, with its cardioinhibitory and vasodepressor reflexes, can be identified by an electrocardiogram that is conducted while the carotid sinus is massaged.

Subclavian steal syndrome must be ruled out because its symptoms are caused by basilar artery insufficiency. However, syncopal episodes are precipitated by exertion of the upper extremity. With the subclavian steal syndrome, occlusion occurs at the portion of the subclavian artery that

---

ORTHOPEDIC GAMUT 3-16

VERTEBRAL ARTERY PATENCY TESTS

Several variations of the vertebral artery patency tests include:
1. Houle test
2. DeKleyn test
3. Smith and Estridge maneuver (see Note 1 below)
4. Modified Adson maneuver
5. Extension rotation test
6. Maigne test (see Note 1 below)
7. Wallenberg test
8. Reclination test (see Note 2 below)

---

is proximal to the origin of the VA. Because of this occlusion, blood flow is diverted from the opposite VA into the artery on the obstructed side, which results in perfusion of the distal subclavian bed with blood that was intended for cerebral circulation.

Note 1: Maigne Maneuver and Smith and Estridge Maneuver

The patient's head is maintained for several seconds in a position of rotation and extension. The patient is asked to comment on the development of any symptoms of vertebrobasilar insufficiency, and the examiner observes for nystagmus. If vertebrobasilar insufficiency signs or symptoms occur, the head is immediately returned to a neutral position.

Note 2: Reclination Test (Sitting)

With the patient sitting, the examiner moves the patient's head into extreme positions of extension and rotation. If

ORTHOPEDIC GAMUT 3-17

POTENTIAL SITES OF COMPRESSION OR INJURY DURING SPINAL MOVEMENT

At least eight potential sites have been identified in the cervical spine at which arterial structures can be compressed or injured by spinal movement:

1. Between C1–C2 transverse processes (Rotation tends to produce stretching of the VA at this site.)
2. At the level C2–C3 as a result of compression of the VA by the superior articular facet of C3 on the ipsilateral side to head rotation
3. By the C1 transverse process compressing the internal carotid artery
4. At the C4–C5 or C5–C6 level as a result of osteoarthrosis of the uncovertebral joints, which can displace the VA anteriorly and laterally (Compression of the artery is ipsilateral to the side of head rotation.)
5. As a result of compression before entering the C6 transverse process, by traction over a prominent longus colli muscle, or by tissue communicating between the longus colli and scalenus anticus muscles
6. By constriction of the VA by the ventral ramus of the second cervical nerve during head rotation
7. At the atlantooccipital aperture, on extension:
   - By compression between the posterior arch of atlas and the foramen magnum
   - By folding of the atlantooccipital joint capsule anteriorly and the atlantooccipital membrane posteriorly
8. By compression by the oblique capitis inferior muscle or intertransversarii muscle between the transverse foramina of C1 and C2

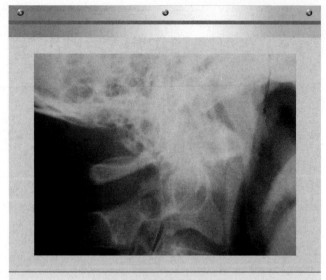

AT THE VIEWBOX

Adult male with neck pain, headache, and dizziness. No trauma or other common cause of C1 transverse ligament laxity. Spina bifida occulta of C1 (note absent spinolaminar junction line) and anterior C1–2 subluxation. This is an uncommon cause of C1–2 subluxation and instability. An enlarged C2 transverse foramen raises question of vertebral artery aneurysm or tortuosity versus a normal variant. Vertebral artery compromise may result form any cause of anterior C1–2 subluxation, including os odontoideum, unstable dens fracture, and chronic inflammatory arthritis. Follow-up imaging with magnetic resonance angiography (MRA) or other dedicated vascular imaging helps distinguish a normal variant from vertebral artery tortuosity producing the expanded transverse foramen. Advanced imaging is appropriate when there is clinical evidence of vertebrobasilar artery compromise. Radiographs may be negative or may demonstrate findings that are not clearly related to the clinical findings. (From the teaching file of Timothy Mick, DC, DACBR)

threatening signs or symptoms occur, the head is returned to the neutral position.

Normally, even if these maneuvers occlude one VA, no symptoms occur because adequate brainstem blood flow occurs through the opposite VA. These tests, when positive, indicate only that rotation has produced brainstem ischemia, possibly resulting from compression of one VA and in-adequate patency of the opposite artery. Additionally, these tests do not necessarily indicate any underlying arteriopathy that would predispose the patient to arterial wall damage and vertebrobasilar syndrome.

PROCEDURE

- With the patient in the supine position and the patient's head off the table, the examiner instructs the patient to hyperextend and rotate the head and hold this position for 15 to 45 seconds (Fig. 3-64).
- The patient repeats this maneuver with the head rotated and extended to the opposite side.
- Vertigo, blurred vision, nausea, syncope, and nystagmus are signs of a positive test.

Next Steps/Procedures

Hautant test, George screening procedure, Underburg test, Hallpike maneuver, vertebrobasilar artery functional maneuver, Barré-Liéou sign, vascular assessment, vascular imaging, and MRI

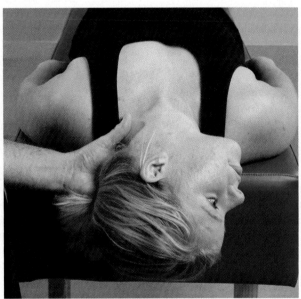

FIG. 3-64 The patient is supine with the head extending off the end of the examination table. The patient rotates and hyperextends the neck to one side and holds this position for 15 to 45 seconds. The examiner may provide minimal support for the weight of the skull. The maneuver is repeated for the opposite side. The production of vertigo, visual disturbance, nausea, syncope, or nystagmus suggests vertebrobasilar circulation compromise.

Assessment for Cervical Nerve Root Compression, Intervertebral Foraminal Encroachment, and Facet Capsulitis

Comment

Cervical spondylotic radiculopathy is a common degenerative problem associated with neck and arm pain. The pathogenesis of spondylotic radiculopathy often relates to foraminal narrowing resulting from uncovertebral and facet joint hypertrophy, as well as disc height collapse (Jenis et al, 2002).

Synovial folds (menisci) from Z joints project into the Z joints at all levels of the cervical spine.

When the individual vertebrae are united, the articular process of each side of the cervical spine forms an articular pilar that bulges laterally at the pediculolaminar junction (Fig. 3-66).

The cervical articular pillars support the weight of the head and neck. Therefore, weight bearing in the cervical region is carried out by a series of three longitudinal columns: one anterior column, which runs through the vertebral bodies, and two posterior columns, which run through the right and left articular pillars.

Articular pillar fracture is fairly common in the cervical spine and often goes undetected. This type of fracture is usually a chip fracture of a superior articular facet. The patient often experiences transient radicular pain, which is usually followed by mild to intense neck pain. Persistent radiculopathy in such patients indicates displacement of the fractured facet onto the dorsal root as it exits the intervertebral foramen.

The complaints of patients with chronic or degenerative conditions of the cervical disc are quite different from those of patients with acute conditions. Patients with chronic conditions experience intermittent episodes of pain, discomfort, and muscle spasm. Exacerbations come from exertion. Pain and stiffness may result from weather changes or unexplained causes. Radiculopathy is not always present. Hyporeflexia, motor weakness, and sensory disturbance (especially paresthesia) are common (Table 3-7).

In cervical spine hyperflexion or hyperextension injuries, significant indirect signs of trauma can be observed (Table 3-8). These signs are evident on typical plain-film radiographic studies.

Whiplash injuries are commonly, but not exclusively, associated with road traffic accidents (RTAs). A rear-end RTA usually involves a sudden acceleration then deceleration with resultant hyperflexion, hyperextension and, possibly, lateral flexion or torsional forces to the cervical spine. Most RTAs are not fatal and result in a sprain or strain type of injury to the muscles, ligaments, soft tissues, intervertebral discs, and facet joints of the cervical spine. This type of injury leads to local tissue inflammation, edema, muscle spasm, stiffness, and nociception as a result of altered cervical facet joint biomechanics together with proprioceptive dysfunction. In more severe cases, radicular arm pain caused by nerve root traction or discal lesion may also be present or, indeed, myelopathy as a result of spinal cord damage. Patients may also complain of headaches, dizziness, blurred vision, dysphagia, paresthesia, shoulder girdle pain, temporomandibular joint dysfunction, and cognitive difficulties after a whiplash-type injury. These related symptoms are known as whiplash-associated disorders and were classified in 1995 by the Quebec Task Force study (Alpass, 2004).

Whiplash injuries from motor-vehicle crashes, although common, remain a poorly understood clinical entity. Most individuals recover within a few weeks of injury, but a significant proportion (14% to 42%) will develop persistent ongoing pain, with 10% reporting constant severe pain. These people with persistent symptoms are the ones who contribute substantially to the significant economic costs related to this condition (Sterling, 2004).

ORTHOPEDIC GAMUT 3-18

Z JOINT MENISCI

Four distinct types of cervical Z joint menisci exist (Fig. 3-65):

Type I: Menisci are thin and protrude far into the Z joints, covering approximately 50% of the joint surface (found only in children).

Type II: Menisci are relatively large wedges that protrude a significant distance into the joint space (found almost exclusively at the lateral C1–C2 Z joints).

Type III: Folds are rather small nubs (found throughout the C2–C3 to C6–C7 cervical Z joints of most healthy adults).

Type IV: Menisci are quite large and thick (found in degenerative Z joints).

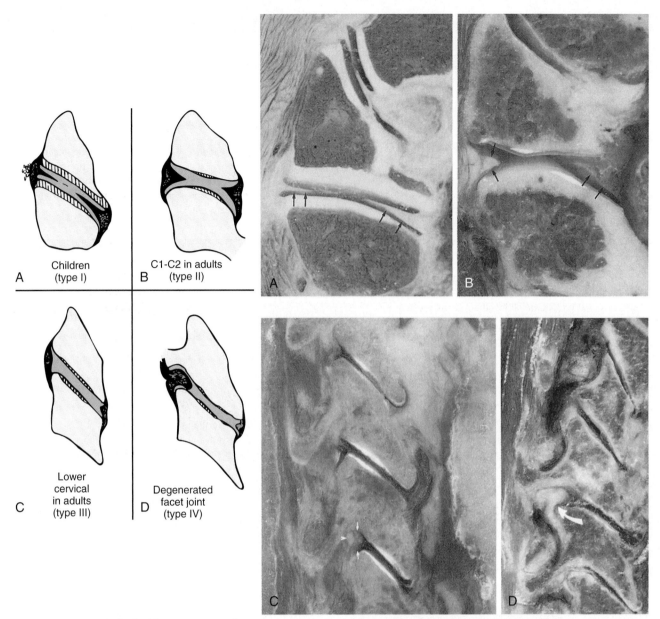

FIG. 3-65 Four types of menisci (*left* and *right*). **A,** Type I. **B,** Type II. **C,** Type III. **D,** Type IV. (From Yu et al: *Brain,* vol 109, Oxford, UK, 1986, Oxford University Press.)

TABLE 3-7

COMMON CLINICAL FEATURES OF CERVICAL DISC SYNDROMES

Disc	Pain	Sensory Change	Motor Weakness, Atrophy	Reflex Change
C4–C5 (C5 root)	Base of neck, shoulder, anterolateral aspect of arm	Numbness in deltoid region	Deltoid, biceps	Biceps
C5–C6 (C6 root)	Neck, shoulder, medial border of scapula, lateral aspect of arm, dorsum of forearm	Dorsolateral aspect of thumb and index finger	Biceps, extensor pollicis longus	Biceps, brachioradialis
C6–C7 (C7 root)	Neck, shoulder, medial border of scapula, lateral aspect of arm, dorsum of forearm	Index and middle fingers, dorsum of hand	Triceps	Triceps

Adapted from Mercier LR: *Practical orthopedics*, ed 4, St Louis, 1995, Mosby.

TABLE 3-8

CLINICAL PRESENTATIONS IN CERVICAL RADICULOPATHIES

	C5	C6	C7	C8
Pain	To parascapular area, shoulder, and upper arm	To shoulder, arm, forearm, and thumb/index finger	To posterior arm, forearm, and index/middle fingers	To medial arm, forearm, and little/ring fingers
Sensory	Upper arm	Lateral arm, forearm, and thumb/index fingers	Index and middle fingers	Medial arm, forearm, and little finger
Motor	Scapular fixators, shoulder abduction, and elbow flexion	Shoulder abduction, elbow flexion, and forearm pronation	Elbow extension, wrist and fingers extension	Hand intrinsics, long flexors and extensors of fingers
Hyporeflexia/areflexia	Biceps and/or brachioradialis reflexes	Biceps and/or brachioradialis reflexes	Triceps reflex	None

Adapted from Katirji B: *Electromyography in clinical practice: a case study approach*, St Louis, 1998, Mosby.

ORTHOPEDIC GAMUT 3-19

INDIRECT SIGNS OF CERVICAL TRAUMA OR INJURY

Abnormal Soft Tissue

Hemorrhage caused by injury of the paracervical soft tissues displaces certain physiologic spaces that are appreciated radiographically, representing a space-occupying lesion:

1. Widened retropharyngeal space (in excess of 7 mm)
2. Widened retrotracheal space (in excess of 21 mm)
3. Displacement of the prevertebral fat stripe
4. Tracheal deviation and laryngeal dislocation

Abnormal Vertebral Alignment

Injury of soft tissue (a strain or sprain of muscle, tendon, ligament, and capsule) produces spasm, identified by the following:

1. Loss of lordosis
2. Acute kyphotic hyper angulation
3. Torticollis
4. Widened interspinous space
5. Rotation of vertebral bodies (one spinous process significantly rotated, suggests unilateral facet dislocation)
6. Widened middle atlantoaxial joint (the atlantodental interspace) (in excess of 2 mm in adults or 5 mm in children)
7. Abnormal intervertebral disc
8. Widening of apophyseal joints

PROCEDURE

- With the patient seated, the examiner exerts upward pressure on the patient's head (Figs. 3-67 and 3-68).
- This pressure removes the weight of the patient's head from the neck.
- Generalized, increased pain indicates muscle spasm.
- Relief of pain indicates intervertebral foraminal encroachment or facet capsulitis.
- The examiner continues the distraction for up to 30 to 60 seconds to relax the involved tissues completely (Fig. 3-69).
- This test provides some prediction of the effect of cervical spine traction in relieving pain or paresthesia.
- Nerve root compression may be relieved, with disappearance of the symptoms and signs, if the intervertebral foramina are opened or the disc spaces extended.
- Pressure on the joint capsules of the apophyseal joints is also decreased by distraction.

Next Steps/Procedures

Bakody sign, maximum foraminal encroachment test, shoulder depression test, brachial plexus tension test, Bikele sign, Jackson cervical compression test, Spurling test, reflexes, and diagnostic imaging

CLINICAL PEARL

The distraction test not only indicates the nature of the patient's complaint but also identifies the merit of cervical traction in the treatment regimen. Notably, the higher the poundage of *static* cervical traction required for relief is, the more unstable the nerve compression syndrome will be. Indeed, the higher poundage requirement is often an indicator of the need for surgical resolution.

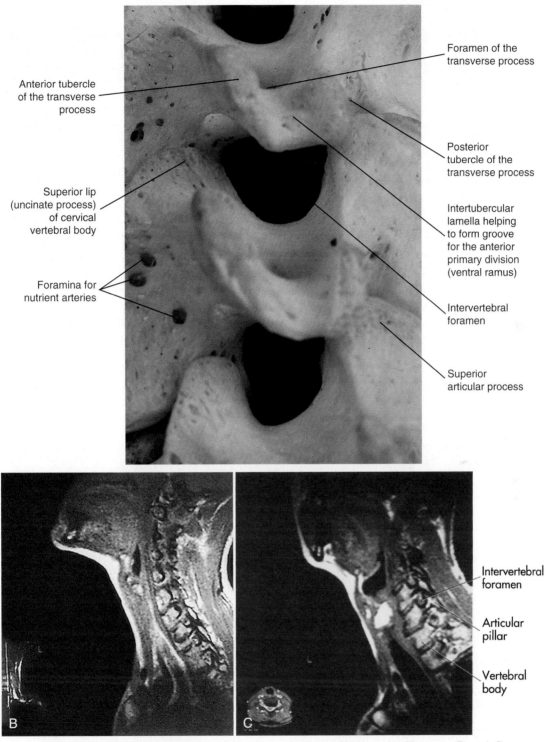

FIG. 3-66 Obliquely oriented cervical intervertebral foramina. **A,** Close-up. **B** and **C,** Standard magnetic resonance imaging scans. (From Cramer GD, Darby SA: *Basic and clinical anatomy of the spine, spinal cord, and ANS,* St Louis, 1995, Mosby.)

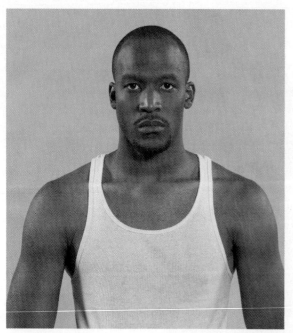

FIG. 3-67 The patient is seated comfortably, with the spine erect and the head and neck in a neutral position.

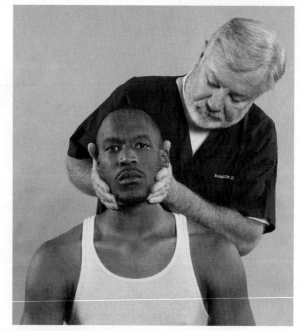

FIG. 3-68 With the hands cupping the patient's mandible and occiput, the examiner lifts the patient's head. A positive finding is the relief of the patient's localized or radicular pain. The sign is confirmed if the symptoms return when the weight of the head is returned to the neck.

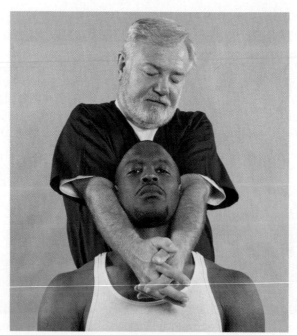

FIG. 3-69 Alternatively, the examiner can lift the patient's head by clasping the forearms under the patient's mandible. In this procedure the back of the patient's head is fixed against the examiner's chest. In both methods the lift or distraction is maintained for as many seconds as possible but not beyond patient tolerance.

Assessment for Cervical Nerve Root Encroachment

Comment

Cervical radiculopathy (CR) is a disorder that is painful and often disabling. Limited work has been performed to determine the prevalence and incidence of CR; however, Radhakrishnan and colleagues estimated the average annual age-adjusted incidence in Rochester, Minnesota, to be 83.2 per 100 000 people. Whether an increased incidence exists by sex is unclear. The most common levels affected are C6 and C7, with conflicting evidence as to which of these two levels is most commonly involved. The most common causes of CR are lateral canal stenosis and cervical disk herniation (CDH). Lateral canal stenosis involves encroachment on the intervertebral foramen from osteophytes from the vertebral body or the Z joint or ligamentum flavum hypertrophy (or both). CDH involves herniation of disk material into the intervertebral foramen. In both cases, nerve root pain and dysfunction can occur (Murphy et al, 2006).

Radiculopathy can result from disc or osteophyte encroachment on one or several cervical nerve roots, especially C6 (C5–C6 disc) and C7 (C6–C7 disc). Such encroachment may result in pain or paresthesias affecting the upper limb dermatomes at the involved levels, with weakness and hyporeflexia (Fig. 3-70).

Approximately one fifth of the intervertebral foramen in the cervical region is filled by the dorsal and ventral roots (medially) or the spinal nerve (laterally). When the spine is in the neutral position, the dorsal and ventral roots are located in the inferior portion of the foramen at or below the disc level. Hypertrophy of the superior and inferior articular processes secondary to degeneration (osteoarthritis) of the Z joints may result in compression of the dorsal rootlets, dorsal root, or dorsal root ganglion.

The outer fibers of the annulus fibrosis of the cervical intervertebral discs are richly supplied with sensory receptors from which impulses are transmitted by way of the sinuvertebral nerve. When the anterior fibers of each of the cervical discs from C3 to C7 are stimulated on one side of the midline, pain is referred to the vertebral border of the scapula on the ipsilateral side (doorbell sign). Pain from the upper cervical discs develops a more cephalad level along the inner border of the scapula. Pain from the lower disc develops at a more caudad level. When the anterior peripheral fibers are stimulated in the midline, pain develops in the interscapular area.

If the disc is ruptured in a posterior or posterolateral direction, the resulting pain is of three types: discogenic, neurogenic, or myelogenic.

In *discogenic* pain, the disc rupture extends to but not through the peripheral fibers. Pain develops first at the medial scapular border and then spreads to the shoulder and down the posterior surface of the arm as far as the elbow. This type of disc rupture produces a sometimes severe deep, dull, aching sensation that usually subsides in 5 to 10 minutes.

In *neurogenic* pain, the peripheral fibers of the disc are lacerated with or without herniation of disc fragments into the spinal canal. Fluid pressure is transmitted through the defect resting against the nerve root and spinal cord. Neurogenic pain that is the result of nerve root irritation has a sharper, more intense quality that is described as an electric shock or a hot burning sensation. This type of pain shoots into the arm, forearm, and hand along a dermatome distribution.

Myelogenic pain results from a central posterior defect, which permits a midline protrusion and spinal cord compression, allowing the pressure of the disc to be transmitted to the spinal cord. This pain produces a momentary shocklike sensation (Lhermitte's sign) that shoots downward along the spine and that may spread into one or several extremities. An electrodiagnostic study (EDX) is useful in discriminating pain origins.

In the population of patients with upper-limb and neck symptoms referred for an EDX, the medical history and physical examination are helpful in predicting the outcome of an EDX when they show positive findings. A normal physical examination does not, however, rule out the possibility of an abnormal EDX, and electromyography is still necessary to differentiate those patients with true versus false negative physical examination findings (Lauder et al, 2000).

ORTHOPEDIC GAMUT 3-20

INTERVERTEBRAL FORAMEN

An intervertebral foramen may enlarge as a result of various pathologic conditions:

1. Neurofibroma (most common)
2. Meningioma
3. Fibroma
4. Lipoma
5. Herniated meningocele
6. Tortuous VA
7. Congenital absence of the pedicle with malformation of the transverse process
8. Chordoma

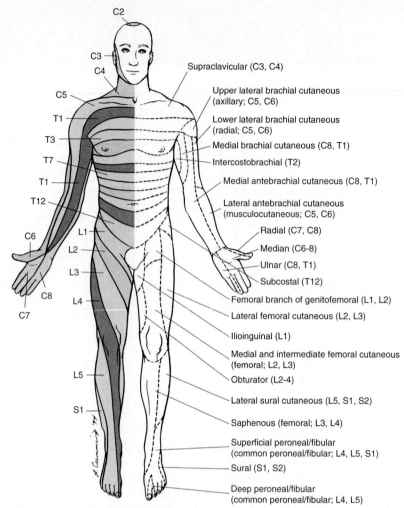

FIG. 3-70 **A,** Anterior view of the body showing its cutaneous innervation. *Left:* Dermatomal pattern. *Right:* Areas of cutaneous peripheral nerve distributions.

PROCEDURE

- With the patient in the seated position, the examiner rotates the patient's neck while exerting strong downward pressure on the head (Figs. 3-71 to 3-73). Pressure is first applied with the head in a neutral position, and then with the head rotated to the side of complaint.
- The test is then repeated bilaterally (Fig. 3-74).
- When the neck is rotated and downward pressure is applied, closure of the intervertebral foramen occurs.
- Localized pain indicates foraminal encroachment.
- Radicular pain indicates pressure on the nerve root.
- If nerve root involvement is suspected, the neurologic level must be evaluated.

Next Steps/Procedures

Bakody sign, maximum foraminal encroachment test, shoulder depression test, distraction test, brachial plexus tension test, Bikele sign, Jackson cervical compression test, Spurling test, reflex and sensory testing, electrodiagnosis, and diagnostic imaging

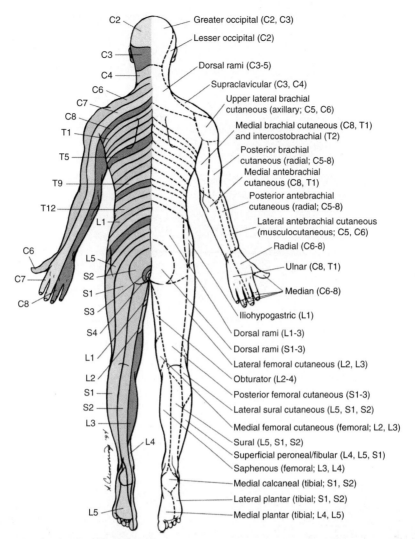

C2
Greater occipital (C2, C3)
Lesser occipital (C2)
C3
Dorsal rami (C3-5)
C4
Supraclavicular (C3, C4)
C6
Upper lateral brachial
cutaneous (axillary; C5, C6)
C7
C8
Medial brachial cutaneous (C8, T1)
and intercostobrachial (T2)
T1
Posterior brachial
cutaneous (radial; C5-8)
T5
Medial antebrachial
cutaneous (C8, T1)
T9
Posterior antebrachial
cutaneous (radial; C5-8)
T12
Lateral antebrachial cutaneous
(musculocutaneous; C5, C6)
L1
Radial (C6-8)
C6
Ulnar (C8, T1)
L5
C7
S2
Median (C6-8)
S1
C8
S3
Iliohypogastric (L1)
S4
Dorsal rami (L1-3)
L1
Dorsal rami (S1-3)
L2
Lateral femoral cutaneous (L2, L3)
S1
Obturator (L2-4)
S2
Posterior femoral cutaneous (S1-3)
L3
Lateral sural cutaneous (L5, S1, S2)
Medial femoral cutaneous (femoral; L2, L3)
L4
Sural (L5, S1, S2)
Superficial peroneal/fibular (L4, L5, S1)
Saphenous (femoral; L3, L4)
Medial calcaneal (tibial; S1, S2)
Lateral plantar (tibial; S1, S2)
L5
Medial plantar (tibial; L4, L5)

FIG. 3-70, CONT'D **B,** Posterior view of the body showing its cutaneous innervation. *Left:* Dermatomal pattern. *Right:* Areas of cutaneous peripheral nerve distributions. (From Cramer GD, Darby SA: *Basic and clinical anatomy of the spine, spinal cord, and ANS,* St Louis, 1995, Mosby.)

CLINICAL PEARL

This test, as well as other compression maneuvers, often produces a *cervical collapse sign* in addition to radicular complaints. In the presence of capsular sprain with radicular components, compression overcomes the modicum of muscular strength that remains in the neck and is required for postural control. This condition means that the neck will collapse or buckle during the test. This collapse is found in grade II or greater sprain syndromes.

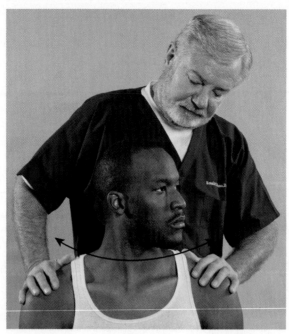

FIG. 3-71 The seated patient actively rotates the head from side to side. Localization of any discomfort is noted. Alternatively, the examiner can passively rotate the patient's head from side to side, while exerting strong downward pressure on the head.

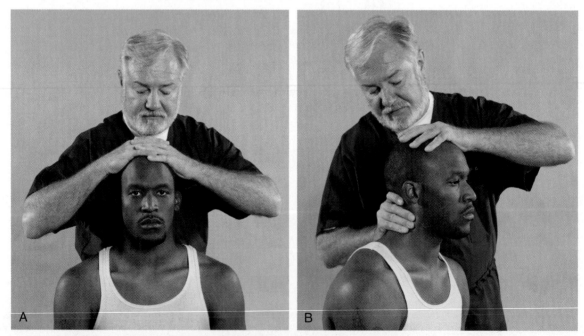

FIG. 3-72 With the head and neck returned to a neutral position, the examiner exerts progressively increasing downward pressure (compression) on the head and neck. Symptoms may lateralize and localize at this point.

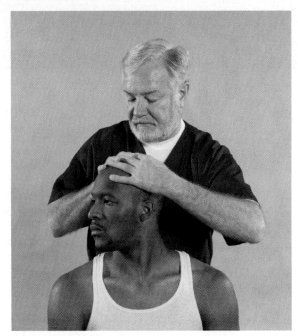

FIG. 3-73 The head is rotated toward the side of complaint and similar compression is applied. Reproduction of the complaint is a positive finding and suggests foraminal encroachment.

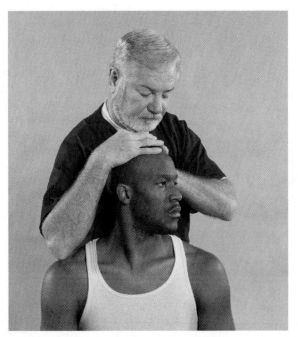

FIG. 3-74 The maneuver is repeated for the opposite side.

Assessment for Vertebrobasilar Artery Insufficiency

Comment

Rotation of the cervical spine to the extent of 45 to 50 degrees occurs chiefly at the atlantoaxial joint. This rotation is approximately one half of the total cervical spine rotation. The VA is held fast at the C1 and C2 transverse foramina by fibrous tissue. During head rotation, the VA is stretched, compressed, and torqued. Decreased flow or even cessation of flow through one VA (the vertebrobasilar artery [VBA]) can occur when the head is turned. The atlantoaxial joint is the probable site of vessel compression (Fig. 3-75).

> The VBA system provides blood flow to the hind brain (i.e., brainstem, medulla oblongata, pons, cerebellum, vestibular apparatus). The left and right VAs arise from the subclavian arteries and pass through the transverse foramina of C6 to C1. When they exit the atlas, the vessels make a sharp posteromedial turn to pass along the posterior mass of the atlas. They then enter the skull through the foramen magnum of the occiput. The vessels are *tethered* at various points along

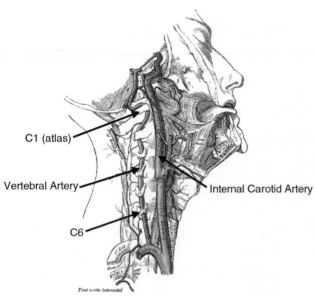

FIG. 3-75 Course of the vertebral and internal carotid arteries through the cervical spine. Considering this anatomy of the upper cervical spine, it is easy to appreciate how, during rotation, the contralateral vessel may be stretched therefore potentially affecting flow. This principle is the basis for the *VBI tests* that have commonly been advocated for VBI screening. (From Kerry R, Taylor AJ: Cervical arterial dysfunction assessment and manual therapy, *Man Ther* 11[4]:243-253, 2006.)

this route, namely C2 transverse foramina, C1 transverse foramina, and at the atlantooccipital membrane (Kerry, Taylor, 2006).

The blood flow in the VAs fluctuates during normal daily activities, but symptoms do not occur because of adequate circulation from the opposite VA. Occlusion of one VA does not necessarily reduce the arterial supply to the posterior fossa via the basilar or posterior cerebellar arteries. Compression or spasm of a VA from C1–C2 rotation will induce symptoms only if flow in the contralateral VA is already compromised.

In cerebral transient ischemic attacks, the symptoms vary according to which area of the brain is ischemic. Two main groups of symptoms are those associated with partial or total ischemia of a cerebral hemisphere and those associated with ischemia of the brainstem. The symptoms most often include transient contralateral weakness of the lower face, fingers, hand, arm, or leg. Such patients may also experience fleeting sensory symptoms, such as tingling, paresthesia, or numbness, in parts of the body contralateral to the ischemia. Ischemia in the dominant hemisphere may cause dysphasia, with impairment of speech and, at times, a transient lack of understanding.

Patients with ischemia in the portion of the brain that is supplied by the posterior cerebral artery may experience blurred vision or may notice transient hemianopic or altitudinal visual field defects or impairment of visual acuity.

Ischemia or insufficiency resulting from internal carotid artery stenosis often produces transient retinal ischemia, which results in monocular blindness or reduced acuity on the side of the stenosis combined with contralateral weakness of the face, arm, or leg.

Although the symptoms of vertebrobasilar artery ischemia vary, they tend to occur in combinations that aid in diagnosis. Vertigo, ataxia, dysarthria, paresthesia, diplopia, tinnitus, and dysphagia, as well as focal weakness of the face, jaw, or pharynx tend to coexist, although not always in the same sequence or combination. Another grouping of symptoms is that of unilateral or bilateral weakness of the extremities with drop attacks and diplopia. The reason for these differences in symptom combinations can be found by referring to any diagram of the blood supply of the brainstem. Ischemia of the dorsal and lateral portions of the brainstem, which are supplied by the circumferential arteries, produces the first group of symptoms. Ischemia of the more ventral portions, supplied by the medial perforating arteries, causes the second group of symptoms.

Several less common spinal cord syndromes may result from direct injury to the cervicomedullary junction and upper cervical segments or from vertebral artery occlusion secondary to severe hyperextension. The *posteroinferior*

3

ORTHOPEDIC GAMUT 3-21
COMMON VERTEBROBASILAR ARTERIAL ISCHEMIC SYMPTOMS

Ischemic attacks that involve the section of the brain that is supplied by the vertebral and basilar arteries have an extremely wide range of symptoms:

- Vertigo
  - Dizziness is the most common complaint with transient ischemic attacks that are caused by vertebrobasilar insufficiency. However, dizziness is commonly associated with other physiologic disturbances and is rarely the only symptom of brainstem ischemia.
- Tinnitus
  - Tinnitus, hearing loss, and ataxia may be present.
- Diplopia

- Dysarthria
- Dysphagia
- Dysphonia
- Patients may complain of unilateral or bilateral face, arm, and leg weakness and unilateral or bilateral sensations of numbness and tingling in the face, arms, or legs.
- In addition, patients with brainstem ischemia experience drop attacks in which they suddenly lose postural tone and fall to the ground without losing consciousness; they then immediately regain postural control and rise quickly.

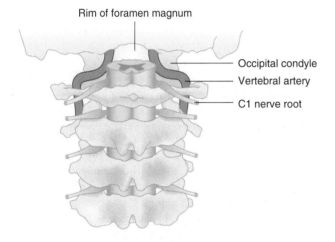

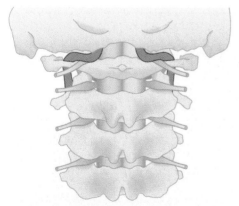

FIG. 3-76 Mechanism of vertebral artery injury in extension injuries of the cervical spine. (From Marx: *Rosen's emergency medicine: concepts and clinical practice*, ed 6, St Louis, 2006, Mosby.)

cerebellar artery syndrome may produce dysphagia, dysphonia, hiccups, nausea, vomiting, dizziness or vertigo, and cerebellar ataxia. The *Dejeune onion skin pattern* of analgesia of the face is caused by damage to the spinal trigeminal tract. *Horner syndrome* results from damage to the cervical sympathetic chain and is characterized by ipsilateral ptosis, miosis, and anhidrosis (Figs. 3-76 and 3-77).

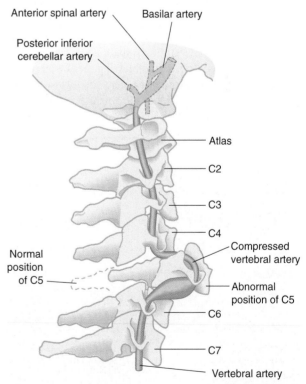

FIG. 3-77 Mechanism of vascular injury of the spinal cord resulting from cervical vertebral injury. (From Marx: *Rosen's emergency medicine: concepts and clinical practice*, ed 6, St Louis, 2006, Mosby.)

PROCEDURE

- The Hallpike maneuver is an enhanced DeKleyn test and must be performed with extreme caution.
- The patient lies in the supine position, with the head extending off the end of the examination table.
- The examiner provides support for the weight of the patient's skull (Fig. 3-78).
- The examiner brings the patient's head into positions of reclination (extension), rotation, and lateral flexion (Fig. 3-79).
- The patient's eyes are open so that the examiner may look for nystagmus and other neurovascular signs (Fig. 3-80).
- The test is repeated for the opposite side (Fig. 3-81).
- These positions are held for 15 to 45 seconds.
- In a final maneuver, the patient's head is allowed to hang freely in extreme extension (hyperextension) off the end of the examination table (Fig. 3-82).
- Vertigo, blurred vision, nausea, syncope, and nystagmus are signs of a positive test.

Next Steps/Procedures

Barré-Liéou sign, vertebrobasilar artery functional maneuver, Hautant test, DeKleyn test, Underburg test, vascular assessment, and vascular imaging (MRI)

CLINICAL PEARL

Cervical spine manipulation and adjunctive therapeutic techniques are safe to use. Nevertheless, the patient's welfare is always of prime concern, and screening tests will help identify patients who may be predisposed to cerebrovascular problems. During these procedures, symptoms of vertigo, nystagmus, dizziness, fainting, nausea, vomiting, visual blurring, headache (onset), or other sensory disturbances may identify a possible vertebrobasilar insufficiency. Problems in the cervical spine apart from the VAs may cause the same signs and symptoms. In suspected VA constriction, resisted neck extension may be painful, and prolonged cervical extension may produce a feeling of faintness. The transverse processes of the atlas are often tender on the side of involvement. These symptoms may improve significantly by using manipulative procedures. Therefore, manipulation should not necessarily be abandoned; rather, the manipulative technique should be modified so that simultaneous extension and rotation are not used.

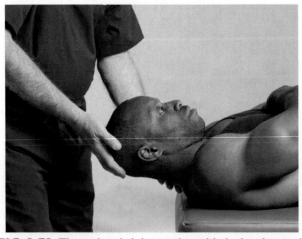

FIG. 3-78 The patient is lying supine with the head extending off the end of the examination table. The examiner provides support for the weight of the skull.

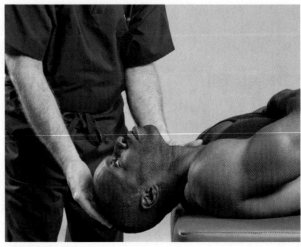

FIG. 3-79 The examiner brings the patient's head into the reclination (extension) position.

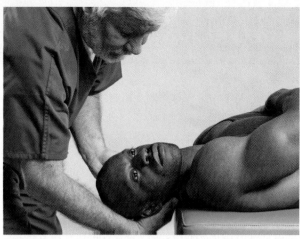

FIG. 3-80 The examiner then moves the patient's head into rotation and lateral flexion. The patient's eyes are open so that the examiner may look for nystagmus and other neurovascular signs.

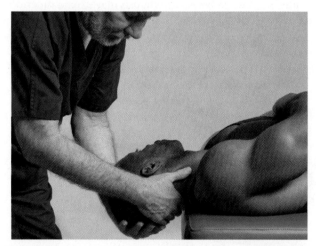

FIG. 3-81 The test is repeated for the opposite side. These positions are held for 15 to 45 seconds.

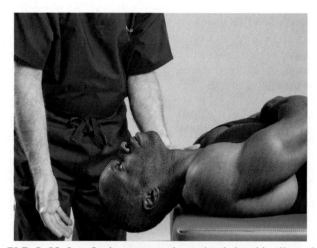

FIG. 3-82 In a final maneuver the patient's head is allowed to hang freely in extreme extension (hyperextension) off the end of the examination table. Vertigo, blurred vision, nausea, syncope, and nystagmus are signs of a positive test. The test indicates vertebral, basilar, or carotid artery stenosis or compression.

Assessment for Vertebral Artery Syndrome

Comment

VA syndrome often occurs as a result of spondylotic changes in the cervical spine. Osteophyte formation in combination with reduced cervical height and a forward head position may cause encroachment on the vertebral foramina. This encroachment, which may be further irritated by cervical position, results in decreased blood flow through the VA to the brain.

The atlantoaxial joints (C1–C2) constitute the most mobile articulations of the spine. Flexion and extension involve a move of approximately 10 degrees and lateral flexion involves a move of approximately 5 degrees. Rotation, which involves a move of approximately 50 degrees, is the primary movement of these joints. During rotation, the height of the cervical spine decreases (because of the shape of the facet joints) as the vertebrae approximate. The odontoid process of C2 acts as a pivot point for the rotation. This middle, or median, joint is classified as a pivot (trochoidal) type of joint. The lateral atlantoaxial, or facet, joints are classed as plane joints. If a patient can talk and chew, some motion is probably occurring at C1–C2. Rotation of the cervical spine past 50 degrees to one side may lead to kinking of the contralateral VA. The ipsilateral VA may kink at 45 degrees of rotation. This kinking of the ipsilateral VA may lead to vertigo, nausea, tinnitus, drop attacks, visual disturbances, stroke, or death.

If an osteophyte developing on the neurocentral joint extends laterally, the VA foramen may be encroached, and the VA may become significantly compressed. Minor degrees of VA compromise may be responsible for the so-called *VA syndrome*. Occasionally, a neurocentral osteophyte may produce severe kinking of the artery, which eventually results in VA thrombosis. Thrombosis may extend superiorly and involve the posteroinferior cerebellar artery. Occlusion of this artery leads to the development of Wallenberg syndrome.

The VA is particularly vulnerable to obstruction in patients with atlantoaxial dislocation (AAD) in whom an abnormal translational movement exists between the atlas and axis (Fig. 3-83). The clinical manifestations in AAD are mainly caused by compression of the thecal sac and spinal cord and

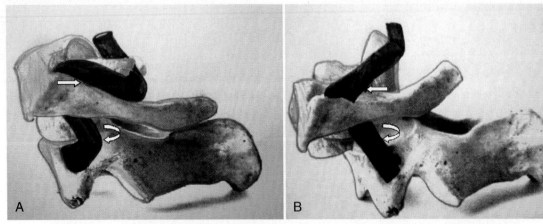

FIG. 3-83 Schematic diagrams showing C: normal C1 through C2 orientation and the third segment of VA with its normal proximal (curved arrow) and distal (straight arrow) loops, and D: showing AAD with opening of the distal loop of VA as it emerges from the C1 foramen transversarium and traverses on the dorsum of C1 posterior arch (straight arrow) and by a shortened and stretched portion of VA forming the proximal loop after emerging from the C2 foramen transversarium (curved arrow). The complete diagnostic protocol for evaluation of AAD should include a DSA or MRA. The presence of a "straight loop sign" of VA may be a valuable pointer toward an impending VBI. (Adapted from Sawlani V et al: "Stretched loop sign" of the vertebral artery: a predictor of vertebrobasilar insufficiency in atlantoaxial dislocation, *Surg Neurol* 66[3]:298-304, 2006.)

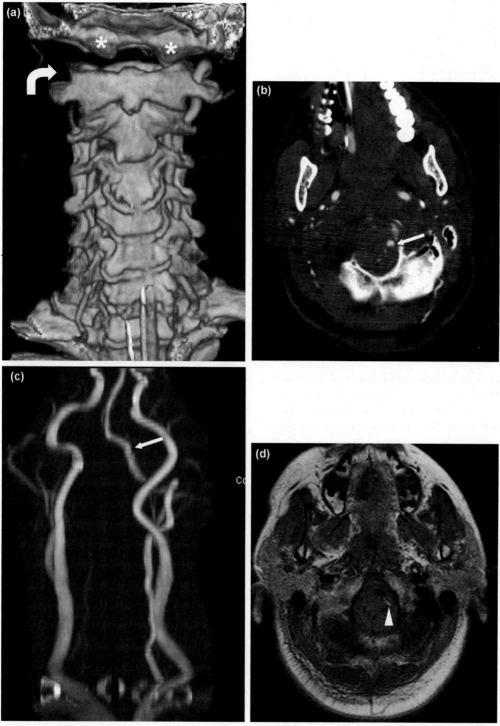

FIG. 3-84 An 82-year old woman with atlanto-occipital dissociation and bilateral vertebral artery injuries following motor vehicle collision. 3-D volume rendered (a) and axial
images (b) obtained with whole-body multidetector computed tomography (WB-MDCT)
protocol. Magnetic resonance angiogram (MRA) (c) and T1 weighted spin echo magnetic
resonance image (MRI) (d). WB-MDCT demonstrates right vertebral artery segmental
occlusion from C1 to foramen magnum (curved arrow), focal left vertebral artery central
narrowing from intramural hematoma at level of foramen magnum, and bare occipital
condyles (asterisks). MRA demonstrates absent flow in distal right vertebral artery with
focal narrowing of injured left vertebral artery (arrow). Left vertebral artery high T1 signal
(arrowhead) indicates intramural hematoma from dissection. (From Sliker CW, Mirvis SE:
Imaging of blunt cerebrovascular injuries, *Eur J Radiol* 64(1):3-14, 2007.)

ORTHOPEDIC GAMUT 3-22

WALLENBERG SYNDROME

Wallenberg syndrome characteristics:

1. Dysphagia, ipsilateral palatal weakness, and vocal cord paralysis (involvement of the nucleus ambiguous of the vagus)
2. Impairment of sensation to pain and temperature on the same side of the face (involvement of the descending root and nucleus of the fifth cranial nerve)
3. Horner syndrome in the homolateral eye (involvement of the descending sympathetic fibers)
4. Nystagmus (involvement of the vestibular nuclei)
5. Cerebellar dysfunction in the ipsilateral arm and leg (interference of the function of the midbrain and cerebellum)
6. Impairment of sensation to pain and temperature on the side of the body opposite (involvement of the spinothalamic tract)

rarely caused by vertebrobasilar territory infarction. In the conventional evaluation of the craniovertebral junction anomalies, however, the bony anomalies are investigated thoroughly, whereas VA often remains unevaluated because digital subtraction arteriography or magnetic resonance angiography does not form a part of the conventional radiologic investigative protocol (Sawlani et al, 2006).

Dizziness, nystagmus, nausea, and unilateral pupil dilation are positive indicators that VA syndrome can be differentially diagnosed from vestibular dysfunction if the provocative posture, rather than movement, of the head reproduces the symptoms.

PROCEDURE

- While seated, the patient extends the arms out in front with the palms up (Figs. 3-85 and 3-86).
- With eyes closed, the patient extends and rotates the head to one side (Fig. 3-87).
- The patient repeats this maneuver with the head extended and rotated to the opposite side.
- Drifting of the arms, vertigo, blurred vision, nausea, syncope, and nystagmus are signs of a positive test.
- The test indicates vertebral, basilar, or carotid artery stenosis or compression.

Next Steps/Procedures

Barré-Liéou sign, vertebrobasilar artery functional maneuver, DeKleyn test, Hallpike maneuver, Underburg test, vascular testing or imaging, and diagnostic imaging

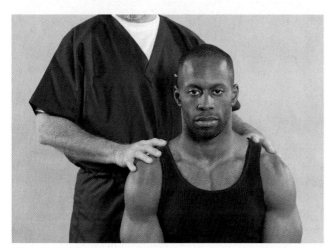

FIG. 3-85 The patient is seated comfortably with the head and neck in a neutral position.

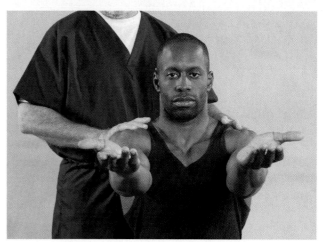

FIG. 3-86 The patient extends the arms forward and elevates them to shoulder level. The hands are supinated. The patient maintains this position for a few seconds.

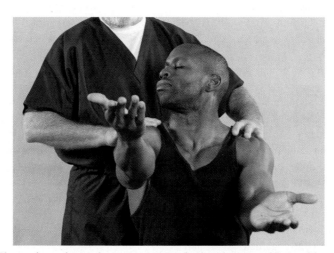

FIG. 3-87 The patient closes the eyes, rotates the head to one side, and hyperextends the neck. The examiner observes for any significant drifting of the arms from their original position. Drifting of the arms is a positive sign for vertebrobasilar vascular compromise.

Assessment for Cervical Nerve Root Compression Resulting From a Space-Occupying Lesion, Subluxation, Inflammatory Edema, Exostosis of Degenerative Joint Disease, Tumor, or Intervertebral Disc Herniation

Comment

Degenerative processes affecting the cervical spine are a common affliction. The secondary effects of degeneration may include degenerative disc disease, primarily leading to effects on the adjacent end-plates and central canal. Degeneration affecting the facet and unco-vertebral articulations may lead to osteophyte formation, synovial cysts, and soft-tissue effects, including ligamentum flavum hypertrophy. Stenosis (central, lateral, or both) may be the result of either *hard* degenerative changes such as osteophyte formation or *soft* degenerative changes affecting the soft-tissue structures such as the ligamentum flavum or facet joint capsule, both of which can hypertrophy. MRI may be also used to demonstrate complications such as spinal cord edema and additional spinal cord lesions (Wessely, 2004).

Patients who are symptomatic for cervical disc degeneration usually have compression of a nearby nerve root or the spinal cord. Acute herniation of degenerated disc material produces such compression and resembles an acute lumbar disc herniation. The various syndromes related to chronic disc degeneration, with herniation and insidious compression or degenerative subluxation, make the condition difficult to diagnose during clinical presentation. Typical of the confusion surrounding the problem of chronic disc degeneration are its many partial synonyms: osteoarthritis, chronic herniated disc, chondroma, spur formation, and others. The term *cervical spondylosis* has recently gained favor and may be used interchangeably for *chronic cervical disc degeneration.*

From C3 through C7 the average AP measurement of the cervical canal is 17 mm. Spinal cord compression will occur only if the canal is reduced to 11 mm or less. In cervical spondylosis, some reduction will usually take place in the AP diameter of the spinal canal, and when associated with a canal that is initially small, myelopathy can occur.

The dorsal and ventral nerve roots pass through the subarachnoid space and converge to form the spinal nerve at approximately the level of its respective intervertebral foramen.

Root pain may awaken the patient after several hours of sleep and may be relieved approximately 15 to 30 minutes after the patient sits up. The patient may learn to prevent the pain by sleeping in a chair. However, in contrast to peripheral neuritis, the antalgic position is the important determining factor. If the patient lies down for awhile during the day, the pain would occur as it does during the night. This feature of root pain occurs because the spinal column lengthens when the patient lies down and shortens when the patient sits up. Because the length of the spinal cord remains the same regardless of the patient's position, the lengthening of the spinal column results in a tensing of, or traction on, the nerve roots.

At each intervertebral foramen, a mixed spinal nerve is formed by the fusion of the dorsal (afferent, sensory) and ventral (efferent motor, sympathetic) roots (Fig. 3-88). The Z joints share this innervation (Fig 3-89).

Because the Z joints are replete with pain-sensitive structures, any deviation from its normal physiologic function caused by degenerative disorders or trauma may lead to facet-induced pain in the head, neck, and shoulders, depending on the level at which integrity of the joint is compromised (Yoganandan, Kumaresan, Pintar, 2001).

In the cervical spine, each cervical root exits above the vertebra that shares the same numeric designation. That is, the C5 root exits above the C5 vertebra (i.e., between the C4 and C5 vertebrae). Because the region has seven cervical vertebrae but eight cervical roots, the C8 roots exist between the C7 and T1 vertebrae (Fig. 3-90).

CR is often the result of a herniated intervertebral disc, or it can be caused by osteophytic spondylitic changes that result in mechanical compression of the cervical root.

Despite the variability in sensory and motor presentations of cervical radiculopathies, certain classic symptoms and signs exist and are extremely helpful in localizing the compressed root (Table 3-9).

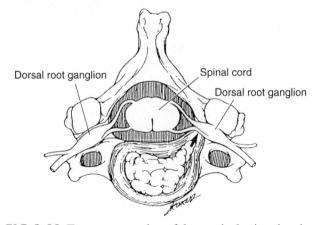

FIG. 3-88 Transverse section of the cervical spine showing the usual site of root injury in cervical radiculopathy caused by disc herniation. (From Brown WF, Bolton CF: *Clinical electromyography,* ed 2, Boston, 1993, Butterworth-Heinemann.)

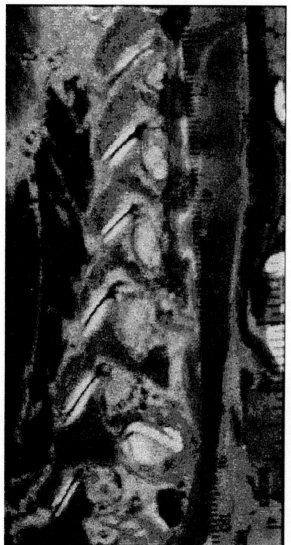

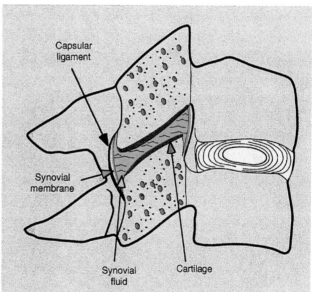

FIG. 3-89 *Left:* Sagittal frozen anatomic section of the human cervical spine showing the Z joint. *Right:* Illustration of Z joint in magnified view. The components of the Z joint such as the articular cartilage, synovial fluid, and synovial membrane were included in the finite element model based on the details obtained from these anatomic sections. (From Yoganandan N, Kumaresan S, Pintar FA: Biomechanics of the cervical spine. Part 2. Cervical spine soft tissue responses and biomechanical modeling, *Clin Biomech* 16[1]:1-27, 2001.)

TABLE 3-9

MODIFIED QUEBEC TASK FORCE CLASSIFICATION SYSTEM FOR ACUTE WHIPLASH ASSOCIATED DISORDERS (WAD)

Proposed classification grade	Physical and psychological impairments present
WAD 0	No complaint about neck pain
	No physical signs
WAD I	Neck complaint of pain, stiffness or tenderness only
	No physical signs
WAD II A	Neck pain
	Motor Impairment
	Decreased ROM
	Altered muscle recruitment patterns (CCFT)
	Sensory Impairment
	Local cervical mechanical hyperalgesia
WAD II B	Neck pain
	Motor Impairment
	Decreased ROM
	Altered muscle recruitment patterns (CCFT)
	Sensory Impairment
	Local cervical mechanical hyperalgesia
	Psychological impairment
	Elevated psychological distress (GHQ-28, TAMPA)
WAD II C	Neck pain
	Motor Impairment
	Decreased ROM
	Altered muscle recruitment patterns (CCFT)
	Increased JPE
	Sensory Impairment
	Local cervical mechanical hyperalgesia
	Generalised sensory hypersensitivity (mechanical, thermal, BPPT)
	Some may show SNS disturbances
	Psychological Impairment
	Psychological distress (GHQ-28, TAMPA)
	Elevated levels of acute posttraumatic stress (IES)
WAD III	Neck pain
	Motor Impairment
	Decreased ROM
	Altered muscle recruitment patterns (CCFT)
	Increased JPE
	Sensory Impairment
	Local cervical mechanical hyperalgesia
	Generalised sensory hypersensitivity (mechanical, thermal, BPPT)
	Some may show SNS disturbances
	Psychological Impairment
	Psychological distress (GHQ-28, TAMPA)
	Elevated levels of acute posttraumatic stress (IES)
	Neurological signs of conduction loss including:
	Decreased or absent deep tendon reflexes
	Muscle weakness
	Sensory deficits
WAD IV	Fracture or dislocation

BPPT, Brachial plexus provocation test; *CCFT*, craniocervical flexion test; *IES*, impact of events scale; *TAMPA*, Tampa scale of kinesio phobia; *JPE*, joint positioning error; *GHQ-28*, general health questionnaire.

Adapted from Sterling M. A proposed new classification system for whiplash associated disorders—implications for assessment and management, *Man Ther* 9(2):60-70, 2004.

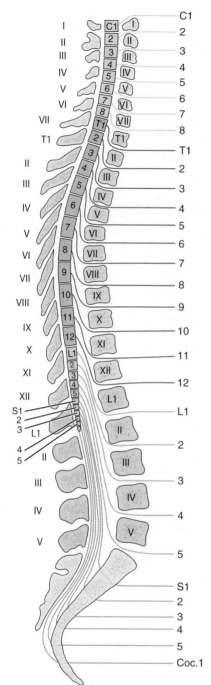

FIG. 3-90 Alignments of spinal segments and roots to vertebrae. (From Katirji B: *Electromyography in clinical practice: a case study approach,* St Louis, 1998, Mosby.)

ORTHOPEDIC GAMUT 3-23

CERVICAL NERVE ROOT COMPRESSION SYNDROME

Clinical axioms regarding cervical nerve root compression syndrome:

1. When sensory manifestations occur in C7 radiculopathy, the index or middle finger is always involved.
2. When sensory manifestations occur in C8 radiculopathy, the little or ring finger is always involved.
3. The thumb is never involved exclusively in C7 radiculopathy.
4. Significant triceps weakness is seen only in C7 radiculopathy.
5. Significant supraspinatus and infraspinatus weakness is seen only in C5 radiculopathy.
6. Significant interossei and hand intrinsic weakness is seen only in C8 radiculopathy.

PROCEDURE

- Cervical compression is commonly performed by having the patient sit up and bend the head obliquely backward while the examiner applies downward pressure on the vertex (Figs. 3-90 and 3-91).
- However, with the Jackson cervical compression test, the head is only slightly rotated to the involved side (Fig. 3-92).
- In either case, the sign is positive if localized pain radiates down the arm.
- A positive sign indicates nerve involvement from a space-occupying lesion, subluxation, inflammatory swelling, exostosis of degenerative joint disease, tumor, or disc herniation.

Next Steps/Procedures

Bakody sign, maximum foraminal encroachment test, shoulder depression test, distraction test, brachial plexus tension test, Bikele sign, Spurling test, foraminal compression test, reflexes, sensory testing, and diagnostic imaging

CLINICAL PEARL

Closure of the intervertebral foramina occurs on the side of flexion in this maneuver. This test should be performed without excessive discomfort. The *cervical collapse sign* may be present.

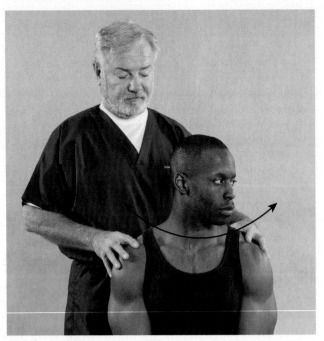

FIG. 3-91 While seated, the patient rotates the head from side to side. Localization of any complaint is noted.

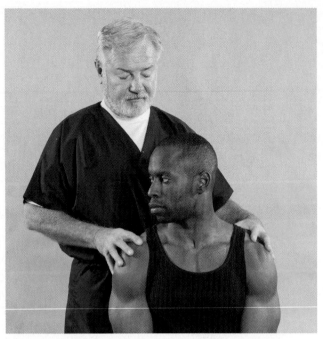

FIG. 3-92 Pain on the side opposite of rotation suggests muscular strain, whereas pain on the side of rotation suggests facet or nerve root involvement.

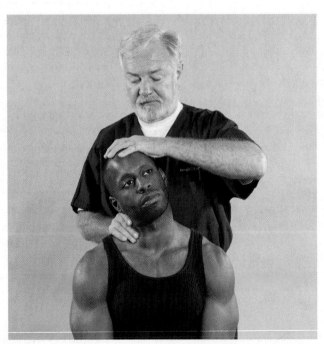

FIG. 3-93 The head is laterally flexed in an attempt to approximate the ear to the shoulder. This position is held, and the examiner exerts downward pressure on the patient's head. An exacerbation of the local or radicular pain indicates a positive test.

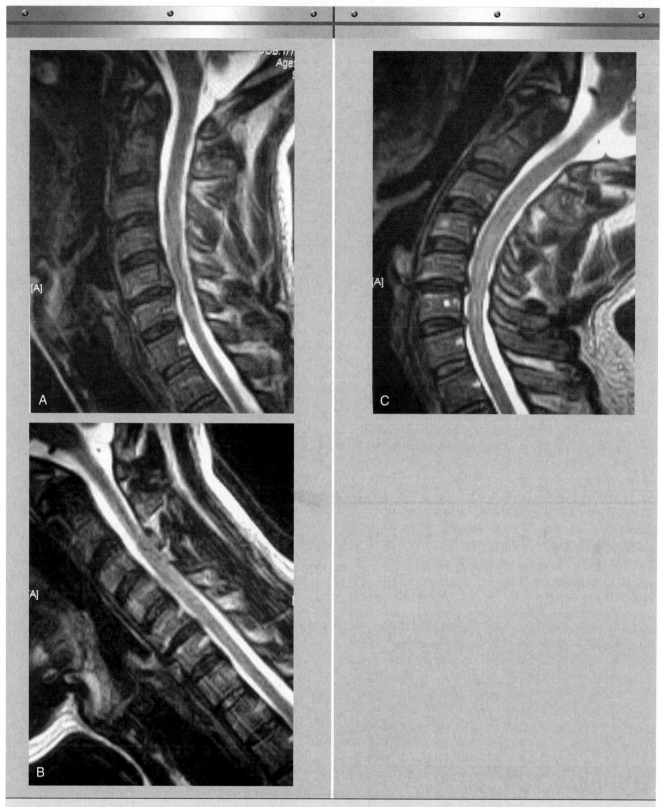

AT THE VIEWBOX

The dynamic component of disc lesions and other space-occupying masses producing neural compression can now be more fully assessed with upright MRI. In this case, there was no neural impingement on neutral images from a small protruded (contained) disc herniation at C5–6 **(A)**. The herniation is not evident on flexion **(B)**.

On extension, there is increased prominence of the C5–6 disc herniation and a second, previously occult herniation at C6–7 **(C)**. Hypermobility of C5 on C6 is present. The appearance of cord deformation on the neutral sagittal image is related to slice plane artifact. (From the teaching file of Timothy Mick, DC, DACBR)

LHERMITTE SIGN

Assessment for Myelopathy of the Cervical Spine

Comment

Cervical myelopathy results from spinal cord injury caused by a cervical spine pathologic condition, such as spondylitic spurs, central disc herniation, tumors, and dislocation of the cervical spine.

Cervical myelopathy refers to disease of a cervical segment of the spinal cord consisting of lesions of descending and ascending tracts and of anterior and posterior horns of the gray medullary substance. The cord damage leads to hyperreflexia and spasticity of legs and arms with positive Babinski sign, to a spastic gait, in an advanced state to muscular atrophy of the arms and hands, to severe spastic paresis of the legs, reduced depth and superficial sensitivity, and rarely to bladder and bowel disfunction (Payer, Hodler, Benini, 2004).

Increasing age, progressive disc dehydration, and altered biomechanics may lead to spondylosis, with osteophytosis at the discovertebral junction, enthesopathy and calcification of the anterior and posterior longitudinal ligaments, hypertrophy of the ligamentum flavum, and joint-space narrowing, hypertrophy, and osteophytosis of the uncovertebral and facet joints. These progressive changes have the potential to narrowing of the spinal canal, lateral recess, and neural foramina. Compression of vascular and neural elements can lead to ischemia and demyelination of ascending and descending spinal pathways. Changes in the lateral columns, especially the corticospinal tract, the anteromedial portion of the posterior columns, and the nerve roots, are more prevalent than changes in the anterior spinal tracts (Salvi, Jones, Weigert, 2006).

Examining for cervical myelopathy is of paramount importance in evaluating every patient with a spinal problem. Key historical and physical examination factors should be noted. During the history, every patient should be asked about a gait disturbance. Questioning patients about sports activities can reveal the key aspects of loss of balance and control, pointing to potential cervical myelopathy. Questions concerning numbness and tingling in the legs, numbness in the hands, loss of agility in the hands, inability to fasten small buttons, deterioration in handwriting, loss of ability to stand on one foot, and a decrease in bowel, bladder, or sexual function should be asked of every patient with cervical pain.

When the history and physical examination suggest the presence of cervical myelopathy, the appropriate diagnostic tests with indication of abnormality are MRI or a contrast computed tomographic (CT) scan of the cervical spine. With significant neurologic symptoms, an electromyogram (EMG) and nerve-conduction study can also be ordered to rule out radiculopathy.

Peripheral neuropathy is a disorder that affects the peripheral motor, sensory, or autonomic nerves to a variable degree. If only one nerve is affected, the dysfunction is considered a mononeuropathy. If several nerves are involved in a distal symmetric or asymmetric fashion, it is considered a polyneuropathy. If multiple, single-peripheral nerves or their branches are involved, this pattern is considered mononeuritis multiplex (Table 3-10).

Patients with any form of peripheral neuropathy often describe their symptoms similarly, using words such as *prickling*, *burning*, or *jabbing*. These symptoms often indicate whether disease exists in the peripheral nerves.

In most patients with polyneuropathy, distal weakness is more prominent than proximal weakness, and an accompanying sensory abnormality is usually present. With mononeuropathy, muscles innervated by a single peripheral nerve are weak and atrophic. This pattern must be differentiated from that in a patient with a radiculopathy, in which only the muscles supplied by a single root are affected. The pattern must also be differentiated from that of a patient with a plexopathy, in which the pattern of motor and sensory dysfunction is in a multiple root or peripheral nerve distribution.

ORTHOPEDIC GAMUT 3-24

CAUSES OF PROGRESSIVE DEGENERATIVE NARROWING OF THE CERVICAL SPINAL CANAL

- Osteophytic growth from the edge of the end-plates of the vertebral bodies
- Disc herniation

ORTHOPEDIC GAMUT 3-25

OTHER COMMON CAUSES OF CERVICAL MYELOPATHY

- A focus of multiple sclerosis
- Intra- and extraaxial tumor
- Huge cervical disc herniation
- Hydrosyringomyelia

TABLE 3-10

CLINICAL SIGNS OF CERVICAL RADICULOPATHY AND MYELOPATHY

	Cervical Radiculopathy	Myelopathy
Muscle wasting	Path, unilateral	Path, bilateral
Sensory deficit radicular	Path	Norm
Vibratory sense diminished	Norm	Path, lower extremities
Muscle stretch reflexes	Path (weak)	Path (hyper)
Abdominal reflexes	Norm	Path (absent)
Spurling	Path	Norm
Babinski sign	Norm	Path
Hypertonicity	Norm	Path
Gait	Norm	Path

Classic findings include limitations in cervical range of motion, spasticity (with increased muscle tendon reflexes below the level of canal compromise), a positive Babinski sign, absent abdominal reflexes, decreased joint position and vibratory sensation, and an abnormal gait *Norm*, Normal; *path*, pathologic.
Adapted from Salvi FJ, Jones JC, Weigert BJ: The assessment of cervical myelopathy, *Spine* 6(6, suppl 1):S182-S189, 2006.

ORTHOPEDIC GAMUT 3-26

NEUROPATHY

Neuropathy evolving over many weeks or months suggests several possibilities:
1. Exposure to toxic agents or drugs
2. Nutritional deficiencies
3. Chronically abnormal metabolic state
4. Remote effect of a malignant disease
5. Genetic polyneuropathy, which may have an insidious onset at any age

Neuropathies that develop abruptly and that are associated with pain are usually of an ischemic origin, such as in rheumatoid arthritis and polyarteritis nodosa. Neuropathies that evolve over a few days may be caused by industrial intoxications, such as those associated with the use of thallium or triorthocresyl phosphate.

The spinal canal can be compromised in many ways. The canal may be congenitally stenotic; anomalies in the canal or even a smaller-than-usual canal can leave the person vulnerable to later injury. Cervical spine stenosis can also occur as a result of trauma or repetitive injury.

The signs and symptoms of cervical canal stenosis range from simple paresthesia to myelopathy to transient quadriplegia (Fig. 3-94).

Developmental stenosis of the cervical spine has been associated with cervical cord neurapraxia (CCN), transient quadriplegia, chronic intervertebral disc disease, and ligamentous instability. Secondary myelopathy of the cervical cord may occur after severe neck injury in patients with a stenotic cervical canal.

The anteroposterior diameter of the vertebral canal (or sagittal developmental diameter) has been identified as a predictor for the development of cervical myelopathy, as well as spinal cord injury. The ratio of the sagittal diameter of the cervical canal to that of the vertebral body was first proposed by Torg and colleagues as an indicator of the degree of developmental canal narrowing. This ratio excludes magnification error resulting from nonstandardized film-tube distances. Reduced Torg ratios have been demonstrated in patients with cervical spondylotic myelopathy compared with nonspondylotic, nonmyelopathic controls. A ratio of less than 0.80 has been shown to have a high sensitivity for transient CCN in athletes and is strongly correlated with further episodes of CCN (Lim, Wong, 2004).

The Torg ratio is the ratio of the width of the canal to the AP width at the midpoint of the corresponding vertebral body; a ratio of less than 4:5 (i.e., 0.80) indicates spinal stenosis (Fig. 3-95). An AP dimension of 13 mm or less may be indicative of cord compression. The interpediculate spacing is less significant in the cervical region than in the dorsolumbar spine.

Primary diseases of muscle are not usually confused with peripheral neuropathies, but in some cases, an EDX is required for differentiation. Distal symmetric or asymmetric paresthesia in the extremities without a significant component of muscle weakness should be differentiated from multiple sclerosis, cervical spondylitic myelopathy, or occasionally extradural tumors of the cervical cord. Constant and severe pain in the neck or pain while flexing the neck (Lhermitte sign) usually indicates cervical cord disease. Symptoms or signs of spasticity may occur later in these myelopathies, which can create a problem in diagnosis. Electrophysiologic testing usually resolves the issue.

The prevalence of multiple sclerosis varies with location; it can be as high as 122 in 100,000 individuals (Olmsted County, Minnesota) or as low as 2 in 100,000 persons (Seoul, South Korea). With ageing the prevalence of degenerative changes in the cervical spine increases, and cervical spondylosis is prevalent in 50% of people older than 50 years and 75% of people older than 65 years. Sixty percent of people older than 50 years have some spondylotic-related neurologic abnormality if examined thoroughly. Therefore and not surprisingly the practicing neurologist will inevitably encounter patients in whom the two conditions coexist, particularly primary progressive multiple sclerosis and spondylotic myelopathy (Ronthal, 2006).

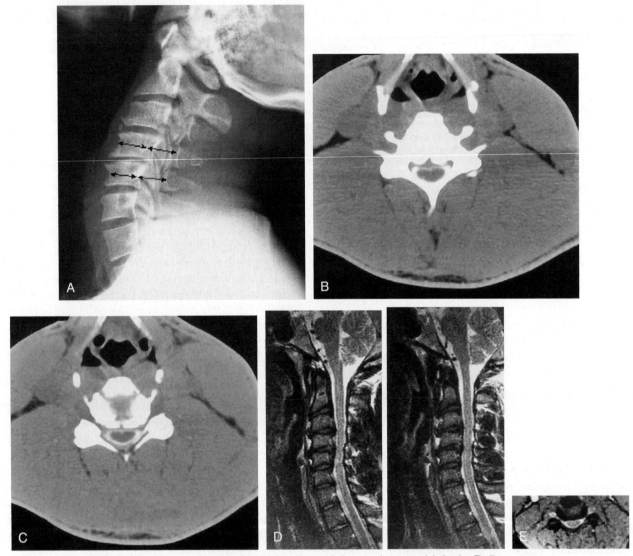

FIG. 3-94 **A,** Lateral cervical spinal radiograph in transient quadriplegia. **B,** Postcontrast CT scan at C5. **C,** Postcontrast CT scan opposite C4-C5 disc space. **D,** Sagittal T2-weighted MRI scans. **E,** Axial MRI scan opposite C4-C5. (From Nicholas JA, Hershman EB: *The lower extremity and spine in sports medicine,* vol 2, St Louis, 1995, Mosby.)

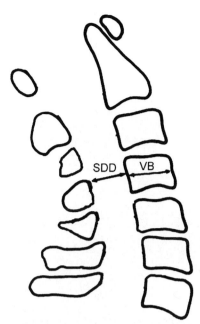

FIG. 3-95 Torg Ratio Assessment. (1) sagittal developmental diameter of the cervical canal (SDD). The distance between the cephalocaudal midpoint of the posterior aspect of the vertebral body to the nearest point on the corresponding spinal laminar line. (2) Anteroposterior diameter of the vertebral body (VB). The distance between the cephalocaudal midpoints of the anterior and posterior surfaces of the vertebral body. (3) Torg ratio (SDD/VB). Derived from the ratio of the sagittal developmental diameter of the canal (SDD) to the anteroposterior diameter of the vertebral body (VB). (Adapted from Lim J-K, Wong H-K: Variation of the cervical spinal Torg ratio with gender and ethnicity, *Spine J* 4(4):396-401, 2004)

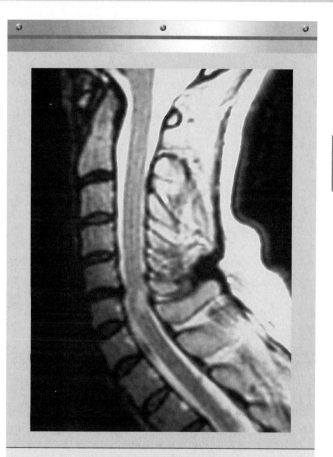

AT THE VIEWBOX

There are numerous potential sources of dural irritation, including blood products from trauma, inflammatory processes such as arachnoiditis, and degenerative disease of the spine with osteophytes. This 47-year-old female fell from a ski lift, with cervical spine MRI demonstrating a cord contusion at the level of a C5–6 disc herniation. Focal bright signal in the cord on fluid-weighted (e.g., T2 or gradient echo) images is a nonspecific finding and, depending on the clinical setting, may indicate a demyelinating process, vascular lesion, cord tumor, or traumatic lesion, as in this case. Incidentally noted is a cerebrospinal fluid (CSF) flow artifact with focal low signal ventral to the cord at the C7–T1 level, along with normal basivertebral venous plexus structures (high signal) at multiple levels in the dorsal vertebral bodies. (From the teaching file of Timothy Mick, DC, DACBR)

PROCEDURE

- The patient is seated on the examining table (Fig. 3-96).
- The patient's head is passively flexed (Fig. 3-97).
- A sharp pain radiating down the spine and into the upper or lower limbs is a positive finding (Fig. 3-98).
- Dural irritation in the spine is indicated.
- The test is similar to a combination of other meningeal irritation challenges.

Next Steps/Procedures
Soto-Hall sign, reflexes and sensory testing, electrodiagnosis, and MRI

CLINICAL PEARL

Although Lhermitte sign is often construed as a pathognomonic test for multiple sclerosis, it is not. However, Lhermitte sign does *reveal* or *suggest* myelopathy resulting from multiple sclerosis, stenosis, tumor, or disc herniation.

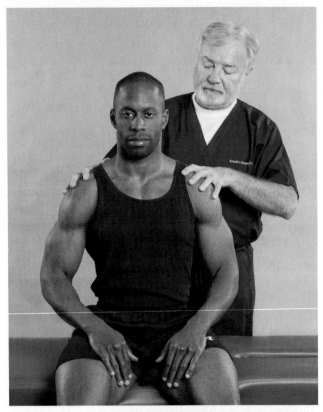

FIG. 3-96 The patient sits comfortably but erect, with the head and neck in the neutral position.

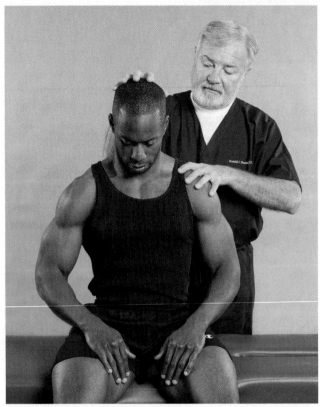

FIG. 3-97 The head and neck are passively flexed toward the patient's chest.

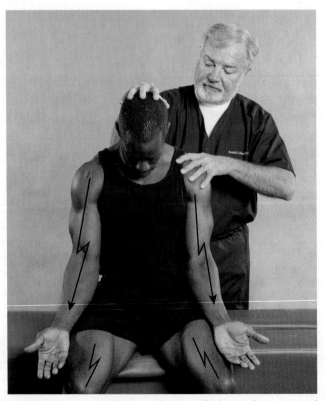

FIG. 3-98 The patient may experience a sharp, radiating pain or paresthesia along the spine and into one or more extremities. The presence of these symptoms suggests myelopathy and constitutes a positive test.

MAXIMAL CERVICAL COMPRESSION TEST

Assessment for Cervical Nerve Root Syndrome or Facet Syndrome (Concave Testing) and Cervical Muscular Strain (Convex Testing)

Comment

Often associated with cervical muscular strain, myofascial trigger points refer dull, aching pain. This deep pain ranges from uncomfortable to incapacitating. Active trigger points are hyperirritable areas of skeletal muscle tissue that cause pain. Latent trigger points cause weakness and restriction of movement but are not painful.

Active trigger points demonstrate a *jump sign*. Stimulation of the affected trigger point will cause the musculature to react.

Myofascial trigger points (MTrPs) are recognized by many clinicians to be one of the most common causes of pain and dysfunction in the musculoskeletal system. They have been detected in the shoulder girdle musculature in nearly one half of a group of young, asymptomatic military personnel and with a similar prevalence in the masticatory muscles of a group of unselected student nurses. Active MTrPs—those causing spontaneous pain—have been diagnosed as the primary source of pain in 74% of 96 patients with musculoskeletal pain seen by a neurologist in a community pain medical center and in 85% of 283 consecutive admissions to a comprehensive pain center. Of 164 patients referred to a dental clinic for chronic head and neck pain, 55% were found to have active MTrPs as the cause of their pain, as were 30% of those with pain at a university primary care internal medicine group practice from a consecutive series of 172 patients. A study of musculoskeletal disorders in villagers from rural Thailand demonstrated myofascial pain as the primary diagnosis in 36% of 431 subjects with pain during the previous 7 days (Cummings, Baldry, 2007).

The anterior, middle, and posterior scalene muscles act to stabilize the cervical spine against lateral movement and elevate the first and second ribs during inspiration. Tightness in these muscles may occlude nerves and blood vessels and compress nerves to the proximal and distal part of the arm. Physical symptoms include morning edema specifically on the radial and dorsal aspect of the hand.

The vulnerability to injury of the cervical region is so great that even low- to moderate-intensity trauma can compromise a multitude of systems. As a result, a variety of signs and symptoms may develop. As is known, the secondary effects of whiplash are sometimes as disabling, if not more so, than the soreness and muscular stiffness of the initial symptoms (Table 3-11 and Fig. 3-99).

TABLE 3-11

SYMPTOMS EXPERIENCED WITH CERVICAL ACCELERATION/DECELERATION SYNDROMES

Symptom	Lesion Site
Headache	Suboccipital muscles, greater occipital nerve, myofascial trigger points, facet point irritation
Disorientation, irritability	Brain
Visual disturbances	Vertebrobasilar artery network, brainstem, cervical spinal cord
Memory and concentration disturbances	Brain
Vertigo	Cervical sympathetic nerves, vertebral artery, inner ear
Arm and hand numbness	Brachial plexus, scalenes
Thumb, index finger, middle finger numbness; weakness; temperature changes	Median nerve, carpal tunnel
Difficulty swallowing	Pharynx
Ringing in ears	Temporomandibular joint, vertebral and basilar arteries, cervical sympathetic chain, inner ear
Dizziness, light-headedness	Cervical sympathetic nerves, brain, inner ear
Neck and shoulder pain	Paravertebral muscles, apophyseal joints, cervical nerve roots, cervical disc
Poor balance, proprioception, and posture	Inner ear

Adapted from Brier SR: *Primary care orthopedics*, St Louis, 1999, Mosby.

ORTHOPEDIC GAMUT 3-27

MYOFASCIAL INVOLVEMENT

Two common areas of myofascial involvement of the cervical spine are:
1. Levator scapulae
2. Scalenes

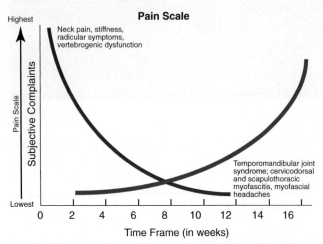

FIG. 3-99 Clinical picture of moderate to severe whiplash trauma. (From Brier SR: *Primary care orthopedics,* St Louis, 1999, Mosby.)

ORTHOPEDIC GAMUT 3-28

Three tests that help in differentiating other thoracic outlet syndrome causes from the scalene trigger point hyperirritability are:

1. *The cramp test:* The patient fully rotates the head to the affected side and drops the chin to the clavicle. The test is positive if a firm contraction or cramp of the scalene muscles occurs.
2. *The finger-flexion test:* A positive finding is present when all of the medial fingertips cannot press tightly against the metacarpophalangeal joints when the proximal phalanges are extended.
3. *The scalene relief test:* Elevation of the arm and clavicle lifts the clavicle from the underlying scalenes. To do this the patient places the forearm of the involved side across the forehead (similar to reverse Bakody sign); this produces pain relief within minutes.

Acute injury (sprain) of a joint produces synovial effusion, histamine release, capsular or ligamentous stretching or tearing, bleeding, and associated clinical disabilities. Some of these conditions are visible and palpable in joints of the extremities but not the spine. With repetition of the traumatic process or with chronic stress on the joint from shearing and other forces, a chronic synovial reaction is established. This reaction extends to the underlying articular cartilage. The cartilage softens and then becomes rough and eroded. Stresses in the capsule and periosteum result in marginal osteophytosis, which may encroach on the underlying nerve root. A loose body may develop in the joint cavity, or an osteophytic process may fracture and lie free or loosely attached in or near the foramen. The facetal bone may thicken or become hypertrophic, and the laminae may do so as well. Degenerative enlargement of facets with irritative compression of one or more cervical roots may also occur.

Trauma to the cervical spine may injure the nervous tissue and related structures in several ways. During the hyperextension phase of an injury, nerve roots may suffer a compression injury at the point of exit from the neural foramina. The nerve root may become contused enough to produce actual disruption of axons and resulting axonotmesis. However, because the internal structure is fairly well preserved, recovery is spontaneous. Neurapraxic injury is more common and is clinically associated with the transient paresthesia that is seen most often approximately a week after the trauma occurred. The spinal cord, dura, and arachnoid may also be contused. During the hyperflexion phase traction injury may occur.

The nerve supply to the capsular and ligamentous structures of the cervical spine is of significance in the interpretation of painful conditions. The capsules of the atlantoaxial joints and those of the posterior or apophyseal joints are supplied by the capsular branches of the medial divisions of the posterior primary rami of the cervical spine nerves. The posterior longitudinal ligament and the capsular structures of the lateral interbody joints receive their nerve supply from the recurrent spinal meningeal nerves (the sinuvertebral nerves), which contain afferent somatic sensory fibers and efferent sympathetic fibers.

> Whiplash injury is a frequent mechanism for chronic neck pain and accounts for one half of all patient-care expenses from motor-vehicle accidents. Despite the frequency and costs of whiplash, little is known about the injury mechanism in these painful neck injuries. The cervical facet joint has been identified as a source of neck pain and is a likely candidate for mechanical injury caused by the bony motions of the spine during neck loading. The capsular ligament in the lower cervical facet joints can, in some cases, exceed its physiologic limit because of an altered spinal kinematic during whiplash (Quinn, Winkelstein, in press).

Chronic cervical strain is the most common cause of neck pain that mimics cervical spondylosis. This mimicry has led to unnecessary myelography because the associated patterns of referred pain and neuralgia are so similar between the two conditions (Fig. 3-100).

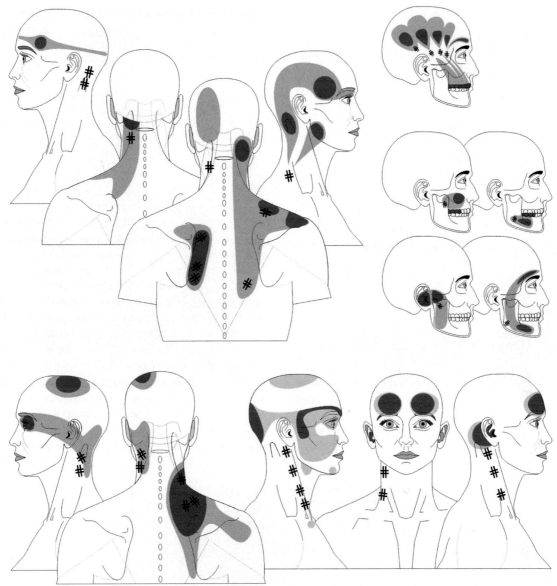

FIG. 3-100 Common myofascial trigger point sites (#) in the head and neck and their respective pain patterns. (From Cummings M, Baldry P: Regional myofascial pain: diagnosis and management, *Best Pract Res Clin Rheum* 21[2]:367-387, 2007.)

PROCEDURE

- While in the seated position, the patient is instructed to approximate the chin to the shoulder and extend the neck (Figs. 3-101 to 3-103).
- The test is performed bilaterally.
- Pain on the concave side indicates nerve root or facet involvement.
- Pain on the convex side indicates muscular strain.

Next Steps/Procedures

Dejerine sign, swallowing test, Valsalva maneuver, Naffziger test, Bakody sign, shoulder depression test, distraction test, brachial plexus tension test, Bikele sign, Jackson cervical compression test, Spurling test, foraminal compression test, reflexes, sensory testing, and diagnostic imaging

CLINICAL PEARL

The patient with lower cervical nerve root compression syndrome has already discovered that looking up or down with the head rotated is uncomfortable and produces neck and arm pain. If these positions are already producing pain, then attempts to use manipulative procedures incorporating these positions will be difficult for the patient to tolerate.

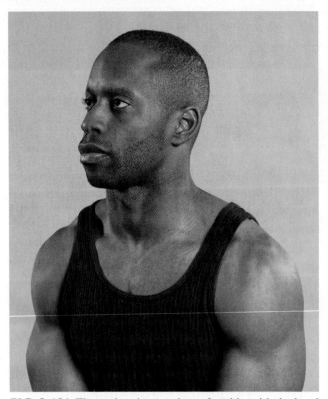

FIG. 3-101 The patient is seated comfortably with the head and neck in the neutral position.

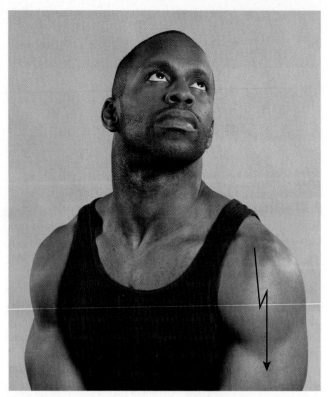

FIG. 3-102 The patient actively rotates the head and hyperextends the neck toward the side of radicular complaint. Reproduction of symptoms suggests foraminal encroachment. The maneuver is repeated for the opposite side.

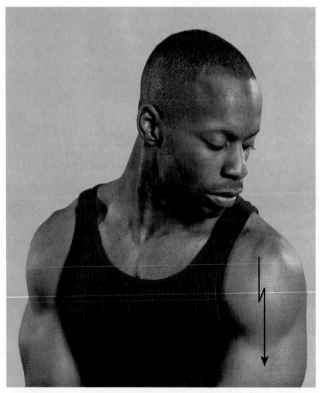

FIG. 3-103 A slight variation of this test requires rotation and maximal flexion of the neck toward the side of radicular complaint, as if looking into a shirt pocket. Reproduction of the radicular complaint suggests foraminal encroachment of a nerve root.

NAFFZIGER TEST

Assessment for Space-Occupying Mass in the Cervical Spine or Canal

Comment

A herniated cervical disc causing nerve root compression that is unresponsive to conservative treatment may require surgery. Disc herniation commonly occurs at the high-motion segments of C4–C5, C5–C6, and C6–C7. As the intradiscal contents leave the annulus, they may migrate around the adjacent nerve root, resulting in radiculopathy. If the herniated disc displaces into the epidural space, cord compression may result. Free fragments of disc material may occasionally be found in the epidural space. Patients usually complain of severe radicular pain involving the upper extremity and shoulder girdle area. Disc herniation of C4–C5 results in numbness around the shoulder and weakness of the deltoid muscle. Deep-tendon reflexes are not altered. With C5–C6 disc herniation, the patient loses the biceps reflex and biceps muscle strength. Numbness along the dorsal aspect of the thumb and index finger is typical. Herniations of the C6–C7 disc cause depression of the triceps reflex, weakness of the triceps muscle, and numbness of the long and ring fingers.

Although spinal cord tumors are rare, they are always a part of the differential diagnosis of neck pain. These tumors arise within the spinal cord from cells that may be metastatic. Such tumors can be primary or secondary and extradural or intradural. Intradural tumors require further sorting into extramedullary or intramedullary.

Of the intradural tumors, 71% are extramedullary; 32% of these are meningiomas, and 38% are schwannomas. The remaining tumors found in this location are sarcomas, angiomas, chordomas, lymphomas, lipomas, epidermoids, melanomas, and neuroblastomas. Other kinds of lesions occur very rarely. Virtually any kind of tumor may metastasize to the intradural space, but such spread is distinctly unusual.

> Congenital cervical cord and posterior fossa lipomas can masquerade during first few months after birth as the floppy infant syndrome. Tetraparesis and inability to stand and walk during the first few years of life indicate cervical cord involvement. Opisthotonos and respiratory involvement are suggestive of intracranial extension and brainstem compression (Naimur et al, 2006).

Of meningiomas, 15% are either completely extradural or both intradural and extradural, and 85% are intradural and extramedullary. Meningiomas are found in the cervical region in approximately 13% of the patients. The tumors are usually nodular, well circumscribed, and less well encapsulated than neurofibromas. The histology of cervical meningiomas is not different from that of meningiomas elsewhere,

and malignant tumors are very rare. The tumors begin growing at the dorsal root entry zone and are clinically indistinguishable from neurofibromatosis. The pain is rarely localized. An unusual meningioma involves the upper cervical area, as well as the intracranial cavity, and is called a *foramen magnum tumor*. Tumors in this area are difficult to diagnose and are most commonly meningiomas (Fig. 3-104).

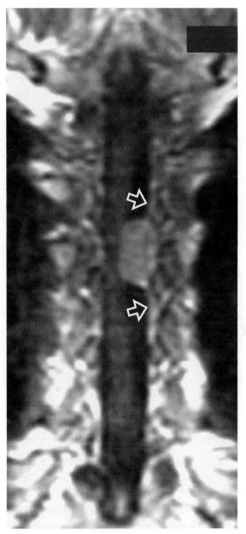

FIG. 3-104 Enhancing dural thickening (dural tail sign) is noted cranial and caudal to the meningioma *(open arrows)* for a distance that is almost equal to the longitudinal diameter of the meningioma. (From Alorainy IA: Dural tail sign in spinal meningiomas, *Eur J Radiol* 60[3]:387-391, 2006.)

The enhancing dural thickening adjacent to meningioma on MRI has been called *dural tail sign*, *flare sign*, or *meningeal sign*. This sign is seen in 52% to 72% of cranial meningiomas (Alorainy 2006).

Symptoms of meningiomas are bizarre and often variable. Patients with these tumors often have their complaints dismissed as psychiatric. A nondescript headache is an early complaint. Weakness and paresthesia in the lower extremities may occur, but the complaints and locations often vary from examination to examination. Muscular atrophy and fibrillation in the hands and forearms are common and probably result from compression of the anterior spinal arteries. A mistaken diagnosis of lower motor neuron disease in the cervical region is common. The course of the illness is relentlessly progressive, and the nature of the disease often becomes apparent only when quadriparesis is evident.

Changing position, coughing, or sneezing or a rise in cerebrospinal fluid pressure results in increased pain.

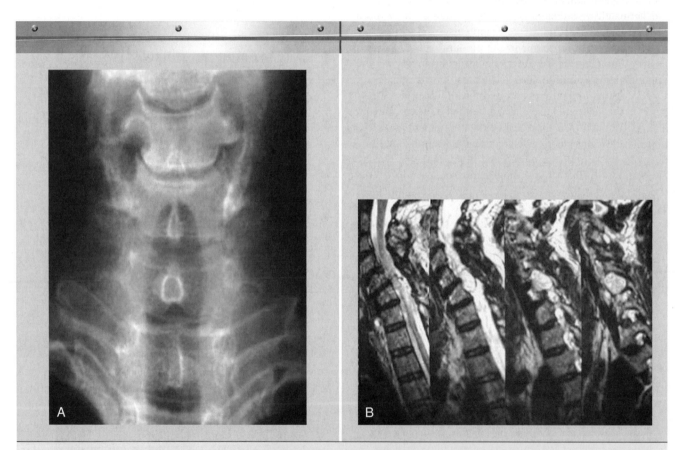

AT THE VIEWBOX

History of long-standing right upper extremity radicular symptoms not responding to conservative management. Plain films demonstrate erosion and expansion of the right C5–6 intervertebral foramen (IVF). Follow-up MRI reveals a neural tumor causing the IVF remodeling **(A)**. Neurofibromas and Schwannomas account for the majority of these types of intradural/extramedullary tumors with extension into the nerve root canal, often with a so-called "dumb-bell" configuration. However, low-grade malignant neural tumors may have a similar appearance. Minimally, serial MRI is appropriate to follow-up; in cases that are managed nonsurgically to ensure stability of the lesion over time **(B)**. (From the teaching file of Timothy Mick, DC, DACBR)

PROCEDURE

- The Naffziger compression test is performed by having the patient sit erect while the examiner holds digital pressure over the jugular veins for 30 to 40 seconds (Fig. 3-105).
- The patient is then instructed to cough deeply.
- Pain along the distribution of a nerve may indicate nerve root compression (Fig. 3-106).
- Although this test is more commonly used for lower back involvement, cervical or thoracic root compression may also be aggravated.
- Local pain in the spine does not positively indicate nerve compression but may indicate the site of a strain or sprain injury or other lesion.
- The sign is always positive in the presence of cord tumors, particularly spinal meningiomas.
- The resulting increased spinal fluid pressure above the tumor causes the growth to compress or pull on certain sensory nerve structures, which produces radicular pain.
- *The test is contraindicated for a geriatric patient, and extreme care should be taken when performing this test on anyone suspected of having atherosclerosis.*
- In all cases, the patient should be alerted that jugular pressure may result in light-headedness or dizziness.

Next Steps/Procedures

Dejerine sign, swallowing test, Valsalva maneuver, Barré-Liéou sign, vertebrobasilar artery functional maneuver, Hautant test, DeKleyn test, Hallpike maneuver, Underburg test, and vascular assessment

CLINICAL PEARL

This test is *not* a good one for a geriatric or atheromatous patient to endure. The resulting increase in cerebrospinal fluid pressure is uncomfortable, and the momentary circulatory obstruction may result in significant syncope.

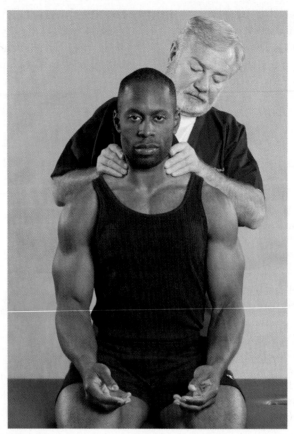

FIG. 3-105 With the patient seated comfortably, the examiner occludes the jugular veins bilaterally for 30 to 40 seconds.

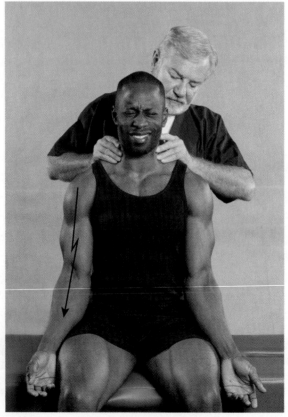

FIG. 3-106 The patient may experience radicular pain or localized pain in the spine. The finding is nonspecific but suggests a space-occupying mass in the spinal column.

Assessment for Cervical Muscular Strain (Isometric) and Cervical Ligamentous Sprain (Passive Range of Motion)

Comment

Patients with whiplash frequently remark on their belief that significance exists to their head position at the time of impact. Some believe that the fact that they "saw it coming" because they were looking to their right at the time of a right lateral impact, for example, protected them from more serious injury. Others believe that having their neck *twisted* at the time of impact is the reason they have unilateral neck pain (Kumar, Ferrari, Narayan, 2005).

The clinical syndrome of whiplash injury includes neck pain, upper thoracic pain, cervicogenic headache, and tightness, and dizziness, restriction of cervical range of motion, tinnitus, and blurred vision. The exact nature of these symptoms is not clearly understood, although the pain is attributed to musculoskeletal disorders (i.e., it involves the soft tissues and facet-joint dysfunction caused by the impact). Moreover, experimental research involving human cadavers has demonstrated that a variety of musculoskeletal injuries can occur during whiplash, such as muscle and ligament sprains. Several theories have been postulated to explain these symptoms, including VA insufficiency and injury of the cervical sympathetic chain, in relation to visual disturbances and dizziness, C1-C2 facet joint injury in relation to headaches, and paraspinal muscle spasm in relation to neck pain. Moreover, some authors have reported that people suffering from whiplash injury display signs of both central and peripheral sensitization (Fernandez de las Penas, Palomeque del Cerro, Fernandez Carnero, 2005).

Examination of whiplash injuries requires evaluation of entities such as fracture, instability, and spinal cord or nerve root compression. These entities are readily apparent on routine clinical and radiologic assessment. However, many more serious bony, articular, and ligamentous injuries can occur in whiplash (Fig. 3-107). These injuries may be undetectable on plain films, CT, or MRI, especially injuries to the cervical Z joints. Furthermore, the intervertebral discs have the potential to cause chronic symptoms with no obvious clinical or radiologic findings.

Most patients with cervical strain complain of paraspinal muscular aches and stiffness that may extend as far cephalad as the suboccipital region (Table 3-12). Chronic muscular strain of the cervical spine can affect distant organ systems. Pain may be referred to the head, orbits, or scapula.

A strain is damage to a muscle or tendon as a direct result of a sudden forcible contraction or violent stretching. Muscle strain includes those cases of overuse and overstretching that are just short of actual muscular rupture.

In all varieties of strain, contraction of the muscle against resistance will increase pain. This response is a characteristic finding of strains and differentiates the injury from sprains. A sprain is an injury to a ligamentous tissue that

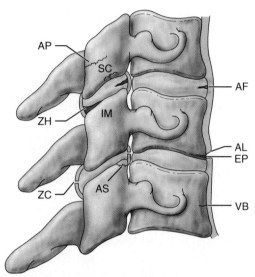

FIG. 3-107 Sites for clinical consideration following cervical spine acceleration-deceleration trauma. *AF,* Annulus fibrosus tear; *AL,* articular longitudinal tear; *AP,* articular pillar fracture; *AS,* articular surface fracture; *EP,* end-plate avulsion; *IM,* intraarticular meniscus contusion; *SC,* subcoronal plate fracture; *VB,* vertebral body fracture; *ZC,* zygapophyseal capsule tear; *ZH,* zygapophyseal hemarthrosis. (Adapted from *Spine: State of the Art Reviews,* 1993;7. In Klippel JH, Dieppe PA: *Rheumatology,* vol 1-2, ed 2, London, 1998, Mosby.)

TABLE 3-12	
CERVICAL STRAIN ASSESSMENT	
Physical examination findings	Paravertebral muscle tenderness
	Intermittent stiffness
	Loss of cervical mobility
	Headaches and alterations of postural reflexes in chronic sufferers
	Normal neurologic signs
	No instability; screening for postural distortion
	Intersegmental posterior joint dysfunction
X-ray finding	Findings generally normal
	Possible decrease in cervical lordosis

Adapted from Brier SR: *Primary care orthopedics,* St Louis, 1999, Mosby.

ORTHOPEDIC GAMUT 3-29

CERVICAL SPINE MUSCULAR INJURY

The mechanism of cervical spine muscular injury is usually one of the following:

1. Athletic participation, which is by far the most frequent means of sustaining a strain injury
2. Overuse
3. Overstretching
4. Contraction of the muscle against resistance
5. Direct blow

ORTHOPEDIC GAMUT 3-31

SPRAINS

Sprains are divided into four categories according to the severity of the ligamentous injury:

1. A mild sprain describes an injury in which only a few of the ligamentous fibers are severed.
2. A moderate sprain is a more severe tearing but less than a complete separation of the ligament.
3. A severe sprain is a complete tearing of a ligament from its attachments or a complete separation within its substance.
4. A sprain-fracture has occurred when the ligamentous attachment pulls loose with a fragment of bone (avulsion).

ORTHOPEDIC GAMUT 3-30

STRAINS

Strains are divided into three categories according to the degree of muscle tissue damage:

1. A mild strain is a low-grade inflammatory reaction accompanied by no appreciable hemorrhage, minimal amounts of swelling and edema, and some disruption of adjacent fibers.
2. A moderate strain involves laceration of fibers and appreciable hemorrhaging into the surrounding tissue (hematoma), followed by an inflammatory reaction with swelling and edema.
3. A severe strain is the consequence of a single, violent incident that results in complete disruption of the muscle unit. These strains occur when a tendon is torn from the bone or pulled apart, when the musculotendinous junction ruptures, or when the muscle ruptures through its belly.

ORTHOPEDIC GAMUT 3-32

CERVICAL ACCELERATION-DECELERATION INJURY

The five types of cervical acceleration-deceleration injury:

Type I: Patients can have severe injuries as a result of seemingly small degrees of acceleration trauma. The symptoms include mild discomfort and stiffness of the cervical spine and loss of small increments in range of motion.

Type II: Injury palpable muscle splinting, restriction of motion, and mild to moderate spasm. No neurologic deficits or evidence of radiculopathy is observed.

Type III: Injury symptoms include moderate ligamentous sprain, advanced muscle swelling, and muscle spasm. Loss of range of motion in all planes is observed.

Type IV: Injury produces radicular symptoms that may be bilateral or unilateral. Motor and reflex changes are common.

Type V: Injury usually produces signs of neurologic instability. Cervical fracture or facet dislocation are common. Myelopathy and frank disc herniation commonly occur. Swelling and disc fragmentation are possible at the level of the spinal canal.

---

results in some degree of damage to the fibers of the ligament or its attachments.

Fundamentally, motion that exceeds the tolerance of a ligament is sufficient to produce a sprain. The extent of damage depends on the amount and duration of the applied force. As the abnormal force is applied, the ligament becomes tense and gives way at one or more of its attachments or at a point within its substance. A sprain may also involve injury to the periosteum, muscles, tendons, blood vessels, supporting soft tissue, and nerves in the adjacent area.

The examination of a sprain will initially reveal discomfort when an attempt is made to stretch the ligament or the mechanism of injury is repeated. This one maneuver, when positive, will differentiate a sprain from a strain.

Separating various grades of cervical whiplash injury is possible according to the degree of external trauma, orthopedic, and neurologic findings, as well as patient disability (Table 3-13).

TABLE 3-13

CERVICAL ACCELERATION/DECELERATION INJURY TYPES

	Type I	Type II	Type III	Type IV	Type V
Physical examination findings	Cervical stiffness or discomfort No motor or sensory deficits No nerve root traction signs No instability Intersegmental fixation, spinal subluxation Results of compression tests normal	Palpable tenderness and muscle guarding No motor or sensory deficits Sympathetic nerve irritation (mild) consisting of headache, dizziness, or light-headedness intermittent for the first week Mild instability Mild to moderate muscle spasm	Swelling and spasm Loss of range of motion in all planes Sympathetic nerve injury with deficit for 7-10 days Moderate signs of instability Possible radiculopathy without motor or reflex loss Results of orthopedic testing abnormal Evaluation for cervical disc lesion and craniomandibular injury	Pain, spasm, and disability Severe restriction of motion in all planes Sympathetic nerve injury involving head, face, and eye disturbances Moderate to severe instability Concomitant disk and articular and soft-tissue injury Severe generalized pain and spasm produced by orthopedic testing; abnormal nerve root traction signs Unilateral or bilateral radicular symptoms	Severe spinal trauma, frank disc herniation with fragmentation common Loss of motor function common Myelopathy and spinal cord compromise Multiple injury sites, often with deformity
X-ray findings	Normal	Unremarkable, except for hypolordosis	Soft-tissue swelling and loss of lordotic curve No osseous abnormality	Secondary soft-tissue swelling Loss of lordotic curve Need to rule out ligamentous disruption, fracture, and anatomic subluxation (anterior vertebral translation)	Ligamentous instability usually seen on lateral projection Need to rule out fracture or facet dislocation Immediate follow-up with CT scan to evaluate for occult fractures, disc injury, and spinal cord compromise

CT, Computed tomography.
Adapted from Brier SR: *Primary care orthopedics*, St Louis, 1999, Mosby.

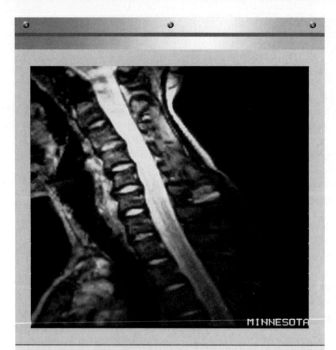

MINNESOTA

AT THE VIEWBOX

History of recent hyperflexion injury with antalgia and muscle guarding. Midline sagittal fluid-weighted MR images demonstrate disruption of the C6–7 interspinous ligament. This represents a grade 3 ligamentous injury, associated with instability. Isolated disruption of a single ligamentous structure in the spine is uncommon and warrants careful review of all other structures to exclude other high-grade soft tissue injury and fracture. (From the teaching file of Timothy Mick, DC, DACBR)

PROCEDURE

- While the patient is sitting, the cervical spine is actively moved through resisted range of motion and then through passive range of motion (Fig. 3-108).
- Pain during resisted range of motion, or isometric contraction, signifies muscle strain (Fig. 3-109).
- Pain during passive range of motion signifies ligamentous sprain (Fig. 3-110).

Next Steps/Procedures
Soto-Hall sign, spinal percussion test, and diagnostic imaging

CLINICAL PEARL

This maneuver can be applied to any joint or series of joints to determine ligamentous or muscular movement. By remembering that resisted range of motion stresses mainly muscles and passive range of motion stresses mainly ligaments, the examiner should be able to differentiate between strain and sprain and should be able to determine whether a combination of both is present.

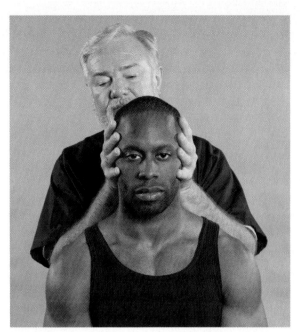

FIG. 3-108 The patient is seated comfortably, with the head and neck in the neutral position. The examiner grasps the patient's head with both hands.

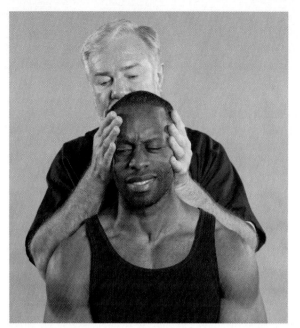

FIG. 3-109 The patient *actively* attempts rotation of the head to one side against isometric resistance. Pain production at this stage suggests muscular strain of the activated musculature. The test is repeated for the opposite side.

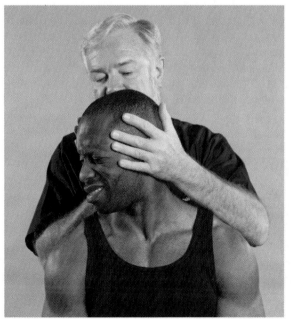

FIG. 3-110 If isometric testing is negative, the examiner *passively* rotates the patient's head and neck to one side to the limit of joint play. Pain produced in this maneuver suggests ligamentous injury. The maneuver is performed bilaterally.

Assessment for Severe Cervical Spine Sprain, Upper Cervical Rheumatoid Arthritis, Upper Cervical Spine Fracture, and Severe Upper Cervical Spine Subluxation

Comment

Of the three areas in the upper cervical spine in which fractures can be identified, the most common is the odontoid fracture, followed by the so-called hangman's fracture and by Jefferson fracture. Anatomic areas, such as transverse processes, spinous processes, and lamina and lateral masses, may also be injured. Compression fractures of the upper three vertebral bodies occur, but these fractures are uncommon. Upper cervical fractures are usually associated with injury to the head or face and not to the neck itself. Most patients with upper cervical vertebral fractures sustain minimal neurologic damage because a severe spinal cord injury results in death from respiratory arrest before the patient can be treated. Pathologic fractures of the upper cervical spine occur in osteomyelitis, tuberculosis, osteogenic sarcoma, and metastatic carcinoma, as well as in association with nasopharyngeal infections (Grisel disease). Untreated fractures of the upper cervical spine may produce serious neurologic sequelae.

A lateral radiograph of the upper cervical spine should be obtained in all trauma patients who complain of neck pain; have evidence of head, fascial, or neck trauma; or have altered consciousness. A lateral radiograph of the cervical spine will detect approximately 85% of injuries to the cervical spine and should be adequate to assess alignment from the skull to the T1 vertebral body.

Type II odontoid process fractures may be displaced anteriorly or posteriorly. The potential for neurologic injury is greater with posterior displacement. Type III odontoid process fractures may be displaced or undisplaced.

A quick and accurate diagnosis in the traumatized spinal patient is essential. Assessing whether the injury is stable or unstable is also essential. Because 5% to 10% of spinal cord injuries occur in the postinjury period because of patient mishandling, any cervical spine motion should be limited until proper examination is performed to exclude any catastrophic fracture. This task is usually accomplished with plain-film radiography in the AP, lateral, and open-mouth projections. Because spasm or voluntary guarding may occur as a result of pain, significant ligamentous injury may be masked on the initial X-ray films, thereby necessitating further evaluation with flexion and extension views.

An acute flexion injury may result in a fracture of the dens with the ligament remaining intact (Fig. 3-112). CT and MRI can easily demonstrate the fracture on images in the coronal projection.

Flexion fractures in the lower cervical spine occur typically at the C5–C6 intervertebral disc level, the most mobile segment of the cervical spine. The common *teardrop* fracture refers to a triangular piece of bone from the anterosuperior end-plate of the compressed vertebral body. With more significant force, the posterior ligamentous complex may be disrupted, resulting in complete bony failure with severe compression and comminution of the vertebral body (Fig. 3-113). This *burst* type of fracture usually involves a sagittal component of the vertebral body, as well as fractures of the posterior arch. Bony fragments are often displaced posteriorly into the spinal canal, resulting in spinal cord compression and causing severe neurologic damage. CT is excellent in demonstrating any retropulsed bony fragments within the spinal canal (Fig. 3-114).

Most patients with upper cervical spine fractures have sustained the trauma from motor-vehicle accidents, diving injuries, or falls. A large percentage of patients exhibit neck rigidity and complain of painful torticollis that is sometimes out of proportion to the injury. Such complaints, either immediately after an injury or as long as several weeks later, should alert the physician to the possibility of an upper cervical spine fracture. Examination reveals neck rigidity, and tenderness is often felt over the upper cervical spine and occasionally paraparesis or quadriparesis. The symptoms and signs may be puzzling and atypical. For instance, sleep attacks have been described.

Cervical myelopathy in the presence of significant underlying rheumatoid cervical spine disease is likely the result

---

ORTHOPEDIC GAMUT 3-33

ODONTOID PROCESS FRACTURES

The Anderson/D'Alonzo classification of odontoid process fractures:

Type I: Fractures of the odontoid are thought to represent an avulsion injury of the tip of the dens by the alar ligament. This injury is very rare, and because it is located above the transverse ligament, no associated atlantoaxial instability occurs (Fig. 3-111).

Type II: Fractures through the body or base of the odontoid have a reported prevalence of nonunion of up to 64%.

Type III: Fractures that extend into the cancellous bone of the axis have an excellent prognosis with adequate reduction and external immobilization.

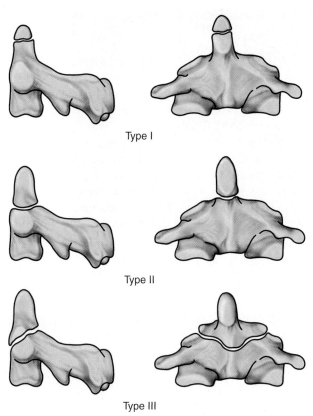

Type I

Type II

Type III

FIG. 3-111 Fractures of the odontoid are classified into three types depending on the line of the fracture through the odontoid. (From Bucholz RW: *Orthopaedic decision making*, ed 2, St Louis, 1996, Mosby.)

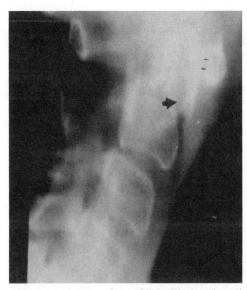

FIG. 3-112 Lateral X-ray film of C1–C2 showing displaced fracture at the base of the odontoid process with a normal atlantoaxial space, suggesting integrity of the transverse ligament. (From Watkins RG: *The spine in sports*, St Louis, 1996, Mosby.)

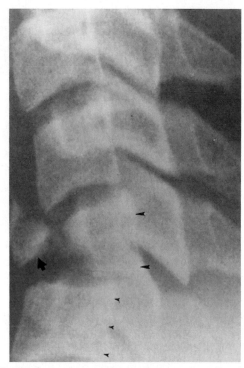

FIG. 3-113 Lateral view of a cervical teardrop fracture with posterior displacement of the remaining body into the spinal canal. (From Watkins RG: *The spine in sports*, St Louis, 1996, Mosby.)

of significant spinal cord or brainstem compression. The clinical features are the result of white or gray matter injury. There is usually central cord necrosis, long tract demyelinization and gliosis, and hypoxic changes in both anterior and posterior horn cells. An unusual clinical phenomenon known as *cruciate paralysis* may be present, which represents selective injury to the decussating corticospinal tracts of the upper extremities at the level of the cervicomedullary junction, and which may occur with C1–2 instability.

Atlantoaxial (C1–C2) instability, or *subluxation*, is the most common form of radiographic instability encountered in the **rheumatoid cervical spine**. Erosive pannus formation at the level of the C1–C2 articulation antecedes the destruction of its skeletal and ligamentous supports. The odontoid process (dens) can be partially or totally destroyed by erosive synovitis involving the atlantodental articulation. Progression of the disease process results in incompetence of surrounding ligamentous supports (transverse, alar, and apical ligaments) and articular capsular supports at C1–C2. With loss of normal static bony and ligamentous supports, some degree of atlantoaxial subluxation follows in 50% to 70% of patients, most commonly anterior subluxation (70%) of C1 on C2, although lateral, posterior, rotational, and vertical subluxation can also occur (Gurley, Bell, 1997).

Atlantoaxial subluxation is the most common and significant manifestation of rheumatoid involvement of the cervical spine. Long duration of disease, advanced patient age, and peripheral joint erosive instability are associated with more common and severe C1–C2 instabilities affecting the activities of daily living (Tables 3-14 and 3-15).

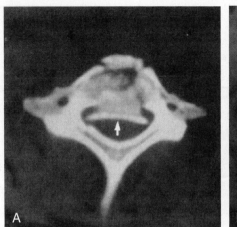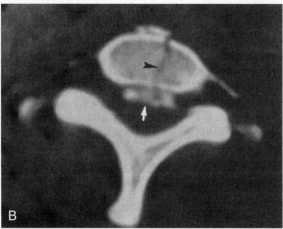

FIG. 3-114 Axial CT images demonstrating the posteriorly displaced bony fragments, as well as a sagittal cleavage fracture, through the vertebral body. (From Watkins RG: *The spine in sports,* St Louis, 1996, Mosby.)

TABLE 3-14				
NURICK CLASSIFICATION GRADES OF MYELOPATHIC DISABILITY				
Grade	**Root Involvement**	**Cord Involvement**	**Ambulatory Status**	**Employable**
Grade 0	Present	Absent	Normal	Yes
Grade I	Present	Present	Normal	Yes
Grade II	Present	Present	Mildly abnormal	Yes
Grade III	Present	Present	Severely abnormal	No
Grade IV	Present	Present	Assist dependent	No
Grade V	Present	Present	Nonambulatory	No

Based on the patient's ability to ambulate and perform daily activities.
Adapted from Gurley JP, Bell GR: The surgical management of patients with rheumatoid cervical spine disease, *Rheum Dis Clin North Am* 23(2):317-332, 1997.

TABLE 3-15				
ZEIDMAN AND DUCKER MODIFICATION OF NURICK CLASSIFICATION				
Grade	**Root Involvement**	**Cord Involvement**	**Ambulatory Status**	**Hand Function**
Grade 0	Present	Absent	Normal	Normal
Grade I	Present	Present	Normal	Slightly abnormal
Grade II	Present	Present	Mildly abnormal	Abnormal, functional
Grade III	Present	Present	Severely abnormal	Unable to button
Grade IV	Present	Present	Assist dependent	Severe dysfunction
Grade V	Present	Present	Nonambulatory	Useless

Adapted from Gurley JP, Bell GR: The surgical management of patients with rheumatoid cervical spine disease, *Rheum Dis Clin North Am* 23(2):317-332, 1997.

The instability pattern of rheumatoid involvement of the atlantoaxial joint complex is usually one of two types: anterior atlantoaxial subluxation or upward translocation of the odontoid, which is also called *superior migration, vertical subluxation,* and *downward luxation of the atlas on the axis.* Posterior subluxation of the atlantoaxial joint does not occur in rheumatoid arthritis without an associated fracture of the odontoid or nearly complete arthritic erosion and destruction of the odontoid. The anterior and posterior contact points of the odontoid are true synovial joints. Synovitis destruction of the front or back of the odontoid on the anterior arch of C1 produces some instability.

In atlantoaxial instability caused by rheumatoid arthritis, pain in the cervical area is common and usually of moderate severity. Subjective symptoms include paresthesia in the hands, *electric shock* sensations, and feelings of weakness. Joint crepitus and instability in the upper cervical spine may be felt upon palpation. The crepitus is often in the form of

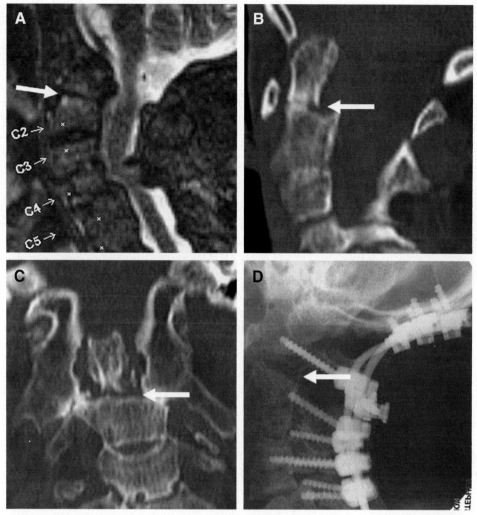

FIG. 3-115 The patient is a 78-year-old male with a long-standing history of rheumatoid arthritis. Studies showed a previously unrecognized odontoid fracture. **A,** T2-weighted sagittal magnetic resonance imaging scan. **B,** Computed tomographic sagittal reformat. **C,** Coronal reformat. **D,** Postoperative X-ray showing posterior occiput to C5 reconstruction. (From Lewandrowski K-U et al: Atraumatic odontoid fractures in patients with rheumatoid arthritis, *Spine J* 6(5):529-533, 2006.)

ORTHOPEDIC GAMUT 3-34
ATLANTOAXIAL INSTABILITY

Atlantoaxial instability caused by rheumatoid arthritis results from a combination of the following:

1. Local arthritic and mechanical instability and pain
2. Neurologic dysfunction of brainstem, cord, and peripheral nerve (root)
3. VA insufficiency

a *clunk* as C1 subluxation forward on C2. This even produces an increased prominence of C2 posteriorly. Described as the **Sharp and Purser test**, this *clunk test* or phenomenon is to be *avoided* in early examination of the patient (Fig. 3-115 and 3-116).

Sudden death caused by severe rheumatoid cervical spine disease has been reported. Mikulowski reported autopsy results in 104 patients with rheumatoid arthritis; 7 of the 11 patients (10%) with significant C1-C2 subluxation and cord compression died suddenly. Webb also reported sudden death from VA thrombosis. These reports indicate that sudden death may be the first and only clinical manifestation of significant underlying spinal disease (Gurley, Bell, 1997).

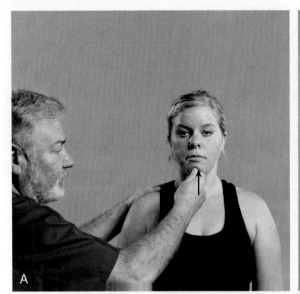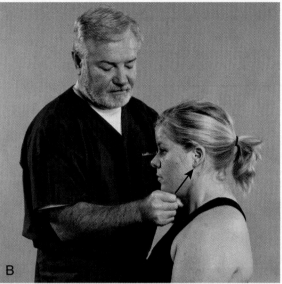

FIG. 3-116 Sharp and Purser testing. **A,** Crepitus is often in the form of a *clunk* as C1 subluxation forward on C2, when the patient resists the examiner's attempt to push the head vertically, using the chin as the fulcrum point. **B,** This can produce an increased prominence of C2 posteriorly. This *clunk test* or phenomenon is to be *avoided* in early examination of the patient.

PROCEDURE

If the patient spontaneously grasps the head with both hands when lying down or when arising from a recumbent position, this is a positive sign that indicates severe sprain, rheumatoid arthritis, fracture, or severe cervical subluxation (Figs. 3-117 and 3-118).

Next Steps/Procedures
Diagnostic imaging

CLINICAL PEARL

*N*o other physical finding is as important or as revealing as Rust sign. The presence of this sign mandates that (1) no further passive or active testing be undertaken, (2) imaging be performed immediately, and (3) the neck be adequately supported by using a cervical collar. *Rust sign has never been observed in conditions of minor consequence.*

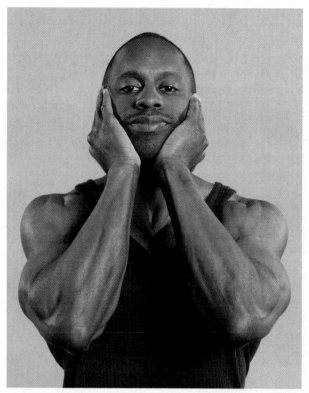

FIG. 3-117 The patient exhibits a markedly splinted cervical spine and holds the weight of the head with both hands. Removal of this support cannot be tolerated, which implies gross instability of the upper cervical spine as a result of fracture or severe sprain.

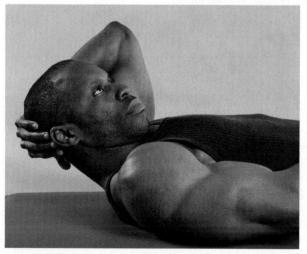

FIG. 3-118 No less significant is the patient who cannot rise from the supine position without lifting the head manually, suggesting gross upper cervical spine instability as a result of fracture or severe sprain.

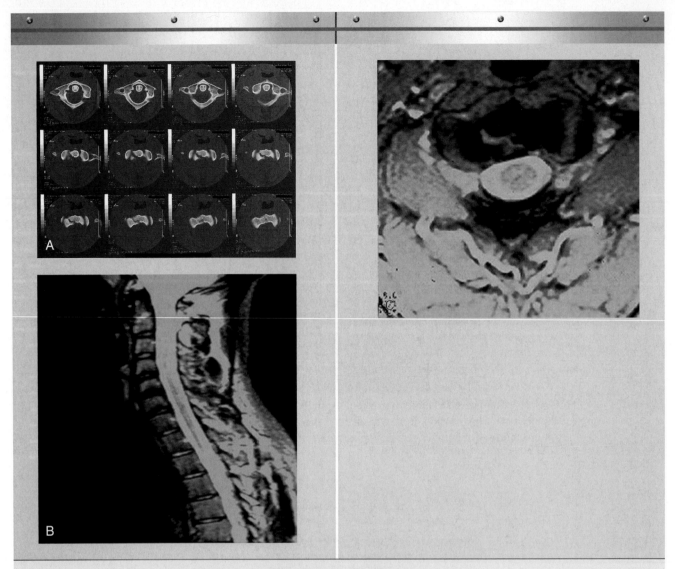

AT THE VIEWBOX

18-year-old male with recent motor vehicle accident. Emergency room films with immobilized cross-table lateral view were reported as negative and a diagnosis of cervical sprain-strain was made. Postural radiographs performed by the patient's chiropractor revealed subtle evidence of minimal anterior angulation of the dens as the only sign suggesting a C2 fracture. Clinical findings were suspicious for upper cervical fracture. Follow-up axial CT (**A**) and sagittal and axial MR images (**B** and **C**) demonstrate acute fracture of the dens, extending minimally into the C2 body (type 3 fracture), with some encroachment upon the central spinal canal. Note linear high signal near the base of the dens on fluid-weighted MR images, corresponding to lucent (low attenuation) fracture line on CT images. Careful clinical–radiographic correlation and appropriate advanced imaging follow-up avoided potentially catastrophic effects of conservative management and prompted immediate neurosurgical consultation, with a positive long-term outcome. (From the teaching file of Timothy Mick, DC, DACBR)

Assessment for Cervical Dural Sleeve Adhesion (Nerve Root) and Shoulder Adhesive Capsulitis

Comment

After trauma, scar formation (epidural fibrosis) occurs with regularity around the dura and nerve root.

Epidural fibrosis is one of the contributing factors that have led to chronic pain after spinal surgery or spinal cord injuries. The dense scar formation on the dura surrounding the neural elements has been described as the *laminectomy membrane*. Separate from potential neurologic compromise, it makes subsequent spine surgery technically difficult (Massey et al, 2002).

Epidural fibrosis may be associated with processes of tissue damage mediated by inflammation and cellular adhesion molecules (CAMs). Specifically, CAMs have been implicated with scar or adhesion formation and in the pathogenesis of different diseases, including pulmonary fibrosis, peritoneal sclerosis, cystic fibrosis, respiratory insufficiency, liver fibrosis in chronic hepatitis, interstitial pneumonia, renal interstitial fibrosis, and sarcoidosis (Sabuncuoglu et al, in press).

The reasons epidural fibrosis causes symptoms in one patient and not in others are not well understood. One explanation is that the scar tissue can act as a tethering force, as well as a constricting force, around the nerve roots. A direct traumatic insult to the nerve roots causes inflammation in the dural sleeves and perineural tissues. This inflammation may result in fibrosis, and adhesions may occur between the dural sleeves and the adjacent capsular structures. Normally the nerve roots are free in the intervertebral canals and can be moved approximately $\frac{1}{4}$ to $\frac{1}{2}$ of an inch. Nerve roots that have been injured or compressed by capsular thickening or bony encroachments cannot move within the intervertebral canals.

Nerve roots that are subjected to compressive forces by osteophytic encroachments have varying degrees of distortion and perineural fibrosis.

Postlaminectomy scar formation, termed *laminectomy membrane*, is a nonspecific postsurgical inflammatory process that causes recurrent pain after lumbar disc surgery. Recurrent pain might be induced by restriction of mobility of the nerve roots in the canal resulting from adhesions. The recurrence of pain after an initial pain-free period after spinal surgery appears in some cases to be related to the formation of fibrous tissue (Sabuncuoglu et al, in press).

The typical *burner* or *stinger* can result from different injury mechanisms. History, physical examination, and appropriate diagnostic studies help differentiate brachial plexus from cervical nerve root lesions.

Brachial plexus injuries are more likely to occur in younger patients with less well-developed neck

---

ORTHOPEDIC GAMUT 3-35

ADHESION DEGREES BETWEEN DURA MATER AND FIBROUS TISSUE

- Grade 0: when the dura mater is free of the fibrous tissue
- Grade 1: when only a thin fibrous band or bands between dura mater and fibrous tissue is observed
- Grade 2: when continuous adherence is observed but less than two thirds of the laminectomy defect
- Grade 3: when fibrous tissue adherence is large, more than two thirds of the laminectomy defect, or extends to the nerve roots

---

ORTHOPEDIC GAMUT 3-36

MATERIALS USED FOR PREVENTION OF EPIDURAL FIBROSIS

- Fat grafts
- Steroid application and injection
- Silastic membrane and polytetrafluoroethylene barrier
- Polyvinyl alcohol hydrogen membrane
- Polylactic acid membrane
- Vicryl mesh
- Sodium hyaluronate
- Methyl methacrylate
- Gel recombinant tissue plasminogen activator
- Gelatin
- Aprotinin e
- Dextran 70
- Gore-Tex
- Urokinase
- Gel foam and microfibrillar collagen
- Dexamethasone
- Fibrin glue
- CO_2 laser
- Mitomycin-c

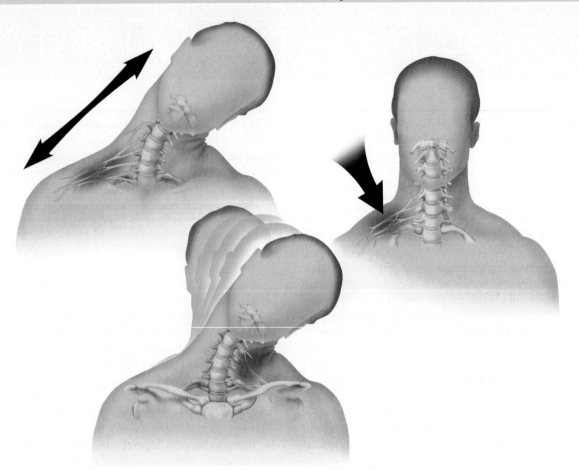

FIG. 3-119 Spurling maneuver. (From Torg JS, Shepard RJ: *Current therapy in sports medicine,* ed 3, St Louis, 1995, Mosby.)

musculature. Brachial plexus injuries are usually traction injuries resulting from lateral neck flexion away from the side of involvement. Ipsilateral shoulder depression is also a component. Pain and paresthesias involving the arm and shoulder are transient. In this injury, the Spurling test is negative (Fig. 3-119). Weakness involves the deltoid, supraspinatus, infraspinatus, and biceps.

Root lesions result from compression of the nerve root or dorsal root ganglion (or both) in the intervertebral foramen. Hyperextension or hyperextension with lateral neck flexion are the common mechanisms of injury. Neck pain and a decreased cervical range of motion may be present. Spurling test is positive.

PROCEDURE

- With the patient seated, the examiner depresses the patient's shoulder on the affected side and laterally flexes the cervical spine away from that shoulder (Figs. 3-120 and 3-121).
- This sign is positive if radicular pain is produced or aggravated.
- A positive sign indicates adhesions of the dural sleeves, spinal nerve roots, or adjacent structures of the joint capsule of the shoulder.

Next Steps/Procedures

Bakody sign, maximum foraminal encroachment test, distraction test, brachial plexus tension test, Bikele sign, Jackson cervical compression test, Spurling test, foraminal compression test, reflexes, sensory testing, and diagnostic imaging

CLINICAL PEARL

As with cervical distraction testing, this maneuver helps predict the viability of cervical traction in therapy. A sharply positive finding usually means that the patient will not tolerate cervical traction. The traction may aggravate the dural sleeve adhesion instead of relieving it.

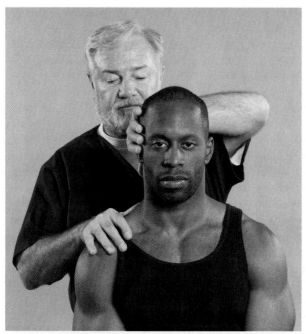

FIG. 3-120 The patient is seated, and the head and neck are in the neutral position. On the side of complaint, the examiner uses the contact points of the lateral skull and superior shoulder.

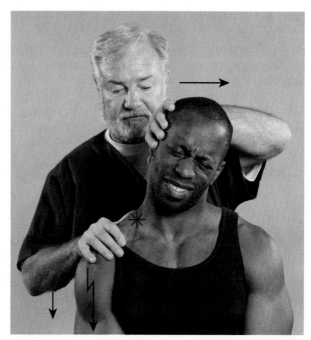

FIG. 3-121 In a slow, controlled fashion, the examiner depresses the shoulder while flexing the head toward the opposite shoulder. Reproduction of symptoms suggests a brachial plexitis or dural sleeve adhesion.

SOTO-HALL SIGN

Assessment for Cervical Spine Subluxation, Exostoses, Intervertebral Disc Lesion, Muscular Strain, Ligamentous Sprain, Vertebral Fracture, or Meningeal Irritation (Febrile)

Comment

The neck is at risk for injury in contact sports because of the inability to pad, brace, or protect the cervical spine while maintaining its function. The cervical spine must be flexible enough to allow the head and eyes to move to the right place at the right time. The spine also serves as a conduit for the central nervous system. The spinal cord and the cervical nerve roots pass through the cervical spine, making injury to the neck a potentially catastrophic event.

Even noncontact sports can be responsible for traumatic spinal injuries. Although fractures with spinal cord injuries are common, fractures without neurologic deficits are more common (Figs. 3-122 and 3-123).

Most local cervical spinal pain is secondary to involvement of the vertebral bodies, intervertebral discs, and ligamentous structures and the associated spasms of the paravertebral muscles. Too often, the symptoms of neck pain are translated into evidence for diagnosis of arthritis or disc disease without adequate examination of the patient or full consideration of the various possible causes of this symptom (Fig. 3-124).

Hereditary multiple exostosis is the most common form of bone dysplasia. This entity is also known as diaphyseal aclasis, hereditary deforming chondrodysplasia, multiple hereditary exostoses, multiple osteochondromatosis, multiple cartilaginous exostosis, dyschondroplasia, and Ehrenfried disease. It is an inherited autosomal-dominant disease with a male predominance and a benign condition characterized by the presence of multiple exostosis or osteochondromas arising from long and flat bones. However, spinal cord compression resulting from vertebral osteochondroma is a rare complication (Giudicissi-Filho et al, 2006).

During infancy and childhood, neck pain is uncommon, but when it occurs, the possibilities are intriguing. Discitis is an important consideration when it occurs as a local bacterial infection of the disc space in the cervicothoracic region and is accompanied by X-ray changes that are characteristic but late to develop. Meningismus, or meningitis, particularly in infants and very young children (whose sensorium may be difficult to evaluate) can be associated with neck pain caused by meningeal inflammation and associated muscle spasm. Lymphomatous infiltration or an abscess in the epidural space may become painful long before neurologic symptoms are evident. A herniated disc may also be symptomatic.

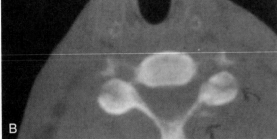

FIG. 3-122 A fractured lamina and facet of this kind can occur with head trauma. (From Watkins RG: *The spine in sports,* St Louis, 1996, Mosby.)

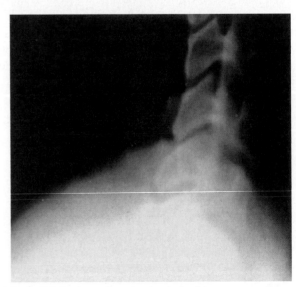

FIG. 3-123 A facet fracture healed with nonoperative care and produced a stiff but stable segment. (From Watkins RG: *The spine in sports,* St Louis, 1996, Mosby.)

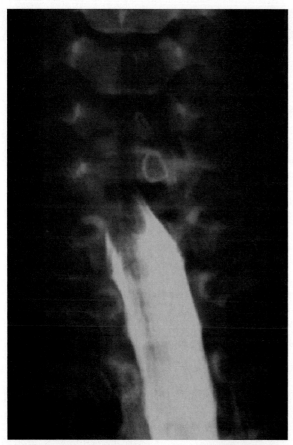

FIG. 3-124 Myelography showing an extradural mass causing a block at C7 level. (From Giudicissi-Filho M et al: Cervical spinal cord compression due to an osteochondroma in hereditary multiple exostosis: case report and review of the literature, *Surg Neurol* 66[suppl 3]:S7-S11, 2006.)

Although infections in the cervical spine are rare, the consequences of failing to diagnose such infections are so ominous that infection is a necessary consideration even in instances of slightly aberrant cervical spine syndromes. Approximately 15% of bone infections involve the spine, but the spine is the most common site of tuberculosis of bone. Of the entire spine—cervical, thoracic, lumbar, and sacral—the cervical spine is the most uncommon site for infection. Although all age groups may have infections in the spine, people in their teens or 40s and older have the highest rates of incidence.

> Bacterial meningitis is a significant problem among hospitalized patients. Patients with nosocomial meningitis have been described as a patient group distinct from community-acquired meningitis by atypical clinical presentation, unusual bacterial pathogens and a high rate of adverse outcome (Weisfelt et al, 2007)

ORTHOPEDIC GAMUT 3-37

RISK FACTORS FOR NOSOCOMIAL MENINGITIS

1. History of neurosurgery
2. Cerebrospinal fluid leakage or recent head trauma
3. Distant focus of infection
4. An immunocompromised state

ORTHOPEDIC GAMUT 3-38

GLASGOW OUTCOME SCALE

- 1: Death
- 2: Vegetative state
- 3: Severe disability
- 4: Moderate disability
- 5: Mild or no disability

PROCEDURE

- The patient is placed supine (Fig. 3-125).
- The examiner places one hand on the sternum of the patient and exerts slight pressure so that no flexion can take place at either the lumbar or thoracic regions of the spine (Fig. 3-126).
- The examiner places the other hand under the patient's occiput and flexes the head toward the chest (Fig. 3-127).
- The test is used primarily when fracture of a vertebra is suspected.
- The flexion of the head and neck on the sternum progressively produces a pull on the posterior spinous ligaments.
- When the spinous process of the injured vertebra is reached, the patient experiences a noticeable local pain.
- A positive result indicates subluxation, exostoses, disc lesion, sprain or strain, vertebral fracture, or meningeal irritation (an elevated temperature must exist for corroboration) (Fig. 3-128).

Next Steps/Procedures

O'Donoghue maneuver, spinal percussion, Lhermitte sign, Dejerine sign, swallowing test, Valsalva maneuver, Naffziger test, reflexes, sensory testing, and diagnostic imaging

CLINICAL PEARL

Soto-Hall sign is often misapplied in the assessment of fractures and sprains for the entire spine. The sign is a nonspecific test with limited capacity to localize conditions of the cervical and upper thoracic spine. The use of this sign to draw conclusions below T8 is largely guesswork.

With the Kernig-Brudzinski phenomena in this test, the patient's temperature must be assessed. A febrile patient with Kernig or Brudzinski sign—a variation of Soto-Hall sign—is a high-risk candidate for meningitis.

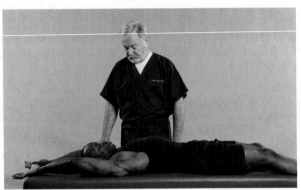

FIG. 3-125 The patient rests on the examining table in a supine position with the legs fully extended and the arms extended over the head.

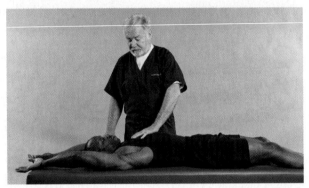

FIG. 3-126 The examiner supports the patient's head with one hand while stabilizing the patient's chest with the other hand.

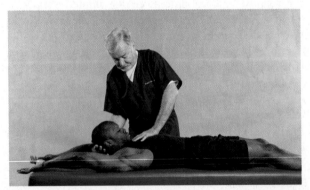

FIG. 3-127 The head and neck are sharply and passively flexed, approximating the patient's chin to the chest. Any tendency for the shoulders to rise from the table is countered with downward sternal pressure. Pain that is localized to the cervicothoracic spine suggests subluxation, exostoses, disc lesion, sprain, strain, or fracture of vertebrae.

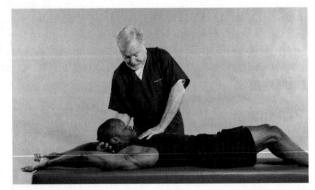

FIG. 3-128 While the head is flexed toward the chest, a reflex flexion of the knees and thighs may be produced. This reflex is equivalent to a Kernig or Brudzinski sign and suggests meningitis.

SPINAL PERCUSSION TEST

Assessment for Osseous or Soft-Tissue Injury

Comment

Compression fractures resulting from axial loading may be stable or unstable. Stability depends on the degree of displacement and associated soft-tissue injury. Axial cervical burst fractures are usually unstable and result in neurologic damage. Dislocation of the cervical facet joints may occur unilaterally or bilaterally in association with forward displacement of a vertebral body on the one below. Injuries to the upper cervical spine may result in C1–C2 instabilities as a result of rupture to the transverse and alar ligaments. These ligaments stabilize or fix the odontoid process to C1.

Isolated fractures of the posterior arch of the atlas are secondary to hyperextension with or without axial loading of the upper cervical spine. In this circumstance, the chance that some other cervical injury is also present is approximately a 50%.

The Jefferson (or burst) fracture may involve four fractures: two anterior and two posterior to the lateral masses. Because of the spreading of the lateral masses and the arch, neurologic compromise rarely occurs.

Transverse ligament ruptures occur from direct blows to the occiput. If the distance between the anterior ring of C1 and the anterior cortex of the odontoid process on the lateral flexion radiograph is more than 5 mm, a transverse ligament rupture is present. If the distance is more than 9 to 10 mm, additional ruptures of the alar ligaments and apical ligaments of the odontoid process are present.

Pain or discomfort that is nonarticular may be myofascial in origin. The patient with myofascial pain typically has multiple sites of trigger points that refer pain to a distant site (Table 3-16).

Vehicular accidents are a common source of trauma to the lower cervical spine and may cause a wide variety of fractures and dislocations. Compression fractures at the anterior edge of the vertebral bodies may be caused by a hyperflexion motion alone or in combination with a vertical compression. The stability of these fractures depends on the degree of vertebral compression and the presence of posterior ligamentous damage. (Fig. 3-129)

ORTHOPEDIC GAMUT 3-39

ATLANTOAXIAL INJURIES

The radiographic signs of atlantoaxial injuries are often subtle:

1. The prevertebral soft-tissue shadow on the lateral radiograph should be less than 5 mm wide at C2 and 5 to 10 mm wide in front of the ring of the atlas.
2. The lateral cervical spine view will reveal fractures of the posterior ring of the atlas.
3. The open-mouth odontoid view helps in detecting subtle displacement of the lateral masses in relation to the facets of the axis.

ORTHOPEDIC GAMUT 3-40

CERVICAL SPINE FLEXION-EXTENSION RADIOGRAPHS

The following are prerequisites for cervical spine flexion-extension radiographs:

1. A neurologically intact patient
2. Performance of all movements actively by the patient
3. No altered state of consciousness (including intoxication)
4. Direct physician supervision of the radiographic study

TABLE 3-16

REFERRAL ZONES ASSOCIATED WITH TRIGGER POINTS IN MYOFASCIAL PAIN SYNDROME

Localized Trigger Points	Referral Zone
Suboccipital muscles	Temporal region
	Vertex of head
	Temporalis muscle via greater occipital nerve
Levator scapula	Inferior or superior scapula border, occiput
Greater or lesser rhomboid muscles	Cervical spine, shoulder, or scapula region
Infraspinous or teres minor muscles	Arm, shoulder, hand
Sternocleidomastoid muscles	Supraorbital region
	Temporal region
	Forehead, ear
Scalene muscles	Shoulder, arm or hand, chest, scapula
Masseter muscle	Ear, suboccipital region, temporal region
Trapezius muscle	Suboccipital region, shoulder, orbit or temporal area

From Brier SR: *Primary care orthopedics*, St Louis, 1999, Mosby.

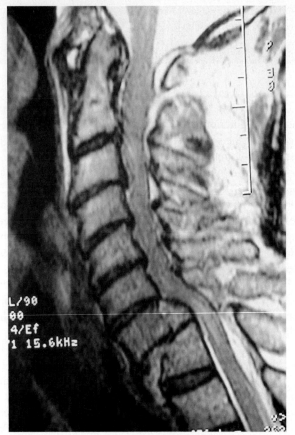

FIG. 3-129 C7–T1 dislocation under an osteoarthritic block. Fractures of the cervicothoracic junction are a rare entity but must be monitored systematically, particularly in intubated poly-traumatized cases. This injury is associated with severe neurologic and vital prognosis. (Adapted from Lenoir T et al: Neurological and functional outcome after unstable cervicothoracic junction injury treated by posterior reduction and synthesis, *Spine* 6[5]:507-513, 2006.)

The cervicothoracic junction is a complex anatomical region. Injuries in this area are associated with serious clinical problems regarding the anatomic diagnosis of the lesion, the choice of surgical treatment to perform, and the clinical outcome. Diagnosis is often difficult to make. X-ray examination provides little help because the cervicothoracic junction is often difficult to see; therefore CT scan or MRI imaging is needed. Diagnosing spinal fractures is not always easy. Diagnosis is even more difficult when the subjects are suffering from multiple trauma, are unconscious, or are sedated. Indeed, in most cases, despite such aids as arm

traction or swimmer's position, it is often best seen in profile than on the superior end-plate of C7, particularly when the subject is elderly or obese. Facial positions may give elements of orientation, particularly when either transverse processes or the first costal arches are fractured (Lenoir et al, 2006).

Traumatic injuries of the cervical spine are among the most common causes of severe disability and death after trauma. These injuries are often not diagnosed in the emergency room situation. Approximately one third of the injuries to the cervical spine result from motor-vehicle accidents, one third from falling, and the remaining one third from some type of athletic injury or wound inflicted by a missile or falling object.

The incidence of cervical spine injuries peaks during adolescence, young adulthood, and again during the sixth and seventh decades. Because of the nature of accidents resulting in cervical spine injuries, most involve young, healthy persons who are very active. This group includes people who engage in physically dangerous activities and occasionally those who exhibit sociopathic personality traits. People in their fifth and sixth decades make up the second largest group of cervical spinal injury patients. Cervical spondylosis and a preexisting narrow spinal canal are closely associated with injury in this age group. Lesser forces may result in severe spine and spinal cord injury in this group.

PROCEDURE

- With the patient seated and the head slightly flexed, the examiner percusses the spinous processes and associated musculature of each of the cervical vertebra with a neurologic reflex hammer (Fig. 3-130).
- Evidence of localized pain indicates a possible fractured vertebra.
- Evidence of radicular pain indicates a possible disc lesion.
- Because of the nonspecific nature of this test, other conditions will also elicit a positive pain response.
- A ligamentous sprain will cause pain when the spinous processes are percussed.
- Percussing the paraspinal musculature will elicit a positive sign for muscular strain (Fig. 3-131).

Next Steps/Procedures
Soto-Hall sign, O'Donoghue test, Dejerine sign, swallowing test, Valsalva maneuver, Naffziger test, Lhermitte sign, and diagnostic imaging

CLINICAL PEARL

When soft-tissue percussion reproduces the pain, the examiner may expect the same phenomenon from applications of ultrasound to the tissue. This pain represents spasmophilia, and the uses of such therapies may need to be delayed until the soft tissue is no longer reactive to percussion.

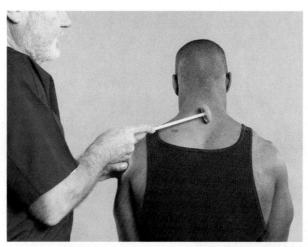

FIG. 3-130 In the seated position, the patient flexes the cervical spine forward, exposing the spinous processes as much as possible. The examiner percusses the spinous processes of each vertebra. Localized pain is evidence of a fracture or severe sprain. Radiating pain suggests an intervertebral disc syndrome.

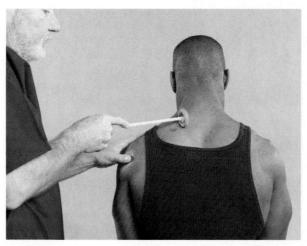

FIG. 3-131 The paravertebral tissues are percussed. Pain elicited in the soft tissues suggests muscular strain and highly sensitive MTrPs.

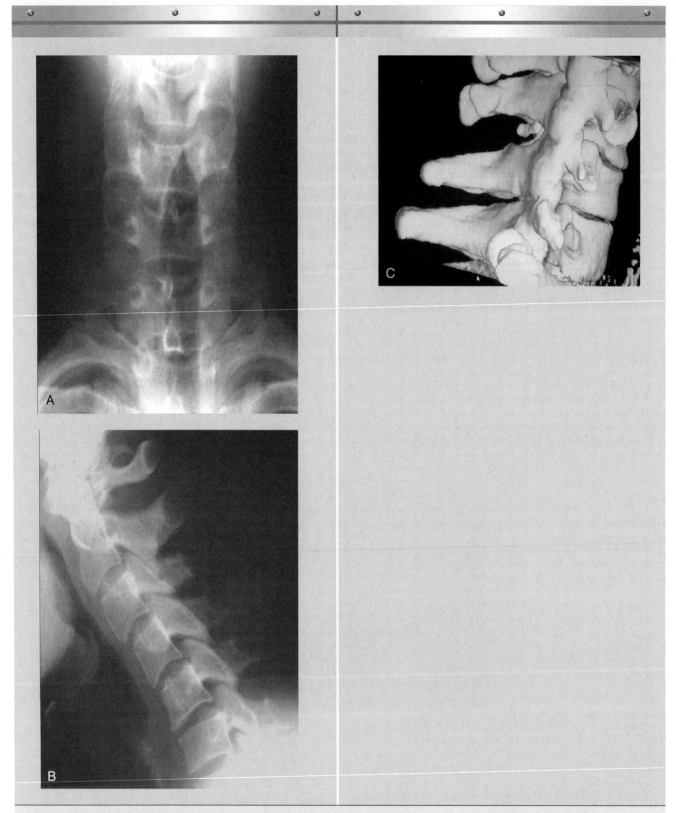

AT THE VIEWBOX

18-year-old male with history of neck pain after motor vehicle accident. Plain films (**A** and **B**) demonstrate a widened interspinous space at C6–7 with flexion and anterolisthesis of C6 on C7. An interspinous space exceeding 1.5 times the spaces above and below repre-sents a sign of instability. There is a subtle C6–7 laminar avulsion fracture on plain films, more obvious on cervical spine CT with 3-D reconstruction (**C**). There is also evi-dence of a minimal compression fracture of C7. (From the teaching file of Timothy Mick, DC, DACBR)

SPURLING TEST

Assessment for Cervical Nerve Root Compression Syndrome

Comment

Cervical radiculopathy is a dysfunction of a cervical spinal nerve. It is usually associated with neck and upper extremities pain and a combination of sensory, motor or reflex changes in the affected nerve-root distribution. Neoplastic processes are infrequent etiologic causes for nerve impingement and commonly seen as extradural spinal metastasis because the dura mater provides a relative barrier for metastatic disease. Extranodal presentations of lymphoma account for 15% to 30% of all lymphoma cases, and it can occur in sites outside lymphatic structures. The incidence of spinal cord or root compression caused by epidural Hodgkin lymphoma is less than 5% and usually seen in the setting of advanced disease. Radicular syndromes as a first sign of lymphoma are exceptional (Al-Khayat et al, 2007).

Narrowing of the intervertebral foramina, pressure and shearing forces on the Z joint surfaces, intervertebral disc compression, and pressure on stiff ligamentous and muscular structures may all cause pain (Fig. 3-132). A pain pattern may be perfectly reproduced, which allows for identification of the neurologic level. If radicular pain or paresthesia with referral to the upper extremity occurs, nerve root irritation is present. If the pain is confined to the neck, soft, connective tissues or joints are more likely to be the pain-sensitive structures.

Cervical radicular pain affects approximately 1 in 1000 adults per year and has a high impact on the patient's quality of life. It is most commonly caused by an irritation or injury of the cervical spinal roots as a result of herniated intervertebral disc or narrowing of the intervertebral foramen (Van Zundert et al, 2007). Root pain may be aggravated by spinal motions that narrow the intervertebral foramen through which the diseased nerve root passes. In cervical nerve root disease, simultaneous extension and lateral flexion of the neck toward the affected side or a blow to the vertex of the head (**Spurling Bonk test**) may result in sudden aggravation of neck and dermatomal arm pain, paresthesia, or both. This test is sometimes of value in the diagnosis of a laterally herniated intervertebral disc in the cervical spine.

All patients who sustain sufficient injury to the cervical spine to make the examiner suspect cervical disc compromise should have a standard three-view plain-film x-ray series (Table 3-17).

Patients with persistent radiculopathy with or without motor loss for at least 4 to 8 weeks should undergo electrodiagnostic testing after MRI. Electrodiagnostic tests can document any central denervating disorder or concomitant peripheral entrapment neuropathy.

TABLE 3-17		
CERVICAL DISC SYNDROMES		
	Acute	**Chronic**
Type	Herniated cervical disc	Degenerative disc disease
Physical examination findings	Paravertebral myospasm	Chronic cervical stiffness, hypertonicity
	Limited range of motion with signs of instability	Upper extremity referral
	Radicular signs with possible arm, hand, or scapula referral	Possible bilateral or unilateral intermittent radiculopathy, progressive motor changes or atrophy, prolonged cervical instability
	Often motor, sensory, or reflex changes	
	Nerve root traction signs	Possible nerve root traction signs
	Abnormal results on compression tests	Abnormal results on compression tests
X-ray findings	Standard three-view series (i.e., anteroposterior, open-mouth, lateral) if antecedent trauma	Same as for acute conditions, plus oblique films, if neuroforaminal pathologic abnormality or fracture suspected
	Decreased intervertebral disc spacing or spondylosis possible	Decreased intervertebral disc space, osteophytes, possible anterior subluxation secondary to anterior longitudinal ligament buckling
	Altered cervical lordosis	Hypolordosis
Secondary diagnoses	Cervical radiculopathy, radiculitis; cervical myelopathy; cervical spinal stenosis; acute cervical myospasm	Cervical radiculopathy, radiculitis; cervical myelopathy; cervical spinal stenosis; acute cervical myospasm

Adapted from Brier SR: *Primary care orthopedics*, St Louis, 1999, Mosby.

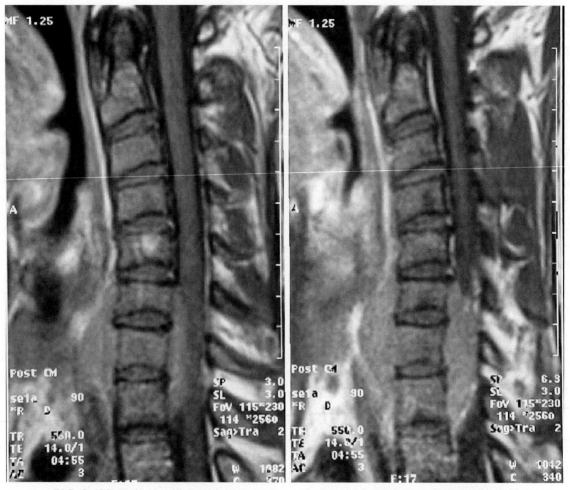

FIG. 3-132 Patients with lymphoma may have discrete epidural masses (MRI of paraspinal masses above) that compress the spinal cord, causing long tract signs, or they may infiltrate and compress exiting nerve roots, causing the symptoms of pure radiculopathy. In addition, radiculopathy can be the result of autoimmune inflammatory conditions or infectious etiology commonly caused by herpes zoster infections or the effects of radiation therapy. In general, radiation plexopathy is much less painful than malignant plexopathy. A latency of 6 months or more typically occurs from the time of radiation, and affected patients usually have experienced higher doses of radiation. (From Al-Khayat H et al: Cervical radiculopathy secondary to Hodgkin's lymphoma, *Surg Neurol* 67[5]:540-543, 2007.)

ORTHOPEDIC GAMUT 3-41

MRI SCANS

Follow-up with an MRI scan of the cervical spine is appropriate for the following patients:

1. Patients who do not respond to conservative measures of care within 2 to 4 weeks and have abnormal neurologic findings
2. Patients who have persistent radiculopathy and loss of motion in multiple planes

3. Patients who exhibit signs of myelopathy and stenosis
4. Patients who have progressive symptoms with motor or sensory deficits
5. Patients who have a cervical spinal canal of questionable patency
6. Patients who have equivocal findings on routine radiography

---

PROCEDURE

- The test is performed with the patient seated (Fig. 3-133).
- The examiner places one hand on top of the patient's head and gradually increases downward pressure (Fig. 3-134).
- The patient notes any pain or paresthesia and the distribution thereof.
- Pressure may also be applied while the head is laterally flexed to either side and extended (Fig. 3-135).
- Pressure should be maintained.
- This maneuver closes the intervertebral foramina on the side of the flexion and reproduces the familiar pain or paresthesia (Fig. 3-136).

Next Steps/Procedures

Bakody sign, maximum foraminal encroachment test, shoulder depression test, distraction test, brachial plexus tension test, Bikele sign, Jackson cervical compression test, foraminal compression test, reflex and sensory testing, electrodiagnosis, and diagnostic imaging

---

CLINICAL PEARL

Spurling test is an aggressive cervical compression test, and the patient should be informed of each step as it is introduced. However, the examiner should not cue the patient for pain responses. Spurling test elicits *cervical collapse sign* quite easily.

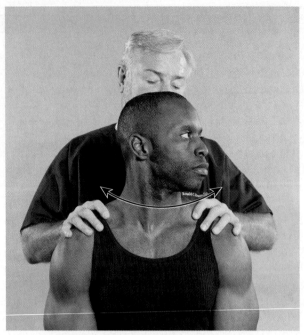

FIG. 3-133 While seated comfortably and with an erect posture, the patient actively rotates the head from side to side. Localization of pain is noted.

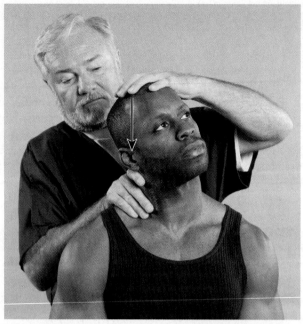

FIG. 3-134 The patient's head is laterally flexed toward the side of complaint. The examiner applies gradually progressive downward pressure to the head and neck. Reproduction of symptoms or collapse sign at this point constitutes a positive test. The balance of the test should not be completed.

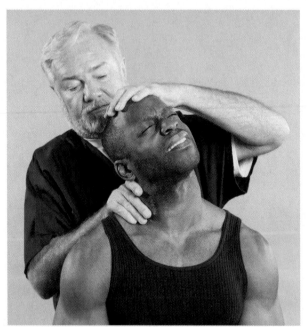

FIG. 3-135 From the laterally flexed position, the neck is extended as far as the patient can tolerate. The examiner applies progressive downward pressure. Reproduction of radicular symptoms suggests nerve root compression. Localized spinal pain suggests facet involvement.

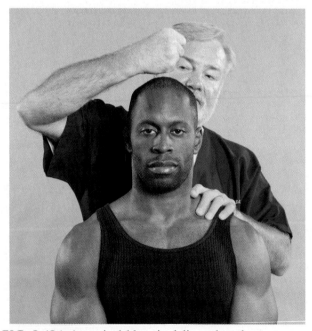

FIG. 3-136 A vertical blow is delivered to the uppermost portion of the cranium. The examiner may wish to interpose a hand between the concussing hand and the patient's skull. The head and neck are first in a neutral position for this procedure and then positioned into lateral flexion and extension for a repeated procedure. The test will stimulate any nerve root irritation or other pain-sensitive structures related to disc disease and cervical spondylosis. Use of this modification should not be a surprise to the patient.

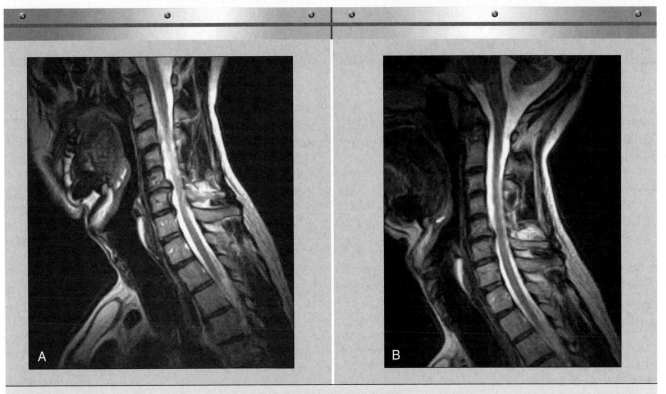

AT THE VIEWBOX

Upright MRI now allows assessment of the dynamic (position-dependent) component of abnormality of the multijoint complex of the spine in sagittal, axial, and coronal planes. In this instance, the full impact of the right posterolateral disc herniation and the associated right spondylophyte-uncinate osteophyte formation on the subjacent neural structures is best assessed on the axial image performed with extension and right rotation (**A**). Compare this with the axial image in the neutral posture (**B**). This patient had right radicular symptoms only when in a position of extension and right rotation, which produced maximal compromise of the right nerve root canal and right half of the central canal. (From the teaching file of Timothy Mick, DC, DACBR)

SWALLOWING TEST

Assessment for Space-Occupying Mass, Ligamentous Sprain, Muscular Strain, Fracture, Cervical Intervertebral Disc Lesion, Tumor, or Osteophyte at the Anterior Portion of the Cervical Spine

Comment

Dysphagia may be of prognostic significance and is often indicative of esophageal injury, pharyngeal hemorrhage or edema, or retropharyngeal hemorrhage (Fig. 3-137).

Retropharyngeal hemorrhage is an uncommon occurrence but can have serious consequences. If the hematoma is contained locally, it can cause airway obstruction as a result of external compression of the larynx or trachea. This circumstance has been reported in both traumatic and spontaneous retropharyngeal hematomas. Although laryngeal compression can occur rapidly and be life threatening, theories suggest that the majority of cases can be managed safely by observation. Less frequently documented is the potential for large volume blood loss, as illustrated by this case report. The majority of reported cases of retropharyngeal hemorrhage occur as a result of trauma. Although some of these are from major trauma, a surprisingly large number are from relatively minor head injuries, usually involving hyperextension of the neck and often involving an elderly patient. Retropharyngeal hemorrhage has also been reported as a complication of infection, foreign body, polycythemia rubra vera, and anticoagulation (Newton 2006).

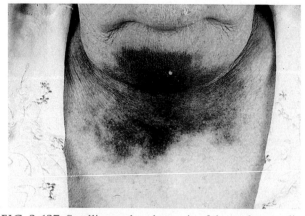

FIG. 3-137 Swelling and ecchymosis of the neck extending onto the upper chest wall associated with extensive hematoma of the posterior pharyngeal wall but no laryngeal swelling or compression. (Adapted from Newton AI: Spontaneous retropharyngeal hematoma: an unusual presentation of thoracic aortic dissection, *J Emerg Med* 31[1]:45-48, 2006.)

Dysphagia may also result from severe muscle spasm. When dysphagia is present, the examiner should look for ligamentous disruption, dislocation, subluxation, or fracture and should make thorough use of cineradiography, tomography, and CT or bone scanning to uncover the true nature and extent of the injuries.

Anterior osteophytes from the cervical vertebrae, particularly C5, C6, and C7, may compress the posterior wall of the esophagus and irritate the tissues and smooth muscle. The symptom may be either dysphagia or simply an annoying awareness of swallowing.

Ossification of anterior longitudinal ligament is associated with diffuse idiopathic skeletal hyperostosis, which is characterized by extensive spinal osteophyte formation and ossification of tendons, ligaments, and fasciae. Huge ossification of cervical anterior longitudinal ligament may cause dysphagia by compressing the cervical esophagus. Symptoms of dysphagia are subjective (Terai et al, 2006).

True disc herniation is relatively uncommon in older adults because of the decreased water content of the nucleus pulposus. When disc herniation does occur, it is usually triggered by some form of trauma. Symptoms may include sudden and severe neck and arm pain, as well as paresthesia along the involved nerve root. Neck movements, especially lateral flexion toward the affected side, will typically aggravate the pain (Fig 3-138).

Intervertebral CDH is a relatively common disorder, affecting approximately 5.5 in 100,000 individuals within the United States. CDH affects primarily the C5-C6 or C6-C7 disc and affects men slightly more than women in the fourth and fifth decades of life. CDH leads to degenerative disorders throughout the cervical spine, which may portend the risk of rupture of the posterior longitudinal ligament, disc fragmentation, and, potentially, central canal encroachment. Central canal encroachment is a hallmark of cervical spondylitic myelopathy, the most common form of spinal cord dysfunction in individuals over the age of 55 (Braga-Baiak et al, in press).

PROCEDURE

- While seated, the patient is instructed to swallow (Fig. 3-139).
- Presence of pain or difficulty swallowing indicates a space-occupying lesion, ligamentous sprain, muscular strain, or fracture, such as disc protrusion, tumor, or osteophyte at the anterior portion of the cervical spine.

Next Steps/Procedures
Dejerine sign, Valsalva maneuver, Naffziger test, Lhermitte sign, reflexes and sensory testing, and diagnostic imaging

CLINICAL PEARL

Dysphagia is often observed after hyperextension trauma of the cervical spine. Coupled with other sympathetic nervous system phenomena, the patient attributes the sore throat or hoarseness to a cold. The dysphagia is fleeting but serves as a more conclusive sign as to the extent of soft-tissue involvement in the injury.

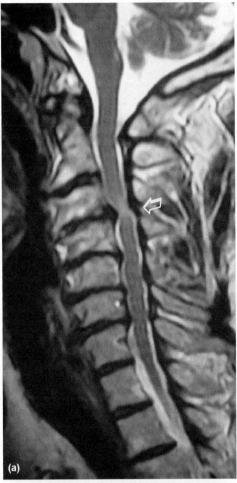

(a)

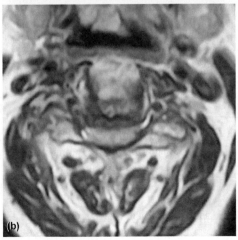

(b)

FIG. 3-138 Sagittal T2-weighted image of a 71-year-old woman demonstrates diffuse disc desiccation, and disc space narrowing at C2–C3, C3–C4, C4–C5, C5–C6, and C6–C7. A severe diffuse disc extrusion is observed at the C3–C4 level *(arrow)* with spinal cord compression and spinal cord high T2 SI (myelomalacia). (Adapted from Braga-Baiak A et al: Intra- and inter-observer reliability of MRI examination of intervertebral disc abnormalities in patients with cervical myelopathy, *Eur J Radiol* 65[1]:91–98, 2008.)

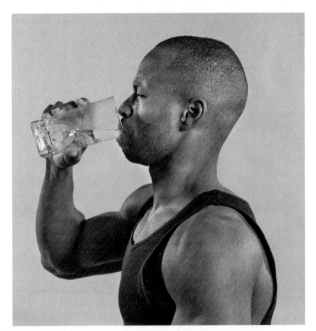

FIG. 3-139 The patient is instructed to swallow. A beverage or small food item may be needed to induce this activity. The presence of pain indicates esophageal irritation caused by direct trauma or a retroesophageal space–occupying mass.

Assessment for Vertebrobasilar Artery Syndrome

Comment

The blood supply of the vital neck structures, including bony spine, spinal cord, nerve roots, coverings, and posterior cranial fossa and cerebral visual cortex, is derived from the VAs. The tortuous course these arteries take and the susceptibility of their intimate coverings to structural change places them in a vulnerable position. In most instances, the protective mechanism is amazingly adequate. However, when changes such as atheromatous cracks develop within the vessels, circulation may be compromised or temporarily obstructed. Doppler examination is useful in establishing changes in vertebrobasilar arterial flow (Fig. 3-140).

The artery is intimately related to the Luschka joints medially and the apophyseal joint posterolaterally; thus osteophyte formation at either site may encroach on the artery's usual course. The efficiency of the VA system is related to the anastomosis at the circle of Willis with the internal carotid system. A weak point in one area may influence the other.

Contrast studies have been used to show that head and neck movement, primarily involving rotation, may alter blood flow in the VA. Pathologic changes in the VA may favor ischemia. The flow between C6 and C2 may be diminished on the side to which the head and neck is turned, and the flow may be increased in the opposite vessel at the point where the artery twists over the arch of the atlas. Changes in such a mechanism would explain transient attacks of vertigo that are attributed to vertebrobasilar ischemia.

Vertebrobasilar insufficiency (VBI) is a condition caused by insufficient blood supply to certain parts of the brain, leading to various temporary and permanent symptoms. Symptoms can be quite varied, including vertigo or dizziness, gait disturbances, impaired vision, position-related nystagmus, difficulty talking, and weakness or numbness on one or both sides of the body. Among these symptoms, vertigo is the most common symptom in patients with VBI. Arteriosclerosis, embolic incidents, and compressive effects of cervical spondylosis play most important roles in the etiology of VBI. Different noninvasive imaging techniques can quantify blood flow volume among which only sonography and MR phase-contrast flow quantification allow the assessment of individual vessels. Doppler examination of the extracranial arteries has become a widely available and reliable tool in the evaluations of patients with suspected VBI (Acar et al, 2005).

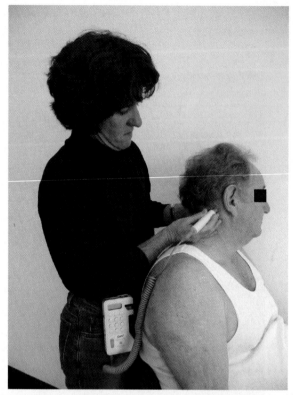

FIG. 3-140 Protocol for ultrasonographic examination of the VA at the suboccipital and the C1–C2 level; a velocimeter is used to determine the status of VA blood flow at rest and to examine flow velocity changes when the head and neck have been rotated. As changes in flow velocity may occur with vessel stenosis and can be identified by changes in pitch of the audible signal (or amplitude of the digital display), a change in audible signal may give an indication of the biomechanical forces imparted to the artery by cervical spine positioning. (Adapted from Thomas LC, Rivett DA, Bolton PS: Pre-manipulative testing and the use of the velocimeter, *Man Ther* 13[1]:29-36, 2008.)

ORTHOPEDIC GAMUT 3-42

BRAINSTEM ISCHEMIA

In vertebrobasilar artery insufficiency, brainstem ischemia is the result of:
1. Trauma to the arterial wall producing damage to the arterial wall
2. Trauma to the arterial wall producing vasospasm

ORTHOPEDIC GAMUT 3-43

ARTERIAL WALL (INTIMAL) DAMAGE

In vertebrobasilar syndrome, damage to the artery wall is the result of:

1. Compression or stretching (or both) of the VA wall that applies enough force to disrupt the vaso vasorum, resulting in subintimal hematoma. VA blood flow is decreased by occlusion of the lumen.
2. The intima is the most likely tissue to tear when the vessel is stretched, compressed, or both. Exposure of the subendothelial tissue leads to the cascade mechanism, resulting in clot formation (thrombosis). The clot remains adherent to the tear and may lead to vessel occlusion.
3. The propagating clot extends into the lumen. The blood flow may *break off* part of the clot and form an embolus. The embolus causes arterial occlusion distally, leading to infarction.
4. When blood dissects the intima and the internal elastica, a dissecting aneurysm is formed.

ORTHOPEDIC GAMUT 3-44

VASOSPASM

Arterial wall intimal trauma producing vasospasm follows the Virchow triad:

1. Change in vessel wall within the VBA system: Neck rotation causes the artery to be momentarily compressed or stretched, which may result in spasm, without VA damage.
2. Change in blood flow within the VBA system: Even after the removal of the arterial compression, the spasm may persist, which reduces the blood supply to tissue. Blood flow may stagnate within the involved vessel.
3. Change in blood constituents within the VBA system: The VAs can be sufficiently compromised (stasis) to initiate a propagating thrombus and subsequent embolism.

PROCEDURE

- The patient is standing and is instructed to outstretch the arms, supinate the hands, and close the eyes (Figs. 3-141 to 3-143).
- The patient marches in place and extends and rotates the head while continuing to march (Fig. 3-144).
- The test is repeated with the head rotated and extended to the opposite side.
- The examiner watches for a loss of balance, dropping of the arms, and pronation of the hands.
- If any of these events occurs, the examiner should suspect vertebral, basilar, or carotid artery stenosis or compression.

Next Steps/Procedures

Barré-Liéou sign, vertebrobasilar artery function test, Hautant test, DeKleyn test, Hallpike maneuver, vascular diagnosis, and diagnostic imaging

CLINICAL PEARL

If the patient loses equilibrium at any time while the eyes are closed, cerebellar circulation must be evaluated. In this procedure the patient may lose equilibrium as soon as the head is rotated to one side. The examiner must be prepared to prevent the patient from falling.

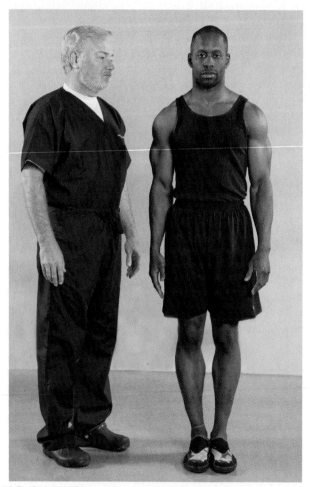

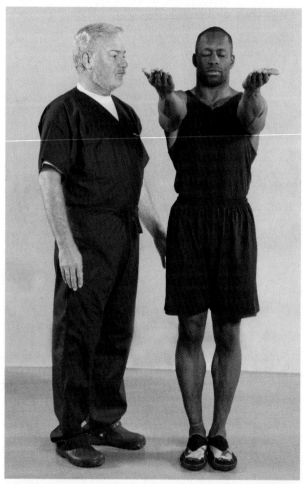

FIG. 3-141 The patient stands with the eyes open and the arms resting at the sides. The postural base is narrowed. The examiner observes for any equilibrium difficulty. The examiner should remain close to the patient throughout this procedure.

FIG. 3-142 The patient closes the eyes and elevates the extended arms forward to shoulder level. The patient's hands are fully supinated. While the patient maintains this position with the narrowed postural base, the examiner observes for loss of equilibrium or drift of the arms and pronation of the hands.

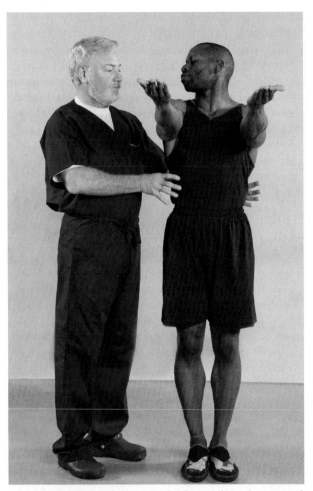

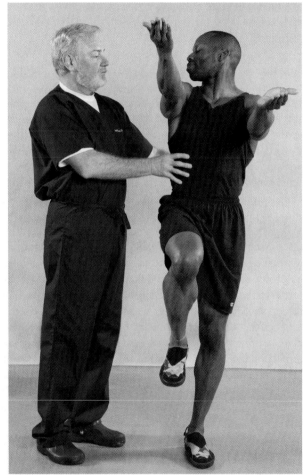

FIG. 3-143 The patient extends the neck and rotates the head to one side while maintaining a narrowed postural base, elevating the arms, and supinating the hands. The eyes remain closed. The examiner observes for difficulty in the performance of each segment of the test.

FIG. 3-144 The patient attempts to maintain the head and neck rotation or extension, arm elevation, and hand supination while marching in place. Loss of balance, dropping or drifting of the arms, or pronation of the hands is indicative of vertebrobasilar or carotid artery stenosis or compression. The test is repeated with the head and neck rotated to the opposite side.

NEURO-ORTHOPEDIC APPLICATION

Assessment for Space-Occupying Lesion, Tumor, Intervertebral Disc Herniation, or Osteophytes

Comment

More than 90% of disc lesions in the cervical spine occur at the C5 and C6 levels. As degeneration of a disc occurs, two different types of lesions can produce very similar symptoms. The first type is the soft disc protrusion or nuclear herniation. In this lesion, a mass of nucleus pulposus bulges outward, commonly posterolaterally (Fig. 3-145). Complete extrusion of disc material may occur. With acute rupture of a cervical disc, immediate compression of the nerve root occurs. Compression results in nerve root symptoms and radicular pain.

The second lesion results from chronic disc degeneration with subsequent narrowing of the disc space. This abnormality is cervical *spondylosis* and occurs primarily in the older age group. As narrowing and collapse of the disc proceeds, the vertebrae become more closely approximated, which leads to spur formation along the disc edges and at the joints of Luschka. Mild subluxation of the facet joint may also occur. All of these changes decrease the size of the intervertebral foramen, which results in pressure on the nerve root. Mild inflammation and swelling are usually present in conjunction with osteophyte formation, which further contributes to the narrowing of the foramen and nerve root

compression. Coughing, sneezing, and straining can accentuate the pain, which may radiate into the shoulder and arm and along the radial aspect of the forearm (Fig. 3-146).

Spondylosis in the cervical spine may occasionally produce symptoms referable to the lower extremities (cervical spondylotic myelopathy). These symptoms occur as a result of pressure of posterior osteophytes on the anterior portion of the cervical spinal cord. The symptom complex appears as a combination of cervical root and cord symptoms (rhizalgia).

In most cases the diagnosis is clear without further testing. Neck, interscapular, arm pain, or any combination that is aggravated by neck motion is typical (Figs. 3-147 and 3-148).

ORTHOPEDIC GAMUT 3-45
CERVICAL SPINE SPONDYLOSIS

Assessment of cervical spine spondylosis includes the following:
1. Plain-film roentgenograms are usually obtained first, within the first few weeks of onset of symptoms. AP and lateral views are sufficient.
2. Myelography, sometimes followed by CT, will demonstrate loss of the normal root *sleeve*, and indentation of the dural sac is often seen.
3. MRI is performed.
4. Electromyography and discography are performed. However, the diagnosis can usually be well established based on the history, physical examination, and myelographic examination alone.

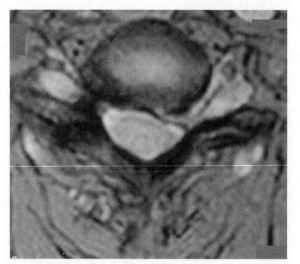

FIG. 3-145 Disc herniation causing nerve root compression. (From Mercier LR, Pettid FJ: *Practical orthopedics,* ed 4, St Louis, 1995, Mosby.)

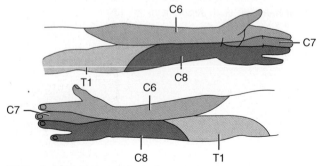

FIG. 3-146 Volar and dorsal dermatome pattern of the forearm and hand. (From Mercier LR, Pettid FJ: *Practical orthopedics,* ed 4, St Louis, 1995, Mosby.)

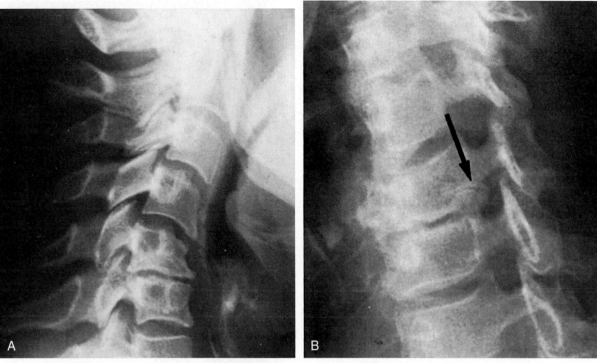

FIG. 3-147 Lateral (**A**) and oblique (**B**) radiographs showing degenerative disc disease at the C5–C6 level. (From Mercier LR, Pettid FJ: *Practical orthopedics,* ed 4, St Louis, 1995, Mosby.)

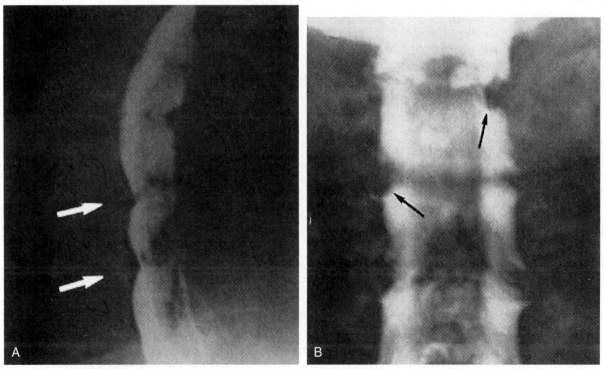

FIG. 3-148 Myelographic findings in cervical disc disease. **A,** Lateral view. **B,** Antero-posterior view. (From Mercier LR, Pettid FJ: *Practical orthopedics,* ed 4, St Louis, 1995, Mosby.)

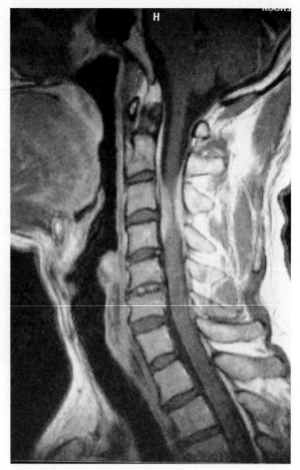

FIG. 3-149 Contrast-enhanced mid-sagittal T1-weighted MRI showing enhancing tumor extending up to the C1 level. (From Takeuchi H et al: Cervical extradural meningioma with rapidly progressive myelopathy, *J Clin Neurosci* 13[3]:397-400, 2006.)

Disc compression of the nerve root is influenced by changes in volume and consistency of the disc, as well as changes in position of the motion segment. These factors form the basis for several diagnostic measures. During infantile and adult stages, the intervertebral disc is not stiff and inflexible; rather, the disc is a connective tissue structure, which can physiologically change its form and volume by loading and unloading. The remaining parts of the motion segment, including the nerve fibers, adjust themselves to these changes. Space between the dural sac and its nerve roots is sufficient in relation to the posterior part of the intervertebral disc. Changes in the form of the disc, as well as changes in the position of the nerve roots during spinal movement, will not influence the spinal nerves. The epidural space, which is filled with fatty tissue and venous plexus, varies in width. As a rule, the intervertebral foramen is large enough to allow ample space for the passage of nerves. When the spinal space becomes diminished by disc protrusions, osteophytes, engorged vessels, or stenosis (a narrowing of the spinal canal), the nerve roots come under pressure. When the nerve roots come in contact with a disc surface that has undergone physiologic changes, the nerve roots can no longer alter their position, making them more sensitive to the mechanical influence.

Symptoms of extramedullary lesions may include local tissue destruction, radicular involvement by space-occupying mass or bony compression, or spinal cord compression secondary to bony collapse or tumor (Fig. 3-149). Radicular pain is common, and the spinal cord level is usually discrete. Sensory loss is uniform, and motor loss is often uniform.

Malignant neoplasms such as metastases or lymphoma are common in the spinal extradural space. However, meningiomas are uncommon in this location, being more commonly an intradural extramedullary neoplasm. From the literature, the incidence of entirely extradural spinal meningioma ranges from 2.6% to 10% of spinal meningiomas. However, as many reports use differing criteria to distinguish between partially and totally extradural lesions, the actual frequency of these lesions is unknown, and the explicit clinical features of these lesions are not described. A suggestion has been offered that extradural lesions may be more common than intradural meningiomas in children and men (Takeuchi et al, 2006).

Radicular complaints follow the roots involved and are similar to those associated with disc herniation.

PROCEDURE

- The patient takes a deep breath and holds it while bearing down abdominally (Figs. 3-150 and 3-151).
- A positive test is indicated by increased pain caused by increased intrathecal pressure.
- Increased intrathecal pressure is usually caused by a space-occupying lesion (herniated disc, tumor, osteophytes).
- The test should be performed with care and caution because the patient may become dizzy and pass out while or shortly after performing this test because the procedure can block the blood supply to the brain.

Next Steps/Procedures

Dejerine sign, swallowing test, Naffziger test, Bakody sign, maximum foraminal encroachment test, shoulder depression test, distraction test, brachial plexus tension test, Bikele sign, Jackson cervical compression test, Spurling test, foraminal compression test, reflexes and sensory testing, and diagnostic imaging

3

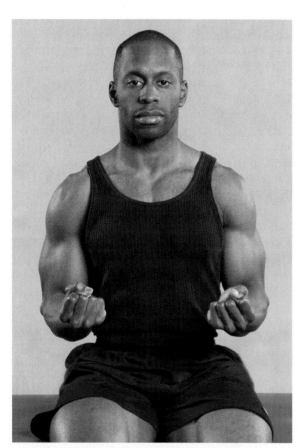

FIG. 3-150 The patient is seated comfortably. The arms may be slightly flexed at the elbows. The patient is instructed to take a deep breath and hold it.

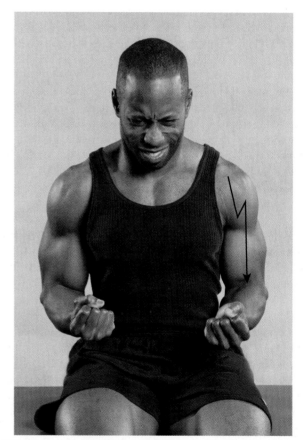

FIG. 3-151 While holding the deep breath, the patient bears down to create greater intraabdominal pressure. Reproduction of radicular pain is indicative of nerve root compression by a space-occupying mass in the spine.

VERTEBROBASILAR ARTERY FUNCTIONAL MANEUVER

Assessment for Vertebral, Basilar, or Carotid Artery Stenosis or Compression

Comment

The VAs are vulnerable to injury in the foramina of the lower cervical vertebra, at the junction between C1 and C2, and as they pass over the arch of C1 through the atlantooccipital membrane. Intimal disruption may lead to acute, complete thrombotic occlusion, subintimal hematoma, dissection of the artery, or pseudoaneurysm formation. Obviously, atlantooccipital dislocation usually causes total disruption of the vertebrobasilar system and results in death.

The mechanism of injury seems to be cervical hyperextension accompanied by excessive rotation. Severely diminished flow in one of the VAs may lead to occlusion of the posterior inferior cerebellar artery on that side, resulting in a lateral medullary infarction (Wallenberg syndrome). This syndrome is characterized by the ipsilateral loss of cranial nerves V, IX, X, and XI and by cerebellar ataxia, Horner syndrome, and contralateral loss of pain and temperature sensation.

With increasing severity of injury, vascular involvement can ascend to the basilar, superior cerebellar, and posterior cerebral arteries. Sudden death, quadriplegia, or locked-in syndrome (quadriplegia accompanied by the loss of lower cranial nerves, which allows eye blinking only) can ensue. These symptoms should alert the examiner to the possibility of vascular injury, which means that immediate cerebral arteriography is recommended to obtain an accurate diagnosis.

Symptoms of vertebrobasilar insufficiency include paroxysmal symptoms induced by certain head movements, mainly rotation, extension, and lateral flexion. Dizziness, diplopia, drop attack, syncope, and spinal stroke increase in frequency and intensity with increasing magnitudes of cervical osteoarthritis, atheromatosis in vessels, and advanced age. Manipulation of the neck in patients with these characteristics is hazardous.

The time between the VA trauma and the onset of ischemic symptoms and signs can vary from immediate to several days later. The interval is probably related to the mechanism of injury. When brainstem ischemia is caused by vasoconstriction, symptoms are immediate; ischemia symptoms (other than the pain of dissection) resulting from thrombus embolus become symptomatic only after some time.

Dizziness is the most common symptom of vertebrobasilar insufficiency and may be unaccompanied by any other symptoms or signs.

Marked pathophysiologic involvement occurs of the Luschka and Z joints when encroachment of the VA occurs, especially at the occipitoatlantoaxial level, but this involvement may occur at any level. Atheromatous plaques with calcification may be noted in the carotid artery (specifically at the siphon) and in the walls of the VA. Occasionally a rare aneurysm of the vertebral or carotid artery may develop in the cervical spine. Angiography discloses varying magnitudes of obstruction or complete obstruction such as that caused by thrombosis.

In patients suspected of having carotid occlusive disease, a thorough physical examination that includes blood pressure measurements in both arms and careful auscultation of the heart should be performed. In the absence of a precordial murmur a bruit at the carotid bifurcation suggests carotid bifurcation arthrosclerosis either in the internal or external artery or both. Cholesterol embolization can occur, especially following great vessel endovascular procedures (Fig. 3-152).

No physical finding differentiates which of these sites is involved (Fig. 3-153).

Cholesterol embolization (CE) from ulcerated atherosclerotic plaques is an uncommon phenomenon and it is reported mainly after juxtarenal and infrarenal aneurysm surgery. The embolization is predominantly distal, primarily to the

---

ORTHOPEDIC GAMUT 3-47

VERTEBROBASILAR INSUFFICIENCY

The major signs and symptoms of vertebrobasilar insufficiency are as follows:

1. Dizziness, vertigo, giddiness, light-headedness
2. Drop attacks, loss of consciousness
3. Diplopia (or other visual problems, amaurosis fugax)
4. Dysarthria (speech difficulties)
5. Dysphagia
6. Ataxia of gait (walking difficulties, incoordination of the extremities, ataxia, falling to one side)
7. Nausea (with possible vomiting)
8. Numbness on one side of the face or body
9. Nystagmus

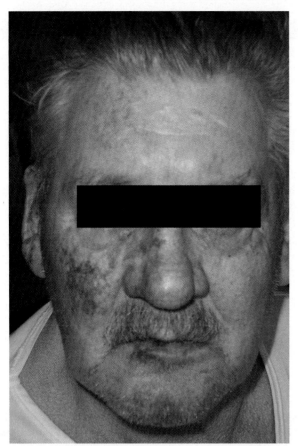

FIG. 3-152 Photograph showing purpuric lesions surrounded with livedo racemosa at the level of the right hemi face (face), suggesting that the diagnosis of ipsilateral carotid artery stenosis should be considered. (From El Idrissi R et al: Facial cutaneous cholesterol embolism revealing a tight carotid stenosis: a case report, *Eur J Vasc Endovasc Surg* 33[1]:62-64, 2007.)

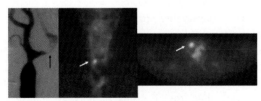

FIG. 3-153 Stenosis of carotid diameter. (From Lynch TG, Hobson RW: *Vascular surgery: principles and practice,* New York, 1987, McGraw-Hill.)

lower limb, with an estimated incidence of 3%. This phenomenon is usually triggered by endovascular procedures involving wire and catheter manipulation through the infra-renal aorta. Other territories of CE may involve kidneys, bowel, brain, and retina. To our knowledge, spontaneous cholesterol embolization of the face deriving from atherosclerotic plaque of the carotid artery bifurcation has not previously been described (El Idrissi et al, 2007). The examiner should listen over the supraclavicular region, where a bruit suggests subclavian or innominate artery ste-

ORTHOPEDIC GAMUT 3-48

DIFFERENTIAL DIAGNOSES OF FACIAL PURPURA

Bilateral (usual):
- Traumatic origin
- Viral infection
- Scurvy

Unilateral:
- Sneddon syndrome characterized by the association of livedo racemosa and ischemic neurologic events (requires neurologic deficit and abnormal brain CT)
- Harlequin syndrome (autonomic dysfunction affecting sweating and flushing of the face and less commonly the upper limb and upper chest) (Fig. 3-154)

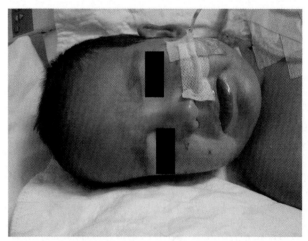

FIG. 3-154 Postoperative photograph showing flushing of the right side of the face with clear transition at the midline. (From Darvall JN, Morsi AW, Penington A: Coexisting harlequin and Horner syndromes after paediatric neck dissection: a case report and a review of the literature, *J Plastic Reconstr Aesthat Surg* 2007 June 5 [E-pub ahead of print].)

nosis. A significant difference in blood pressure between the two extremities confirms the presence of subclavian artery obstruction.

Sneddon syndrome (SS) is a disorder characterized by livedo racemosa and ischemic cerebrovascular lesions and is defined by clinical criteria associated with the presence of a widespread noninflammatory arteriopathy involving small and medium-size arteries. Some patients with SS, even in familial forms, may have positive antiphospholipid antibodies; therefore a broad definition of this syndrome includes these cases, which are otherwise identical in clinical and pathologic features to antiphospholipid-negative cases. SS is then divided into idiopathic, autoimmune, and thromboembolic subsets or in systemic lupus erythematosus–associated SS, antiphospholipid syndrome–associated SS, and primary forms. The etiopathogenesis of this disorder is still unknown (Lousa et al, 2007).

ORTHOPEDIC GAMUT 3-49

VERTEBROBASILAR ISCHEMIA

Three types of vertebrobasilar ischemia:

1. Transient ischemic attacks (TIAs) are brief episodes of neurologic dysfunction most commonly caused by embolic showers from an atheromatous carotid artery to the ipsilateral cerebral hemisphere. Patients experience paresthesia or anesthesia in an arm or leg. When a motor abnormality is prominent, weakness, paralysis, or incoordination on the involved side of the body is present. Brief aphasic or dysphasic symptoms occur with involvement of the dominant hemisphere. Attacks are brief, lasting for a few seconds to minutes. Rarely do the attacks extend beyond 3 hours. TIAs occur on the side opposite the involved area of the brain and carotid artery.

2. Reversible ischemia neurologic deficits (RINDs) persist for longer than 24 hours and disappear completely. When the symptoms of RINDs occur and are identical to those of TIA, the patient may have sustained a small area of cerebral infarction. Neurologic symptoms that persist for long periods are diagnosed as a completed stroke.

3. *Stroke in evolution* and crescendo TIAs may occur. A patient with a stroke in evolution experiences acute neurologic deficit, which progresses over hours or days and ultimately results in a fixed deficit caused by cerebral infarction. Crescendo carotid TIAs is a syndrome of multiple TIAs occurring within a short time. Each attack is followed by complete recovery. These syndromes indicate high-grade carotid artery stenosis with embolization and are an urgent indication for further evaluation.

ORTHOPEDIC GAMUT 3-50

RESIDUAL EFFECT OF CAROTID OCCLUSION

When serious residual effects of carotid occlusion occur, the symptoms will conform to one of the following syndromes:

1. Wallenberg syndrome (occlusion of the posterior inferior cerebral artery)
2. Locked-in syndrome (occlusion of the VBA)
3. Other brainstem syndromes
4. Occipital lobe injury
5. Cerebellar injury
6. Thalamus injury

harlequin side represents the normally innervated half of the face. The pathologic appearance is caused by an inability on the ipsilateral affected side to mount a vasomotor response to sympathetic stimuli, resulting in unequal flushing on the contralateral side of the face (Darvall, Morsi, Penington, in press).

PROCEDURE

- With the patient in a seated position, the examiner palpates the carotid and subclavian arteries and auscultates for pulsations and bruits (Fig. 3-155).
- If neither of these possibilities exists, the patient is instructed to rotate and hyperextend the head to one side and then the other (Fig. 3-156).
- This second maneuver should be performed only if initial palpation and auscultation did not reveal bruits or pulsations.
- The test is considered positive if either maneuver reveals pulsations or bruits.
- The rotation and hyperextension portion of this test places motion-induced compression on the VAs.
- Vertigo, dizziness, visual blurring, nausea, faintness, and nystagmus are all signs of a positive test, which indicates vertebral, basilar, or carotid artery stenosis or compression.

Next Steps/Procedures

Barré-Liéou sign, Hautant test, DeKleyn test, Hallpike maneuver, Underburg test, reflex and sensory testing, vascular assessment, vascular imaging, and MRI

The sudden presentation of hemifacial flushing and sweating was first termed *harlequin syndrome* by Lance and colleagues in 1988, named after the similar though separate physiologic flushing response occasionally seen in newborns in the dependent half of the body. Since then, the syndrome has been well represented in the literature. Acquired harlequin syndrome caused by sympathetic denervation has been associated with central autonomic disruption in cases of stroke, as well as linked to more peripheral autonomic denervation caused by trauma, anesthesia, and tumors. An important factor to recognize is that the flushed

3

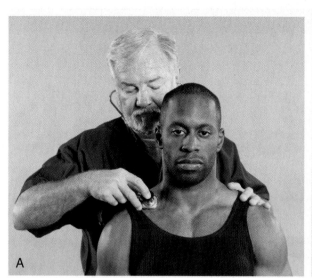
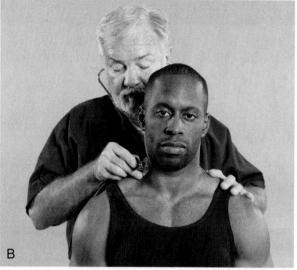

FIG. 3-155 While the patient is in a seated position, the subclavian (**A**) and then the carotid (**B**) arteries are auscultated for bruits. This assessment is followed by palpation of the arteries for pulse assessment. If bruits are present, the balance of the test is not completed, and the test is considered positive.

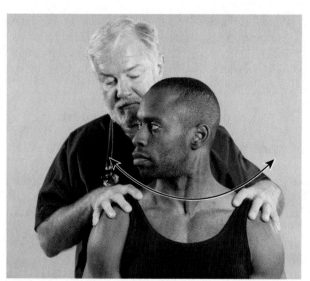

FIG. 3-156 If bruits are not found, the patient rotates and hyperextends the head and neck, both to the right and left. The production of vertigo, visual disturbances, nausea, syncope, or nystagmus is indicative of vertebral, basilar, or carotid artery stenosis or compression.

CRITICAL THINKING

1. What artery has an intimate relationship with the cervical spine and serves as the major source of blood to the cervical cord and cervical spine?

2. Why is the atlantoaxial joint (C1, C2) an unstable joint?

3. The teardrop fracture of the cervical spine is caused by what type of injury: hyperflexion, hyperextension, or compression?

4. In cervical trauma, what radiograph should be obtained, before any other measure is taken, to evaluate the stability of the cervical spine?

5. When the fracture is not obvious on a lateral radiograph of the cervical spine, what is initially evaluated to help in determining whether fracture has occurred?

6. What is the most common congenital abnormality found in patients with quadriplegia caused by a football injury?

7. Multiple types of fractures and dislocations occur in the cervical spine. Name the six most common types of cervical spine fractures and dislocations according to the type of forces implied.

8. Name a common anatomic finding associated with compressive extension injuries.

9. Give the most common signs and symptoms of hangman's fracture.

10. Where is the most common injury to the cervical spine in children?

11. In C4 quadriplegia, with the lesion between C4 and C5 vertebrae, what changes in motor function, sensory function, or reflexes are expected?

12. In C5 quadriplegia, what motor, sensation, and reflex changes are expected?

13. In C6 quadriplegia, what motor functions, sensations, and reflexes would remain intact?

14. In C7 quadriplegia, what motor functions, sensations, and reflexes remain intact?

15. What is the most common pain pattern of herniated cervical disc?

16. Provocative tests of the cervical spine not only tests range of motion but which specific anatomical structures?

17. A prevalent complaint of patients suffering from spinal cord injury is chronic and intractable pain. How is the pain characterized when it emanates from the site of injury?

18. The most common area of lax ligaments with increased spinal motion in children occurs at what spinal level?

19. How many millimeters of movement should be considered within normal limits?

20. Name two conditions of the cervical spine in adulthood that can result in compressive myelopathy and how it occurs.

21. What imaging study would you order to evaluate this area?

22. What cranial nerve supplies cervical muscles?

23. Which muscle and how does the clinician test this muscle?

24. Describe the symptoms that distinguish nerve root compression from those of complex regional pain syndrome or reflex sympathetic dystrophy or neurovascular compression syndromes.

25. Which orthopedic test helps to define nerve root compression versus neurovascular compression?

26. The brachial plexus tension test is helpful in the assessment of compression of which cervical nerve root?

27. What is the subclavian steal syndrome?

28. Why is subclavian steal syndrome significant?

29. Indirect signs of cervical trauma that occurs in the soft tissue of the cervical spine may be visualized radiographically. Name four areas and signs that might indicate soft-tissue hemorrhage.

30. What is the average AP measurement of the cervical canal between C3 through C7?

31. Spinal cord compression will occur only if the canal is reduced by what measurement?

32. Describe the sleep cycle with someone that has root pain from myelopathy.

33. Lhermitte sign is one of the tools for assessment for cervical myelopathy. Describe the characteristic positive finding.

34. In addition to cervical stenosis from osteophytic growth (spondylitic spurs), name four additional conditions that may give a positive sign.

35. Why is Naffziger test not recommended for the geriatric patient or a younger patient with known atherosclerotic plaques?

36. Reporting the correct extent of injury is expected from the clinician. What defines a strain from sprain injury?

37. What are the three classifications of strain and describe each?

38. Describe four classifications of sprain.

39. Why is the Rust sign so important?

40. How is the test performed?

41. What is the significance of a febrile patient with a positive Soto-Hall sign?

BIBLIOGRAPHY

Abrams WB, Berkow R: *The Merck manual of geriatrics*, Rahway, NJ, 1990, Merck Sharp & Dohme Research Laboratories.

Adams JC, Hamblen DL: *Outline of orthopaedics*, ed 11, Edinburgh, 1990, Churchill Livingstone.

Alario AJ: *Practical guide to the care of the pediatric patient*, St Louis, 1997, Mosby.

Alexander E Jr, Davis CH: Reduction and fusion of fracture of the odontoid process, *J Neurosurg* 31:580, 1969.

Allen BL et al: A mechanistic classification of closed indirect fractures and dislocations of the lower cervical spine, *Spine* 7:1, 1982.

Allison D, Strickland N: *Acronyms & synonyms in medical imaging*, Oxford, UK, 1996, ISIS Medical Media.

American Medical Association: *Guides to the evaluation of permanent impairment*, ed 4, Chicago, 1993, American Medical Association.

American Medical Association: *How to use guides to the evaluation of permanent impairment*, ed 4, Falmouth, Colo, 1993, SEAK.

Ames MD, Schut L: Results of treatment of 171 consecutive myelomeningoceles, *Pediatrics* 50:466, 1972.

Amyes EW, Anderson FM: Fracture of the odontoid process of the axis, *J Bone Joint Surg* 56A:1663, 1974.

Anderson KN, Anderson LE: *Mosby's pocket dictionary of medicine, nursing, & allied health*, ed 2, St Louis, 1994, Mosby.

Apley AG, Solomon L: *Concise system of orthopaedics and fractures*, London, 1988, Butterworth-Heinemann.

Askenasy HM, Braham MJ, Kosary IZ: Delayed spinal myelopathy after atlanto-axial fracture dislocation, *J Neurosurg* 17:1100, 1960.

Ba AM, LoTempio MM, Wang MB: Pharyngeal diverticulum as a sequela of anterior cervical fusion, *Otolaryngol Head Neck Surg* 131(2):P256-P257, 2004.

Bailey RW, Badgley CE: Stabilization of the cervical spine by anterior fusion, *J Bone Joint Surg* 42A:565, 1960.

Barkauskas VH et al: *Health & physical assessment*, ed 2, St Louis, 1998, Mosby.

Barnsley L, Lord S, Bogduk N: Whiplash injury, *Pain* 59:283, 1994.

Barnsley L et al: The prevalence of chronic cervical zygapophyseal joint pain after whiplash, *Spine* 10:20, 1995.

Barré JA: Le syndrome sympathique cervical posterieur et sa cause frequente, l'artherite cervicale, *Rev Neurol (Paris)* 33:1246, 1926.

Bateman JE: *The shoulder and neck*, Philadelphia, 1972, WB Saunders.

Bernstein EF: *Vascular diagnosis*, ed 4, St Louis, 1993, Mosby.

Berquist T: *MRI of the musculoskeletal system*, ed 3, Philadelphia, 1996, JB Lippincott.

Bettmane EH, Neudorfer RJ: Cervical disc pathology resulting in dysphagia in an adolescent boy, *N Y State J Med* 60:2465, 1960.

Bland JH: *Disorders of the cervical spine diagnosis and medical management*, Philadelphia, 1987, WB Saunders.

Bland JH: Rheumatoid arthritis of the cervical spine, *J Rheumatol* 1:319, 1974.

Bocchi L, Orso CA: Whiplash injuries of the cervical spine, *Ital J Orthop Traumatol* 9:171, 1983.

Bohlman HH: Indications for late anterior decompression and fusion for cervical spinal cord injuries. In Tator CH, editor: *Early management of acute cervical spinal cord injury*, New York, 1982, Raven Press.

Bohlman HH et al: Spinal cord monitoring of experimental incomplete cervical spinal cord injury, *Spine* 6:428, 1981.

Bohlman HH, Ducker TB, Lucas JT: Spine and spinal cord injuries. In Rothman RH, Simeone FA, editors: *The spine*, ed 2, Philadelphia, 1982, WB Saunders.

Bohlman HH, Eismont FJ: Surgical techniques of anterior decompression and fusion for spinal cord injuries, *Clin Orthop* 138:154, 1981.

Bohlman HH, Riley L Jr, Robinson RA: Anterolateral approaches to the cervical spine. In Ruge D, Wiltse LL, editors: *Spinal disorders*, Philadelphia, 1977, Lea & Febiger.

Bohlman HH: Late anterior decompression and fusion for the spinal cord injuries: review of 100 cases with long term results, *Orthop Trans* 4:42, 1980.

Bohlman HH: The neck. In D'Ambrosia R, editor: *Regional examination and differential diagnosis of musculoskeletal disorders*, Philadelphia, 1977, JB Lippincott.

Bradley JP, Tibone JE, Watkins RC: History, physical examination, and diagnostic tests for neck and upper extremity problems. In Watkins RG, editor: *The spine in sports*, St Louis, 1996, Mosby.

Brain WR: Some unsolved problems in cervical spondylosis, *Br Med Bull* 1:711, 1963.

Brieg A: *Biomechanics of the central nervous system*, Chicago, 1960, Mosby.

Brieg A, Turnbull IM, Hassler O: Effects of mechanical stresses in the spinal cord in cervical spondylosis, *J Neurosurg* 25:45, 1966.

Brier SR: *Primary care orthopedics*, St Louis, 1999, Mosby.

Brooks M, Evans R, Fairclough J: *Sports injuries*, ed 2, London, 1992, Gower Medical.

Brotzman SB: *Clinical orthopaedic rehabilitation*, St Louis, 1996, Mosby.

Brown DE, Neumann RD: *Orthopedic secrets*, Philadelphia, 1995, Hanley & Belfus.

Bucholz RW: *Orthopaedic decision making*, ed 2, St Louis, 1996, Mosby.

Bunker TD, Schranz PJ: *Clinical challenges in orthopaedics: the shoulder*, Oxford, UK, 1998, ISIS Medical Media.

Cailliet R: *Head and face pain syndromes*, Philadelphia, 1992, FA Davis.

Campbell JB, Campbell JM: *Mosby's survival guide to medical abbreviations & acronyms prefixes & suffixes symbols Greek alphabet*, St Louis, 1995, Mosby.

Canale ST: *Campbell's operative orthopaedics*, vol 1-4, ed 9, St Louis, 1998, Mosby.

Carver G, Willits J: Comparative study and risk factors of a CVA, *J Am Chiropractic Assoc* 32:65, 1996.

Cashley MAP: Basilar artery migraine or cerebral vascular accident? *J Manip Physiol Ther* 16:112, 1993.

Cervical Spine Research Society: *The cervical spine*, Philadelphia, 1983, JB Lippincott.

Chapman S, Nakielyn R: *Aids to radiological differential diagnosis*, ed 3, London, 1995, Bailliere Tindall.

Chobanian AV, Gavras H: *Hypertension, Clinical Symposia, January*. Summit, Colo, 1990, CIBA Pharmaceutical.

Choi IS et al: Clinical characteristics of brachial plexopathy, *Clin Neurophysiol* 117(suppl 1):188-189, 2006.

Cipriano JJ: *Photographic manual of regional orthopaedic and neurological test*, ed 3, Baltimore, 1997, Williams & Wilkins.

Cloward RB: The clinical significance of the sinu-vertebral nerve or the cervical spine in relation to the cervical disc syndrome, *J Neurol Neurosurg Psychiatry* 23:321, 1960.

Cohn RE: *Impairment rating examination and disability evaluation*, ed 3, Wilkesboro, NC, 1994, R Ernest Cohn.

Conlon PW, Isdale IC, Rose BS: Rheumatoid arthritis of the cervical spine: an analysis of 333 cases, *Ann Rheum Dis* 25:120, 1966.

Cramer GD, Darby SA: *Basic and clinical anatomy of the spine, spinal cord, and ANS*, St Louis, 1995, Mosby.

Crellin RQ, MacCabe JJ, Hamilton EB: Surgical management of the cervical spine in rheumatoid arthritis, *J Bone Joint Surg* 52B:244, 1970.

Dambro MR, Griffith JA: *Griffith's 5 minute clinical consult*, Baltimore, 1997, Williams & Wilkins.

D'Ambrogio KJ, Roth GB: *Positional release therapy assessment & treatment of musculoskeletal dysfunction*, St Louis, 1997, Mosby.

D'Ambrosia RD: *Musculoskeletal disorders: regional examination and differential diagnosis*, Philadelphia, 1977, JB Lippincott.

Dandy DJ: *Essential orthopaedics and trauma*, Edinburgh, 1989, Churchill Livingstone.

Daniels L, Worthington C: *Muscle testing: techniques of manual examination*, Philadelphia, 1980, WB Saunders.

Darby S, Cramer G: Pain generators and pathways of the head and neck. In Curl D, editor: *Chiropractic approach to head pain*, Baltimore, 1994, Williams & Wilkins.

Davidson RI, Dunn EJ, Metzmaker W: The shoulder abduction test in the diagnosis of radicular pain in cervical extradural compressive monoradiculopathies, *Spine* 6:441, 1981.

De Hertogh WJ et al: The clinical examination of neck pain patients: the validity of a group of tests, *Man Ther* 12(1):50-55, 2007.

de Kleyn A, Nieuwenhuyse P: Schwindelanfaelle und nystagmus bei einer bestimmten stellung des dopfes, *Acta Otolaryng* 11:155, 1927.

de Kleyn A, Versteegh C: Uber verschledene formen von nemieres syndrome, *Dtsch Z Nervenheilkd* 132:157, 1933.

DeJong RH: *The neurologic examination*, ed 3, New York, 1967, Harper & Row.

Deltoff MN, Kogon PL: *The portable skeletal x-ray library*, St Louis, 1998, Mosby.

Demeter SL, Andersson GBJ, Smith GM: *Disability evaluation*, St Louis, 1996, Mosby.

Deshpande JK, Tobias JD: *The pediatric pain handbook*, St Louis, 1996, Mosby.

Dettenmeier PA: *Radiographic assessment for nurses*, St Louis, 1995, Mosby.

Doherty M: *Color atlas and text of osteoarthritis*, London, 1994, Wolfe.

Doherty M, Doherty J: *Clinical examination in rheumatology*, London, 1992, Wolfe.

Doherty M, George E: *Self-assessment picture tests in rheumatology*, London, 1995, Mosby-Wolfe.

Dossett AB, Watkins RG: Stinger injuries in football. In Watkins RG, editor: *The spine in sports*, St Louis, 1996, Mosby.

Dreyfus P, Michaelsen M, Fletcher D: Atlanto-occipital and atlantoaxial joint pain patterns, *Spine* 19:1125, 1994.

Durrett LC: Management of patients with vertebrobasilar ischemia, *Chiro Technique* 6:95, 1994.

Elliott J et al: MRI study of the cross-sectional area for the cervical extensor musculature in patients with persistent whiplash associated disorders (WAD), *Man Ther* (in press, corrected proof).

Elster AD: *Questions and answers in magnetic resonance imaging*, St Louis, 1994, Mosby.

Epstein O et al: *Clinical examination*, ed 2, London, 1997, Mosby.

Ernst CW et al: Prevalence of annular tears and disc herniations on MR images of the cervical spine in symptom free volunteers, *Eur J Radiol* 55(3):409-414, 2005.

Esposito MD et al: Thoracic outlet syndrome in a throwing athlete diagnosed with MRI and MRA, *J Magn Reson Imaging* 7:598, 1997.

Eyigor S, Durmaz B, Karapolat H: Monoparesis with complex regional pain syndrome-like symptoms due to brachial plexopathy caused by the Varicella zoster virus: a case report, *Arch Phys Med Rehabil* 87(12):1653-1655, 2006.

Farrar WE: *Atlas of infections of the nervous system*, London, 1993, Wolfe.

Fayssoux RS et al: Spinal injuries after falls from hunting tree stands, *Spine* (in press, uncorrected proof).

Feipel V, Berghe MV, Rooze MA: No effects of cervical spine motion on cranial dura mater strain, *Clin Biomech* 18(5):389-392, 2003.

Feldmann E: *Current diagnosis in neurology*, St Louis, 1994, Mosby.

Ferezy JS: *The chiropractic neurological examination*, Gaithersburg, Md, 1992, Aspen.

Fernandez-de-las-Penas C et al: Referred pain from trapezius muscle trigger points shares similar characteristics with chronic tension type headache, *Eur J Pain* 11(4):475-482, 2007.

Fessler RG, Khoo LT: Minimally invasive posterior cervical microendoscopic foraminotomy: an initial clinical experience, *Neurosurgery* 51(5 Suppl):S37-S45, 2002.

Fisher M: Basilar artery embolism after surgery under general anesthesia: a case report, *Neurology* 43:1856, 1993.

Ford JS: *Posttraumatic headache*, Chicago, 1985, Med Recertification Associates.

Foreman SM, Croft AC: *Whiplash injuries: the cervical acceleration/deceleration syndrome*, Baltimore, 1992, Williams & Wilkins.

Fornage B: *Musculoskeletal ultrasound*, New York, 1995, Churchill Livingstone.

Frank ED et al: *Merrill's atlas of radiographic positioning and procedures*, ed 11, St Louis, 2007, Mosby.

Ganguly DN, Roy KKS: A study on the craniovertebral joint in man, *Anat Anz* 114:433, 1964.

Garcia JH: *Neuropathology the diagnostic approach*, St Louis, 1997, Mosby.

Gargan MF, Fairbank JCT: Anatomy of the spine. In Watkins RG, editor: *The spine in sports*, St Louis, 1996, Mosby.

Goldie BS: *Orthopaedic diagnosis and management: a guide to the care of orthopaedic patients*, ed 2, Oxford, UK, 1998, ISIS Medical Media.

Gowers WR: *Diseases of the nervous system*, ed 2, London, 1969, Churchill.

Gracovetsky S: Biomechanics of the spine. In White A, Scholfferman JA, editors: *Spine care: diagnosis and treatment*, St Louis, 1994, Mosby.

Greenspan A, Montesano P: *Imaging of the spine in clinical practice*, London, 1993, Wolfe.

Greenstein GM: *Clinical assessment of neuromusculoskeletal disorders*, St Louis, 1997, Mosby.

Grossman ZD, et al: *Cost-effective diagnostic imaging the examiner's guide*, ed 3, St Louis, 1995, Mosby.

Hall CW, Danoff D: Sleep attacks-apparent relationship to atlantoaxial dislocation, *Arch Neurol* 32:57, 1975.

Hammer WI: *Functional soft tissue examination and treatment by manual methods the extremities*, Gaithersburg, Md, 1991, Aspen.

Hann CL: Retropharyngeal-tendinitis, *AJR Am J Roentgenol* 130:1137, 1978.

Harrison DE et al: Cervical coupling during lateral head translations creates an S-configuration, *Clin Biomech* 15(6):436-440, 2000.

Hartley A: *Practical joint assessment upper quadrant*, ed 2, St Louis, 1995, Mosby.

Hastings D, McNab I, Lawson V: Neoplasms of the atlas and axis, *Can J Surg* 11:290, 1968.

Hawkins RJ: *An organized approach to musculoskeletal examination and history taking*, St Louis, 1995, Mosby.

Helliwell PS, Evans PF, Wright V: The straight cervical spine: does it indicate muscle spasm? *J Bone Joint Surg (Br)* 76:103, 1994.

Hinkle CZ: *Fundamentals of anatomy & movement a workbook and guide*, St Louis, 1997, Mosby.

Howard RP et al: Head, neck, and mandible dynamics generated by 'whiplash,' *Accid Anal Prev* 30(4):525-534, 1998.

Howe JR, Taren JA: Foramen magnum tumors: pitfalls in diagnosis, *JAMA* 225:1060, 1973.

Huntoon MA: Anatomy of the cervical intervertebral foramina: vulnerable arteries and ischemic neurologic injuries after transforaminal epidural injections, *Pain* 117(1-2):104-111, 2005.

Isdale IC, Corrigan B: Backward luxation of the atlas, *Ann Rheum Dis* 29:6, 1970.

Jablonski S: *Dictionary of medical acronyms & abbreviations*, ed 3, Philadelphia, 1998, Hanley & Belfus.

Jackson R: *The cervical syndrome*, ed 3, Springfield, Ill, 1966, Charles C Thomas.

Jenis L et al: Complex cervical reconstruction: the effect of posterior cervical distraction on foraminal dimensions using a screw-rod system, *Spine* 2(5, suppl 1):53, 2002.

Jonsson HJ et al: Findings and outcome in whiplash-type neck distortions, *Spine* 19:2733, 1994.

Kanner R: *Pain management secrets*, Philadelphia, 1997, Hanley & Belfus.

Katirji B: *Electromyography in clinical practice: a case study approach*, St Louis, 1998, Mosby.

Katz WA: *Rheumatic diseases diagnosis and management*, Philadelphia, 1977, JB Lippincott.

Keats TE: *Atlas of roentgenographic measurement*, ed 6, St Louis, 1990, Mosby.

Keats TE: *Atlas of normal roentgen variants*, ed 6, St Louis, 1996, Mosby.

Keiser RP, Grimes HA: Intervertebral disc space infections in children, *Clin Orthop* 30:163, 1963.

Kendall HO, Kendall FP, Wadsworth GE: *Muscles testing and function*, ed 2, Baltimore, 1971, Williams & Wilkins.

Kettenbach G: *Writing S.O.A.P. notes*, Philadelphia, 1990, FA Davis.

Keuter EJW: Non-traumatic atlanto-axial dislocation associated with nasopharyngeal infections (Grisel's disease), *Acta Neurochirurg* 21:11, 1969.

Kim H-A, Lee S-R, Lee H: Acute peripheral vestibular syndrome of a vascular cause *J Neurol Sci* 254(1-2):99-101, 2007.

Kleinrensink GJ et al: Upper limb tension tests as tools in the diagnosis of nerve and plexus lesions: anatomical and biomechanical aspects, *Clin Biomech* 15(1):9-14, 2000.

Klippel JH, Dieppe PA: *Rheumatology*, vol 1-2, ed 2, London, 1998, Mosby.

Koenigsberg R: *Churchill's illustrated medical dictionary*, New York, 1989, Churchill Livingstone.

Kramer J: *Intervertebral disc diseases*, Chicago, 1981, Mosby.

Kuan T-S et al: The spinal cord connections of the myofascial trigger spots, *Eur J Pain* 11(6):624-634, 2007.

Kumar R et al: Innervation of the spinal dura, myth or reality? *Spine* 21:18, 1996.

Kumar S, Narayan Y, Amell T: Analysis of low velocity frontal impacts, *Clin Biomech* 18(8):694-703, 2003.

Lambert EH, Rooke ED: Myasthenic state and lung cancer. In Brain RL, Norris FH, editors: *The remote effects of cancer on the nervous system*, New York, 1965, Grune & Stratton.

Lavy CBD, Barrett DS: *Questions and answers on Apley's concise system of orthopaedics and fractures*, Oxford, UK, 1991, Butterworth-Heinemann.

Lerner AJ: *The little black book of neurology*, ed 3, St Louis, 1995, Mosby.

Levick JR: An investigation into the validity of subatmospheric pressure recordings from synovial fluid and their dependence on joint angle, *J Physiol* 289:55, 1979.

Lewis CB, Knortz KA: *Orthopedic assessment and treatment of the geriatric patient*, St Louis, 1993, Mosby.

Lhermitte J: Etude de la commotion de la moelle, *Rev Neurol (Paris)* 1:210, 1932.

Lhermitte J, Bollak P, Nicholas M: Les douleurs a type de decharge electrique dans la sclerose en plaques, un cas e forme sensitive de la sclerose multiple, *Rev Neurol (Paris)* 2:56, 1924.

Liéou YC: *Syndrome sympathique cervical posterieur et arthrite cervicale chronique: etude clinique et radiologique*, Strasbourg, Germany, 1928, Schuler and Minh.

Liesegang TJ: Ross syndrome plus: beyond Horner, Holmes-Adie, and harlequin. In Shin RK et al, *Neurology* 2000;55:1841-1846; *Am J Ophthal* 131(6):826, 2001.

Lipson SJ: Fractures of the atlas associated with fractures of the odontoid process and transverse ligament ruptures, *J Bone Joint Surg* 59A:940, 1977.

Lorber J: Spina bifida cystica, *Arch Dis Child* 47:854, 1972.

Loth TS: *Orthopedic boards review II: a case study approach*, St Louis, 1996, Mosby.

Lynch JM, Hennessy MJ: Third nerve palsy: harbinger of basilar artery thrombosis and locked-in syndrome? *J Stroke Cerebrovasc Dis* 14(1):42-43, 2005.

Macnab I: Acceleration extension injuries of the cervical spine. In Rothmann RH, Simeone FA, editors: *The spine*, vol 2, ed 2, Philadelphia, 1982, WB Saunders.

Magee DJ: *Orthopedic physical assessment*, ed 3, Philadelphia, 1997, WB Saunders.

Maitland GD: *Vertebral manipulation*, London, 1973, Butterworths.

Malone TR, McPoil TG, Nitz AJ: *Orthopedic and sports physical therapy*, ed 3, St Louis, 1997, Mosby.

Marchiori DM: *Clinical imaging with skeletal, chest, and abdomen pattern differentials*, St Louis, 1999, Mosby.

Markhashov AM: Variations in the arterial blood supply of the spine, *Vestn Khir* 94:64, 1965.

Martel W: The occipito-atlanto-axial joints in rheumatoid arthritis and ankylosing spondylitis, *AJR Am J Roentgenol* 86:233, 1961.

Martin JH: *Neuroanatomy text and atlas*, ed 2, Stamford, Conn, 1996, Appleton & Lange.

Mathers LH, et al: *Clinical anatomy principles*, St Louis, 1996, Mosby.

Mayo Clinic & Mayo Foundation: *Clinical examination in neurology*, Philadelphia, 1981, WB Saunders.

Mazion JM: *Illustrated manual of neurological reflexes/signs/tests, part I; orthopedic signs/tests/maneuvers for office procedure, part II*, Orlando, Fla, 1980, Daniels.

McRae R: *Clinical orthopaedic examination*, ed 3, Edinburgh, 1990, Churchill Livingstone.

Medical Economics Books: *Patient care flow chart manual*, ed 3, Ordell, NJ, 1982, Medical Economics Books.

Mellion MB: *Office sports medicine*, ed 2, St Louis, 1996, Mosby.

Mellion MB: *Sports medicine secrets*, Philadelphia, 1994, Hanley & Belfus.

Mengel MB, Schwiebert LP: *Ambulatory medicine the primary care of families*, ed 2, Stamford, Conn, 1996, Appleton & Lange.

Mennell JM: *The musculoskeletal system differential diagnosis from symptoms and physical signs*, Gaithersburg, Md, 1992, Aspen.

Mercier LR, Pettid FJ: *Practical orthopedics*, ed 4, St Louis, 1995, Mosby.

Michelow BJ, et al: The natural history of obstetrical brachial plexus palsy, *Plast Reconstr Surg* 93:675, 1994.

Miller B: Manual therapy treatment of myofascial pain and dysfunction. In Rachlin ES, editor: *Myofascial pain and fibromyalgia*, St Louis, 1994, Mosby.

Modic MT, Masaryk TJ, Ross JS: *Magnetic resonance imaging of the spine*, ed 2, St Louis, 1994, Mosby.

Mosby-Year Book, Inc: *Expert 10-minute physical examination*, St Louis, 1997, Mosby.

Nettina SM: *The Lippincott manual of nursing practice*, ed 6, Philadelphia, 1996, Lippincott.

Newton RW: *Color atlas of pediatric neurology*, St Louis, 1995, Mosby-Wolfe.

Nicholas JA, Hershman EB: *The lower extremity & spine in sports medicine*, vol 1-2, ed 2, St Louis, 1995, Mosby.

Nordin M, Andersson GBJ, Pope MH: *Musculoskeletal disorders in the workplace: principles and practice*, St Louis, 1997, Mosby.

Norris SH, Watt I: The prognosis of neck injuries resulting from rear-end vehicle collisions, *J Bone Joint Surg* 65B:608, 1983.

O'Connor CE, Pekow PS, Klingersmith MT: Brachial plexus injury (burners) incidence and risk factors in collegiate football players: a prospective study, *J Athl Train* 33(suppl):5, 1998.

O'Donoghue DH: *Treatment of injuries to athletes*, ed 3, Philadelphia, 1976, WB Saunders.

Oh VMS: *Brain infarction and neck calisthenics*, Lancet 342:739, 1993.

Olson WH et al: *Handbook of symptom-oriented neurology*, ed 2, St Louis, 1994, Mosby.

Omer GE, Spinner M: *Management of peripheral nerve problems*, Philadelphia, 1981, WB Saunders.

O'Young B, Young MA, Stiens SA: *PM&R secrets*, Philadelphia, 1997, Hanley & Belfus.

Pagana KD, Pagana TJ: *Mosby's manual of diagnostic and laboratory tests*, St Louis, 1998, Mosby.

Patten J: *Neurological differential diagnosis*, ed 2, London, 1996, Springer.

Payne EE, et al: The cervical spine, *Brain* 80:571, 1957.

Peterson CK et al: Prevalence of hyperplastic articular pillars in the cervical spine and relationship with cervical lordosis, *J Manipulative Physiol Ther* 22(6):390-394, 1999.

Pheasant S: *Ergonomics, work and health*, Gaithersburg, Md, 1991, Aspen.

Prineas J: Polyneuropathies of undetermined cause, *Acta Neurol Scand* 46(suppl 44):1, 1970.

Przybyla A et al: Outer annulus tears have less effect than endplate fracture on stress distributions inside intervertebral discs: relevance to disc degeneration, *Clin Biomech* 21(10):1013-1019, 2006.

Przybylski G, Marion DW: Injury to the vertebrae and spinal cord. In Moore EE, Mattox KL, Feliziano DV, editors: *Trauma*, ed 3, Stanford, Conn, 1996, Appleton & Lange.

Rachlin ES: *Myofascial pain and fibromyalgia trigger point management*, St Louis, 1994, Mosby.

Radnovc BP, Sturzenegger M, Stefano GD: Long-term outcome after whiplash injury: a two-year follow-up considering features of injury mechanism and somatic, radiologic, and psychosocial factors, *Medicine* 74:281, 1995.

Rana NA, et al: Upward translocation of the dens in rheumatoid arthritis, *J Bone Joint Surg* 55B:471, 1973.

Ranawat CS, et al: Cervical spine fusion in rheumatoid arthritis, *J Bone Joint Surg* 61A:1003, 1979.

Ravel R: *Clinical laboratory medicine clinical application of laboratory data*, ed 6, St Louis, 1995, Mosby.

Resnick D, Niwayama G: *Diagnosis of bone and joint disorders*, Philadelphia, ed 3, 1995, WB Saunders.

Robbins SL: Blood vessels. In Robbins SL, editor: *Pathologic basis of disease*, Philadelphia, 1974, WB Saunders.

Rolak LA: *Neurology secrets*, ed 2, Philadelphia, 1998, Hanley & Belfus.

Rothman RH, Simeone FA: *The spine*, vol 1, Philadelphia, 1975, WB Saunders.

Rowell RM, Stites J, Stone-Hall K: A case report of an unstable cervical spine fracture: parallels to the thoracolumbar chance fracture, *J Manipulative Physiol Ther* 29(7):586-589, 2006.

Rumack CM, Wilson SR, Charboneau JW: *Diagnostic ultrasound*, vol 1-2, ed 2, St Louis, 1998, Mosby.

SAL JA, Dillingham MF: Nonoperative treatment and rehabilitation of disc, facet, and soft tissue injuries. In Nicholas JA, Hershman EB, editors: *The lower extremity and spine in sports medicine*, vol 2, St Louis, 1995, Mosby.

Saidoff DC, McDonough AL: *Critical pathways in therapeutic intervention*, St Louis, 1997, Mosby.

Schneider RC, Livingston KE, Cave AJE: "Hangman's fracture" of the cervical spine, *J Meirpsirg* 22:141, 1965.

Schumacher HR, Klippel JH, Koopman WJ: *Primer on the rheumatic diseases*, ed 10, Atlanta, 1993, Arthritis Foundation.

Scott NW: *Office Orthopedic Practice: The orthopedic clinics of North America*, vol 13, Philadelphia, 1982, WB Saunders.

Seidel HM: *Mosby's guide to physical examination*, ed 4, St Louis, 1999, Mosby.

Shankman GA: *Fundamental orthopedic management for the physical therapist assistant*, St Louis, 1997, Mosby.

Sharp J, Purser DW: Spontaneous atlanto-axial dislocation in ankylosing spondylitis and rheumatoid arthritis, *Ann Rheum Dis* 20:47, 1961.

Silberstein SD, Lipton RB, Goadsby PJ: *Headache in clinical practice*, Oxford, UK, 1998, ISIS Medical Media.

Simons DG: Clinical and etiological update of myofascial pain from trigger points, *J Musculoskel Pain* 4:93, 1996.

Sledge CB, Poss R: *The year book of orthopedics 1997*, St Louis, 1997, Mosby.

Smith PH, Benn RT, Sharp J: Natural history of rheumatoid cervical luxations, *Ann Rheum Dis* 31:431, 1972.

Specht NT, Russo RD: *Practical guide to diagnostic imaging*, St Louis, 1998, Mosby.

Sprou G: Basilar artery insufficiency secondary to obstruction of left subclavian artery, *Circulation* 28:259, 1963.

Spurling RG, Scoville WB: Lateral rupture of the cervical intervertebral discs, *Syn Gyn Obstet* 78:350, 1944.

Starlanyl D, Copeland ME: *Fibromyalgia & chronic myofascial pain syndrome: a survival manual*, Oakland, Calif, 1996, New Harbinger.

Stedman TL: *Stedman's medical dictionary*, ed 25, Baltimore, 1990, Williams & Wilkins.

Stewart DL, Abeln SH: *Documenting functional outcomes in physical therapy*, St Louis, 1993, Mosby.

Stoller DW: *Magnetic resonance imaging in orthopaedics & sports medicine*, Philadelphia, 1993, JB Lippincott.

Sutton D, Young JWR: *A concise textbook of clinical imaging*, ed 2, St Louis, 1995, Mosby.

Tan JC, Horn SE: *Practical manual of physical medicine and rehabilitation*, St Louis, 1998, Mosby.

Tan JC, Nordin M: The role of physical therapy in the treatment of cervical disc disease, *Orthop Clin North Am* 23:435, 1992.

Taybi H, Lachman RS: *Radiology of syndromes, metabolic disorders, and skeletal dysplasias*, ed 4, St Louis, 1996, Mosby.

Tehranzadeh J, Palmer S: Imaging of cervical spine trauma, *Semin Ultrasound CT MRI* 17(2):93-104, 1996.

Terrett AGJ: *Malpractice avoidance for chiropractors*, West Des Moines, Iowa, 1996, National Chiropractic Mutual Insurance Company.

Tettenborn B, et al: Postoperative brainstem and cerebellar infarcts, *Neurology* 43:471, 1993.

Theisler CW: *Migraine headache disease diagnostic and management strategies*, Gaithersburg, Md, 1990, Aspen.

Thibodeau GA, Patton KT: *Anatomy & physiology*, ed 3, St Louis, 1996, Mosby.

Thibodeau GA, Patton KT: *Pocket reference to accompany anatomy & physiology*, ed 3, St Louis, 1996, Mosby.

Thomas LC, Rivett DA, Bolton PS: Pre-manipulative testing and the use of the velocimeter, *Man Ther* (in press, corrected proof).

Thompson AJ, Polman C, Hohlfeld R: *Multiple sclerosis: clinical challenges and controversies*, St Louis, 1997, Mosby.

Thompson JM: *Clinical outlines for health assessment*, St Louis, 1997, Mosby.

Thompson RE, Pearcy MJ, Barker TM: The mechanical effects of intervertebral disc lesions, *Clin Biomech* 19(5):448-455, 2004.

Thurston SE: *The little black book of neurology*, Chicago, 1987, Mosby.

Toghill PJ: *Examining patients: an introduction to clinical medicine*, London, 1990, Edward Arnold.

Tollison CD, Satterthwaite JR, Tollison JW: *Handbook of pain management*, ed 2, Baltimore, 1994, Williams & Wilkins.

Torg JS, et al: The relationship of development narrowing of the cervical spinal canal to reversible and irreversible injury of the cervical spinal cord in football players, *J Bone Joint Surg Am* 78:1308, 1996.

Torg JS, Shepard RJ: *Current therapy in sports medicine*, ed 3, St Louis, 1995, Mosby.

Turek SL: *Orthopaedics principles and their applications*, ed 3, Philadelphia, 1977, JP Lippincott.

Van Beusekom GT: The neurological syndrome associated with cervical luxations in rheumatoid arthritis, *Acta Orthop Belg* 58:38, 1972.

Van Holsbeeck M, Introcaso JH: *Musculoskeletal ultrasound*, St Louis, 1991, Mosby.

Wakefield TS, Frank RG: *The examiner's guide to neuromusculoskeletal practice*, Abbotsford, Wisc, 1995, Allied Health of Wisconsin, S.C.

Watkins RG: *The spine in sports*, St Louis, 1996, Mosby.

Weigang E et al: Incidence of neurological complications following overstenting of the left subclavian artery, *Eur J Cardiothorac Surg* 31(4):628-636, 2007.

Weineck J: *Functional anatomy in sports*, ed 2, St Louis, 1990, Mosby.

Weinstein SL, Buckwalter JA: *Turek's orthopaedics principles and their application*, ed 5, Philadelphia, 1994, JB Lippincott.

Weinstein SM: Assessment and rehabilitation of the athlete with a "stinger": a model for the management of noncatastrophic athletic cervical spine injury, *Clin Sports Med* 17(1):127-135, 1998.

White A: Biomechanical stability of the cervical spine, *Clin Orthop* 109:85, 1975.

White AH, Schofferman JA: *Spine care*, vol 1-2, St Louis, 1995, Mosby.

White G: *Levene's color atlas of dermatology*, ed 2, London, 1997, Mosby-Wolfe.

White G: *Regional dermatology*, London, 1994, Mosby-Wolfe.

Whitmore I, Willan PLT: *Multiple choice questions in human anatomy*, London, 1995, Mosby.

Whitmore RG et al: Bow hunter's syndrome caused by accessory cervical ossification: posterolateral decompression and the use of intraoperative Doppler ultrasonography, *Surg Neurol* 67(2):169-171, 2007.

Wickstrom J, LaRocca H: Trauma: head and neck injuries from acceleration-deceleration forces. In Ruge D, Wiltse LL, editors: *Spinal disorders: diagnosis and treatment*, Philadelphia, 1977, Lea & Febiger.

Wiegand R et al: Cervical spine geometry correlated to cervical degenerative disease in a symptomatic group, *J Manipulative Physiol Ther* 26(6):341-346, 2003.

Wilkinson M: The anatomy and pathology of cervical spondylosis, *Proc Roy Soc Lond (Belg)* 57:159, 1964.

Windsor RE, Lox DM: *Soft tissue injuries: diagnosis and treatment*, Philadelphia, 1998, Hanley & Belfus.

Yashon D: *Spinal injury*, New York, 1978, Appleton-Century-Crofts.

Yochum T, Rowe L: *Essentials of skeletal radiology*, ed 2, Baltimore, 1996, Williams & Wilkins.

Yousem DM: *Case review head and neck imaging*, St Louis, 1998, Mosby.

Zatouroff M: *Diagnosis in color physical signs in general medicine*, ed 2, London, 1996, Mosby-Wolfe.

Ziadeh MJ, Richardson JK: Arnold-Chiari malformation with syrinx presenting as carpal tunnel syndrome: a case report, *Arch Phys Med Rehabil* 85(1):158-161, 2004.

Zitelli BJ, Davis HW: *Atlas of pediatric physical diagnosis*, ed 2, London, 1992, Wolfe.

CITATIONS

Acar M et al: Comparison of vertebral artery velocity and flow volume measurements for diagnosis of vertebrobasilar insufficiency using color duplex sonography, *Eur J Radiol* 54 (2):221-224, 2005.

Al-Khayat H et al: Cervical radiculopathy secondary to Hodgkin's lymphoma, *Surg Neurol* 67 (5):540-543, 2007.

Alorainy IA: Dural tail sign in spinal meningiomas, *Eur J Radiol* 60 (3):387-391, 2006.

Alpass L: Chiropractic management of 'intractable' chronic whiplash syndrome, *Clin Chiropr* 7(1):16-23, 2004.

Balster SM, Jull GA: Upper trapezius muscle activity during the brachial plexus tension test in asymptomatic subjects, *Man Ther* 2(3):144-149, 1997.

Beric A: Post-spinal cord injury pain states, *Anesthesiol Clin North Am* 15(2):445-463, 1997.

Braga-Baiak A et al: Intra- and inter-observer reliability of MRI examination of intervertebral disc abnormalities in patients with cervical myelopathy, *Eur J Radiol* (in press, corrected proof).

Crown ED et al: Upregulation of the phosphorylated form of CREB in spinothalamic tract cells following spinal cord injury: relation to central neuropathic pain, *Neurosci Lett* 384(1-2):139-144, 2005.

Cummings M, Baldry P: Regional myofascial pain: diagnosis and management, *Best Pract Res Clin Rheum* 21(2):367-387, 2007.

Darvall JN, Morsi AW, Penington A: Coexisting harlequin and Horner syndromes after paediatric neck dissection: a case report and a review of the literature, *J Plast Reconstr Aesthet Surg* (in press, corrected proof).

El Idrissi R et al: Facial cutaneous cholesterol embolism revealing a tight carotid stenosis: a case report, *Eur J Vasc Endovasc Surg* 33(1):62-64, 2007.

Fernandez de las Penas C, Palomeque del Cerro L, Fernandez Carnero J: Manual treatment of post-whiplash injury, *J Bodywork Move Ther* 9(2):109-119, 2005.

Giudicissi-Filho M et al: Cervical spinal cord compression due to an osteochondroma in hereditary multiple exostosis: case report and review of the literature, *Surg Neurol* 66(suppl 3):S7-S11, 2006.

Gurley JP, Bell GR: The surgical management of patients with rheumatoid cervical spine disease, *Rheum Dis Clin North Am* 23(2):317-332, 1997.

Jenis L et al: Complex cervical reconstruction: the effect of posterior cervical distraction on foraminal dimensions using a screw-rod system, *Spine* 2(5, suppl 1):53, 2002.

Kerry R, Taylor AJ: Cervical arterial dysfunction assessment and manual therapy, *Man Ther* 11(4):243-253, 2006.

Kumar S, Ferrari R, Narayan Y: Cervical muscle response to head rotation in whiplash-type right lateral impacts, *J Manipulative Physiol Ther* 28(6):393-401, 2005.

Lauder TD et al: Predicting electrodiagnostic outcome in patients with upper limb symptoms: are the history and physical examination helpful? *Arch Phys Med Rehabil* 81(4):436-441, 2000.

Laureys S et al: The locked-in syndrome: what is it like to be conscious but paralyzed and voiceless? In *Progress in brain research*, vol 150, St Louis, 2005, Elsevier.

Lenoir T et al: Neurological and functional outcome after unstable cervicothoracic junction injury treated by posterior reduction and synthesis, *Spine* 6(5):507-513, 2006.

Lim J-K, Wong H-K: Variation of the cervical spinal Torg ratio with gender and ethnicity, *Spine* 4(4):396-401, 2004.

Lousa M et al: Histocompatibility class I and II antigens in extensive kindred with Sneddon's syndrome and related hypercoagulation disorders, *Human Immunol* 68(1):26-29, 2007.

Massie J et al: Antifibrotic gels versus a barrier sheet in the prevention of epidural fibrosis postlaminectomy, *Spine* 2(2, suppl 1):35, 2002.

Murphy DR et al: A nonsurgical approach to the management of patients with cervical radiculopathy: a prospective observational cohort study, *J Manipulative Physiol Ther* 29(4):279-287, 2006.

Naimur R et al: Intramedullary lipoma of the cervicodorsal spinal cord with intracranial extension: case report, *Surg Neurol* 65(5):486-489, 2006.

Newton AI: Spontaneous retropharyngeal hematoma: an unusual presentation of thoracic aortic dissection, *J Emerg Med* 31(1):45-48, 2006.

Nomura M et al: A patient with Wallenberg's syndrome induced by severe cough, *J Clin Neurosci* 11(2):179-182, 2004.

Oliphant D, Frayne R, Kawchuk G: A new method of creating intervertebral disc disruption of various grades, *Clin Biomech* 21(1):21-25, 2006.

Park SM, Kim E-S, Sung DH: Cervical radiculopathy caused by neural foraminal migration of a herniated calcified intervertebral disk in childhood: a case report, *Arch Phys Med Rehabil* 86(11):2214-2217, 2005.

Payer M, Hodler J, Benini A: Surgical treatment of cervical myelopathy of unclear aetiology, *J Clin Neurosci* 11(2):159-162, 2004.

Quinn KP, Winkelstein BA: Cervical facet capsular ligament yield defines the threshold for injury and persistent joint-mediated neck pain, *J Biomech* (in press, corrected proof).

Ronthal M: On the coincidence of cervical spondylosis and multiple sclerosis, *Clin Neurol Neurosurg* 108(3):275-277, 2006.

Sabuncuoglu H et al: Attenuation of postlaminectomy epidural fibrosis with monoclonal antibodies against intercellular adhesion molecule-1 and CD-18, *Spine* (in press, corrected proof).

Salvi FJ, Jones JC, Weigert BJ: The assessment of cervical myelopathy, *Spine* 6(6, suppl 1):S182-S189, 2006.

Sarikaya S et al: Magnetic resonance neurography diagnosed brachial plexitis: a case report, *Arch Phys Med Rehabil* 86(5):1058-1059, 2005.

Sasai K et al: Two-level disc herniation in the cervical and thoracic spine presenting with spastic paresis in the lower extremities without clinical symptoms or signs in the upper extremities, *Spine* 6(4):464-467, 2006.

Sathornsumetee S, Morgenlander JC: Friday night palsy: an unusual case of brachial plexus neuropathy, *Clin Neurol Neurosurg* 108(2):191-192, 2006.

Sawlani V et al: "Stretched loop sign" of the vertebral artery: a predictor of vertebrobasilar insufficiency in atlantoaxial dislocation, *Surg Neurol* 66(3):298-304, 2006.

Sterling M: A proposed new classification system for whiplash associated disorders—implications for assessment and management, *Man Ther* 9(2):60-70, 2004.

Takeuchi H et al: Cervical extradural meningioma with rapidly progressive myelopathy, *J Clin Neurosci* 13(3):397-400, 2006.

Terai H et al: Evaluation of dysphagia caused by ossification of anterior longitudinal ligament of cervical spine, *Spine* 6(5, suppl 1):114S, 2006.

Van Zundert J et al: Pulsed radiofrequency adjacent to the cervical dorsal root ganglion in chronic cervical radicular pain: a double blind sham controlled randomized clinical trial, *Pain* 127(1-2):173-182, 2007.

Velat GJ et al: Intraoperative dynamic angiography to detect resolution of bow hunter's syndrome: technical case report, *Surg Neurol* 66(4):420-423, 2006.

Weisfelt M et al: Nosocomial bacterial meningitis in adults: a prospective series of 50 cases, *J Hosp Infect* 66(1):71-78, 2007.

Wessely M: Cervical MRI. Part II: common disorders affecting the cervical spine, *Clin Chiropractic* 7(1):31-39, 2004.

Wight S, Osborne N, Breen AC: Incidence of ponticulus posterior of the atlas in migraine and cervicogenic headache, *J Manipulative Physiol Ther* 22(1):15-20, 1999.

Yoganandan N, Kumaresan S, Pintar FA: Biomechanics of the cervical spine. Part 2. Cervical spine soft tissue responses and biomechanical modeling, *Clin Biomech* 16(1):1-27, 2001.

AXIOMS IN ASSESSING THE SHOULDER

- Shoulder motion involves four primary articulations: the glenohumeral, acromioclavicular, sternoclavicular, and scapulothoracic.
- Common shoulder disorders include rotator cuff tendinopathy, rotator cuff tears, capsulitis (frozen shoulder), glenohumeral arthritis, and acromioclavicular syndromes.
- In early capsulitis and glenohumeral arthritis, all active and passive motions are painful, resisted motion produces no pain, and passive motion is decreased.

INTRODUCTION

The shoulder is a system of joints, and many movements of this system involve the neck. Completely independent action of the shoulder is possible, but independent, simultaneous action of the shoulder and neck is not.

The glenohumeral joint may be affected as part of widespread joint disease (i.e., a polyarthropathy such as rheumatoid arthritis, crystal deposition disease arthropathy, other inflammatory arthropathies, generalized osteoarthritis). Periarticular conditions can be grouped into categories with and without capsulitis. In the absence of capsular involvement, passive joint motion is largely unaffected, whereas active movement may be limited by pain, weakness, or both. In the presence of capsulitis, multidirectional restriction of passive motion is seen. Clinical and radiologic studies differentiate these conditions from articular conditions (Tables 4-1 and 4-2).

Referred pain to the shoulder can occur with cervical disorders, Pancoast tumor of the lung (a subphrenic pathologic condition), entrapment neuropathies, myofascial pain syndromes, and brachial neuritis (Table 4-3).

> Non–small-cell lung carcinomas (NSCLCs) of the superior sulcus, frequently termed Pancoast tumors, are some of the most challenging thoracic malignant diseases to treat because they generally invade adjacent vital structures, including the brachial plexus, subclavian vessels, and spine. Originally described by a radiologist, Henry Pancoast, in 1932, superior sulcus NSCLCs were deemed universally fatal until the 1950s, when the strategy of induction radiotherapy and en-bloc resection was shown to be potentially curative (Rusch, 2006).

Identifying the primary cause of shoulder pain is not always easy. Referred pain to the shoulder girdle region occurs from multiple sources other than the neck. With diaphragmatic irritation, pain is referred along the phrenic nerve to the supraclavicular region, the trapezius, and the superomedial angle of the scapula. Gastric and pancreatic diseases may refer pain to the interscapular region. The rare superior sulcus lung tumor, or Pancoast tumor, occasionally coincident with Horner syndrome, may have shoulder pain as its initial symptom (Figs. 4-2 and 4-3).

The arm as a lever is useless unless it has a fixed base. The fixed base comes largely from the layers of flat muscles

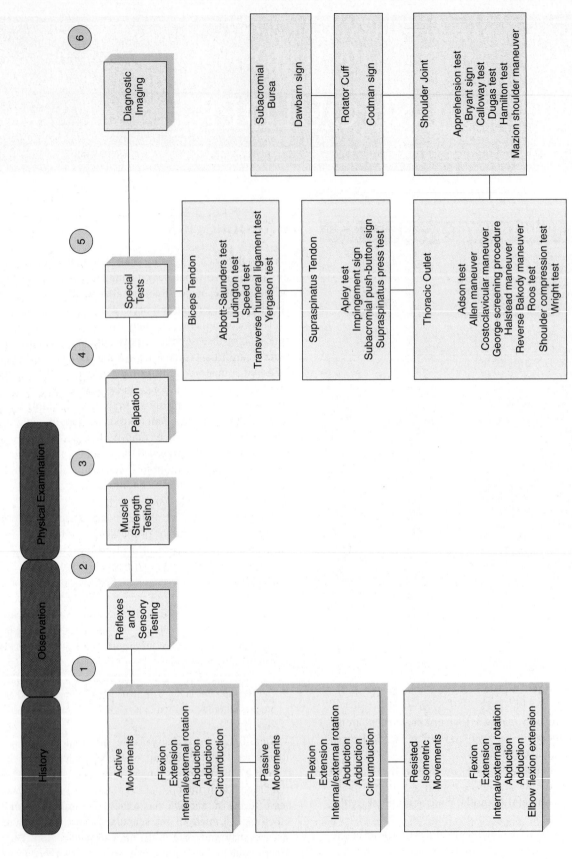

FIG. 4-1 Shoulder joint assessment.

TABLE 4-1

SHOULDER JOINT CROSS-REFERENCE TABLE BY ASSESSMENT PROCEDURE

Shoulder Joint / Test/Sign	Biceps Tendon	Scalenus Anticus Syndrome	Thoracic Outlet Syndrome	Rotator Cuff	Anterior Dislocation	Posterior Dislocation	Supraspinatus Tendon	Subacromial Bursa	Subclavian Arterial Stenosis	Adhesive Capsulitis	Transverse Humeral Ligament
Abbott-Saunders test	•										
Adson test		•	•								
Allen maneuver			•								
Apley test				•							
Apprehension test					•	•					
Bryant sign					•	•					
Calloway test					•	•					
Codman sign					•		•				
Costoclavicular maneuver			•								
Dawbarn sign								•			
Dugas test					•	•					
George screening procedure									•		
Halstead maneuver			•								
Hamilton test					•	•					
Impingement sign	•						•				
Ludington test	•										
Mazion shoulder maneuver				•	•	•				•	
Reverse Bakody maneuver		•	•								
Roos test			•								
Shoulder compression test			•						•		
Speed test	•										
Subacromial push-button sign					•			•			
Supraspinatus press test								•			
Transverse humeral ligament test	•										•
Wright test			•								
Yergason test	•										•

piled one on top of another and attached to all surfaces of the scapula.

Paralytic disorders implicating these muscles come into clinical focus when weakness in the fixation mechanism is demonstrated. The serratus anterior, when paralyzed, allows the scapula to swing backward and loosen its attachment to the chest. The trapezius allows the scapula to spin in the manner of a pinwheel, which contributes to the loss of fixation.

The mobility of this part of the body results from the configuration of the bony parts and the mechanically advantageous attachment of the multiple muscles. The shallow socket and ball head favor frictionless spinning, and the main joint has four accessory articulating zones that compliment and enhance the action of the shoulder.

Everyday activities are made up of acts such as lifting, holding, pushing, turning, and shoving. Through such common and accepted motions, clinical disorders are exhibited. These motions are combined pattern motions with contributions from many parts of the shoulder complex. Individual joint and muscle contribution may be analyzed in these acts to aid localization and understanding of injury and disease. Consideration must also be given to the part that the elbow and hand play in shoulder function. Shoulders are used unconsciously during actions of the hand, wrist, and elbow. Injury or disease may hamper normal action of any

TABLE 4-2

SHOULDER JOINT CROSS-REFERENCE TABLE BY SYNDROME OR TISSUE

Adhesive capsulitis	Mazion shoulder maneuver	Scalenus anticus syndrome	Adson test and Reverse Bakody maneuver
Anterior dislocation	Apprehension test Bryant sign Calloway test Dugas test Hamilton test Mazion shoulder maneuver	Subacromial bursa	Dawbarn sign
Biceps tendon	Abbott-Saunders test Impingement sign Ludington test Speed test Transverse humeral ligament test Yergason test	Subclavian arterial stenosis	George screening procedure Shoulder compression test
Posterior dislocation	Apprehension test Bryant sign Calloway test Dugas test Hamilton test Mazion shoulder maneuver	Supraspinatus tendon	Codman sign Impingement sign Subacromial push-button sign Supraspinatus press test
Rotator cuff	Apley test Codman sign Mazion shoulder maneuver Subacromial push-button sign	Thoracic outlet syndrome	Adson test Allen maneuver Costoclavicular maneuver Halstead maneuver Reverse Bakody maneuver Roos test Shoulder compression test Wright test
		Transverse humeral ligament	Transverse humeral ligament test Yergason test

TABLE 4-3

COMMON CAUSES OF SHOULDER PAIN

Periarticular Disorders	Regional Disorders	Glenohumeral Disorders

Rotator cuff tendinitis/impingement syndrome
Calcific tendinitis
Rotator cuff tear
Bicipital tendinitis
Acromioclavicular arthritis
	Cervical radiculopathy
	Brachial neuritis
	Nerve entrapment syndromes
	Sternoclavicular arthritis
	Reflex sympathetic dystrophy
	Fibrositis
	Neoplasms
	Miscellaneous
	  Gallbladder disease
	  Splenic trauma
	  Subphrenic abscess
	  Myocardial infarction
	  Thyroid disease
	  Diabetes mellitus
	  Renal osteodystrophy
		Inflammatory arthritis
		Osteoarthritis
		Osteonecrosis
		Cuff arthropathy
		Septic arthritis
		Glenoid labrum tears
		Adhesive capsulitis
		Glenohumeral instability

From Kelley WN et al: *Textbook of rheumatology*, ed 5, Philadelphia, 1997, WB Saunders.

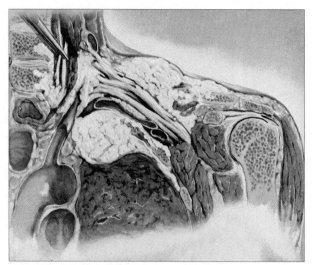

FIG. 4-2 Superior sulcus lung carcinoma (Pancoast tumor). Cancer is shown invading structures of the thoracic inlet, including brachial plexus, subclavian vessels, and ribs. (From Rusch VW: Management of pancoast tumours, *Lancet Oncol* 7[12]:997-1005, 2006.)

ORTHOPEDIC GAMUT 4-1

DIRECT SHOULDER TRAUMA

Direct trauma to the shoulder consists of:
1. Posterior dislocations of the sternoclavicular joint
2. Acromioclavicular subluxations or dislocations after a fall on the posterior superior shoulder
3. Direct blows to the supraclavicular brachial plexus at the base of the neck or axillary nerve as it courses under the deltoid
4. Clavicular fractures
5. Muscle contusions

4

ORTHOPEDIC GAMUT 4-2

MECHANISMS OF AXILLARY ARTERY INJURY CAUSED BY BLUNT TRAUMA (FIG. 4-5)

- Compression with contusion
- Forceful repeated stress
- Direct trauma by a sharp bony fragment
- Avulsion
- Traction

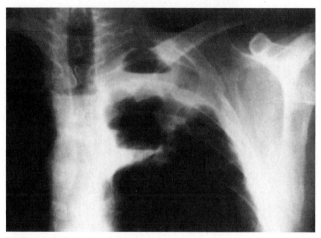

FIG. 4-3 Pancoast tumor. (From Nicholas JA, Hershman EB, editor: *The upper extremity in sports medicine,* St Louis, 1990, Mosby.)

of these areas; thus increased replacement effort is sought from the shoulder. For example, loss of rotatory range, as in arthrodesis of the wrist or elbow, unconsciously results in increased rotation at the shoulder. Weakness or disorder of one muscle group evokes replacement effort in another group. For example, the hunching motion by the trapezius that follows attempted abduction is a replacement effort associated with paralysis of the deltoid. Scrutiny of these purposeful patterns is of great help in understanding disability in this region.

Chronic overuse syndromes with repetitive stretching, as in rowing, swimming, or throwing, are injuries of repetitive microtrauma. Atraumatic disorders generally result from ligamentous laxity or congenital hypoplasia of the glenoid. Impact injuries may be divided into direct and indirect trauma. For direct trauma, the injury force is in direct contact with the shoulder complex. Indirect forces injuring the shoulder usually pass up through the hand, wrist, or elbow and result in a rotational or longitudinal force directed along the humerus.

Indirect trauma results in muscle, tendon, ligament, and brachial plexus stretch, strain, rupture, and bony fractures. Glenohumeral subluxations are usually caused by indirect forces (Fig. 4-4).

Patients with periclavicular trauma should be examined for vascular injury. Because of extensive collateral circulation of the upper limb, all patients with a shoulder or axillary injury who have an axillary hematoma or a specific neurologic injury should be assessed for need of digital substrate angiography even if pulses are present. Because of the high morbidity of axillary vascular injuries, early diagnosis, hemostasis, and prompt restoration of blood flow are critical (Ersel et al, 2007).

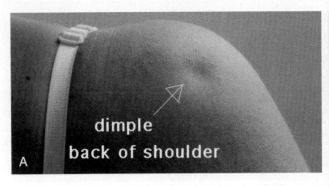

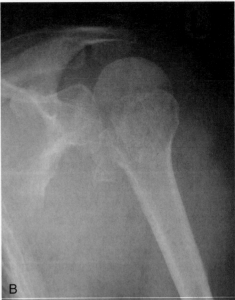

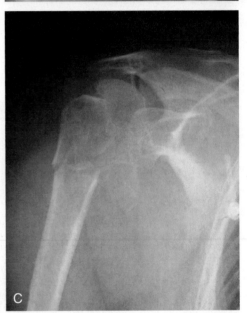

FIG. 4-4 **A,** The posterior aspect of the shoulder showing the typical dimple or skin tether associated with positional posterior dislocation of the shoulder. Posterior positional dislocation is a form of atraumatic posterior dislocation commonly presenting in late teenage years in either sex. This dimple is not seen in other shoulder disorders, and appears to be specific to this condition. (From Von Raebrox A et al: The association of subacromial dimples with recurrent posterior dislocation of the shoulder, *J Shoulder Elbow Surg* 15[5]:591-3, 2006). **B and C,** A 63-year-old male, retired electrician, presented to accident and emergency following electric shock. He had bilateral burns to the hands, full thickness in places and painful, stiff shoulders. There was no other injury noted at that time and no neurovascular deficit was documented. X-rays of the shoulders showed bilateral, comminuted, displaced proximal humeral fractures. (From Cooke SJ, Hackney RG: Bilateral posterior four-part fracture-dislocations of the shoulders following electric shock: a case report and literature review, *Injury Extra* 36[4]:90-95, 2005.)

ESSENTIAL ANATOMY

The shoulder joint is a ball-and-socket joint that is the articulation of the humerus and the glenoid fossa of the scapula (Fig. 4-6). To describe the anatomy of the shoulder joint, the term *shoulder joint complex* may be more accurate. The shoulder joint complex really consists of four joints: (1) the glenohumeral, (2) the acromioclavicular, (3) the sternoclavicular, and (4) the scapulothoracic articulation (Fig. 4-7). The acromioclavicular joint is formed by the lateral end of the clavicle and acromion. The acromioclavicular joint is reinforced by the surrounding capsule and ligaments, containing an anterior, posterior, superior, and inferior component, in addition to the coracoclavicular ligaments, which are made up of two individual ligaments: the coracoid and

trapezoid ligaments (Fig. 4-8). The short head of the biceps arises with the coracobrachialis from the scapular coracoid process and runs down the medial side of the long head of the biceps. The two bellies join as a common distal tendon just above the elbow joint as a flattened tendon, only to separate into two distal insertions (Fig. 4-9).

The serratus anterior muscle extends from the deep surface of the scapula to the upper eight or nine ribs. When this muscle does not function, the scapula is not held tightly against the chest wall and protrudes outward or *wings*. The most common cause is injury to the long thoracic nerve, which innervates the serratus anterior.

As is the case with most parts of the body, the shoulder region has a set of deep veins, usually accompanying the major arterial trunks, and a set of superficial veins, draining

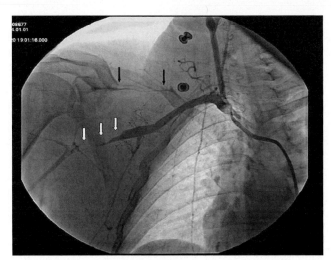

FIG. 4-5 The dissection *(white arrows)*, which completely occluded the third segment of right axillary artery, and displaced fracture of the clavicle *(black arrows)*. (From Ersel M et al: Axillary artery dissection due to blunt shoulder trauma, *Am J Emerg Med* 25[2]:242-243, 2007.)

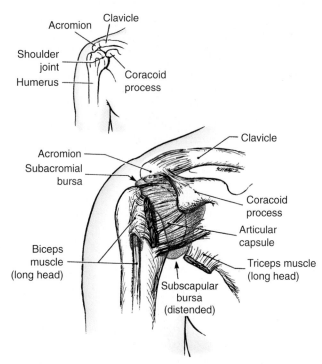

FIG. 4-6 Shoulder joint. (From Barkauskas VH et al: *Health & physical assessment,* ed 2, St Louis, 1998, Mosby.)

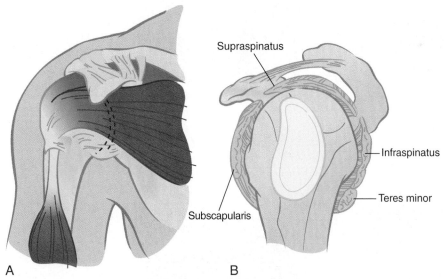

FIG. 4-7 **A,** Anterior-posterior and **(B)** lateral cross-sectional drawings of the shoulder demonstrate the relationship of the rotator cuff muscles (supraspinatus, infraspinatus, teres minor, and subscapularis) to the bony structure of the shoulder. (From Rakel: *Textbook of family medicine,* ed 7, St Louis, Saunders, 2007 Saunders.)

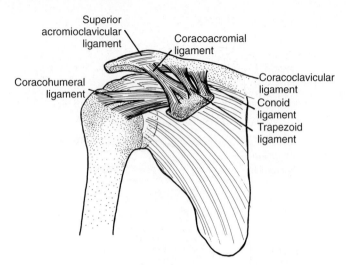

FIG. 4-8 Glenohumeral, acromioclavicular, and sternoclavicular joints. Thoracoscapular joint is between anterior scapular surface and chest wall. (From Noble: *Textbook of primary care medicine*, ed 3, St Louis, 2001, Mosby.)

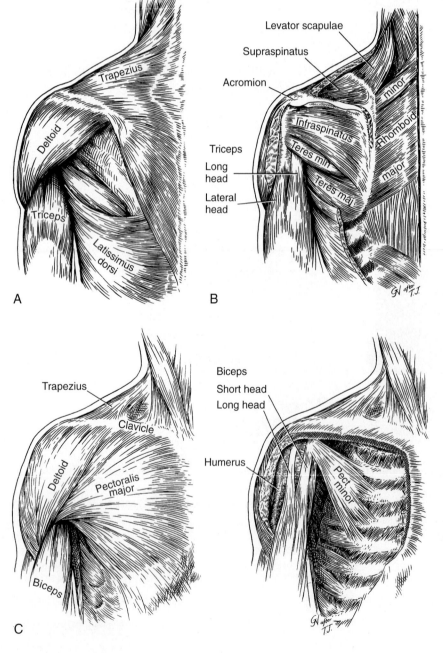

FIG. 4-9 A, Posterior view of the shoulder surface muscles, all groups. **B,** Rotator cuff; subscapularis not shown (medial rotator). Rhomboids and levator scapula displace scapula medially toward midline, while scapulohumeral group rotates humerus laterally. **C,** Interior view of the shoulder surface muscles and deep layer of muscles. (From Noble: *Textbook of primary care medicine*, ed 3, St Louis, 2001, Mosby.)

the skin and subcutaneous tissues (Fig. 4-10). The brachial and axillary veins and their tributaries represent the deep veins of the shoulder.

The nerve supply to the shoulder joint complex (Fig. 4-11) arises mainly fr om the fifth through the seventh cervical nerve roots via its formation into the brachial plexus.

The brachial plexus is the major structure for innervation of the shoulder area (Fig. 4-12).

On the lateral aspect of the shoulder, extending inferiorly from acromion to mid humerus, the skin is innervated by a cutaneous branch of the axillary nerve (C5 to C6) (Fig. 4-13).

The axillary artery is the central structure of the axilla (Fig. 4-14).

ESSENTIAL MOTION ASSESSMENT

Shoulder motion is interpreted through excursion of the arm from the body and is recorded according to the anatomic planes (Fig. 4-15).

The shoulder's total range of external and internal rotation is described as 180 degrees (external rotation of 108

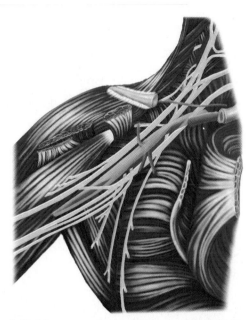

FIG. 4-11 Neurovascular supply to the shoulder joint complex. (From Nicholas JA, Hershman EB, editors: *The upper extremity in sports medicine,* St Louis, 1990, Mosby.)

ORTHOPEDIC GAMUT 4-3

SHOULDER MOVEMENTS

Primary shoulder movements are:

1. Elevation in the coronal (frontal) plane (abduction and adduction)
2. Flexion and extension in the sagittal plane (Figs. 4-16 and 4-17)
3. Horizontal adduction and abduction in the transverse (horizontal) plane (Figs. 4-18 and 4-19)
4. Internal and external rotation (torque around the humerus) (Figs. 4-20 and 4-21)

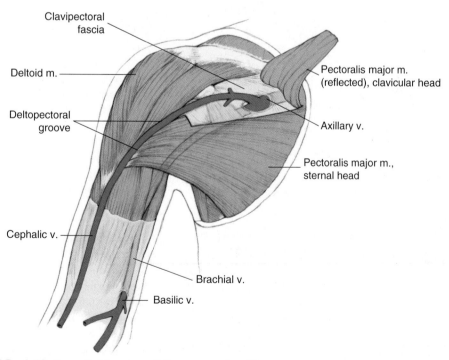

FIG. 4-10 Superficial veins of the arm and axilla. (From Mathers LH et al: *Clinical anatomy principles,* St Louis, 1996, Mosby.)

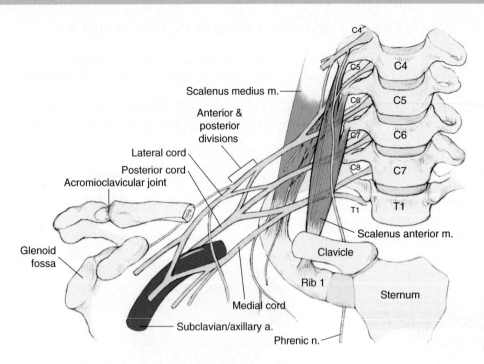

FIG. 4-12 Brachial plexus with relationships of nearby structures. (From Mathers LH et al: *Clinical anatomy principles,* St Louis, 1996, Mosby.)

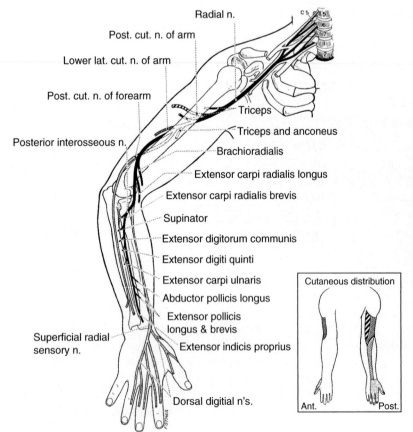

FIG. 4-13 Anatomy of the radial nerve. The radial nerve is derived from the posterior cord of the brachial plexus. In the proximal arm, the radial nerve first gives off the posterior cutaneous nerve of the arm, lower lateral cutaneous nerve of the arm, and the posterior cutaneous nerve of the forearm, followed by muscular branches to the triceps brachii and anconeus. The nerve then wraps around the humerus, descending into the region of the elbow, where muscular branches are given off to the brachioradialis, extensor carpi radialis long head, and supinator. More distally, the nerve bifurcates into the superficial radial sensory and posterior interosseous nerves. The posterior interosseous nerve supplies the remainder of the wrist and finger extensors, as well as the supinator and abductor pollicis longus. *Inset*: Sensory territories supplied by the radial nerve. (Adapted from W Haymaker, B Woodhal: *Peripheral nerve injuries.* Philadelphia, 1953, Saunders.) (From Katirji: *Neuromuscular disorders in clinical practice*, Philadelphia, 2002, Butterworth-Heinemann.)

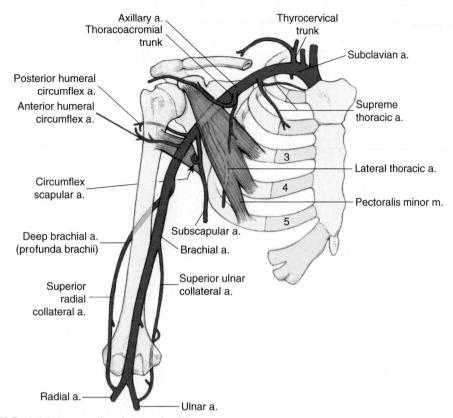

FIG. 4-14 Pectoralis minor and axillary artery. (From Mathers LH et al: *Clinical anatomy principles,* St Louis, 1996, Mosby.)

degrees [60%] and internal rotation of 72 degrees [40%]) with the arm placed at anatomic position. With the arm at 90 degrees of abduction, the total rotational arc is 120 degrees (more internal rotation), and at full flexion, minimal internal and external rotation is possible.

Inflammation caused by injury to any of the anatomic structures located between the acromion and the ascending humeral head during shoulder abduction will cause a painful arc between 60 and 120 degrees (Fig. 4-22).

The deltoid muscle is hinged at its origin and therefore exerts a shear force that forces the humerus upward on the glenoid labrum at abduction. In elevation to 90 degrees, the deltoid's shear forces are converted to a compressive force that places the humerus directly into the glenoid cavity (Fig. 4-23). With a weak or damaged supraspinatus tendon, the loss of the rotational force component results in painful impingement attributable to the imbalance of normal compressive forces (Fig. 4-24).

Adhesive capsulitis, also called *frozen shoulder*, is characterized by decreased shoulder range of motion, pain, capsular inflammation, fibrous synovial adhesions, and reduction of the joint cavity (Fig. 4-25).

ORTHOPEDIC GAMUT 4-4

MUSCLES OF THE SHOULDER JOINT COMPLEX

Muscles of the shoulder joint complex fall into three categories:
1. Those attaching to the scapula with their origin from the axial skeleton
2. Those that have their origin from the scapula and insert onto the humerus
3. Those that have their origin from the axial skeleton and insert onto the humerus

ESSENTIAL MUSCLE FUNCTION ASSESSMENT

The muscles surrounding the shoulder joint complex provide the ability to generate motion while simultaneously providing dynamic stability to the glenohumeral joint.

Text continued on p. 222

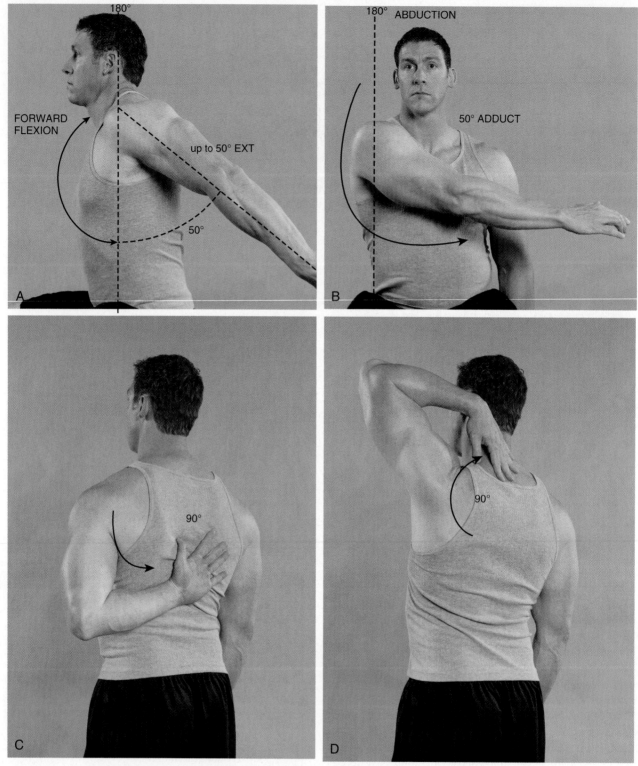

FIG. 4-15 Range of motion of the shoulder. **A,** Forward flexion and hyperextension. **B,** Abduction and adduction. **C,** Internal rotation. **D,** External rotation.

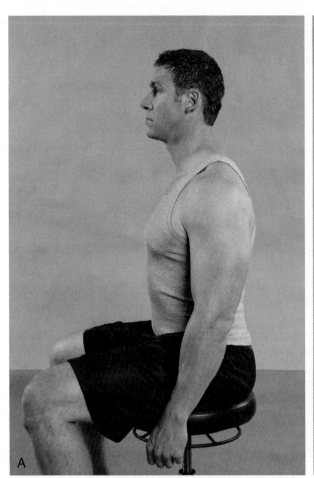
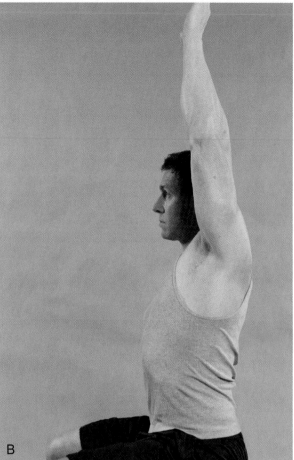

FIG. 4-16 **A,** The patient sits with the shoulder in a neutral position and the arm hanging straight at the side. **B,** The arm may be flexed 110 degrees at the shoulder and carried on up to 180 degrees in circumduction flexion. In this movement, the head of the humerus does not encounter the same obstructions from the coracoacromial arch that occurs during abduction. The scapula is fixed to the chest initially and then moves forward around the chest wall during the 90 degrees of elevation, ending up farther in front than during the motion of abduction. Flexion is accomplished by the anterior deltoid, pectoralis major, coracobrachialis, and biceps. A retained flexion range of motion that is 160 degrees or less is an impairment of the shoulder in the activities of daily living.

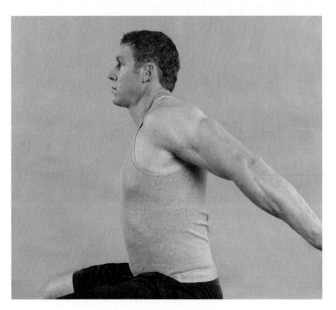

FIG. 4-17 The arm may be extended at the shoulder behind the line of the body for 50 degrees. In this action, the clavicle rotates downward a little on its long axis and moves backward, with the sternoclavicular joint as the fulcrum. The scapula shifts backward and tilts upward a little on the chest wall. Extension is accomplished by the posterior deltoid, latissimus, teres major and minor, infraspinatus, and triceps muscles. Adhesive joint disorders and arthritis in the glenohumeral joint interfere with extension. Forty degrees or less of retained extension range of motion is an impairment of the shoulder in the activities of daily living.

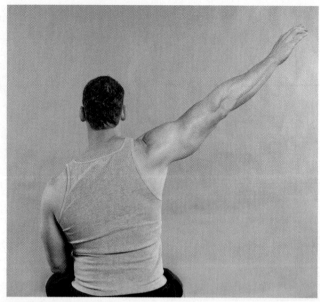

FIG. 4-18 Abducting the arm from the side of the body to over the head is a complex procedure. The normal range of motion is 180 degrees and is accomplished largely at the glenohumeral joint, but all of the axillary joints contribute. The muscles chiefly concerned are the trapezius, the serratus anterior, and the deltoid and rotator cuff group. Less than 160 degrees of retained abduction range of motion is an impairment of the shoulder in the activities of daily living.

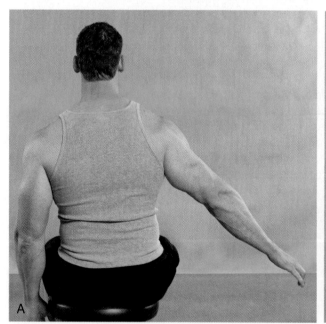

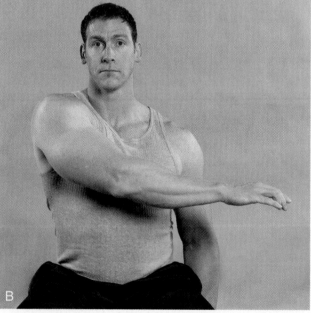

FIG. 4-19 From 180 degrees circumduction, the arm may be pulled down to the side (**A**), and at the end of the excursion the arm can be adducted in front of the chest 50 degrees farther (**B**). This action takes place with the assistance of gravity, and when resistance is added, the latissimus dorsi, teres major, and pectoralis major are the movers. As the arm descends from 180 degrees circumduction, the clavicle rotates downward on its long axis. The scapula moves on the chest wall during the middle 90 degrees, starting at 45 degrees from the top and stopping at 45 degrees from the bottom. The motion is largely at the glenohumeral joint, as the head of the humerus rotates internally and follows a linear arc from the bottom to the top of the glenoid. This motion reverses the route taken during abduction. A retained adduction range of motion of 30 degrees or less is an impairment of the shoulder in the activities of daily living.

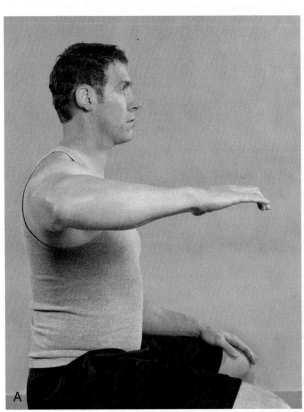
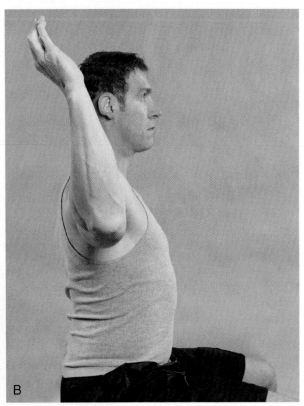

FIG. 4-20 From the mid position, which involves horizontal abduction of the arm at the side (**A**), the shoulder may be externally rotated almost 90 degrees (**B**). Nearly all of this movement occurs at the glenohumeral joint. When the arm is at the side, this action is accomplished by the infraspinatus, teres minor, and posterior deltoid. When the arm is horizontal, the supraspinatus also contributes. External rotation is the most important action, and when this rotation is lost, shoulder action is seriously compromised. Sixty degrees or less of retained external rotation is an impairment of the shoulder in the activities of daily living.

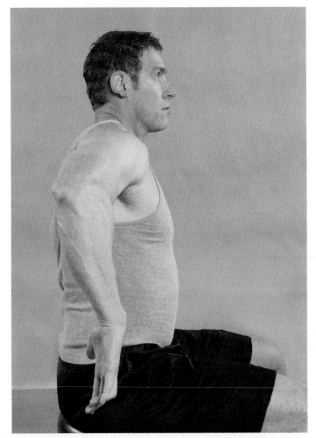

FIG. 4-21 The arm may be turned inward a little more than 90 degrees in both horizontal and vertical planes. This movement occurs chiefly at the glenohumeral joint and is powered by the subscapularis, pectoralis major, latissimus dorsi, and teres major muscles. The motion is an action that synchronizes with adduction as a striking blow and is hindered mainly by paralytic deformities. Sixty degrees or less of retained internal rotation is an impairment of the shoulder in the activities of daily living.

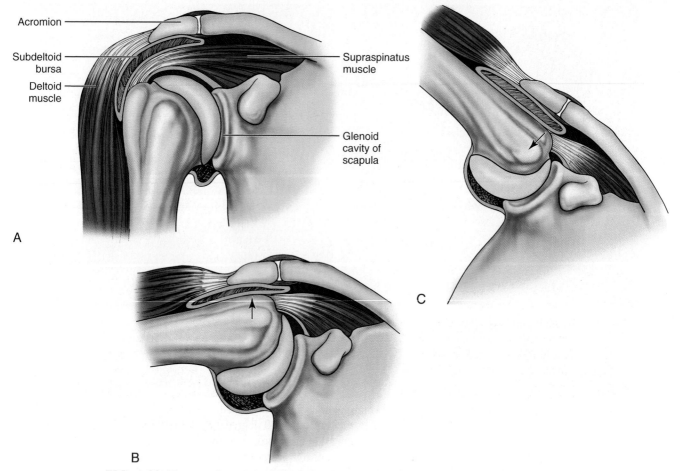

FIG. 4-22 The translatory motion of the glenohumeral joint during shoulder abduction. **A,** The shoulder in anatomic position. **B,** At 90 degrees. **C,** At 170 degrees. (Adapted from Greenstein GM: *Clinical assessment of neuromusculoskeletal disorders,* St Louis, 1997, Mosby.)

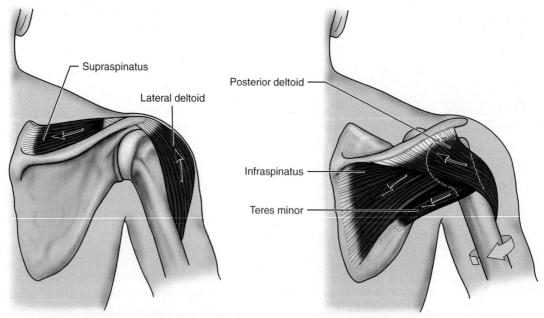

FIG. 4-23 The rotator cuff and deltoid muscle forces at the onset of abduction (0 degrees) and with the arm elevated 90 degrees. (Adapted from Saidoff DC, McDonough AL: *Critical pathways in therapeutic intervention,* St Louis, 1997, Mosby.)

4

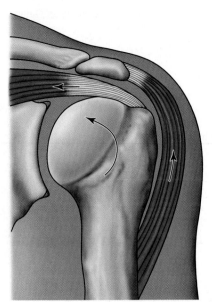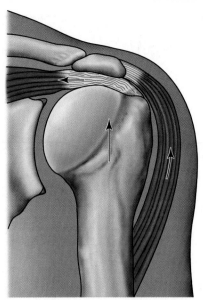

FIG. 4-24 Supraspinatus, exerting a rotational force, works in synergy with the deltoid, which yields a compressive force. **A,** Working together, both muscles facilitate shoulder elevation. **B,** Deep surface tearing of the supraspinatus weakens the cuff's ability to hold the humeral head down and away from the underside of the acromion, resulting in impingement. (Adapted from Saidoff DC, McDonough AL: *Critical pathways in therapeutic intervention,* St Louis, 1997, Mosby.)

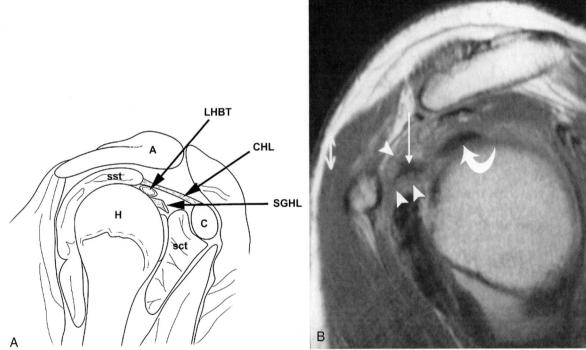

FIG. 4-25 The rotator interval subtends a medially based triangular space bordered superiorly by the leading edge of the supraspinatus tendon, inferiorly by the superior aspect of the subscapularis tendon, medially by the base of the coracoid process and laterally by the long head of biceps tendon and its sulcus. **A,** Line drawing of the rotator interval in sagittal section. (A) acromion process; (C) coracoid process; (H) humeral head; (LHBT) long head of biceps tendon; (CHL) coracohumeral ligament; (SGHL) superior glenohumeral ligament; (sst) supraspinatus tendon; (sct) subscapularis tendon. Sagittal oblique T1W fast spin-echo MR image demonstrating enhancing soft-tissue (arrowheads) surrounding the coracohumeral ligament (straight arrow), extending towards the intra-articular portion of long head of biceps tendon (curved arrow). Coracohumeral ligament thickness greater than 4 mm on sagittal oblique MR arthrographic images is a specific sign of adhesive capsulitis. **B,** In *adhesive capsulitis* and *disturbances affecting the rotator interval*, MRI may also show thickening of the rotator interval capsule and exuberant synovitis surrounding the coracohumeral ligament, which may enhance after intravenous gadolinium injection. (From Lee JC et al: MRI of the rotator interval of the shoulder, *Clin Radiol* 62(5):416-423, 2007.)

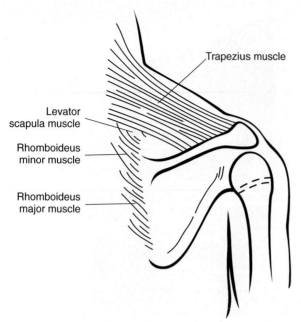

FIG. 4-26 The posterior periscapular musculature, including the trapezius, the levator scapulae, and the rhomboids. (From DeLee: *DeLee and Drez's orthopaedic sports medicine*, ed 2, St Louis, 2003, Saunders.)

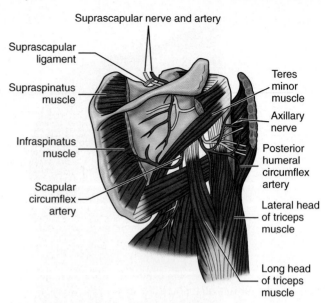

FIG. 4-27 Posterior view of shoulder with quadrangular space containing the axillary nerve and posterior humeral circumflex artery and the triangular space containing the scapular circumflex artery. (From Nicholas JA, Hershman EB, editors: *The upper extremity in sports medicine,* St Louis, 1990, Mosby.)

ORTHOPEDIC GAMUT 4-5
MUSCLE ATTACHMENTS

The scapula to spine muscle attachments are as follows:
1. Trapezius
2. Levator scapula
3. Rhomboid major
4. Rhomboid minor
5. Serratus anterior

Muscles, particularly those attaching to the scapula with their origin from the axial skeleton, include the trapezius, levator scapula, rhomboid major and minor, and serratus anterior (Fig. 4-26).

The trapezius is innervated by the spinal accessory nerve, which travels along its undersurface. The levator scapula originates from the posterior tubercles of the transverse processes of the first through fourth cervical vertebrae. It receives its innervation from the cervical plexus and occasionally from the dorsal scapular nerve.

The rhomboids also lie deep to the trapezius, with the rhomboid minor arising from the spinous processes of the seventh cervical and thoracic vertebrae and the intervening supraspinous ligament. Both rhomboids are supplied by the dorsal scapular nerve.

The serratus anterior arises from the outer surface of the first eight ribs and follows the curvature of the ribs to insert along the medial aspect of the scapula on its costal surface. The serratus anterior is supplied by the long thoracic nerve.

The subscapularis muscle arises from the costal surface of the scapula, with its muscles converging into an anterior tendon that inserts onto the lesser tuberosity of the humerus. It is innervated by the subscapularis nerve.

The supraspinatus muscle arises from the supraspinous fossa and passes laterally under the coracoacromial arch to attach to the greater tuberosity. It is supplied by the suprascapular nerve and vessels that travel on its undersurface.

The infraspinatus muscle arises from the infraspinous fossa and travels laterally to insert on the posterior aspect of the greater tuberosity. It is also supplied by the suprascapular nerve and vessels.

The teres minor muscle arises from the central third of the lateral border of the scapula below the scapular neck to pass behind the long head of the triceps and insert onto the lower posterior aspect of the greater tuberosity.

The teres major muscle arises from the lower third of the lateral border of the scapula and travels around the anterior aspect of the humerus and in front of the long head of the triceps to insert onto the crest of the lesser tubercle (Fig. 4-27). The teres minor and deltoid receive their innervation by the axillary nerve, whereas the teres major is supplied by the lower subscapular nerve (Figs. 4-28 to 4-33).

ESSENTIAL IMAGING

The shoulder girdle consists of the two bones that attach the upper limb to the thoracic wall: the scapula and clavicle. The glenoid fossa of the scapula forms the articulation of the shoulder girdle with the head of the humerus (Figs. 4-34 and 4-35).

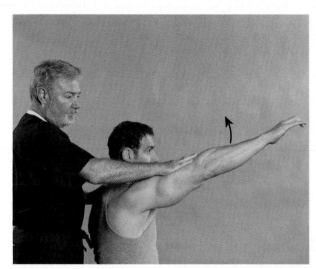

FIG. 4-28 The prime movers of flexion of the shoulder are the anterior portion of the deltoid muscle (axillary nerve, C5, and C6) and the coracobrachialis muscle (musculocutaneous nerve, C5, and C6). The accessory muscles to flexion are the middle fibers of the deltoid, the clavicular fibers of the pectoralis major, and the biceps brachii. To test flexion of the shoulder, the examiner immobilizes the patient's scapula on the side being tested. The examiner achieves immobilization by grasping and holding the lower border with one hand. The patient flexes the arm anteriorly to 90 degrees while the forearm is pronated and the elbow slightly flexed. The examiner's free hand provides graded resistance just above the elbow. Rotation, adduction, or abduction of the arm should be prevented while flexion is being tested.

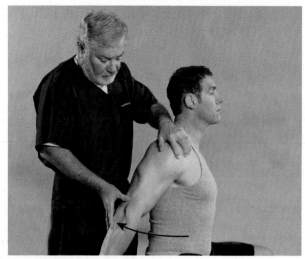

FIG. 4-29 The prime movers involved in shoulder extension are the latissimus dorsi (thoracodorsal nerve and C6 through C8), teres major (lowest subscapular nerve, C5, and C6), and deltoid (axillary nerve, C5, and C6) muscles. The teres minor and the long head of the triceps muscles are accessory to this motion. Extension of the shoulder is tested with the patient's elbow straightened and the forearm fully pronated (palm posterior) to prevent lateral rotation and adduction. The examiner fixes the scapula as described for testing flexion, and the patient extends the arm posteriorly through the range of motion. The examiner's other hand, which is placed just above the elbow, provides graded resistance.

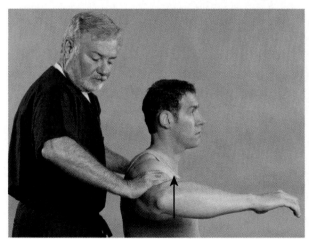

FIG. 4-30 The prime movers involved in abduction are the middle fibers of the deltoid (axillary nerve, C5, and C6) and the supraspinatus (suprascapular nerve and C5) muscles. The accessory muscles involved in abduction are the anterior and posterior fibers of the deltoid and serratus anterior muscles. The latter muscle functions by direct action of the scapula. Abduction of the shoulder is tested while the patient's arm is at the side, while the forearm is between pronation and supination (palm medial), and while the elbow is flexed a few degrees. The examiner stabilizes the scapula as described for flexion. The patient abducts the arm to 90 degrees. This abduction occurs against graded resistance applied by the examiner's other hand, which is placed proximal to the patient's elbow.

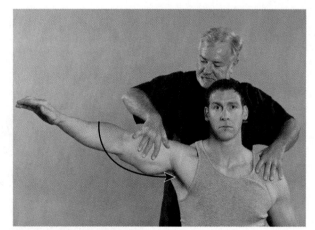

FIG. 4-31 The prime mover involved in adduction of the shoulder is the pectoralis major muscle (medial and lateral pectoral nerves, C5 through C8, and T1). The anterior fibers of the deltoid muscle are accessory to this motion. Adduction also occurs mainly at the glenohumeral joint and is assessed with the patient's arm abducted to 90 degrees. The patient adducts the arm anteriorly through the horizontal plane of motion and against graded resistance. This resistance is applied by the examiner's other hand, which is placed over the front of the arm and proximal to the patient's elbow.

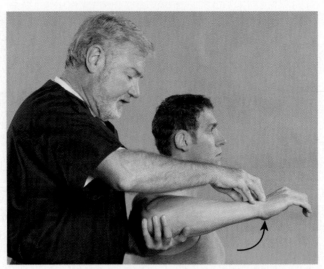

FIG. 4-32 The prime movers involved in external rotation are the infraspinatus (supra-scapular nerve, C5, and C6) and teres minor (axillary nerve and C5). The posterior fibers of the deltoid muscle are accessory to this motion. The external rotation of the shoulder is assessed with the patient's arm abducted to 90 degrees (or at the patient's side if abduction is not possible), with the elbow flexed to 90 degrees, and with the hand and fingers pointing forward. The examiner supports the patient's elbow by holding it with one hand while the patient rotates the arm upward (or outward if shoulder abduction is not possible) against graded resistance that is applied by the examiner's other hand, which is placed on the patient's forearm proximal to the wrist.

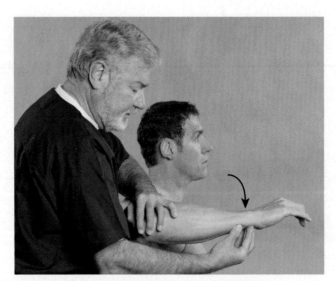

FIG. 4-33 The prime movers of internal rotation of the shoulder are the subscapularis (upper and lower subscapular nerves, C5, and C6), pectoralis major (medial and lateral pectoral nerves, C5 through C8, and T1), and teres major (lowest subscapular nerve, C5, and C6) muscles. The anterior fibers of the deltoid muscle are accessory to this motion. Internal rotation of the shoulder is tested with the arm abducted to 90 degrees (or at the side if abduction is not possible), the elbow flexed to 90 degrees, and the hand pointed forward. The examiner supports the patient's elbow with one hand, as described previously, while the patient rotates the arm downward (or inward if the shoulder abduction is not possible) against graded resistance that is applied by the examiner's other hand, which is placed on the patient's forearm proximal to the wrist.

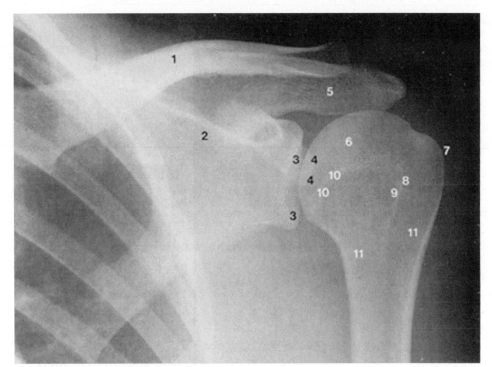

FIG. 4-34 Shoulder joint. Anteroposterior plain-film radiograph. *1,* Clavicle; *2,* scapula; *3,* glenoid fossa; *4,* humeral head, articular surface; *5,* acromion; *6,* head of humerus; *7,* greater tubercle of humerus; *8,* intertubercular groove; *9,* lesser tubercle of humerus; *10,* anatomic neck; *11,* surgical neck. (From Mathers LH et al: *Clinical anatomy principles,* St Louis, 1996, Mosby.)

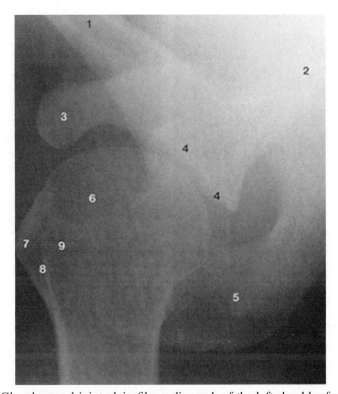

FIG. 4-35 Glenohumeral joint plain-film radiograph of the left shoulder from cephalad. *1,* Clavicle; *2,* spine of scapula; *3,* coracoid process; *4,* glenoid fossa; *5,* acromion; *6,* head of humerus; *7,* lesser tubercle; *8,* intertubercular groove; *9,* greater tubercle. (From Mathers LH et al: *Clinical anatomy principles,* St Louis, 1996, Mosby.)

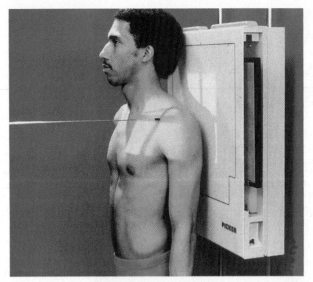

FIG. 4-36 Anteroposterior shoulder with neutral rotation of the humerus. (From Frank ED, et al: *Merrill's atlas of radiographic positioning and procedures,* vol 1-3, ed 11, St Louis, 2007, Mosby.)

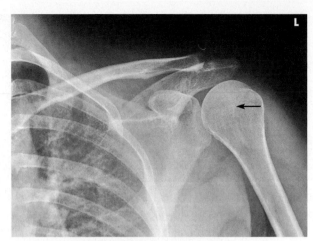

FIG. 4-37 Anteroposterior shoulder in neutral rotation of the humerus. (From Frank ED, et al: *Merrill's atlas of radiographic positioning and procedures,* vol 1-3, ed 11, St Louis, 2007, Mosby.)

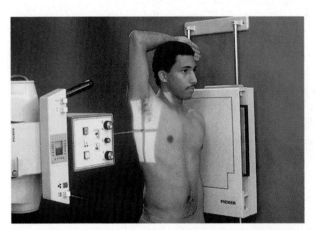

FIG. 4-38 Upright transthoracic lateral shoulder. (From Frank ED, et al: *Merrill's atlas of radiographic positioning and procedures,* vol 1-3, ed 11, St Louis, 2007, Mosby.)

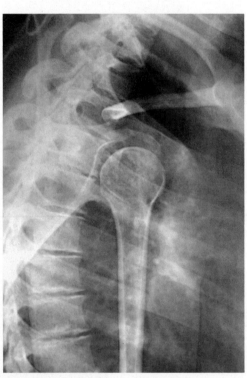

FIG. 4-39 Transthoracic lateral shoulder. (From Frank ED, et al: *Merrill's atlas of radiographic positioning and procedures,* vol 1-3, ed 11, St Louis, 2007, Mosby.)

The most important films to obtain are the true antero-posterior (AP) (Figs. 4-36 and 4-37) and the modified West Point views (Figs. 4-38 to 4-41). Both of these projections provide an excellent view of a glenohumeral joint. The examiner is able to appreciate the characteristic posterior glenoid wear (Fig. 4-42). The acromioclavicular joint can be radiographically evaluated and correlated with the physical examination. The AP view should include the proximal two thirds of the humeral shaft so that the physician can safely estimate the appropriate humeral component diameter (Figs. 4-43 and 4-44). When clinically indicated, the radiographic examination of the shoulder must include a cervical spine series.

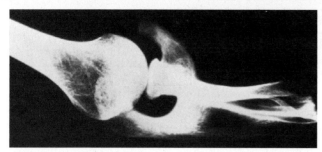

FIG. 4-40 Radiographic appearance of the modified West Point view. (From Nicholas JA, Hershman EB, editors: *The upper extremity in sports medicine,* St Louis, 1990, Mosby.)

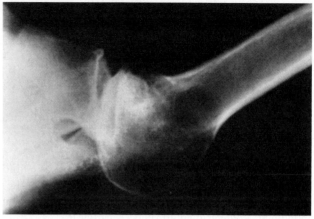

FIG. 4-42 Modified West Point view shows the marked posterior subluxation and migration. (From Nicholas JA, Hershman EB, editors: *The upper extremity in sports medicine,* St Louis, 1990, Mosby.)

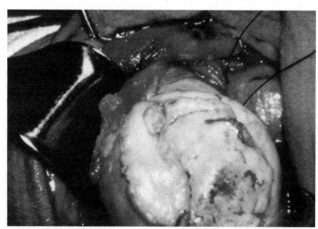

FIG. 4-43 Intraoperative view demonstrating the circumferential nature of the osteophytes on the humeral head. (From Nicholas JA, Hershman EB, editors: *The upper extremity in sports medicine,* St Louis, 1990, Mosby.)

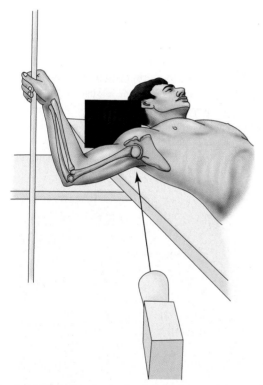

FIG. 4-41 Technique of obtaining the supine modified West Point view. With the patient laying supine and holding onto a support, the X-ray tube is angled 20 degrees upward from the floor and 20 degrees away from the long axis of the patient's body. (From Nicholas JA, Hershman EB, editors: *The upper extremity in sports medicine,* St Louis, 1990, Mosby.)

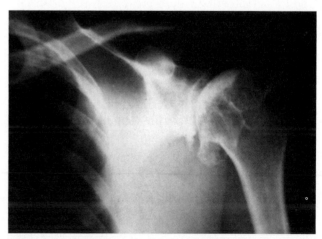

FIG. 4-44 Characteristic inferior glenoid osteophyte seen with loss of sphericity of the humeral head. (From Nicholas JA, Hershman EB, editors: *The upper extremity in sports medicine,* St Louis, 1990, Mosby.)

4

Assessment for Biceps Tendinopathy

Comment

Rotator cuff tears may be acute or chronic, partial or full thickness. Partial tears may occur in any age group after trauma. A full-thickness (or complete) tear is rarely seen in individuals younger than 40 years. A partial tear can result from a fall or explosive shoulder movement and is characterized very much as a rotator cuff tendinopathy. Full active range of motion may be preserved. The acute complete rupture after trauma should be easily diagnosed. Chronic full-thickness tears are found incidentally in approximately 27% of patients at autopsy.

Examination of rotator cuff tears reveals many of the features of rotator cuff tendinopathy. The patient is often unable to maintain the arm in abduction when lowering it from the elevated position. Subacromial crepitus and pain on impingement testing are present. A common clinical finding is atrophy of the infraspinatus.

Subluxation of the tendon of the long head may be isolated and result from attrition but is often concomitant with moderate to massive tears extending into the anterior portion of the cuff.

When an excessive load is applied to the arm in the position of abduction and external rotation, the line of pull of the long bicipital tendon is placed in the coronal plane and presses against the medial wall of the groove but is restrained from bowstringing by the lesser tuberosity acting as a simple pulley (Fig. 4-45).

Rupture or stretching of the fascial covering of the bicipital groove permits the tendon to subluxate from the groove, which may occur as an acute injury. The predisposing factor for this condition is a congenitally shallow bicipital groove. The intertubercular groove may be not only shallow, but also broader than normal. This feature permits the tendon to flatten out and slide back and forth within the groove itself. The patient complains of a snap that occurs anteriorly in the shoulder and is accompanied by pain. The pain is followed by residual soreness along the bicipital groove. The soreness is elicited by the same motions that cause pain with tenosynovitis. Rupture or stretching of the fascial covering of the bicipital groove is indistinguishable from tenosynovitis. In a muscular patient, palpating the subluxing tendon may be difficult. If the condition becomes chronic as a result of a defect in the roof of the groove with redundant tissue chronic synovitis usually occurs. Movement of the shoulder results in painful snapping as the tendon slips back and forth out of the groove, particularly during rotation of the arm.

According to Gilcreest, rupture of the long head occurs in 50% of biceps ruptures. The author also noted that an acute, traumatic rupture of this tendon occurs most often when a person is raising a weight of 68 kg or more. Ruptures of the long head of the biceps tendon are commonly caused

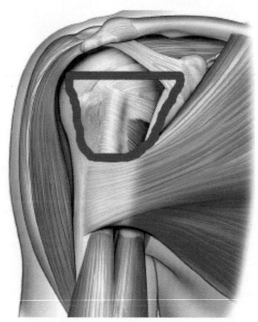

FIG. 4-45 The boundaries of the subdeltoid space include the greater tuberosity superiorly, the long head of the biceps tendon laterally, the pectoralis major tendon inferiorly, and the conjoint tendon medially. The anterior deltoid forms the roof and the anterior shoulder capsule forms the floor of this space. (From O'Brien SJ, Miller AN, Drakos MC: Arthroscopic subdeltoid approach to the biceps transfer, *Oper Tech Sports Med* 15[1]:20-26, 2007.)

ORTHOPEDIC GAMUT 4-6
BICEPS TENDON

The biceps tendon may luxate medially out of the groove and over the lesser medial tuberosity in one of two patterns:
1. Rupture of the transverse ligament and subluxation of the biceps tendon out of the groove, with the tendon lying anterior to the subscapularis muscle
2. Tendon subluxation beneath the subscapularis muscle belly (Fig. 4-46)

The long tendon returns into the groove once the upper arm is rotated medially and then laterally while the forearm is flexed at the elbow (Yergason test) (Fig. 4-47).

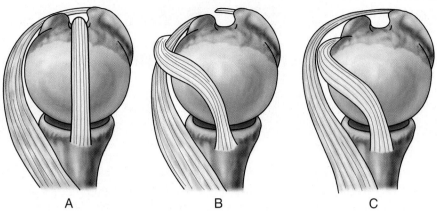

FIG. 4-46 **A,** The normal relationship of the biceps tendon in the groove covered by the transverse humeral ligament. **B,** Rupture of the transverse ligament and subluxation of the biceps tendon out of the groove with the tendon lying anterior to the subscapularis muscle. **C,** Intertendinous disruption of the subscapularis commonly occurs when the subscapularis insertion degenerates and the tendon subluxates beneath the muscle-tendon belly. (Adapted from Saidoff DC, McDonough AL: *Critical pathways in therapeutic intervention,* St Louis, 1997, Mosby.)

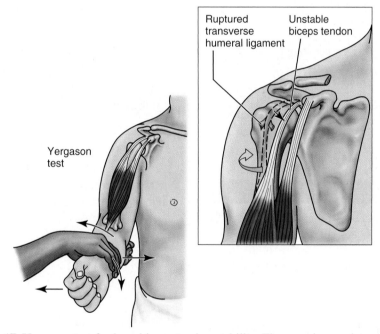

FIG. 4-47 Yergason test for long biceps tendon stability. The examiner resists supination as the patient simultaneously externally rotates the shoulder against resistance. (Adapted from Saidoff DC, McDonough AL: *Critical pathways in therapeutic intervention,* St Louis, 1997, Mosby.)

by degenerative changes within the tendon and are associated with diseases of the subacromial space. Degenerative changes in the tendon, characterized by disorganized collagen fibers and large mucoid deposits, occur mainly in the distal bicipital groove. The common site of rupture occurs within the groove; this occurs predominantly in men in their sixth or seventh decade of life as a result of the weakening of the tendon by the degenerative process. The other commonly recognized site of traumatic tears occurs at the

biceps anchor on the labrum (superior labrum AP lesions), but these do not lead to complete rupture of the tendon. Less commonly, ruptures have been reported in weightlifters at the musculotendinous junction and within the muscle belly. The abuse of anabolic steroids, however, accelerates the natural history of tears, and they are seen in a much younger population; this is a result of changes within the tendon structure itself by the anabolic steroids (Cope et al, 2004).

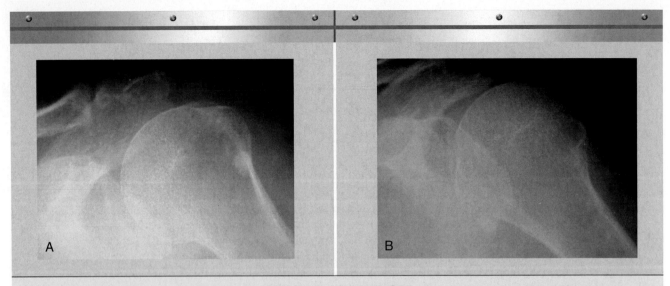

AT THE VIEWBOX

Adult male with shoulder pain, especially with flexion and internal rotation. Positive orthopedic tests for tenosynovitis of the biceps-subscapularis tendon complex, with focal pain with palpation at the bicipital groove. A globular focus of calcification maintains its relationship with the bicipital groove with external **(A)** versus internal **(B)** rotation, findings characteristic of calcium hydroxyapatite deposition disease (HADD/calcific tendinitis) of the biceps-subscapularis tendon complex. Rotator cuff calcific tendinitis most commonly involves the supraspinatus tendon insertion superolateral to this at the greater tuberosity. With symptoms of tenosynovitis of the shoulder, plain films are most often negative for intrinsic abnormality of the rotator cuff and biceps tendon. Ongoing symptoms with conservative management warrants MRI to follow-up. (From the teaching file of Timothy Mick, DC, DACBR)

PROCEDURE

- With the patient in the seated position, the examiner fully abducts and externally rotates the patient's arm (Figs. 4-48 and 4-49).
- The examiner then lowers the arm to the patient's side (Fig. 4-50).
- A palpable or audible click indicates a subluxation or dislocation of the biceps tendon.
- While the examiner's finger or fingers palpate for the point of maximal tenderness within the bicipital groove, the shoulder is alternately rotated.
- A positive test occurs in biceps tendinopathy when the patient feels pain as the tendon glides beneath the examiner's finger.

Next Steps/Procedures
Ludington test, Speed test, transverse humeral ligament test, and Yergason test

CLINICAL PEARL

The biceps tendon will not rupture or dislocate under ordinary stresses unless it is already weak. The predisposing factor to rupture or dislocation is age degeneration, which is probably accelerated by often-repeated friction and angulation at the point where the tendon enters the bicipital groove of the humerus.

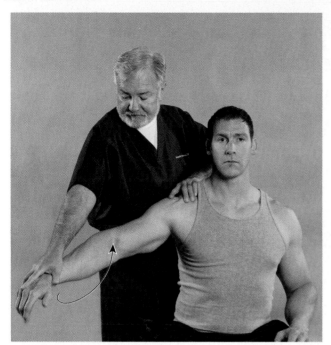

FIG. 4-48 With the patient in the seated position, the examiner fully abducts the patient's arm.

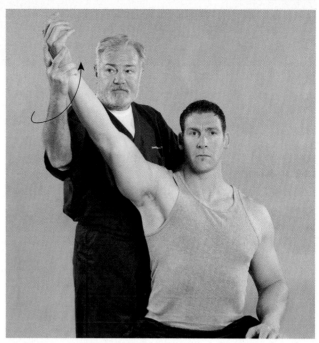

FIG. 4-49 The examiner externally rotates the patient's arm when the arm is at the top of the abduction maneuver.

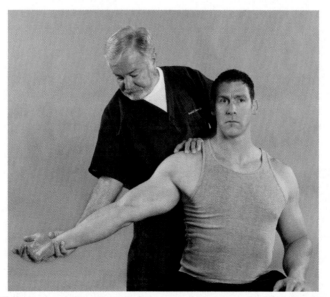

FIG. 4-50 While maintaining the arm in external rotation, the examiner then lowers the arm to the patient's side. A palpable or audible click is a positive finding, which indicates a subluxation or dislocation of the biceps tendon.

4

ALSO KNOWN AS SCALENE MANEUVER AND SCALENUS ANTICUS TEST

Assessment for Neurovascular Compression of the Subclavian Artery and Brachial Plexus Caused By Scalenus Anticus or Cervical Rib Thoracic Outlet Syndromes

Comment

Anatomic anomalies of cervicothoracic structures include the presence of a cervical rib (Fig. 4-51), unusually long transverse processes of the seventh cervical vertebra, and an anomalous fibrous band. Cervical ribs, which articulate with the seventh cervical vertebra (Fig. 4-52), are present in 1% of the population.

The brachial plexus and the subclavian artery can be compressed as they pass between the anterior and medial scalene muscles and the first rib, yielding a characteristic neurovascular syndrome: the anterior scalene syndrome.

All three scalene muscles originate from the transverse processes of the cervical vertebrae and insert on the first and second ribs. The anterior and medial scalene muscles insert on the respective tubercles on the first rib and sandwich the subclavian artery into a sulcus. The posterior scalenus muscle is fixed to the second rib. A variable scalenus minimus muscle may exist and insert between the anterior and medial scalenus muscles. The scalene muscles raise the first and second rib during inspiration. Unilateral contraction inclines the head to the side of action and turns the face to the opposite side. Bilateral contraction flexes the cervical spine. The anterior and medial scalene muscles form one side of the scalene foramen, with the sternocleidomastoid muscle and the first rib forming the other sides. Bounded by the anterior scalene muscle, the first rib, and the medial scalene muscle, the posterior scalene foramen admits the brachial plexus and the subclavian artery to the costoclavicular space. The posterior foramen can range from 0.4 to 3.5 cm in width.

The subclavian artery bends over and passes through a sulcus in the first rib. Made up of nerve roots from C5–C8 and T1, the brachial plexus represents the innervation of the entire upper extremity and lies tautly stretched and without bony protection in this region.

Neurovascular compression can occur when disease or anatomic variations narrow a tight foramen. In the development of the anterior scalene syndrome, some anatomic variations are very important (Figs. 4-53 and 4-54).

The anterior scalene syndrome has many similarities with the costoclavicular syndrome, also known as the *syndrome of the cervical rib*.

Under normal circumstances, enough room exists in the posterior scalene foramen of the brachial plexus and the subclavian artery. However, many anatomic variations and consequent changes in the functional anatomic features of the shoulder and upper extremity can cause the development of the clinical symptoms. Many embryologic, anatomic, and physiologic factors create a disposition for development of compression in the posterior scalene foramen.

Thoracic outlet syndrome (TOS) results from impending thoracic outlet pressure on the neurovascular bundle exiting the thoracic cavity and entering the upper extremity. The pressure is created by several factors, including the first rib and accessory or cervical ribs. Associated surrounding hypertrophic muscles, namely the scalene and the subclavius with their corresponding tendons, will also contribute to this local pressure syndrome (Barkhordarian, 2007).

The neurovascular symptoms depend on the frequency, duration, and degree of compression of the subclavian artery and the brachial plexus. The lower roots of the brachial plexus (C8–T1) are at higher risk than the more superior roots because of their location in the plexus. The symptoms include pain in the fingers, hand, forearm, arm, and shoulder and paresthesia and hyperesthesia, especially in the eighth cervical and first thoracic nerve root dermatomes. Numbness occurs most often in the fingers, hand, and forearm. Depending on the degree of arterial compression, ischemic symptoms of numbness, cold, weakness, and skin color changes appear.

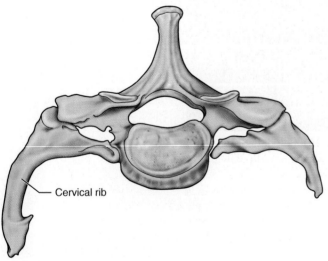

FIG. 4-51 Cervical rib. (From Saidoff DC, McDonough AL: *Critical pathways in therapeutic intervention,* St Louis, 1997, Mosby.)

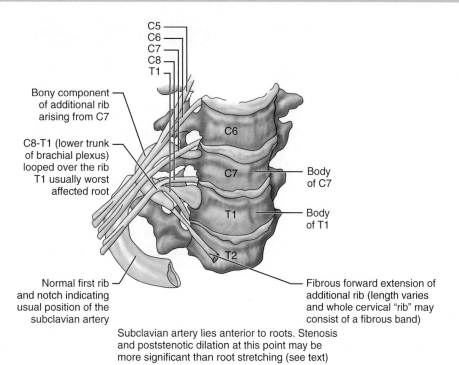

C5
C6
C7
C8
T1

Bony component
of additional rib
arising from C7

C8-T1 (lower trunk
of brachial plexus)
looped over the rib
T1 usually worst
affected root

C6

C7

T1

T2

Body
of C7

Body
of T1

Normal first rib
and notch indicating
usual position of the
subclavian artery

Fibrous forward extension of
additional rib (length varies
and whole cervical "rib" may
consist of a fibrous band)

Subclavian artery lies anterior to roots. Stenosis
and poststenotic dilation at this point may be
more significant than root stretching (see text)

FIG. 4-52 Relation of the cervical rib to its surrounding structures. (From Saidoff DC, McDonough AL: *Critical pathways in therapeutic intervention,* St Louis, 1997, Mosby.)

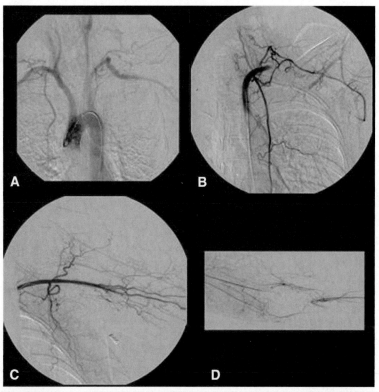

FIG. 4-53 Arteriogram of left upper extremity. **A,** The mid-left subclavian artery is very tortuous and irregular, with a short focal 50% stenosis at its mid-distal aspect. **B,** In hyperabduction of the left arm the subclavian artery is compressed by the cervical rib and arterial flow is interrupted. **C,** Embolic occlusion of the proximal mid-humerus brachial artery with reconstitution. **D,** Second embolic occlusion of the distal brachial artery with reconstitution to the interosseous artery. (From Hugl B et al: Unusual etiology of upper extremity ischemia in a scleroderma patient: thoracic outlet syndrome with arterial embolization, *J Vasc Surg* 45(6):1259-1261, 2007.)

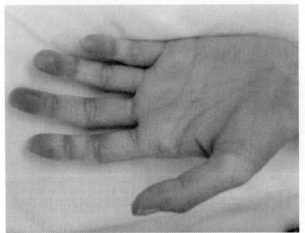

FIG. 4-54 A 47-year-old woman with diffuse systemic scleroderma (ANA positive) with an ischemic left third distal finger. Six days prior, she awakened during the early morning with pain in her left third distal phalanx which persisted, and her finger became cyanotic. On examination, she had an absent left radial, ulnar, and brachial pulse. She had a bruit in the left infraclavicular area. An upper extremity angiogram, demonstrated a tortuous and irregular mid-left subclavian artery with a short focal 50% stenosis at its mid-distal aspect (Fig. 4-53). (From Hugl B et al: Unusual etiology of upper extremity ischemia in a scleroderma patient: thoracic outlet syndrome with arterial embolization, *J Vasc Surg* 45(6):1259-1261, 2007.)

ORTHOPEDIC GAMUT 4-7

THORACIC OUTLET SYNDROME

Even though the first thoracic rib forms the floor of the thoracic compression compartment, trapping or scissoring the brachial plexus and subclavian vessels between the first ribs, other local structures contribute to the problem:

- The clavicle
- A cervical rib
- A anomalous cervical band from an elongated C7 transverse process
- The subclavius muscle
- Bony callous or exostosis

PROCEDURE

- The examiner locates the radial pulse of the involved extremity (Fig. 4-55).
- The patient's head is rotated to the involved extremity (Fig. 4-56).
- The patient extends the neck as the examiner externally rotates and extends the patient's shoulder.
- The patient takes a deep breath and holds it (Fig. 4-57).
- Loss of the pulse is a positive test.
- If the test is negative, it is repeated by having the patient rotate the head to the uninvolved extremity.

Next Steps/Procedures

Allen maneuver, costoclavicular maneuver, George screening procedure, Halstead maneuver, reverse Bakody maneuver, Roos test, shoulder compression test, and Wright test

---

CLINICAL PEARL

Radiographic demonstration of a cervical rib does not prove that it is the cause of the symptoms. The condition has to be distinguished (1) from other causes of pain and paresthesia in the forearm and hand, (2) from other causes of muscle atrophy in the hand, and (3) from other causes of peripheral vascular changes in the upper extremity

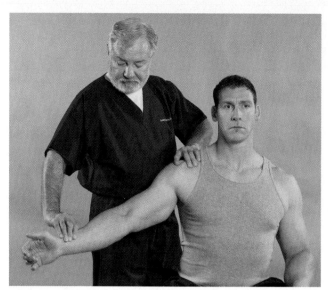

FIG. 4-55 The patient is seated comfortably with the arms at the sides. The examiner slightly abducts the affected arm and palpates the radial pulse.

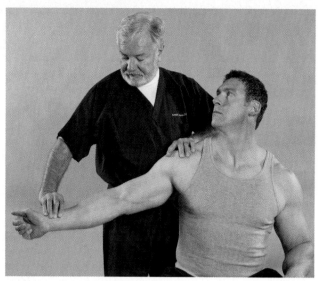

FIG. 4-56 The patient rotates the head toward the affected shoulder. The patient then extends the head, and the examiner externally rotates and extends the shoulder slightly.

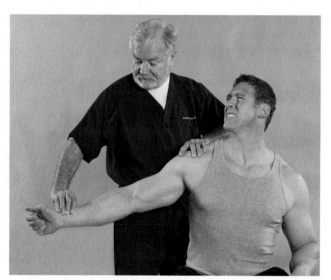

FIG. 4-57 The patient takes a deep breath and holds it. Loss of the pulse is a positive test. If the test is negative, it is repeated with the patient turning the head to the uninvolved side (modified Adson test).

ALLEN MANEUVER

Assessment for Thoracic Outlet Syndrome

Comment

Multiple etiologic possibilities, complex anatomic considerations, and a variety of neurogenic and vascular symptoms engage the interest of many disciplines that encounter the thoracic outlet neurovascular compression syndromes. Static and dynamic anatomic relationships within the thoracic outlet dictate morbid aberrations in blood perfusion and neural function.

Usually a contributory anatomic element that underlies each of the compression syndromes can be identified. Therefore, the usual clinical maneuvers used to bracket the level of compression can be equivocal. Patients do not often have one single complaint or set of complaints that unfailingly point to a compression syndrome. In fact, symptoms of several compression syndromes may be similar.

The anatomic areas of potential neurovascular compression are the interscalene space (near the thoracic rib), the costoclavicular space, and the axilla between the coracoid process and pectoralis minor tendon.

Sensory disturbances can occur in either a dermatomal (root) distribution or in the distribution of peripheral nerves (Fig. 4-58). If spinal cord lesions are suspected, the examiner should evaluate all sensory functions, including light touch, temperature, vibration, position sense, and pain (pinprick).

Pulses can be evaluated at the wrist for both the radial and the ulnar arteries. The Allen maneuver should be performed if vascular injuries are suspected at the wrist. The brachial artery is easily palpated at the elbow, just medial to the lacertus fibrosus. Obliteration of the pulse implies a vascular problem proximally in the axillary or subclavian region. Venous tone and patterns should be observed. In axillary-vein thrombosis, the venous pattern of the involved extremity is increased, and the dorsal hand veins do not collapse when raised to the level of the heart (Fig. 4-59).

Additional considerations exist that may affect these levels of compression. Movement of the head and neck, deep inspiration, and clavicular, scapular, and humeral movement, when performed in concert, can simultaneously alter structural relationships at one level or several levels and can cause impingement of nerves and vessels. Muscle hypertrophy resulting from occupational stress and obesity may compromise otherwise patent spaces. Loss of muscle tone and strength from a variety of causes, pain from unrelated but adjacent structures, chest deformity as a result of emphysema, postural portrayal of depressed mental status, poor working posture, and middle-age disuse atrophy (either singly or in combination) may alter potential spaces through sagging or displacement of the anatomic members.

Clavicular fractures with excessive callus or residual displacement of fragments and subacromial humeral luxation, blunt trauma to the upper thorax, postirradiation fibrosis, and the use of vibrating tools may either stretch part of the brachial plexus or damage vessel walls, and result in thrombotic vessel wall complications. The following may contribute to compression symptoms: a cervical rib with or without a

---

ORTHOPEDIC GAMUT 4-8

THORACIC OUTLET SYNDROME (TOS) CLASSIFICATIONS

TOS is categorized in three types:

- Vascular TOS (vTOS): Unilateral arm swelling without thrombosis, when not caused by lymphatic obstruction, may be caused by subclavian vein compression at the costoclavicular ligament because of compression by either that ligament or the subclavius tendon most often because of congenital close proximity of the vein to the ligament. Patients with compression of the subclavian artery and vein are classified into two other groups as vTOS: arterial TOS or venous TOS.

- Neurogenic TOS (nTOS): nTOS compromises the majority of these symptomatic individuals with brachial plexus and T1 nerve palsy. Neck trauma is also the most common cause of nTOS in patients with abnormal ribs. Involvement of the brachial plexus causes the nTOS that comprises two groups: one corresponding to patients harboring the true or classic signs and symptoms and electromyographic (EMG) findings (nTOS) and the other corresponding to patients with nonspecific clinical and EMG findings (nonspecific nTOS).

- Disputed neurogenic TOS (dnTOS): Upper extremity arterial compromise caused by this compacted thoracic outlet may also occur with a resulting limb ischemia. Patients often complain of a painful upper extremity after exercise, albeit limb claudication symptoms. Discolored, pale, underperfused arms with absent or decreased arterial pulse is a common finding in these individuals with an arterial form of TOS. This group includes patients with signs and symptoms of posttraumatic neurovascular compression (Paget-Schroetter syndrome).

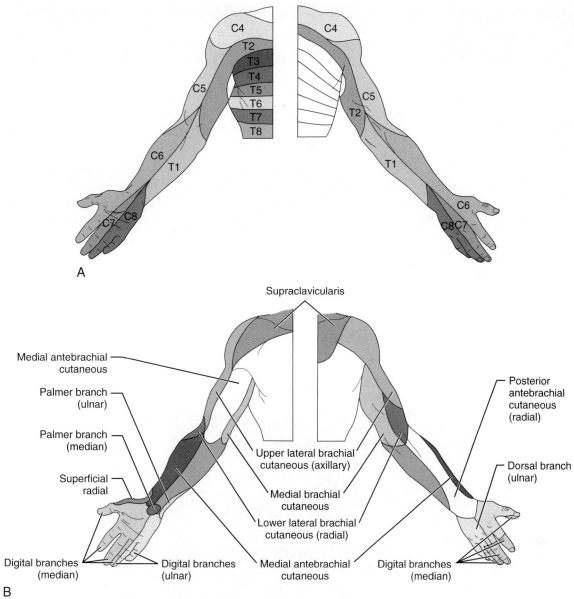

FIG. 4-58 Sensory distribution. **A,** Root dermatomes. **B,** Peripheral nerve distribution.
(From Nicholas JA, Hershman EB, editors: *The upper extremity in sports medicine,* St Louis, 1990, Mosby.)

prefixed brachial plexus, a bifid clavicle, abnormal bony protuberances from the first thoracic rib, a fibrous remnant of the scalenus minimus muscle, abnormal scalene insertions on the first rib, and abnormal splitting of the scalenus medius by all or part of the brachial plexus (Fig. 4-60). Postural, dynamic, traumatic, or arteriosclerotic factors must be added to precipitate patient symptoms. Adson test may be helpful in the diagnosis of TOS.

Although Paget-Schroetter syndrome (PSS) occurs infrequently and accounts for only approximately 1% to 4% of all deep-vein thromboses, affected patients are often young and otherwise healthy. Major morbidity can develop in this patient population and can lead to long-term disability if PSS is not promptly diagnosed and treated. If the condition is poorly managed, these patients may experience chronic

arm swelling, pain, and early exercise fatigue that can severely limit function. The exact pathophysiologic mechanism of this condition is poorly understood, but several well-established features have lent practitioners at least a theory. The typical history includes a strenuous, repetitive overhead activity, most often involving the dominant arm. Reproducibly observed are venographic and surgical evidence of chronic scarring around and within the vein where it courses among the clavicle, first rib, and anterior scalene muscle. The mechanical, traumatic nature of PSS involves a misalignment of musculoskeletal elements surrounding the subclavian vein such that a characteristic motion of these elements results in chronic constrictive trauma to the vein, with attendant endothelial damage, progressive stenosis, and ultimately a thrombotic tendency (Lee et al, 2006).

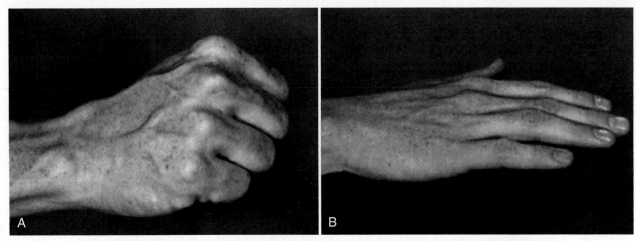

FIG. 4-59 Evaluation of hand veins. **A,** Engorged veins in dependent hand. **B,** Collapsed veins in elevated hand if the axillary vein is patent. If the venous tone remains prominent in the elevated position, axillary vein thrombosis is suspected. (From Seidel HM et al: *Mosby's guide to physical examination,* ed 4, St Louis, 1999, Mosby.)

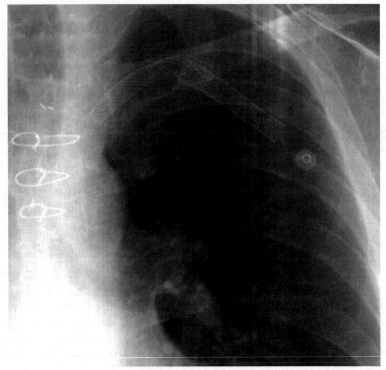

FIG. 4-60 A crushed stent is seen in the subclavian vein, with damage in the area of compression by the clavicle over the first rib. (From Lee JT et al: Long-term thrombotic recurrence after nonoperative management of Paget-Schroetter syndrome, *J Vasc Surg* 43[6]:1236-1243, 2006.)

PROCEDURE

- The patient's elbow is flexed to 90 degrees (Fig. 4-61).
- The shoulder is abducted and externally rotated.
- As the examiner palpates the radial pulse, the patient rotates the head away from the involved extremity (Fig. 4-62).
- If the pulse disappears when the head is rotated, it is a positive test result for TOS.

Next Steps/Procedures

Adson test, costoclavicular maneuver, George screening procedure, Halstead maneuver, reverse Bakody maneuver, Roos test, shoulder compression test, and Wright test

4

CLINICAL PEARL

Altered relative position of the shoulder girdle to the neurovascular bundle, or vice versa, is a common element of TOS. However, a group of symptoms may be separated, in which a static or gradual process may be underway that appears as a more general development without specific, separate, irritating incidents. Such a condition is labeled *postural* because of the alteration of the normal girdle relationship to the rest of the body.

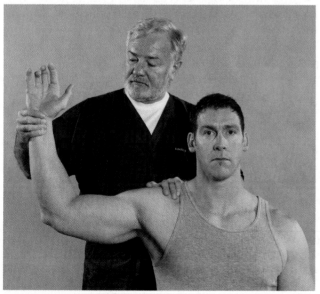

FIG. 4-61 The patient is seated. The examiner abducts the affected shoulder to 90 degrees. The patient's elbow is flexed to 90 degrees, and the shoulder is externally rotated. The radial pulse is located and recorded.

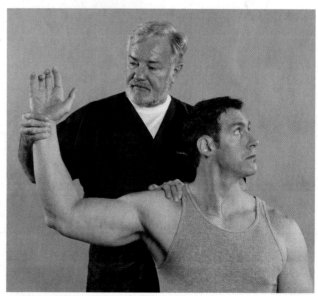

FIG. 4-62 The patient rotates the head to the opposite side. If the pulse disappears during this maneuver, the test is positive. The test is significant for TOS.

ALSO KNOWN AS APLEY SCRATCH TEST

Assessment for Degenerative Tendinopathy of One of the Tendons of the Rotator Cuff, Usually the Supraspinatus Tendon

Comment

In healthy individuals, approximately 120-degree shoulder elevation is attributable to the glenohumeral joint. The remaining motion occurs at the scapulothoracic joint at a 2 : 1 ratio. Considerable individual deviation from this 2 : 1 glenohumeral-scapulothoracic ratio exists among the general populace. Limitation at the glenohumeral joint leads to compensatory movement at the scapulothoracic joint during attempted elevation, which results in an altered or reverse scapulothoracic rhythm or ratio and is observed as a shoulder-hike or girdle-hunching maneuver (Fig. 4-63).

Supraspinatus tendinopathy is the most common type of tendinopathy in the upper limb. This condition occurs most often in swimmers and tennis players or in other athletes who engage in sports that require repeated overhead movement of the arm.

The supraspinatus tendon passes beneath the acromion and inserts on the greater tubercle of the humerus, passing beneath the coracoacromial ligament that forms a fibrous arch over the tendon. Between the tendon and the overlying structures is the subacromial bursa.

Repeated abduction of the shoulder, unless it is maintained in external rotation, causes impingement of the tendon within the very narrow space between the humerus and the overlying acromion and ligament. This disorder is often called *impingement syndrome*. It has also been called *swimmer's shoulder*.

> Anterior rotator cuff tears are not uncommon in throwing athletes, and a concealed type of tear was a representative lesion. Different mechanisms may be involved in the development of anterior and posterior rotator cuff tears resulting from throwing injuries. Posterior capsular tightness might influence the occurrence of anterior tears (Nakagawa et al, 2006).

The microvasculature of the supraspinatus tendon is reduced where the tendon is wrung out by pressure during abduction. This site corresponds to that of tears in the supraspinatus tendon of geriatric patients. These tears may be the result of poor healing because of impaired circulation. Although tears are not as common in younger patients, the area affected is the same. Calcification sometimes occurs at this site.

The cause of this tendinopathy is well defined and can be confirmed by horizontally adducting the patient's arm across the body. This move causes further impingement and reproduces the painful symptoms. The belly-off sign is observable with the arm in this position (Figs. 4-64 and 4-65).

> Rupture of the subscapularis tendon is rare in patients with ruptures of the rotator cuff; the incidence had been reported as 4% to 8%. Rupture typically occurs traumatically through forced abduction or external rotation. The injury may occur in isolation or combined with rupture of the supraspinatus. The rupture of the supraspinatus may preexist or may occur at the time of the injury or as a degenerative secondary development. Without treatment, rupture of the subscapularis leads to pain, loss of function, and weakness. In the long term, dynamic anterior instability can lead to the development of glenohumeral arthrosis (Flury et al, 2006).

Different clinical signs and diagnostic tests have been published in the literature to evaluate the integrity of the musculotendinous unit of the subscapularis. With the lift-off

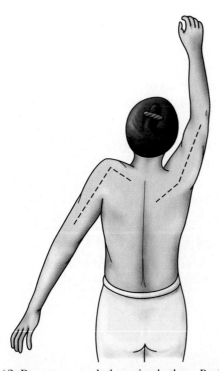

FIG. 4-63 Reverse scapulothoracic rhythm. *Broken lines* indicate the position of the scapular spine and humeral axis on each side, showing little or no movement of the left shoulder. This *shoulder hiking* attempt at abduction elevates rather than depresses the humeral head. (From Saidoff DC, McDonough AL: *Critical pathways in therapeutic intervention*, St Louis, 1997, Mosby.)

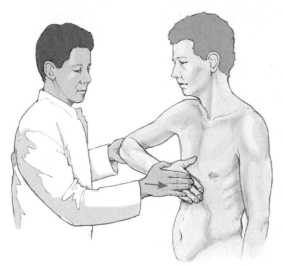

FIG. 4-64 Starting position for the evaluation of the belly-off sign. The affected arm of the patient is passively brought into flexion and maximal internal rotation with the elbow flexed to 90 degrees. The elbow of the patient is supported by one hand of the examiner while the other hand places the palm on the abdomen. (From Scheibel M et al: The belly-off sign: a new clinical diagnostic sign for subscapularis lesions, *Arthroscopy* 21[10]:1229-1235, 2005.)

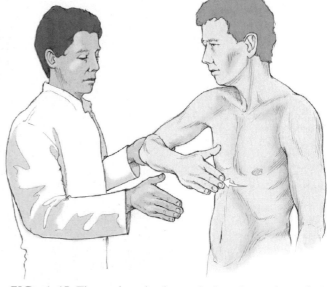

FIG. 4-65 The patient is then asked to keep the wrist straight and actively maintain the position of internal rotation as the examiner releases the wrist while maintaining support at the elbow. If the patient cannot maintain this position, the hand lifts off the abdomen resulting in the belly-off sign. (From Scheibel M et al: The belly-off sign: a new clinical diagnostic sign for subscapularis lesions, *Arthroscopy* 21[10]:1229-1235, 2005.)

test, described by Gerber and Krushell, the affected arm of the patient is internally rotated and extended, placing the hand on the lumbar region. The test is considered positive if the patient is unable to raise the arm posteriorly off the back. The presence of an internal rotation lag sign, as described by Hertel and colleagues, is evaluated from the same starting position. The affected arm of the patient is held by the examiner at almost maximal internal rotation. The dorsum of the hand is passively lifted away from the body until almost full internal rotation is reached. The patient is than asked to maintain this position actively. The sign is considered positive when lag occurs and the magnitude can be judged in degrees (Scheibel et al, 2005).

PROCEDURE

- The patient is seated and is instructed to place the affected hand behind the head and touch the opposite superior angle of the scapula (Fig. 4-66).
- The patient is then instructed to place the hand behind the back and attempt to touch the opposite inferior angle of the scapula (Fig. 4-67).
- Exacerbation of the patient's pain indicates degenerative tendinopathy of one of the tendons of the rotator cuff, usually the supraspinatus tendon.

Next Steps/Procedures
Impingement sign, subacromial push-button sign, and supraspinatus test

CLINICAL PEARL

Apley inferior is a useful test of internal rotation and extension. With severe restriction, the patient will not be able to get the hand behind the back at all. This movement is commonly affected in adhesive capsulitis.

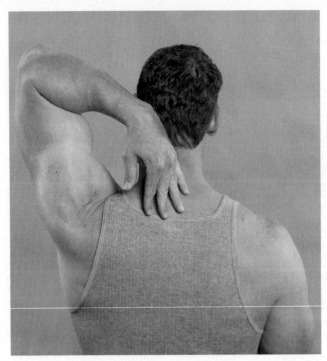

FIG. 4-66 The patient is seated and is instructed to place the hand of the affected arm behind the head and touch near the opposite scapula *(Apley scratch superior)*.

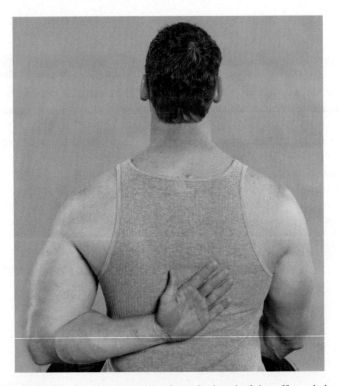

FIG. 4-67 The patient is then instructed to place the hand of the affected shoulder behind the back and attempt to touch near the opposite scapula *(Apley scratch inferior)*. If either position exacerbates the patient's pain, this indicates degenerative tendinitis of one of the tendons, usually the supraspinatus, of the rotator cuff.

APPREHENSION TEST

Assessment for Anterior Shoulder Dislocation Trauma and Posterior Dislocation of the Humerus

Comment

Glenohumeral joint stability is provided by several mechanisms: bony surfaces, the capsuloligamentous structures, the glenoid labrum, the negative intraarticular pressure, and active centering of the humerus mainly by the rotator cuff muscles (concavity compression). The subscapularis muscle has been reported to be the main muscular stabilizer of the abducted and externally rotated humerus, a position known to be critical for shoulders with anteroinferior instability. This contention is supported by electromyographic findings (Werner, Favre, Gerber, 2007).

Dislocation of the shoulder follows the loss of function of the restraining structures around the shoulder. This dislocation is a result of the same mechanism that causes subluxations. The most common type of dislocation of the shoulder in young patients is anteroinferior, which is pure dislocation, unaccompanied by fracture. As age advances, the ligaments become firmer and the bone less strong; thus the dislocation may be accompanied by avulsion fracture, rather than a tear of the ligament. In the young patient, the ligament or muscle always gives way. As the arm is forced into abduction and external rotation, the humeral head is thrust against the anterior portion of the glenohumeral joint. The coracoacromial ligament forces the humeral head downward, and it then emerges anteriorly and inferiorly into the redundant area of the capsule, which is protected by the glenohumeral ligaments. These ligaments give way when they are torn from the glenoid labrum because of avulsion of the labrum or actual disruption of the ligaments. The head of the humerus slips over the glenoid rim and immediately slides forward to lodge between the rim of the glenoid and coracoid process, and the arm drops toward the side but not against it. This circumstance is the classic dislocation of the shoulder in young patients. The damage to the ligament may be a transverse tear across the capsule; in addition, the capsular reinforcements known as the *glenohumeral ligaments* may split, with one passing above the humeral head and the other below it. In some instances the ligaments actually grasp the humeral head to impede its reduction.

> The term *terrible triad of the shoulder* was coined by Groh and Rockwood to describe the association of anterior glenohumeral dislocation, rotator cuff tear, and neurologic injury.

The posterior-inferior capsule seems to be the primary posterior stabilizer of the glenohumeral joint with the arm in flexion and internal rotation, the position of posterior apprehension. Severe posterior translation typically results in tearing or shredding of the posterior labrum, and disruption of the lateral region of the posterior-inferior capsule is rare (Bhatia et al, 2007).

Posterior dislocation of the shoulder is uncommon. Such dislocation is caused by a direct driving force against the lower end of the humerus with the arm flexed forward. This force is transmitted up the arm, driving the head out posteriorly. No gross deformity of the shoulder is evident. The patient resists any motion of the shoulder, and on careful palpation, the examiner can feel less fullness of the humeral head in front and some increased fullness behind. Prominence of the coracoid is also increased. Such a dislocation is readily determined only if it is palpated very early because within a short time the swelling that is around the shoulder and that occurs from this extremely disabling injury will mask any physical findings.

> Posterior glenohumeral dislocation associated with a massive rotator cuff tear and neurologic injury represents the *reverse terrible triad of the shoulder*. Additional lesions, such as biceps tendon dislocation, anterior capsular tear, and humeral avulsion of the inferior glenohumeral ligament, result in a circumferential pattern of injury (Bhatia et al, 2007).

Dislocations and subluxations (partial dislocation) of the glenohumeral joint often occur after indirect trauma with the arm abducted, extended, and externally rotated (anterior dislocation) and with the arm abducted, flexed, and internally rotated (posterior dislocation) (Fig. 4-68).

Two associated injuries may occur as a result of acute glenohumeral dislocation and instability. Because the shoulder is the most mobile joint in the body, bony restrictions do not provide substantial restraints. Rather, the fibrocartilaginous glenoid labrum deepens the articulation between the humeral head and the bony glenoid fossa (Fig. 4-69). When forces are great enough to dislocate the humerus from its confines within the glenoid, injury to the labrum occurs (Bankart lesion). A *Bankart lesion* is an avulsion of the capsule and glenoid labrum off of the anterior rim of the glenoid (Fig. 4-70).

The head of the humerus is subject to injury as a result of the anterior shoulder instability (Hill-Sachs lesion). The *Hill-Sachs* lesion is a compression or *impaction fracture* of the posterolateral aspect of the humeral head (Fig. 4-71).

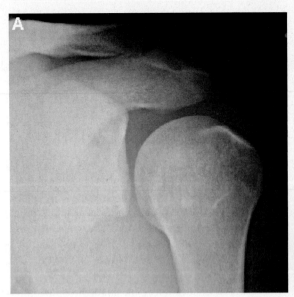
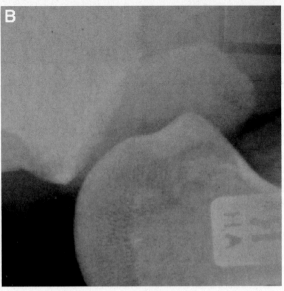

FIG. 4-68 A 22-year-old professional rugby player fell onto his right elbow with the arm adducted, internally rotated, and flexed to 90° while 2 players landed forcefully on him, loading his posterior thorax on the right side. The injury resulted in a posterior dislocation of the right glenohumeral joint and acute, severe pain radiating along the arm, forearm, and hand. The posterior dislocation reduced spontaneously, but the radiating pain and a feeling of lameness of the arm persisted. Clinical examination revealed increased posterior translation of the humeral head suggestive of posterior instability; inability to elevate, abduct, or externally rotate the arm actively; weak internal rotation; and paresthesia over the lateral aspect of the upper arm and medial aspect of the forearm and hand. Radiographic examination of the right shoulder showed an "empty glenoid" sign on the anteroposterior view and posterior subluxation of the humeral head on the axillary view. (From Bhatia DN et al: The reverse terrible triad of the shoulder: circumferential glenohumeral musculoligamentous disruption and neurologic injury associated with posterior shoulder dislocation, *J Shoulder Elbow Surg* 16(3):e13-e17, 2007.)

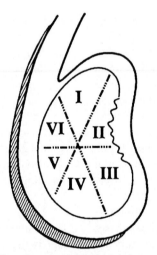

FIG. 4-69 To aid in localizing the site of labral injury, the glenoid labrum has been divided into six areas: (I) the superior labrum, (II) the anterior labrum above the midglenoid notch, (III) the anterior labrum below the midglenoid notch, (IV) the inferior labrum, (V) the posteroinferior labrum, and (VI) the posterosuperior labrum. Several mechanisms of injury have been postulated, such as compression, avulsion, traction, shear, and chronic degenerative changes. The tear pattern can be described by its arthroscopic appearance, similar to meniscal tears in the knee. Common tear types include flap, bucket handle, split nondetached, degenerative, and SLAP lesions. Lesions located above the equator of the glenoid (a line drawn between the 3 o'clock and 9 o'clock positions on the glenoid) often are associated with rotator cuff or biceps disease. Lesions located below the equator, most commonly split, nondetached lesions, both anteriorly and posteriorly, are highly suggestive of shoulder instability. (From Canale: *Campbell's operative orthopaedics,* ed 10, St Louis, 2003, Mosby.)

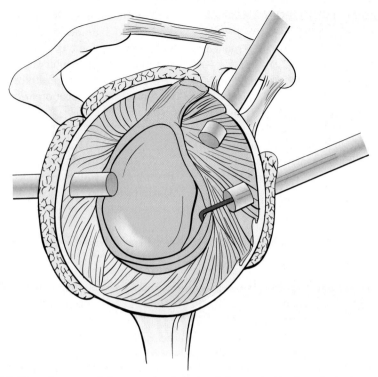

FIG. 4-70 Detachment of the anterior inferior labrum (a Bankart lesion). (From Rakel: *Textbook of family medicine*, ed 7, St Louis, 2007, Saunders.)

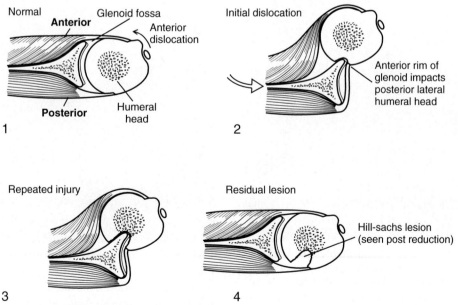

FIG. 4-71 With repeated anterior shoulder dislocations, a Hill-Sachs lesion may form. During the dislocation the humeral head is damaged by the sharp anterior rim of the glenoid *(2)*. With repeated dislocation the lesion, called the "hatchet sign" develops *(3)*. On the reduction film the lesion is apparent *(4)*. (From Roberts: *Clinical procedures in emergency medicine,* ed 4, St Louis, 2004, Saunders.)

PROCEDURE

- The patient's shoulder is abducted and externally rotated (Fig. 4-72).
- If the patient shows apprehension or alarm and resists further motion, the test is positive (Fig. 4-73).
- This test may elicit a feeling that resembles the pain felt when the shoulder was previously dislocated.
- This test is performed slowly and cautiously; performed too quickly, dislocating the humerus may be possible.
- Anterior shoulder dislocation trauma is suggested by a positive test.

- To evaluate posterior shoulder dislocation, the shoulder is flexed and internally rotated (Fig. 4-74).
- A posterior force is applied on the patient's elbow.
- If the patient exhibits apprehension and resists further motion, the test is positive.
- A posterior dislocation of the humerus is suggested by a positive test.

Next Steps/Procedures

Bryant sign, Calloway test, Dugas test, Hamilton test, Mazion shoulder maneuver, and diagnostic imaging.

CLINICAL PEARL

These maneuvers are also known as the *drawer tests of Gerber and Ganz*. Any movements, clicks, or patient apprehension support the diagnosis of recurrent shoulder dislocation. Axial diagnostic images are made to confirm the diagnosis.

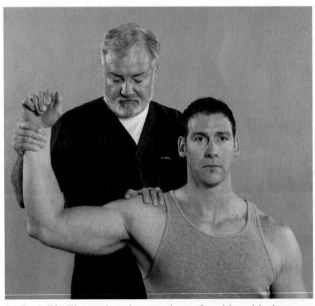

FIG. 4-72 The patient is seated comfortably with the arms at the sides. The shoulder is slowly abducted and externally rotated.

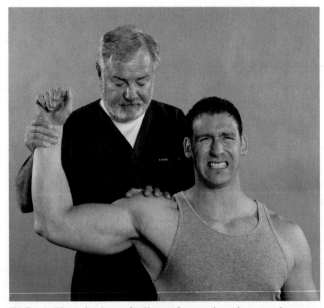

FIG. 4-73 A look or feeling of apprehension or alarm on the patient's face is the positive finding. The patient will resist further motion. This maneuver may also duplicate the feeling of an imminent dislocation. If performed too briskly, the humerus can dislocate. A positive test suggests anterior shoulder dislocation trauma.

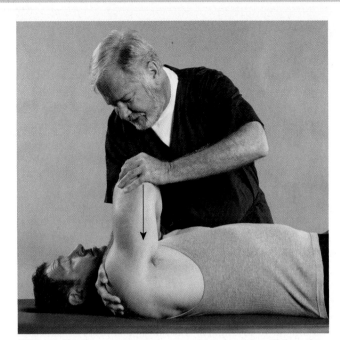

FIG. 4-74 For evaluating posterior shoulder dislocation, the patient should be supine. The shoulder is flexed and internally rotated. A posterior force is applied on the patient's elbow (forcing the humeral head posterior on the glenoid). A look of apprehension is a positive finding. The patient will resist further motion. A positive test suggests posterior dislocation of the humerus.

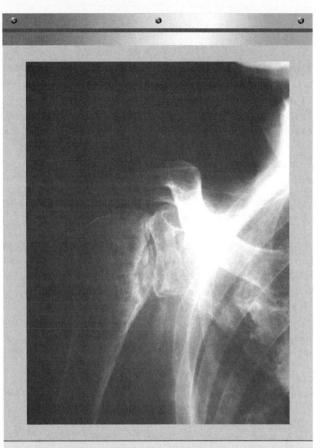

AT THE VIEWBOX

84-year-old female with shoulder pain and loss of range of motion for 10 months, after being lifted from bed by her husband, following total hip arthroplasty. Radiography demonstrates an impacted fracture of the anteromedial aspect of the humeral head, producing a "trough sign" and diagnostic of a posterior glenohumeral dislocation, which remains non-reduced. Glenohumeral dislocations are much more often anterior, in which case associated fractures are classically at the posterosuperior aspect of the humeral head (Hill-Sachs lesion) and the inferior glenoid labrum or glenoid margin (Bankart lesion variants). (From the teaching file of Timothy Mick, DC, DACBR)

4

Assessment for Dislocation of the Glenohumeral Articulation

Comment

The shoulder is the most commonly dislocated joint in the body. The typical mechanism of injury is abduction, extension, and external rotation, which results in an anterior dislocation. Axial loading of the internally rotated and extended arm, violent trauma, electrical shock, or convulsions can produce posterior dislocations. Severe trauma with hyperabduction forces on the upper extremity can produce an inferior dislocation. Because of the bony anatomy of the shallow glenoid and the round humeral head, initial dislocations can become locked by a wedge-shaped impression defect in the humeral head.

The humerus is most commonly dislocated anteriorly (95%) or, in practice, anteriorly, medially, and inferiorly, coming to lie inferior to the coracoid process (Fig. 4-75). This circumstance may cause a cortical impaction of both the superior posterior aspect of the humerus (Hill-Sachs, or *hatchet*, deformity) and the inferior aspect of the glenoid (Bankart lesion) or detachment of the anterior portion of the glenoid labrum.

Glenohumeral, AP, axillary lateral, and transscapular radiographs are necessary to document the direction and degree of instability. A Hill-Sachs lesion is best demonstrated by an AP view in internal rotation or the Stryker notch view. An osseous Bankart or glenoid rim fracture is best demonstrated by the axillary West Point view.

Although posterior dislocations may be difficult to appreciate, they should not be missed. In general, they can be appreciated on the AP view by persistent internal rotation of the humerus and asymmetry of the glenohumeral joint (Fig. 4-76). An axillary view may be impossible to obtain, but a transthoracic *(swimmer's view)* or oblique view will confirm the diagnosis.

An unusual inferior dislocation, luxatio erecta, is caused by severe hyperabduction of the arm, whereby the humeral head impinges on the acromion. The acromion then acts as a fulcrum and thus causes an inferior displacement of the humeral head with the arm *locked* in abduction (Fig. 4-77).

Thorough and early inspection in the acute dislocation injury reveals flattening and loss of the normal curvature of the shoulder, but swelling obliterates these findings later. Diagnostic imaging is needed to confirm the diagnosis. When shoulder dislocation is suspected, an axillary view is paramount to distinguish the exact position of the head of the humerus in relation to the glenoid process.

Dislocations of the shoulder are occasionally accompanied by injury to the axillary nerve with resulting loss of function of the deltoid muscle. With shoulder dislocations, the function of the deltoid and any sensory disturbance in the skin overlying the deltoid must be ascertained. The area over the deltoid is innervated by the axillary nerve, and assessment of the skin sensation will aid in predicting the recovery of the nerve. Dislocations of the shoulder rarely result in injury to other nerves and vessels of the upper extremity (Fig 4-78), but injuries of the posterior cord of the brachial plexus are possible.

Anterior glenohumeral joint dislocation is relatively common and results when the arm is forcibly abducted and externally rotated. Although it is not associated with a high vascular complication rate (less than 1% of cases), evidence suggests that, after the popliteal artery, the axillary artery is the most frequently damaged by severe trauma. One reason for this proclivity is its anatomic position and lack of protective sheath distally leaving it more vulnerable to injury (Whittam et al, in press).

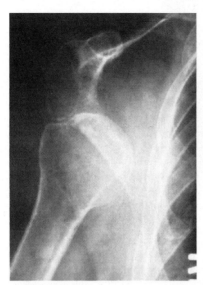

FIG. 4-75 Anterior dislocation of the right humerus. (From Sutton D, Young JWR: *A concise textbook of clinical imaging,* ed 2, St Louis, 1995, Mosby.)

ORTHOPEDIC GAMUT 4-10
AXILLARY PSEUDOANEURYSM

Accurate detection and diagnosis of axillary pseudoaneurysm after anterior glenohumeral joint dislocation presents difficulties:

- Limited abduction of the arm, as a result of pain and muscle spasm, prevents appropriate and full clinical examination of the axillary region.
- The gradual onset of clinical changes and the delayed radiologic evidence of a pseudoaneurysm may prevent attribution of clinical findings being associated with traumatic glenohumeral joint dislocation.
- An axillary hematoma may be concealed by bone and muscle tissue or bruising mistakenly attributed to the dislocation itself.
- Pulsation of the pseudoaneurysm may be obscured by overlying tissues.
- The motor and sensory disturbances related to ischemia may be mistakenly attributed to brachial plexus damage, which is a more common complication of glenohumeral joint dislocation.
- The robust collateral circulation may maintain the radial pulse allowing ischemia to go undetected.
- When recurrent dislocation is experienced, limited hemorrhage may result as a result of scar tissue from a previous dislocation.

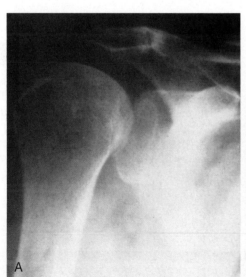
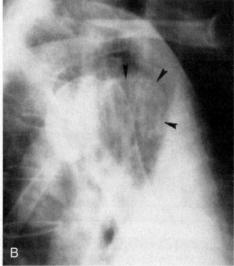

FIG. 4-76 **A,** Posterior dislocation of the humerus. **B,** A *swimmer's view.* (From Sutton D, Young JWR: *A concise textbook of clinical imaging,* ed 2, St Louis, 1995, Mosby.)

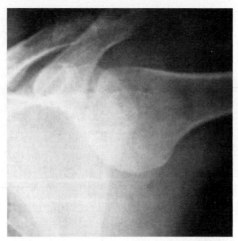

FIG. 4-77 Luxatio erecta. (From Sutton D, Young JWR: *A concise textbook of clinical imaging,* ed 2, St Louis, 1995, Mosby.)

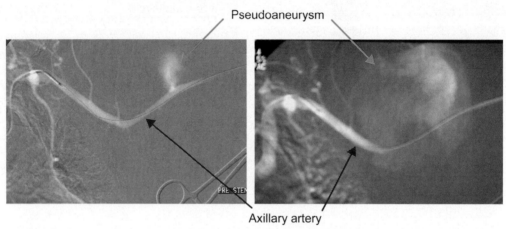

FIG. 4-78 Left axillary pseudoaneurysm. (Adapted from Whittam K, Hardy M: A case study of an axillary artery pseudoaneurysm following anterior dislocation of the glenohumeral joint: a rare presentation on plain film radiographs, *Radiography* 13[3]:221–228, 2007.)

ORTHOPEDIC GAMUT 4-9
SHOULDER DISLOCATIONS

Shoulder dislocation classification relative to:
1. The degree of instability (dislocation or subluxation)
2. The cause of the instability (traumatic or atraumatic)
3. The direction of the instability (anterior, posterior, or multidirectional)

PROCEDURE

The examiner views the characteristic lowering of the axillary fold (anterior and posterior pillars of the armpit) that is seen after trauma when dislocation of the glenohumeral articulation ensues (Figs. 4-79 and 4-80).

Next Steps/Procedures
Apprehension test, Calloway test, Dugas test, Hamilton test, Mazion shoulder maneuver, and diagnostic imaging

CLINICAL PEARL

With dislocations of the shoulder, the axillary nerve may be injured. The patient is unable to contract the deltoid muscle, and a small patch of anesthesia may be present over the muscle. This anesthesia is usually a neurapraxia, which recovers spontaneously after a few weeks or months. The posterior cord of the brachial plexus is occasionally injured. This occurrence is somewhat alarming, but it usually recovers with time.

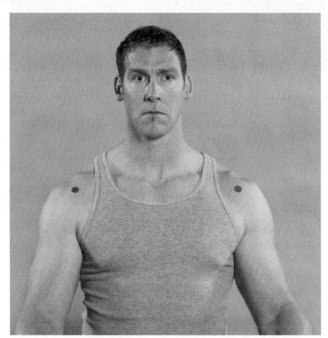

FIG. 4-79 The patient is seated with the arms comfortably at the sides.

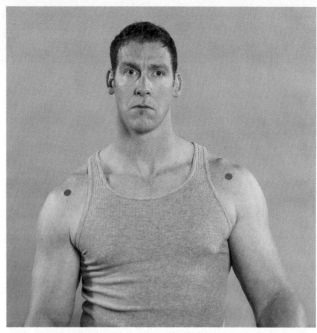

FIG. 4-80 If the sign is present, a characteristic lowering of the axillary fold (anterior and posterior pillars of the armpit) occurs on the affected side. The sign is present when dislocation of the glenohumeral articulation has occurred.

4

Assessment for Dislocation of the Humerus

Comment

Shoulder dislocation at the glenohumeral joint occurs anteriorly in 95% of the cases. The remaining 5% dislocate posteriorly. The incidence of anterior dislocation is attributed to the anatomic weakness of the anterior aspect of the joint.

The joint capsule is thin and loose. The capsule is reinforced by folds called *glenohumeral ligaments*. These ligaments attach from the humerus and fan out to attach to the superior anterior aspect of the glenoid fossa, partly to the glenoid labrum, and partly to a portion of the bone of the scapula. An opening in the capsule often exists between the superior and middle glenohumeral ligaments. This opening is called *Weitbrecht foramen*. The opening may be a frank perforation or may be covered by a thin layer of the capsule. The articular cavity connects with the subscapular fossa through Weitbrecht foramen. The humeral head dislocates through this opening, and dislocations may recur as a result of fraying or actual destruction of the middle glenohumeral ligament.

With dislocations, the glenoid labrum may be partially or completely detached and a tear may occur in the anteroinferior aspect. The glenoid labrum contains no fibrocartilage and is a redundant fibrous fold of the anterior capsule that disappears when the humerus is externally rotated. This pouch invites dislocation. The humeral head can protrude into this pouch, especially if an anatomic variant of the middle humeral ligament exists.

Five types of dislocation have been identified, and the most common is the subcoracoid dislocation. The subclavicular and subglenoid types are less common and may be a progression of the subcoracoid type. All anterior types of dislocations can change into any of the other anterior types. The fifth type of dislocation, the posterior, or subspinous, is rare. The type of dislocation is determined by the location of the humeral head in relation to the glenoid seat when the diagnosis is made. More uncommon is a form of glenohumeral dislocation caused by hyperabduction of the affected extremity or, less commonly, by a direct axial load to the extremity, in which the arm is locked in a hyperabducted position (*luxatio erecta*) (Fig 4-81).

Primary anterior dislocations occur with equal frequency regardless of age, but recurrence of a dislocation is highest in the young and decreases after age 45. Recurrence is less in cases in which the primary dislocation was severe and resulted in greater hemorrhage and therefore greater scar formation in healing.

The sulcus sign is often present in shoulder instability. Grading of the sulcus sign is based on the distance between the inferior margin of the lateral acromion and the humeral head when a downward traction force is applied to the adducted arm (Fig. 4-82, *A*). Less than 1 cm of distance represents a 1+ sulcus; 1 to 2 cm indicates a 2+ sulcus; and more than 2 cm is a 3+ sulcus. A 3+ sulcus sign reflects laxity of the superior glenohumeral ligament and inferior glenohumeral ligament and is indicative of inferior instability. It is pathognomonic of multidirectional instability.

Apprehension tests are designed to induce anxiety and protect muscular contraction as the shoulder is brought to a position associated with instability. The anterior apprehension test is performed with the arm abducted and externally rotated. The examiner progressively increases the degree of external rotation and notes the development of patient apprehension. The posterior stress test (Fig. 4-82, *B*) is performed with the arm internally rotated and forward flexed to 90 degrees. Apprehension is unusual in this position, but pain or a palpable jump may be noted as the humerus is loaded in an AP direction and progressively adducted across the chest.

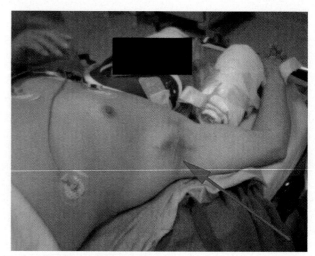

FIG. 4-81 Hyperabducted shoulder with bulging of axillary skin by inferior displacement of the humeral head (*arrow*). (From Begaz T, Mycyk MB: Luxatio erecta: inferior humeral dislocation, *J Emerg Med* 31[3]:303-304.)

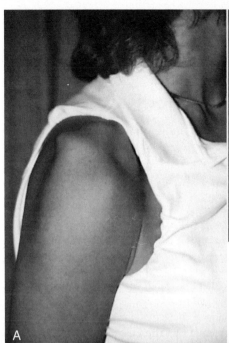
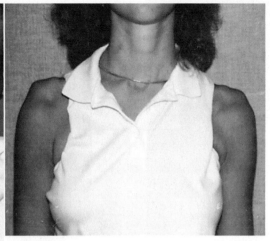

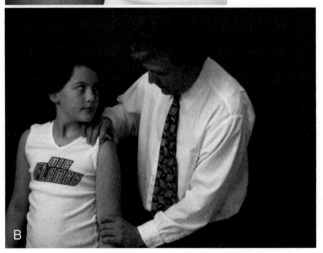

FIG. 4-82 **A,** "Sulcus sign" in patient with multidirectional shoulder instability and unilateral complaints. **B,** The sulcus test is then done with the arm in both 0 degrees and 45 degrees of abduction. This test is done by pulling distally on the extremity and observing for a sulcus or dimple between the humeral head and the acromion. The distance between the humeral head and acromion should be graded from 0 to 3 with the arm in 0 degrees and 45 degrees of abduction, with 1+ indicating subluxation less than 1 cm, 2+ indicating 1 to 2 cm of subluxation, and 3+ indicating more than 2 cm of inferior subluxation. Subluxation at 0 degrees of abduction is more indicative of laxity at the rotator interval, and subluxation at 45 degrees is indicative of laxity of the inferior glenohumeral ligament complex. The presence or absence of a sulcus sign is evaluated by distracting the arm inferiorly in an attempt to sublux the humeral head out of the socket in an inferior direction. If a sulcus is appreciated as the glenoid is emptied of the humeral head, suspicion of multidirectional instability should be entertained. (From Canale: *Campbell's operative orthopaedics,* ed 10, St Louis, 2003, Mosby.)

Ligamentous laxity is commonly associated with shoulder instability and can be measured objectively on physical examination. The degree of thumb hyperabduction with the wrist volar flexed can be noted by the distance between the thumb and volar forearm. If the thumb reaches the forearm, the test is considered positive. An assessment is also made for index metacarpophalangeal hyperextension in excess of 90 degrees, elbow hyperextension, and knee hyperextension *(Beighton hypermobility assessment)* (Fig. 4-83).

Luxatio erecta is an uncommon form of glenohumeral dislocation caused by hyperabduction of the affected extremity or, less commonly, by a direct axial load to the extremity. Classically, the arm is held in a hyperabducted *overhead* position and any movement from this position is painful.

Luxatio erecta has a high propensity for associated injuries. In one series, 80% of patients had an associated greater tuberosity fracture or rotator cuff tear, and 60% had some neurologic compromise, with the axillary nerve most commonly affected. Of all types of glenohumeral dislocation, *luxatio erecta* has the highest incidence of vascular compromise (3.3%). Therefore the evaluating physician should readily obtain Doppler blood flow studies or observe the patient for an extended period. Radiographically, *luxatio erecta* can sometimes be confused with subglenoid anterior dislocation of the humerus, but the two entities can be differentiated by clinical observation of a hyperabducted arm and by radiographic observation of the abducted humerus seen in *lux erect* (Begaz, Mycyk, 2006).

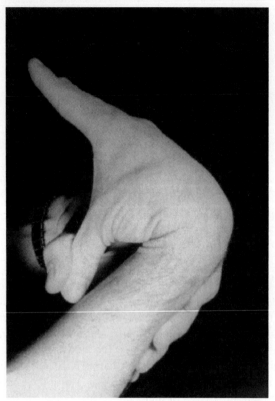

FIG. 4-83 Generalized ligamentous laxity is a patient with shoulder instability. (From Nicholas JA, Hershman EB, editors: *The upper extremity in sports medicine,* St Louis, 1990, Mosby.)

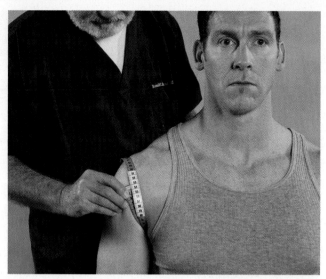

FIG. 4-84 The patient is seated comfortably with the arms at the sides. The examiner loops a flexible tape measure through the axilla and measures the girth of the affected shoulder at the acromial tip. The girth of the affected shoulder is compared with the girth of the unaffected shoulder. In a positive test, the girth of the affected joint is increased. The test is significant for dislocation of the humerus.

PROCEDURE

- The test consists of measuring the girth of the shoulder joints bilaterally.
- This test is helpful in the examination of obese patients.
- The examiner loops a flexible tape measure through the axilla (Fig. 4-84).
- The girth is measured at the acromial tip.
- In a positive test, the girth of the affected joint is increased.
- The test is significant for dislocation of the humerus.

Next Steps/Procedures

Apprehension test, Bryant sign, Dugas test, Hamilton test, Mazion shoulder maneuver, and diagnostic imaging

CLINICAL PEARL

S houlder dislocation results in severe pain. The patient supports the arm with the opposite hand and is hesitant to permit any kind of examination. The lateral outline of the shoulder may be flattened, and if the patient is not too muscular, a small bulge may be seen and felt just below the clavicle. The arm must always be examined for nerve and vessel injury.

CODMAN SIGN

ALSO KNOWN AS DROP ARM TEST

Assessment for Tear in the Rotator Cuff Complex

Comment

Full-thickness supraspinatus tears are common in elderly patients, often occurring with clinical symptoms of chronic subacromial impingement. The associated functional restriction and morbidity is significant and well known. In contrast, subcoracoid impingement of the subscapularis tendon is less frequently identified and rarely considered as a potential cause of pain when symptoms persist after supraspinatus tendon repair. The progression of subacromial impingement from bursitis through to tendinopathy is a well-described cause of supraspinatus tendinopathy. However, the origin of subscapularis tendinopathy is relatively unclear. It is thought to occur through a variety of mechanisms: intrinsic tendon degeneration, by extension of a supraspinatus tear through the rotator interval, and trauma. Subscapularis tendinopathy is also postulated to occur secondary to acquired subcoracoid impingement, though this notion is poorly understood and controversial. Goldthwait first recognized the changes associated with impingement on the coracoid process in 1909. The term *subcoracoid impingement syndrome* is used to describe entrapment of the subscapularis muscle and tendon between the coracoid process and lesser tubercle of the humerus (MacMahon et al, 2007).

The long head of the biceps (LHB) tendon originates at the supraglenoid tubercle, runs intraarticularly, and exits the glenohumeral joint through the bicipital groove between the greater and lesser tuberosity. Immediately before entering the bicipital groove, the LHB is stabilized by a sling formed by the insertion of the supraspinatus and subscapularis tendons and by the humeral insertion of the superior glenohumeral and coracohumeral ligaments. This complex structure merits detailed consideration. In 1928, Meyer already emphasized in an anatomic study the importance of the capsular attachments to the bone in the region of the bicipital groove for anterior stability of the LHB (Lafosse et al, 2007).

Sudden biceps tendon rupture in the shoulder results in immediate sharp pain. An audible pop is sometimes heard in the shoulder. Mild swelling and ecchymosis of the upper anterior arm and a change of contour of the biceps muscle occur. Contraction of the musculature fibers takes the appearance of a firm ball of muscle that is more distal than normally expected and is palpable as a soft hump. This deformity will persist and is sometimes called the *Popeye sign* after the well-known cartoon character (Fig. 4-85).

Rotator cuff tear is a common lesion that occurs with increasing frequency with advancing age. Cadaveric studies have shown an incidence of full-thickness tears of up to 30% (Lahteenmaki et al, in press).

One of the major functions of the rotator cuff is humeral head depression, although this function is progressively compromised during the evolution of the rotator cuff disorder. With progressive loss of this mechanism, the humeral head rises higher and higher as a result of the unrelenting upward pull of the deltoid. In the event of a major defect in the rotator cuff, the humeral head migrates even further proximally by protruding through the defect. A boutonniere deformity, just as in the finger, victimizes the buttonholed

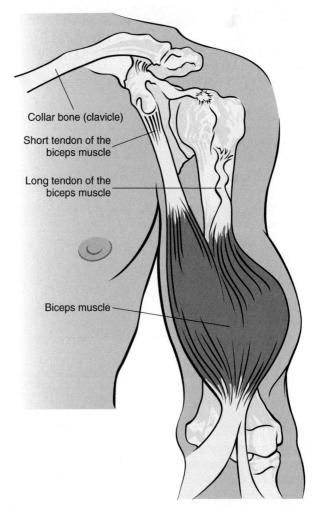

FIG. 4-85 Proximal long tendon biceps rupture with retraction of torn tendon ends. (From Saidoff DC, McDonough AL: *Critical pathways in therapeutic intervention,* St Louis, 1997, Mosby.)

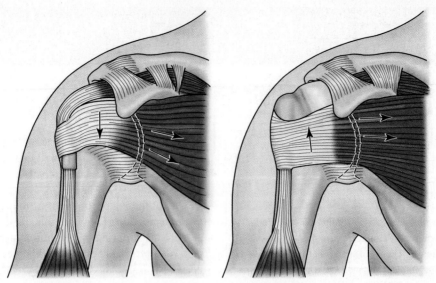

FIG. 4-86 Major cuff failure and retraction allow the humeral head to protrude upward through the cuff defect, creating a boutonniere lesion. (Adapted from Saidoff DC, McDonough AL: *Critical pathways in therapeutic intervention,* St Louis, 1997, Mosby.)

ORTHOPEDIC GAMUT 4-11

CLASSIFICATION OF LONG HEAD OF THE BICEPS INSTABILITY

- Direction of instability
  - Anterior
  - Posterior
  - Anteroposterior
- Extent of instability
  - None
  - Subluxation
  - Dislocation
- Lesion grade
  - 0 (normal)
  - I (minor lesion)
  - II (major lesion)
- Rotator cuff tear/lesion
  - A (intact)
  - B (partial thickness)
  - C (full thickness)

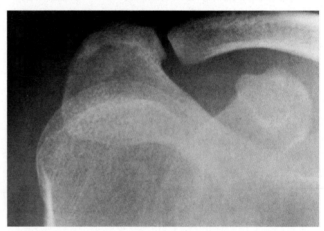

FIG. 4-87 Normal right acromioclavicular (AC) joint. (From Nicholas JA, Hershman EB, editors: *The upper extremity in sports medicine,* St Louis, 1990, Mosby.)

---

cuff by changing its line of pull so as to convert balancing forces into unbalancing forces (Fig. 4-86).

The thickness of the supraspinatus is approximately 6 mm. Diminution of the interval between the humeral head and the acromion, which is occupied by the supraspinatus and its surrounding soft tissues, suggests rupture of the rotator cuff. The interval diminishes with age in men only. A space of less than 6 mm is abnormal in a middle-age person (Fig. 4-87). Upward subluxation of the humeral head is almost always more pronounced on external than on internal rotation views (Fig. 4-88).

The acromiohumeral interval bears prognostic importance. Patients whose acromiohumeral distance is less than 7 mm often have larger tears and less strength and motion than others after cuff repair.

The pathogenesis of rotator cuff tears has not been fully elucidated. Codman suggested that the cause of the cuff tear was degenerative. Ozaki and colleagues suggested that intrinsic tendon degeneration was dominant in a study of 200 cadavers; however, most of these theories were derived from postmortem studies. The complaints of the patient, the patient's profession or daily activity, and the history of shoulder injury were not considered, and these might have influenced the interpretation of their observations. Neer, however, indicated the importance of impingement by the subacromial surface and coracoacromial ligament because of the good results achieved with a combined procedure of

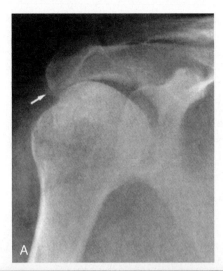

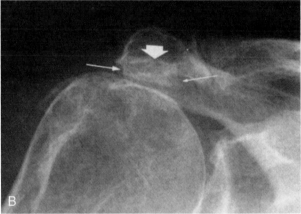

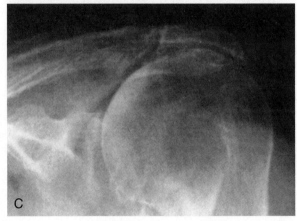

FIG. 4-88 Rotator cuff disease and impingement. **A,** Right shoulder; both the greater tuberosity and the acromion process are sclerotic. Hypertrophic changes of the peripheral margin of the acromion are also evident *(arrow)*. **B,** Right shoulder. Bone formation *(long arrows)* is observed along the undersurface of the acromion process *(large arrow)*. This formation occupies the subacromial space and is conformed to the humeral head contour. **C,** Left shoulder. Superior migration of the humeral head is evident. (From Nicholas JA, Hershman EB, editors: *The upper extremity in sports medicine,* St Louis, 1990, Mosby.)

cuff repair and anterior acromioplasty. Bigliani and colleagues popularized the theory of extrinsic subacromial impingement and described three types of acromial shape. However, some cases of articular side tears of the rotator cuff did not show degenerative changes of the acromion (Ko et al, 2006).

Complete tears of the tendinous cuff must be distinguished from incomplete tears. The clinical effects of the tears are different. An incomplete tear is one cause of the painful arc syndrome, and a complete tear seriously impairs the patient's ability to abduct the shoulder.

The tendon gives way under a sudden strain, usually caused by a fall or by overexertion. Age attrition of the tendon is a predisposing factor.

The cause of rotator cuff tears is multifactorial, but decreased tensile strength of the tendon and the force applied to it may be the most important factors. Preexisting degenerative changes of the tendon, in association with microtrauma, seem to have a major effect on the tear. Although rotator cuff tears are mostly degenerative lesions, trauma is often associated. In previous reports, 64% to 88% of the patients with cuff lesions had a history of trauma (Lahteenmaki et al, in press).

A tear of the tendinous cuff is mainly of the supraspinatus tendon, but it may extend into the adjacent subscapularis or infraspinatus tendons. Such a tear is close to the insertion of the tendons and usually involves the capsule of the joint into which the tendons are blended. The edges of the rent retract, leaving a gaping hole that establishes a communication between the shoulder joint and the subacromial bursa.

With complete tears of the supraspinatus tendon, the patient is usually a man who is older than 60. After a strain or fall, the patient's complaints include pain at the tip of the shoulder and down the upper arm and an inability to raise the arm.

Examination reveals local tenderness below the margin of the acromion. When the patient attempts to abduct the arm, no movement occurs at the glenohumeral joint, but a range of 45 to 60 degrees of abduction can be achieved entirely by scapular movement. However, the range of passive movement is full. If the arm is abducted with assistance beyond 90 degrees, the patient can sustain the abduction by deltoid action. The essential and characteristic feature in cases of torn supraspinatus tendon is the inability to initiate glenohumeral abduction. The usual explanation is that the early stages of abduction demand combining the action of the supraspinatus with the action of the deltoid muscle. This feature-combined action supplies the main abduction force and the supraspinatus action that stabilizes the humeral head in the glenoid fossa.

A complete tear of the tendinous cuff must be distinguished from other causes of impaired glenohumeral abduction, especially the painful arc syndrome and paralysis of the abductor muscles (poliomyelitis or nerve injury). Inability to initiate glenohumeral abduction accompanied by enough power to sustain abduction once the limb has been raised passively is characteristic of a widely torn supraspinatus. With the painful arc syndrome, the power of abduction is retained, but the movement is painful. In a case of complete tear, arthrography will demonstrate communication between the joint and the subacromial bursa. The tear also may be visualized by ultrasound scanning.

PROCEDURE

- The patient's arm is passively abducted (Figs. 4-89 and 4-90).
- The examiner suddenly removes support at some point above 90 degrees, which makes the deltoid contract suddenly (Fig. 4-91).
- If shoulder pain occurs and a hunching of the shoulder occurs because rotator cuff function is absent, the sign is present for rotator cuff tear or, more specifically, rupture of the supraspinatus tendon.
- In a modification of Codman sign, the patient's shoulder is abducted to 90 degrees passively.
- The patient tries to lower the arm slowly to the side in the same arc of movement.
- If the patient is unable to return the arm to the side slowly or has severe pain, the test is positive.
- A positive test suggests a tear in the rotator cuff complex.

Next Steps/Procedures
Apley scratch test, impingement sign, subacromial push-button sign, and supraspinatus test

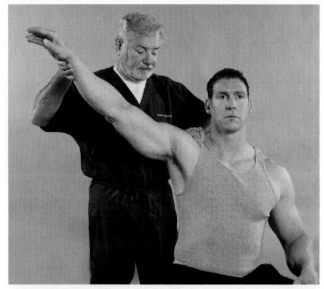

FIG. 4-90 The passive abduction is carried to a range slightly above 90 degrees.

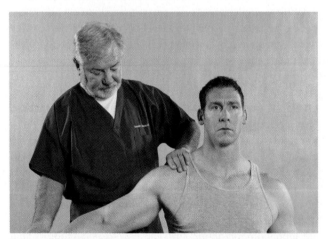

FIG. 4-89 The patient is seated. The examiner passively abducts the patient's affected arm.

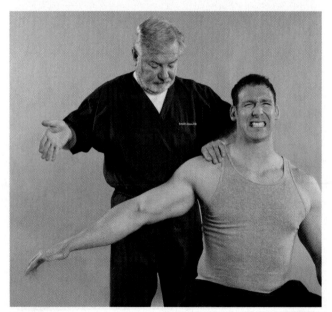

FIG. 4-91 The examiner suddenly removes support, making the deltoid contract suddenly. If the sign is present, shoulder pain and a hunching of the shoulder occur because rotator cuff function is absent. The sign is significant for rotator cuff tear (rupture of the supraspinatus tendon).

CLINICAL PEARL

The cardinal sign of cuff rupture is persistent weakness. The patient may be conscious of this weakness, but the examiner must often point it out. Sometimes the weakness is easily overlooked. The patient may be able to lift the arm into full abduction or beyond the point of a full-thickness cuff tear. However, if this action is resisted a little, sometimes by as little as the pressure of one finger, even a very strong patient may be unable to abduct or flex the shoulder well.

COSTOCLAVICULAR MANEUVER

Assessment for Thoracic Outlet Syndrome

Comment

Thoracic outlet compression syndrome refers to a common condition in which nerves or vessels or both are compressed between the root of the neck and axilla. Two clearly defined forms of this condition have been described. One is a neurologic syndrome that involves the lower trunk of the brachial plexus and is caused by abnormal nerve stretch or compression. The other is a vascular form that involves the subclavian artery and vein and is more common in men than in women.

> Pseudoaneurysm of the axillary artery was first described in 1975. The pathogenesis of axillary artery injury is poorly understood. Historically, the majority of these cases affect individuals over the age of 50 years. Atherosclerotic change in the vessels makes them less elastic and less resistant to shearing forces. Vessels of the younger patient are more elastic and compliant, being less vulnerable to injury during dislocation. The anatomic position of the vessel is thought to play a role in its susceptibility to trauma. Theories initially suggested that injury may arise as a consequence of the position of the axillary artery, fixed between the anterior and posterior circumflex arteries and the subscapular arteries. Another theory purports that movement of the humeral head into hyperabduction compresses and distorts the vessel against pectoralis minor. The majority of injuries occur within the lower third of the artery distal to this muscle. The axillary artery displays a degree of anatomic variation in its course, which may contribute further to its susceptibility to injury by enveloping structures (McCann, Barakat, Wand, 2006).

The neurologic form of TOS often occurs in women of slim build and drooping shoulders. Presenting symptoms include aching pain in the side or back of the neck that extends across the shoulder and down along the inner aspect of the arm and paresthesias in the ulnar aspect of the hand. The sensory findings extend more proximally than an ulnar nerve lesion, whereas the motor findings include thenar and intrinsic muscle weakness and wasting.

An important sign reproduces the patient's symptoms by abducting and laterally rotating the arm at the shoulder with a flexed elbow while palpating the pulses at the wrist (*Wright maneuver*).

The overhead exercise test may elicit symptoms of aching and fatigue in patients with TOS after 20 to 30 seconds of rapidly flexing and extending the fingers as the arm is held overhead (*Roos test*).

As the neurovascular bundle enters the axillary canal, it runs through a narrow cleft beneath the clavicle and on top of the first rib. This cleft is a slitlike aperture over which the subclavius muscle arches, sometimes with a sharp, fusiform lower margin. Alterations and abnormalities in this cleft can compress the neurovascular bundle. Because the vein is the most medial structure running into the arm and lies in the narrowest part of the cleft, it suffers the most from any narrowing that develops. Abnormalities, fractures, and dislocations of the medial third of the clavicle or fractures of the first rib followed by excessive callus formation can constrict this space. The resulting symptoms are a sense of fullness in the hand and fingers and an aching, crampy pain in the forearm and hand. Vague shoulder or shoulder-arm discomfort may be mentioned, but the radiating pain is emphasized. The hand may be intermittently swollen, and sometimes superficial veins around the shoulder are engorged. Shoulder movement is not limited, which contrasts with shoulder-arm-hand syndrome, in which gross shoulder immobilization is prominent and hand symptoms are present. The radiating discomfort has the typically diffuse vascular pattern, which means the discomfort is not localized to nerve root or peripheral nerve distribution.

> Unilateral arm swelling without thrombosis, when not caused by lymphatic obstruction, may be caused by subclavian vein compression at the costoclavicular ligament because of compression either by that ligament or the subclavius tendon most often because of congenital close proximity of the vein to the ligament. Arm symptoms of neurogenic TOS pain and paresthesia often accompany venous TOS, whereas neck pain and headache, which are other common symptoms of neurogenic TOS, are infrequent (Sanders, Hammond, 2005).

In addition to patients with obvious abnormality of the rib and clavicle, some patients develop this disturbance from a sagging shoulder girdle and atonic musculature. Normally, encroaching on the neurovascular bundle beneath the clavicle is difficult, but conceivably, some sagging occurs, and

---

ORTHOPEDIC GAMUT 4-12

THORACIC OUTLET SYNDROME

Depending on the mechanism and level of compression, several disorders are included under the title of thoracic outlet syndrome:

1. Cervical rib syndrome
2. Scalenus-anticus syndrome
3. Wright hyperabduction syndrome
4. Pectoralis minor syndrome
5. Costoclavicular syndrome

ORTHOPEDIC GAMUT 4-13

SYMPTOMS OF SUBCLAVIAN VENOUS OBSTRUCTION

- Swelling
- Cyanosis
  - Intermittent blueness over the hand, arm, and often the upper chest wall is a common symptom, although it is seldom significant enough to be a major complaint.
  - This cyanosis is different than the color changes that are frequently seen in neurogenic TOS and are associated with increased sympathetic activity.
  - The color changes in neurogenic TOS are rubor, pallor, and some cyanosis and are usually limited to the hand.
- Arm pain
- Paresthesia
- Neck pain and occipital headache

no scalene or supraclavicular tenderness is noted. The diagnostic images are different because no cervical rib is present. Arterial symptoms are occasionally prominent, but most of the disturbance is the result of venous obstruction. Costoclavicular compression can be differentiated from postural compression by the absence of any significant relation to body position either at work or while sleeping.

Costoclavicular compression is also clearly differentiated from hyperabduction compression by the lack of significant correlation to shoulder movement.

PROCEDURE

- The radial pulse is palpated while the patient's shoulders are drawn down and in extension (Fig. 4-92).
- The cervical spine is flexed maximally (Figs. 4-93 and 4-94).
- If the pulses are lost, the test is positive.
- TOS is suggested by a positive test.

when tension in the bundle and enveloping sheath is added, the vessels may be compressed.

This costoclavicular disturbance can be separated from scalene and cervical rib disturbances by several findings.

No relationship to cervical spine movements exists, and

Next Steps/Procedures
Adson test, Allen maneuver, George screening procedure, Halstead maneuver, reverse Bakody maneuver, Roos test, shoulder compression test, and Wright test

CLINICAL PEARL

Radiating discomfort from neurovascular compression can be associated with sleep or recumbency. This discomfort is a common disturbance that has many descriptive terms applied to it, including *Wartenberg nocturnal dysesthesia, sleep tetany, waking numbness, nocturnal palsy,* and *morning numbness.*

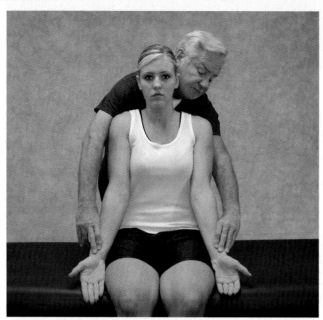

FIG. 4-92 The patient is seated comfortably with the arms at the sides. The examiner bilaterally palpates the radial pulse.

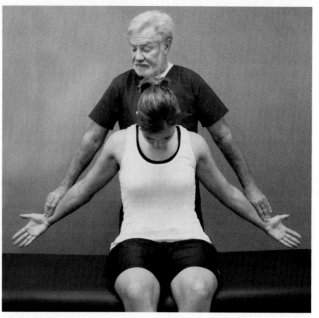

FIG. 4-93 The examiner extends the patient's shoulders as the patient flexes the cervical spine (chin to chest). The test is positive if the radial pulse of the affected arm disappears. A positive test indicates TOS.

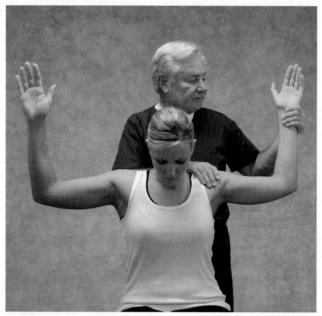

FIG. 4-94 An alternative is to have the patient actively abduct the shoulders and flex the elbows to 90 degrees. The examiner palpates the radial pulse of the affected arm and externally rotates the arm. The test is positive if the pulse disappears. A positive test indicates TOS. Before the arm is externally rotated in this position, a subtle sign of TOS may occur. This sign involves blanching of the hand of the affected arm. The examiner should use the unaffected side as a control.

Assessment for Subacromial Bursitis

Comment

As is the case with many other important joints, many of the major muscles surrounding the shoulder joint are *cushioned* by a bursal sac, which minimizes friction and subsequent irritation associated with movement. The most clinically significant bursae at the shoulder joint are the deltoid bursa and the subacromial bursa (Fig. 4-95).

A painful shoulder is a complaint that is common to all age groups and both sexes. To treat these patients effectively, the exact cause must be determined in each case. The use of *bursitis* as an all-inclusive term denoting the diagnosis and basis for therapy in the painful shoulder syndrome is irrational. Most of the body's bursae exist in or around the shoulder complex.

Excluding traumatic causes, shoulder pain may radiate from a lesion of the cervical spine or may be the result of irritation from some other organ, such as the gallbladder or heart. However, shoulder pain most often originates as some derangement of the subacromial mechanism in the shoulder joint proper.

The subacromial mechanism of the shoulder joint is bounded above by the acromion and the coracoacromial ligament and below by the humeral head. The component structures of the shoulder include the subacromial, or subdeltoid, bursa; the musculotendinous, or rotator, cuff; the articular capsule of the shoulder joint; and the tendon sheath gliding mechanism of the LHB brachii muscle.

Most patients with shoulder pain will have some lesion involving a component of this mechanism. The use of the blanket term *bursitis* to explain all of the derangements of the subacromial mechanism is the most important factor against successful management of the painful or stiff shoulder. All lesions of the subacromial mechanism may secondarily involve the subdeltoid bursa. True primary subdeltoid

---

ORTHOPEDIC GAMUT 4-14

BURSAE LOCATIONS

The most commonly present bursae locations are (Fig. 4-96):
1. Subacromial and subdeltoid
2. Between the coracoid and the glenohumeral joint capsule
3. Summit of the acromion
4. Between the infraspinatus and the joint capsule
5. Between the teres major and the long head of the biceps
6. Between the subscapularis and the joint capsule
7. Anterior and posterior to the tendinous insertion of the latissimus dorsi
8. Behind the coracobrachialis muscle

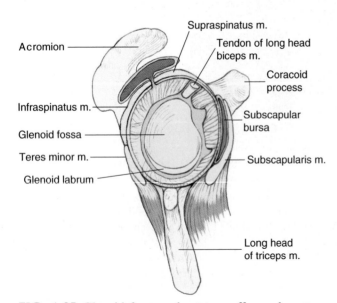

FIG. 4-95 Glenoid fossa and rotator cuff muscles. (From Mathers LH et al: *Clinical anatomy principles*, St Louis, 1996, Mosby.)

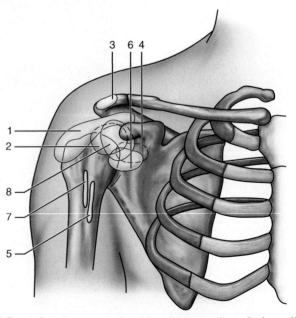

FIG. 4-96 Common shoulder bursae. (See Orthopedic Gamut 4-14 for number key.) (From Saidoff DC, McDonough AL: *Critical pathways in therapeutic intervention*, St Louis, 1997, Mosby.)

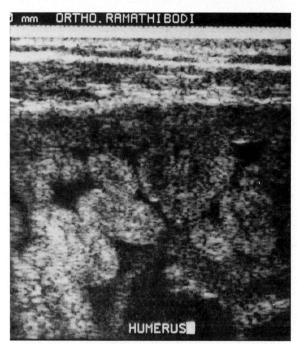

FIG. 4-97 While shoulder radiographs may show soft-tissue swelling with osteopenia, in tuberculous subacromial bursitis, ultrasonography of the bursa demonstrates a large cystic mass with hyperechoic contents resembling rice bodies. (From Pookarnjanamorakot C, Sirikulchayanonta V: Tuberculous bursitis of the subacromial bursa, *J Shoulder Elbow Surg* 13[1]:105-107, 2004.)

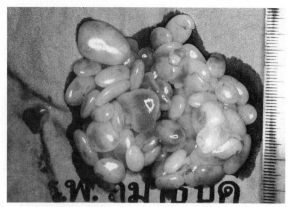

FIG. 4-98 Rice bodies. (From Pookarnjanamorakot C, Sirikulchayanonta V: Tuberculous bursitis of the subacromial bursa, *J Shoulder Elbow Surg* 13[1]:105-107, 2004.)

bursitis is rarely encountered. The most common derangements of the subacromial mechanism that cause shoulder pain are calcific deposits in the musculotendinous cuff, bicipital tendinopathy, lesions of the acromioclavicular joint, adhesive capsulitis of the shoulder joint, and infection (Figs. 4-97 and 4-98).

Infection originating in a deep bursa is rare and should be differentiated from infected bursitis extending from the nearby septic joint. The number of reported cases of septic subacromial bursitis caused by nonspecific organisms and rare cases caused by a tuberculous process is considerable. These reported cases of tuberculous bursitis in this location were mainly secondarily extended from the shoulder joint (Pookarnjanamorakot, Sirikulchayanonta, 2004).

PROCEDURE

- With the patient's arm comfortably at the side, deep palpation of the shoulder by the examiner elicits a well-localized, tender area (Fig. 4-99).
- With the examiner's finger still on the painful spot, the patient's arm is passively abducted by the examiner's other hand.
- The sign is present if the painful spot under the examiner's nonmoving finger disappears as the arm is abducted (Fig. 4-100).
- The sign is significant for subacromial bursitis.

Next Steps/Procedures
Diagnostic imaging

CLINICAL PEARL

Subacromial bursitis is not common as a primary condition. The condition may be caused by a direct blow over the shoulder. This blow causes an inflammatory reaction that is aggravated by further motion. Bursitis is usually a secondary reaction. The examiner should search for a primary lesion before beginning treatment.

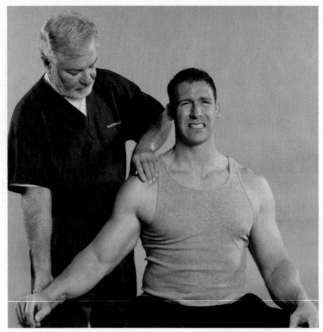

FIG. 4-99 The patient is seated with the arms comfortably at the side. The examiner palpates the affected shoulder deeply. A well-localized, tender area at the subacromial bursa is found.

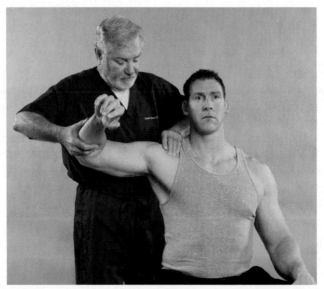

FIG. 4-100 While the examiner's finger is still on the painful spot, the patient's arm is passively abducted by the examiner's other hand. The sign is present when, as the arm is abducted, the painful spot disappears under the examiner's nonmoving finger. The sign is significant for subacromial bursitis.

Assessment for Shoulder Dislocation

Comment

Anterior dislocation is by far the most common pattern of shoulder dislocation. This type of dislocation occurs when the head of the humerus slips off and in front of the glenoid when the arm is abducted and extended.

Once off the glenoid, the head slips medially when the arm is lowered. This slipping produces the characteristic profile of a dislocated shoulder. Because the head of the humerus is not lying in its normal position, the shoulder has a flatter appearance than usual and the elbow points outward. If the tip of the acromion and the lateral epicondyle can be joined by a straight line (Hamilton test), the shoulder is dislocated.

This appearance and the observation that the patient supports the injured arm with the other hand enables the examiner to diagnose a dislocated shoulder from the other end of the examination room. A similarly flattened contour is also seen in patients with atrophied deltoid muscles and in displaced fractures of the surgical neck. However, in these patients, the humeral head is still in its normal position, and the ruler test is negative.

Damage to the axillary nerve that occurs as it runs around the neck of the humerus causes partial or complete paralysis of the deltoid. The axillary nerve should be examined with an electromyogram (EMG) 3 and 6 weeks after the injury. If the examiner finds no change in pathologic findings between the two examinations, the nerve has been damaged, and specific treatment may be necessary.

Brachial plexus injuries also occur if a violent abduction strain has occurred. If dislocation occurs and causes neurologic damage, the results are often poor.

The axillary artery can be damaged by traction at the time of injury or by pressure from the humeral head. The radial pulse should be checked, and its presence should be recorded.

The humeral head occasionally buttonholes through the subscapularis. This action makes reduction impossible.

Chronic recurrent posterior subluxations are often demonstrable by the patient either by positioning the arm or by selected muscle contracture. It may be unilateral after trauma

---

ORTHOPEDIC GAMUT 4-16

CHRONIC RECURRENT DISLOCATIONS

Four subsets of chronic recurrent dislocations are:
1. Voluntary habitual (emotionally disturbed)
2. Voluntary
3. Not willful (muscular control)
4. Involuntary positional and involuntary unintentional (not demonstrable by patient)

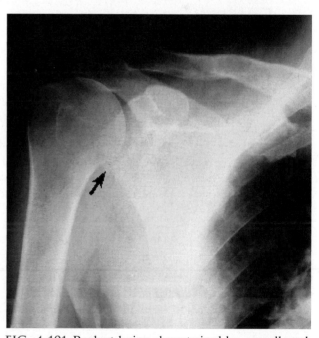

FIG. 4-101 Bankart lesion characterized by a small avulsion fragment of the inferior glenoid rim at the site of the triceps insertion *(arrow).* (From Deltoff MN, Kogon PL: *The portable skeletal x-ray library,* St Louis, 1998, Mosby.)

ORTHOPEDIC GAMUT 4-15

ANTERIOR SHOULDER DISLOCATION

Radiographic appearances of anterior shoulder dislocation:
1. Bankart lesion, which is an avulsion of a small fragment of the glenoid rim at the site of the triceps insertion (Fig. 4-101)
2. Flap fracture, an avulsion of the greater tuberosity (Fig. 4-102)
3. Hill-Sachs (hatchet) deformity, an impaction fracture of the posterosuperior surface of the humeral head produced by repetitive traumatization by the inferior glenoid rim after recurrent anterior glenohumeral joint dislocation

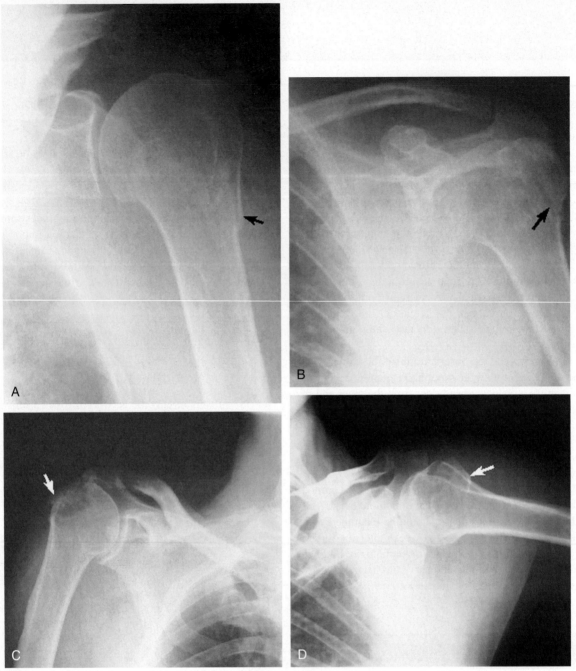

FIG. 4-102 **A** and **B,** Avulsion fracture of the greater tuberosity *(arrow).* **C,** Flap fracture featuring an avulsion of the greater tuberosity *(arrow).* **D,** The greater tuberosity demonstrates avulsion *(arrow).* (From Deltoff MN, Kogon PL: *The portable skeletal x-ray library, St Louis,* 1998, Mosby.)

or bilateral with pain only on one side, with or without a precipitating traumatic event.

The usual history is one of gradual onset in which subluxation of both shoulders can occur posteriorly either by contracture of the anterior deltoid and pectoralis (Fig. 4-103) or by arm position with the arm forward flexed (Fig. 4-104,*A*). Extension of the arm causes a sudden snap with a concomitant reduction (Fig. 4-104,*B*). Although apprehension is common for anterior instability, it is not reliable for posterior instability. The Castagna test is useful in identifying minor shoulder dislocation instability (Fig. 4-105).

Patients with minor shoulder instability complain of pain in the posterior-superior aspect of the affected, generally dominant, shoulder. Sometimes the pain radiates toward the arm. The pain is often diffuse and difficult to pinpoint. Patients describe snapping and popping, *dead arm*, painful subluxation, or transient locking (Castagna et al, 2007).

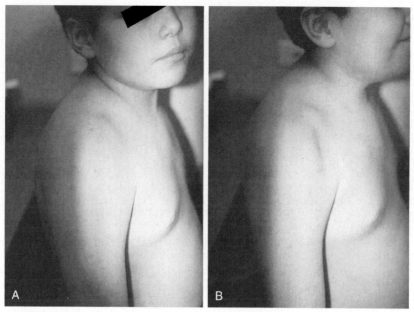

FIG. 4-103 **A** and **B,** A 10-year-old boy with voluntary instability of the shoulder. Voluntary instability can be accomplished in patients with multidirectional laxity by conscious firing of certain muscle groups while their antagonists are inhibited and combining these muscle manipulations with certain arm positions that lead to subluxation of the glenohumeral joint. A most notable finding in cases of voluntary instability is the lack of pain associated with the subluxation or dislocation. Pathologic voluntary instability can be associated with psychological or emotional instability. (From DeLee: *DeLee and Drez's orthopaedic sports medicine,* ed 2, St Louis, 2003, Saunders.)

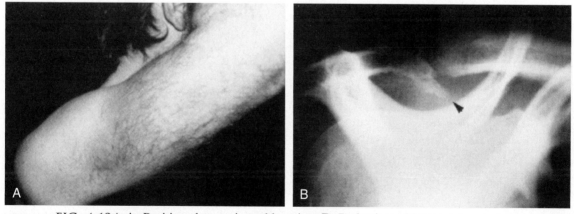

FIG. 4-104 **A,** Positioned posterior subluxation. **B,** Reduction with snap. (From Nicholas JA, Hershman EB, editors: *The upper extremity in sports medicine,* St Louis, 1990, Mosby.)

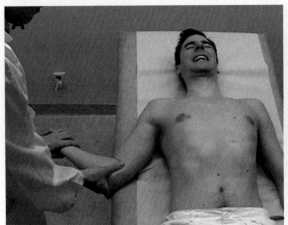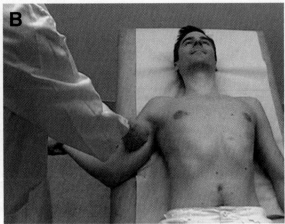

FIG. 4-105 The Castagna test for minor instability. The patient is positioned with 45 degrees of glenohumeral abduction. The arm is maximally externally rotated. Posterior-superior pain is associated with a loose anterior joint capsule and middle glenohumeral ligament. **A,** If pain is relieved with relocation, this represents a positive Castagna test. **B,** The Castagna test is similar to the *Jobe relocation test* except that the *Jobe test* is performed with the arm at 90 degrees abduction. (From Castagna A et al: Minor shoulder instability, *Arthroscopy* 23[2]:211-215, 2007.)

PROCEDURE

- The patient places the hand of the affected shoulder on the opposite shoulder and attempts to touch the chest with the elbow (Fig. 4-106).
- The test is positive if the patient cannot touch the chest wall with the elbow (Fig. 4-107).
- The test is positive in shoulder dislocation.

Steps/Procedures
Apprehension test, Bryant sign, Calloway test, Hamilton test, Mazion shoulder maneuver, and diagnostic imaging

CLINICAL PEARL

In exceptional circumstances, the humeral head can become jammed below the glenoid with the arm pointing directly upward (luxatio erecta), presenting a spectacular appearance sometimes mistaken for hysteria. This condition is a true inferior dislocation. In contrast to anterior dislocation, the humeral head in this situation lies against the vessels and can cause ischemia. The rotator cuff is always damaged.

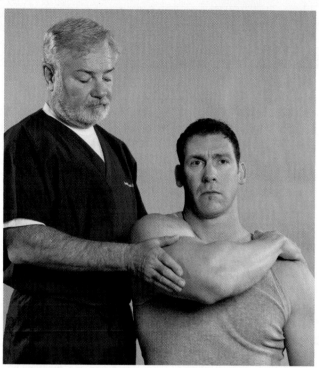

FIG. 4-106 The patient is seated comfortably with the arms at the sides. The patient places the hand of the affected shoulder on the opposite shoulder and attempts to touch the chest with the elbow.

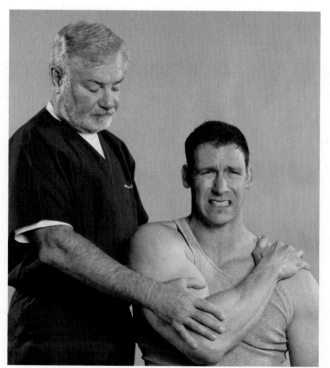

FIG. 4-107 If the patient cannot actively touch the chest wall with the elbow, the examiner passively confirms this by gently applying pressure to the elbow, attempting to approximate the elbow to the chest. Inability to move the elbow or increased pain is a positive sign. The presence of the sign indicates shoulder subluxation or dislocation.

Assessment for Subclavian Artery Stenosis or Occlusion

Comment

The vascular form of TOS is uncommon. It is characterized by a well-developed cervical rib producing stenosis and poststenotic dilation of the subclavian artery. The initial symptoms may vary from intermittent blanching of the hand and fingers as a result of embolization from a thrombus in the subclavian artery to a sudden catastrophic occlusion.

The *Adson test* can be used to reproduce the symptoms by abducting and externally rotating the arm and raising the hand above the head. If the radial pulse disappears, a lesion of the subclavian artery should be considered. An important point to remember is that approximately 80% of healthy people demonstrate a positive Adson test. Another provocative test is to have the patient raise both arms overhead and rapidly open and close the hand; this causes cramping very quickly if vascular TOS is present *(Roos test)*.

Paget-Schroetter syndrome (PSS) or *effort thrombosis* (ET) affects young, active adults who are engaged in sports activities or whose professions require repetitive arm move-ments causing trauma to the axillary-subclavian vein and leading to deep-vein thrombosis (DVT) (Fig. 4-108). This abnormality is a form of TOS accounting for fewer than 2% of all reported incidents of DVT.

In the past, spontaneous upper extremity DVT accounted for 1% to 2% of all DVT cases or was reported as occurring in 2 in 100,000 patients each year. The increase has been dramatic with the advent of central venous catheterization, accounting for 2% to 16% of the 5 to 20 million cases of DVT that occur yearly in the United States.

ET has important short-term ramifications, such as severe disability and pulmonary embolism, reported to occur in 12% of patients with subclavian-vein thrombosis.

PSS is now considered synonymous with ET because it presents after a venous injury occurring after acute or repetitive venous compression by the musculoskeletal components of the thoracic outlet (Shebel, Marin 2006). Most school-age children and young adults use backpacks to tote heavy books that are often slung over one shoulder, placing excessive weight on the shoulder structures. Theories suggest that the repetitive shoulder and arm motion may cause microintimal tears that trigger the coagulation cascade, thus precipitating a thrombotic event. Prolonged venous compression is known to cause vein wall irritation, injury, and fibrosis (Shebel, Marin, 2006).

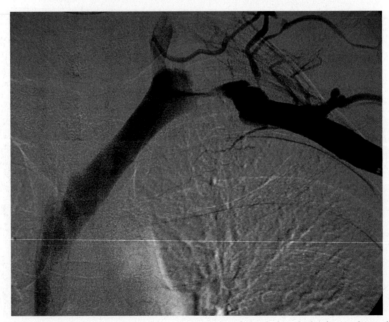

FIG. 4-108 Venogram reveals significant stenosis of the left subclavian vein as it passes through the costoclavicular space. (From Shebel ND, Marin A: Effort thrombosis (Paget-Schroetter syndrome) in active young adults: current concepts in diagnosis and treatment, *J Vasc Nurs* 24[4]:116-126, 2006.)

ORTHOPEDIC GAMUT 4-17

PRECIPITATING FACTORS IN PAGET-SCHROETTER SYNDROME OR *EFFORT THROMBOSIS*

- Playing tennis
- Golf
- Baseball
- Throwing a ball
- Rowing a boat
- Swimming
- Gymnastics
- Weightlifting
- Wrestling

ORTHOPEDIC GAMUT 4-18

INDIVIDUALS PREDISPOSED TO PAGET-SCHROETTER SYNDROME OR *EFFORT THROMBOSIS*

- Professional athletes
- Beauticians, painters
- Mechanics

The symptoms and disability of ET may persist for a prolonged period in 68% to 75% of patients. Although most cases result from trauma or use of cervical venous catheters, a small portion of the cases are related to various activities that require shoulder abduction.

The clinical presentation of ET varies dramatically from intermittent, nonspecific symptoms that consist of a generalized aching of the arm, with a degree of fullness and swelling, to a dramatically swollen, painful arm with dependent rubor. Typically, this presentation occurs in boys and men 15 to 40 years of age, often after a particular physical activity. The symptoms may appear immediately or up to 2 weeks later. The most common symptom noted with time is increased swelling of the arm, which responds to elevation (venous tone assessment). Swelling may be accompanied by abnormal subcutaneous vein distension, which worsens if the arm is exercised.

In ET, a venogram demonstrates occlusion of the axillary and subclavian veins, although the study itself may result in extension of the thrombosis. Doppler studies are useful in distinguishing intermittent compression from thrombosis. Other noninvasive methods of evaluation include duplex scanning and impedance plethysmography.

TOS describes the signs and symptoms resulting from proximal compression of the neurovascular structures supplying the upper limb.

The normal anatomy of the thoracic outlet, which extends from the intervertebral foramina and superior mediastinum to the axilla, must be considered not only in one plane, but also in three dimensions to appreciate the potential mechanisms of compression.

The scalene muscles, which are the flexors and rotators of the neck, were formerly considered major causes of compression. This belief led not only to the term *scalenus anticus syndrome*, but also to therapy directed solely at the release of these structures (scalenotomy). This method of therapy is a simple procedure with a high failure rate.

With many potential causes for compression, the three structures at risk—the subclavian artery, the vein, and the lower trunk of the brachial plexus—may be affected to significantly different degrees. The typical patient is likely to be a woman between the ages of 20 and 40. The ratio of women with TOS to men with the syndrome is 5:1. Complaints are often vague and hard to define.

Scleroderma causes thickened skin and varying degrees of organ dysfunction resulting from small-vessel vasculopathy and immune-mediated fibrosis. Bilateral Raynaud phenomenon is common in these patients and causes recurrent painful attacks and frequent digital ischemic lesions. Raynaud phenomenon in scleroderma is fundamentally different than the primary form of this disorder, because the digital artery closures affect not only the thermoregulatory vessels, but also the nutritional vessels. In combination with sustained vasospasm, progressive tissue ischemia occurs and tissue necrosis or ulceration can develop. Patients with primary Raynaud disease lack evidence of structural vessel disease and, despite vasospasm, maintain a certain nutritional flow in the arterioles to avoid ischemic lesions. TOS, which is caused by compression or irritation of the neurovascular bundle at the level of the costo-clavicular passage, is an unusual cause of arm pain and often difficult to diagnose. Upper extremity ischemia is caused by TOS in less than 5% of patients (Hugl et al, 2007).

PROCEDURE

- With the patient seated, the examiner assesses the patient's blood pressure bilaterally and records it (Fig. 4-109).
- The examiner also assesses the character of the patient's radial pulse bilaterally (Fig. 4-110).
- A difference of 10 mm Hg between the two systolic blood pressure readings and a feeble or absent radial pulse suggest possible subclavian artery stenosis or occlusion on the side of the feeble or absent pulse.
- If the test is negative, the examiner places a stethoscope over the supraclavicular fossa and auscultates the subclavian artery for bruits (Fig. 4-111).
- If bruits are present, subclavian artery stenosis or occlusion is suspected.

Next Steps/Procedures

Adson test, Allen maneuver, costoclavicular maneuver, Halstead maneuver, reverse Bakody maneuver, Roos test, shoulder compression test, and Wright test

CLINICAL PEARL

The shoulder joint can be linked with the hand in a symptom complex presenting the features of a reflex sympathetic disturbance. The shoulder symptoms may caused, in part, by the neurovascular upset that develops as a result of sympathetic stimulation. The shoulder complaint is usually secondary to some other factor, but the reflex dystrophy phenomenon has become so predominant that it is mislabeled as the cause when it is actually a result.

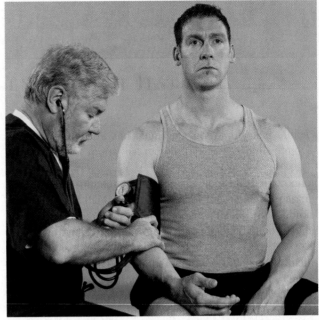

FIG. 4-109 The patient is seated. The examiner bilaterally assesses the patient's blood pressure and records the findings.

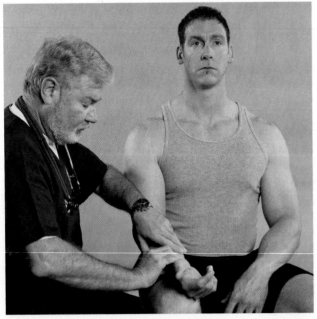

FIG. 4-110 The examiner bilaterally determines the character of the patient's radial pulse. A difference of 10 mm Hg between the two systolic blood pressures and a feeble or absent radial pulse suggests subclavian artery stenosis or occlusion on the side of the feeble or absent pulse.

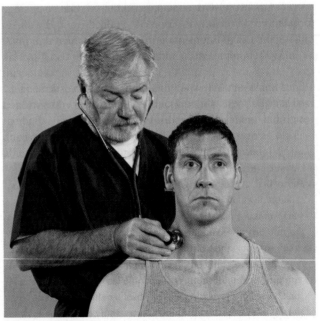

FIG. 4-111 If the first two procedures are negative, the examiner places a stethoscope over the supraclavicular fossa and auscultates the subclavian artery for bruits. If bruits are present, the screening procedure suggests a possible subclavian artery stenosis or occlusion.

Assessment for Thoracic Outlet Syndrome

Comment

Farther outward from the spinal cord, the nerve roots are grouped into trunks and cords that become intimately associated with the vascular bundle of the arm. The union takes place above the clavicle at a point where an additional cervical rib or tight scalenus anterior muscle may partially block the combined neurovascular bundle.

Compression of this bundle results in radiating discomfort and shoulder pain. However, the character of the pain changes from a well-defined neural pattern to a broad, vaguer discomfort because of the vascular association. The general properties of both of these pain conditions should be appreciated. Both conditions produce an aching neck, shoulder pain, a feeling of numbness, and tingling down the arm to the fingers. The inner aspect of the forearm and hand is the site usually involved, as opposed to the outer aspect of the thumb and index finger in the common cervical root lesions. The tingling that occurs often involves all of the fingers and produces a sense of fullness in the hand. If motor and sensory signs develop, they typically involve the ulnar supply because of pressure on the medial cord of the plexus. The small muscles of the hand may be involved, but either median or ulnar groups are singled out.

Entrapment neuropathy results from increased pressure on a nerve as it passes through an enclosed space. A nerve is most vulnerable to compression as it traverses a fibro-osseous canal, where a disproportion of contents and capacity exists. Nerves that have previously been affected by a neuropathic process, as with diabetes or alcoholism, appear to be even more vulnerable to entrapment.

The signs and symptoms that accompany thoracic outlet nerve entrapment at times may be subtle and easily confused with other orthopedic disorders (i.e., Raynaud syndrome or phenomenon) (Fig. 4-112).

TOS is a term that encompasses several clinical entities. The syndrome results from compression of one or more of the neurovascular elements that pass through the superior thoracic aperture. In most cases, neurogenic entrapment accounts for the symptoms; an isolated vascular lesion is rare.

Patients usually experience sensory symptoms as the first manifestation of TOS. Paresthesias are common, which follow the ulnar nerve distribution along the medial aspect of the arm and forearm and then to the fourth and fifth fingers. Aching pain radiating to the neck, shoulder, and arm is common, often being more diffuse than the paresthesias. Carrying heavy objects, persistent abduction of the shoulder, and work that requires using the arms over the head may

exacerbate these symptoms. TOS is also more likely to occur in individuals with poor posture and drooping shoulders.

Signs of motor weakness, if they appear, usually follow the sensory complaints. Patients may describe a feeling of weakness or clumsiness in using the hand. Wasting of the thenar, hypothenar, and intrinsic muscles of the hand may be noted.

This distribution of atrophy, following a definite peripheral nerve pattern, is in contrast to progressive muscular atrophy, in which generalized involvement occurs that does not follow a specific pattern.

Shoulder and arm movements are not particularly involved in either cervical rib or scalenus anticus disorders. Points of tenderness and soreness may be identified in the supraclavicular region away from the shoulder area proper and lying above the clavicle. When neck pain is present, it tends to be at the front, which is in contrast to the posterior discomfort of fibrositis and postural disorders.

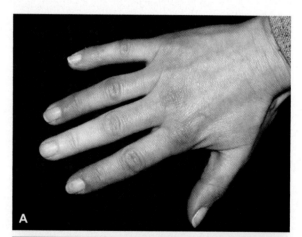
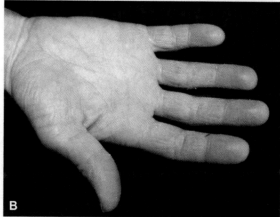

FIG. 4-112 **A** and **B,** Ischemic and hyperemic phases of Raynaud phenomenon. (From Gayraud M: Raynaud's phenomenon, *Joint Bone Spine* 74[1]:e1-e8, 2007.)

ORTHOPEDIC GAMUT 4-19

SUBTLE SYMPTOMS OF NEUROGENIC THORACIC OUTLET SYNDROME

Sixteen moderate and mild clinical symptoms and signs suggestive of disputed neurogenic thoracic outlet syndrome:

1. Paresthesias in the whole hand
2. Paresthesias in median digits
3. Paresthesias in ulnar digits
4. Nocturnal paresthesias
5. Diurnal paresthesias
6. Pain in hand
7. Pain in forearm
8. Pain in shoulder
9. Pain in head
10. Pain after pressure of upper trapezius muscle
11. Pain after pressure on Erb point
12. Pain after shoulder mobilization
13. Roos test (3 min)
14. Roos test (paresthesias)
15. Adson maneuver
16. Radial pulse suppression after abduction/external rotation of the shoulder and various positions of the cervical spine

In 1862, Maurice Raynaud described a paroxysmal phenomenon that included three phases: (1) ischemia, with pallor of the digits caused by vasoconstriction of the digital arteries, precapillary arteries, and cutaneous arteriovenous shunts; (2) hyperemia with redness of the digits; and (3) a return to normal. Whereas the ischemic phase is required for the diagnosis, the hyperemic phase may be lacking. The abnormalities usually spare the thumb but involve most of the other digits, although they may start in a limited number of digits. The nose, ears, and tongue may be affected. The attack resolves within an hour after the end of cold exposure. Raynaud phenomenon is associated with migraine and chest pain (usually from the chest wall, an association with spastic angina being controversial) (Gayraud, 2007).

PROCEDURE

- As the radial pulse of the affected arm is palpated, downward traction is applied on the extremity (Fig. 4-113).
- The neck is hyperextended (Fig. 4-114).
- Loss or diminution of the pulse suggests a positive test.
- If the test is negative, it is repeated with the patient rotating the head to the opposite side.
- TOS is suggested by a positive test.

Steps/Procedures

Adson test, Allen maneuver, costoclavicular maneuver, George screening procedure, reverse Bakody maneuver, Roos test, shoulder compression test, and Wright test

CLINICAL PEARL

Raynaud disease, acroparesthesia, and thromboangiitis obliterans *may be confused* with thoracic outlet compression syndromes, but the former three conditions actually differ profoundly from outlet compression syndromes because Raynaud disease, acroparesthesia, and thromboangiitis obliterans are not accompanied by shoulder discomfort, have no correlation to arm or shoulder movement, and are not affected by body posture.

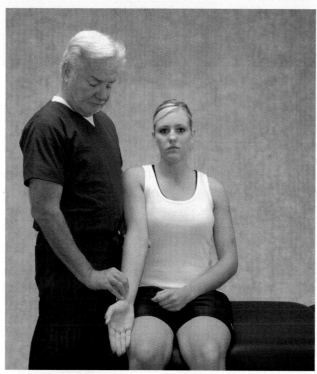

FIG. 4-113 The patient is seated comfortably with the arms at the sides. The examiner palpates the radial pulse of the affected arm.

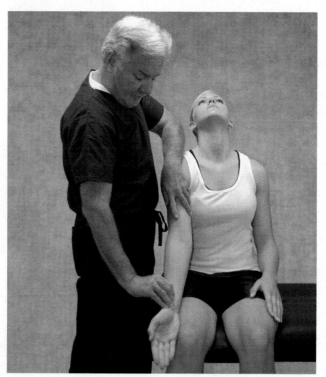

FIG. 4-114 The examiner applies downward traction on the affected extremity while the patient hyperextends the neck. Disappearance of the pulse is a positive test. A positive test indicates TOS. If the pulse does not disappear, the test is repeated with the patient's head rotated to the opposite side.

HAMILTON TEST

Assessment for Dislocation of the Shoulder

Comment

One of the consequences for superb mobility of the shoulder is frequent dislocation. A dislocated shoulder is an injury of the young, in whom it occurs more often than fracture of the neck of the humerus. Solid, healthy bone withstands abduction and twisting strain, but the weak capsule of the young gives way. Later in life, the bone becomes soft, and the capsule contracts; therefore, abduction and twisting result in shaft breaks while the joint remains intact. Young adults suffer this injury often. The most common accident that causes a dislocated shoulder is a fall with the arm outstretched for protection. The contributions of the elbow and body weight have been somewhat overlooked in explaining the mechanism of this injury. The essential episode is that the head of the humerus is forced against the weak anterior or anteroinferior capsule. In a fall, the outstretched hand absorbs the impact while the elbow is extended. As long as this extension is retained, a solid strut transmits the force to the superior or posterosuperior joint structures. The weight of the body alters this situation. As full weight is applied, momentary giving way or buckling of the elbow is inevitable. This action breaks the solid strut, and the elbow must flex, which tilts the upper end of the humerus downward and forward. As the fall continues, the head slips off the glenoid rim easily. At this point, the extremity is in abduction and external rotation, exposing the posterosuperior part of the humeral head to the glenoid rim. The rim usually gets cut or creased. Understandably, with repeated similar trauma, less and less force is needed to dislocate the humeral head. The humeral head commonly comes to lie at the front of the glenoid, resting on the rib. Occasionally, the humeral head lies higher, just below the clavicle.

In evaluating chronic laxity of the shoulder ligaments, the examiner first asks the patient to reproduce subluxation of the shoulder voluntarily to demonstrate laxity. Then provocative maneuvers to reproduce glenohumeral subluxations or dislocations can be performed with the patient sitting, lying supine, or standing.

With the patient sitting, the examiner stabilizes the scapula by placing one finger on the coracoid and resting the body of the hand and forearm on the scapula. With the other hand, the index and middle fingers grasp the anterior humeral head and the thumb grasps the posterior head. A force is directed anteriorly and inferiorly (Fig. 4-115). Subluxation of the head over the anteroinferior glenoid rim is estimated as to degree. Pain may preclude this testing.

With the patient seated, abduction and external rotation of the involved arm and a force directed in an anteroinferior direction from behind may cause a palpable subluxation, labral crepitation, or frank dislocation (Fig. 4-116). The patient is most apprehensive and resists this maneuver when

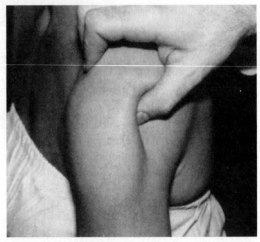

FIG. 4-115 Anteroinferior subluxation creates a void under the posterior acromion and a slight bulge below the coracoid. (From Nicholas JA, Hershman EB, editors: *The upper extremity in sports medicine,* St Louis, 1990, Mosby.)

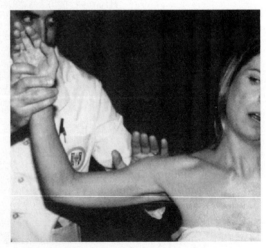

FIG. 4-116 Positive apprehension test. Attempts at anteroinferior subluxation of the abducted and externally rotated arm are exacerbated by forceful pressure on the proximal posterior humerus directed anteriorly. (From Nicholas JA, Hershman EB, editors: *The upper extremity in sports medicine,* St Louis, 1990, Mosby.)

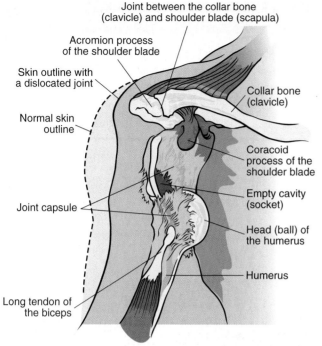

Joint between the collar bone
(clavicle) and shoulder blade (scapula)

Acromion process
of the shoulder blade

Skin outline with
a dislocated joint

Collar bone
(clavicle)

Normal skin
outline

Coracoid
process of the
shoulder blade

Joint capsule

Empty cavity
(socket)

Head (ball) of
the humerus

Humerus

Long tendon of
the biceps

FIG. 4-117 Subcoracoid (anteroinferior) dislocation of the glenohumeral joint with tear of the glenoid labrum and joint capsule. (From Saidoff DC, McDonough AL: *Critical pathways in therapeutic intervention,* St Louis, 1997, Mosby.)

ORTHOPEDIC GAMUT 4-20

CAUSES OF NONTRAUMATIC SHOULDER OSTEOARTHRITIS

- Gout
- Septic arthritis
- Rheumatoid arthritis
- Juvenile rheumatoid arthritis
- Alkaptonuria
- Acromegaly
- Epiphyseal dysplasia
- Crystal-induced arthritis
- Apatite deposition disease (Milwaukee shoulder)
- Hemophilia
- Ankylosing spondylitis
- Massive rotator cuff tear
- Steroid-induced avascular necrosis
- Idiopathic avascular necrosis
- Avascular necrosis caused by sickle cell disease
- Lupus erythematosus
- Gaucher disease

Anterior (subcoracoid) glenohumeral joint dislocation (Fig. 4-117) is the most common (90%) of all four possible glenohumeral dislocations. The shoulder joint is the most commonly dislocated major body joint.

Compared with weight-bearing joints, primary osteoarthritis of the shoulder is uncommon. It usually occurs in older adults, although most of these occurrences are asymptomatic. On the other hand, secondary osteoarthritis is more common. This condition is divided into two groups: nontraumatic and posttraumatic (Ogawa, Yoshida, Ikegami, 2006).

ORTHOPEDIC GAMUT 4-21

CAUSES OF POSTTRAUMATIC OSTEOARTHRITIS

- Fracture of the humeral head or glenoid and traumatic dislocation
- Osteoarthritis caused by dislocation is sometime called
  - Postdislocation osteoarthritis
  - Dislocation arthropathy
  - Dislocation-induced arthropathy

PROCEDURE

- If a straight edge (ruler or yardstick) can rest simultaneously on the acromial tip and the lateral epicondyle of the elbow, the test is positive (Fig. 4-118).
- The positive test is significant for dislocation of the shoulder.

Next Steps/Procedures

Apprehension test, Bryant sign, Calloway test, Dugas test, and Mazion shoulder maneuver

---

the arm is abducted to approximately 120 degrees and externally rotated. The patient's subjective apprehension that the shoulder may slip out of joint is considered a positive apprehension finding, whether actual joint subluxation occurs or not.

CLINICAL PEARL

Fractures of the humeral head that result in several fragments are usually accompanied by dislocation. Fracture dislocations of the humeral head present several problems: (1) The fragment may obstruct reduction and make open reduction necessary, (2) the reduction will be very unstable, (3) soft-tissue damage and hemorrhage into and around the shoulder lead to joint stiffness, and (4) avascular necrosis of the humeral head can follow fractures through the anatomic neck.

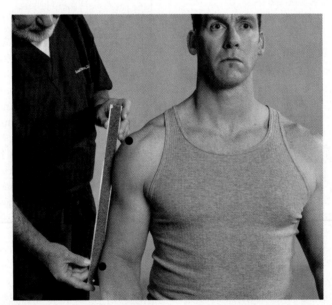

FIG. 4-118 The patient is seated comfortably with the arms at the sides. The examiner places a straight edge at the lateral border of the affected shoulder from the acromion to the elbow. The test is positive if the straight edge can rest simultaneously on the acromial tip of the shoulder and the lateral epicondyle of the elbow (*dots*). The test is significant for dislocation of the shoulder.

Assessment for Overuse Injury to the Supraspinatus or Biceps Tendons

Comment

The most common shoulder disorders are relatively easy to diagnose with thorough history taking, structured clinical examination, and plain-film radiographs. The increasing availability of specialist imaging and arthroscopy have enabled a more accurate assessment of shoulder disorders than was previously possible (Frost, Michael Robinson, 2006).

The terms used for impingement lesions had led to confusion. Many names and causes for this condition have been cited, including *bursitis, tendinopathy, acute trauma, overuse, instability, aging, tendon degeneration, vascular deficiencies,* and *mechanical impingement* (Table 4-4). The rotator cuff is the only tendon situated between two bones.

ORTHOPEDIC GAMUT 4-22

IMPINGEMENT SYNDROME

The four stages of impingement syndrome are as follows:

Phase 1: Edema and swelling (correlated with overuse tendonitis from activities requiring repetitive overhead arm action)

Phase 2: Thickening and fibrosis (correlated with incomplete thickness rotator cuff tears)

Phase 3: Comprises complete thickness tearing and bone changes (Fig. 4-119)

Phase 4: Cuff tear arthropathy (occurs in a small percentage of neglected cuff tears) (Fig. 4-120)

The clinical presentations with impingement syndrome are recognized in young patients involved in activities using repetitive overhead arm motion. They become sore, and at times, a patient is unable to continue because of the pain that accompanies use of the arm at the level of the shoulder.

The differential diagnosis of rotator cuff impingement is adhesive capsulitis, nerve compression (C5–C6 disc) (Fig. 4-121), suprascapular neuropathy or other brachial plexus lesions, and shoulder instability.

The subacromial space is the most common site for impingement syndrome of symptoms in older active adults. This condition is usually associated with degenerative changes in the rotator cuff (Fig. 4-122,*A*).

Phase-2 impingement occurs more commonly in patients who are 35 to 50 years of age. Evidence of degeneration and fibrosis of the supraspinatus tendon and biceps tendon is noted (Fig. 4-122,*B*). Calcium salt deposition can and often does occur within the still intact supraspinatus tendon (Fig. 4-123).

Phase-3 impingement involves a complete tear of the rotator cuff, most commonly the supraspinatus tendon (Fig. 4-122,*C*), less commonly the subscapularis tendon.

Deposition of calcium salts occurs within the intact supraspinatus tendon in calcific tendonitis. Usually occurring in middle age, calcific tendonitis produces severe pain over the anterolateral aspect of the shoulder, which may be refractory even to potent analgesics. Pain is aggravated by shoulder movements, and secondary impingement may be present. Pain may cause global restriction of active movement in the acute phase, though passive movements are preserved. Calcium deposits seen on plain-film radiographs are diagnostic (Frost, Michael Robinson, 2006).

Tenosynovitis of the LHB is a common cause of shoulder pain in adults older than 40. This condition also may occur in young athletes from repeated strains, such as those caused

---

TABLE 4-4

CLINICAL PRESENTATIONS OF THE MOST COMMON SHOULDER CONDITIONS

Disorder	Age Group Affected	Key Diagnostic Features
Rotator cuff impingement	Middle age	Painful arc within full ROM
Rotator cuff tear	Middle age and older adults	Selective weakness of supraspinatus/infraspinatus
Frozen shoulder	Middle age	Restriction of passive ROM/external rotation
Calcific tendonitis	Middle age	Severe pain; full passive ROM; calcific deposit on radiograph
Acromioclavicular osteoarthrosis	Middle age and older adults	Pain over joint; radiographic changes
Glenohumeral osteoarthrosis	Middle age and older adults	Loss of passive ROM; radiographic changes
Shoulder instability	<40 yrs	Recurrent dislocation or subluxation symptoms Clinical signs of instability

ROM, Range of motion.
Adapted from Frost A, Michael Robinson C: The painful shoulder, *Surgery (Oxford)* 24(11):363-367, 2006.

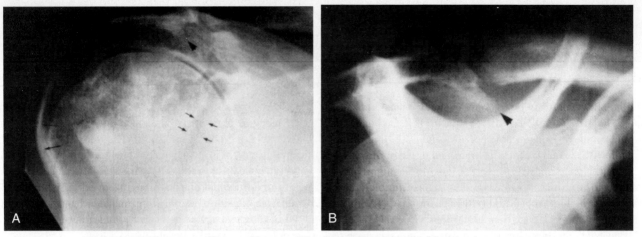

FIG. 4-119 Rotator cuff tear with stage III impingement. **A,** Calcification is seen extending into the superior portion of the coracoacromial ligament. **B,** This type III hooked acromion is the most common shape associated with tearing of the rotator cuff. (From Nicholas JA, Hershman EB, editors: *The upper extremity in sports medicine,* St Louis, 1990, Mosby.)

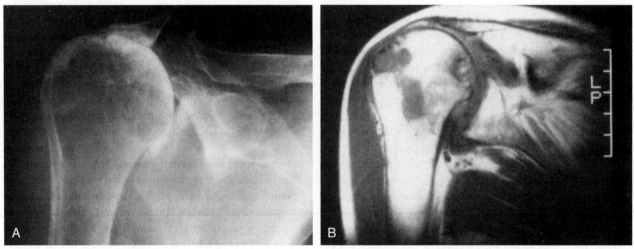

FIG. 4-120 Rotator cuff tear arthropathy with loss of the supraspinatus and superior migration of the humeral head. **A,** The humeral head thins out the acromion as a new facet is formed superiorly. The humeral head can no longer be fixed within the glenoid for adequate elevation or use of the intact deltoid. **B,** Magnetic resonance imaging demonstrates roughening and necrosis of the subchondral bone. (From Nicholas JA, Hershman EB, editors: *The upper extremity in sports medicine,* St Louis, 1990, Mosby.)

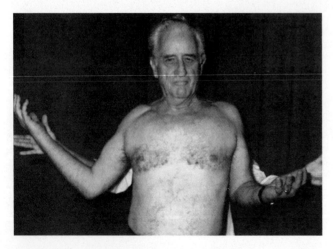

FIG. 4-121 Herniated C5–C6 disc resulting in external rotation weakness mimics rotator cuff tear of the left shoulder. Once the arms are released, the left arm falls in toward the stomach, demonstrating passive but not active external rotation. (From Nicholas JA, Hershman EB, editors: *The upper extremity in sports medicine,* St Louis, 1990, Mosby.)

4

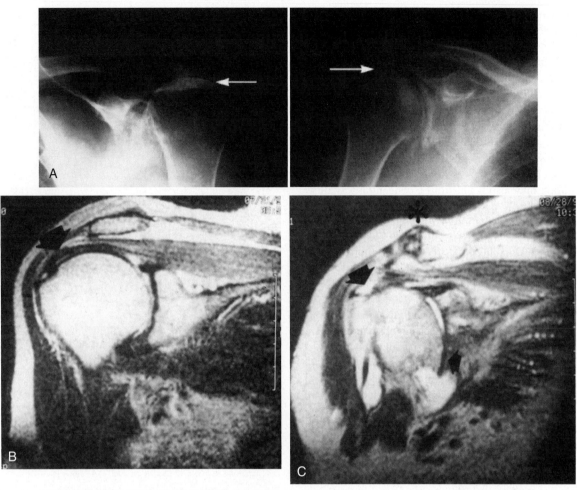

FIG. 4-122 **A,** Normal magnetic resonance imaging (MRI) scan of the shoulder. **B,** MRI of the shoulder showing a partial rotator cuff tear. **C,** MRI of the shoulder showing a complete tear of the rotator cuff. (From Lewis CB, Knortz KA: *Orthopedic assessment and treatment of the geriatric patient,* St Louis, 1993, Mosby.)

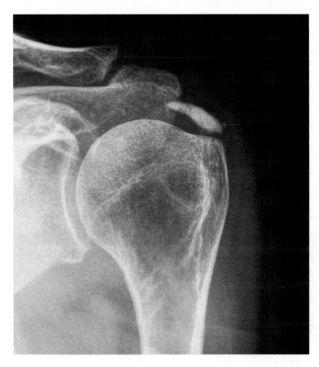

FIG. 4-123 Radiograph (anteroposterior view) of a calcific deposit within the supraspinatus tendon *(arrow).* (From Frost A, Michael Robinson C: The painful shoulder, *Surgery (Oxford)* 24[11]:363-367, 2006.)

by the throwing motion. The basic lesion is an inflammation of the tendon and its sheath in the bicipital groove. The disorder may be primary or secondary to disease of the overlying rotator cuff.

The biceps tendon may rupture as a result of advanced degeneration from chronic tendinopathy. The rupture is usually complete and may follow a forceful contraction of the biceps muscle.

The biceps tendon may occasionally dislocate from the bicipital groove. The usual cause is a tear in the overlying subscapularis tendon as the result of degenerative changes. The condition may also result from a congenitally shallow groove. The disorder may also occur in the young patient after forceful external rotation and abduction of the shoulder. Recurrences are common and may be reproducible by the patient. Tenosynovitis often develops, leading to pain and stiffness.

PROCEDURE

- The patient's arm is slightly abducted and moved fully through flexion (Figs. 4-124 to 4-126).
- This move causes a jamming of the greater tuberosity into the anteroinferior acromial surface.
- A positive result is pain in the shoulder.
- A positive test suggests injury to the supraspinatus and sometimes to the biceps tendons.

Next Steps/Procedures

Apley test, subacromial push-button sign, supraspinatus press test, and Codman sign

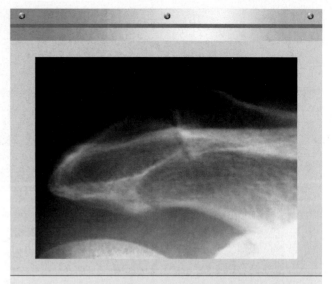

AT THE VIEWBOX

Adult male with clinical evidence of subacromial impingement syndrome. On an AP view of the right shoulder, a large subacromial osteophyte narrows the acromiohumeral interval to below the lower limits of normal (7.0 mm). This typically results in chronic impingement upon the rotator cuff, especially the supraspinatus tendon. This plain film finding is a sign of a full thickness supraspinatus tendon tear which would be directly visualized with MRI. (From the teaching file of Timothy Mick, DC, DACBR)

CLINICAL PEARL

The archaic concept of the hunching girdle rhythm as the telltale mark of supraspinatus rupture needs to be discarded. Without resistance, a decrease in the range of motion may not be apparent. Motion must always be assessed against resistance. The presence of consistent weakness helps differentiate a tear from simple chronic tendinopathy.

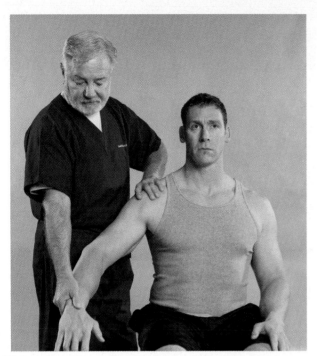

FIG. 4-124 The patient is seated comfortably with the arms at the sides. The examiner slightly abducts the patient's affected arm moving it through forward flexion.

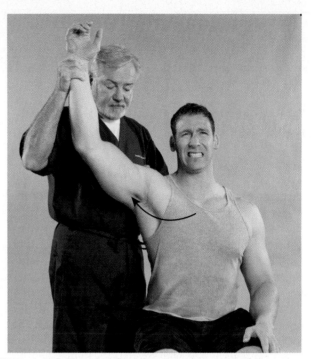

FIG. 4-125 Forward flexion causes jamming of the greater tuberosity against the anteroinferior acromial surface. Pain in the shoulder is a positive result. A positive test indicates an overuse injury to the supraspinatus and sometimes the biceps tendon.

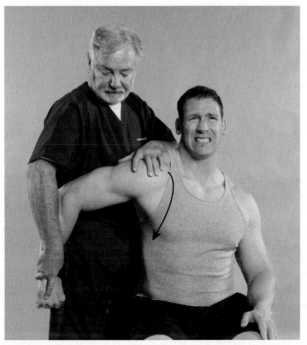

FIG. 4-126 As an alternative, the examiner can internally rotate the affected shoulder. This rotation occurs while the shoulder is abducted to 90 degrees and flexed at the elbow. The arm also can be moved into flexion, which will produce the same jamming effect.

LUDINGTON TEST

Assessment for Rupture of the Long Head of the Biceps Tendon

Comment

Although commonly diagnosed, bicipital tendinopathy is not often seen in isolation and usually occurs in association with rotator cuff tendinopathy or impingement or with glenohumeral instability. The bicipital tendon acts as a secondary stabilizer of the humeral head, and the translational movement seen with glenohumeral laxity can place increased stress on the tendon, leading to tendinopathy.

Pain is usually felt over the anterior aspect of the shoulder, often radiating into the biceps muscle with well-localized tenderness over the tendon as it runs in the bicipital groove. Pain is felt with overhead activities and often with shoulder extension and elbow flexion. Examination may reveal features of impingement, rotator cuff tendinopathy, and instability, all of which are important in determining the cause of bicipital tendinopathy. Pain may be reproduced with resisted elbow flexion, supination, and shoulder flexion. Passive shoulder extension stretches the biceps and may be painful. Rupture of the tendon is evident with the characteristic deformity of the upper arm with bunching up of the lateral muscle belly of the biceps best seen with resisted elbow flexion and supination.

Acute rupture of the transverse humeral ligament can result in subluxation or dislocation of the tendon. This circumstance can produce symptoms similar to bicipital tendinopathy, but often a more specific complaint is made of catching and a clicking sensation at the shoulder. Clinical examination may demonstrate subluxation of the tendon, which is felt as the arm is passively moved through internal and external rotation while in the 90-degree abducted position. Medial dislocation of the tendon is often found in association with tears of the subscapularis tendon.

The tendon of the LHB may be involved at several sites: its attachment to the superior glenoid labrum, which may be injured in a fall or throwing action (superior labrum anteroposterior lesion); as it runs across the glenohumeral joint (intraarticular); or as it runs in the bicipital groove (extraarticular). The transverse humeral ligament stabilizes the tendon in the bicipital groove, and if this mechanism is disrupted, subluxation or dislocation of the tendon can result, which tends to occur as the arm is rotated in the abducted position. The tendon can become inflamed, thickened, and fibrotic in chronic cases. Older patients may have attenuation and thinning of the tendon, and rupture may eventually ensue (Fig. 4-127). This latter presentation is almost always indicative of underlying rotator cuff degeneration as the bicipital tendon appears to become stressed in its attempt to

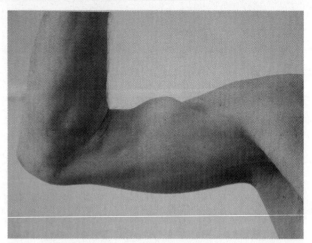

FIG. 4-127 Rupture of the long head of biceps *(Popeye sign)*. (Source: David Potter, Northern General Hospital, Sheffield, UK. From Frost A, Michael Robinson C: The painful shoulder. *Surgery (Oxford)* 24[11]:363-367, 2006.)

act as a humeral head depressor in cases of rotator cuff incompetence. In addition, the presence of a complete rotator cuff tear exposes the intraarticular portion of the bicipital tendon to the overlying acromion and further impingement.

Acute rupture of the LHB tendon may occur in older patients, which causes a characteristic visible lump over the mid biceps *(Popeye sign)*. The rupture is usually managed conservatively in elderly patients, although early surgical repair should be considered in younger athletes (Frost, Michael Robinson, 2006).

PROCEDURE

- The patient clasps both hands behind the head.
- The biceps tendons are in resting positions.
- The patient alternately contracts and relaxes the biceps muscles.
- As the patient contracts the muscles, the examiner palpates the biceps tendons (Fig. 4-128).
- The tendon will be felt to contract on the uninvolved side but not on the affected side.
- A positive test result is the loss of tendon contraction.
- A positive test suggests rupture of the LHB tendon.

Next Steps/Procedures

Abbott-Saunders test, Speed test, transverse humeral ligament test, and Yergason test

CLINICAL PEARL

A double defect sometimes occurs, with the cuff giving way from the tuberosity on both sides of the tendon. Cuff laxity at this point seriously interferes with biceps function, and the tendon may slip medially over the lesser tuberosity and off the head.

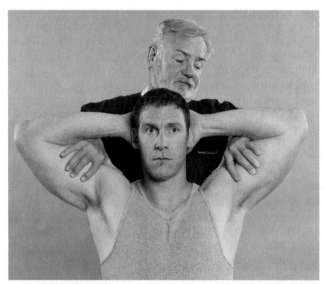

FIG. 4-128 Seated, the patient clasps both hands behind the head. The patient contracts and relaxes the biceps muscles. During this action, the examiner palpates the biceps tendons. The test is positive if tendon contraction is absent on the affected side. A positive test suggests a rupture of the long head of the biceps tendon.

ALSO KNOWN AS SHOULDER ROCK TEST

Assessment for Significant Pathologic Process of the Shoulder

Comment

Pain felt in the cervicobrachial area may extend from the occiput to the arm or, at times, to the upper anterior chest and back.

Muscle strain and nerve root compression often follow this distribution. Tendinopathy, arthritis, and trigger points usually cause a more localized discomfort that enables the patient to pinpoint the source of the pathologic process. One notable exception is the pain of acute subdeltoid bursitis. In this condition, the patient thinks that the discomfort can be located precisely in the musculature of the upper arm, but tenderness is always over the inflamed area, several centimeters higher, and beneath the acromion. Having the patient characterize the onset of the pain, including whether it was precipitated by acute or repeated trauma to the shoulder and neck, narrows the differential diagnosis. For example, continuous use of the arm above the head predisposes it to bursitis or tendinopathy. Acute injury, of course, can result in obvious fractures or dislocations. Lacerations of the rotator cuff may be more elusive. Sudden lifting of a heavy object is all that is needed to tear the subacromial tendons.

Shoulder pain brought on by exertion, especially if the upper extremities are not being used, is more apt to be caused by coronary insufficiency than by a localized pathologic process.

The clinical history may be the key to diagnosis. For example, adhesive capsulitis follows immobilization of the joint, shoulder-arm-hand syndrome is a complication of myocardial infarction, and fibromyositis is associated with emotional tension. Shoulder pain of arthritis and polymyalgia rheumatica is insidious at the onset. The pain from both of the conditions is worse in the morning when the patient arises from sleep. Other disorders may be worse during the day. The temporal relationships of the pain are important to the diagnosis. Pain severity, constancy, and migratory nature are also important.

The most common complaint of patients with arthritis of the shoulder is pain (Figs. 4-129 and 4-130). Typically, the pattern of pain is worsened with activities and somewhat relieved by rest. Patients often complain of night pain during recumbency. The examiner should inquire about a medication history with particular attention to oral steroids, which may cause osteonecrosis. Patients with rheumatoid arthritis are affected by mechanical changes from rotator cuff dys-

function, as well as joint destruction in the glenohumeral joint. A general history combined with a physical examination should allow the examiner to limit the number of ancillary diagnostic tests to determine the cause of the arthritic condition. Patients should be examined in a relaxed atmosphere with full visualization of the entire upper trunk. Observation of range of motion with notation of scapulothoracic rhythm is helpful in determining what portion of the range is coming from the glenohumeral joint. Muscle examination includes strength measurement and examination for wasting or atrophy. Rotator cuff integrity, stability, and the patient's ability to perform activities such as combing hair, reaching the buttock, and dressing are assessed. Particular attention should be paid to loss of rotation.

Synovial cysts (or ganglions) are benign cystic tumors originating from articular joints or tendon sheaths. They are typically located in the back of the wrist and foot, but they can occur in other locations as the knee, coxofemoral, and glenohumeral joints. Acromioclavicular juxtaarticular cysts have been described in association with full-thickness rotator cuff tears and a degenerated acromioclavicular joint. These cysts often present as a supraclavicular mass (Moratalla, Gabarda, in press).

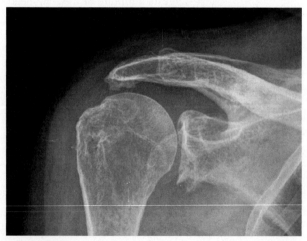

FIG. 4-129 X-ray demonstrated acromioclavicular sclerosis, osteophytes in the inferior aspect of the acromion, subchondral geodes in the humeral head, elevation of the humeral head, decrease of the subacromial space, glenohumeral sclerosis, and glenoid osteophytes. (From Moratalla MB, Gabarda RF: Acromioclavicular joint ganglion, *Eur J Radiol Extra* 63[1]:21–23, 2007.)

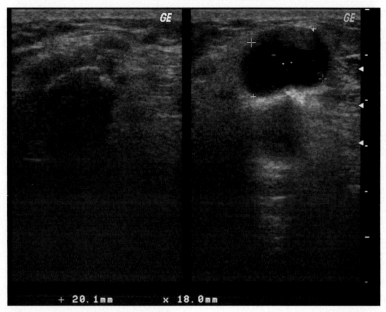

FIG. 4-130 Ultrasound of same shoulder shows a supraclavicular mass of 2 cm of diameter, cystic and well-delimitated, adjacent to acromioclavicular joint. (Adapted from Moratalla MB, Gabarda RF: Acromioclavicular joint ganglion, *Eur J Radiol Extra* 63[1]:21–23, 2007.)

PROCEDURE

- While standing or sitting, the patient places the palm of the affected upper limb over the top of the opposite clavicle (Fig. 4-131).
- From this position, the patient moves the elbow from the chest to the forehead, giving it an inferior to superior rocking motion (Figs. 4-132 and 4-133).
- The maneuver is positive if this action produces or aggravates shoulder or arm pain on the ipsilateral side.
- The pain of any significant pathologic process of the shoulder will be intensified and localized by this maneuver.

Next Steps/Procedures

Apprehension test, Bryant sign, Calloway test, Dugas test, Hamilton test, and diagnostic imaging

CLINICAL PEARL

Adhesive capsulitis is a common but poorly understood affliction of the glenohumeral joint. Capsulitis is characterized by pain and uniform limitation of all movements but without radiographic change and with a tendency to a slow spontaneous recovery. No evidence of inflammatory or destructive change has been found.

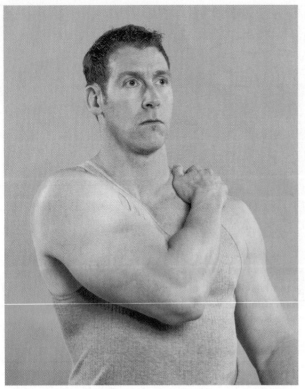

FIG. 4-131 While seated, the patient places the palm of the hand of the affected shoulder over the top of the opposite clavicle.

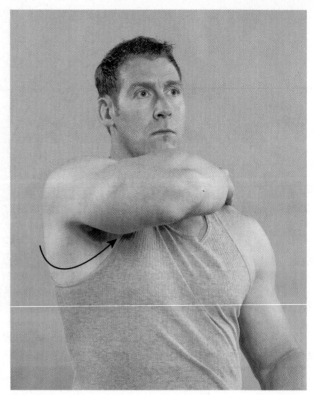

FIG. 4-132 The patient moves the elbow of the affected side from the chest toward the forehead.

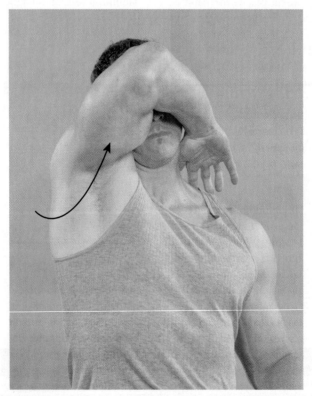

FIG. 4-133 This movement provides an inferior to superior rocking motion. The maneuver is positive if this action produces or aggravates shoulder or arm pain on the ipsilateral side. This maneuver will intensify and localize the pain of any significant shoulder disease.

Assessment for Cervical Foraminal Compression and Interscalene Compression

Comment

TOS is a disorder characterized by compression of the subclavian artery, vein, or brachial plexus separately or, rarely, in combination. This compression results in a vascular or neurogenic syndrome, depending on which structure is involved. Neurogenic TOS is a neurologic syndrome caused by compression of the lower brachial plexus.

True, or classic, neurogenic TOS is usually caused by a congenital band that originates from the tip of the rudimentary cervical rib and inserts into the first rib. In this form, objective clinical and electrophysiologic evidence peripheral nerve fiber injury can be found that is usually limited to the lower trunk of the plexus. The typical patient is a young woman with weakness of the hand and wasting of the thenar more than the hypothenar eminence who experiences variable pain and paresthesia in the medial aspect of the upper extremity. Symptoms commonly are exacerbated by upper extremity activity. Multiple compression sites have been described, resulting in many *syndromes* (Fig. 4-134).

Electrodiagnostic examination is the most useful and objective diagnostic procedure in the diagnosis of neurogenic TOS. The compression results in a chronic, axon-loss, lower trunk brachial plexopathy (Fig. 4-135). Because all ulnar sensory fibers, all ulnar motor fibers, and the C8–T1 median fibers course the lower trunk, they are among the most obviously noted abnormalities on routine nerve conduction study.

A cervical rib is a congenital overdevelopment, bony or fibrous, of the costal process of the seventh cervical vertebra. A cervical rib often exists without causing symptoms, especially in the young. However, in adults, the tendency for gradual drooping of the shoulder girdle may lead to neurologic or vascular disturbance in the upper limb.

The overdeveloped costal process may be unilateral or bilateral, and it can range in size from a small bony protrusion, often with a fibrous extension, to a complete supernumerary rib. The subclavian artery and the lowest trunk of the brachial plexus arch over the rib. In some cases, the nerve trunk suffers damage at the site of pressure against the rib, which accounts for the neurologic manifestations. The vascular changes are accounted for by local damage to the subclavian artery, from which thrombotic emboli may be repeatedly discharged into the peripheral vessels of the upper limb.

A cervical rib is often symptomless. When symptoms occur, they usually begin during adult life. They may be neurologic, vascular, or combined.

Congenital fibrous band linking cervical ribs or elongated transverse process of C7 to the first rib is considered to be the cause of compression or stretching of the C7–T1 or lower trunk of the brachial plexus in patients with true neurogenic TOS. Patients with nonspecific neurogenic TOS may exhibit anomalies of the first rib that are considered by the advocates of this syndrome to be the common denominator on which many compressive factors can act (Colli et al, 2006).

ORTHOPEDIC GAMUT 4-23

OTHER ANATOMOPATHOLOGIC CAUSES IN NEUROGENIC THORACIC OUTLET SYNDROME

- Anomalous first rib
- Sibson fascia
- Small branches of the subclavian artery or thyrocervical trunk
- Scalene muscles

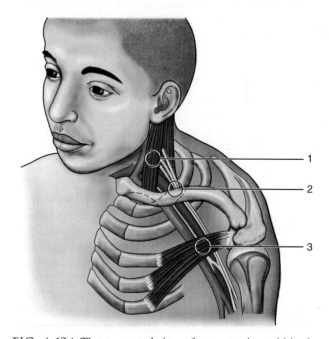

FIG. 4-134 The presumed sites of compression within the cervicoaxillary canal for the *scalenus anticus syndrome: 1,* Interscalene triangle, the costoclavicular syndrome; *2,* between the first rib and the clavicle; and *3,* the hyperabduction syndrome, beneath the pectoralis minor tendon. (Adapted from Katirji B: *Electromyography in clinical practice: a case study approach,* St Louis, 1998, Mosby.)

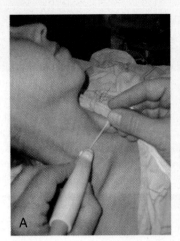
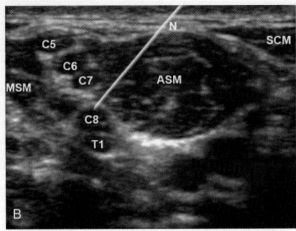

FIG. 4-135 Ultrasound-guided interscalene block. **A,** In this example, the needle is introduced from an antero-medial to postero-lateral direction, in-plane with the transducer, which is held in an axial oblique orientation. **B,** Ultrasound scan of real-time needle guidance during interscalene block. (N) needle (enhanced with photo editing for emphasis); (C5–T1) cervical and first thoracic nerve roots; (ASM) anterior scalene muscle; (MSM) middle scalene muscle; (SCM) sternocleidomastoid muscle. (From Orebaugh SL, Bigeleisen P: Ultrasound imaging in brachial plexus blockade, *Semin Anesth Periop Med Pain* 26(4):180-188, 2007.)

ORTHOPEDIC GAMUT 4-24

UPPER EXTREMITY NEUROGENIC SYNDROMES

The important alternative causes of upper extremity neurogenic syndromes include:

1. Central lesions (tumors involving the spinal cord or its roots)
2. Plexus lesions (tumors at the thoracic inlet Pancoast tumor)
3. Distal nerve lesions (friction neuritis of the ulnar nerve at the elbow)
4. Pressure on the median nerve in the carpal tunnel

The sensory symptoms are pain and paresthesia in the forearm and hand. These symptoms are most marked toward the medial (ulnar) side and are often relieved temporarily by changing the position of the arm. The motor symptoms include increasing weakness of the hand with difficulty carrying out the finer movements.

Usually an area of sensory impairment and sometimes complete anesthesia occurs in the forearm and hand. The affected area does not correspond in distribution to any of the peripheral nerves but may be related to the lowest trunk of the brachial plexus. Atrophy of the muscles of the thenar eminence or of the interosseous and hypothenar muscles may be present.

The vascular changes observed range from dusky cyanosis of the forearm and hand to gangrene of the fingers. The radial pulse may be weak or absent.

Occasionally the neurologic manifestations characteristic of a cervical rib occur without a demonstrable skeletal deformity. The manifestations may have been ascribed to trapping of the nerves between the first rib and the clavicle (costoclavicular compression) or between the first rib and the scalenus anterior muscle or to stretching of the lowest trunk of the brachial plexus over the normal first rib. They are more often caused by a tough fibrous band in the scalenus medius muscle that may lead to kinking of the lowest trunk of the brachial plexus. The symptoms are easily confused with those from a prolapsed intervertebral disc between C7 and T1.

PROCEDURE

- While in the seated position, the patient actively places the palm of the affected extremity on top of the head, raising the elbow to a height approximately level with the head (Fig. 4-136).
- By elevating the arm, interscalene compression increases.
- The sign is present when the radiating pain appears or is worsened with this maneuver (Fig. 4-137).
- The sign helps differentiate between cervical foraminal compression and interscalene compression.

Next Steps/Procedures

Adson test, Allen maneuver, costoclavicular maneuver, George screening procedure, Halstead maneuver, Roos test, shoulder compression test, and Wright test

CLINICAL PEARL

Radiographs will show the abnormal rib. If it is small, the abnormal rib is clearly observed in the oblique projections. In cases of suspected vascular obstruction, arteriography is required.

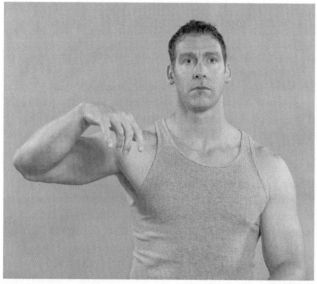

FIG. 4-136 While seated, the patient abducts and externally rotates the affected shoulder, moving the hand toward the top of the head.

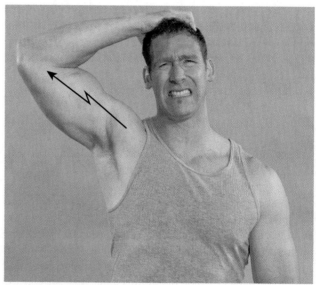

FIG. 4-137 The hand is placed on top of the head. The increase of pain in this position is a positive sign and indicates interscalene compression of the lower branches of the brachial plexus.

ROOS TEST

Assessment for Thoracic Outlet Syndrome

Comment

TOS produces many well-known neurologic complications. Sympathetic nervous system problems of the upper extremities such as vasomotor changes, complex regional pain syndrome and hyperhidrosis may be observed as a result of the compression of the sympathetic nerve fibers of the brachial plexus. However, sympathetic nervous system of the heart may also be affected in these patients (Kaymak et al, 2004).

TOS complex refers to a series of neurovascular compression syndromes in the shoulder region. TOS is recognized as an entrapment compression vasculopathy of the subclavian vessels, which more commonly involves the lower trunk or medial cord of the brachial plexus at any one of four sites (Fig. 4-138).

Costoclavicular syndrome occurs with compression of the subclavian artery, subclavian vein, and brachial plexus as they pass between the clavicle and the first rib. This syndrome is separate from the anterior scalene syndrome because of the vascular involvement.

The triangular costoclavicular space connects the cervical spine with the upper extremity and is called the *canalis cervico axillaris*. The boundaries of this space are as follows: anteriorly, the medial third of the clavicle and the subclavius muscle; posteriorly, the upper margin of the scapula; and posteromedially, the anterior third of the first rib and the insertions of the anterior and medial scalene muscles. The neurovascular bundle runs in the medial angle of this triangle. The subclavian vein lies medially in front of the anterior scalenus insertion on the first rib and deep to the costoclavicular ligament and thickening of the clavipectoral fascia, which extends from the coracoid process to the first rib (costocoracoid ligament). The subclavian artery briefly enters this space via the posterior scalene foramen to lie lateral to the subclavian vein. Passing between the anterior and medial scalene muscles, the brachial plexus joins the vascular bundle in the costoclavicular space.

When the costoclavicular space becomes narrowed by disease or dynamic compression, the neuromuscular struc-

---

ORTHOPEDIC GAMUT 4-25

COSTOCLAVICULAR NEUROVASCULAR SPACE

The following actions narrow the costoclavicular neurovascular space:
1. Raising the arm rotates the clavicle posteriorly into the space.
2. Displacing the shoulder posteriorly and interiorly rotates the clavicle posteriorly.
3. Inhaling deeply raises the first rib into the space because the clavicle does not rise with inspiration.

---

tures are compromised. Although congenital anomalies are associated with TOS, functional or dynamic anatomy predominates as a cause for clinical disease.

Patients with costoclavicular syndrome have subjective complaints similar to those of the anterior scalene syndrome (scalenus anticus syndrome). Although the neurologic complaints of pain, paresthesia, and hyperesthesia dominate in the anterior scalene syndrome, vascular symptoms dominate in the costoclavicular syndrome. Vein compression leads to temporary or permanent edema.

Clinical examination relies on the radial pulse evaluation, which occurs when the patient thrusts the chest forward and posteriorly and interiorly pulls the shoulders. Typically, the pulse weakens or disappears.

Roos test causes narrowing of the costoclavicular space and tightening of the cervical muscles, including scalenus anterior; thus, compression of the stellate ganglion that is localized in this space or the postganglionic efferent fibers that innervate the heart may cause cardiac arrhythmias according to the affected side. Stimulation of the right stellate ganglion results in an increase in the heart rate causing sinus tachycardia. On the other hand, when the left stellate ganglion is exposed to stimulation, a transient increase occurs in the heart rate; at the same time Q-T interval is prolonged and it causes cardiac arrhythmia (Kaymak et al, 2004).

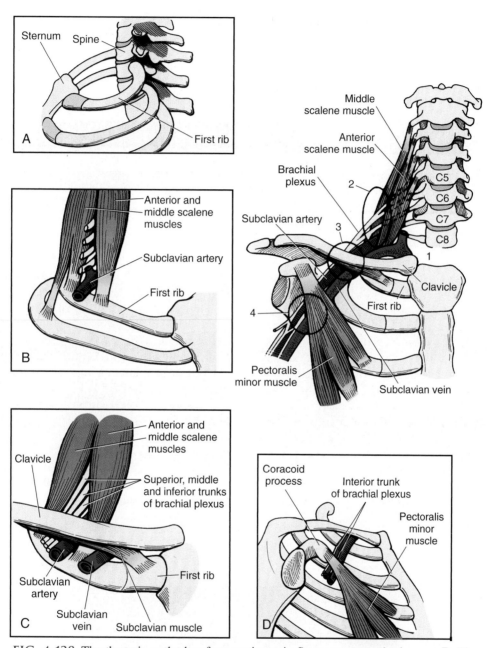

FIG. 4-138 The thoracic outlet has four sections. **A,** Sternocostovertebral space. **B,** The scalene triangle. **C,** The costoclavicular space. **D,** The coraco pectoral space. (From Saidoff DC, McDonough AL: *Critical pathways in therapeutic intervention,* St Louis, 1997, Mosby.)

PROCEDURE

- While in the seated position, the patient positions both arms at 90 degrees and abducts and externally rotates them (Fig. 4-139).
- The patient repeatedly opens and closes the fists for up to 3 minutes (Fig. 4-140).
- If this maneuver reproduces the usual symptoms of discomfort, the patient probably has TOS (Fig. 4-141).

Next Steps/Procedures

Adson test, Allen maneuver, costoclavicular maneuver, George screening procedure, Halstead maneuver, reverse Bakody maneuver, shoulder compression test, and Wright test

CLINICAL PEARL

Because all of the neurologic, arterial, and venous symptoms are consistently aggravated by both exercise and arm elevation, the most reliable test for the diagnosis of TOS is the 3-minute elevated-arm stress test (EAST).

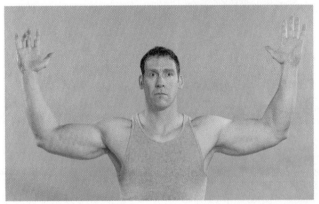

FIG. 4-139 While in the seated position, the patient places both arms in the 90-degree abducted and externally rotated position.

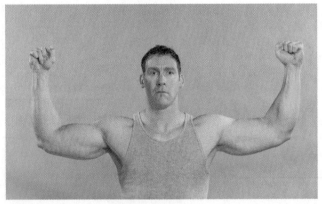

FIG. 4-140 The patient repeatedly opens and closes the fists slowly for 3 minutes.

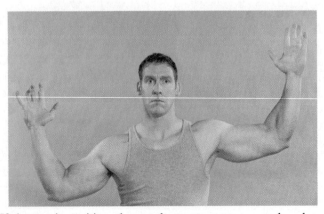

FIG. 4-141 If the test is positive, the usual symptoms are reproduced and the affected arm weakens. A positive test indicates TOS.

Assessment for Hyperabduction Type of Thoracic Outlet Syndromes

Comment

The diagnosis of TOS is a clinical one that is largely reached by exclusion.

Vessels and nerves that travel from the thoracocervical region to the axilla must run between the anterior and middle scalene muscle, through the costoclavicular space, and under the pectoralis minor tendon. Several anatomic or functional characteristics can produce further narrowing of these three channels during elevation of the upper limbs, causing compression of the vessels and nerves. This entrapment syndrome has become known as TOS. The clinical spectrum of TOS is extremely broad, ranging from severe compression with permanent vascular or nervous lesions (or both) to intermittent postural symptoms without organic damage. This milder picture is probably the more common. TOS is readily recognized when electrophysiologic studies or vascular evaluation by ultrasonography or angiography show a permanent proximal lesion (Gillard et al, 2001).

Ulnar nerve entrapment is suggested by nocturnal numbness, but patients never have sensory loss in the proximal or middle portions of the forearm. In addition, patients with ulnar nerve entrapment have no atrophy of the intrinsic muscles innervated by the median nerve in the thenar eminence. Carpal tunnel syndrome also can cause thenar atrophy, but the sensory loss, if present, occurs in the first two digits. Carpal tunnel syndrome is also differentiated from TOS by electrophysiologic studies indicating distal, not proximal, compression. In C8 cervical radiculopathy, compression occurs with an almost identical pattern of T1 nerve fibers as in TOS. Neck pain, triceps weakness, reduced triceps reflex, and weakness of finger extensors provide a clue toward involvement of the C8 nerve root. Intramedullary or extramedullary spinal cord process such as syringomyelia, glioma of the spinal cord, extramedullary cervical tumor, infarction of the spinal cord, or meningioma in the foramen magnum may mimic TOS.

Pancoast tumor, also known as *pulmonary superior sulcus tumor*, is accompanied by rapid and severe weakness of all of the small muscles of the hand and, in advanced cases, results in radiographically visible cancerous erosion of the first and second ribs, as well as possible hoarseness attributable to paralysis of one vocal cord.

Clavipectoral compression syndrome is a disorder that produces shoulder and other radiating symptoms but does not belong to the cervical root or scalenus or cervical rib classes. The syndrome resembles the latter because the findings suggest a vascular or neurovascular cause.

Many forms of clavipectoral compression have been erroneously called *scalene* or cervical rib lesions. However, further distinguishing features separate these conditions. The complete cause and pathologic features have not been firmly established; thus, classification relies largely on clinical attributes.

The symptom common to the group as a whole is paresthesia, or numbness and tingling, in the hand and fingers. Paresthesia develops after vague shoulder discomfort. The peripheral portion of the extremity, forearm, hand, and fingers quickly becomes the seat of the prominent discomfort, and the shoulder symptoms fade. The paresthesia follows no well-defined distribution, and the pattern is indistinct, particularly compared with the pain or numbness of peripheral nerve lesions. Both sides are often involved. The vascular contribution is exhibited by coldness, cyanotic hue, and crampy pain on effort. Writer's cramp is an example. Many of the symptoms and disorders have a striking relation to the position of the arm or the head. In many instances, the abducted position of the arm at work or rest is a potent irritant.

The fundamental pathologic process common to the group is stretching and compression of the neurovascular bundle at some point in the periclavicular, not clavicular, course. This possibility above the clavicle has been acknowledged in cervical rib and scalene lesions, but the fact that a similar disturbance may arise behind and below the clavicle as well has not been generally recognized. Pressure on the neurovascular bundle along the cervicoaxillary canal may develop directly behind the clavicle, below the clavicle, or behind the pectoralis minor. The bundle lies on a firm bed along its entire course, but the structures on top of it move in three separate zones. Superiorly, the clavicle rolls up and down and may pinch vessels on the first rib. Lower down, the costocoracoid membrane, as a remnant of the precoracoid primitive form, may tighten on the bundle through its connections with the enveloping fascia. Still more distally,

---

ORTHOPEDIC GAMUT 4-26

THORACIC OUTLET

The following signs generally do not implicate the thoracic outlet:

1. Long tract signs such as brisk reflexes or extensor plantar response
2. Loss of tendon reflexes in the arms
3. Horner syndrome
4. Weakness of the upper arm or shoulder

the sharp edge of the pectoralis minor may become the compressing force or fulcrum. A soft bundle on a hard bed is easily crushed by these structures. Several special types of compression may be recognized: costoclavicular, postural, and hyperabduction. These conditions are to be differentiated from carpal tunnel syndrome, in which no shoulder involvement occurs, and the numbness and tingling are clearly confined to the median nerve distribution.

Patients with hyperabduction syndrome are usually young males of short, stocky stature who work long hours with the arms held above the shoulder level. Shoulder pain and finger paresthesia develop. In some instances, the discomfort appears without extreme abduction. Some patients are more prone than others to develop these symptoms. Patients prone to this condition are easily separated from the rest by their medical history, their youth, and the characteristically easy obliteration of the pulse during abduction.

PROCEDURE

- While the patient is seated upright, the examiner palpates the distal apex of the coracoid process and marks it with a flesh pencil (Fig. 4-142).
- With a hypothenar contact, the examiner applies downward pressure over the marked area (Fig. 4-143).
- Production of symptoms that are similar to neurovascular compression of the subclavian artery and brachial plexus constitutes a positive test.
- The test is significant for coracoid pressure syndrome, which is identical to the hyperabduction type of TOSs.

Next Steps/Procedures
Adson test, Allen maneuver, costoclavicular test, George screening procedure, Halstead maneuver, reverse Bakody maneuver, Roos test, and Wright test

CLINICAL PEARL

The neurovascular bundle may be compressed in the zone distal to the clavicle as the bundle passes beneath the costocoracoid membrane and pectoralis minor. The pectoralis minor has a particular contribution in this process and is a significant factor in creating the shoulder and radiating symptoms. A patient's degree of skeletal maturation has a great influence on the type of fracture that may result from trauma and the concern physicians have about the sequelae of such injuries. First, the relative softness of the bones of newborns and toddlers increases the likelihood of trauma producing a *greenstick fracture* rather than an ordinary fracture completely separating the two bone fragments. Another crucial consideration in the evaluation of fractures in children is the possible involvement of the epiphyseal plates of the bone in the fracture. If the line of a fracture crosses one of these areas of bone growth, the post–healing alignment of the bone on opposite sides of the plate is disturbed, and the subsequent growth and development of the bone will be asymmetric.

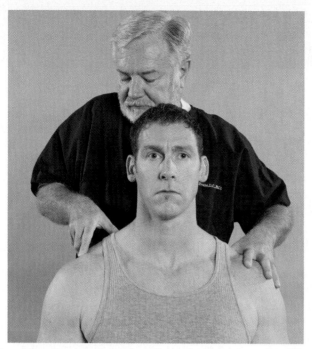

FIG. 4-142 The patient is seated comfortably with the arms at the sides. The examiner palpates the distal apex of the coracoid process and marks it.

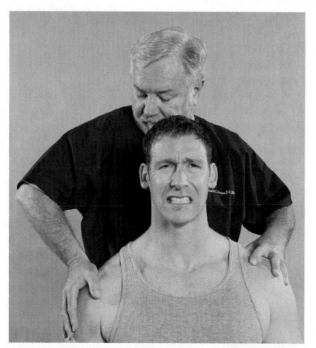

FIG. 4-143 With a hypothenar contact, the examiner applies downward pressure over the marked area. If the symptoms produced are similar to neurovascular compression of the subclavian artery and brachial plexus, this constitutes a positive test. The test is significant for coracoid pressure syndrome, which is identical to the hyperabduction type of TOSs.

Assessment for Bicipital Tendinopathy

Comment

The bicipital groove is between the greater and lesser tuberosities and lies along the anterior aspect of the surface of the humerus. The bicipital groove demonstrates varying configurations, depending on the height of the medial wall of the groove, formed by the lesser tuberosity (Fig. 4-144).

The LHB arises by a long, narrow tendon from the supraglenoid tubercle of the scapula. The long head passes through the shoulder joint and emerges from it to lie in the intertubercular sulcus (bicipital groove), where it is restrained by the transverse humeral ligament. The LHB is subject to the same type of impingement as the supraspinatus tendon, which can produce biceps tendon instability or subluxation (or both) from the bicipital groove (Fig. 4-145). Differentiating between impingement of the LHB tendon and impingement of the supraspinatus tendon is initially difficult. One distinguishing feature relates to internal and external rotation of the shoulder. In cases of bicipital tendinopathy, rotation during abduction is usually painful, especially if the examiner applies slight pressure to the tendon in its groove while the patient's arm is passively maneuvered (the *biceps passive test*) (Fig. 4-146). In patients with supraspinatus tendinopathy, the internally rotated position may be painful. However, this pain will disappear when the humerus is rotated outward because the greater tubercle of the humerus no longer impinges on the acromion process *(Anguin test)*.

The slight difference in the mechanics of these two types of tendinopathy means that bicipital tendinopathy occurs more often in patients who participate in activities involving throwing or paddling. Of course, bicipital tendinopathy may occur in swimmers or other patients as well. Bicipital ten-

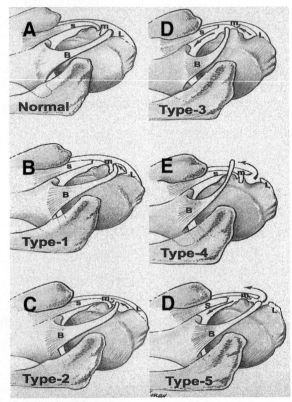

FIG. 4-145 Biceps Subluxation/Instability Classification (*s*, subscapularis; *m*, medial head coracohumeral ligament; *B*, biceps; *L*, lateral head coracohumeral ligament; arrows represent biceps subluxation/instability direction). *Type 1:* with tears of the intraarticular subscapularis tendon without involvement of the medial head of the coracohumeral ligament. *Type 2:* without tears of the intraarticular subscapularis tendon with involvement of the medial head of the coracohumeral ligament. *Type 3:* with tears of the intraarticular subscapularis tendon and with involvement of the medial head of the coracohumeral ligament. *Type 4:* with tears of the supraspinatus and the lateral head of the coracohumeral ligament. *Type 5:* with tears of the intraarticular subscapularis tendon with medial and lateral head of the coracohumeral ligament including the leading edge of the supraspinatus tendon. (From Bennett WF: Arthroscopic bicipital sheath repair: two-year follow-up with pulley lesions, *Arthroscopy* 20[9]:964-973, 2004.)

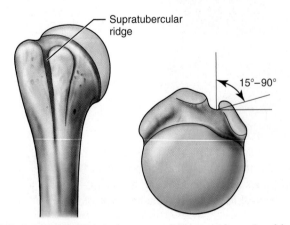

FIG. 4-144 **A,** Bicipital groove with supratubercular ridge. **B,** Angle of inclination of medial wall. (Adapted from Nicholas JA, Hershman EB, editors: *The upper extremity in sports medicine,* St Louis, 1990, Mosby.)

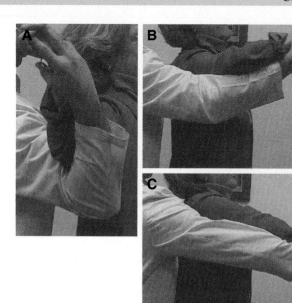

FIG. 4-146 *Biceps passive test.* The arm is cradled in the examiner's arm and brought from a position of 90 degrees of abduction with full external rotation to cross-body adduction and internal rotation while decreasing the amount of shoulder flexion. The arm and shoulder should be relaxed. The test is positive if, during the midrange of motion, the patient complains of catching, popping, or the feeling of something slipping or loose inside associated with pain. The test is not positive at the extremes of motion as pain at the extremes may indicate something different than the biceps tendon's movement in an untoward medial-lateral direction. Also, care should be taken to avoid forcing cross-body adduction. (From Bennett WF: Arthroscopic bicipital sheath repair: two-year follow-up with pulley lesions, *Arthroscopy* 20[9]:964-973, 2004.)

dinopathy is sometimes secondary to supraspinatus tendinopathy because the latter may be accompanied by inflammation that involves the nearby biceps.

PROCEDURE

- Shoulder flexion by the patient is restricted (Fig. 4-147).
- The patient further resists forearm supinating and elbow extension.
- A positive test is indicated by increased tenderness in the bicipital groove (Fig. 4-148).
- A positive test suggests bicipital tendinopathy.

Next Steps/Procedures

Abbott-Saunders test, Ludington test, transverse humeral ligament test, and Yergason test

CLINICAL PEARL

Tenosynovitis in the bicipital groove may develop into complete adherence of the tendon, which interdicts any extensive range of motion of the shoulder. The shoulder motion may remain restricted, or the biceps may rupture proximal to the groove.

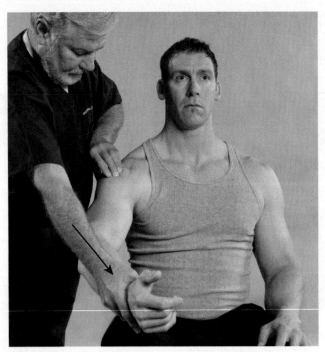

FIG. 4-147 While seated, the patient flexes the affected shoulder. The examiner then provides resistance.

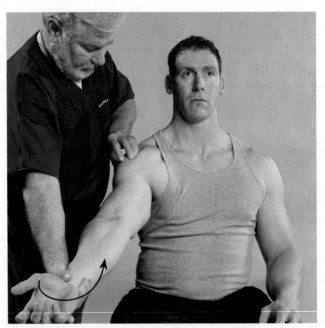

FIG. 4-148 While flexing the shoulder, the patient supinates the forearm and completely extends the elbow. A positive test elicits increased tenderness in the bicipital groove and indicates bicipital tendinitis.

SUBACROMIAL PUSH-BUTTON SIGN

ALSO KNOWN AS MAZION CUFF MANEUVER

Assessment for Rotator Cuff Tear of the Supraspinatus Tendon

Comment

Ruptures of the rotator cuff result from continued deterioration and degeneration (Table 4-5). The tear may be partial or complete.

If the rupture is partial, the clinical findings are similar to those seen in chronic tendinopathy. Even with complete rupture, the shoulder may have a full range of motion because of continued function of the other rotator muscles. Usually, however, with both partial and complete ruptures, some weakness in abduction or flexion is observed. The weakness is usually most severe in abduction because the muscle most commonly torn is the supraspinatus. If the tear is more anterior into the subscapularis, forward flexion will be weak. Actively abducting the arm more than 45 or 50 degrees may be impossible, after which further abduction is obtained by scapulothoracic motion. A painful *catch* may be noted on passive motion between 50 and 100 degrees, at which point compression of the swollen tissues between the tuberosity and the overlying arch occurs. Tenderness at the site of the tear is a common finding, and with complete ruptures, a defect in the cuff may be palpated through the deltoid muscle. Passive range of motion is often normal in the pain-free shoulder.

Atrophy of the cuff muscles is often present, and the *drop-arm* test may be positive.

Acute hemarthrosis and prominent ecchymosis down the arm may occasionally accompany longstanding rotator cuff tears, especially those with cuff-tear arthropathy, which is probably the result of further rupture with bleeding of remaining rotator cuff musculature. Chronic subdeltoid swelling usually means synovial fluid has escaped from the glenohumeral joint to the subacromial space and indicates a large rotator cuff rupture.

The rotator cuff is an almost complete tissue annulus that is attached to the humerus in the region of the anatomic neck and is formed by the fusion of the joint capsule with the musculotendinous insertions of the subscapularis in front, the supraspinatus above, and the teres minor and infraspinatus behind. The most important of these structures is the supraspinatus, which runs through a tunnel formed by the acromion and the coracoacromial ligament. The supraspinatus is separated from the acromion by part of the subdeltoid bursa.

The rotator cuff may suffer a large tear as a result of sudden traction to the arm. Such a tear occurs most readily in middle-age patients because of degenerative changes in the rotator cuff. Most commonly, the supraspinatus region is involved, and the patient has difficulty initiating abduction of the arm. In other cases, a torn or inflamed rotator cuff impinges the acromion during abduction, causing a painful arc of movement. Although the range of passive movement is not disturbed initially, limitation of rotation supersedes, so many of these cases become indistinguishable from adhesive capsulitis.

Any condition that decreases the functional space between the rotator cuff tendons and the rigid subacromial arch can cause impingement. Ultrasonography has some popularity in the evaluation of the rotator cuff. It is safe and noninvasive and is most accurate in large and moderately large tears. Magnetic resonance imaging (MRI) now plays a major role in diagnosing rotator cuff disease.

Most rotator cuff tears are associated with type-3 acromion.

TABLE 4-5	
GOUTALLIER GRADING SYSTEM OF FATTY DEGENERATION OF MUSCLE	
Stage	**Findings (MRI/CT)**
Stage 0	Normal muscle; no fatty streaking
Stage 1	Occasional fatty streaking
Stage 2	Fat < 50% of cross-sectional area (fat < muscle)
Stage 3	Fat = 50% of cross-sectional area (fat = muscle)
Stage 4	Fat > 50% of cross-sectional area (fat > muscle)

CT, Computed tomography; *MRI*, magnetic resonance imaging.

ORTHOPEDIC GAMUT 4-27
ACROMION CHANGES
Three types of acromion changes observed in impingement syndrome: • Type 1: flat   • Type 2: curved   • Type 3: hooked

Arthroscopic rotator cuff repair in patients with grade-3 or grade-4 fatty degeneration (≥50%) can provide significant functional improvement. Those with 50% to 75% fatty degeneration show a much greater degree of improvement than those with more than 75% fatty degeneration. However, clinical improvement was observed for some patients having more than 75% fatty degeneration and for all patients in the 50% to 75% group (Burkhart et al, 2007).

PROCEDURE

- The patient is seated with the upper extremities hanging limply at the sides.
- The examiner exerts strong finger or thumb pressure toward the midline at the clavicle, at a point even with the scapular spine (Fig. 4-149).
- The production or increase of shoulder pain indicates a positive test.
- The test is significant for rotator cuff tear of the supraspinatus tendon.

Next Steps/Procedures

Apley test, impingement sign, supraspinatus press test, and Codman sign

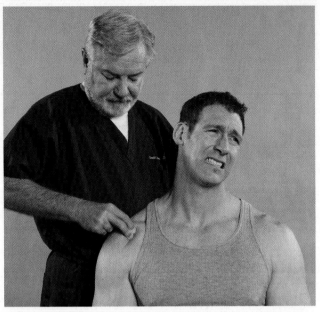

FIG. 4-149 The patient is seated with the upper extremities hanging limply at the sides. The examiner exerts strong finger or thumb pressure toward the midline of the clavicle, at a point even with the scapular spine. The production or increase of shoulder pain is a positive test. The test is significant for a rotator cuff tear, specifically a tear of the supraspinatus tendon.

CLINICAL PEARL

Degenerative changes in the supraspinatus tendon may be accompanied by the local deposition of calcium salts. This process may continue without symptoms, although radiographic changes are obvious. However, the calcified material sometimes causes inflammatory changes in the subdeltoid area and results in sudden, severe, and incapacitating pain. When this event occurs, the shoulder is acutely tender and is often swollen and warm to the touch.

Assessment for Tear of the Supraspinatus Tendon or Muscle

Comment

Supraspinatus syndrome (painful arc syndrome) is characterized by pain in the shoulder and upper arm during mid-range abduction of the glenohumeral joint with freedom from pain at the extremes of the range. The syndrome is common to five distinct shoulder lesions: (1) supraspinatus tendon tear, (2) supraspinatus tendon inflammation, (3) calcific deposits in the supraspinatus tendon, (4) subacromial bursitis, and (5) undisplaced fracture of the greater tuberosity.

> Calcifying tendinitis is a common disorder of the rotator cuff. Bosworth reported an incidence rate of 2.7% among asymptomatic office workers. Although investigators do not agree on the causes of calcification of the rotator cuff, it may be linked to hypoxia of the tissue. The initial phase of formation of the calcification is rarely symptomatic. The acute-phase symptoms are usually associated with the resorptive phase, in which vascular invasion and influx of phagocytic cells occur together with edema that raise the intratendinous pressure. The pain may be exacerbated by a secondary impingement caused by the increased volume of the tendon. Symptoms may become chronic (Seil et al, 2006).

The pain is produced mechanically by nipping of a tender structure between the tuberosity of the humerus and the acromion process and coracoacromial ligament.

Even in the normal shoulder, the clearance between the upper end of the humerus and the acromion process is small during abduction between 45 and 160 degrees. If a swollen and tender structure is present beneath the acromion, pain occurs during the arc of movement because the clearance is so small. In the neutral position and in full abduction, the clearance is greater and pain is less marked or absent.

The two classic views to rule out calcific tendinopathy are AP views: with the arm in internal and external rotation.

In internal rotation, the Hill-Sachs posterior lateral humeral head impression fracture is seen as a straight line inside the most lateral portion of the head (Fig. 4-150). The Stryker notch view, a supplemental view, images the defect when the patient places a hand on top of the head.

If the greater tuberosity avulsed and is a fragment, it is not seen over the top of the humeral head. It is usually hidden in the AP view behind the humeral head and glenoid. The fragment is visualized either on the lateral scapular view or axillary view (Fig. 4-151).

A plain-film radiograph will identify and localize the calcific deposit to a particular tendon, usually the supraspi-

natus. In the formative phase of calcification, the deposit is well defined and homogeneously dense. In the resorptive phase, usually presenting as the acute condition, the deposit is less well defined, is irregular, and has a fluffy, less dense appearance (Fig. 4-152).

Whatever the primary cause, the clinical syndrome has the same general features, although they vary in degree.

With the arm dependent, pain is absent or minimal. During abduction of the arm, pain begins at approximately 45 degrees and persists up to 160 degrees of movement. Above 160 degrees, the pain lessens or disappears. Pain is experienced again during descent from full elevation in the middle arc of the range. The patient will often twist or circumduct the arm grotesquely to lower it as painlessly as possible. The severity of the pain varies from case to case. When the calcified deposit is in the supraspinatus tendon, the pain may be so intense that the patient is scarcely able to move the shoulder and is driven to seek emergency treatment.

> Codman described the natural history of calcific tendinitis as degeneration of the supraspinatus tendon followed by calcification and eventually rupture into the subacromial bursa. The model used most frequently for the pathogenesis

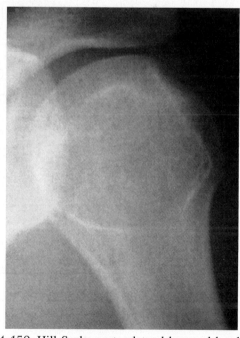

FIG. 4-150 Hill-Sachs posterolateral humeral head defect often is seen as a straight line on an internal rotation anteroposterior view. (From Nicholas JA, Hershman EB, editors: *The upper extremity in sports medicine*, St Louis, 1990, Mosby.)

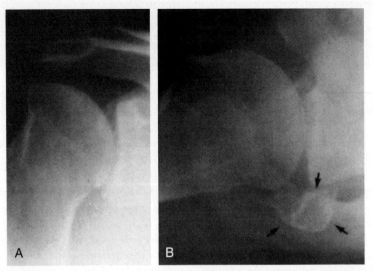

FIG. 4-151 External rotation and axillary view of a patient with a missed tuberosity avulsion. (From Nicholas JA, Hershman EB, editors: *The upper extremity in sports medicine,* St Louis, 1990, Mosby.)

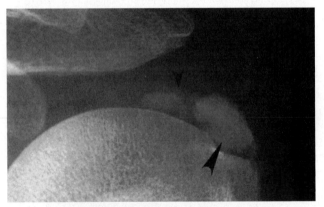

FIG. 4-152 Calcific tendinitis: formative stage *(large arrow)* and resorptive phase *(small arrow).* (From Klippel JH, Dieppe PA: *Rheumatology,* vol 1-2, ed 2, London, 1998, Mosby.)

ORTHOPEDIC GAMUT 4-28

SUPRASPINATUS SYNDROME

Variations of degeneration that lead to supraspinatus syndrome include the following:

1. In minor tearing of the supraspinatus tendon, tearing or strain of a few degenerate tendon fibers causes an inflammatory reaction with local swelling. Power is not as significantly impaired as it is after a complete tear of the rotator cuff.
2. With supraspinatus tendinopathy, an inflammatory reaction is provoked by the degeneration of the tendon fibers.
3. Calcific deposits in the supraspinatus tendon occur when a white, chalky deposit forms within the degenerate tendon, and the lesion is surrounded by an inflammatory reaction. Pain occurs when the calcified material bursts into the surrounding tissue.
4. With subacromial bursitis, the bursal walls are inflamed and thickened by mechanical irritation.
5. With injury to the greater tuberosity, a contusion or undisplaced fracture of the greater tuberosity is a common cause.

of calcific tendinitis of the supraspinatus tendon is that of a degenerative process with secondary calcification within the tendon fibers. The localization of the calcific deposits in the supraspinatus tendon is thought to most likely occur as a result of one of two causes: (1) an early impingement syndrome and longstanding impingement leading to the degeneration of the tendon fibers, which then leads to calcification, or (2) in patients without an impingement syndrome, the localization of the calcium deposit may be related to the blood supply of the region (Gimblett, Saville, Ebrall, 1999).

PROCEDURE

- The patient abducts the shoulders to 90 degrees.
- The examiner resists the abduction (Fig. 4-153).
- The shoulders are medially rotated and angled 30 degrees forward (the patient's thumbs point to the floor) (Fig. 4-154).
- The examiner again resists abduction.
- If the patient exhibits weakness or experiences pain, the test is positive.
- Weakness and pain indicate a tear of the supraspinatus tendon or muscle.

Next Steps/Procedures
Apley test, Codman sign, impingement sign, and subacromial push-button sign

4

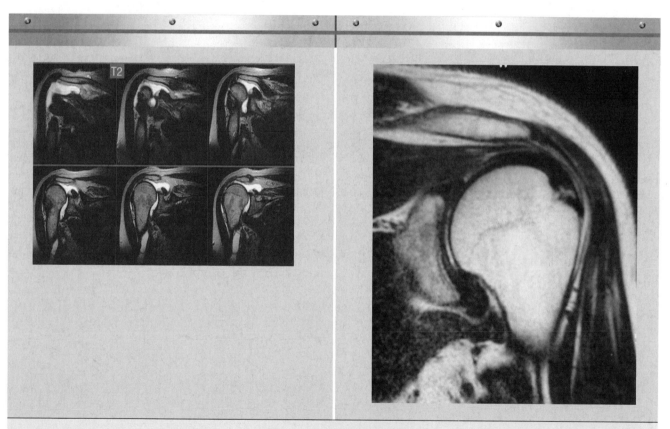

AT THE VIEWBOX

Large, full thickness supraspinatus tendon tear, with marked retraction of the proximal tendon margin and marked atrophy of the supraspinatus muscle. Note the fluid within the subacromial-subdeltoid bursa, characteristically seen with full thickness supraspinatus tendon tears, along with joint effusion. Superior subluxation of the humerus is related to forces from the deltoid muscle unopposed by the supraspinatus, with marked narrowing of the acromiohumeral interval. **(A)** MRI of a second patient with shoulder pain and weakness with abduction and external rotation demonstrates a high grade, partial thickness articular surface tear (focal region of high signal intensity) at the insertional zone of the supraspinatus tendon. (arrow) There is only a thin strand of the tendon still intact across the superior margin of the defect. **(B)** (From the teaching file of Timothy Mick, DC, DACBR)

CLINICAL PEARL

Painful arc syndrome is sometimes confused with arthritis of the acromioclavicular joint, which also causes pain during a certain phase of the abduction arc. However, with acromioclavicular arthritis, the pain begins later in abduction (not below 90 degrees) and increases, rather than diminishes, as full elevation is achieved.

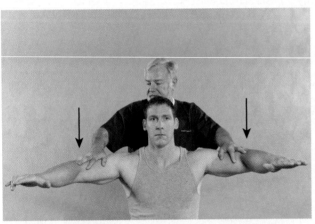

FIG. 4-153 While the patient is seated, the shoulders are abducted to 90 degrees with the arm in a neutral rotation. The examiner provides resistance to abduction.

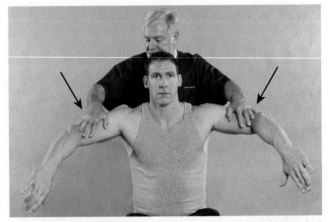

FIG. 4-154 The shoulders are internally rotated and angled 30 degrees forward so that the patient's thumbs point to the floor. The examiner again provides resistance to abduction. A positive test is indicated by pain or weakness in the affected shoulder, compared with the unaffected side. A positive test indicates a tear of the supraspinatus tendon or muscle.

TRANSVERSE HUMERAL LIGAMENT TEST

Assessment for Torn Transverse Humeral Ligament

Comment

Below and medial to the coracoacromial ligament, the long head of the biceps may be palpated beneath the capsule. The long head of the biceps is held in the groove by the transverse humeral ligament, a thickened prolongation of the capsule extending between the lesser and greater tuberosities.

The bicipital retinaculum (Fig. 4-155) serves to hold the tendon of the LHB against the proximal humerus within the bicipital groove. The functional significance of this becomes apparent during shoulder elevation, which limits biceps contribution to either flexion or abduction by tethering of the long tendon within the bicipital groove. The retinaculum prevents the biceps from deflecting away from the humerus during contraction by keeping it straddled between the two tuberosities, thus limiting its leverage as a significant elevator.

No identifiable transverse humeral ligament exists. Rather, the fibers covering the intertubercular groove are composed of a sling formed by fibers from the subscapularis and supraspinatus tendons. Dislocations of the LHB must disrupt fibers from this annular sling created by the anterior rotator cuff tendons (Bond, Pasque, 2005).

Dimensions of the groove vary widely. Deep narrow apertures favor constriction of the tendon, and shallow flat grooves allow slipping and subluxation of the tendon (Fig. 4-156). If the cuff zone at the top of the groove is torn, the tendon may slip out of the groove, particularly if the arm is

---

ORTHOPEDIC GAMUT 4-29

BICEPS LONG HEAD STRUCTURE

Critical zones in the biceps long head structure:
1. The point at which the tendon arches over the humeral head
2. The point where the floor on which the tendon glides changes from bony cortex to articular cartilage

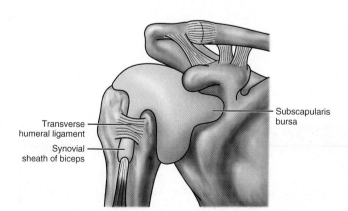

Transverse humeral ligament

Synovial sheath of biceps

Subscapularis bursa

FIG. 4-155 Transverse humeral ligament. (Adapted from Saidoff DC, McDonough AL: *Critical pathways in therapeutic intervention,* St Louis, 1997, Mosby.)

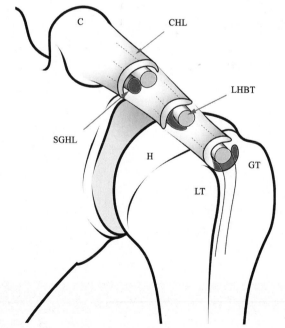

FIG. 4-156 Diagrammatic representation of the biceps reflective pulley system. *CHL,* Coracohumeral ligament; *SGHL,* superior glenohumeral ligament; *C,* coracoid process; *LHBT,* long head of biceps tendon; *H,* humeral head; *GT,* greater tuberosity; *LT,* lesser tuberosity. (From Lee JC et al: MRI of the rotator interval of the shoulder, *Clin Radiol* 62[5]:416-423, 2007.)

abducted and externally rotated. Similarly, if strong force is applied while the arm is abducted and externally rotated, the tendon may be wrenched out of the groove.

The rotator interval of the shoulder joint is located between the distal edges of the supraspinatus and subscapularis tendons and contains the insertions of the coracohumeral and superior glenohumeral ligaments. These structures form a complex pulley system that stabilizes the LHB tendon as it enters the bicipital groove of the humeral head. The rotator interval is the site of a variety of pathologic processes, including biceps tendon lesions, adhesive capsulitis, and anterosuperior internal impingement (Lee et al, 2007).

PROCEDURE

- The patient's affected shoulder is passively abducted and internally rotated (Figs. 4-157 and 4-158).
- The examiner's fingers are placed on the bicipital groove.
- The patient's shoulder is passively externally rotated (Fig. 4-159).
- If a tendon snap in and out of the groove is felt as the external rotation occurs, the test is positive.
- A positive test suggests a torn transverse humeral ligament.

Next Steps/Procedures
Abbott-Saunders test, Ludington test, Speed test, and Yergason test

CLINICAL PEARL

Conditions involving the bicipital tendon and the bicipital groove are particularly pertinent to athletes because many sports involve the throwing motion of the arm. These athletes include baseball pitchers, football quarterbacks, batters, and tennis players. The throwing motion is especially inhibited by bicipital tendon problems. Recognizing if the defect is an adhesive tenosynovitis, fraying of the tendon, or subluxation or dislocation of the tendon is especially pertinent.

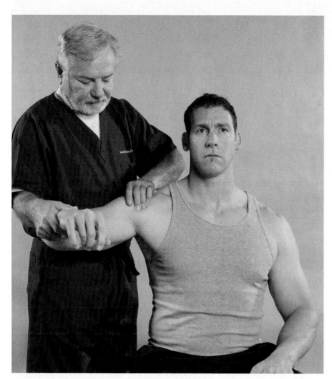

FIG. 4-157 The patient's shoulder is passively abducted with the elbow flexed to 90 degrees.

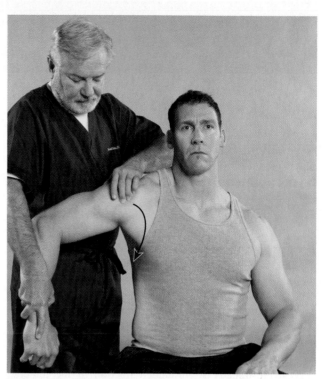

FIG. 4-158 The examiner's fingers are placed on the bicipital groove. The patient's shoulder is passively internally rotated.

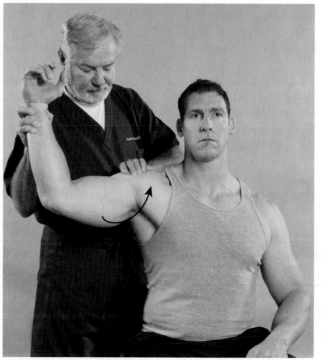

FIG. 4-159 While maintaining palpation of the bicipital groove, the shoulder is externally rotated passively. Tendon snap in and out of the groove as the external rotation occurs is a positive finding. A positive test suggests a torn transverse humeral ligament.

ALSO KNOWN AS HYPERABDUCTION MANEUVER

Assessment for Neurovascular Compromise of the Axillary Artery as Seen in the Hyperabduction Thoracic Outlet Syndromes

Comment

The Adson, hyperabduction, and costoclavicular maneuvers are provocative movements and postures that attempt to reproduce pain, paresthesias, a change in radial pulse, or a supraclavicular bruit.

The *Hunter test* is begun with the shoulder abducted to 90 degrees and the elbow flexed to 90 degrees. The arm is then straightened. A positive sign results in a painful shooting sensation down the arm in the distribution of the involved nerves, presumably from sudden traction of the tethered medial cord of the brachial plexus. Similar tension tests may be performed to stretch the ulnar and radial nerve tracts. The appropriate limb postures may be extrapolated when the various joints of the upper extremity are positioned to stretch each tract in relation to the axis of the joints it crosses (Fig. 4-160).

The *Elvey upper extremity tension test* determines the mobility of the brachial plexus and nerve root, particularly the median nerve. Similar to the straight leg raising test in the lower extremities, this test may determine whether any restrictions of the nerve roots or plexus have occurred in those structures stretched by a sequence of upper extremity movements.

With repetitive or prolonged hyperabduction of the arm, the neurovascular bundle in the axilla can be stretched under the pectoralis minor tendon and the coracoid process, resulting in symptoms of neurovascular compression.

> Direct injury to the axillary artery is a relatively rare occurrence, representing 15% to 20% of the arterial injuries to the upper limb. Ninety-four percent of such injuries are caused by penetrating trauma, with only 6% caused by blunt trauma.

ORTHOPEDIC GAMUT 4-30

ELVEY TEST MOVEMENTS

The three superimposed component movements of Elvey test are as follows:
1. Shoulder abduction and lateral rotation and extension behind the coronal plane
2. Forearm supination and elbow extension
3. Wrist and finger extension (Fig. 4-161)

Fracture-dislocation of the glenohumeral joint accounts for the majority of blunt injuries, and less than 1% have dislocation without associated fracture. In excess of 200 cases of vascular injury secondary to anterior shoulder dislocation have been reported in the literature (Kelley, Hinsche, Hossain, 2004).

When leaving the costoclavicular space, the three cords of the brachial plexus, the subclavian artery, and the subclavian vein pass under the insertion of the pectoralis minor muscle on the coracoid process. As this neurovascular bundle enters the axillary fossa, the artery and vein become known as the *axillary artery* and the *axillary vein*. As the upper extremity is abducted to 180 degrees, the neurovascular bundle is stretched around a fulcrum, which consists of the tendon of the pectoralis minor, the coracoid process, and the humeral head. The bundle almost reaches an angle of 90 degrees around the fulcrum. Unfortunately, the neurovascular bundle's course remains fixed, allowing no motion of the bundle. Compression at the fulcrum and tension along its components is the only way the bundle can compensate. Abduction of the arm produces a 30-degree elevation and a 35-degree posterior displacement of the clavicle, thereby narrowing the costoclavicular tunnel. The tunnel's anterior wall, consisting also of the pectoralis minor muscle, the subclavius muscle, and the costoclavicular ligament (the thickening of the clavipectoral fascia), is stretched and brought posteriorly further, pushing the neurovascular bundle against the fulcrum.

Two critical anatomic points exist where compression of the neurovascular bundle may occur when the arm is hyperabducted. The first point is where the bundle passes through the costoclavicular tunnel, or slit. The second point is where the bundle passes under the pectoralis minor tendon at its insertion on the coracoid process. During abduction of the arm, the fixed neurovascular bundle can be compressed by the tendon of the pectoralis minor muscle, as well as by the humeral head. The characteristic position that produces this compression is 180 degrees abducted and elbow flexion. This position commonly occurs during sleep or in certain occupations, such as that of electricians, painters, bricklayers, dry-wall hangers, or masons.

Pain, paresthesia, and numbness develop first in the fingers and later in the hand. In some patients, transitory ischemia and edema develop. These symptoms may resemble Raynaud disease and are present in 38% of the patients with hyperabduction syndrome. Neurologic symptoms are usually absent in hyperabduction syndrome because as paresthesia and pain develop, the patient corrects the arm position, and thus the nerve compression only lasts for a short

THE MOST COMMONLY ENCOUNTERED CAUSES OF DAMAGE AT THE VARIOUS SITES ARE INDICATED

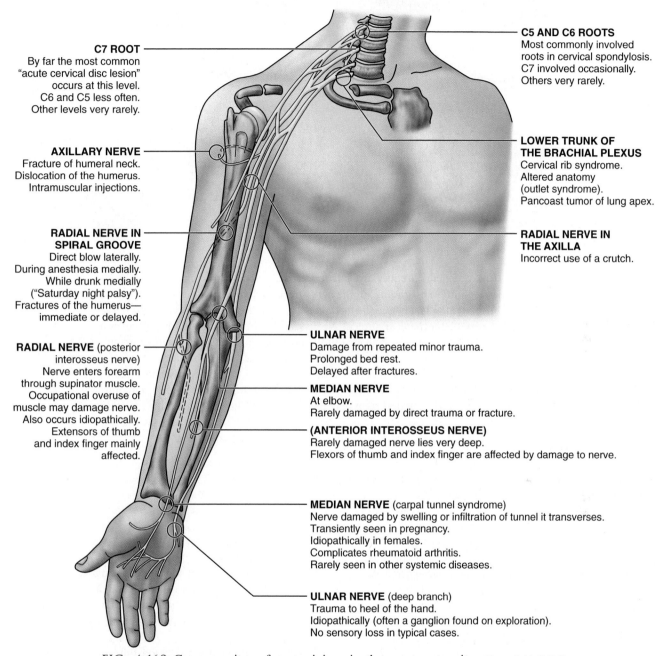

C7 ROOT
By far the most common "acute cervical disc lesion" occurs at this level. C6 and C5 less often. Other levels very rarely.

C5 AND C6 ROOTS
Most commonly involved roots in cervical spondylosis. C7 involved occasionally. Others very rarely.

AXILLARY NERVE
Fracture of humeral neck. Dislocation of the humerus. Intramuscular injections.

LOWER TRUNK OF THE BRACHIAL PLEXUS
Cervical rib syndrome. Altered anatomy (outlet syndrome). Pancoast tumor of lung apex.

RADIAL NERVE IN SPIRAL GROOVE
Direct blow laterally. During anesthesia medially. While drunk medially ("Saturday night palsy"). Fractures of the humerus—immediate or delayed.

RADIAL NERVE IN THE AXILLA
Incorrect use of a crutch.

RADIAL NERVE (posterior interosseus nerve)
Nerve enters forearm through supinator muscle. Occupational overuse of muscle may damage nerve. Also occurs idiopathically. Extensors of thumb and index finger mainly affected.

ULNAR NERVE
Damage from repeated minor trauma. Prolonged bed rest. Delayed after fractures.

MEDIAN NERVE
At elbow. Rarely damaged by direct trauma or fracture.

(ANTERIOR INTEROSSEUS NERVE)
Rarely damaged nerve lies very deep. Flexors of thumb and index finger are affected by damage to nerve.

MEDIAN NERVE (carpal tunnel syndrome)
Nerve damaged by swelling or infiltration of tunnel it transverses. Transiently seen in pregnancy. Idiopathically in females. Complicates rheumatoid arthritis. Rarely seen in other systemic diseases.

ULNAR NERVE (deep branch)
Trauma to heel of the hand. Idiopathically (often a ganglion found on exploration). No sensory loss in typical cases.

FIG. 4-160 Common sites of nerve injury in the upper extremity. (From Saidoff DC, McDonough AL: *Critical pathways in therapeutic intervention,* St Louis, 1997, Mosby.)

time. If the arm is abducted to 180 degrees in patients with hyperabduction syndrome, symptoms can increase. The radial artery pulse may weaken or disappear. However, just as tests for the anterior scalene syndrome or costoclavicular syndrome can be positive in a normal position, the same results can be found when testing for hyperabduction syndrome.

Sports-related injuries have been described in the subclavian artery, axillary artery, and their associated branches. Injury

at the subclavian artery level can result because of compression from a cervical rib, the underlying first rib, or from extrinsic compression from the anterior scalene muscle. Injuries in this location are typical of arterial thoracic outlet lesions that are seen in nonathletes. Isolated injury of the subclavian artery can affect the adjacent segment of the first portion of the axillary artery. The second portion of the axillary artery, immediately deep to the pectoralis minor muscle, can also become compressed, resulting in injury. Three such

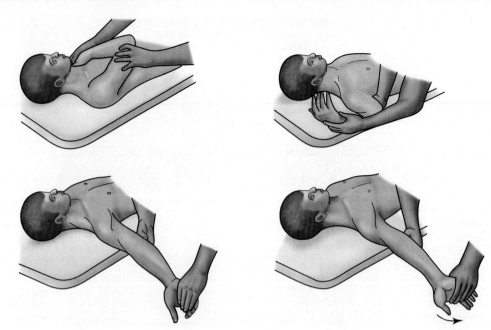

FIG. 4-161 Elvey upper extremity tension test is a provocative sequence of motions that determines mobility (i.e., gliding) of the nerve tract, including the brachial plexus and nerve root. This particular test biases the median nerve and the anterior interosseous nerve for tension by way of mechanical stretch. **A,** First, the arm and scapula are place in a resting position. **B,** Next, the arm is placed in the position of 90 degrees shoulder abduction, lateral rotation, and elbow flexion with the forearm pronated. (From Saidoff DC, McDonough AL: *Critical pathways in therapeutic intervention,* St Louis, 1997, Mosby.) **C,** The elbow and forearm are then extended and supinated. **D,** The wrist is then extended to reproduce symptoms. Cervical lateral flexion to the left or right may then be added. The examiner must maintain each posture before superimposing the next position in this sequence. (Adapted from Saidoff DC, McDonough AL: *Critical pathways in therapeutic intervention,* St Louis, 1997, Mosby.)

cases were described by McCarthy and associates. The third portion of the axillary artery is perhaps most prone to sports-related injury. Extrinsic compression and stretching from the underlying humeral head predisposes to axillary artery trauma in this location. Such injuries can result in stenosis, thrombotic occlusion, aneurysmal degeneration, or any combination of the three (Jackson, 2003).

PROCEDURE

- Before this test is started, the Allen maneuver at the wrist is performed to establish patency of the radial arteries.
- The patient is seated, with both arms hanging at the sides.
- The examiner palpates the patient's radial pulse (Fig. 4-162).
- Both arms, in turn, are passively abducted to 180 degrees (Fig. 4-163).
- The examiner notes the angle of abduction at which the radial pulse diminishes or disappears on the affected side (Fig. 4-164).

- The examiner compares the results with those on the unaffected side.
- The test is significant for neurovascular compromise of the axillary artery, as seen in hyperabduction TOSs.
- Many patients have cessation of the radial pulse on abduction without hyperabduction syndrome being present.
- If the nonaffected limb demonstrates radial pulse dampening or cessation at the same approximate degree of abduction as the affected side, the test is not positive for hyperabduction syndrome.

Next Steps/Procedures
Adson test, Allen maneuver, costoclavicular maneuver, George screening procedure, Halstead maneuver, reverse Bakody maneuver, Roos test, and shoulder compression test

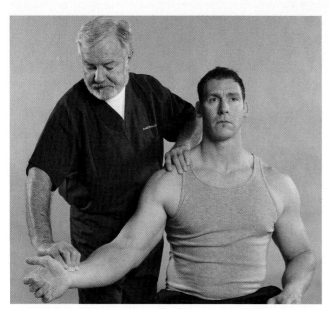

FIG. 4-162 The patient is seated with both arms hanging at the sides. The examiner palpates the radial pulse of the affected arm.

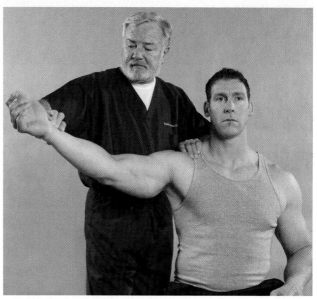

FIG. 4-163 The examiner abducts the affected arm to 180 degrees.

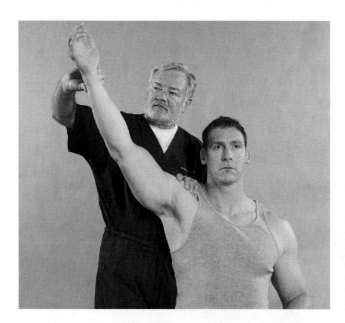

FIG. 4-164 The examiner notes the angle of abduction at which the radial pulse on the affected side diminishes or disappears. This angle is compared with the angle obtained on the unaffected side. The test is significant for neurovascular compromise of the axillary artery, as seen in hyperabduction TOSs. If the nonaffected arm demonstrates radial pulse dampening or cessation at the same approximate angle of abduction, the test is not positive for hyperabduction syndrome.

CLINICAL PEARL

In most instances of compression hyperabduction of the shoulder, the radial pulse is obliterated; but obliteration of the radial pulse also may occur in the normal extremity. However, a difference exists. On the affected side, the marginal position is reached sooner than on the normal side. The marginal position is the level of abduction just below that which produces obliteration of the pulse. The patient is often aware of the exact level of abduction at which the symptoms occur.

Assessment for Tenosynovitis or Involvement of the Transverse Humeral Ligament

Comment

The LHB follows a tortuous and hemmed-in course from its origin in the muscle belly to the supraglenoid tubercle. The type of trauma that usually produces tenosynovitis in the wrist, resulting in constrictive adhesions, is not the mechanism commonly encountered at the LHB. The bicipital tendon area is not nearly so vulnerable to direct trauma; therefore, tendinopathy and tenosynovitis may develop gradually without definite acute episodes of injury.

The gliding of the LHB tendon is guided by the coracohumeral ligament (Fig. 4-165). The ligament runs through the interval between the subscapularis and supraspinatus tendons, known as *the rotator interval*, and reinforces the glenohumeral joint capsule at that locale.

After an activity such as the first game of the season for badminton or tennis or after a jerking strain after lifting with outstretched arms, discomfort is noted in the shoulder. Initially, the ache is indefinite and is not plainly related to motions that use the biceps tendon. Later, more acute pain develops, and the patient avoids lifting and keeps the arm at the side with the elbow flexed (this is the position of maximal comfort). As a prolonged condition or posture of the arm, this results in an imbalance between capillary filtra-

tion and lymphatic drainage (Fig. 4-166). The extra fluid can flood the subcutaneous tissue space. Although this circumstance sets the stage for upper extremity lymphedema, limitations in joint movement, the increase in weight, and the advancing edema may itself result in or perpetuate rotator cuff tendonitis.

Examination reveals tenderness at the top and front of the shoulder. This tenderness is related to the tendon course across the upper end of the humerus. The tenderness follows into the bicipital groove and along the tendon into the arm. Deep palpation at the medial border of the deltoid delineates tenderness when pressure is applied along the tendon as the arm is rotated externally and internally. Flexion of the elbow and supination of the hand against resistance may produce pain that is referred to the front and inner aspects of the shoulder. In all shoulder lesions in which involvement of the biceps mechanism is suspected, diagnostic images that show the groove in profile should be acquired. With tendinopathy or tenosynovitis, bony abnormalities are not unusual, but any abnormal contour of the groove may predispose the patient to development of the condition. If the groove is too flat or shallow, the tendon may slip out. If the groove is too deep, the tendon is roughened and squeezed. If spur formation is present, the tendon may become frayed.

Lymphedema results from an imbalance between capillary filtration and lymphatic drainage that causes an accumulation of protein-rich fluid in the interstitium. Early in the

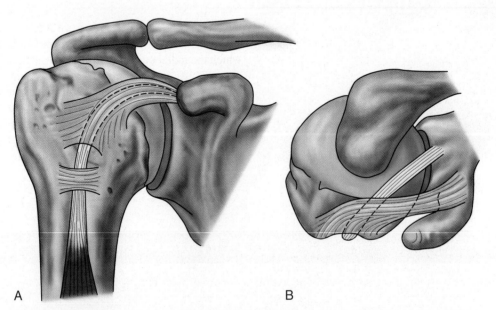

A

B

FIG. 4-165 The coracohumeral ligament thickens the rotator interval, inserts on either side of the bicipital groove, and is an important stabilizer of the biceps tendon. **A,** Anterior view. **B,** Superior view. (Adapted from Saidoff DC, McDonough AL: *Critical pathways in therapeutic intervention,* St Louis, 1997, Mosby.)

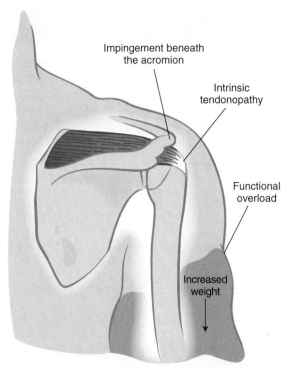

FIG. 4-166 Posterior view of lymphedematous arm and supraspinatus muscle with three possible causes of rotator cuff tendonitis. (From Herrera JE, Stubblefield MD: Rotator cuff tendonitis in lymphedema: a retrospective case series, *Arch Phys Med Rehabil* 85[12]:1939-1942, 2004.)

ORTHOPEDIC GAMUT 4-32

SUPRASPINATUS TEST: *EMPTY CAN TEST*

In the supraspinatus test:
- The patient's shoulder is abducted to 90 degrees with neutral rotation, and the examiner provides resistance to abduction.
- The shoulder is then medially rotated and angled forward 30 degrees so that the patient's thumb points toward the floor.
- Resistance to abduction is given while the examiner looks for weakness or pain, which reflects a positive result.

ORTHOPEDIC GAMUT 4-33

NEER IMPINGEMENT TEST

In Neer impingement test:
The patient's arm is forcibly elevated through forward flexion by the examiner while the scapula is depressed, causing compression of the greater tuberosity against the anteroinferior acromial surface. Discomfort as a result of this maneuver reflects a positive test result.

ORTHOPEDIC GAMUT 4-31

HAWKINS IMPINGEMENT TEST

For the Hawkins impingement test:
- The patient stands while the examiner forward flexes the shoulder to 90 degrees, flexes the elbow to 90 degrees, and forcibly internally rotates the shoulder.
- This movement pushes the supraspinatus tendon against the anterior surface of the coracoacromial ligament.
- Pain indicates a positive test for rotator cuff tendonitis.

---

disease process, the extra fluid flows freely in the subcutaneous tissue space. During this period, the lymphedema responds well to decongestive physical therapy. As the disease progresses, tissues become more fibrotic, and the fluid moves less freely. At this time, the edema becomes brawny and is less likely to improve significantly from decongestive treatment. The increasing fluid tension in the subcutaneous tissues can result in decreased joint range of motion. Furthermore, the weight and size of the arm may hinder function. Limitations in joint movement, the increase in weight, and arm edema especially around the shoulder may result in rotator cuff tendonitis (Herrera, Stubblefield, 2004).

PROCEDURE

- The patient flexes the elbow.
- The patient attempts to supinate the hand against resistance (Fig. 4-167).
- The patient then resists efforts to extend the elbow (Fig. 4-168).
- If pain over the intertubercular groove develops or is aggravated, the test is positive.
- A positive sign suggests tenosynovitis of the transverse humeral ligament.

Next Steps/Procedures
Abbott-Saunders test, Ludington test, Speed test, and transverse humeral ligament test

CLINICAL PEARL

The concept that the biceps tendon moves up and down the groove during motion at the glenohumeral joint is questionable. With the bicipital tendon and groove exposed under anesthesia, the biceps tendon remains fixed in the groove during motion. However, the head of the humerus glides up and down the tendon. Contraction of the biceps muscle, by supinating the forearm or flexing the elbow, makes the tendon taut but produces no motion of the tendon in the groove. All movements of the shoulder joint, regardless of the plane in which the arm is elevated, are accompanied by gliding motions of the humerus on the tendon.

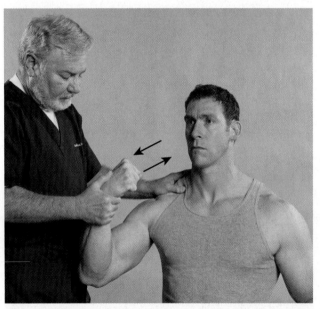

FIG. 4-167 The patient flexes the affected elbow. The patient resists efforts to extend the arm.

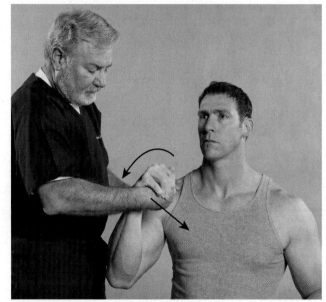

FIG. 4-168 The patient attempts to supinate the forearm against resistance. Pain over the intertubercular groove is a positive finding. A positive test suggests biceps tenosynovitis or involvement of the transverse humeral ligament.

CRITICAL THINKING

1. What is the cause of rotator cuff tears?
2. How is the strength of the supraspinatus and infraspinatus tested?
3. What is the function of the long head of the biceps tendon?
4. What are the most important capsule ligaments?
5. What is a Bankart lesion?
6. What is a Hill-Sachs lesion?
7. What are the most common mechanisms for production of anterior and posterior shoulder dislocations?
8. What physical findings are typical of an unreduced posterior dislocation?
9. Describe the basis and techniques for the sulcus tests.
10. What is the function of the rotator cuff muscles?
11. What is the impingement syndrome?
12. How does a rotator cuff tear differ from impingement?
13. Explain how bicipital tendinopathy relates to impingement.
14. What articulations comprise the shoulder joint?
15. Many causes of shoulder pain have been identified. Name five periarticular disorders that cause shoulder pain.
16. Name five systemic conditions or diseases that may refer pain to the shoulder.
17. The innervation of the shoulder joint arises from what nerve roots?
18. What is the greatest *predisposing factor* for a subluxation or dislocation of the biceps tendon?
19. Adson test is one of the maneuvers the clinician will use to determine if the upper extremity symptoms the patient exhibits are spinal or extraspinal in origin. What artery is compressed within the thoracic outlet?
20. What nerve root branches *are at higher risk of compression* as they pass through this outlet?
21. Which muscle has the most common tendinopathy in the upper extremity?
22. Supraspinatus tendinopathy occurs most commonly in individuals that are repetitively doing what movement?
23. Describe the *reverse terrible triad of the shoulder*.
24. The shoulder is the most commonly dislocated joint in the body. What is the typical mechanism of injury?
25. Which artery is most susceptible to injury with trauma to the shoulder?
26. What is the cardinal sign of rotator cuff rupture in the senior patient?
27. What is the distinguishing factor between a partial tear versus a complete tear of the cuff?
28. What orthopedic test is best described by the examiner holding the arm out and suddenly releasing the support?
29. What is thought to be the number one cause of rupture of the supraspinatus tendon in the senior patient?
30. Depending on the mechanism and level of compression, several disorders are included under the title of TOS. Name five of these disorders.
31. A positive Castagna test indicates what shoulder problem is likely present in the patient?
32. Describe how the test is done.
33. What is different from how it is performed from the Jobe test?
34. TOS encompasses several clinical entities. What is usually the first manifestation of a TOS experienced by the patient?
35. Muscular atrophy can occur with chronic TOS because of nerve compression. What muscles show early atrophy, and why?
36. What key diagnostic features differ in a patient with calcific tendinopathy versus glenohumeral osteoarthritis of the shoulder?
37. What conditions would you consider in the differential diagnosis of rotator cuff impingement?
38. Shoulder flexion by the patient is restricted and you further have the patient resist the forearm supinating and elbow extension. This maneuver produces an increased tenderness in the bicipital groove. What is the name of this positive test, and what condition is present?

BIBLIOGRAPHY

Abrams WB, Berkow R: *The Merck manual of geriatrics*, Rahway, NJ, 1990, Merck Sharp & Dohme Research Laboratories.

Adams JC, Hamblen DL: *Outline of orthopaedics*, ed 11, Edinburgh, 1990, Churchill Livingstone.

Ahmad CS et al: Factors affecting dropped biceps deformity after tenotomy of the long head of the biceps tendon, *Arthroscopy* 23(5):537-541, 2007.

Alario AJ: *Practical guide to the care of the pediatric patient*, St Louis, 1997, Mosby.

Allen AA, Warner JJP: Management of the stiff shoulder, *Oper Tech Orthop* 5(3):238-247, 1995.

Allison D, Strickland N: *Acronyms & synonyms in medical imaging*, Oxford, UK, 1996, ISIS Medical Media.

Altchek DW et al: Arthroscopic acromioplasty: technique and results, *J Bone Joint Surg* 72A:1198, 1990.

American Medical Association: *Guides to the evaluation of permanent impairment*, ed 4, Chicago, 1993, American Medical Association.

American Medical Association: *How to use guides to the evaluation of permanent impairment*, ed 4, Falmouth, Colo, 1993, SEAK, Inc.

Anderson KN, Anderson LE: *Mosby's pocket dictionary of medicine, nursing, & allied health*, ed 2, St Louis, 1994, Mosby.

Apley AG, Solomon L: *Concise system of orthopaedics and fractures*, London, 1988, Butterworth-Heinemann.

Arntz CT, Jackins S, Matsen FA III: Prosthetic replacement of the shoulder for the treatment of defects in rotator cuff and the surface of the glenohumeral joint, *J Bone Joint Surg* 75A:485, 1993.

Arrigoni P, Brady PC, Burkhart SS: Calcific tendonitis of the subscapularis tendon causing subcoracoid stenosis and coracoid impingement, *Arthroscopy* 22(10):1139.e1-1139.e3, 2006.

Barabis J: Therapist's management of thoracic outlet syndrome. In Hunter JM et al, editors: *Rehabilitation of the hand: surgery and therapy*, ed 3, St Louis, 1990, Mosby.

Barkauskas VH et al: *Health & physical assessment*, ed 2, St Louis, 1998, Mosby.

Bateman JE: The diagnosis and treatment of ruptures of the rotator cuff, *Surg Clin North Am* 43:1523, 1963.

Bateman JE: *The shoulder and neck*, ed 2, Philadelphia, 1978, WB Saunders.

Bateman JE: *Trauma to nerves in limbs*, Philadelphia, 1962, WB Saunders.

Bennett WF: Arthroscopic bicipital sheath repair: two-year follow-up with pulley lesions, *Arthroscopy* 20(9):964-973, 2004.

Bergfeld JA: Acromioclavicular complex. In Nicholas JA, Hershman EB, editors: *The upper extremity in sports medicine*, St Louis, 1990, Mosby.

Berquist T: *MRI of the musculoskeletal system*, ed 3, Philadelphia, 1996, JB Lippincott.

Bland JH, Merrit JA, Boushey DR: The painful shoulder, *Semin Arthritis Rheum* 7:21, 1977.

Bloom RA: The active abduction view: a new maneuver in the diagnosis of rotator cuff tears, *Skeletal Radiol* 20:255, 1991.

Boileau P, Chuinard C: Arthroscopic biceps tenotomy: technique and results, *Oper Tech Sports Med* 15(1):35-44, 2007.

Bozyk Z: Shoulder-hand syndrome in patients with antecedent myocardial infarctions, *Revmatologiia (Mosk)* 6:103, 1968.

Brems JJ: Degenerative joints disease of the shoulder. In Nicholas J, Hershman E, editors: *The upper extremity in sports medicine*, St Louis, 1990, Mosby.

Brooks M, Evans R, Fairclough J: *Sports injuries*, ed 2, London, 1992, Gower Medical.

Brotzman SB: *Clinical orthopaedic rehabilitation*, St Louis, 1996, Mosby.

Brown DE, Neumann RD: *Orthopedic secrets*, Philadelphia, 1995, Hanley & Belfus.

Bucholz RW: *Orthopaedic decision making*, ed 2, St Louis, 1996, Mosby.

Bunker TD: Frozen shoulder, *Curr Orthop* 12(3):193-201, 1998.

Bunker TD, Schranz PJ: *Clinical challenges in orthopaedics: the shoulder*, Oxford, UK, 1998, ISIS Medical Media.

Burkhart SS: Arthroscopic treatment of massive rotator cuff tears, *Clin Orthop* 26:45, 1991.

Bush LH: The torn shoulder capsule, *J Bone Joint Surg* 57A:256, 1975.

Butler D: *Mobilisation of the nervous system*, Melbourne, 1991, Churchill Livingstone.

Cailliet R: *Shoulder pain*, Philadelphia, 1966, FA Davis.

Campbell JB, Campbell JM: *Mosby's survival guide to medical abbreviations & acronyms prefixes & suffixes symbols Greek alphabet*, St Louis, 1995, Mosby.

Canale ST: *Campbell's operative orthopaedics*, vol 1-4, ed 9, St Louis, 1998, Mosby.

Castelli P et al: Endovascular repair of traumatic injuries of the subclavian and axillary arteries, *Injury* 36(6):778-782, 2005.

Chandler TJ et al: Shoulder strength, power and endurance in college tennis players, *Am J Sports Med* 20:455, 1992.

Chansky HA, Iannotti JP: The vascularity of the rotator cuff, *Clin Sports Med* 10:807, 1991.

Chappman S, Nakielny R: *Aids to radiological differential diagnosis*, ed 3, London, 1995, Bailliere Tindall.

Chard MD et al: Shoulder disorders in the elderly: a community survey, *Arthritis Rheum* 34:766, 1991.

Cinquegranao D: Chronic cervical radiculitis and its relationship to "chronic bursitis," *Am J Phys Med Rehabil* 47:23, 1968.

Cipriano JJ: *Photographic manual of regional orthopaedic and neurological test*, ed 3, Baltimore, 1997, Williams & Wilkins.

Clark J, Sidles JA, Matsen FF: The repair of the glenohumeral joint capsule to the rotator cuff, *Clin Orthop* 254:29, 1990.

Codman EA: *The shoulder*, Boston, 1934, Author.

Cofield R: Degenerative and arthritic problems of the glenohumeral joint. In Rockwood C, Matsen F, editors: *The shoulder*, Philadelphia, 1990, WB Saunders.

Cohn RE: *Impairment rating examination and disability evaluation*, ed 3, Wilkesboro, NC, 1994, R Ernest Cohn.

Colli BO et al: Neurogenic thoracic outlet syndromes: a comparison of true and nonspecific syndromes after surgical treatment, *Surg Neurol* 65(3):262-271, 2006.

Cooper DE et al: Anatomy, histology and vascularity of the glenoid labrum, *J Bone Joint Surg* 74A:46, 1992.

Copeland SA et al: *Joint stiffness of the upper limb*, St Louis, 1997, Mosby.

Curwin S, Stanish WD: *Tendinitis: its etiology and treatment*, Lexington, KY, 1984, Collamore Press.

Dalton S et al: Human shoulder tendon biopsy samples in organ culture produce procollagenase and tissue inhibitor of metalloproteinases, *Ann Rheum Dis* 54:571, 1995.

Dambro MR, Griffith JA: *Griffith's 5 minute clinical consult*, Baltimore, 1997, Williams & Wilkins.

D'Ambrogio KJ, Roth GB: *Positional release therapy assessment & treatment of musculoskeletal dysfunction*, St Louis, 1997, Mosby.

D'Ambrosia RD: *Musculoskeletal disorders: regional examination and differential diagnosis*, Philadelphia, 1977, JB Lippincott.

Dandy DJ: *Essential orthopaedics and trauma*, Edinburgh, 1989, Churchill Livingstone.

Dawson DM, Hallet M, Millender LH: *Entrapment neuropathies*, ed 2, Boston, 1990, Little, Brown.

Debeyre J, Patte D, Elmelik E: Repair of ruptures of the rotator cuff of the shoulder, *J Bone Joint Surg* 47B:36, 1965.

Deltoff MN, Kogon PL: *The portable skeletal x-ray library*, St Louis, 1998, Mosby.

Demeter SL, Andersson GBJ, Smith GM: *Disability evaluation*, St Louis, 1996, Mosby.

DePalma AF: *Surgery of the shoulder*, ed 2, Philadelphia, 1973, JB Lippincott.

Deshpande JK, Tobias JD: *The pediatric pain handbook*, St Louis, 1996, Mosby.

Dettenmeier PA: *Radiographic assessment for nurses*, St Louis, 1995, Mosby.

Doherty M, Doherty J: *Clinical examination in rheumatology*, London, 1992, Wolfe.

Doherty M, George E: *Self-assessment picture tests in rheumatology*, London, 1995, Mosby-Wolfe.

Doherty M: *Color atlas and text of osteoarthritis*, London, 1994, Wolfe.

Elster AD: *Questions and answers in magnetic resonance imaging*, St Louis, 1994, Mosby.

Engelman RM: Shoulder pain as a presenting complaint in upper lobe bronchogenic carcinoma: report of 21 cases, *Conn Med* 30:273, 1966.

Epstein O et al: *Clinical examination*, ed 2, London, 1997, Mosby.

Farin PU et al: Shoulder impingement syndrome; sonographic evaluation, *Radiology* 176:845, 1990.

Feldmann E: *Current diagnosis in neurology*, St Louis, 1994, Mosby

Ferezy JS: *The chiropractic neurological examination*, Gaithersburg, Md, 1992, Aspen.

Finke J: Neurologic differential diagnosis: the lower cervical region, *Dutsch Med Wochenschr* 90:1912, 1965.

Flores LP, Carneiro JZ: Peripheral nerve compression secondary to adjacent lipomas, *Surg Neurol* 67(3):258-262, 2007.

Fornage B: *Musculoskeletal ultrasound*, New York, 1995, Churchill Livingstone.

Frank ED et al: *Merrill's atlas of radiographic positioning and procedures*, vol 1-3, ed 11, St Louis, 2007, Mosby.

Gabriel DA, Basford JR, An K-N: Vibratory facilitation of strength in fatigued muscle, *Arch of Phys Med Rehabil* 83(9):1202-1205, 2002.

Garn AN, Thorsen H, Lonnberg F: The effect of low-level laser therapy on musculoskeletal pain: a meta-analysis, *Pain* 52:63, 1993.

Garth W: Evaluating and treating brachial plexus injuries, *J Musculoskel Med* 11(10):55-67, 1994.

Gartsman GM: Arthroscopic acromioplasty for lesions of the rotator cuff, *J Bone Joint Surg* 72A:169, 1990.

Gascon J: A current problem: diagnosis of the shoulder pain syndrome, *Union Med Can* 94:463, 1965.

Gerard JA, Kleinfield SL: *Orthopaedic testing*, New York, 1993, Churchill Livingstone.

Gerber C, Krushell FJ: Isolated rupture of the tendon of the subscapularis muscle: clinical features in 16 cases, *J Bone Joint Surg* 73B:389, 1991.

Geven LI, Smit AJ, Ebels T: Vascular thoracic outlet syndrome: longer posterior rib stump causes poor outcome, *Eur J Cardiothorac Surg* 30(2):232-236, 2006.

Gilula LA, Yin Y: *Imaging of the wrist and hand*, Philadelphia, 1996, WB Saunders.

Godfrey J et al: Reliability, validity, and responsiveness of the simple shoulder test: psychometric properties by age and injury type, *J Shoulder Elbow Surg* 16(3):260-267, 2007.

Gohlke F, Essigkrug B, Schmiz F: The pattern of the collagen fiber bundles of the capsule of the glenohumeral joint, *J Shoulder Elbow Surg* 3:111, 1994.

Goldie BS: *Orthopaedic diagnosis and management: a guide to the care of orthopaedic patients*, ed 2, Oxford, UK, 1998, ISIS Medical Media.

Goldie I: Calcified deposits in the shoulder joint produced by calciphylaxis and their inhibition by triamcinolone: an experimental model, *Bull Soc Int Chir* 23:91, 1965.

Greenspan A: *Orthopedic radiology*, ed 2, Philadelphia, 1992, JB Lippincott.

Greenspan A, Montesano P: *Imaging of the spine in clinical practice*, London, 1993, Wolfe.

Greenstein GM: *Clinical assessment of neuromusculoskeletal disorders*, St Louis, 1997, Mosby.

Grossman ZD et al: *Cost-effective diagnostic imaging the clinician's guide*, ed 3, St Louis, 1995, Mosby.

Guanche CA, Jones DC: Clinical testing for tears of the glenoid labrum, *Arthroscopy* 19(5):517-523, 2003.

Halbach JW, Tank RT: The shoulder. In Gould JA, editor: *Orthopaedic and sports physical therapy*, ed 2, St Louis, 1990, Mosby.

Hale MS: *A practical approach to arm pain*, Springfield, Ill, 1971, Charles C Thomas.

Hammer WI: *Functional soft tissue examination and treatment by manual methods the extremities*, Gaithersburg, Md, 1991, Aspen.

Harryman DJ et al: The role of the rotator internal capsule in passive motion and stability of the shoulder, *J Bone Joint Surg* 74A:53, 1992.

Harryman DT II et al: Repairs of the rotator cuff, *J Bone Joint Surg* 73A:982, 1991.

Harryman DT, Matsen FA, Sidles JA: Arthroscopic management of refractory shoulder stiffness, *Arthroscopy* 13(2):133-147, 1997.

Hartley A: *Practical joint assessment lower quadrant*, ed 2, St Louis, 1995, Mosby.

Hawkins RJ: *An organized approach to musculoskeletal examination and history taking*, St Louis, 1995, Mosby.

Hawkins RJ, Bokor D: Clinical evaluation of shoulder problems. In Rockwood C, Matshe F, editors: *The shoulder*, Philadelphia, 1990, WB Saunders.

Hawkins RJ, Kennedy JC: Impingement syndrome in athletics, *Am J Sports Med* 8:141, 1980.

Hawkins RJ, Mohtadi N: Rotator cuff problems in athletes. In DeLee JC, Drez D, editors: *Orthopaedic sports medicine: principals and practice*, vol 1, Philadelphia, 1994, WB Saunders.

Hijioka A et al: Degenerative change and rotator cuff tears: an anatomical study in 160 shoulders of 80 cadavers, *Arch Orthop Trauma Surg* 112:61, 1993.

Hinkle CZ: *Fundamentals of anatomy & movement a workbook and guide*, St Louis, 1997, Mosby.

Holtby R, Razmjou H: Accuracy of the Speed's and Yergason's tests in detecting biceps pathology and SLAP lesions: comparison with arthroscopic findings, *Arthroscopy* 20(3):231-236, 2004.

Hornberger JP: *Exercise physiology therapeutic exercise*, Sarasota, Fla, 1991, Author.

Hsu HC et al: Calcific tendinitis and rotator cuff tearing; a clinical and radiographic study, *J Shoulder Elbow Surg* 3:159, 1994.

Hurley J: Anatomy of the shoulder. In Nicholas J, Hershman E, editors: *The upper extremity in sports medicine*, St Louis, 1990, Mosby.

Iannotti JP et al: Magnetic resonance imaging of the shoulder: sensitivity specificity and predictive value, *J Bone Joint Surg* 73A:17, 1991.

Itamura J et al: Analysis of the bicipital groove as a landmark for humeral head replacement, *J Shoulder Elbow Surg* 11(4):322-326, 2002.

Itoi E et al: Dynamic anterior stabilizers of the shoulder with the arm in abduction, *J Bone Joint Surg* 76B:834, 1994.

Jablonski S: *Dictionary of medical acronyms & abbreviations*, ed 3, Philadelphia, 1998, Hanley & Belfus.

Jafarnia K, Gabel GT, Morrey BF: Triceps tendinitis, *Oper Tech Sports Med* 9(4):217-221, 2001.

Jehl J, Crummy P: *Essentials of radiologic surgery*, ed 6, Philadelphia, 1993, JB Lippincott.

Jobe C: Gross anatomy of the shoulder. In Rockwood C, Matsen F, editors: *The shoulder*, Philadelphia, 1990, WB Saunders.

Jobe FW et al: The shoulder in sports. In Rockwood CA Jr, Matsen FA III, editors: *The shoulder*, Philadelphia, 1992, WB Saunders.

Kamkar A, Irrgang J, Whitney SL: Nonoperative management of secondary shoulder impingement syndrome, *J Orthop Sports Phys Ther* 17:21, 1993.

Kanner R: *Pain management secrets*, Philadelphia, 1997, Hanley & Belfus.

Kasdan ML: *Occupational hand & upper extremity injuries & diseases*, ed 2, Philadelphia, 1998, Hanley & Belfus.

4

Kaspar S, Mandel S: Acromial impression fracture of the greater tuberosity with rotator cuff avulsion due to hyperabduction injury of the shoulder, *J Shoulder Elbow Surg* 13(1):112-114, 2004.

Katirji B: *Electromyography in clinical practice: a case study approach*, St Louis, 1998, Mosby.

Katz WA: *Rheumatic diseases diagnosis and management*, Philadelphia, 1977, JB Lippincott.

Keats TH: *Atlas of normal roentgen variants*, ed 6, St Louis, 1996, Mosby.

Kendall HO, Kendall FP, Wadsworth GE: *Muscles testing and function*, ed 2, Baltimore, 1971, Williams & Wilkins.

Kenter K et al: Dynamic and passive analysis of anterior capsular contractures of the glenohumeral joint, *J Shoulder Elbow Surg* 7(3):302, 1998.

Kessel L, Watson M: The painful arc syndrome: clinical classification as a guide to management, *J Bone Joint Surg* 59B:166, 1977.

Kircher MT, Cappuccino A, Torpey BM: Muscular violence as a cause of humeral fractures in pitchers, *Contemp Orthop* 26:475, 1993.

Kisner C, Colby LA: *Therapeutic exercise; foundations and techniques*, ed 2, Philadelphia, 1990, FA Davis.

Klippel JH, Dieppe PA: *Rheumatology*, vol 1-2, ed 2, London, 1998, Mosby.

Kronberg M, Nemeth G, Brostrom LA: Muscle activity and coordination in the normal shoulder: an electromyographic study, *Clin Orthop Rel Res* 257:76, 1990.

Kursuaogu-Brahme S, Gandry CR, Resnick D: Advanced imaging of the wrist, *Radiol Clin North Am* 228:307, 1990.

Lain TM: The military brace syndrome: a report of 16 cases of Erb's palsy occurring in military cadets, *J Bone Joint Surg* 51A:557, 1969.

Lavy CBD, Barrett DS: *Questions and answers on Apley's concise system of orthopaedics and fractures*, Oxford, UK, 1991, Butterworth-Heinemann.

Leffert RD: Neurological problems. In Rockwood CA, Matsen FA, editors: *The shoulder*, vol 1, Philadelphia, 1990, WB Saunders.

Leffert RD et al: Infra-clavicular brachial plexus injuries, *J Bone Joint Surg* 47B:9, 1965.

Legan JM et al: Tears of the glenoid labrum: MR imaging of 88 arthroscopically confirmed cases, *Radiology* 179:241, 1991.

Lerner AJ: *The little black book of neurology*, ed 3, St Louis, 1995, Mosby.

Lewis CB, Knortz KA: *Orthopedic assessment and treatment of the geriatric patient*, St Louis, 1993, Mosby.

Lippitt S, Matsen F: Mechanisms of glenohumeral joint stability, *Clin Orthop* 291:20, 1993.

Litchfield R et al: Rehabilitation of the overhead athlete, *J Orthop Sports Phys Ther* 18:433, 1993.

Loth TS: *Orthopedic boards review II: a case study approach*, St Louis, 1996, Mosby.

Lucas DB: Biomechanics of the shoulder joint, *Arch Surg* 107:425, 1973.

Magee DJ: *Orthopedic physical assessment*, ed 3, Philadelphia, 1997, WB Saunders.

Malen WJ, Bassett FH III, Goldner RD: Luxatio erecta: the inferior glenohumeral dislocation, *J Orthop Trauma* 4:19, 1990.

Malone TR, McPoil TG, Nitz AJ: *Orthopedic and sports physical therapy*, ed 3, St Louis, 1997, Mosby.

Marchiori DM: *Clinical imaging with skeletal, chest, and abdomen pattern differentials*, St Louis, 1999, Mosby.

Markey KL, DiBenedetto M, Curl WW: Upper trunk brachial plexopathy, *Am J Sports Med* 21:650, 1993.

Martin DR, Gaith WP: Results of orthoscopic debridement of glenoid labral tears, *Am J Sports Med* 23:4, 1995.

Martin JH: *Neuroanatomy text and atlas*, ed 2, Stamford, Conn, 1996, Appleton & Lange.

Mathers LH et al: *Clinical anatomy principles*, St Louis, 1996, Mosby.

Matsen F, Arntz C: Rotator cuff failure. In Rockwood C, Matsen F, editors: *The shoulder*, Philadelphia, 1990, WB Saunders.

Matsen F, Arntz C: Subacromial impingement. In Rockwood C, Matsen F, editors: *The shoulder*, Philadelphia, 1990, WB Saunders.

Matsen FA III, Arntz CT: Rotator cuff tendon failure in the shoulder. In Matsen FA III, Rockwood CA Jr, editors: *The shoulder*, Philadelphia, 1990, WB Saunders.

Mazion JM: *Illustrated manual of neurological reflexes/signs/tests, part I; orthopedic signs/tests/maneuvers for office procedure, part II*, Orlando, Fla, 1980, Daniels Publishing.

McLaughlin HL: The "frozen" shoulder, *Clin Orthop* 20:126, 1961.

McMahon PJ et al: Glenohumeral translations are increased after a type II superior labrum anterior-posterior lesion: a cadaveric study of severity of passive stabilizer injury, *J Shoulder Elbow Surg* 13(1):39-44, 2004.

McRae R: *Clinical orthopaedic examination*, ed 3, Edinburgh, 1990, Churchill Livingstone.

McRae R: *Practical fracture treatment*, ed 3, New York, 1994, Churchill Livingstone.

Medical Economics Books: *Patient care flow chart manual*, ed 3, Oradell, NJ, 1982, Medical Economics Books.

Mellion MB: *Office sports medicine*, ed 2, St Louis, 1996, Mosby.

Mellion MB: *Sports medicine secrets*, Philadelphia, 1994, Hanley & Belfus.

Mendoza RX, Nicholas JA, Sands A: Principals of shoulder rehabilitation in the athlete. In Nicholas JA, Hershman EB, editor: *The upper extremity in sports medicine*, St Louis, 1990, Mosby.

Mengel MB, Schwiebert LP: *Ambulatory medicine the primary care of families*, ed 2, Stamford, Conn, 1996, Appleton & Lange.

Mennell JM: *The musculoskeletal system differential diagnosis from symptoms and physical signs*, Gaithersburg, Md, 1992, Aspen.

Mercier LR, Pettid FJ: *Practical orthopedics*, ed 4, St Louis, 1995, Mosby.

Merle D'Aubigne R: Nerve injuries in fractures and dislocations of the shoulder, *Surg Clin North Am* 43:1685, 1963.

Miller MD: *Review of orthopaedics*, Philadelphia, 1992, WB Saunders.

Mirvis SE, Young JWR: *Imaging in trauma and critical care*, Baltimore, 1991, Williams & Wilkins.

Misamore GW, Woodward C: Evaluation of degenerative lesions of the rotator cuff: a comparison of arthrography and ultrasonography, *J Bone Joint Surg* 73A:704, 1991.

Moore KL: *Clinically oriented anatomy*, ed 3, Baltimore, 1992, Williams & Wilkins.

Morrey BF, An K: *Biomechanics of the shoulder*, Philadelphia, 1990, WB Saunders.

Mosby-Year Book, Inc: *Expert 10-minute physical examination*, St Louis, 1997, Mosby-Year Book.

Moseley HF: *Shoulder lesions*, ed 3, Baltimore, 1969, Williams & Wilkins.

Moseley JB et al: EMG analysis of the scapular muscles during a shoulder rehabilitation program, *Am J Sports Med* 10:128, 1992.

Murnaghan JP: Frozen shoulder. In Rockwood C, Matsen F, editors: *The shoulder*, Philadelphia, 1990, WB Saunders.

Neer CS II: *Shoulder reconstruction*, Philadelphia, 1990, WB Saunders.

Neer CS: Anterior acromioplasty for the chronic impingement syndrome in the shoulder, *J Bone Joint Surg* 54A:41, 1972.

Nettina SM: *The Lippincott manual of nursing practice*, ed 6, Philadelphia, 1996, Lippincott.

Neviaser JS: Musculoskeletal disorders of the shoulder region causing cervicobrachial pain: differential diagnosis and treatment, *Surg Clin North Am* 43:1703, 1963.

Newton RW: *Color atlas of pediatric neurology*, St Louis, 1995, Mosby-Wolfe.

Nielsen KD, Wester JU, Lorensten A: The shoulder impingement syndrome: the results of surgical decompression, *J Shoulder Elbow Surg* 3:12, 1994.

Nordin M, Andersson GBJ, Pope MH: *Musculoskeletal disorders in the workplace: principles and practice*, St Louis, 1997, Mosby.

Nordt WE, Garretson RB, Plotkin E: The measurement of subacromial contact pressure in patients with impingement syndrome, *Arthroscopy* 15(2):121-125, 1999.

Norris T: Treatment and physical examination of the shoulder. In Nicholas J, Hershman E, editors: *The upper extremity in sports medicine*, St Louis, 1990, Mosby.

O'Brien SJ, Miller AN, Drakos MC: Arthroscopic subdeltoid approach to the biceps transfer, *Oper Tech Sports Med* 15(1):20-26, 2007.

O'Brien SJ et al: The anatomy and histology of the inferior glenohumeral ligament complex of the shoulder, *Am J Sport Med* 18:449, 1990.

O'Donoghue DH: *Treatment of injuries to athletes*, ed 3, Philadelphia, 1976, WB Saunders.

Olson WH et al: *Handbook of symptom-oriented neurology*, ed 2, St Louis, 1994, Mosby.

Omer GE, Spinner M: *Management of peripheral nerve problems*, Philadelphia, 1980, WB Saunders.

O'Young B, Young MA, Stiens SA: *PM&R secrets*, Philadelphia, 1997, Hanley & Belfus.

Ozel SK, Kazez A: Horner syndrome due to first rib fracture after major thoracic trauma, *J Pediatr Surg* 40(10):e17-e19, 2005.

Pagana KD, Pagana TJ: *Mosby's manual of diagnostic and laboratory tests*, St Louis, 1998, Mosby.

Pagnani MJ, Galinat BJ, Warren RF: Glenohumeral instability. In Nicholas JA, Hershman EB, editors: *The upper extremity in sports medicine*, St Louis, 1990, Mosby.

Parsons TA: The snapping scapula and subscapular exostosis, *J Bone Joint Surg* 55B:345, 1963.

Patten J: *Neurological differential diagnosis*, ed 2, London, 1996, Springer.

Pecina MM, Krmpotic-Nemanic J, Markiewitz AD: *Tunnel syndromes*, Boca Raton, Fla, 1991, CRC Press.

Pheasant S: *Ergonomics, work and health*, Gaithersburg, Md, 1991, Aspen.

Polley HF, Hunder GG: *Rheumatologic interviewing and physical examination of the joints*, ed 2, Philadelphia, 1978, WB Saunders.

Pollock RG et al: The use of arthroscopy in the treatment of resistant frozen shoulder, *Clin Orthop* 304:30, 1994.

Pradhan S: Shank sign in myotonic dystrophy type-1 (DM-1), *J Clin Neurosci* 14(1):27-32, 2007.

Pronsati MP: Treatment of thoracic outlet syndrome comes under scrutiny, *Adv Physical Therapists* Sept:14, 1991.

Quigley TB: The nonoperative treatment of symptomatic calcareous deposits in the shoulder, *Surg Clin North Am* 43:1495, 1963.

Rachlin ES: *Myofascial pain and fibromyalgia trigger point management*, St Louis, 1994, Mosby.

Ravel R: *Clinical laboratory medicine clinical application of laboratory data*, ed 6, St Louis, 1995, Mosby.

Rayan G, Jensen C: Thoracic outlet syndrome: provocative examination maneuvers in a typical population, *J Shoulder Elbow Surg* 4(2):113-117, 1995.

Reilly PJ, Torg JS: Athletic injury to the cervical nerve roots and brachial plexus, *Op Tech Sports Med* 1:231, 1993.

Relwani JG et al: Luxatio erecta in an adolescent with axillary artery and brachial plexus injury, *Injury Extra* (in press, corrected proof).

Resnick D, Niwayama G: *Diagnosis of bone and joint disorders*, Philadelphia, 1995, WB Saunders.

Riley GP et al: Glycosaminoglycans of human rotator cuff tendons: changes with age and in chronic rotator cuff tendinitis, *Ann Rheum Dis* 53:367, 1994.

Riley GP et al: Tendon degeneration and chronic shoulder pain; changes in the collagen composition of the human rotator cuff tendons in rotator cuff tendinitis, *Ann Rheum Dis* 53:359, 1994.

Rizk TE, Pinals RS, Talaiver AS: Corticosteroid injections in adhesive capsulitis; investigation of their value and site, *Arch Phys Med Rehabil* 72:20, 1991.

Rockwood CA, Young DC: Disorders of the acromioclavicular joint. In Rockwood CA, Matsen FA, editors: *The shoulder*, vol 2, Philadelphia, 1990, WB Saunders.

Rodosky MW, Harner CD, Fu FH: The role of the long head of the biceps muscle and superior glenoid labrum in anterior stability of the shoulder, *Am J Sport Med* 22:121, 1994.

Rogers LR: *Radiology of skeletal trauma*, ed 2, London, 1992, Churchill Livingstone.

Rolak LA: *Neurology secrets*, ed 2, Philadelphia, 1998, Hanley & Belfus.

Roos DB et al: Thoracic outlet syndrome, *Arch Surg* 93:71, 1966.

Rumack CM, Wilson SR, Charboneau JW: *Diagnostic ultrasound*, vol 1-2, ed 2, St Louis, 1998, Mosby.

Ruwe PA et al: Can MR imaging effectively replace diagnostic arthroscopy? *Radiology* 183;335, 1992.

Saidoff DC, McDonough AL: *Critical pathways in therapeutic intervention*, St Louis, 1997, Mosby.

Sano H, Wakabayashi I, Itoi E: Stress distribution in the supraspinatus tendon with partial-thickness tears: an analysis using two-dimensional finite element model, *J Shoulder Elbow Surg* 15(1):100-105, 2006.

Sarris I, Sotereanos DG: Distal biceps tendon ruptures, *J Am Soc Surg Hand* 2(3):121-128, 2002.

Saxena K, Stavas J: Inferior glenohumeral dislocation, *Ann Emerg Med* 12(11):718-720, 1983.

Schamblin ML, Safran MR: Injury of the distal biceps at the musculotendinous junction, *J Shoulder Elbow Surg* 16(2):208-212, 2007.

Schumacher HR, Bomalski JS: *Case studies in rheumatology for the house officer*, Baltimore, 1990, Williams & Wilkins.

Schumacher HR, Klippel JH, Koopman WJ: *Primer on the rheumatic diseases*, ed 10, Atlanta, 1993, Arthritis Foundation.

Seikaly H et al: The clavipectoral osteomyocutaneous free flap, *Otolaryngol Head Neck Surg* 117(5):547-554, 1997.

Selye H: The experimental production of calcified deposits in the rotator cuff, *Surg Clin North Am* 43:1483, 1963.

Seror P: Symptoms of thoracic outlet syndrome in women with carpal tunnel syndrome, *Clin Neurophysiol* 116(10):2324-2329, 2005.

Shankman GA: *Fundamental orthopedic management for the physical therapist assistant*, St Louis, 1997, Mosby.

Silliman JF, Dean MT: Neurovascular injuries to the shoulder complex, *J Orthop Sports Phys Ther* 18:442, 1993.

Silliman JF, Hawkins RJ: Classification and physical diagnosis of instability of the shoulder, *Clin Orthop* 291:7, 1993.

Silliman JF, Hawkins RJ: Current concepts and recent advances in the athlete's shoulder, *Clin Sports Med* 10:693, 1991.

Skyhar MJ, Warren RF, Altchek DW: Instability of the shoulder. In Nicholas JA, Hershman EB, editors: *The upper extremity in sports medicine*, St Louis, 1990, Mosby.

Snyder SJ et al: Partial thickness rotator cuff tears: results of arthroscopic treatment, *Arthroscopy* 7:1, 1991.

Snyder SJ, Karzel RP, Del Pizzo W: SLAP lesions of the shoulder, *Arthroscopy* 6:274, 1990.

Sobel J, Pettrone F, Nirschl R: Prevention and treatment of upper extremity sports injuries. In Nicholas J, Hershman E, editors: *The extremity in sports medicine*, St Louis, 1990, Mosby.

Soslowsky LJ et al: Articular geometry of the glenohumeral joint, *Clin Orthop* 285:181, 1992.

Specht NT, Russo RD: *Practical guide to diagnostic imaging*, St Louis, 1998, Mosby.

Stedman TL: *Stedman's medical dictionary*, ed 25, Baltimore, 1990, Williams & Wilkins.

Steinbrocher O: The painful shoulder. In Hollander JL, McCarty DJ, editors: *Arthritis and allied conditions*, ed 8, Philadelphia, 1972, Lea & Febiger.

Stewart DL, Abeln SH: *Documenting functional outcomes in physical therapy*, St Louis, 1993, Mosby.

Stiles RG, Otte MT: Imaging of the shoulder, *Radiology* 188:603; 1993.

Stoller DW: *Magnetic resonance imaging in orthopaedics & sports medicine*, Philadelphia, 1993, JB Lippincott.

Strege D: Upper extremity. In Loth T, editor: *Orthopaedic boards review*, St Louis, 1993, Mosby.

Sutton D: *A textbook of radiology and imaging*, ed 5, London, 1993, Churchill Livingstone.

Sutton D, Young JWR: *A concise textbook of clinical imaging*, ed 2, St Louis, 1995, Mosby.

4

Tan JC, Horn SE: *Practical manual of physical medicine and rehabilitation*, St Louis, 1998, Mosby.

Taybi H, Lachman RS: *Radiology of syndromes, metabolic disorders, and skeletal dysplasias*, ed 4, St Louis, 1996, Mosby.

Taylor CJ, Bansal R, Pimpalnerkar A: Acute distal biceps tendon rupture—a new surgical technique using a de-tensioning suture to brachialis, *Injury* 37(9):838-842, 2006.

Thein LA: Rehabilitation of shoulder injuries. In Prentice WE, editor: *Rehabilitation techniques in sports medicine*, ed 2, St Louis, 1994, Mosby.

Thibodeau GA, Patton KT: *Anatomy & physiology*, ed 3, St Louis, 1996, Mosby.

Thibodeau GA, Patton KT: *Pocket reference to accompany anatomy & physiology*, ed 3, St Louis, 1996, Mosby.

Thompson JM: *Clinical outlines for health assessment*, St Louis, 1997, Mosby.

Ticker J, Beam G, Warner JP: Recognition and treatment of refractory posterior capsular contracture of the shoulder, *Arthroscopy* 12(3):353-354, 1996.

Toghill PJ: *Examining patients: an introduction to clinical medicine*, London, 1990, Edward Arnold.

Tollison CD, Satterthwaite JR, Tollison JW: *Handbook of pain management*, ed 2, Baltimore, 1994, Williams & Wilkins.

Torg JS, Shepard RJ: *Current therapy in sports medicine*, ed 3, St Louis, 1995, Mosby.

Townsend H et al: Electromyographic analysis of the glenohumeral muscles during a baseball rehabilitation program, *Am J Sports Med* 19:264, 1991.

Turek SL: *Orthopaedics principles and their application*, ed 3, Philadelphia, 1977, JB Lippincott.

Uhthoff H, Sarkar K: Calcifying tendinitis. In Rockwood C, Matsen F, editors: *The shoulder*, Philadelphia, 1990, WB Saunders.

Van Holsbeeck M, Introcaso JH: *Musculoskeletal ultrasound*, St Louis, 1991, Mosby.

Vanderstraeten G, Ozcakar L, Verstraete K: Thoracic outlet syndrome portending Klippel-Feil syndrome, *Joint Bone Spine* 73(6):763-764, 2006.

Verma NN, Drakos M, O'Brien SJ: Arthroscopic transfer of the long head biceps to the conjoint tendon, *Arthroscopy* 21(6):764.e1-764.e5, 2005.

Wakefield TS, Frank RG: *The clinician's guide to neuro musculoskeletal practice*, Abbotsford, Wisc, 1995, Allied Health of Wisconsin.

Warner JJP et al: Arthroscopic release of chronic, refractory capsular contracture of the shoulder, *J Shoulder Elbow Surg* 5(2, part 2):S7-S354, 1996.

Warner JP, Ticker JB, Beim GM: Recognition and treatment of refractory posterior capsular contracture of the shoulder, *J Shoulder Elbow Surg* 5(2, part 2):S113-S354, 1996.

Wasilewski SA, Frankel U: Rotator cuff pathology, *Clin Orthop* 267:65, 1991.

Weineck J: *Functional anatomy in sports*, ed 2, St Louis, 1990, Mosby.

Weinstein SL, Buckwalter JA: *Turek's orthopaedics principles and their application*, ed 5, Philadelphia, 1994, JB Lippincott.

Whitenack SH et al: Thoracic outlet syndrome complex: diagnoses and treatment. In Hunter JM et al, editors: *Rehabilitation of the hand: surgery and therapy*, ed 3, St Louis, 1990, Mosby.

Williams GR, Rockwood CA: Fractures of the scapula. In DeLee JC, Drez D, editors: *Orthopaedic sports medicine: principals and practice*, vol 1, Philadelphia, 1994, WB Saunders.

Williams GR, Rockwood CA: Injuries to the acromioclavicular joint. In DeLee JC, Drez D, editors: *Orthopaedic sports medicine: principals and practice*, vol 1, St Louis, 1994, WB Saunders.

Williams MM, Snyder SJ, Buford D Jr: The Buford complex, the cord-like middle glenohumeral ligament and absent anterosuperior labrum complex; a normal anatomic capsulolabral variant, *Arthroscopy* 10:2417, 1994.

Windsor RE, Lox DM: *Soft tissue injuries: diagnosis and treatment*, Philadelphia, 1998, Hanley & Belfus.

Winter D: *Biomechanics and motor control of human movement*, ed 2, New York, 1990, Wiley-Interscience.

Wright IS: Neurovascular syndrome produced by hyperabduction of the arms, *Am Heart J* 29:1, 1945.

Wright IS: *Vascular diseases in clinical practice*, Chicago, 1948, Mosby.

Wright IS et al: The subclavian steal and other shoulder girdle syndromes, *Trans Am Clin Climatol Assoc* 76:13, 1964.

Wright V: The shoulder-hand syndrome, *Rep Rheum Dis* 24:1, 1966.

Wuelker N, Plitz W, Roetman B: Biomechanical data concerning the shoulder impingement syndrome, *Clin Orthop* 303:242, 1994.

Yahara ML: Shoulder. In Richardson JK, Iglarsh ZA, editors: *Clinical orthopaedic physical therapy*, Philadelphia, 1994, WB Saunders.

Yergason RM: Supination sign, *J Bone Joint Surg* 12:160, 1931.

Yochum T, Rowe L: *Essentials of skeletal radiology*, ed 2, Baltimore, 1996, Williams & Wilkins.

Young DC, Rockwood CA: Fractures of the clavicle. In DeLee JC, Drez D, editors: *Orthopaedic sports medicine: principals and practice*, vol 1, Philadelphia, 1994, WB Saunders.

Young JWR, Mirvis SE, editors: *Imaging in trauma and critical care*, Baltimore, 1991, Williams & Wilkins.

Zitelli BJ, Davis HW: *Atlas of pediatric physical diagnosis*, ed 2, London, 1992, Wolfe.

CITATIONS

Barkhordarian S: First rib resection in thoracic outlet syndrome, *J Hand Surg* 32(4):565-570, 2007.

Begaz T, Mycyk MB: Luxatio erecta: inferior humeral dislocation, *J Emerg Med* 31(3):303-304, 2006.

Bhatia DN et al: The reverse terrible triad of the shoulder: circumferential glenohumeral musculoligamentous disruption and neurologic injury associated with posterior shoulder dislocation, *J Shoulder Elbow Surg* 16(3):e13-e17, 2007.

Bond JL, Pasque C: The transverse humeral ligament: a distinct entity or a continuation of the rotator cuff? (SS-48), *Arthroscopy* 21(6, suppl 1):e23-e24, 2005.

Burkhart SS et al: Arthroscopic repair of massive rotator cuff tears with stage 3 and 4 fatty degeneration, *Arthroscopy* 23(4):347-354, 2007.

Castagna A et al: Minor shoulder instability, *Arthroscopy* 23(2):211-215, 2007.

Colli BO et al: Neurogenic thoracic outlet syndromes: a comparison of true and nonspecific syndromes after surgical treatment, *Surg Neurol* 65(3):262-271, 2006.

Cope MR et al: Biceps rupture in bodybuilders: three case reports of rupture of the long head of the biceps at the tendon-labrum junction. *J Shoulder Elbow Surg* 13(5):580-582, 2004.

Ersel M et al: Axillary artery dissection due to blunt shoulder trauma, *Am J Emerg Med* 25(2):242-243, 2007.

Flury MP et al: Rupture of the subscapularis tendon (isolated or in combination with supraspinatus tear): when is a repair indicated? *J Shoulder Elbow Surg* 15(6):659-664, 2006.

Frost A, Michael Robinson C: The painful shoulder, *Surgery (Oxford)* 24(11):363-367, 2006.

Gayraud M: Raynaud's phenomenon, *Joint Bone Spine* 74(1):e1-e8, 2007.

Gillard J et al: Diagnosing thoracic outlet syndrome: contribution of provocative tests, ultrasonography, electrophysiology, and helical computed tomography in 48 patients, *Joint Bone Spine* 68(5):416-424, 2001.

Gimblett PA, Saville J, Eball P: A conservative management protocol for calcific tendinitis of the shoulder, *J Manipulative Physiol Ther* 22(9):622-627, 1999.

Herrera JE, Stubblefield MD: Rotator cuff tendonitis in lymphedema: a retrospective case series, *Arch Phys Med Rehabil* 85(12):1939-1942, 2004.

Hugl B et al: Unusual etiology of upper extremity ischemia in a scleroderma patient: thoracic outlet syndrome with arterial embolization, *J Vasc Surg* 45(6):1259-1261, 2007.

Jackson MR: Upper extremity arterial injuries in athletes, *Semin Vasc Surg* 16(3):232-239, 2003.

Kaymak B et al: A novel finding in thoracic outlet syndrome: tachycardia, *Joint Bone Spine* 71(5):430-432, 2004.

Kelley SP, Hinsche AF, Hossain JFM: Axillary artery transection following anterior shoulder dislocation: classical presentation and current concepts, *Injury* 35(11):1128-1132, 2004.

Ko J-Y et al: Pathogenesis of partial tear of the rotator cuff: a clinical and pathologic study, *J Shoulder Elbow Surg* 15(3):271-278, 2006.

Lafosse L et al: Anterior and posterior instability of the long head of the biceps tendon in rotator cuff tears: a new classification based on arthroscopic observations, *Arthroscopy* 23(1):73-80, 2007.

Lahteenmaki HE et al: Repair of full-thickness rotator cuff tears is recommended regardless of tear size and age: a retrospective study of 218 patients, *J Shoulder Elbow Surg* (in press, corrected proof).

Lee JC et al: MRI of the rotator interval of the shoulder, *Clin Radiol* 62(5):416-423, 2007.

Lee JT et al: Long-term thrombotic recurrence after nonoperative management of Paget-Schroetter syndrome, *J Vasc Surg* 43(6):1236-1243, 2006.

MacMahon PJ et al: Contribution of full-thickness supraspinatus tendon tears to acquired subcoracoid impingement, *Clin Radiol* 62(6):556-563, 2007.

McCann PA, Barakat MJ, Wand JS: Delayed brachial plexus compression secondary to anterior shoulder dislocation—the late consequence of an axillary artery pseudoaneurysm: a case report, *Injury Extra* 37(12):458-461, 2006.

Moratalla MB, Gabarda RF: Acromioclavicular joint ganglion, *Eur J Radiol Extra* (in press, corrected proof).

Nakagawa S et al: Throwing shoulder injury involving the anterior rotator cuff: concealed tears not as uncommon as previously thought, *Arthroscopy* 22(12):1298-1303, 2006.

Ogawa K, Yoshida A, Ikegami H: Osteoarthritis in shoulders with traumatic anterior instability: preoperative survey using radiography and computed tomography, *J Shoulder Elbow Surg* 15(1):23-29, 2006.

Pookarnjanamorakot C, Sirikulchayanonta V: Tuberculous bursitis of the subacromial bursa, *J Shoulder Elbow Surg* 13(1):105-107, 2004.

Rusch VW: Management of Pancoast tumours, *Lancet Oncol* 7(12):997-1005, 2006.

Sanders RJ, Hammond SL: Subclavian vein obstruction without thrombosis, *J Vasc Surg* 41(2):285-290, 2005.

Scheibel M et al: The belly-off sign: a new clinical diagnostic sign for subscapularis lesions, *Arthroscopy* 21(10):1229-1235, 2005.

Seil R et al: Arthroscopic treatment of chronically painful calcifying tendinitis of the supraspinatus tendon, *Arthroscopy* 22(5):521-527, 2006.

Shebel ND, Marin A: Effort thrombosis (Paget-Schroetter syndrome) in active young adults: current concepts in diagnosis and treatment, *J Vasc Nurs* 24(4):116-126, 2006.

Werner CML, Favre P, Gerber C: The role of the subscapularis in preventing anterior glenohumeral subluxation in the abducted, externally rotated position of the arm, *Clin Biomech* 22(5):495-501, 2007.

Whittam K, Hardy M: A case study of an axillary artery pseudoaneurysm following anterior dislocation of the glenohumeral joint: a rare presentation on plain film radiographs, *Radiography* (in press, corrected proof).

CHAPTER FIVE

ELBOW

INDEX OF TESTS

AXIOMS IN ASSESSING THE ELBOW

- The elbow is a complex hinge joint.
- The elbow is essential to the positioning and full use of the hand.
- Soft-tissue lesions such as lateral epicondylitis and olecranon bursitis occur more often than joint disease.
- Diagnosis of elbow conditions is largely based on pain, location of swelling, presence of point tenderness, and the results of range-of-motion studies.

INTRODUCTION

Although the number of diseases that affect the elbow with any degree of frequency is small, examining the joint often provides clues to diagnosis of specific neuromuscular disease. Pain is the symptom that focuses attention on this joint and prompts the patient to visit the physician. Although it usually reflects a localized process at the elbow, the pain may be referred from the hand and wrist or from the shoulder and neck. Most abnormal actions of the elbow can be compensated by the shoulder; therefore even moderate compromises of motion, provided they are painless, do not result in disability. Subtle flexion contractures may develop over years without the patient even being aware of the changes or range-of-motion losses. In contrast, significant pain at the elbow incapacitates the entire arm. Sleeves of clothing often cover the elbows; thus swellings and deformities become cosmetically important only when they are exaggerated. The examiner should note whether swelling is intracapsular or extracapsular, intramuscular or intermuscular. The earliest sign of joint effusion is induration of the capsule around the

ORTHOPEDIC GAMUT 5-1

ISOSCELES TRIANGLE OF THE ELBOW

If the angles of the isosceles triangle of the elbow are abnormal, the following may exist:
- Posterior elbow dislocation (Fig. 5-2)
- Fracture of the epicondyle
- Intracondylar fracture
- Fracture of the olecranon

TABLE 5-1

ELBOW JOINT CROSS-REFERENCE TABLE BY SYNDROME PROCEDURE

Elbow Test/Sign	Lateral Epicondylitis	Radiohumeral Bursitis	Cubital Tunnel Syndrome	Medial Epicondylitis	Neuropathy	Sprain
Cozen test	•	•				
Elbow flexion test			•			
Golfer elbow test				•		
Kaplan sign	•					
Ligamentous instability test						•
Mills test	•					
Tinel sign at the elbow					•	

olecranon or epicondyles. In the flexed position, the hollows of the indurated synovium are totally filled.

When the elbow is extended, the epicondyles and the tip of the olecranon should be at the same level. In normal elbow configuration, when a line is drawn between the epi-

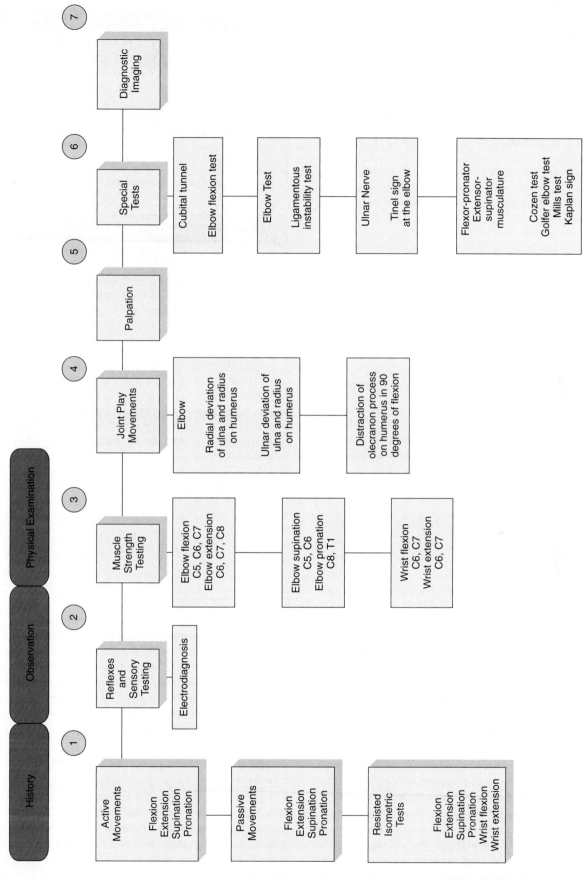

FIG. 5-1 Protocol of elbow joint assessment.

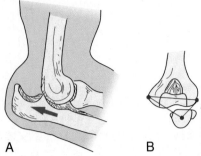

FIG. 5-2 A, Posterior elbow dislocation. **B,** Posterior view of elbow dislocation demonstrating the bony alignment. (From Hartley A: *Practical joint assessment upper quadrant*, ed 2, St Louis, 1995, Mosby.)

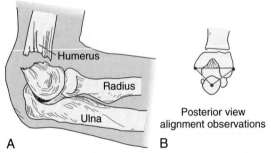

FIG. 5-3 A, Supracondylar fracture with olecranon impingement. **B,** Posterior view demonstrating the bony misalignment. (From Hartley A: *Practical joint assessment upper quadrant*, ed 2, St Louis, 1995, Mosby.)

condyles, the olecranon should bisect and be on the center of the line. When the normal elbow is flexed to an angle of 90 degrees, the tip of the olecranon should be directly below to the line joining the epicondyles. If a line from the olecranon is drawn to each epicondyle, the three prominences and line should form an isosceles triangle.

If the triangle is normal, but abnormal in relation to the shaft of the humerus, the patient might have a supracondylar fracture in which the three bony landmarks are displaced posteriorly (Fig. 5-3).

> The combination of posterior dislocation of the elbow and fractures of the radial head and coronoid process is often called the *terrible triad of the elbow* because of the propensity for complications related to instability, arthrosis, and stiffness. Notably, the fractures of the coronoid that occur in association with the terrible-triad pattern of injury are nearly always transverse fractures of the tip that include the insertion of the anterior elbow capsule, but the height of these fragments is debated. The fracture morphology and injury pattern are more important than the classification of the coronoid fracture according to height. The vast majority of terrible-triad injuries have a transverse fracture of the coronoid process that is less than 50% of the coronoid height. These fragments may seem small on radiographs but are very important to elbow stability by virtue of both the con-

---

ORTHOPEDIC GAMUT 5-2
PRIMARY FUNCTIONS OF THE ELBOW
1. Aids in positioning the hand in appropriate locations
2. Adjusts height and length of the limb
3. Stabilizes the upper extremity for power and fine motor work activities
4. Provides fulcrum for the arm in lifting

ORTHOPEDIC GAMUT 5-3
ELBOW JOINTS
The elbow consists of a complex set of joints that require thorough assessment. The articulations of the joint are as follows:
1. Humeroulnar
2. Humeroradial
3. Proximal radioulnar

TABLE 5-2

ELBOW JOINT CROSS-REFERENCE TABLE BY SYNDROME

Cubital tunnel syndrome	Elbow flexion test
Lateral epicondylitis	Cozen test
	Kaplan sign
	Mills test
Medial epicondylitis	Golfer elbow test
Neuropathy	Tinel sign at the elbow
Radiohumeral bursitis	Cozen test
Sprain	Ligamentous instability test

tribution to an anterior bony buttress against posterior elbow dislocation and the stability of the anterior capsular insertion (Doornberg, van Duijn, Ring, 2006).

The examination of the elbow must be preceded by a precise history to allow emphasis to be placed on particular areas. Complaints usually consist of pain, loss of movement, weakness, clicking, or locking. The patient may complain of sharply localized pain, typical of extraarticular disease, deep joint pain, or the poorly localized pain of ulnar neuropathy with or without typical paresthesia extending to the hand (Fig. 5-4). The functional interplay among the elbow, shoulder, and wrist means that examination of all of these joints may be necessary (Table 5-3). Referred pain in the elbow, especially from the neck or shoulder, is usually diffuse. Examination must include comparison of right and left arms.

Pain of lateral elbow origin is usually diagnosed as radiohumeral bursitis, epicondylitis, or tennis elbow (Fig. 5-5).

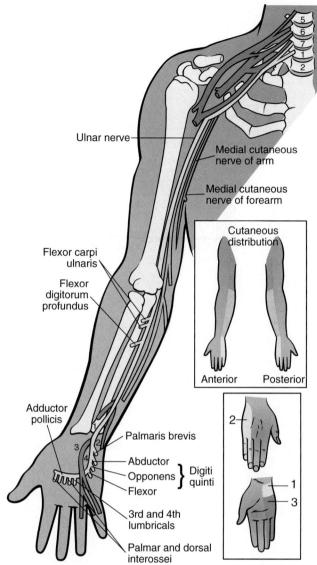

FIG. 5-4 The course of the ulnar nerve. (From Katirji B: *Electromyography in clinical practice: a case study approach*, St Louis, 1998, Mosby.)

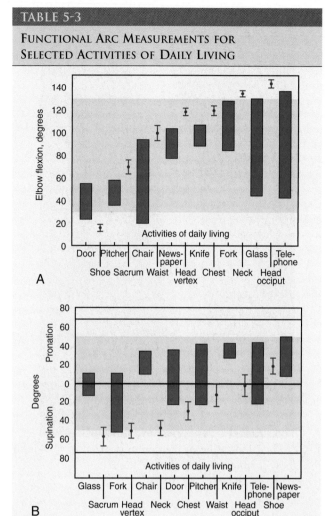

TABLE 5-3

FUNCTIONAL ARC MEASUREMENTS FOR SELECTED ACTIVITIES OF DAILY LIVING

From Kelley WN et al: *Textbook of rheumatology,* ed 5, Philadelphia, 1997, WB Saunders.

This problem involves either the origin of the wrist extensors (tendinopathy) or, occasionally, radial nerve impingement by musculotendinous structures crossing the elbow joint (Fig. 5-6).

A similar problem may occur on the medial elbow epicondyle because all of the wrist flexors and pronators originate from the medial epicondyle. Affected individuals use flexor-pronator muscle groups repetitively, isometrically or isokinetically. This circumstance is unusual because forceful wrist flexor power is seldom used. Most of powerful hand grasping is accomplished in the dorsiflexed wrist position.

Intraarticular abnormalities such as osteochondritis dissecans of the capitellum results in lateral elbow pain (Fig. 5-7).

Osteochondritis dissecans of the elbow is an idiopathic disorder that affects the capitellum of the humerus, with ensuing avascular necrosis. It is usually seen in the dominant arm of adolescent boys, especially those involved in throwing sports (Fig. 5-8). Panner disease is a condition of unclear origin characterized by osteochondrosis of the capitellum. It is seen most often in young boys who complain of tenderness and swelling over the lateral aspect of the elbow with limited extension. Direct trauma or inadequate circulation through the elbow joint has been associated with osteochondritis of the capitellum (Fig. 5-9).

Osteonecrotic lesions have been reported in the trochlea and radial head, as well as the olecranon and olecranon fossa. **Osteochondritis dissecans** generally occurs in athletes ages 11 to 21 years who report a history of overuse. The osteonecrotic lesion involves only a segment of capitellum, located primarily at a central or anterolateral position. Appropriate treatment of this disorder remains controversial. Often treated with benign neglect, this condition is a potentially sport-ending injury for an athlete, with long-term sequelae of degenerative arthritis (Levine, Field, Savoie Iii, 2006).

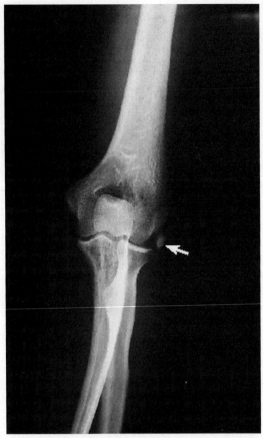

FIG. 5-5 Calcification of the common extensor tendon of the elbow *(arrow).* (From Deltoff MN, Kogon PL: *The portable skeletal x-ray library*, St Louis, 1998, Mosby.)

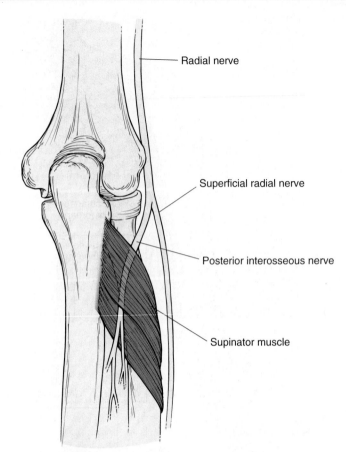

FIG. 5-6 In a posterior view, the radial nerve as it passes through the supinator musculature, travels around the head of the radius, and branches to the posterior interosseous nerves of the elbow. (From Greenstein GM: *Clinical assessment of neuromusculoskeletal disorders*, St Louis, 1997, Mosby.)

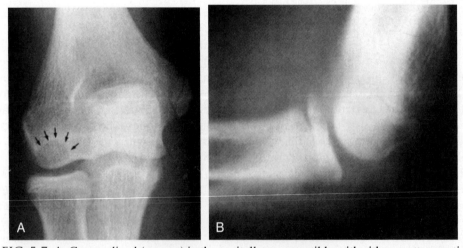

FIG. 5-7 **A,** Cyst outlined *(arrows)* in the capitellum compatible with either posttraumatic osteochondrosis or an osteochondral fracture. **B,** Traumatic osteochondrosis of the radial head. (From Nicholas JA, Hershman EB: *The upper extremity in sports medicine*, ed 2, St Louis, 1995, Mosby.)

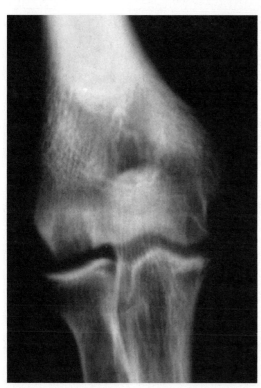

FIG. 5-8 Radiograph of osteochondritis dissecans of the capitellum. (From Nicholas JA, Hershman EB: *The upper extremity in sports medicine*, ed 2, St Louis, 1995, Mosby.)

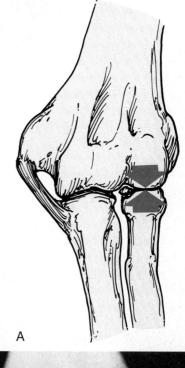

A

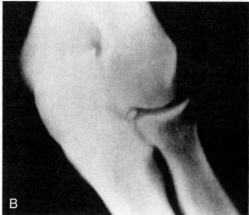

B

FIG. 5-9 **A** and **B,** Demonstration of radial head-capitellum compression and resultant loose bodies. (From Nicholas JA, Hershman EB: *The upper extremity in sports medicine*, ed 2, St Louis, 1995, Mosby.)

ORTHOPEDIC GAMUT 5-4

AVASCULAR NECROSIS OF THE CAPITELLUM

Possible causes of avascular necrosis of the capitellum of the elbow (Panner disease):
1. Bacterial infection
2. Fracture
3. Heredity
4. Vascular insufficiency

An extremely minor fracture of the radial head (chisel fracture) may cause pain that might be confused with tennis elbow (Fig. 5-10). An injury occurring in children and adolescents in whom the medial epicondyle is inflamed with partial separation of the apophysis is *little leaguer's elbow* (Fig. 5-11).

Poorly chosen terms and *umbrella* diagnoses create confusion. The term *little leaguer's elbow* is one such term. To some authorities, it means traction apophysitis of the olecranon; to others, it means medial epicondyle avulsion; and to still others, it means osteochondritis dissecans. Little league elbow now encompasses a series of diagnoses, including (1) medial epicondylar fragmentation and apophysitis, (2) delayed or accelerated apophyseal growth of the medial epicondyle, (3) delayed closure of the medial epicon-

dylar growth plate, (4) osteochondrosis and osteochondritis dissecans of the humeral capitellum, (5) deformation and osteochondritis of the radial head, (6) hypertrophy of the ulna, and (7) olecranon apophysitis (Bradley, Petrie, 2001).

Boxer's elbow (also called *hyperextension overload syndrome* or *olecranon impingement syndrome*) is caused by repetitive valgus extension of the elbow in the boxer's jab or in sports involving throwing (Fig. 5-12). Elbow joint hyperextension injuries usually result from falling on an outstretched arm. The elbow is extended and the forearm supinated (Fig. 5-13).

Pain in the elbow, particularly extending along the entire arm, in the absence of objective findings at the joint suggests psychogenic origins. Other diseases referring pain to the elbow include myocardial infarction, cervical root lesions,

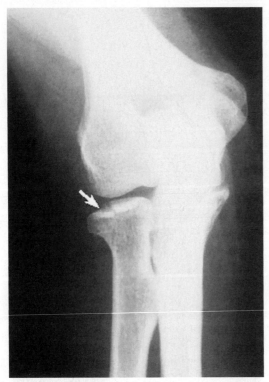

FIG. 5-10 Radial head fracture (chisel) of the lateral radial head *(arrow)*, with inferior displacement of the fragment. (From Deltoff MN, Kogon PL: *The portable skeletal x-ray library*, St Louis, 1998, Mosby.)

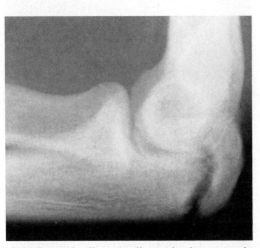

FIG. 5-11 Lateral elbow radiograph demonstrating the widened olecranon apophyseal plate. (From Nicholas JA, Hershman EB: *The upper extremity in sports medicine*, ed 2, St Louis, 1995, Mosby.)

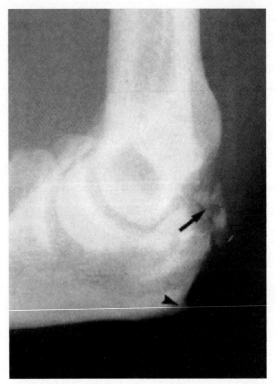

FIG. 5-12 Hypertrophic spurs at the posterior aspect of the olecranon process *(top arrow)*. (From Nicholas JA, Hershman EB: *The upper extremity in sports medicine*, ed 2, St Louis, 1995, Mosby.)

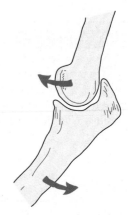

FIG. 5-13 Elbow hyperextension injury mechanism, with olecranon impingement. (From Hartley A: *Practical joint assessment upper quadrant*, ed 2, St Louis, 1995, Mosby.)

thoracic outlet syndromes, or subdeltoid bursitis. Psychogenic origins are further supported with a history of neurosis, strange behavior, or a bizarre and inconsistent complaint history; diagnostic imaging and laboratory tests are as unimpressive as the physical findings. Carpal tunnel syndrome may cause retrograde radiation of pain to the elbow.

Elbow joint complaints usually consist of pain, loss of movement, weakness, clicking, or locking. The patient may complain of sharply localized pain (typical of extraarticular disease), deep joint pain, or poorly localized pain of ulnar neuropathy with or without typical paresthesias extending to the hand. The functional interplay among the elbow, shoulder, and wrist means that examination of all these joints is necessary. Referred pain in the elbow, especially from the neck or shoulder, is usually diffuse (Table 5-4).

True elbow pain can be related to joint disease; however, it is more commonly caused by lesions of the periarticular tissues. Inflammation of the olecranon bursa *(draftsman's elbow)* may be secondary to several conditions, including repetitive or acute trauma, rheumatoid arthritis, gout, and

ORTHOPEDIC GAMUT 5-5

HYPEREXTENSION INJURIES OF THE ELBOW

Structures of the elbow injured with hyperextension forces:

1. Biceps brachii at its point of insertion on the neck of the radius
2. Brachialis at its point of insertion on the ulna
3. Brachioradialis
4. Anterior portion of the medial (ulnar) or lateral (radial) collateral ligaments (The medial collateral ligament is injured more often because of the valgus position of the joint.)
5. Elbow capsular and collateral ligament (They can avulse a piece of the condyle, most commonly the medial epicondyle.)

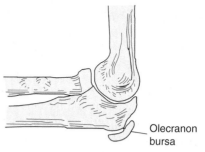

FIG. 5-14 The olecranon bursa. (From Hartley A: *Practical joint assessment upper quadrant*, ed 2, St Louis, 1995, Mosby.)

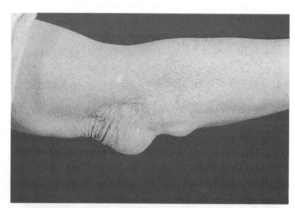

FIG. 5-15 Olecranon bursitis as seen with rheumatoid arthritis; note also the rheumatoid nodule distal to the joint. (From Klippel JH, Dieppe PA: *Rheumatology*, vol 1-2, ed 2, London, 1998, Mosby.)

pseudogout (Fig. 5-14). It is also known as *student's elbow* or *miner's elbow*.

The olecranon bursa is prone to injury by friction or a blow. Additionally, because of its position, swelling occurs easily and is readily visible. It is also a common site involved in crystal arthropathies (gout or, rarely, calcium pyrophosphate arthritis), or in generalized inflammatory arthritis, especially rheumatoid arthritis in which swelling of the olecranon bursa may be seen in association with rheumatoid nodules on the ulnar border of the forearm (Fig. 5-15).

Traumatic or repetitive motion osteochondritis of the radial head occurs in some sports that involve throwing, especially evident in the preadolescent and adolescent athletes. The radioulnar joint is affected by loose bodies and synovial osteochondromatosis. Traumatic partial subluxation of the radial head through the annular ligament occurs in children younger than 8 years (Fig. 5-16).

A *pushed elbow* describes subluxation of the radial head in a proximal direction, which is often seen after a child falls on an outstretched hand. A *pulled elbow* is subluxation of the radial head in a distal direction, which may follow a forceful traction to the forearm.

Pulled elbow is a common injury in preschool children. It is caused by sudden traction on the forearm and is usually characterized by an inability to move the arm with pain. The peak incidence occurs in children aged between 1 and 3 years, and reports indicate that the injury does not occur in older children because the capsular attachment of the annular ligament in older children is thicker and less likely to tear (Kajiwara et al, 2007).

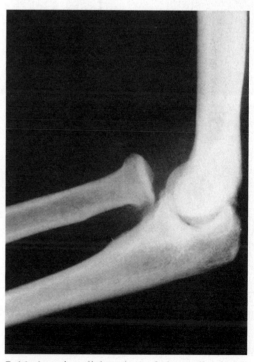

FIG. 5-16 Anterior dislocation of the radial head. (From Nicholas JA, Hershman EB: *The upper extremity in sports medicine*, ed 2, St Louis, 1995, Mosby.)

ESSENTIAL ANATOMY

The elbow acts as a lever system that, along with the other joints, changes the direction of the upper extremity to put the hand in the most effective functional position. The elbow consists of three bones: the distal end of the humerus and the proximal ends of the radius and the ulna (Figs. 5-17 to 5-19). The three articulating surfaces are enclosed in a single synovial cavity. The olecranon bursa is the largest bursa of the elbow, although several smaller bursae are present (Fig. 5-20).

The three major deep nerves of the forearm are the radial, medial, and ulnar nerves. The radial nerve lies anterior to the lateral epicondyle in the arm in its anterior compartment (Fig. 5-21).

The medial nerve enters the forearm by passing between the two heads of pronator teres and descends in the anterior compartment of the forearm, traveling between the flexor digitorum superficialis and flexor digitorum profundus muscles (Fig. 5-22).

At the elbow, the ulnar nerve lies in a groove on the posterior surface of the medial epicondyle of the humerus

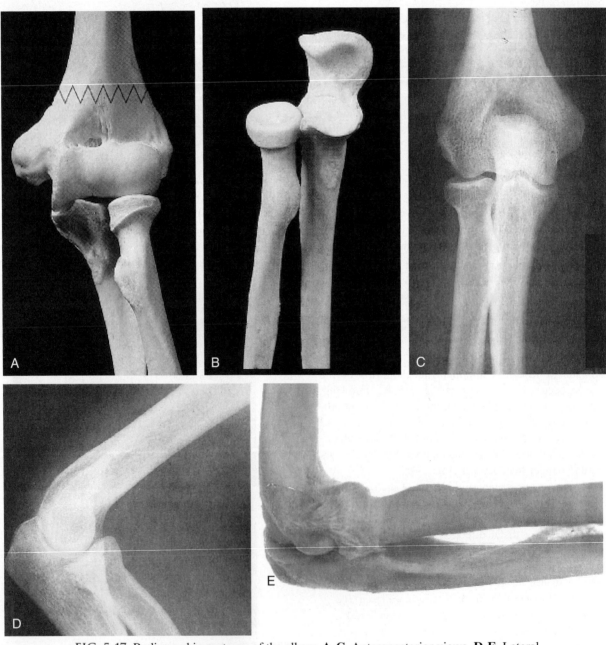

FIG. 5-17　Radiographic anatomy of the elbow. **A-C,** Anteroposterior views. **D-E,** Lateral views. (From Greenstein GM: *Clinical assessment of neuromusculoskeletal disorders*, St Louis, 1997, Mosby.)

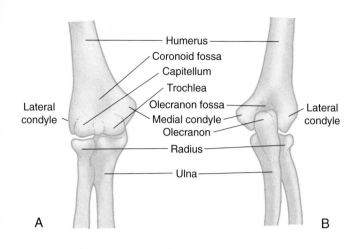

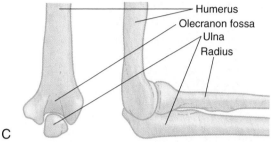

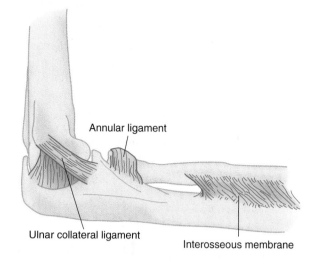

FIG. 5-18 Bony anatomy of distal humerus and elbow region. **A,** Anterior view. **B,** Posterior view. **C,** Posterior view, 90 degrees flexion. **D,** Lateral view. Right elbow is shown. (Modified from Connolly JF: *DePalma's management of fractures and dislocation,* Philadelphia, 1981, WB Saunders; Marx JA, Hockberger RS, Walls RM, et al, eds: *Rosen's emergency medicine: concepts and clinical practice,* ed 6, St. Louis, 2006, Mosby.)

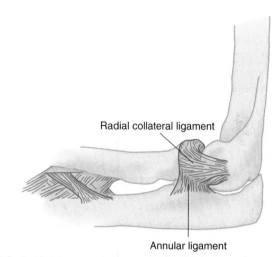

FIG. 5-19 Ligamentous structures of the elbow. (From Simon R, Koenigsknecht S: *Emergency orthopaedics: the extremities,* ed 2, Norwalk, Conn, 1987, Appleton & Lange. In Marx JA, Hockberger RS, Walls RM, et al, eds: *Rosen's emergency medicine: concepts and clinical practice,* ed 6, St. Louis, 2006, Mosby.)

TABLE 5-4

UPPER EXTREMITY PERIARTICULAR SYNDROME DIFFERENTIAL DIAGNOSTIC LIST

Region	Periarticular Syndrome	Monarticular Syndrome
Shoulder	Subacromial bursitis	Pancoast tumor
	Long-head bicipital tendinopathy	Brachial plexopathy
		Cervical nerve root injury
	Rotator cuff tear	
Elbow	**Olecranon bursitis**	**Ulnar nerve entrapment**
	Epicondylitis	
Wrist	Extensor tendinopathy (including de Quervain tenosynovitis)	Carpal tunnel syndrome
	Gonococcal tenosynovitis	
Hand	Palmar fasciitis (Dupuytren contracture)	Ligamentous or capsular injury

Modified from Kelley WN et al: *Textbook of rheumatology,* ed 5, Philadelphia, 1997, WB Saunders.

and travels between the two heads of the flexor carpi ulnaris to enter the forearm (see Fig. 5-22).

Arterial supply to the forearm depends entirely on branches of the brachial artery (Fig. 5-23). The radial artery courses to the lateral side of the forearm and aligns itself with the radius. The ulnar artery is the larger of the two branches of the brachial artery (Fig. 5-24).

ESSENTIAL MOTION ASSESSMENT

Tissue approximation limits elbow flexion to 140 to 150 degrees. Retained flexion motion of 130 degrees or less is impairment in the activities of daily living (Fig. 5-25).

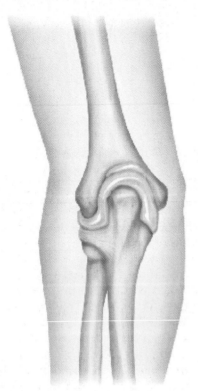

FIG. 5-20 Elbow joint (posterior view). (From Barkauskas VH et al: *Health & physical assessment*, ed 2, St Louis, 1998, Mosby.)

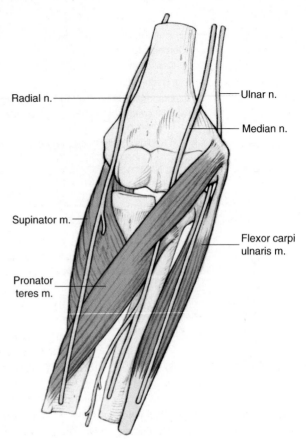

FIG. 5-22 Potential sites for compression of nerves in the proximal forearm (anterior view, right elbow). (From Mathers LH et al: *Clinical anatomy principles*, St Louis, 1996, Mosby.)

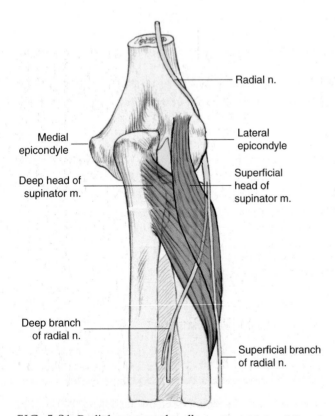

FIG. 5-21 Radial nerve at the elbow. (From Mathers LH et al: *Clinical anatomy principles*, St Louis, 1996, Mosby.)

Elbow extension is 0 degrees. Up to 10 degrees of hyperextension is still within normal limits if the patient has no history of trauma to the joint. The inability to return the elbow to within 10 degrees of the neutral position is impairment in the activities of daily living (Fig. 5-26).

The valgus angle of the elbow ranges from 0 to 15 degrees. This feature allows the forearm to extend beyond the width of the pelvis. The carrying angle enables the forearm to sustain high tensile stresses. Variations in the carrying angle are cubitus valgus (forearm farther than the arm) and cubitus varus (forearm carried more medial) (Fig. 5-27). A *gunstock deformity* is a cubitus varus deformity of the elbow. Gunstock deformities are usually secondary to fractures or epiphyseal injury to the distal humerus. The carrying angle is a normal finding and is not indicative of an elbow occult disease.

Supination of the elbow is limited by tissue stretch to 90 degrees. Retained supination motion of 60 degrees or less is impairment in the activities of daily living (Fig. 5-28).

Elbow pronation is the same as supination, 80 to 90 degrees. Retained pronation motion of 70 degrees or less is impairment in the activities of daily living (Figs. 5-29 and 5-30).

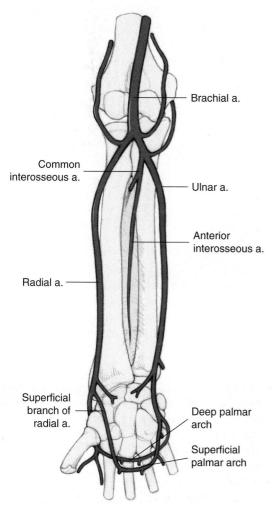

FIG. 5-23 Arterial supply to the forearm (anterior view). (From Mathers LH et al: *Clinical anatomy principles*, St Louis, 1996, Mosby.)

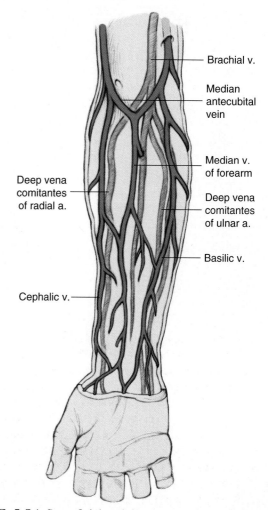

FIG. 5-24 Superficial and deep veins of the forearm (anterior view). (From Mathers LH et al: *Clinical anatomy principles*, St Louis, 1996, Mosby.)

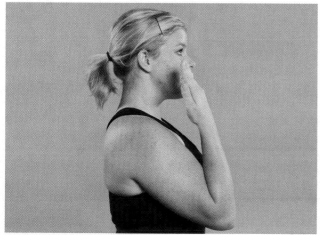

FIG. 5-25 Tissue approximation limits elbow flexion to 140 to 150 degrees. Retained flexion motion of 130 degrees or less is an impairment in the activities of daily living.

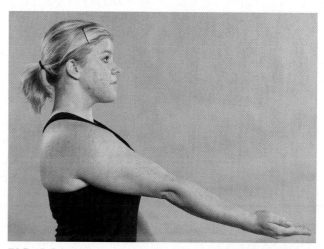

FIG. 5-26 Elbow extension is 0 degrees. Ten degrees of hyperextension is within normal limits if equal bilaterally and in the absence of injury. The inability to return the elbow to within 10 degrees of the neutral position is an impairment in the activities of daily living.

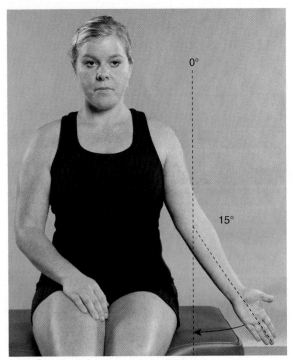

FIG. 5-27 The expected carrying angle of the arm is between 0 and 15 degrees in the adult.

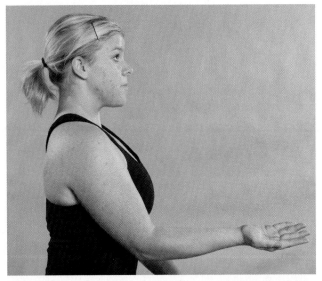

FIG. 5-28 Supination of the elbow is limited, by tissue stretch, to 90 degrees. Retained supination motion of 60 degrees or less is an impairment in the activities of daily living.

ESSENTIAL MUSCLE FUNCTION ASSESSMENT

The arm is divided by fascial septa into anterior and posterior compartments. The lateral and medial intermuscular septa (Figs. 5-31 and 5-32) attach to the humerus and radiate medially and laterally to the skin, dividing the arm.

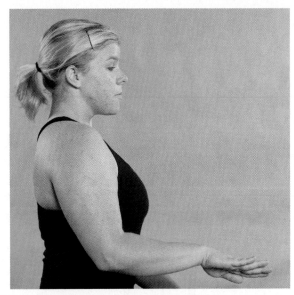

FIG. 5-29 Elbow pronation, 80 to 90 degrees, is the same as supination. Retained pronation motion of 70 degrees or less is an impairment in the activities of daily living.

ORTHOPEDIC GAMUT 5-6

ELBOW JOINT

Plain-film radiographic films demonstrate that the elbow is a compound joint consisting of:
1. Articulation of the trochlea of the humerus with the trochlear notch of the ulna
2. Articulation of the capitulum of the humerus with the superior surface of the radial head

---

The prime movers in flexion of the elbow are the biceps brachii (musculocutaneous nerve, C5, C6), brachialis (musculocutaneous nerve, C5, C6), and brachioradialis (radial nerve, C5, C6) muscles. The flexor muscles of the forearm arising from the medial epicondyle of the humerus are the accessory muscles (Fig. 5-33).

The prime mover in extension of the elbow is the triceps brachii muscle (radial nerve, C7, C8); the anconeus muscle is an accessory. When the arm is horizontally abducted, the long head of the triceps is shortened over the shoulder joint. When the shoulder is flexed, the long head of the triceps is shortened over the elbow joint and elongated over the shoulder joint (Fig. 5-34).

Although the triceps and anconeus act together in extending the elbow joint, the two muscles can be differentiated. The belly of the anconeus muscle is below the elbow joint and is easily distinguished from the triceps by palpation. Paralysis of the anconeus materially reduces the strength of elbow extension (Fig. 5-35).

The primary supinators are the biceps brachii and the supinator. The accessory muscle in this movement is the

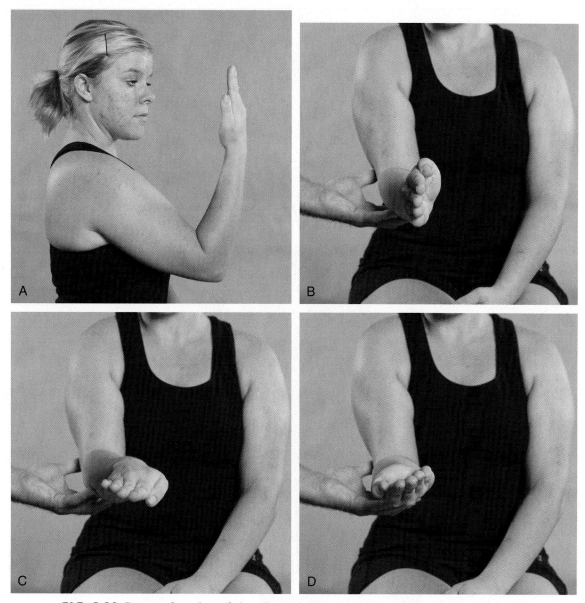

FIG. 5-30 Range of motion of the elbow. **A,** Flexion and extension. **B,** Pronation and supination.

brachioradialis. In addition to its role in supination, the biceps also functions as an elbow flexor. Its total biceps function is well illustrated in the act of twisting a corkscrew into the cork of a bottle and then pulling the cork out of the bottle (Fig. 5-36).

The primary pronators are the pronator teres and the pronator quadratus. The accessory muscle in this movement is the flexor carpi radialis. Pronation and supination are complex movements (Fig. 5-37) that occur simultaneously around an axis best described as an imaginary line between the head of the radius proximally and the medial end of the triangular articular disc distally. In the proximal radioulnar joint, the head of the radius can rotate within the perimeter created by the annular ligament (Fig. 5-38).

ESSENTIAL IMAGING

The elbow position of function is 90 degrees of flexion with the forearm midway between supination and pronation. In this position, the olecranon process of the ulna and the medial and lateral epicondyles of the humerus normally form an isosceles triangle when viewed posteriorly; this position is known as the *triangle sign*. If a fracture, dislocation, or degeneration leading to loss of bone or cartilage occurs, the distance between the apex and base decreases, and the isosceles triangle no longer exists (Fig. 5-39).

Extension of the elbow is limited by the olecranon of the ulna as it contacts the olecranon fossa of the humerus (Figs. 5-40 and 5-41); flexion of the elbow is limited only

PROXIMAL

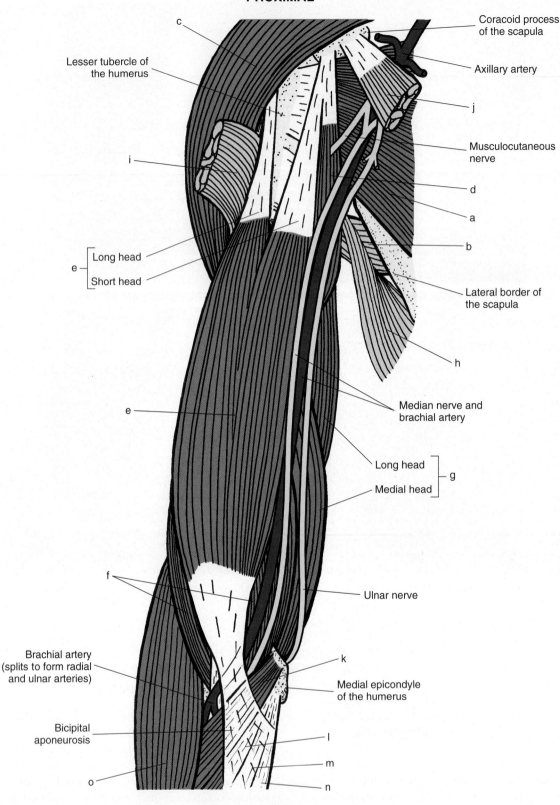

LATERAL

MEDIAL

c

Lesser tubercle of
the humerus

Coracoid process
of the scapula

Axillary artery

j

Musculocutaneous
nerve

d

a

b

i

Long head

Short head

e

Lateral border of
the scapula

h

e

Median nerve and
brachial artery

Long head

Medial head

g

f

Ulnar nerve

Brachial artery
(splits to form radial
and ulnar arteries)

k

Medial epicondyle
of the humerus

Bicipital
aponeurosis

l

m

o

n

DISTAL

FIG. 5-31 Superficial muscles of the anterior aspect of the elbow. (From Muscolino JE: *The
muscular system manual: the skeletal muscles of the human body*, St Louis, 2003, Mosby.)

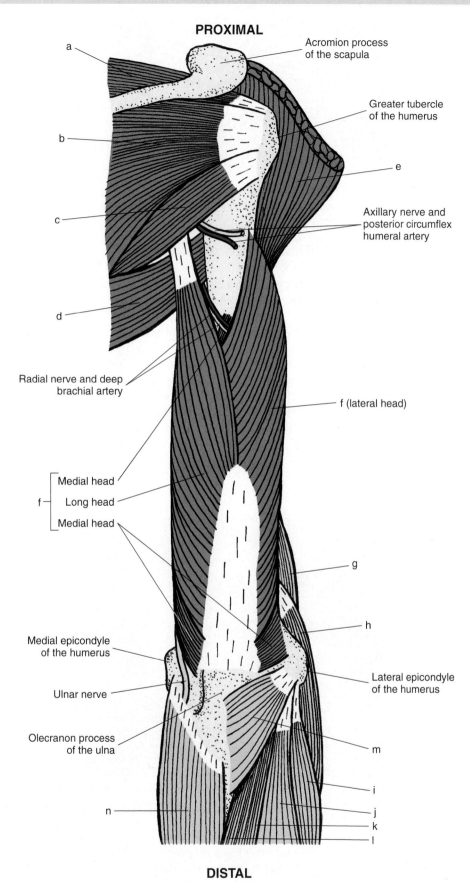

PROXIMAL

a

Acromion process
of the scapula

b

Greater tubercle
of the humerus

c

e

Axillary nerve and
posterior circumflex
humeral artery

d

Radial nerve and deep
brachial artery

MEDIAL

LATERAL

5

f (lateral head)

Medial head
f — Long head
Medial head

g

h

Medial epicondyle
of the humerus

Lateral epicondyle
of the humerus

Ulnar nerve

m

Olecranon process
of the ulna

i

n

j
k
l

DISTAL

FIG. 5-32 Muscles of the posterior aspect of the arm and elbow. (From Muscolino JE: *The muscular system manual: the skeletal muscles of the human body*, St Louis, 2003, Mosby.)

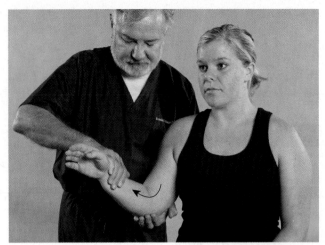

FIG. 5-33 The prime movers in flexion of the elbow are the biceps brachii (musculocutaneous nerve, C5, and C6), brachialis (musculocutaneous nerve, C5, and C6), and brachioradialis (radial nerve, C5, and C6) muscles. The flexor muscles of the forearm that
arise from the medial epicondyle of the humerus are the accessory muscles. For testing
flexion of the elbow, the patient sits with the arm at the side, the elbow slightly flexed,
and the forearm supinated. The examiner stabilizes the patient's arm by grasping it with
one hand. The patient is instructed to flex the elbow through its range of motion against
graded resistance applied by the examiner. The examiner's other hand is just proximal to
the patient's wrist. If the biceps and brachialis are weak, as in a musculocutaneous lesion,
the patient will pronate the forearm before flexing the elbow. With this type of lesion, the
patient is using the brachioradialis, extensor carpi radialis longus, PT, and wrist flexors.

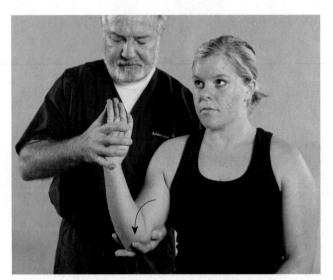

FIG. 5-34 The prime mover in extension of the elbow is the triceps brachii muscle (radial
nerve, C7, and C8), and the anconeus muscle is an accessory. The patient is seated. To
test extension of the elbow, the examiner fixes the patient's arm as described for flexion
and instructs the patient to move the elbow through the range of extension motion while
providing graded resistance with the other hand just proximal to the patient's wrist. When
the arm is horizontally abducted, the long head of the triceps is shortened over the shoulder joint. When the shoulder is flexed, the long head of the triceps is shortened over the
elbow joint and elongated over the shoulder joint.

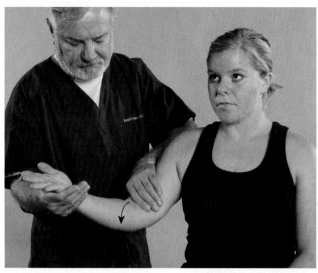

FIG. 5-35 Although the triceps and anconeus act together in extending the elbow joint, the two muscles can be differentiated. The belly of the anconeus muscle is below the elbow joint and is easily distinguished from the triceps by palpation. The branch of the radial nerve that innervates the anconeus arises near the midhumeral level and is long. A lesion can involve only this branch, leaving the triceps unaffected. Paralysis of the anconeus materially reduces the strength of elbow extension. The muscle grade of good in elbow extension strength is actually the result of a normal triceps and a zero anconeus function.

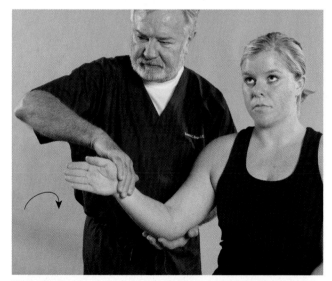

FIG. 5-37 The primary pronators are the PT and the pronator quadratus. The accessory muscle in this movement is the FCR. The examiner stabilizes the patient's elbow just proximal to the joint. This stabilization prevents the substitution of shoulder abduction and internal rotation for pure forearm pronation. The resisting hand is adjusted so that the thenar eminence presses against the volar surface of the hand. This adjustment requires only that the examiner turn the resisting hand from the dorsal to the volar surface of the patient's hand. The patient begins forearm pronation from a position of supination. As the patient moves into pronation, the resistance is increased.

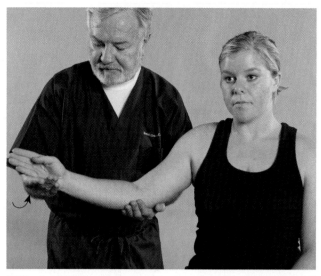

FIG. 5-36 The primary supinators are the biceps brachii and the supinator. The accessory muscle in this movement is the brachioradialis. In addition to its role in supination, the biceps also functions as an elbow flexor. Its total biceps function is well illustrated in the act of twisting a corkscrew into the cork of a bottle and then pulling the cork out of the bottle. In testing supination, the examiner stabilizes and supports the elbow at the side of the patient. This support will prevent the substitution of shoulder adduction and external rotation for forearm supination. The thenar eminence of the examiner's resisting hand is placed on the dorsal surface of the patient's hand and wrist. The patient begins supination from a position of pronation, and as the arm is moved into supination, the resistance is gradually increased.

by the apposition of the muscle masses of the arm and forearm and the bones themselves (Fig. 5-42 and 5-43). Lateral shift of the olecranon process during elbow flexion can result in a medial incongruity of the olecranon-trochlear joint space. A medial incongruity of more than 5 mm is a potential cause of ulnar nerve compression (Figs. 5-44 to 5-47).

Computed tomography (CT) is a successful adjunct to plain-film radiography in demonstrating subtle elbow injury. CT studies are particularly helpful in demonstrating occult fractures and osteochondral injuries, as well as in localizing loose bodies and osteophytes located out of the plane of conventional radiographs (Fig. 5-48).

Muscles in the forearm have a variety of attachments. They are found in two large groupings: the anterior and posterior forearm muscles (Fig. 5-49). Magnetic resonance imaging (MRI) of patients is useful in identifying recalcitrant lateral epicondylitis (Fig. 5-50).

Arthrography of the elbow can be carried out using either single- or double-contrast techniques (Fig. 5-51).

As it crosses the cubital fossa at the elbow, the brachial artery remains superficial, covered only by the bicipital aponeurosis and the median cubital vein (Fig. 5-52).

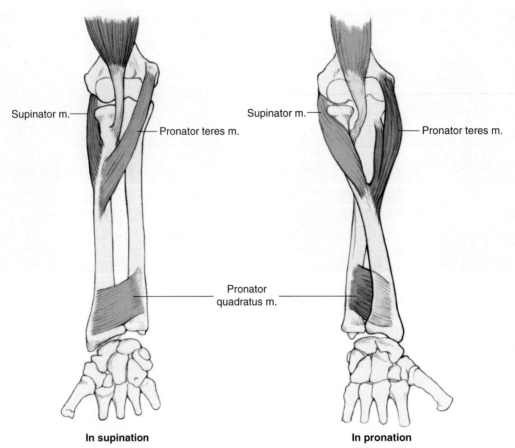

Supinator m.

Pronator teres m.

Supinator m.

Pronator teres m.

Pronator
quadratus m.

In supination

In pronation

FIG. 5-38 Muscles mediating supination (**A**) and pronation (**B**). (From Mathers LH et al: *Clinical anatomy principles*, St Louis, 1996, Mosby.)

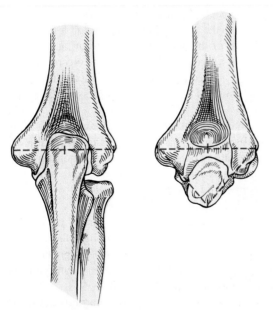

FIG. 5-39 Relationship of the palpable landmarks of the medial and lateral epicondyles of the humerus and the olecranon tip of the ulna. (From Nicholas JA, Hershman EB: *The upper extremity in sports medicine*, ed 2, St Louis, 1995, Mosby.)

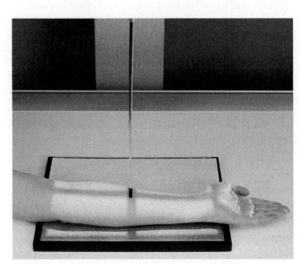

FIG. 5-40 Anteroposterior positioning of the elbow. (From Frank ED, et al: *Merrill's atlas of radiographic positioning and procedures*, vol 1-3, ed 11, St Louis, 2007, Mosby.)

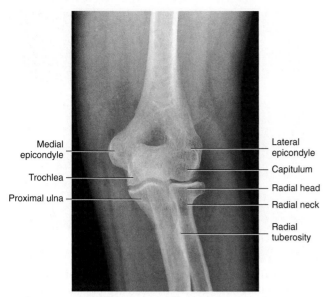

FIG. 5-41 Anteroposterior radiograph of the elbow. (From Frank ED, et al: *Merrill's atlas of radiographic positioning and procedures*, vol 1-3, ed 11, St Louis, 2007, Mosby.)

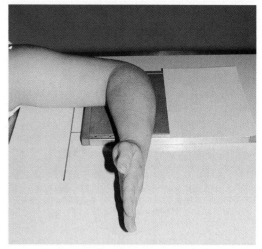

FIG. 5-42 Lateral positioning of the elbow. (From Frank ED, et al: *Merrill's atlas of radiographic positioning and procedures*, vol 1-3, ed 11, St Louis, 2007, Mosby.)

5

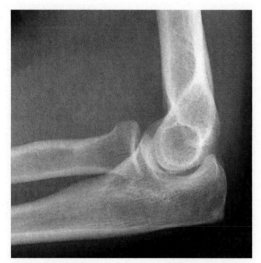

FIG. 5-43 Lateral radiograph of the elbow. (From Frank ED, et al: *Merrill's atlas of radiographic positioning and procedures*, vol 1-3, ed 11, St Louis, 2007, Mosby.)

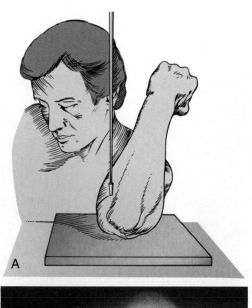

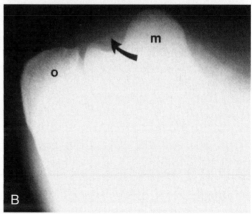

FIG. 5-44 **A,** Cubital tunnel view. **B,** Cubital tunnel radiograph of normal elbow. *Curved arrow,* Cubital tunnel; *m,* medial epicondyle; *o,* olecranon process. (From Nicholas JA, Hershman EB: *The upper extremity in sports medicine*, ed 2, St Louis, 1995, Mosby.)

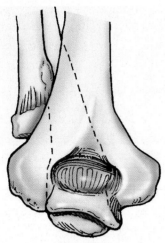

FIG. 5-45 Posteroanterior axial olecranon process. (From Frank ED, et al: *Merrill's atlas of radiographic positioning and procedures*, vol 1-3, ed 11, St Louis, 2007, Mosby.)

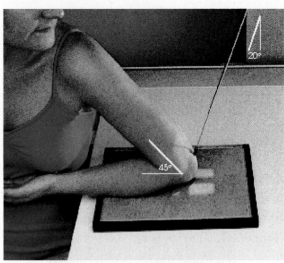

FIG. 5-46 Posteroanterior axial positioning of olecranon process with central ray angled at 20 degrees. (From Frank ED, et al: *Merrill's atlas of radiographic positioning and procedures*, vol 1-3, ed 11, St Louis, 2007, Mosby.)

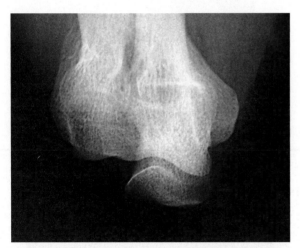

FIG. 5-47 Posteroanterior radiograph of axial olecranon process with central ray angulation at 20 degrees. (From Frank ED, et al: *Merrill's atlas of radiographic positioning and procedures*, vol 1-3, ed 11, St Louis, 2007, Mosby.)

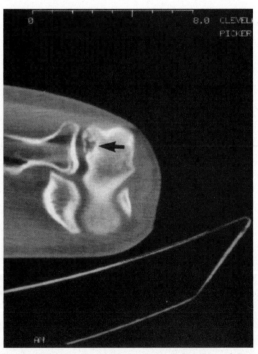

FIG. 5-48 CT scan made through the joint line of the elbow demonstrates osteochondritis dissecans in the subchondral bone of the capitellum. (From Nicholas JA, Hershman EB: *The upper extremity in sports medicine*, ed 2, St Louis, 1995, Mosby.)

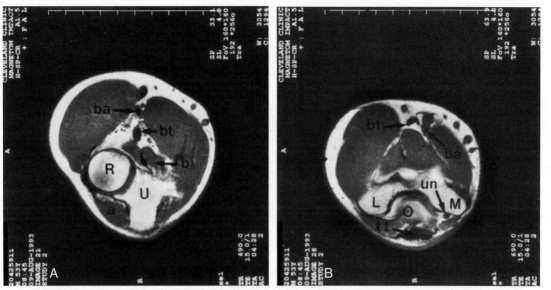

FIG. 5-49 These T1-weighted spin-echo images of a normal elbow demonstrate the signal intensities of normal tissues. **A,** Level of radioulnar articulation. **B,** Level of intercondylar region. (From Nicholas JA, Hershman EB: *The upper extremity in sports medicine*, ed 2, St Louis, 1995, Mosby.)

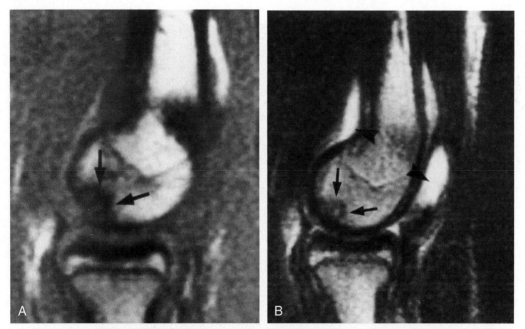

FIG. 5-50 T1-weighted (**A**) and T2-weighted (**B**) spin-echo images of a 12-year-old gymnast documenting the clinically suspected diagnosis of osteochondritis dissecans. (From Nicholas JA, *Hershman EB: The upper extremity in sports medicine*, ed 2, St Louis, 1995, Mosby.)

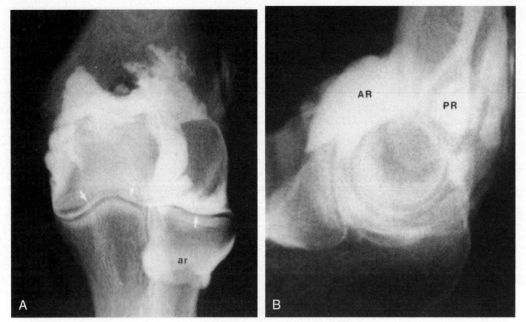

FIG. 5-51 Anteroposterior (**A**) and lateral (**B**) radiographs of the elbow made during a single-contrast elbow arthrogram demonstrate the articular cartilage *(arrows)* with normal filling of the anterior recess *(AR)*, the posterior recess *(PR)*, and the annular recess *(ar)*. (From Nicholas JA, Hershman EB: *The upper extremity in sports medicine*, ed 2, St Louis, 1995, Mosby.)

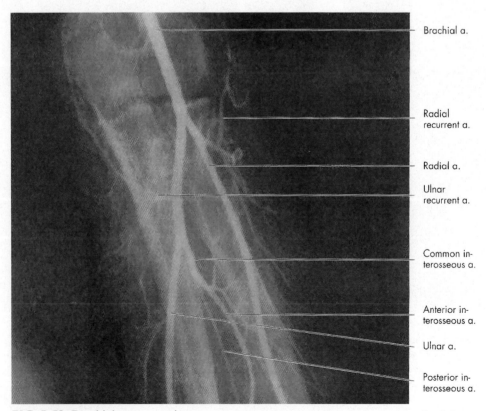

Brachial a.

Radial
recurrent a.

Radial a.

Ulnar
recurrent a.

Common in-
terosseous a.

Anterior in-
terosseous a.

Ulnar a.

Posterior in-
terosseous a.

FIG. 5-52 Brachial artery arteriogram. (From Mathers LH et al: *Clinical anatomy principles, St Louis*, 1996, Mosby.)

COZEN TEST

Assessment for Lateral Epicondylitis and Radiohumeral Bursitis

Comment

Chronic and disabling pain in the elbow, particularly near the radiohumeral articulation, is commonly, and mistakenly, designated tennis elbow rather than epicondylitis or radiohumeral bursitis. Specificity regarding the origin of this type of pain is often lacking. Tennis elbow diagnosis is similar to "shin splints" or "belly ache," having no relationship to the type of injury.

The understanding of the pathoanatomy of *tennis elbow* has been aided significantly by surgical investigations over the last decades. Many concepts advanced by investigators of prior decades have proven flawed, including the terminology.

The histologic evaluation of tennis elbow tendinosis demonstrates a noninflammatory response in the tendon. This histopathology is termed *angio fibroblastic tendinosis* (Fig. 5-53) and is likely the result of a degenerative and avascular process.

The location of elbow tendinosis is classically in the extensor carpi radialis brevis (ECRB) tendon (100%) and the extensor communis (EC) tendon (35%) laterally and in the pronator teres (PT) and the flexor carpi radialis (FCR) (95%) medially.

Because of the proximity of the epicondyle, the radiohumeral joint, and the supinator aponeurosis, diagnosis of exact tissue involvement can be confusing (Fig. 5-54). The conditions are often caused by the same mechanisms: overuse of the elbow joint (Table 5-5).

Lateral epicondylitis generally results from repetitive overuse of the wrist and forearm in patients older than 35 years who have a high activity level or demanding

---

ORTHOPEDIC GAMUT 5-7

EXTENSOR-SUPINATOR APONEUROTIC ATTACHMENT

Conditions on the lateral side of the elbow at the extensor-supinator aponeurotic attachment to the lateral epicondyle are:

1. Radioulnar synovitis, marked by development of a pannus of synovium between the radius and ulna
2. Strain in the aponeurosis itself, often directly over the radial head
3. Radiohumeral bursitis

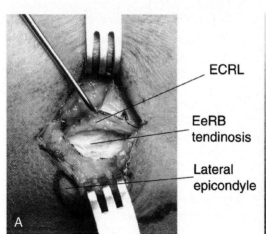
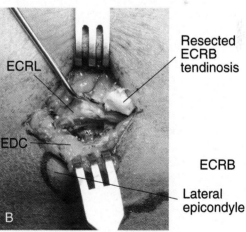

FIG. 5-53 **A,** Although most people respond well to nonoperative treatment of lateral epicondylitis (tennis elbow), some experience chronic symptoms and persistent pain. In such cases, surgery is often recommended. Lateral elbow tendinosis exposure of ECRB. The ECRL is elevated with a skin hook revealing the angiofibroblastic tendinosis of the underlying ECRB tendon. **B,** Resection of angiofibroblastic tendinosis of the ECRB tendon. Note the pathologic tissue displayed on the wound superficially. Also, there is no retraction of the ECRB after tendinosis resection due to retained additional attachments of the tendon. (From Nirschl RP, Davis LD: Mini-open surgery for lateral epicondylitis. In Yahaguchi K et al (eds): *Advanced reconstruction elbow*, Rosemont, IL, 2007, American Academy of Orthopaedic Surgeons.)

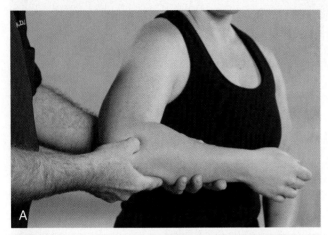

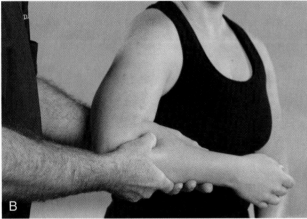

FIG. 5-54 Exact location of the most tender area is important. **A,** Thumb is over the common extensor tendon and radial head. **B,** Thumb is over the supinator and radial nerve.

activity technique and who sometimes have an inadequate fitness level. Although tenderness and swelling occur near the lateral epicondyle, histopathologic studies confirm that the lateral epicondyle of the humerus itself is not injured and that acute inflammation is not the primary problem. Rather, a granulation tissue identified as angiofibroblastic hyperplasia occurs in the ECRB tendon origin as a result of eccentric overload in an area of poor vascularity. Hence the term *tendinopathy* is perhaps more appropriate than *tendinitis*.

TABLE 5-5
CONDITIONS MIMICKING OR CONTRIBUTING TO CHRONIC LATERAL EPICONDYLITIS
Anconeus compartment syndrome
Bursitis
Cervical radiculopathy
Elbow joint components
Hypothyroidism
Lateral epicondyle avulsion
Musculocutaneous nerve entrapment
Non-union of radial neck fracture
Osteoarthritis
Posterior interosseous syndrome
Posterolateral rotatory instability of elbow
Radial nerve traction
Radial tunnel syndrome
Rheumatoid arthritis
Strained lateral collateral ligament
Snapping plicae

Adapted from Greenfield C, Webster V: Chronic lateral epicondylitis: survey of current practice in the outpatient departments in Scotland, *Physiotherapy* 88(10):578-594, 2002.

An objective measurement is infrared thermography of the affected elbow, which shows a discrete localized area of increased heat near the lateral epicondyle in 98% of affected elbows (Fig. 5-55). Analysis of the gradient across the abnormal area reveals a correlation with clinical severity.

PROCEDURE

- The patient clenches a fist tightly, dorsiflexes it, and maintains a pronated position.
- The examiner, while grasping the patient's lower forearm, applies a flexing force to the dorsiflexion posture of the patient's wrist (Fig. 5-56).
- The test is positive if it reproduces acute lancinating pain in the region of the lateral epicondyle.
- The test is significant for epicondylitis or radiohumeral bursitis.

Next Steps/Procedures
Golfer elbow test, Mills test, and Kaplan sign

CLINICAL PEARL

Cozen test is the easiest test to perform for lateral epicondylitis. The patient often has already discovered the pain that accompanies resisted dorsiflexion of the wrist, such as when lifting a gallon of milk. Although the pain of epicondylitis is sometimes exquisite and sharply localized, the condition does not truly differentiate itself from tendinopathy or bursitis.

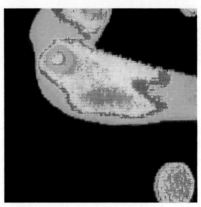

FIG. 5-55 An infrared thermographic pattern in lateral epicondylitis showing localized *hot spot*. (From Klippel JH, Dieppe PA: *Rheumatology*, vol 1-2, ed 2, London, 1998, Mosby.)

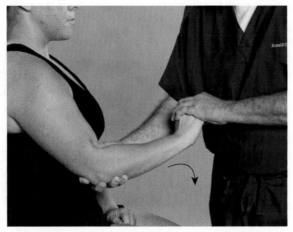

FIG. 5-56 With the patient seated and the affected elbow slightly flexed and pronated, the patient makes a fist. The patient actively dorsiflexes the hand and wrist. The examiner applies steady pressure against the dorsum of the patient's hand in an attempt to flex it. The patient resists this movement. Pain elicited at or near the lateral epicondyle suggests epicondylitis.

ALSO KNOWN AS WADSWORTH ELBOW FLEXION TEST

Assessment for Cubital Tunnel Syndrome and Ulnar Nerve Palsy at the Elbow

Comment

The ulnar nerve may be compressed at a point just distal to the medial epicondyle through the two heads of the flexor carpi ulnaris. The ulnar nerve arises from the brachial plexus in the axilla. While medial to the brachial artery, the nerve passes down the extremity until it reaches the distal third of the arm. At this point, the nerve and the brachial artery diverge, the nerve entering a groove between the medial epicondyle of the humerus and the olecranon. The ulnar nerve passes between the humeral and ulnar heads of the flexor carpi ulnaris muscle and descending to the wrist and hand, along the ulnar aspect of the forearm.

Within the bony groove at the elbow, the nerve is susceptible to compression. The compression can result from direct trauma or changes occurring within the groove, causing gradual impingement. A slow and progressive ulnar palsy is sometimes the delayed result of a fracture or soft-tissue injury at the elbow that has produced scarring. Changes in dimensions of the groove that are caused by osteoarthritis are occasionally seen with ulnar damage. In addition to severe, direct trauma that affects the elbow joint and produces immediate or tardy ulnar palsy, repeated, mild trauma may be an overlooked factor. Habitual leaning on the elbow on a desk or constant use of the elbow as a support at work may cause tardy ulnar palsy.

The restrictive opening that the nerve passes through at the elbow is formed by an aponeurotic arch between the olecranon and the medial epicondyle. The floor of this arch is the medial ligament of the elbow joint. This unyielding passageway is somewhat snug. Tissue edema in this region may produce nerve compression.

If the ulnar nerve lesion is at or below the mid-forearm, clawing of the two fingers innervated by the ulnar nerve can occur. Clawing occurs because the extrinsic muscles producing interphalangeal joint flexion are neurologically spared (Fig. 5-57).

Compression neuropathy of the ulnar nerve as it traverses the elbow is often a complication of local trauma, particularly as a result of fractures of the humerus. Constriction of the nerve in a fibroosseous tunnel is possible.

The osseous portion of the cubital tunnel is formed anteriorly by the medial epicondyle, the fibrous portion by the ulnohumeral ligaments laterally, and the aponeurosis of the

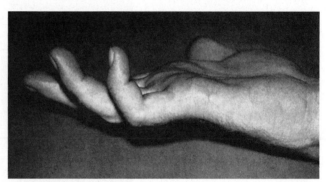

FIG. 5-57 Ulnar claw hand. *(From Katirji B:* Electromyography in clinical practice: a case study approach, *St Louis, 1998, Mosby.)*

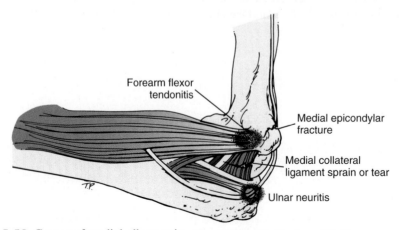

Forearm flexor tendonitis

Medial epicondylar fracture

Medial collateral ligament sprain or tear

Ulnar neuritis

FIG. 5-58 Causes of medial elbow pain. (From Nicholas JA, Hershman EB: *The upper extremity in sports medicine*, ed 2, St Louis, 1995, Mosby.)

two heads of the flexor carpi ulnaris posteromedially (Fig. 5-58). The size of the tunnel is reduced when the elbow is placed in flexion.

Without a history of trauma, identifying a precise cause for cubital tunnel syndrome may be difficult. However, chronic pressure over the ulnar groove, which may be exerted by occupational stress or from unusual elbow positioning, is an etiologic source. Arthritic conditions that result in synovitis at the elbow, or osteophyte production, can also cause compression of the nerve.

Paresthesias are noted in the distribution of the ulnar nerve. The neuropathy is often bilateral. Symptoms are aggravated by prolonged use of the elbow in flexed position. Most patients will demonstrate atrophy of intrinsic muscles and weakness in pinch and grasp (Figs. 5-59 and 5-60). The patient may experience wasting of the hypothenar muscles and slight clawing of the fourth and fifth fingers. A positive *Wartenberg* sign indicates weakness in adduction of the fifth finger.

Differentially, compression of the ulnar nerve can occur at the other locations, including the cervical spine, thoracic outlet, and Guyon canal. Cubital ulnar tunnel syndrome must be differentiated from tardy ulnar palsy. In ulnar palsy, neuropathy develops years after an injury (Fig. 5-61).

Other sites in the forearm for potential compression include the dense fibrous arcade of Struthers and the roof of the cubital tunnel formed by the cubital tunnel retinaculum (Fig. 5-62).

> The test (Wadsworth elbow flexion test) is positive when symptoms of tingling or numbness are initiated or aggravated in the area of the hand confined to the ulnar serve distribution; in positive cases symptoms have been found to appear between 20 seconds and 4 minutes, usually under 2 minutes. Clinical and electromyographic studies demonstrate that the elbow flexion test has a sensitivity of 86%, specificity of 86%, and a predictive value of 86% for male patients and a sensitivity of 25%, specificity of 85% and a predictive value of 20% for female patients (Wadsworth et al, 1995).

ORTHOPEDIC GAMUT 5-8
SITES OF COMPRESSION
Potential sites of compression along the course of the ulnar nerve:
1. The arcade of Struthers
2. The proximal edge of the cubital tunnel retinaculum
3. The cubital tunnel
4. The deep flexor pronator aponeurosis

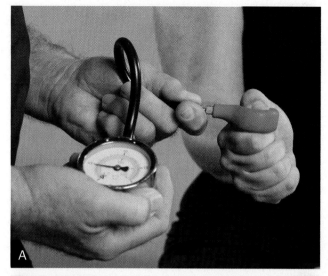
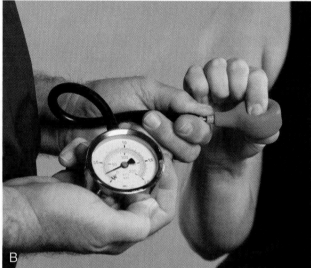
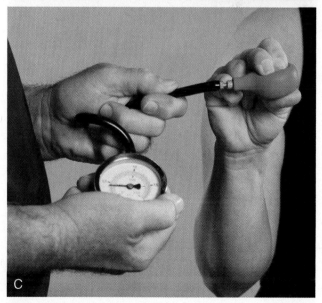

FIG. 5-59 Evaluation of pinch grip. **A,** Assessment of lateral or *key* pinch. **B,** Tip-to-tip pinch. **C,** Chuck pinch.

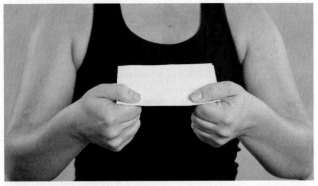

FIG. 5-60 Froment sign in an ulnar nerve lesion. The patient is directed to pull a piece of paper apart using both hands. The affected hand flexes the thumb by using the flexor pollicis longus to prevent the paper from slipping out of the hand. This action masks the weakness of the adductor pollicis.

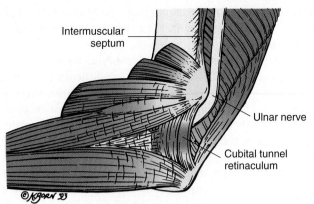

FIG. 5-62 The ulnar nerve passes behind the intermuscular septum and medial condyle. It enters the cubital tunnel beneath the cubital tunnel retinaculum. (From Torg JS, Shepard RJ: *Current therapy in sports medicine*, ed 3, St Louis, 1995, Mosby.)

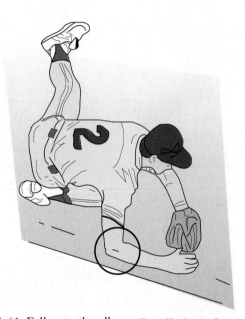

FIG. 5-61 Fall onto the elbow. (From Hartley A: *Practical joint assessment upper quadrant*, ed 2, St Louis, 1995, Mosby.)

PROCEDURE

- The patient completely flexes the elbow.
- The elbow is held in the flexed position for up to 5 minutes (Fig. 5-63).
- If tingling or paresthesia occurs in the ulnar distribution of the forearm and hand, the test is positive.
- A positive finding suggests the presence of cubital tunnel syndrome.

Next Steps/Procedures

Tinel sign at the elbow and electrodiagnosis

CLINICAL PEARL

This test is not only useful for cubital tunnel syndrome, it may also reveal the mechanism that resulted in injury to the ulnar nerve. The fully flexed elbow is a common posture for the arm during sleep, naturally or chemically induced. Patients may wake up with ulnar palsy symptoms that stem from prolonged neural compression and anoxia.

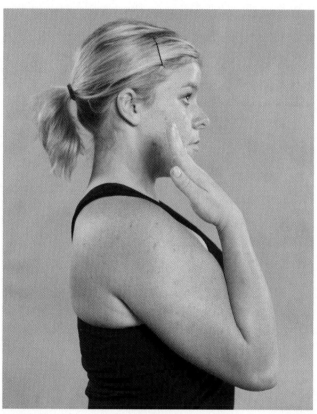

FIG. 5-63 The seated patient maintains a fully flexed elbow for as long as possible. The norm is 5 minutes or longer with no symptoms produced. Ulnar paresthesia developing in less than 5 minutes suggests cubital tunnel syndrome.

Assessment for Medial Epicondylitis

Comment

Epicondylitis is a type of involvement that is peculiar to the elbow and develops along the medial and lateral epicondyles. The extensor-supinator muscles arise along the lateral epicondyle, and the flexor-pronator muscles arise along the medial epicondyle, where they have an aponeurotic attachment.

Epicondylitis occurs either by contusion of the area or, more commonly, by strain (Fig. 5-64). Characteristic irritation develops at the attachment of the aponeurosis to the bone. Pain, which is aggravated by gripping, occurs along the involved epicondyle. When the patient clenches the fist, one of the first phases of action is strong contraction of carpal extensors to fix the wrist. If this contraction did not occur, the wrist would go into flexion, and an ineffective fist would result.

Although epicondylitis may follow an acute strain, it more often results from chronic degenerative changes. These changes are caused by attrition of the aponeurotic fibers at the elbow. If degenerative change occurs, calcification or even spur formation may occur over the epicondyle.

In medial epicondylitis, valgus stress is applied to the elbow while palpating over the medial joint line beneath the ulnar collateral ligament (Fig. 5-65). Occasionally, some patients will have asymptomatic ulnar collateral ligament attenuation and valgus laxity, while others with a significant ligament injury will have no palpable laxity at all (Fig. 5-66).

Valgus stress radiographs, obtained using manual stress or a graded pressure device, document excessive medial joint opening and confirm ligament laxity (Figs. 5-67 and 5-68).

The medial collateral ligament of the elbow is the most important ligament for stability of the elbow joint. It is divided into three bundles according to anatomic location:

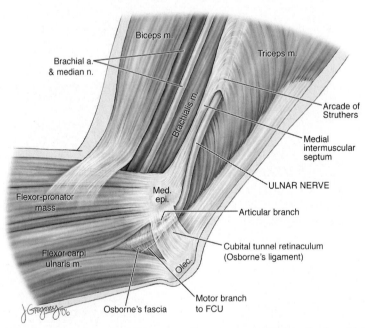

FIG. 5-64 In the upper arm, the ulnar nerve lies posteromedial to the brachial artery. It then traverses the medial intermuscular septum posteriorly, passing through the arcade of Struthers approximately 8 cm proximal to the medial epicondyle. This arcade comprises a band of deep brachial fascia that attaches to the intermuscular septum, has a V-shaped opening, and covers the ulnar nerve for an average length of 5.7 cm Anatomy of the ulnar nerve at the elbow. *a.,* artery; *FCU,* flexor carpi ulnaris; *n.,* nerve; *m.,* muscle; *Med. epi.,* medial epicondyle; *olec.,* olecranon. (From Polatsch DB, Melone Jr CP, Beldner S, et al: Ulnar nerve anatomy, *Hand Clin* 23[3]:283-289, 2007.)

anterior, posterior, and transverse (Fig. 5-69). For simplicity, the medial epicondylar groove is divided into three main zones; the first is proximal to the medial epicondyle, the second is at the medial epicondyle, and the third zone is distal to the medial epicondyle.

When examining for medial epicondylitis, the examiner must consider ulnar neuritis and ulnar collateral ligament instability, especially in the overhead sport athlete. These conditions may coexist, often consequent to the excessive valgus forces imparted to the medial elbow with throwing.

Ulnar neuritis is identified by a positive Tinel sign, as indicated by local pain and numbness or tingling radiating distally with the direct compression of the ulnar nerve at the elbow. A Tinel sign in zone 1 may indicate congenital ulnar nerve subluxation; in zone 2, a Tinel sign may be caused by compression caused by osteophytes, loose bodies, or rheumatoid synovitis changes. A zone 3 Tinel sign implies compression as the ulnar nerve passes through the two heads of the flexor carpi ulnaris (Ciccotti, Schwartz, Ciccotti, 2004).

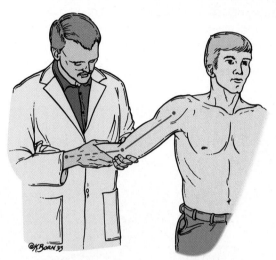

FIG. 5-65 Examination for evaluating medial instability of the elbow. (From Torg JS, Shepard RJ: *Current therapy in sports medicine*, ed 3, St Louis, 1995, Mosby.)

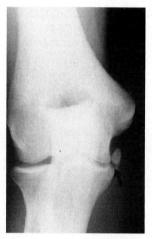

FIG. 5-67 Medial traction spur. (From Nicholas JA, Hershman EB: *The upper extremity in sports medicine*, ed 2, St Louis, 1995, Mosby.)

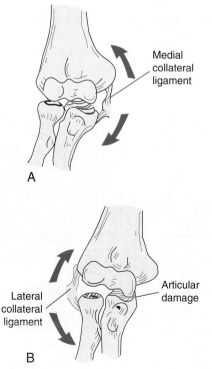

FIG. 5-66 **A,** Valgus overstretch damage to the elbow. **B,** Varus overstretch damage to the elbow. (From Hartley A: *Practical joint assessment upper quadrant*, ed 2, St Louis, 1995, Mosby.)

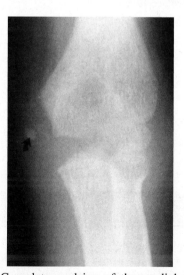

FIG. 5-68 Complete avulsion of the medial epicondylar apophysis *(arrow)* can occur in an acute injury from throwing sports rather than chronic degradation. (From Nicholas JA, Hershman EB: *The upper extremity in sports medicine*, ed 2, St Louis, 1995, Mosby.)

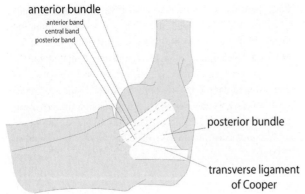

FIG. 5-69 The medial collateral ligament (MCL) complex of the elbow is an important anatomic soft-tissue structure that resists valgus stress of the elbow joint. The MCL complex is composed of 3 major parts: the anterior bundle, the posterior bundle, and the transverse ligament of Cooper. (From Dodson CC, Altchek DW: Management of medial collateral ligament tears in the athlete, *Operat Tech Sports Med* 14(2):75-80, 2006.)

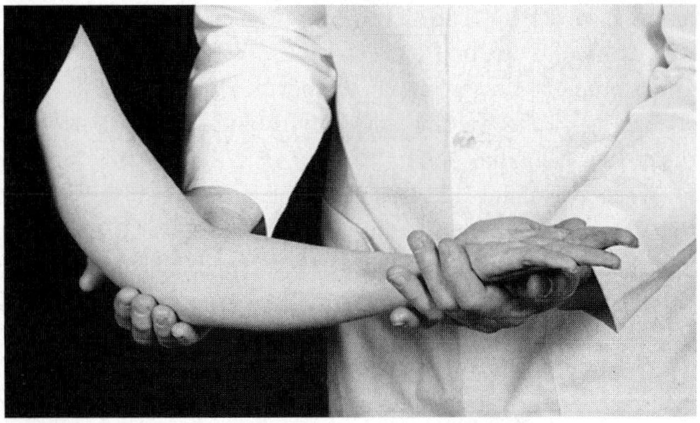

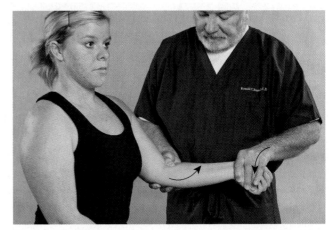

FIG. 5-70 The seated patient slightly flexes the elbow. The hand and wrist are in supination.

PROCEDURE

- The patient is seated, the patient's elbow is flexed slightly, and the hand is supinated (Fig. 5-70).
- The patient flexes the wrist against resistance (Fig. 5-71).
- Medial epicondyle pain suggests epicondylitis.
- In more severe medial epicondylitis, the flexor muscle groups are weakened, and the elbow-wrist mechanism can be extended by the examiner (Fig. 5-72).
- Full extension of the elbow-wrist joint localizes the lesion more sharply in medial aponeurosis contractures.

Next Steps/Procedures
Cozen test, Kaplan sign, and Mills test

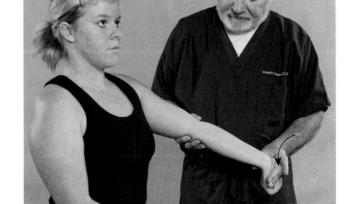

FIG. 5-71 The examiner applies steady pressure to the supinated hand in an attempt to extend the elbow and wrist. The patient resists this movement with active flexion. Pain elicited at the medial epicondyle suggests epicondylitis.

CLINICAL PEARL

This test is a reverse procedure of Cozen test. Cozen test relies on resisted wrist dorsiflexion, but the golfer elbow test relies on resisted elbow-wrist flexion. The pain associated with medial epicondylitis spreads down the forearm and is often confused with carpal tunnel syndrome symptoms.

FIG. 5-72 With severe medial epicondylitis, the examiner is able to overcome the flexor muscle groups and extend the elbow and wrist fully. With aponeurosis contractures present, the full extension of the elbow and wrist localizes the lesion more sharply.

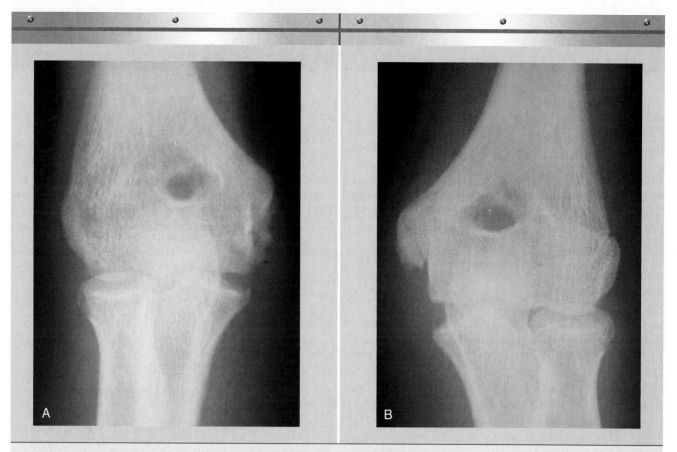

AT THE VIEWBOX

A young female elite gymnast, presenting with medial right elbow pain occurring with any axial weight bearing of the upper extremities. Radiographs demonstrate asymmetric irregularity of the apophyses of the medial epicondyles, much more prominent on the right (**A**). In skeletally immature patients, there is overlap between irregularity as a radiographic normal variation and findings indicating stress related abnormality or avascular necrosis of apophyses and epiphyses. In this case, there is also premature fusion of both the medial and lateral epicondyles of the right distal humerus (**B**). Right hand dominance must be taken into consideration. The clinical-radiographic correlation is compatible with sequelae of stress-related changes of the epicondyles of the right distal humerus, similar to those of Osgood-Schlatter disease of the knee. (From the teaching file of Timothy Mick, DC, DACBR)

Assessment for Lateral Epicondylitis

Comment

Lateral epicondylitis is a symptom complex characterized by pain at the elbow, especially during extension of the wrist or fingers against resistance, and affects 1% to 3% of the population. It is usually caused by a tear in the conjoined tendons of the extensor muscles and is often associated with an osseous avulsion or spur on the lateral epicondyle of the humerus. Direct compression of the dorsal interosseous nerve at or distal to the level of the supinator also exhibits the same symptoms.

On palpation, pain is felt in the area of the lateral epicondyle. This pain continues down the dorsal aspect of the forearm over the wrist extensors and the extensor digitorum communis.

Etiologic factors include direct trauma to the elbow joint in the area of the lateral epicondyle or, more commonly, a muscle strain secondary to athletic activities. If direct trauma is the underlying cause, tangential diagnostic images of the lateral epicondyle should be obtained. The images may demonstrate the presence of small osteophytes within the substance of the conjoined tendon.

The lateral and oblique views, taken at 45 degrees oblique to the anteroposterior view, may reveal characteristic formation of an osteophyte at the tip of the olecranon. The axial view demonstrates the articulation of the olecranon and posteromedial osteophytes with the trochlea (Fig. 5-73).

Although patients do not usually recall a specific traumatic episode, they do admit that symptoms of low-grade pain and morning stiffness were brought on or aggravated by certain repetitive activities, such as tennis, golf, and pipefitting. A grasping motion that stretches the epicondylar muscle attachments will accentuate the pain.

Other pathologic conditions include arthritis of the radiohumeral joint, radiohumeral bursitis, traumatic synovitis of the radiohumeral joint through forced extension and supination, and periostitis or osteitis of the epicondyle (Fig. 5-74).

The presence of immunoglobulin M-rheumatoid factor enzymes and human leukocyte antigen-B27 in cases of epicondylitis suggests that the recurring tenosynovitis (epicondylitis) represents an incomplete form of rheumatoid disease (Fig. 5-75).

Lateral epicondylitis was initially described as an inflammatory condition; however, numerous histologic studies

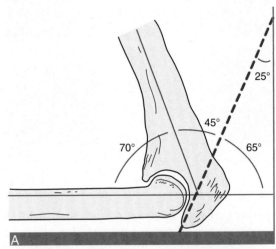

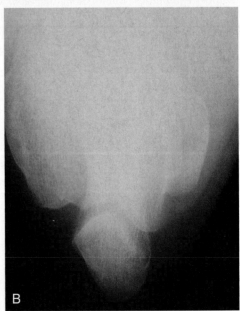

FIG. 5-73 **A,** A diagram demonstrating the radiographic position for the axial (tangential) view of the elbow. (From Torg JS, Shepard RJ: *Current therapy in sports medicine,* ed 3, St Louis, 1995, Mosby.) **B,** Axial view revealing the posteromedial osteophyte and profile of the trochlear articulation.

ORTHOPEDIC GAMUT 5-9
IMAGING OF THE ELBOW

Standard plain-film imaging of the elbow involves five views:
1. Anteroposterior
2. Lateral
3. Medial
4. Lateral obliques
5. Axial

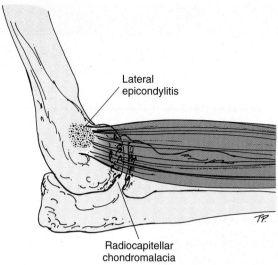

FIG. 5-74 Causes of lateral elbow pain. (From Nicholas JA, *Hershman EB: The upper extremity in sports medicine*, ed 2, St Louis, 1995, Mosby.)

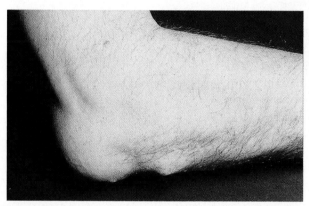

FIG. 5-75 Rheumatoid nodules. (From Epstein O et al: *Clinical examination*, ed 2, London, 1997, Mosby.)

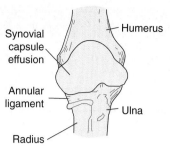

FIG. 5-76 Intracapsular effusion from an anterior view. (From Hartley A: *Practical joint assessment upper quadrant*, ed 2, St Louis, 1995, Mosby.)

ORTHOPEDIC GAMUT 5-10

ELBOW SWELLING

The following are common local swelling locations of the elbow:

1. Olecranon bursa and the radiohumeral bursa
2. Muscle strains or contusions to the tendon, belly, or tenoperiosteal junction
3. Intracapsular effusion

---

have now shown that it is a degenerative process and is not inflammatory. The belief is that these degenerative changes in the tendon are a result of repetitive microtrauma that has failed to heal properly, resulting in angiofibroblastic changes. One of the etiologic factors thought to contribute to the degenerative changes seen in tendinopathies is a relative hypovascular zone seen within the tendon in lateral epicondylitis.

In lateral epicondylitis, a degenerative process takes place with dense populations of fibroblasts and vascular hyperplasia. The vascular structures do not function the same as blood vessels, and the vascular hyperplasia present does not contain patent lumens and thus does not correlate with improved healing. The angiofibroblastic tendinosis that is observed histologically in patients with lateral epicondylitis may occur in response to failed attempts to heal an injury caused by repetitive microtrauma as a result of a lack of adequate blood supply (Bales et al, in press).

Although the radial nerve may be compressed under the brachioradialis muscle, this event is rare and is painful more distally than tennis elbow.

Marked posterior joint swelling is usually olecranon bursitis, whereas anterior and posterior swelling is often caused by intracapsular effusion (Fig. 5-76).

The use of fluoroquinolone antibiotics (ciprofloxacin, ofloxacin, norfloxacin, enoxacin, lomefloxacin) has been implicated in epicondylitis. The intense pain at the epicondyle appears very shortly after administration of the first dose of the drug and is not relieved by conservative treatment. Ultrasonography reveals extensive inflammatory pannus with pseudonecrotic areas. MRI confirms the lesions and demonstrates subclinical abnormality of the adjoining tendons.

PROCEDURE

- While the patient is seated, the affected upper limb is held straight out with the wrist in slight dorsiflexion.
- Grip strength is assessed with a dynamometer (Fig. 5-77).
- This maneuver is repeated as the examiner firmly encircles the patient's forearm with both hands or with a strap placed approximately 1 to 2 inches below the elbow joint line (Fig. 5-78).
- The sign is present if initial grip strength improves and lateral elbow pain diminishes.

Next Steps/Procedures
Cozen test, golfer elbow test, and Mills test

CLINICAL PEARL

K aplan sign is a good test for discerning the efficacy of tennis-elbow support in the management of a patient's condition. Obviously, if the grip does not improve while the brace is in place, the musculature and epicondylar tissues are not being supported adequately. The condition may be so severe that the use of a brace is not helpful.

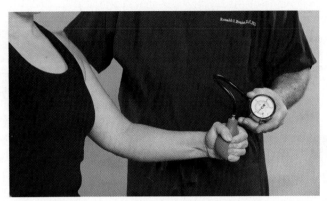

FIG. 5-77 With the elbow flexed slightly and the hand in a position of function, the seated patient grips a dynamometer. The examiner records the findings.

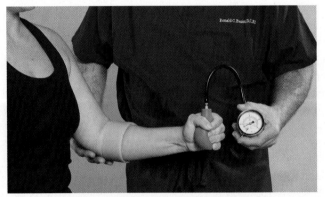

FIG. 5-78 The grip strength is tested again with the elbow supported by either a tennis elbow strap or the examiner's hands. Increased grip strength and decreased elbow pain indicate lateral epicondylitis.

Assessment for Medial or Lateral Collateral Ligament Instability at the Elbow

Comment

Because the elbow is a stable joint, ligament injury is uncommon. Spraining the elbow by excessive flexion is impossible. In excessive extension, the olecranon impinges against the back of the humerus, and the continuing force parts the coronoid from the trochlea of the humerus. This action also results in an injury to the anterior portion of the collateral ligament, particularly on the medial side. This injury may vary from a partial tear to complete rupture of the ligaments and capsule. As the force stops short of complete rupture, the elbow flexes, the tension releases, and no feeling of instability occurs at the elbow joint. Stability is maintained because of the inherent, bony structure of the elbow and because the elbow does not require the same degree of stability for bearing weight that is necessary in the knee.

The patient with an injury of excessive elbow extension has a history of elbow hyperextension with severe pain on the medial and occasionally the lateral side of the elbow. Pain is relieved by flexion. Symptoms at the time of examination vary according to the severity of the injury. Pain is ordinarily not a prominent factor, but localized tenderness will occur at the site of the tear, either along the ulna on the medial side or along the epicondyle. The patient may also experience pain along the lateral collateral ligament at the site of the tear. Any attempt to extend the arm causes pain, and motion is stopped, short of complete extension, as a result of muscle spasm.

Collateral ligaments also may be sprained by lateral motion. Forced abduction of the extended arm damages the medial ligaments (Fig. 5-79). Forced adduction damages the lateral ligaments (Fig. 5-80). Instability is extremely uncommon. Determining whether the rupture of the ligaments is complete is difficult unless complete dislocation of the elbow has occurred. A sprain-fracture (i.e., coronoid fracture) caused by an avulsion of the ligament with a bony fragment is commonly revealed with diagnostic imaging. Symptoms of lateral stresses are localized to the traumatized side and accompanied by the same findings as for hyperextension, including tenderness along the site of the tear, local swelling, and pain during attempts to reproduce the causative force.

Coronoid fractures are uncommon in isolation, typically occurring in the setting of more complex elbow trauma. They commonly occur with injuries to the collateral ligaments and may be associated with the *terrible triad:* elbow dislocation, radial head fracture, and coronoid fracture. Currently, the influence of coronoid fracture size on elbow stability and kinematics, particularly in the setting of concomitant injuries to the ligaments, is not known (Beingessner et al, 2007).

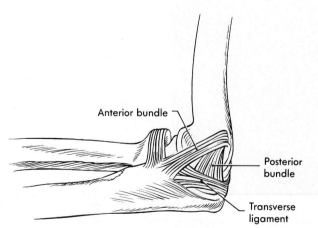

FIG. 5-79 View of the medial collateral ligament bundles. (Adapted from Nicholas JA, Hershman EB: *The upper extremity in sports medicine,* ed 2, St Louis, 1995, Mosby.)

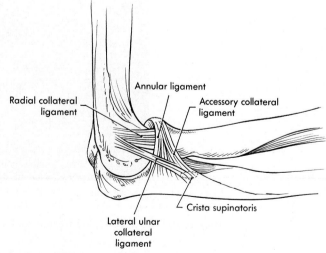

FIG. 5-80 View of lateral collateral and annular ligaments. (Adapted from Nicholas JA, Hershman EB: *The upper extremity in sports medicine,* ed 2, St Louis, 1995, Mosby.)

- The examiner stabilizes the patient's arm with one hand at the elbow, and the other hand is placed at the wrist.
- The patient's elbow is slightly flexed (20 to 30 degrees), and an adduction (varus) force is applied to test the lateral collateral ligament (Fig. 5-81).
- An abduction (valgus) force is then applied to test the medial collateral ligament (Fig. 5-82).

Next Steps/Procedure
Diagnostic imaging

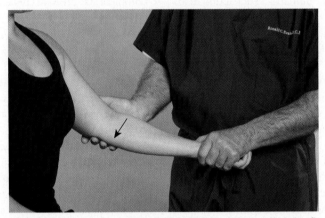

FIG. 5-81 The patient is seated comfortably with the elbow slightly flexed (20 to 30 degrees) and the hand and arm in supination. The examiner stabilizes the elbow while applying an abduction (valgus) force to the distal forearm. This tests the medial collateral ligaments. Pain indicates sprain.

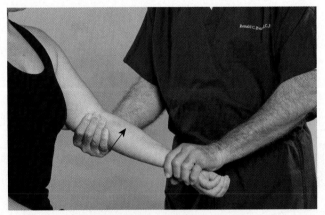

FIG. 5-82 The procedure described in Figure 5-81 is repeated with an adduction (varus) force applied to the distal forearm while the examiner stabilizes the elbow. This procedure assesses the lateral collateral ligaments. Pain indicates sprain.

MILLS TEST

ALSO KNOWN AS MILLS MANEUVER

Assessment for Lateral Epicondylitis

Comment

Used synonymously with the term *tennis elbow*, lateral epicondylitis is one of the most common lesions of the arm. Approximately 1% to 3% of the population is affected by it, mostly persons between 40 and 60 years of age, the dominant arm being affected most frequently. Some 40% to 50% of tennis players suffer with it, mainly older players. It is most often observed in nonathletes, and the majority is not engaged in manual work. Many cannot describe any specific precipitating factors.

More than 25 suggested causes for the condition have been offered, reflecting the use of the diagnosis nonspecifically for lateral elbow pain. The belief is that most cases result from a musculotendinous lesion of the common extensor tendon at the attachment to the lateral epicondyle or nearby, especially that portion derived from ECRB.

Age is an important factor because lateral epicondylitis rarely occurs before the age of 30. Skeletal maturity and continued aging are associated with alterations in the enthesis, including changes in collagen content, reduction in cells and ground substance, and increases in lipids, which then probably predispose it to injury.

Lateral epicondylitis usually arises slowly and apparently spontaneously; a blow or acute traumatic strains are relatively rarely remembered. Pain is localized to the lateral epicondyle but may spread up and down the upper limb. Grip is impaired because of the pain, and this impairment may result in restricted daily activities. Tenderness over the epicondyle is usual, although maximal tenderness is sometimes found at nearby sites. The other cardinal sign is increased pain on resisting wrist dorsiflexion with the elbow in extension.

The examiner must exclude other conditions that produce elbow pain, especially that referred from the cervical spine or shoulder, as well as arthritis of the elbow, although this is usually obvious.

Nerve entrapment around the elbow produces diagnostic confusion. Radial tunnel syndrome or compression of the posterior interosseous nerve causes lateral elbow and upper foramen pain. Compression of the posterior interosseous nerve occurs where it passes through the supinator muscle just below the elbow joint. A well-defined arcade of Frohse is present in 30% of patients, making a compression neuropathy more likely. Diffuse pain, symptoms distal to the lateral epicondyle, and the presence of muscle weakness are useful distinguishing features.

Compression of the radial nerve at the elbow is of moderate frequency compared with the ulnar tunnel syndrome. Compression of the superficial branch at the elbow is relatively rare. Two different manifestations of compression of the deep branch may be (1) radial tunnel syndrome, which is characterized by pain, and (2) posterior interosseous nerve syndrome, which is characterized by painless paralysis. Except for traumatic lesions of the nerve, radial nerve palsy at the elbow is often incomplete and painless. Extrinsic compression is the most important etiologic factor and, in particular, one that is caused by a lipoma. Idiopathic paralysis is often preceded by a short period of pain and is related to forceful repetitive motion, with hourglass-like constrictions of the nerve (Raimbeau, Saint-Cast, 2004).

PROCEDURE

- The patient's forearm, fingers, and wrist are passively flexed (Figs. 5-83 to 5-85).
- The forearm is pronated and extended (Figs. 5-86 and 5-87).
- The test is positive if elbow pain increases.
- A positive test indicates lateral epicondylitis (tennis elbow).

Next Steps/Procedures
Cozen test, golfer elbow test, Kaplan sign, and diagnostic imaging

CLINICAL PEARL

Mills test is also a treatment maneuver. One of the principles of management for lateral epicondylitis is the sectioning of the aponeurosis from the epicondyle. In the final maneuvers of Mills test, this separation is accomplished.

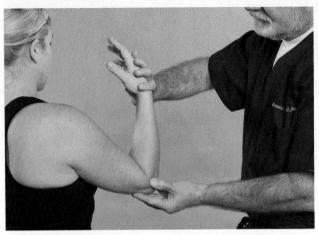

FIG. 5-83 The patient is seated. The examiner passively and fully flexes the elbow.

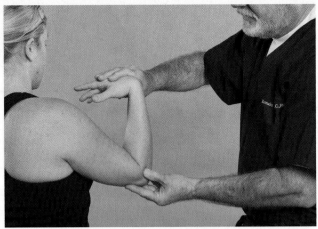

FIG. 5-84 After passively and fully flexing the patient's elbow, the examiner flexes the patient's wrist.

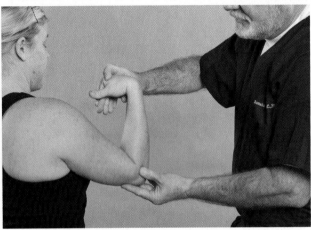

FIG. 5-85 After attaining the position described in Figure 5-84, the patient's fingers are fully flexed. The forearm, wrist, and hand are all fully flexed in supination.

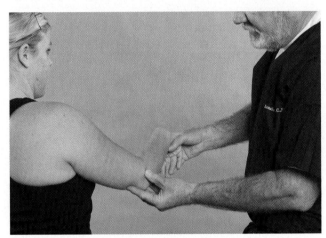

FIG. 5-86 The examiner maintains wrist and finger flexion while extending the patient's elbow.

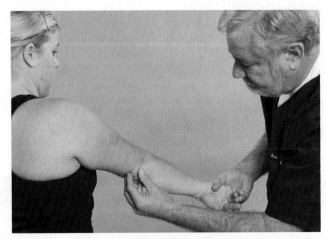

FIG. 5-87 At maximal elbow extension, with the wrist and fingers still flexed, the forearm is pronated. Pain at the lateral epicondyle indicates epicondylitis. All of the movements associated with this procedure should be accomplished in a smooth continuous manner.

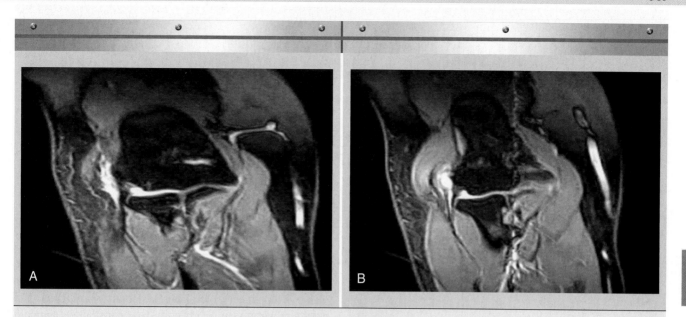

AT THE VIEWBOX

A 52-year-old female presenting with clinical findings of "lateral epicondylitis." **(A)** Fluid-weighted (inversion recovery) MR images demonstrate focal fluid collection at the lateral epicondyle, with evidence of a high grade tear of the common extensor tendon at its origin. **(B)** The lateral collateral ligament is thickened, with some increased intrasubstance signal, consistent with low-grade partial tear. (From the teaching file of Timothy Mick, DC, DACBR)

5

ALSO KNOWN AS FORMICATION SIGN, DISTAL TINGLING ON PERCUSSION (DTP) SIGN, AND HOFFMAN-TINEL SIGN

Assessment for Ulnar or Radial (Posterior Interosseous) Neuropathy at the Elbow

Comment

Nerve roots and peripheral nerves may be injured by a blunt object that causes a contusion or by a sharp object that produces a partial or complete laceration. The nerve also can be injured by a severe stretch, resulting from a traction injury. Additionally, nerves are particularly vulnerable to prolonged ischemia, which can lead to necrosis.

In *neuropraxia,* only slight damage occurs to the nerve with transient loss of conductivity, particularly in its motor fibers. In neuropraxia, wallerian degeneration, which is the breakdown of the myelin sheaths into lipid material and fragmentation of the neurofibrils, does not occur. Complete recovery from neuropraxia may be expected within a few days or weeks.

In *axonotmesis,* the injury damages axons, which are prolongations of the cells in the spinal cord, but does not damage the structural framework of the nerve. Axons distal to the injury undergo wallerian degeneration. Peripheral regeneration of the axons occurs along the intact neural tubes to the appropriate end organs. Regeneration occurs very slowly, approximately 1 mm each day or 3 cm each month (e.g., if axonotmesis in a nerve occurred 9 cm proximal to its site of entrance into a muscle, approximately 3 months would be required for the regenerating axons to reinnervate that muscle).

In the injury of *neurotmesis,* the internal neural structural framework and the enclosed axons are divided, torn, and destroyed. Wallerian degeneration occurs in the distal segment. Because axons in the proximal segment lose their neural tubes, natural regeneration is improbable. Neurofibrils and fibrous elements grow out of the divided end of the nerve, producing a bulbous neuroma. The only hope of recovery lies in excision of the damaged section of the nerve and accurate approximation of the freshened ends. Even under ideal circumstances, recovery is less than complete.

Immediately after nerve injury, the patient experiences a loss of conductivity in motor, sensory, and autonomic fibers. Muscles supplied by the nerve root or peripheral nerve exhibit flaccid paralysis and later undergo atrophy. The loss of cutaneous sensation, deep sensation, and position sense can be detected. Autonomic deficit is characterized by a lack of sweating (anhidrosis) in the cutaneous distribution of the nerve. The patient experiences temporary vasodilation and resultant warm skin, followed by vasoconstriction and cold skin.

The appropriate electrical tests, which include nerve conduction, strength curve, and electromyography can help in the precise diagnosis concerning both the type of injury and its location (Fig. 5-88).

The prognosis depends on the type of injury (neuropraxia, axonotmesis, or neurotmesis). If recovery does take place, it is demonstrated first by return of muscle power in the most proximally supplied muscle. Return of sensation follows a definite pattern, with deep sensation returning first, followed by pain and position sense. As regeneration of axons proceeds along the nerve, the regenerated portion becomes hypersensitive. Tapping over the injured area causes a tingling sensation. Assessing the distal limit of this phenomenon at intervals enables the examiner to determine the progress of regeneration (Fig. 5-89). The violence of injury and the delay between that injury and treatment are two particularly important factors in recovery after nerve repair.

The radial nerve is particularly vulnerable in high energy–transfer injury. It passes obliquely across the axes of the limb. The radial nerve courses along the posterior aspect of the humerus where it lies close to the bone and is tethered by the lateral head of triceps. It is usually composed of only a few bundles or fascicles with a relatively small proportion of supporting connective tissue. The blood supply may also be a contributory factor to its vulnerability. The proximal part of the radial nerve is dependent on the descending profunda artery; and if this artery is ruptured, the upper part of the radial nerve is relatively ischemic. Severe neuropathic pain suggests continuing injury to the nerve and it is a strong indication for surgical intervention.

A strong Tinel sign at the level of the lesion confirms a clinical diagnosis of a degenerative lesion and suggests that the nerve has been ruptured. The sign is usually evident on the day of injury. A diagnosis of conduction block (neurapraxia) is inconsistent with Tinel sign. This important clinical sign is difficult to evaluate in a young child, and it cannot

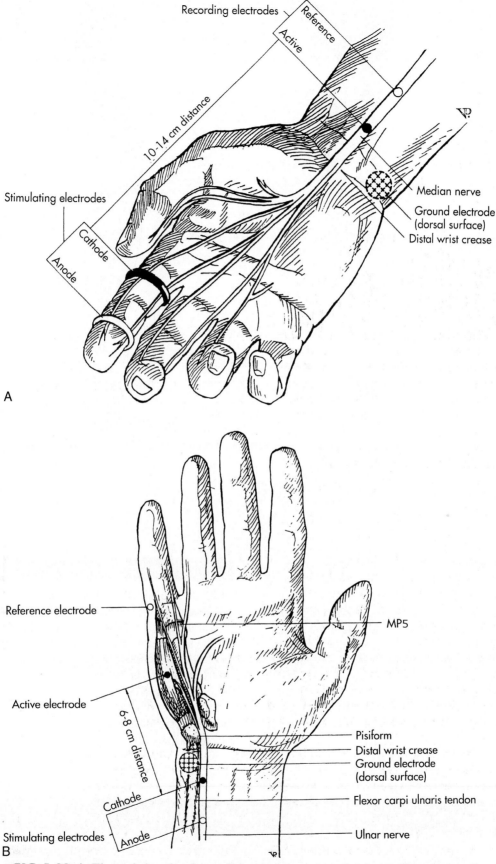

FIG. 5-88 **A,** Electrode location for median sensory nerve conduction. **B,** Electrode location for ulnar motor nerve conduction. (From Umphred DA: *Neurological rehabilitation*, ed 5, St Louis, 2006, Mosby.)

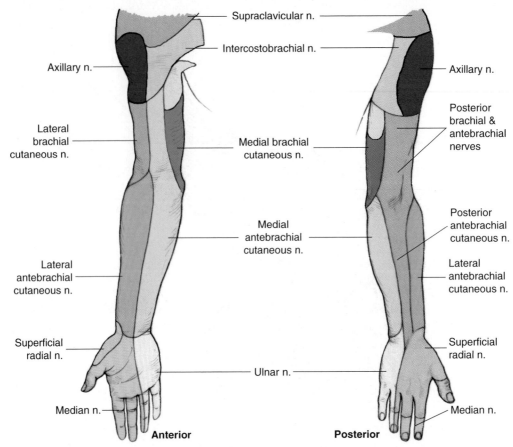

FIG. 5-89 Cutaneous innervation of the upper extremity. (From Mathers LH et al: *Clinical anatomy principles*, St Louis, 1996, Mosby.)

be demonstrated in such deep-seated nerves as the circumflex. A weak but advancing Tinel sign is not necessarily consistent with a favorable prognosis for the nerve. Tinel sign can be evoked by percussion over a relatively small number of regenerating axons even when much of the nerve trunk has been transected or remains entrapped within a fracture. If the sign remains stronger at the level of lesion than at the growing point, then recovery is likely to be poor (Kato, Birch, 2006).

PROCEDURE

- While the patient is seated, the examiner taps the groove between the olecranon process and the lateral epicondyle with a neurologic reflex hammer (Fig. 5-90).
- The same action is repeated for the groove between the olecranon process and the medial epicondyle.
- Hypersensitivity indicates neuritis or neuroma of the respective nerve.

Next Steps/Procedure
Electrodiagnosis

CLINICAL PEARL

An important point to remember is that the tingling elicited by the Tinel sign represents regeneration. Pain and tingling represent injury and degeneration. The more distally the tingling is felt from the site of percussion, the more distally the axons have regenerated.

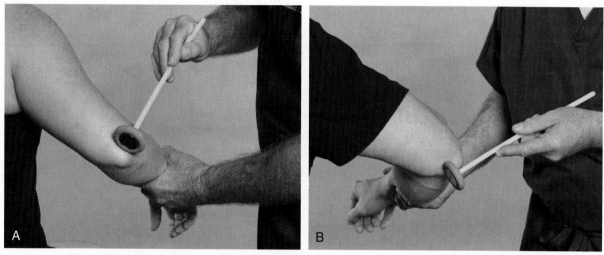

FIG. 5-90 The patient is seated comfortably with the elbow flexed to 90 degrees. The examiner percusses the superficial radial nerve at the lateral epicondylar groove. Tingling that radiates down the lateral forearm indicates regeneration associated with superficial radial nerve palsy. Pain radiating down the lateral forearm is associated with injury and superficial radial nerve degeneration. The same procedure is repeated for the medial epicondylar groove and the ulnar nerve.

CRITICAL THINKING

1. What articulations make up the elbow joint?
2. List the functions of the elbow.
3. Describe the carrying angle of the elbow.
4. What is a gunstock deformity of the arm?
5. What muscles originate from the medial epicondyle?
6. What muscles originate from the lateral epicondyle?
7. List the ligaments of the elbow.
8. What is the normal position of function of the elbow?
9. What is the most common congenital anomaly of the elbow?
10. What is Panner disease?
11. What is osteochondritis dissecans of the elbow?
12. Describe tennis elbow.
13. Describe Cozen test.
14. What is usually responsible for medial epicondylitis, or golfer elbow?
15. How is medial epicondylitis tested?
16. Describe boxer elbow.
17. Describe little leaguer elbow.
18. Where does ulnar nerve entrapment at the elbow typically occur?
19. Describe draftsman elbow.
20. What are *pushed elbow* and *pulled elbow?*
21. Diagnosis of elbow conditions is largely based on what findings?
22. If the isosceles triangle from the olecranon to each epicondyle is abnormal, what are the abnormal possibilities that might contribute to this disruption?
23. Describe the *terrible triad of the elbow.*
24. What ages of athletes are susceptible to osteochondritis dissecans?
25. What are the potential long-term consequences of osteochondritis dessicans in the athlete?
26. What retained elbow flexion motion is considered impairment in the activities of daily living of your patient?
27. What ROM is considered impairment with extension?
28. What is the cause of a gunstock deformity?
29. What are the prime flexors of the elbow?
30. What is the innervation of the prime flexion of the elbow?
31. What is the prime mover in extension of the elbow?
32. What muscle is an accessory to extension?
33. What is the innervation of elbow extension musculature?
34. What sites are the potential areas of compression along the course of the ulnar nerve?
35. Why is Kaplan sign a good test for discerning the efficacy of a tennis-elbow support?
36. How are the radial tunnel syndrome and the posterior interosseous syndrome at the elbow demonstrated?

BIBLIOGRAPHY

Adams JC, Hamblen DL: *Outline of orthopaedics,* ed 11, Edinburgh, 1990, Churchill Livingstone.

Adolfsson L: Ganglion cyst communicating with the elbow joint presenting as a distal forearm tumour, *J Hand Surg* 22(4):552-554, 1997.

American Medical Association: *Guides to the evaluation of permanent impairment,* ed 4, Chicago, 1993, The Association.

American Medical Association: *How to use guides to the evaluation of permanent impairment,* ed 4, Falmouth, Conn. 1993, SEAK.

American Orthopaedic Association: *Manual of orthopaedic surgery,* Chicago, 1972, The Association.

Anderson KN, Anderson LE: *Mosby's pocket dictionary of medicine, nursing, & allied health,* ed 2, St Louis, 1994, Mosby.

Andrews JR, Whiteside JA, Buettner CM: Clinical evaluation of the elbow in throwers, *Oper Tech Sports Med* 4(2):77-83, 1996.

Angelo RL, Soffer SR: Elbow anatomy relative to arthroscopy. In Andrews Jr, Soffer SR, editors: *Elbow arthroscopy,* St Louis, 1994, Mosby.

Aoki M, Okamura K, Yamashita T: Snapping annular ligament of the elbow joint in the throwing arms of young brothers, *Arthroscopy* 19(8):e89-e92, 2003.

Aoki M et al: Magnetic resonance imaging findings of refractory tennis elbows and their relationship to surgical treatment, *J Shoulder Elbow Surg* 14(2):172-177, 2005.

Apfelberg DB, Larson SJ: Dynamic anatomy of the ulnar nerve at the elbow, *Plast Reconstr Surg* 51:76, 1973.

Apley AG, Solomon L: *Concise system of orthopaedics and fractures,* London, 1988, Butterworth-Heinemann.

Barkauskas VH et al: *Health & physical assessment,* ed 2, St Louis, 1998, Mosby.

Bateman JE: *Trauma to nerves in limbs,* Philadelphia, 1962, WB Saunders.

Beals RK: The normal carrying angle of the elbow, *Clin Orthop* 119:194, 1976.

Beetham WP et al: *Physical examination of the joints,* Philadelphia, 1965, WB Saunders.

Benjamin HJ, Hang BT: Common acute upper extremity injuries in sports, *Clin Pediatr Emerg Med* 8(1):15-30, 2007.

Bennett JB, Tullos HS: Acute injuries to the elbow. In Nicholas JA, Hershman EB, editors: *The upper extremity in sports medicine,* St Louis, 1990, Mosby.

Berquist T: *MRI of the musculoskeletal system,* ed 3, Philadelphia, 1996, JB Lippincott.

Blackwell JR, Cole KJ: Wrist kinematics in expert and novice tennis players performing the backhand stoke: implications for tennis elbow, *J Biomech* 27:509, 1994.

Boyd HB, McLeod AC: Tennis elbow, *J Bone Joint Surg* 55A:1183, 1973.

Bradley WG: *Disorders of peripheral nerves,* Oxford, UK, 1974, Blackwell Scientific.

Brooks M, Evans R, Fairclough J: *Sports injuries,* ed 2, London, 1992, Gower Medical.

Brotzman SB: *Clinical orthopaedic rehabilitation,* St Louis, 1996, Mosby.

Brown DE, Neumann RD: *Orthopedic secrets,* Philadelphia, 1995, Hanley & Belfus.

Bucholz RW: *Orthopaedic decision making,* ed 2, St Louis, 1996, Mosby.

Busa R et al: Acute posterior interosseous nerve palsy caused by a synovial haemangioma of the elbow joint, *J Hand Surg* 20(5):652-654, 1995.

Cain EL, Dugas JR: History and examination of the thrower's elbow, *Clin Sports Med* 23(4):553-566, 2004.

Canale ST: *Campbell's operative orthopaedics,* vol 1-4, ed 9, St Louis, 1998, Mosby.

Carson WG, Meyer JF: Diagnostic arthroscopy of the elbow: surgical techniques and arthroscopic portal anatomy. In McGinty JB, editor: *Operative arthroscopy,* New York, 1991, Raven.

Chapman S, Nakielny R: *Aids to radiological differential diagnosis,* ed 3, London, 1995, Bailliere Tindall.

Cipriano JJ: *Photographic manual of regional orthopaedic and neurological tests,* ed 3, Baltimore, 1997, Williams & Wilkins.

Cohn RE: *Impairment rating examination and disability evaluation,* ed 3, Wilkesboro, NC, 1994, R Ernest Cohn.

Colman WW, Strauch RJ: Physical examination of the elbow, *Orthop Clin North Am* 30(1):15-20, 1999.

Conway JE et al: Medial instability of the elbow in throwing athletes: treatment by repair or reconstruction of the ulnar collateral ligament, *J Bone Joint Surg* 74A:67, 1992.

Copeland SA et al: *Joint stiffness of the upper limb,* St Louis, 1997, Mosby.

Dacre JE, Worrall JG: Rheumatological examination, *Medicine* 30(8):6-10, 2002.

Daffner RH: *Clinical radiology, the essentials,* Baltimore, 1993, Williams & Wilkins.

Dambro MR, Griffith JA: *Griffith's 5 minute clinical consult,* Baltimore, 1997, Williams & Wilkins.

D'Ambrosia RD: *Musculoskeletal disorders, regional examination and differential diagnosis,* Philadelphia, 1977, JB Lippincott.

Dandy DJ: *Essential orthopaedics and trauma,* Edinburgh, 1989, Churchill Livingstone.

Dawson DM, Hallett M, Millender LH: Pathology of nerve entrapment. In Dawson DM, Hallett M, Wilbourn A, editors: *Entrapment neuropathies,* ed 2, Boston, 1990, Little & Brown.

Delagi E et al: *An anatomic guide for the electromyographer,* Springfield, Ill, 1975, Charles C Thomas.

Dellon AL, Hament W, Gittelshon A: Nonoperative management of cubital tunnel syndrome: an 8 year prospective study, *Neurology* 43:1673, 1993.

Deltoff MN, Kogon PL: *The portable skeletal x-ray library,* St Louis, 1998, Mosby.

Demeter SL, Andersson GBJ, Smith GM: *Disability evaluation,* St Louis, 1996, Mosby.

Dimitru D: *Electrodiagnostic medicine,* Philadelphia, 1995, Hanley & Belfus.

Doherty M, Doherty J: *Clinical examination in rheumatology,* London, 1992, Wolfe.

Doherty M, George E: *Self-assessment picture tests in rheumatology,* London, 1995, Mosby-Wolfe.

Doherty M: *Color atlas and text of osteoarthritis,* London, 1994, Wolfe.

Edeiken J: *Roentgen diagnosis of diseases of bone,* ed 4, Baltimore, 1990, Williams & Wilkins.

Edelson G et al: Bony changes at the lateral epicondyle of possible significance in tennis elbow syndrome, *J Shoulder Elbow Surg* 10(2):158-163, 2001.

Elattrache NS, Thompson B: Clinical impact of elbow magnetic resonance imaging, *Oper Tech Sports Med* 5(1):33-36, 1997.

Elster AD: *Questions and answers in magnetic resonance imaging,* St Louis, 1994, Mosby.

Epstein O et al: *Clinical examination,* ed 2, London, 1997, Mosby.

Fedorczyk JM: Tennis elbow: blending basic science with clinical practice, *J Hand Ther* 19(2):146-153, 2006.

Feldmann E: *Current diagnosis in neurology,* St Louis, 1994, Mosby.

Folberg CR, Weiss AP, Akelman E: Cubital tunnel syndrome, part 1: presentation and diagnosis, *Orthop Rev* 23:136, 1994.

Fornage B: *Musculoskeletal ultrasound,* New York, 1995, Churchill Livingstone.

Frank ED et al: *Merrill's atlas of radiographic positioning and procedures,* ed 11, St Louis, 2007, Mosby.

Fritz RC, Brody GA: MR imaging of the wrist and elbow, *Clin Sports Med* 14:315, 1995.

Garden RS: Tennis elbow, *J Bone Joint Surg* 43B:100, 1961.

Gardner E: *Fundamentals of neurology,* ed 4, Philadelphia, 1963, WB Saunders.

Gerard JA, Kleinfield SL: *Orthopedic testing,* New York, 1993, Churchill Livingstone.

Gilula LA, editor: *The traumatized wrist and hand: radiographic and anatomic correlation,* Philadelphia, 1992, Saunders.

Gilula LA, Yin Y: *Imaging of the wrist and hand,* Philadelphia, 1996, WB Saunders.

Grant JCB, Basmajian JV: *Grant's method of anatomy,* ed 7, Baltimore, 1965, Williams & Wilkins.

Greenspan A: *Orthopedic radiology,* ed 2, Philadelphia, 1992, JB Lippincott.

Greenstein GM: *Clinical assessment of neuromusculoskeletal disorders,* St Louis, 1997, Mosby.

Grossman ZD et al: *Cost-effective diagnostic imaging: the clinician's guide,* ed 3, St Louis, 1995, Mosby.

Hale MS: *A practical approach to arm pain,* Springfield, Ill, 1971, Charles C Thomas.

Hammer WI: *Functional soft tissue examination and treatment by manual methods the extremities,* Gaithersburg, Md, 1991, Aspen.

Hartley A: *Practical joint assessment upper quadrant,* ed 2, St Louis, 1995, Mosby.

Hawkins RJ: *An organized approach to musculoskeletal examination and history taking,* St Louis, 1995, Mosby.

Hinkle CZ: *Fundamentals of anatomy & movement: a workbook and guide,* St Louis, 1997, Mosby.

Ho CP, Sartoris DJ: Magnetic resonance imaging of the elbow, *Rheum Dis Clin North Am* 17:705, 1991.

Hollinshead WH: *Anatomy for surgeons, the back and limbs,* vol 3, ed 2, New York, 1969, Harper & Row.

Hoppenfeld S: *Physical examination of the spine and extremities,* New York, 1976, Appleton-Century-Crofts.

Jablonski S: *Dictionary of medical acronyms & abbreviations,* ed 3, Philadelphia, 1998, Hanley & Belfus.

Jehl J, Crummy P: *Essentials of radiologic surgery,* ed 6, Philadelphia, 1993, JB Lippincott.

Kaplan EB: Treatment of tennis elbow (epicondylitis) by denervation, *J Bone Joint Surg* 41A:147, 1959.

Kasch MC: Acute hand injuries. In Pedretti LW, Zolton B, editors: *Occupational therapy: practice skills for physical dysfunction,* ed 3, St Louis, 1990, Mosby.

Kasdan ML: *Occupational hand & upper extremity injuries & diseases,* ed 2, Philadelphia, 1998, Hanley & Belfus.

Katirji B: *Electromyography in clinical practice: a case study approach,* St Louis, 1998, Mosby.

Katz WA: *Rheumatic diseases diagnosis and management,* Philadelphia, 1977, JB Lippincott.

Kendall HO, Kendall FP, Wadsworth GE: *Muscles: testing and function,* ed 3, Baltimore, 1992, Williams & Wilkins.

Klippel JH, Dieppe PA: *Rheumatology,* vol 1-2, ed 2, London, 1998, Mosby.

Lavy CBD, Barrett DS: *Questions and answers on Apley's concise system of orthopaedics and fractures,* Oxford, UK, 1991, Butterworth-Heinemann.

LeHuec JC et al: Epicondylitis after treatment with fluoroquinolone antibiotics, *J Bone Joint Surg* 77B:293, 1995.

Lerner AJ: *The little black book of neurology,* ed 3, St Louis, 1995, Mosby.

Lewis CB, Knortz KA: *Orthopedic assessment and treatment of the geriatric patient,* St Louis, 1993, Mosby.

Loth TS: *Orthopedic boards review II: a case study approach,* St Louis, 1996, Mosby.

MacDermid JC, Michlovitz SL: Examination of the elbow: linking diagnosis, prognosis, and outcomes as a framework for maximizing therapy interventions, *J Hand Ther* 19(2):82-97, 2006.

Magee DJ: *Orthopedic physical assessment,* ed 3, Philadelphia, 1997, WB Saunders.

Majima M, Horii E, Nakamura R: Treatment of chronically dislocated elbows: a report of three cases, *J Shoulder Elbow Surg* (in press, corrected proof).

Malmivaara A et al: Rheumatoid factor and HLA antigens in wrist tenosynovitis and humeral epicondylitis, *Scand J Rheumatol* 24:154, 1995.

Malone TR, McPoil TG, Nitz AJ: *Orthopedic and sports physical therapy,* ed 3, St Louis, 1997, Mosby.

Martin JH: *Neuroanatomy text and atlas,* ed 2, Stamford, Conn, 1996, Appleton & Lange.

Martinoli C et al: Ultrasound of the elbow, *Eur J Ultrasound* 14(1):21-27, 2001.

Mathers LH et al: *Clinical anatomy principles,* St Louis, 1996, Mosby.

Mazion JM: *Illustrated manual of neurological reflexes/signs/tests, part 1, orthopedic signs/tests/maneuvers for office procedure, part II,* Orlando, Fla, 1980, Daniels Publishing.

McRae R: *Clinical orthopaedic examination,* ed 3, Edinburgh, 1990, Churchill Livingstone.

Medical Economics Books: *Patient care flow chart manual,* ed 3, Oradell, NJ, 1982, Medical Economics Books.

Mehta JA, Bain GI: Elbow dislocations in adults and children, *Clin Sports Med* 23(4):609-627, 2004.

Mellion MB: *Office sports medicine,* ed 2, St Louis, 1996, Mosby.

Mellion MB: *Sports medicine secrets,* Philadelphia, 1994, Hanley & Belfus.

Melloni P, Valls R: The use of MRI scanning for investigating soft-tissue abnormalities in the elbow, *Eur J Radiol* 54(2):303-313, 2005.

Mennell JM: *The musculoskeletal system differential diagnosis from symptoms and physical signs,* Gaithersburg, Md, 1992, Aspen.

Mercier LR, Pettid FJ: *Practical orthopedics,* ed 4, St Louis, 1995, Mosby.

Meyers JF: Elbow arthroscopy. In Shahriaree H, editor: *O'Connor's textbook of arthroscopic surgery,* Philadelphia, 1992, JB Lippincott.

Miles KA, Lamont AC: Ultrasonic demonstration of the elbow fat pads, *Clin Radiol* 40(6):602-604, 1989.

Miller JH, Beggs I: Detection of intraarticular bodies of the elbow with saline arthrosonography, *Clin Radiol* 56(3):231-234, 2001.

Mills GP: The treatment of tennis elbow, *Dr Med J* 1:12, 1928.

Mitchell SW: *Injuries of nerves and their consequences,* Philadelphia, 1972, JB Lippincott.

Moore KL: *Clinically oriented anatomy,* ed 3, Baltimore, 1992, Williams & Wilkins.

Mosby-Year Book, Inc: *Expert 10-minute physical examination,* St Louis, 1997, Mosby.

Murphy BJ: MR imaging of the elbow, *Radiology* 184:525, 1992.

Nabhan A et al: Simple decompression or subcutaneous anterior transposition of the ulnar nerve for cubital tunnel syndrome, *J Hand Surg* 30(5):521-524, 2005.

Newman JS et al: Detection of soft-tissue hyperemia: value of power Doppler sonography, *Am J Roentgenol* 163:385, 1994.

Nicholas JA, Hershman EB: *The upper extremity in sports medicine,* ed 2, St Louis, 1995, Mosby.

Nirschi RP: Elbow tendinosis/tennis elbow, *Clin Sports Med* 4:851, 1992.

Nirschi RP: Muscle and tendon trauma. In Morrey BF, editor: *The elbow and its disorders,* Philadelphia, 1993, Saunders.

Nirschi RP: Patterns of failed healing in tendon injury. In Buckwalter J, Leadbetter W, Goodwin P, editors: *Sports induced soft tissue inflammation,* Chicago, 1991, American Academy of Orthopedic Surgeons.

Nordin M, Andersson GBJ, Pope MH: *Musculoskeletal disorders in the workplace: principles and practice,* St Louis, 1997, Mosby.

Nordin M, Frankel VH: *Basic biomechanics of the musculoskeletal system,* ed 2, Philadelphia, 1989, Lea & Febiger.

Nourissat G, Kakuda C, Dumontier C: Arthroscopic excision of osteoid osteoma of the elbow, *Arthroscopy* (in press, corrected proof).

O'Donoghue DH: *Treatment of injuries to athletes,* ed 3, Philadelphia, 1976, WB Saunders.

O'Drsicoll SW, Ball DF, Morrey BF: Posterolateral rotary instability of the elbow, *J Bone Joint Surg* 73A:440, 1991.

O'Drsicoll SW et al: The anatomy of the lateral ulnar collateral ligament, *Clin Anat* 5:296, 1992.

O'Dwyer KJ, Howie CR: Medial epicondylitis of the elbow, *Int Orthop* 19:69, 1995.

Omer GE, Spinner M: *Management of peripheral nerve problems,* Philadelphia, 1980, WB Saunders.

Osborne G: Compression neuritis of the ulnar nerve at the elbow, *Hand Clin* 2:10, 1970.

Parkes JC: Overuse injuries of the elbow. In Nicholas JA, Hershman EB, editors: *The upper extremity in sports medicine,* St Louis, 1990, Mosby.

Pecina MM, Krmpotic-Nemanic J, Markiewitz AD: *Tunnel syndromes,* Boca Raton, Fla, 1991, CRC Press.

Peterson AR et al: Variations in dorsomedial hand innervation, electrodiagnostic implications, *Arch Neurol* 49:870, 1992.

Pheasant S: *Ergonomics, work and health,* Gaithersburg, Md, 1991, Aspen.

Polley HF, Hunder GG: *Rheumatologic interviewing and physical examination of the joints,* ed 2, Philadelphia, 1978, WB Saunders.

Pomianowski S et al: The effect of forearm rotation on laxity and stability of the elbow, *Clin Biomech* 16(5):401-407, 2001.

Potter HG et al: Lateral epicondylitis: correlation of MR imaging, surgical, and histophysiologic findings, *Radiology* 196:43, 1995.

Pradhan S: Shank sign in myotonic dystrophy type-1 (DM-1), *J Clin Neurosci* 14(1):27-32, 2007.

Preston DC et al: The median-ulnar latency difference studies are comparable in mild carpal tunnel syndrome, *Muscle Nerve* 17:1469, 1994.

Qureshi F, Stanley D: The painful elbow, *Surgery (Oxford)* 24(11):368-372, 2006.

Regan W et al: Biomechanical study of ligaments around the elbow joint, *Clin Orthop* 271:170, 1991.

Regan W, Lapner PC: Prospective evaluation of two diagnostic apprehension signs for posterolateral instability of the elbow, *J Shoulder Elbow Surg* 15(3):344-346, 2006.

Regan W et al: Microscopic histopathology of chronic refractory lateral epicondylitis, *Am J Sports Med* 20:746, 1992.

Regan WD, Morrey BF: Physical examination of the elbow. In Morrey BF, editor: *The elbow and its disorders,* Philadelphia, 1993, WB Saunders.

Reid DC: *Sports injury assessment and rehabilitation,* New York, 1992, Churchill Livingstone.

Resnick D, Niwayama G: *Diagnosis of bone and joint disorders,* Philadelphia, 1995, WB Saunders.

Roetert EP et al: The biomechanics of tennis elbow, an integrated approach, *Clin Sports Med* 14:47, 1995.

Rompe JD et al: Chronic lateral epicondylitis of the elbow: a prospective study of low-energy shockwave therapy and low-energy shockwave therapy plus manual therapy of the cervical spine, *Arch Phys Med Rehabil* 82(5):578-582, 2001.

Rosenbaum RB, Ochoa JL: *Carpal tunnel syndrome and other disorders of the median nerve,* Boston, 1993, Butterworth-Heinemann.

Rosenberg ZS et al: The elbow: MR features of nerve disorders, *Radiology* 188:235, 1993.

Ruch DS, Papadonikolakis A, Campolattaro RM: The posterolateral plica: a cause of refractory lateral elbow pain, *J Shoulder Elbow Surg* 15(3):367-370, 2006.

Safran M, Ahmad CS, Elattrache NS: Ulnar collateral ligament of the elbow, *Arthroscopy* 21(11):1381-1395, 2005.

Saidoff DC, McDonough AL: *Critical pathways in therapeutic intervention,* St Louis, 1997, Mosby.

Salter RB: *Textbook of disorders and injuries of the musculoskeletal system,* Baltimore, 1970, Williams & Wilkins.

Sandifer PH: *Neurology in orthopaedics,* London, 1967, Butterworths.

Sauser DD, Thodorson SH, Fahr LM: Imaging of the elbow, *Radiol Clin North Am* 28:923, 1990.

Savoie Iii FH, Field LD, Ramsey JR: Posterolateral rotatory instability of the elbow: diagnosis and management, *Oper Tech Sports Med* 14(2):81-85, 2006.

Schamblin ML, Safran MR: Injury of the distal biceps at the musculotendinous junction, *J Shoulder Elbow Surg* 16(2):208-212, 2007.

Schumacher HR, Klippel JH, Koopman WJ: *Primer on the rheumatic diseases,* ed 10, Atlanta, 1993, Arthritis Foundation.

Seddon H: *Surgical disorders of the peripheral nerves,* Baltimore, 1968, Williams & Wilkins.

Smith FM: *Surgery of the elbow,* ed 2, Philadelphia, 1972, WB Saunders.

Spinner M, Spencer PS: Nerve compression lesions of the upper extremity: a clinical and experimental review, *Clin Orthop* 104:46, 1974.

Spinner RJ, Morgenlander JC, Nunley JA: Ulnar nerve function following total elbow arthroplasty: a prospective study comparing preoperative and postoperative clinical and electrophysiologic evaluation in patients with rheumatoid arthritis, *J Hand Surg* 25(2):360-364, 2000.

Stanley J: Radial tunnel syndrome: a surgeon's perspective, *J Hand Ther* 19(2):180-185, 2006.

Stedman TL: *Stedman's medical dictionary,* ed 25, Baltimore, 1990, Williams & Wilkins.

Steinmann SP: Elbow arthroscopy, *J Am Soc Surg Hand* 3(4):199-207, 2003.

Stoller DW: *Magnetic resonance imaging in orthopaedics & sports medicine,* Philadelphia, 1993, JB Lippincott.

Storen G: The radiocapitellar relationship, *Acta Chir Scand* 116:144, 1995.

Stubbs MJ, Field LD, Savoie Iii FH: Osteochondritis dissecans of the elbow, *Clin Sports Med* 20(1):1-9, 2001.

Sunderland S: *Nerves and nerve injuries,* Baltimore, 1968, Williams & Wilkins.

Tan JC, Horn SE: *Practical manual of physical medicine and rehabilitation,* St Louis, 1998, Mosby.

Tashjian RZ et al: Functional outcomes and general health status after ulnohumeral arthroplasty for primary degenerative arthritis of the elbow, *J Shoulder Elbow Surg* 15(3):357-366, 2006.

Timmerman LA, Andrews JR: Undersurface tear of the ulnar collateral ligament in baseball players, *Am J Sports Med* 22:33, 1994.

Toghill PJ: *Examining patients: an introduction to clinical medicine,* London, 1990, Edward Arnold.

Torg JS, Shepard RJ: *Current therapy in sports medicine,* ed 3, St Louis, 1995, Mosby.

Tullos HS, King JW: Lesions of the pitching arm in adolescents, *JAMA* 220:264, 1972.

Turek SL: *Orthopaedics principles and their application,* ed 3, Philadelphia, 1977, JB Lippincott.

Vanderpool DW et al: Peripheral compression lesions of the ulnar nerve, *J Bone Joint Surg* 50B:792, 1968.

Vicenzino B: Lateral epicondylalgia: a musculoskeletal physiotherapy perspective, *Man Ther* 8(2):66-79, 2003.

Wadsworth TG: *The elbow,* New York, 1982, Churchill Livingstone.

Ward WL, Belhobek GH, Anderson TE: Arthroscopic elbow findings: correlation with preoperative radiographic studies, *Arthroscopy* 8:498, 1992.

Warwick R, Williams PL: *Gray's anatomy,* ed 35, Philadelphia, 1973, WB Saunders.

Watchmaker GP, Lee G, Mackinnon SE: Intraneural topography of the ulnar nerve in the cubital tunnel facilitates anterior transposition, *J Hand Surg Am* 19:915, 1994.

Watt I: Magnetic resonance imaging in orthopaedics, *J Bone Joint Surg* 73:534, 1991.

Weinstein SL, Buckwalter JA: *Turek's orthopaedics principles and their application,* ed 5, Philadelphia, 1994, JB Lippincott.

Westkaemper JG, Varitimidis SE, Sotereanos DG: Posterior interosseous nerve palsy in a patient with rheumatoid synovitis of the elbow: a case report and review of the literature. *J Hand Surg* 24(4):727-731, 1999.

Wiens E, Lane S: The anterior interosseous nerve syndrome, *Can J Surg* 21:354, 1978.

Wiesler ER et al: Ultrasound in the diagnosis of ulnar neuropathy at the cubital tunnel, *J Hand Surg* 31(7):1088-1093, 2006.

Wilson FC: *The musculoskeletal system,* Philadelphia, 1975, JB Lippincott.

Windsor RE, Lox DM: *Soft tissue injuries: diagnosis and treatment,* Philadelphia, 1998, Hanley & Belfus.

Winter D: *Biomechanics and motor control of human movement,* ed 2, New York, 1990, Wiley-Interscience.

Yamazaki H et al: The two locations of ganglions causing radial nerve palsy, *J Hand Surg* (in press, corrected proof).

Yochum T, Rowe L: *Essentials of skeletal radiology,* ed 2, Baltimore, 1996, Williams & Wilkins.

Yorgancigil H, Karahan N, Baydar ML: Multiple loose bodies in the joints: from snowstorm to hailstones, *Arthroscopy* 20(8):e113-113e6, 2004.

CITATIONS

Bales CP et al: Microvascular supply of the lateral epicondyle and common extensor origin, *J Shoulder Elbow Surg* (in press, corrected proof).

Beingessner DM et al: The effect of coronoid fractures on elbow kinematics and stability, *Clin Biomech* 22(2):183-190, 2007.

Bradley JP, Petrie RS: Osteochondritis dissecans of the humeral capitellum: diagnosis and treatment, *Clin Sports Med* 20(3):565-590, 2001.

Ciccotti MC, Schwartz MA, Ciccotti MG: Diagnosis and treatment of medial epicondylitis of the elbow, *Clin Sports Med* 23(4):693-705, 2004.

Doornberg JN, van Duijn J, Ring D: Coronoid fracture height in terrible-triad injuries, *J Hand Surg* 31(5):794-797, 2006.

Greenfield C, Webster V: Chronic lateral epicondylitis: survey of current practice in the outpatient departments in Scotland, *Physiotherapy* 88(10):578-594, 2002.

Kajiwara R et al: Irreducible pulled elbow in an adult: a case report, *J Shoulder Elbow Surg* 16(1):e1-e4, 2007.

Kato N, Birch R: Peripheral nerve palsies associated with closed fractures and dislocations, *Injury* 37(6):507-512, 2006.

Levine JW, Field LD, Savoie Iii FH: Arthroscopic management of osteochondritis dissecans of the elbow, *Oper Tech Sports Med* 14(2):60-66, 2006.

Raimbeau G, Saint-Cast Y: Compressions du nerf radial au coude, *Chirurgie de la Main* 23(suppl 1):S86-S101, 2004.

Wadsworth TG et al: The elbow flexion test, *J Shoulder Elbow Surg* 4(1):S20.

CHAPTER SIX

FOREARM, WRIST, AND HAND

ORTHOPEDIC GAMUT 6-1

WRIST CARPAL SYSTEM

The nature of injury of the wrist carpal system is determined by:
1. The type of three-dimensional loading
2. The magnitude and direction of the forces involved
3. The position of the hand at the time of impact
4. The biomechanical properties of the bones and ligaments

AXIOMS IN ASSESSING THE FOREARM, WRIST, AND HAND

- Pain in the wrist and hand may have origin in the bones and joints, periarticular soft tissues, nerve roots, peripheral nerves, and vascular structures.
- Pain in the wrist and hand may also be referred from the cervical spine, thoracic outlet, shoulder, or elbow.

INTRODUCTION

Chronic wrist pain has often been called the *lower back pain of hand conditions.* Both areas offer the clinician significant diagnostic and therapeutic challenges. As in the examination of the lower back, a precise evaluation based on thorough knowledge of regional anatomy is essential to successful management.

The wrist joint is probably the most complicated joint in the body because of its unique arrangement and articulation of the radiocarpal and intercarpal joints. Ligamentous injuries to the carpus can lead to significant and possibly per-

manent disability. Diagnosis may be difficult, with persistent degrees of carpal instability. Definitive treatment modalities have not been perfected. As with most joint injuries, a more thorough understanding of the anatomy and pathogenesis of these injuries is useful.

Carpal injuries represent a spectrum of bony and ligamentous damage. The names given to the various injuries describe the resultant damage apparent only on radiographs, for example, *lunate dislocation, perilunate dislocation, scaphoid fracture, transscaphoid perilunate fracture-dislocation,* and *transscaphoid transtriquetral perilunate fracture-dislocation.* Each injury is not an entity but part of a continuum (Figs. 6-1 through 6-3).

A stable and pain-free wrist is a prerequisite for normal hand function. In contrast, a painful, unstable, or deformed wrist impairs function. The wrist, a common target of rheumatoid arthritis, is adversely affected by the reaction of synovial tissue on capsuloligamentous structures, articular cartilage, and subchondral bone. The mechanical forces of the different muscle groups acting across the wrist also contribute to deformities.

The initial evaluation of a patient with an injured wrist must be thorough and methodical. In recent years, increased understanding of carpal mechanics and instability patterns, with and without fractures, has increased the importance of accurate examination of the wrist. The diagnosis of *sprained wrist* is not adequate in establishing a proper treatment regimen. By taking a complete history, performing an thorough examination, and using appropriate diagnostic aids such as motion views, tomography, bone scans, and arthrography, the clinician can establish an accurate diagnosis of

TABLE 6-1

FOREARM, WRIST, AND HAND CROSS-REFERENCE TABLE BY ASSESSMENT PROCEDURE

Forearm, Wrist, and Hand / Test/Sign	Arterial Stenosis	Rheumatoid Arthritis	Digit Contractures	Carpal Fracture	Sprain	Denervation	Tenosynovitis	Aseptic Necrosis	Ulnar Neuropathy	Neuroma	Colles Fracture	Carpal Tunnel Syndrome	Anterior Interosseous Syndrome
Allen test	•												
Bracelet test		•											
Bunnell-Littler test			•										
Carpal lift sign				•	•								
Cascade sign		•		•									
Dellon moving two-point discrimination test						•			•				
Finkelstein test							•						
Finsterer sign				•				•					
Froment paper sign									•				
Interphalangeal neuroma test										•			
Maisonneuve sign											•		
Phalen sign												•	
Pinch grip test													•
Shrivel test						•							
Test for tight retinacular ligaments			•										
Tinel sign at the wrist									•			•	
Tourniquet test	•								•			•	
Wartenberg sign						•			•				
Weber two-point discrimination test						•			•				
Wringing test													•

wrist injury. Only after an accurate diagnosis is established can a rational, therapeutic regimen be prepared.

As with any other orthopedic problem, assessment of wrist and hand disorders begins with a complete history (Box 6-1). Painful disorders of the forearm, wrist, and hand can be classified based on the tissue of origin of pain and its distribution.

ESSENTIAL ANATOMY

The bones of the hand can be divided into four units: a central fixed unit for stability and three mobile units for dexterity and power. The fixed unit is composed of eight carpal bones tightly bound to the second and third metacarpals (Fig. 6-4).

The carpal bones form a volar concave arch or carpal tunnel. The four bony prominences are joined by the flexor retinaculum (transverse carpal ligament), which forms the

---

ORTHOPEDIC GAMUT 6-2

MOBILE UNITS OF THE WRIST

The three mobile units projecting from the fixed unit of the wrist are:

1. The thumb, for powerful pinch and grasp and fine manipulations
2. The index finger, for precise movements alone or with the thumb
3. The middle, ring, and little fingers, for power grip

---

roof of the carpal tunnel. The flexor retinaculum straps down the flexor tendons as they cross at the wrist. The ulnar nerve, artery, and vein cross over the retinaculum but are sometimes covered by a fibrous band—the superficial part of the transverse carpal ligament—to form the ulnar tunnel, or

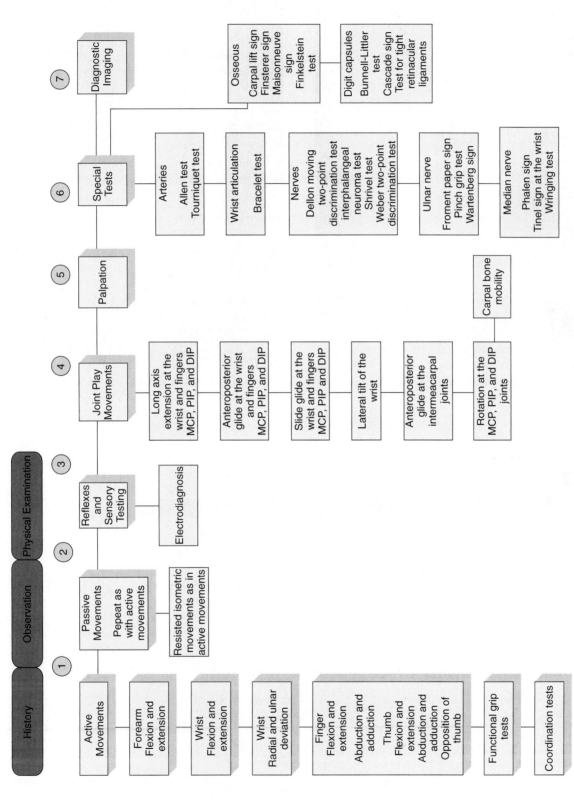

FIG. 6-1 Forearm, wrist, and hand assessment. *DIP,* Distal interphalangeal; *MCP,* metacarpophalangeal; *PIP,* proximal interphalangeal.

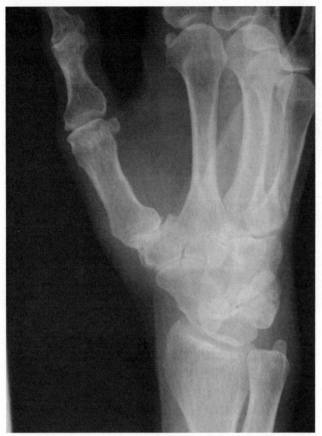

FIG. 6-2 Early trapeziometacarpal joint arthritis. (From Ankarath S: Chronic wrist pain: diagnosis and management, *Curr Orthop* 20[2]:141-151, 2006.)

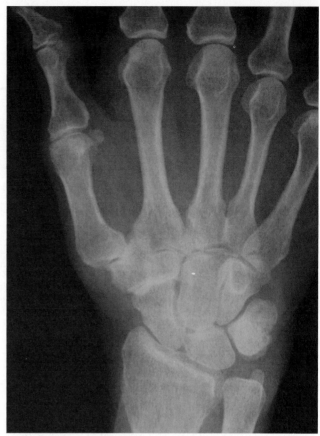

FIG. 6-3 Isolated scaphotrapeziotrapezoid joint arthritis. (From Ankarath S: Chronic wrist pain: diagnosis and management, *Curr Orthop* 20[2]:141-151, 2006.)

TABLE 6-2	
PRINCIPAL DIFFERENTIAL DIAGNOSIS LIST FOR WRIST PAIN	
	Tenosynovitis (de Quervain disease)
	Osteoarthritis of first carpal-metacarpal joint
	Scaphotrapeziotrapezoid osteoarthritis
	Scaphoid non-union
Radial side	Ganglion
Dorsal, central	Kienböck disease
	Scapholunate dissociation
	Scapholunate advanced collapse (SLAC wrist)
	Intraosseous ganglion
	Ganglion
Ulnar side	Ulnar abutment syndrome
	Ulnar impaction syndrome
	Distal radioulnar joint degenerative arthritis/instability
	Ulnar head chondromalacia
	Triangular fibrocartilage complex tear
	Extensor carpi ulnaris tendonitis/subluxation
	Lunotriquetral instability
	Pisotriquetral joint disease
	Midcarpal instability

Adapted from Ankarath S: Chronic wrist pain: diagnosis and management, *Curr Orthop* 20(2):141-151, 2006.

BOX 6-1

Précis of Forearm Wrist and Hand Diagnostic Consideration

Skin and Subcutaneous Tissue
Forearm
Dorsal hand
Palmar hand
Digits

Bones and Joints
Forearm
Wrist
Hand
Digits:
• Metacarpophalangeal joints
• Interphalangeal joints
• Thumb articulations

Flexor Muscle System
Forearm
Carpal tunnel
Palm and digits

Extensor Muscle System
Forearm
Extensor retinaculum
Dorsal hand
Extensor hood mechanism

Nerves
Superficial nerves
Deep nerves
• Radial nerve
• Ulnar nerve
• Median nerve

Vessels
Arteries
Veins
Lymphatics

ORTHOPEDIC GAMUT 6-3

RADIOCARPAL JOINT

The radiocarpal joint consists of the following:
1. The distal surface of the radius
2. The scaphoid and lunate bones
3. The triangular fibrocartilage connecting the medial side of the distal radius with the ulnar styloid process
4. The triquetrum

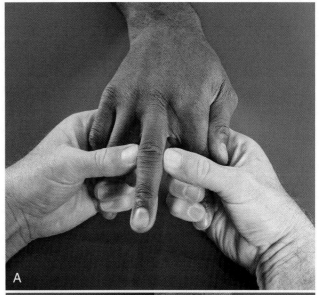
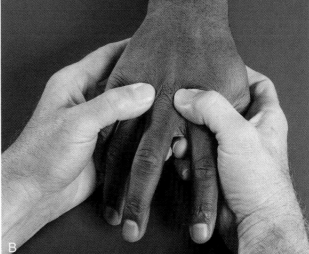
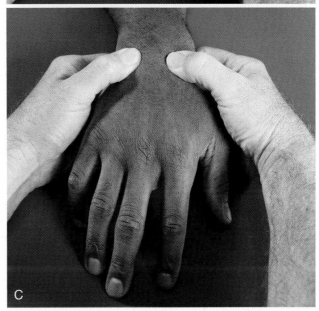

FIG. 6-4 Palpation of joints of the hand and wrist. **A,** Interphalangeal joints. **B,** Metacarpophalangeal joints. **C,** Radiocarpal groove and wrist.

6

Guyon canal. The eight carpals (Fig. 6-5) are arranged in two roughly parallel rows, each row extending from lateral to medial. Each of the carpal bones articulates with adjacent carpal bones by small synovial joints, and small individual ligaments unite adjacent bones (Fig. 6-6).

The wrist transmits force between the hand and forearm. Force (Fig. 6-7) passes through the capitate bone of the distal carpal row, through the scaphoid and lunate bones of the proximal carpal row, and onward to the distal end of the radius. These bones are the ones most likely to be fractured

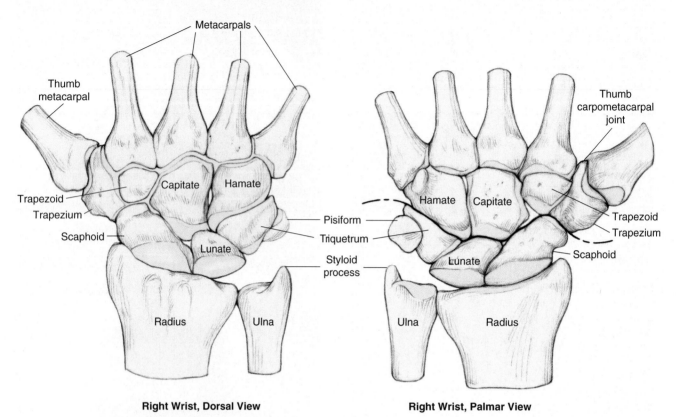

Right Wrist, Dorsal View   **Right Wrist, Palmar View**

FIG. 6-5 Carpal bones, dorsal and palmar views. (From Mathers LH et al: *Clinical anatomy principles,* St Louis, 1996, Mosby.)

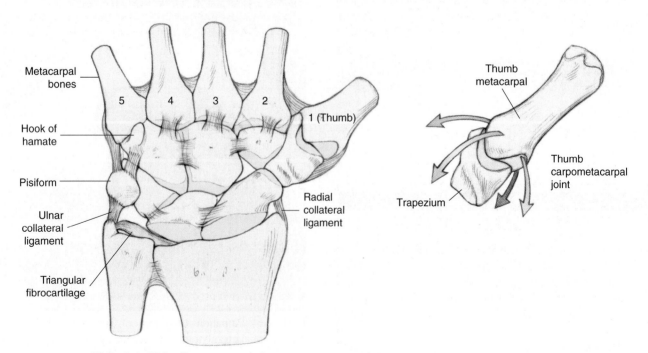

FIG. 6-6 Wrist ligaments and the carpometacarpal joint of the thumb. (From Mathers LH et al: *Clinical anatomy principles,* St Louis, 1996, Mosby.)

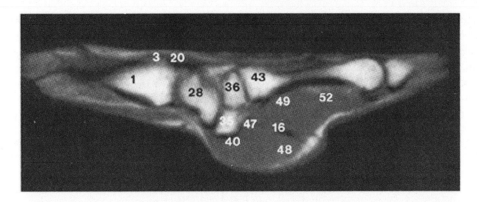

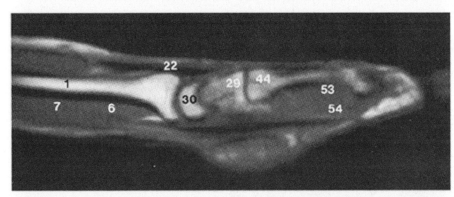

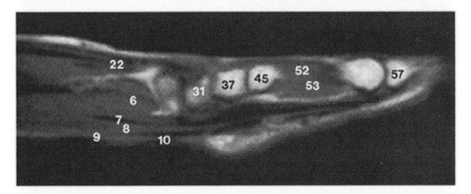

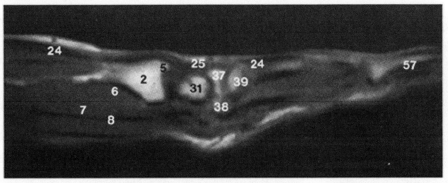

1 Radius
2 Ulna
3 Dorsal tubercle of radius
5 Styloid process of ulna
6 Pronator quadratus muscle
7 Flexor digitorum profundus muscle
8 Tendon of flexor digitorum profundus muscle
9 Flexor digitorum superficialis muscle
10 Tendon of flexor digitorum superficialis muscle
16 Tendon of flexor pollicis longus muscle
20 Tendon of extensor carpi radialis brevis muscle
22 Tendon of extensor digitorum muscle
24 Tendon of extensor digiti minimi muscle
25 Tendon of extensor carpi ulnaris muscle
28 Scaphoid
29 Capitate
30 Lunate
31 Triquetral
35 Trapezium
36 Trapezoid
37 Hamate
38 Hook of hamate
39 Base of fifth metacarpal
40 Abductor pollicis brevis muscle
43 Base of second ⎞
44 Base of third ⎬ metacarpal
45 Base of forth ⎠
47 Opponens pollicis muscle
48 Flexor pollicis brevis muscle
49 Adductor pollicis muscle
52 Dorsal interossei muscles
53 Ventral interossei muscles
54 Lumbrical muscle
57 Shaft of proximal phalanx

FIG. 6-7 Magnetic resonance imaging through the wrist. Sagittal sections. (From Mathers LH et al: *Clinical anatomy principles,* St Louis, 1996, Mosby.)

or dislocated in injury of the hand-wrist mechanism. Of the two long bones of the forearm, only the radius has true articulation with the carpal bones (Fig. 6-8). The carpal fractures often involve the scaphoid. Scaphoid fractures, with typical tenderness at the anatomic snuffbox, can result in chronic wrist pain because of non-union or collapse of the structure following injury (Figs. 6-9 and 6-10). Wrist

radiocarpal trauma can also involve the triangular fibrocartilage complex (Table 6-4).

Tenderness in the anatomic snuffbox and over the tuberosity is sensitive but not a specific test of scaphoid fracture. Plain-film radiographs are helpful not only in confirming a non-union, but also in assessing the other carpal bones for instability. Other imaging modalities such as computed tomog-

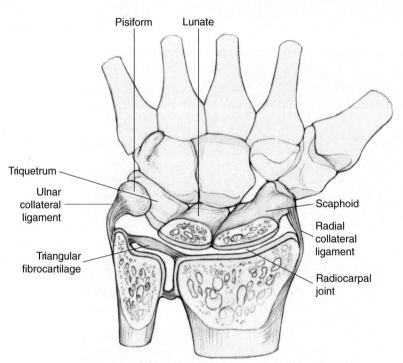

FIG. 6-8 Interior of the radiocarpal joint, anterior view, right wrist. (From Mathers LH et al: *Clinical anatomy principles,* St Louis, 1996, Mosby.)

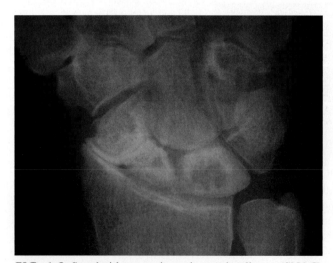

FIG. 6-9 Scaphoid non-union advanced collapse (SNAC) type of degenerative arthritis. (From Ankarath S: Chronic wrist pain: diagnosis and management, *Curr Orthop* 20[2]:141-151, 2006.)

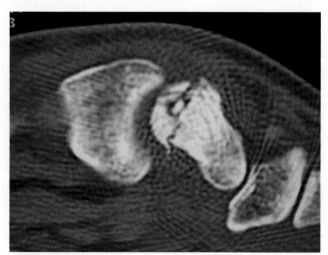

FIG. 6-10 Scaphoid non-union with collapse leading to humpback deformity. (From Ankarath S: Chronic wrist pain: diagnosis and management, *Curr Orthop* 20[2]:141-151, 2006.)

TABLE 6-3

FOREARM, WRIST, AND HAND CROSS-REFERENCE TABLE BY SYNDROME OR TISSUE

Anterior interosseous syndrome	Pinch grip test
Arterial stenosis	Allen test
	Tourniquet test
Aseptic necrosis	Finsterer sign
Carpal fracture	Carpal lift sign
	Cascade sign
	Finsterer sign
Carpal tunnel syndrome	Phalen sign
	Tinel sign at the wrist
	Tourniquet test
	Wringing test
Colles fracture	Maisonneuve sign
Denervation	Dellon moving two-point discrimination test
	Shrivel test
	Weber two-point discrimination test
Digit contractures	Bunnell-Littler test
	Test for tight retinacular ligaments
Neuroma	Interphalangeal neuroma test
Rheumatoid arthritis	Bracelet test
	Cascade sign
Sprain	Carpal lift sign
Tenosynovitis	Finkelstein test
Ulnar neuropathy	Dellon moving two-point discrimination test
	Froment paper sign
	Tinel sign at the wrist
	Tourniquet test
	Wartenberg sign
	Weber two-point discrimination test

TABLE 6-4

TRIANGULAR FIBROCARTILAGE COMPLEX INJURY CLASSIFICATION

Class I: Traumatic	A. Central perforation
	B. Ulnar avulsion
	a. With distal ulnar fracture
	b. Without distal ulnar fracture
	C. Distal avulsion
	D. Radial avulsion
	a. With sigmoid notch fracture
	b. Without sigmoid notch fracture
Class II: Degenerative (ulnocarpal abutment syndrome)	A. Triangular fibrocartilage complex wear
	B. Triangular fibrocartilage complex wear—with lunate or ulnar chondromalacia
	C. Triangular fibrocartilage complex perforation—with lunate or ulnar chondromalacia
	D. Triangular fibrocartilage complex perforation
	a. With lunate or ulnar chondromalacia
	b. With lunotriquetral ligament perforation
	E. Triangular fibrocartilage complex perforation
	a. With lunate or ulnar chondromalacia
	b. With lunotriquetral ligament perforation
	c. With ulnocarpal arthritis

Adapted from Ankarath S: Chronic wrist pain: diagnosis and management, *Curr Orthop* 20(2):141-151, 2006.

6

raphy or magnetic resonance imaging can help in providing further assessment of the degree of collapse and deformity in the scaphoid (Mazet, 1961).

As described earlier, the flexor retinaculum (Fig. 6-11) is a strong fibrous ligament extending across the anterior surface of the wrist, connecting the tubercles of the scaphoid and trapezium laterally with the pisiform and hamulus of the carpal tunnel. On the posterolateral side of the wrists is a triangular region bounded by several tendons, known as the *anatomic snuffbox* (Fig. 6-12). The tendons of extensor carpi radialis longus and brevis lie in the floor of the snuffbox, as do the scaphoid bone and the radial artery.

Two main groups of blood vessels supply the scaphoid. The volar vessels, which are branches of the radial artery entering the distal tubercle, supply the distal 20% to 30% of the bone. The proximal 70% to 80% is supplied by branches of the radial artery entering through the foramina along the dorsal ridge. These vessels run from distal to proximal (Weberet, Chao, 1978).

Various anatomic studies have consistently demonstrated poor blood supply to the proximal pole. An interruption to the dorsal blood vessels may lead to ischemia of the proximal end of the bone. An ulnar-directed force of sufficient magnitude on the radial side of the wrist with the wrist in 95 to 100 degrees of extension has consistently been shown to produce fractures of the scaphoid (Gelberman, Menon, 1980).

With the forearm in supination, the radius lies alongside and parallel to the ulna. On pronation of the forearm, the distal radius moves around the ulna with the radial sigmoid fossa articulating with the ulnar head. This movement results in a relative lengthening of ulna. In people with a positive ulnar variance, this overlengthening of the ulna can cause abutment on the lunate, resulting in pain and discomfort, which happens more often with the wrist in slight ulnar deviation. The triangular fibrocartilage complex can get caught between the lunate and ulna. Over a period, this circumstance may result in a central perforation of the triangular fibrocartilage

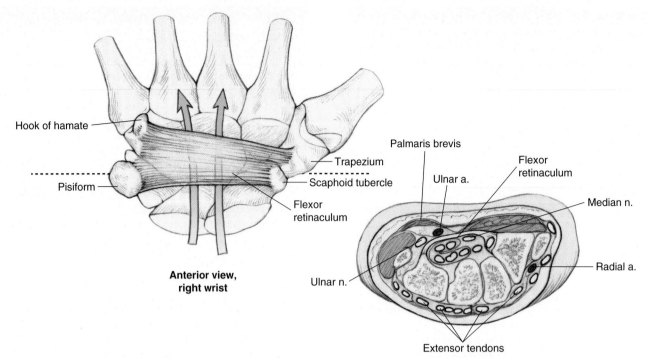

FIG. 6-11 Flexor retinaculum and wrist in cross-section. (From Mathers LH et al: *Clinical anatomy principles,* St Louis, 1996, Mosby.)

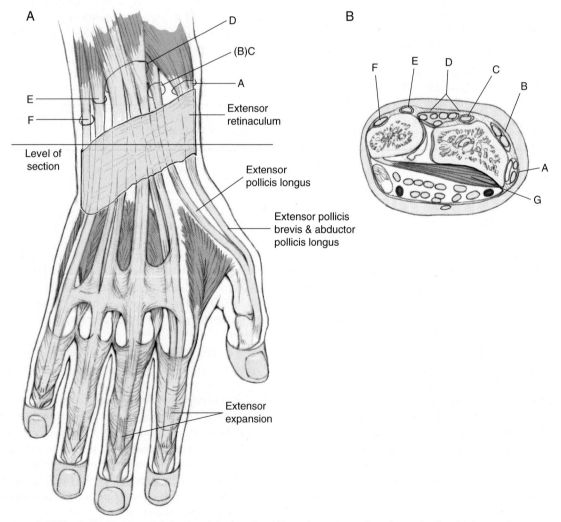

FIG. 6-12 Dorsum of the hand and wrist (**A**) and cross-section through distal ulna and radius (**B**). (From Mathers LH et al: *Clinical anatomy principles,* St Louis, 1996, Mosby.)

complex. This degenerative tear of the triangular fibrocartilage complex is different to the traumatic variety. Patients often complain of a catching sensation on forearm rotation with the wrist in ulnar deviation (Ankarath, 2006).

ESSENTIAL MOTION ASSESSMENT

Movements of the wrist comprise flexion, extension, and ulnar and radial deviation. Flexion-extension movements of the fingers occur at both the metacarpophalangeal (MCP) and the interphalangeal (IP) joints (Fig. 6-13).

Movements of the thumb are described in terms different from those applied to the other digits because the thumb is positioned in a way that is different from the way the fingers are positioned, and the thumb is capable of unique movements not possible in the other digits.

Opposition is a unique capability, possessed only by the thumb. The goal of opposition is to cause the *pulp* surface (i.e., the rounded eminence directly opposite the nail) of the distal phalanx to face the pulp surfaces of the other digits. This capability is essential to realizing the full range of capabilities for grasping and manipulating objects with the hand.

Creating a cup-shaped recess in the palm of the hand requires movement of the other four digits. This recess allows an object to be cradled in the palm before the fingers are closed over it.

For examination of the wrist-hand range of motion, the middle finger is considered midline (Fig. 6-14). Wrist flexion decreases as the fingers are flexed. Movements of flexion and extension are ultimately limited by muscles and ligaments (Figs. 6-15 and 6-16).

Finger abduction is 20 to 30 degrees at the MCP joints. Finger adduction is 0 degrees at the same joint. The loss of finger abduction or adduction has minimal effect on the activities of daily living. Thumb flexion at the carpometacarpal joint is in a range of 45 to 50 degrees. At the MCP joint, the range is 50 to 55 degrees. At the IP joint, thumb flexion is in a range of 80 to 90 degrees. Extension of the thumb at the IP joint is 0 to 5 degrees. Thumb abduction is 60 to 70 degrees. Thumb adduction is 30 degrees. Seventy degrees or less of retained flexion of the thumb at the IP joint and 50 degrees or less retained flexion at the MCP joint are considered impairments of the thumb in the activities of daily living. Zero degrees of extension at the IP joint is considered the sole impairment of extension for the thumb. Forty degrees or less of radial abduction and 25 degrees or less of adduction are considered impairments of the thumb in the activities of daily living (Fig. 6-17).

ESSENTIAL MUSCLE FUNCTION ASSESSMENT

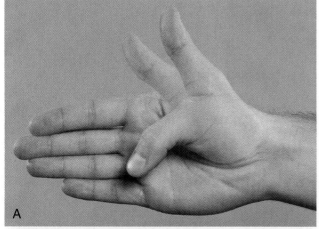
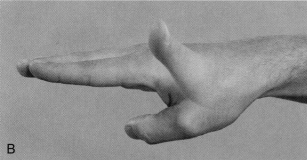
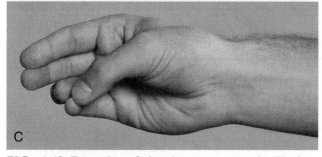

FIG. 6-13 Examples of thumb movements. **A,** Flexion-extension. **B,** Abduction-adduction. **C,** Opposition.

ORTHOPEDIC GAMUT 6-4

MUSCLES OF THE HAND

Muscles controlling movements of the hand are divided into two groups:
1. Extrinsic muscles that originate within the arm and forearm
2. Intrinsic muscles, the origins and insertions of which are entirely within the hand (Figs. 6-18 to 6-22)

ESSENTIAL IMAGING

The importance of routine posteroanterior (PA) and lateral radiographs in neutral position of the wrist cannot be overemphasized.

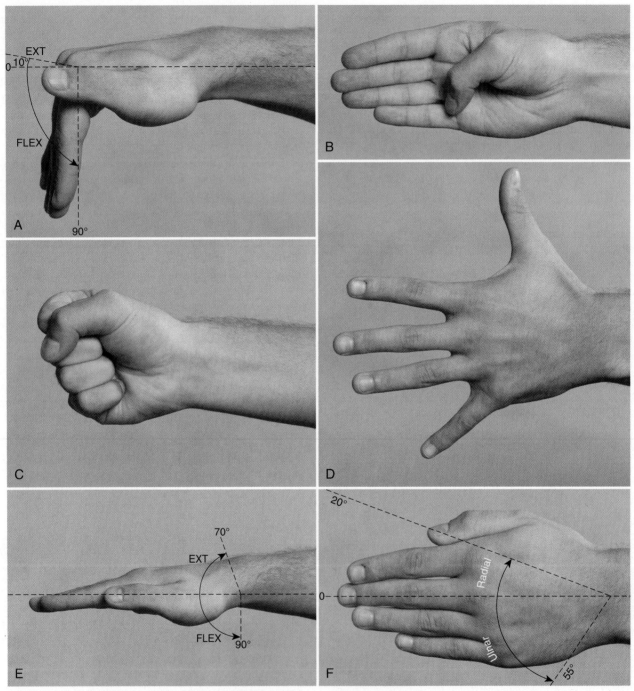

FIG. 6-14 Range of motion of the hand and wrist.

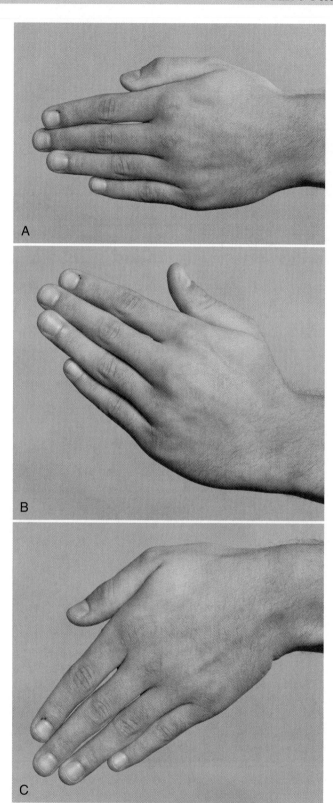

FIG. 6-15 The wrist in a neutral position (**A**). Radial deviation (**B**). Ulnar deviation (**C**). Radial deviation of 15 degrees or less and ulnar deviation of 30 degrees or less are impairments of the forearm in the activities of daily living.

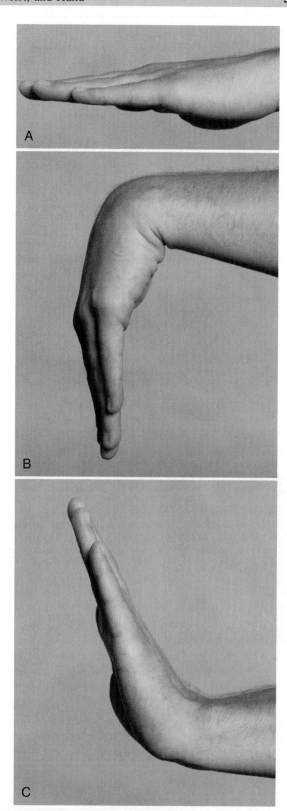

FIG. 6-16 The wrist in a neutral position (**A**). Wrist flexion (**B**). Wrist extension (dorsiflexion) (**C**). Wrist flexion of 50 degrees or less and wrist extension dorsiflexion of 35 degrees or less are impairments of the forearm in the activities of daily living.

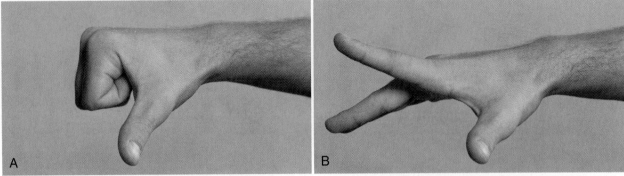

FIG. 6-17 Finger flexion (**A**) at the MCP joints. Extension (**B**) at the MCP joints. Extension of the proximal interphalangeal joints. Retained active finger flexion of 80 degrees or less at the MCP joint, 90 degrees or less at the proximal interphalangeal joint, and 60 degrees or less at the distal interphalangeal joint serve as an impairment of the fingers in the activities of daily living. Retained active extension of 10 degrees or less at the MCP joint serves as the sole impairment of the fingers in the activities of daily living.

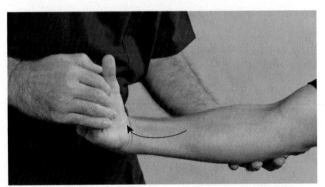

FIG. 6-18 Flexion. The prime movers for flexion of the wrist are the flexor carpi radialis (median nerve, C6, and C7) and the flexor carpi ulnaris (ulnar nerve, C8, and T1) muscles. The palmaris longus muscle is an accessory muscle used for this motion. The patient flexes the wrist against graded resistance provided by the fingertips of the examiner's other hand placed in the patient's palm. The flexor carpi radialis muscle is tested when the examiner provides resistance on the palmar side of the base of the second metacarpal bone in the directions of extension and ulnar deviation. The flexor carpi ulnaris is tested when the examiner applies resistance on the palmar side of the base of the fifth metacarpal bone in the directions of extension and radial deviation.

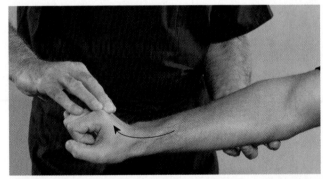

FIG. 6-19 Extension. The prime movers for extension of the wrist are the extensor carpi radialis longus (radial nerve, C6, and C7), extensor carpi radialis brevis (radial nerve, C6, and C7), and extensor carpi ulnaris (radial nerve, C7, and C8) muscles. The patient extends the wrist against graded resistance applied by the examiner's other hand to the dorsal surface of the patient's metacarpals. For testing the extensor carpi radialis longus and brevis muscles, resistance is applied by the examiner to the dorsal surface of the patient's second and third metacarpal bones in the directions of flexion and ulnar deviation. For testing the extensor carpi ulnaris muscle, resistance is applied to the dorsal surface of the fifth metacarpal bone in the directions of flexion and radial deviation.

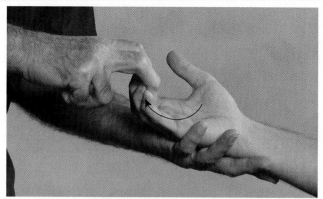

FIG. 6-20 Flexion of the interphalangeal joints of the fingers is accomplished by the long flexor tendons. Of the two long flexor tendons, the flexor digitorum sublimis has its main action on the middle finger joint. To test for sublimis action, the profundus tendon to the finger in question must be put completely out of action by passively flexing the MCP joint and by hyperextending the adjacent fingers. In tests for profundus action, the finger must be held passively and extended at both the proximal and middle finger joints.

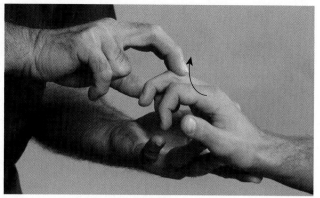

FIG. 6-22 The interosseous and lumbrical muscles are of fundamental importance in the extension of the fingers.

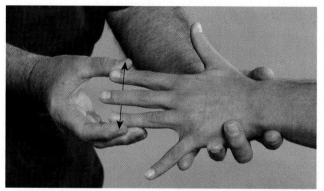

FIG. 6-21 The intrinsic muscles of the hand consist of a central group containing the interossei and lumbricales and the two lateral groups of hypothenar and thenar eminences. Many actions have been attributed to the lumbricales, but they have no powerful individual action of their own and can operate only with the stronger interossei.

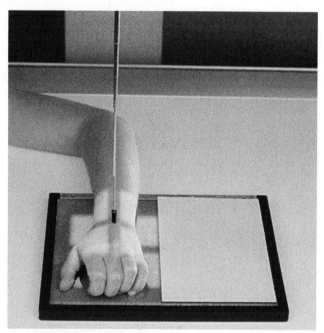

FIG. 6-23 Posteroanterior positioning of the wrist. (From Frank ED, et al: *Merrill's atlas of radiographic positioning and procedures,* ed 11, St Louis, 2007, Mosby.)

With PA wrist radiographs, the scaphoid and the distance between the carpal bones can be assessed (Figs. 6-23 and 6-24). A gap of 3 mm or more between the scaphoid and the lunate is abnormal and indicates a tear in the scapholunate interosseous ligament *(Terry Thomas sign)* (Fig. 6-29). A supinated, clenched-fist anteroposterior (AP) radiograph accentuates this gap. With extreme flexion of the scaphoid, in a PA view of the wrist, the scaphoid tubercle may project in the form of a dense circle or ring over the distal two-thirds of scaphoid (the *signet ring sign*).

A *Watson's shift test* is diagnostic of scapholunate dissociation. The test is performed with the examiner and patient facing each other. The examiner's fingers are placed dorsally on the distal radius, while the thumb is placed on the palmar distal tuberosity of the scaphoid. The examiner's other hand holds the metacarpals. Firm pressure is applied to the palmar tuberosity of the scaphoid while the wrist is moved from ulnar to radial deviation, moving the scaphoid from a position of extension to flexion. The examiner's thumb over the distal tuberosity prevents the scaphoid from

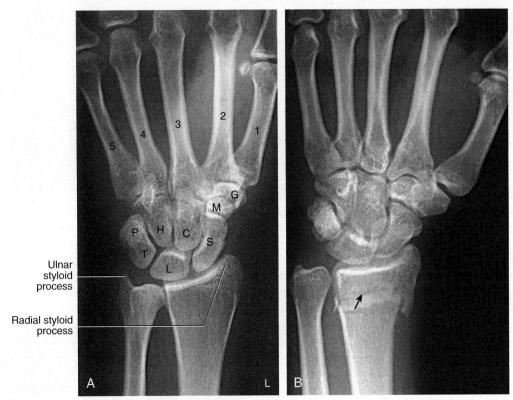

FIG. 6-24 **A,** Posteroanterior radiograph of the wrist. *C,* Capitate; *G,* trapezium; *H,* hamate; *L,* lunate; *M,* trapezoid; *P,* pisiform; *S,* scaphoid; *T,* triquetrum. **B,** Posteroanterior radiograph showing fracture *(arrow).* (From Frank ED et al: *Merrill's atlas of radiographic positioning and procedures,* ed 11, St Louis, 2007, Mosby.)

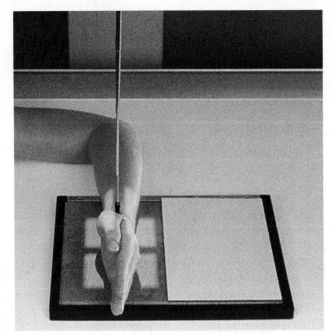

FIG. 6-25 Lateral positioning of wrist with ulnar surfaces to the film. (From Frank ED et al: *Merrill's atlas of radiographic positioning and procedures,* ed 11, St Louis, 2007, Mosby.)

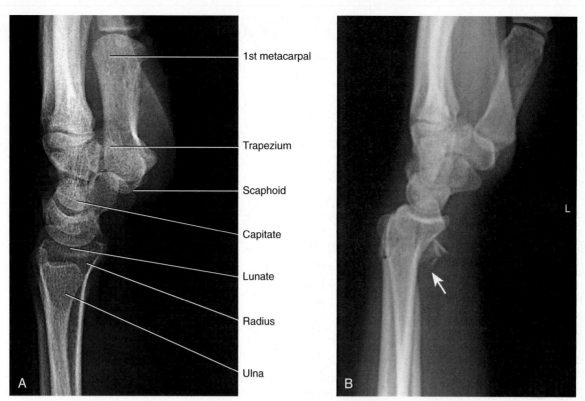

1st metacarpal

Trapezium

Scaphoid

Capitate

Lunate

Radius

Ulna

L

FIG. 6-26 **A,** Lateral wrist radiograph (ulnar surface to film). **B,** Lateral with fracture *(arrow).* (From Frank ED, et al: *Merrill's atlas of radiographic positioning and procedures,* ed 11, St Louis, 2007, Mosby.)

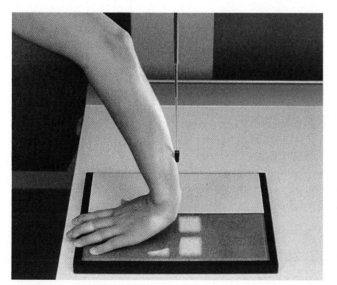

FIG. 6-27 Tangential (superoinferior) carpal canal. (From Frank ED, et al: *Merrill's atlas of radiographic positioning and procedures,* ed 11, St Louis, 2007, Mosby.)

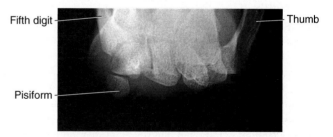

Fifth digit

Thumb

Pisiform

FIG. 6-28 Tangential radiograph of carpal canal (superoinferior). (From Frank ED, et al: *Merrill's atlas of radiographic positioning and procedures,* ed 11, St Louis, 2007, Mosby.)

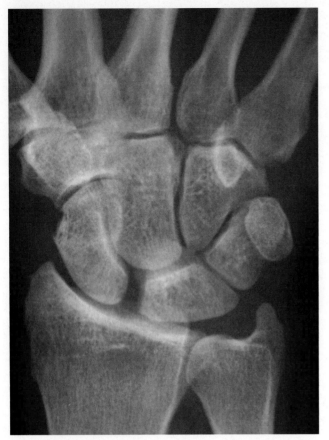

FIG. 6-29 Increased scapholunate gap after injury to the scapholunate ligament (Terry Thomas sign). (From Ankarath S: Chronic wrist pain: diagnosis and management, *Curr Orthop* 20[2]:141-151, 2006.)

ORTHOPEDIC GAMUT 6-5

SCAPHOLUNATE ADVANCE COLLAPSE (SLAC) WRIST GRADING BASED ON THE EXTENT OF THE DEGENERATIVE CHANGES

Stage 1a: Degenerative changes between the scaphoid and the radial styloid

Stage 1b: Degenerative changes involving the whole of the radioscaphoid joint

Stage 2: Degenerative arthritis involving the scapho-capitate (midcarpal) joint

---

oid and lunate as a unit fall into flexion, resulting in a volar intercalated segmental instability. Patients may complain of a painful clunk on ulnar deviation of the wrist. A positive ballottement test, in which the lunate is held firmly by the thumb and index finger of one hand while the pisotriquetral complex is moved dorsally and palmarly with the other, is diagnostic (Hoii et al, 1991; Reagan, Linscheid, Dobyns, 1984).

On the lateral radiograph, an angle between the long axis of the scaphoid and the lunate greater than 70 degrees is abnormal and is consistent with scapholunate dissociation (Figs. 6-25 and 6-26). An angle of 30 degrees or less is also abnormal and could signify ulnocarpal instability.

The most common cause of a scapholunate advance collapse (SLAC) wrist is rotary subluxation of the scaphoid. Other causes include Preiser disease, Kienböck disease, and midcarpal instability, or it can be posttraumatic after injuries involving the radioscaphoid or capitolunate joints.

Special plain-film radiographs can further identify pathologic conditions. A carpal tunnel view, which is a radiograph with the wrist in full extension, fingers extended, and the beam in front of the third metacarpal, helps the examiner visualize fractures of the hook of the hamate (Figs. 6-27 and 6-28). The pisotriquetral area can be better seen with lateral radiographs of the hand and forearm in 10 to 15 degrees of supination.

---

flexing. In cases of scapholunate ligament tears or in patients with a lax wrist, resistance to flexion of the distal pole will cause the scaphoid to move dorsally under the posterior margin of the radius, which can be felt by the examiner's index finger, normally inducing pain. Sometimes this test may only be painful, without any perception of dorsal scaphoid displacement. When pressure over the distal tuberosity of the scaphoid is removed, the scaphoid may go back into position with a clunk.

When disruption of the intrinsic (lunotriquetral) and extrinsic (radiotriquetral) supporting ligaments occurs, the scaph-

Assessment for Peripheral Vascular Obstruction at the Wrist

Comment

Blood supply for the hand is largely anterior or palmar in position. All the arterial supply enters on the proximal volar surface of the wrist, and at least one half of the venous drainage leaves by the same route. Both arterial and venous systems are subject to many variations. Age has some influence on the state of the system. Arteriovenous anastomoses are poorly developed in children. In elderly persons, both the arteries and the veins become elongated, large, and tortuous. In the absence of local vascular trauma, sympathetic dystrophy influence of vascular homeostasis must be considered in evaluating wrist-hand complaints.

> The challenge to understand and successfully manage reflex sympathetic dystrophy (RSD) and complex regional pain syndrome (CRPS) is unparalleled among disorders confronting examiners because of ignorance of cause, pathophysiologic factors, and proper treatment. As such, this task is frustrating and controversial, with an unpredictable incidence and course developing with little or no warning. Consequently, the unsuspecting examiner can easily underrate a patient's severe pain complaints after minor injury or operation only later to be confronted by a dystrophic, functionless hand, now easily diagnosed as RSD-CRPS. Unfortunately, once diagnosis is easy, treatment is not because the dystrophic changes and chronic pain are difficult to reverse (Merritt, 2005).

CRPS and sympathetic-mediated pain dysfunction are the most serious of the complications that can occur after injuries to the wrist.

Sympathetic pain is a diffuse, disabling hypersensitivity in one or more peripheral nerve autonomous zones. The pain initiates with burning pain, cold sensitivity, hyperhidrosis, and painful motion. RSD-CRPS causes an exaggerated response of the tissue to injury, producing intense and prolonged pain, vasomotor disturbance, and associated trophic changes. The pain and discomfort of RSD-CRPS cross several dermatome distributions. Clinical characteristics include protecting and guarding the extremity, holding or carrying the hand and wrist, and limiting use of the limb in pinch, grasp, and daily activities (Fig. 6-30).

Diagnosis of RSD-CRPS is based initially on clinical symptoms and signs for the upper extremity, which includes painful disuse of the hand and wrist with a high degree of awareness. Supportive laboratory testing includes positive bone scans (Fig. 6-31), hypervascularity (thermography), and positive sweat test with autonomic dysfunction and quantitative sudomotor axon reflex test. Later, osteoporosis

---

ORTHOPEDIC GAMUT 6-6

REFLEX SYMPATHETIC DYSTROPHY–COMPLEX REGIONAL PAIN SYNDROME (RSD-CRPS) LIMB PROTECTION

Three stages of RSD-CRPS limb protection by the patient are:

1. Not allowing palpation or percussion or even light touch of the affected tissue
2. Loss of use, stiffness of soft tissues, loss of joint motion, development of contracture, and atrophy of skin; warmth of hypervascularity turns to coldness; strength and function diminish further
3. Shiny, dry skin; degeneration of muscle tone; further joint stiffness; and both joint and muscle contracture

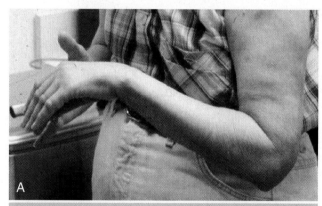

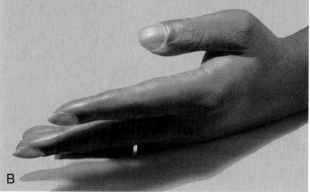

FIG. 6-30 **A,** Disassociation of RSD. This patient developed RSD after a Colles fracture and carried her hand like a foreign object. **B,** Stage II RSD with shiny skin and loss of extension joint wrinkles 3 months after meningitis and septic shock. (From Merritt WH: The challenge to manage reflex sympathetic dystrophy/complex regional pain syndrome, *Clin Plastic Surg* 2005;32[4]:575–604.)

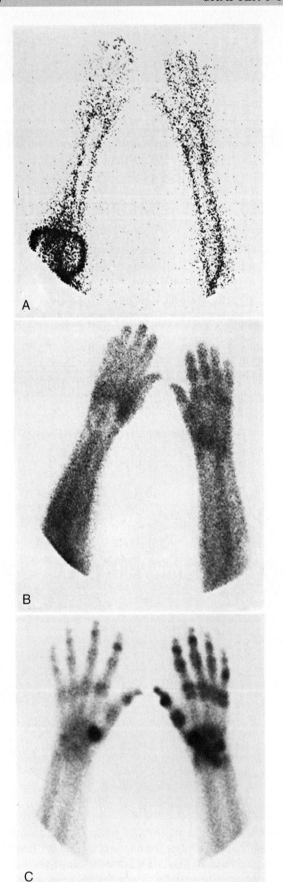

FIG. 6-31 Triphasic bone scan in sympathetic dystrophy. **A,** Injection phase. **B,** Early phase. **C,** Late phase. (From Cooney WP, Linscheid RL, Dobyns JH: *The wrist diagnosis and operative treatment,* vol 1-2, St Louis, 1998, Mosby.)

can help confirm the diagnosis. The sympathetic dystrophy scale is effective in confirming and rating the severity of this syndrome (Boxes 6-2 and 6-3).

CRPS is also defined on purely clinical grounds, with no new diagnostic tests or improved understanding of the cause of this disorder (Manning, 2000).

The superficial and deep palmar arterial arches are so named because of their relationship to the flexor tendons. These arches are connected to the dorsal carpal arterial arch, which lies deep in the extensor tendons, by a proximal and distal row of perforating arteries that pass between the metacarpal shafts.

The extensive anastomoses between the various vessels allow occlusion of an arch within its length without serious risk to the distal blood supply. Even when both the radial and ulnar arteries are occluded at the wrist, the blood supply can usually be maintained through collateral circulation that, in such cases, will pass mainly through the perforating arteries. The digital arteries of a finger are of sufficient caliber to allow survival of the fingertip.

The veins that drain blood from the hand are either superficial or deep systems. The superficial veins start on the dorsum of the fingers and collect their blood from the plexuses on the palmar and lateral sides of the fingers. The superficial veins run in several trunks parallel to the long axis of the fingers and drain into the cephalic and basilic veins via the dorsal venous network. No consistent pattern for this dorsal network exists; however, in general, the cross communications are scanty. The deep veins of the hand and forearm are small and do not drain as much blood as the superficial system.

BOX 6-3

CLASSIFICATION OF COMPLEX REGIONAL PAIN SYNDROME (CRPS)—MAJOR CATEGORIES

I. Sympathetically maintained pain syndrome (type I and type II)

II. Sympathetically independent pain syndrome (type III)
- Category I
- Type I (reflex sympathetic dystrophy) usually follows an initiating noxious event
  - Continuous pain or allodynia and hyperpathia is not limited to the territory of a single peripheral nerve.
  - Disproportionate pain to the inciting event
  - Edema, skin blood flow abnormality
  - Abnormal sudomotor activity
  - Motor dysfunction disproportionate to the inciting event
  - Diagnosis is excluded by the existence of conditions that would otherwise account for the degree of pain and dysfunction.
- Type II (major causalgia)
  - Major nerve injury, more regionally confined presentation (usually), principally involving the territory of the involved nerve
  - Spontaneous pain or allodynia and hyperpathia is usually limited to the area involved but may spread distally or proximally.
  - Edema, blood flow abnormality
  - Abnormal pseudomotor activity is or has been shown in the region of pain subsequent to the inciting event.
  - Motor dysfunction disproportionate to the inciting event
  - Diagnosis is excluded by conditions that otherwise account for the degree of pain and dysfunction.
- Category II
- Type III CRPS (sympathetically independent pain)
  - Disproportionate pain and sensory change, with motor and tissue change that do not respond to sympathetic block

Adapted from Manning DC: Reflex sympathetic dystrophy, sympathetically maintained pain, and complex regional pain syndrome: diagnoses of inclusion, exclusion, or confusion? *J Hand Ther* 13(4):260-268, 2000.

ORTHOPEDIC GAMUT 6-7

PULSES IN THE WRIST

Pulses are palpated at the wrist in three places:
1. The radial artery lying just medial to the radial styloid process, which passes toward the hand
2. The ulnar artery, which passes just lateral (in the anatomic position) to the pisiform bone
3. The deep radial artery, which crosses the floor of the anatomic snuffbox

Occlusion of the ulnar artery at the wrist may produce symptoms similar to those seen with ulnar tunnel syndrome. This disorder usually is secondary to some repetitive trauma to the ulnar aspect of the hand, such as when the hand is used as a mallet (hypothenar hammer syndrome). This disorder produces a thrombosis of the ulnar artery and results in ischemic manifestations such as pain, pallor, paresthesias, and decreased temperature of the affected digits. Local tenderness may be present, and Allen test is often positive.

PROCEDURE

- The patient is seated and instructed to make a tight fist to express blood from the palm. The examiner uses finger pressure to occlude the radial and ulnar arteries (Figs. 6-32 and 6-33).
- The patient opens and closes the fist to express any remaining blood (Fig. 6-34). The examiner releases the arteries one at a time (Fig. 6-35).
- The sign is negative if the pale skin of the palm flushes immediately after an artery is released.
- The sign is positive if the skin of the palm remains blanched for more than 5 seconds. This test, which should be performed before Wright test, Eden test, and the shoulder hyperabduction maneuver, is significant for revealing vascular occlusion of the artery tested.

Next Steps/Procedures
Tourniquet test and vascular assessment

CLINICAL PEARL

This test will often elicit paresthesia when an underlying distal peripheral nerve entrapment syndrome exists (carpal tunnel syndrome). The test is used as an early indicator of other general pathologic conditions only when paresthesia is elicited.

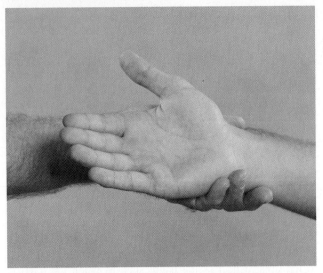

FIG. 6-32 The patient is seated with the elbow of the affected arm flexed and the forearm supinated.

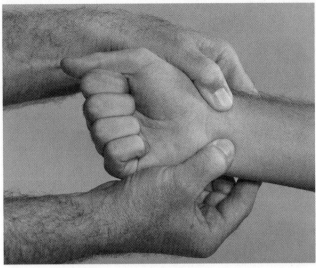

FIG. 6-33 With the patient's arm in the position of that described in Figure 6-27, the radial and ulnar arteries are occluded by the examiner. The examiner will use both hands to occlude the arteries.

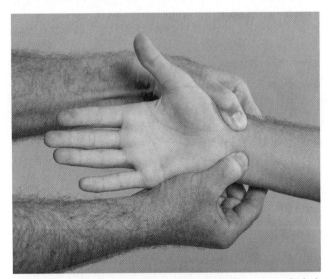

FIG. 6-34 While the radial and ulnar arteries are occluded, the patient opens and closes the hand repeatedly to express the blood from the tissue. Arterial occlusion is maintained.

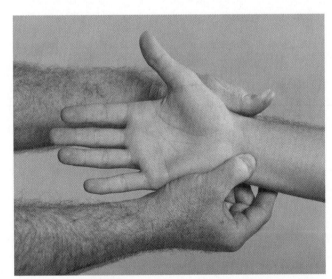

FIG. 6-35 The patient opens the hand, which should be blanched by ischemia. The examiner opens one artery, radial or ulnar. The filling time of the hand is recorded. If circulation fails to return within 5 seconds, vascular compromise is indicated. The test is repeated for the remaining artery.

Assessment for Degenerative Changes of the Wrist Articulations (Rheumatoid Arthritis)

Comment

The hands and wrists are extremely important in the differential diagnosis of orthopedic diseases. Many of these disorders, which number more than 100, affect only the hands, and most of them strike at one time or another. In both hands and both wrists, an examiner may witness more than 60 articulations activated by dozens of muscles, tendons, ligaments, and bones. In a single glance, an examiner may witness the manifestations not only of one joint complex, but also of an entire clinical syndrome.

The hands are in constant motion during the waking hours and even during sleeping hours. The hands are used in most activities of daily living, such as working, eating, and playing; the slightest compromise of function will be quickly bothersome to the patient. Such a disease has an effect psychosocially as well because the hands are often noticed by others and they cannot be concealed for long. Handshaking, dining, and touching have cardinal roles in interpersonal relationships. No orthopedic examination is complete without a thorough assessment of symptoms, physical findings, and functions of the hands.

Osteoarthritis (OA) is a degenerative joint disease characterized by a progressive loss of articular cartilage and formation of new bone at the joint surfaces and subchondral area (Fig. 6-36). When located in the distal interphalangeal (DIP) joints, they are Heberden nodes. When located in the proximal interphalangeal (PIP) joints, they are Bouchard nodes.

Visible evidence of rheumatoid arthritis and clues at the wrist level include the following: early swelling in one or more of the extensor tendon sheaths (Fig. 6-37) dorsally; swelling and tenderness just proximal to the transverse carpal ligament palmarly; or diffuse swelling of the entire wrist joint area, visible medially (Fig. 6-38), dorsally (Fig. 6-39), and laterally (Fig. 6-40); or a combination of these. Inflammation may or may not be visible (Figs. 6-41 and 6-42).

ORTHOPEDIC GAMUT 6-8
RHEUMATOID DEFORMITY

Rheumatoid deformity of the wrist is usually characterized by:

1. Dorsal, distal, and then ulnar displacement of the distal ulna (*caput ulnae syndrome*)
2. Subluxation of the carpus, usually palmarly with supination and radial deviation, leading to a zigzag collapse of the wrist and secondary increased ulnar drift
3. Foreshortening and widening of the carpus
4. End-point deformities in which the patient exhibits subluxation, dislocation, or ankylosis of the wrist
5. Digit stance deformities, particularly extension or flexion stance alterations during cascade testing
6. Signs of neurovascular alterations

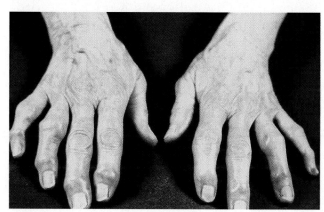

FIG. 6-36 Nodules of the hand associated with OA. (From Barkauskas VH et al: *Health & physical assessment*, ed 2, St Louis, 1998, Mosby.)

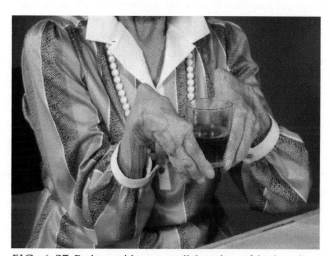

FIG. 6-37 Patient with severe dislocation of both wrists. (From Simmen BR, Kolling C, Herren DB: The management of the rheumatoid wrist, *Curr Orthop* [In Press, Corrected Proof.])

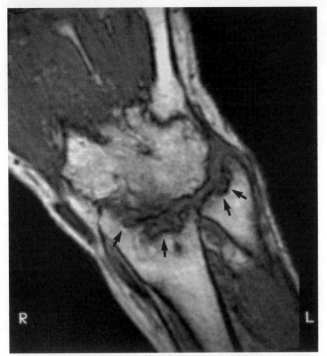

FIG. 6-38 Advanced rheumatoid arthritis. MR coronal T1-weighted gradient echo image. There is complete ankylosis of the carpal bones. Erosions are present at the distal radius and distal ulna (*arrows*), and there is narrowing of the radiocarpal and ulnocarpal joint spaces. (From Brahee DD, Pierre-Jerome C, Kettner NW: Clinical and radiological manifestations of the rheumatoid wrist. A comprehensive review, *J Manip Physiol Ther* 2003;26[5]:323–329.)

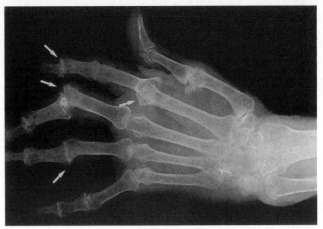

FIG. 6-39 Posteroanterior radiograph of the left hand. Advanced rheumatoid arthritis with soft tissue swelling in the carpals and digits. There is partial collapse of the carpus and joint space narrowing in the carpus and digits. Subluxations of the second metacarpophalangeal joint and of the second, third, and fourth proximal interphalangeal joints (*arrows*). (Courtesy of John A. M. Taylor, DC, DACBR, Seneca Falls, NY.) (From Brahee DD, Pierre-Jerome C, Kettner NW: Clinical and radiological manifestations of the rheumatoid wrist. A comprehensive review, *J Manip Physiol Ther*, 2003;26[5]:323–329.)

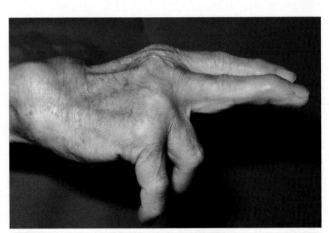

FIG. 6-40 Clinical picture of caput ulnae syndrome with ruptures of the extensor tendons to the small and ring fingers. (From Simmen BR, Kolling C, Herren DB. (iv): The management of the rheumatoid wrist, Curr Orthop [In Press, Corrected Proof].)

Rheumatoid arthritis usually begins in the PIP joints, with development of typical fusiform swelling. At a later stage, the MCP and carpal joints may be affected.

A gradual loss of articular cartilage occurs, as demonstrated by narrowing of the joint spaces, and decalcification of bone occurs, particularly at a point adjacent to the affected joint (Fig. 6-43). Along with these joint changes, the patient may exhibit a weakness of grip as a result of atrophy of the intrinsic muscles. As the disease progresses, increasing deformity occurs with flexion contractures of the MCP joints, ulnar deviation of the fingers, and adduction of the thumb.

The characteristic changes of adult rheumatoid arthritis are found most commonly in the hands. Although arthritis may show as a monarticular process, multiple joints are usually symmetrically affected. The onset of arthritis is usually gradual, and some of the early signs may be morning stiffness, weakness, paresthesia, and relative disability. Uncapping jars and holding a coffee cup may be difficult, and fastening buttons may be frustrating.

Examination of someone with arthritis reveals that the palms are moist and red while the fingers are tremulous. Fist formation, grip strength, and pinching are impaired, especially after prolonged disuse of the hands (Fig. 6-44).

Early in the disease, the latex fixation test is most often negative and only soft-tissue swelling is found when using diagnostic imaging. The test for rheumatoid factor eventually becomes positive in 70% of patients. Subchondral osteoporosis, erosive changes, and joint-space narrowing later appear on the diagnostic images.

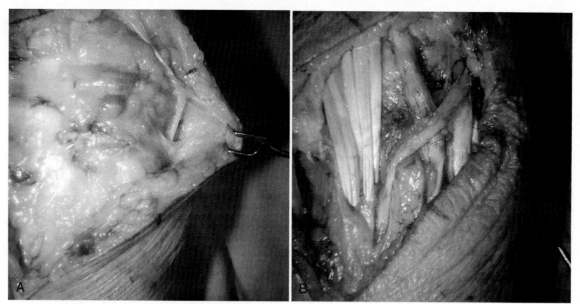

FIG. 6-41 A, Dorsal surface, left wrist at time of dorsal synovectomy. Florid proliferative tenosynovitis is seen. Thumb is at top right. **B,** Same wrist after removal of rheumatoid tenosynovium. Frayed extensor pollicis longus tendon crosses obliquely from bottom left to top right around Lister tubercle and superficial to frayed wrist extensor tendons. (From Canale ST, Beaty JH: *Campbell's operative orthopaedics*, ed 11, Philadelphia, 2007, Mosby.)

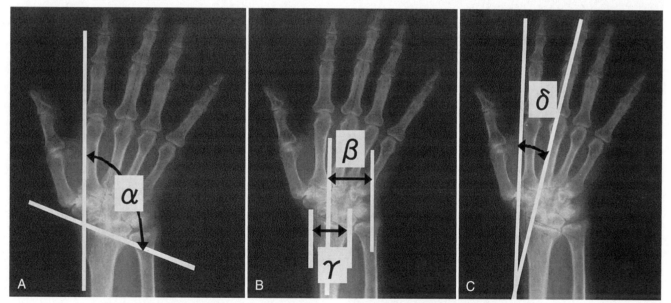

FIG. 6-42 Measurement of radial angulation of wrist, ulnar translocation of carpus, and ulnar drift of the fingers. **A,** Radial angulation of wrist (RAW) is measured as the angle formed between the tangent of the radial border of the second metacarpus and that of the distal end of the radius (α = RAW). **B,** Ulnar translocation of carpus (UTC) was calculated as the ratio of β/γ. β is the distance between the central axis of the radius and the ulnar end of the carpus. γ is the width of the distal end of the radius. **C,** Ulnar drift of fingers (UDF) is defined as the angle between the midline of the third proximal phalanx and the radial tangent of the second metacarpus (δ = UDF). (From Ito J, Koshino T, Okamoto R et al: Radiologic evaluation of the rheumatoid hand after synovectomy and extensor carpi radialis longus transfer to extensor carpi ulnaris, *J Hand Surg* 2003; 28 [4]:585–90.)

ORTHOPEDIC GAMUT 6-9

FINDINGS THAT SUGGEST, BUT ARE NOT PATHOGNOMONIC OF, RHEUMATOID ARTHRITIS

- Symmetric swelling of the PIP joints
- Boutonniere or swan-neck deformities of several pip joints (Fig. 6-45)
- Swelling or tenderness of the MCP joints
- Ulnar deviation or subluxation of these MCP and PIP joints
- Synovitis of the wrist (especially at the distal ulna)
- Tenderness of the distal ulna
- Swelling of the extensor carpi ulnaris tendon

ORTHOPEDIC GAMUT 6-10

MORE THAN ONE OF THESE MAKES RHEUMATOID ARTHRITIS A LIKELY DIAGNOSIS

- The symptom complex of MCP joint swelling with ulnar deviation of the fingers is present.
- Dorsal interosseous muscle atrophy and extensor swelling at the wrist is virtually pathognomonic of rheumatoid arthritis.
- Caput ulnae syndrome also has a high degree of specificity.
- Subcutaneous nodules in the elbow and forearm may point to early diagnosis of this syndrome.
- The skin is moist, warm, lightly mottled, and thin and may be transparent (Fig. 6-46).
- The erythrocyte sedimentation rate is elevated, but a normal value does not rule out the disease.

H.S.1957

FIG. 6-43 Type 3A (ligamentous unstable) rheumatoid wrist that shows complete dislocation of the carpus to the palmar-ulnar side, with preserved bone stock. (From Simmen BR, Kolling C, Herren DB: (iv) The management of the rheumatoid wrist, *Curr Orthop*; [In Press, Corrected Proof].)

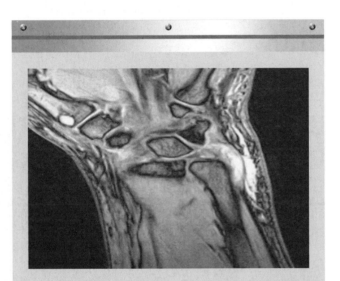

AT THE VIEWBOX

42-year-old male with chronic psoriasis. Fluid-weighted (gradient echo) MR image demonstrates synovial thickening and inflammation over the region of the ulnar styloid process. Tenosynovitis here often produces erosion of the ulnar styloid process in patients with rheumatoid, psoriatic or other inflammatory arthropathies. Note also the erosion (oval focus of bright signal) at the base of the thumb. There was also more generalized carpal and metacarpophalangeal synovial thickening from chronic synovitis. Orthopedic tests were positive for tenosynovitis and there was a positive "bracelet test," classically described in rheumatoid arthritis, but seen in any inflammatory disease of the wrist. (From the teaching file of Timothy Mick, DC, DACBR)

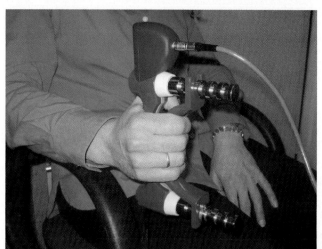

FIG. 6-44 Prehensions tested for strength: power grip *(top)*, index pinch *(bottom left)*, key grip, *(bottom right)*. (From Goodson A et al: Direct, quantitative clinical assessment of hand function: usefulness and reproducibility, *Man Ther* 12[2]:144-152, 2007.)

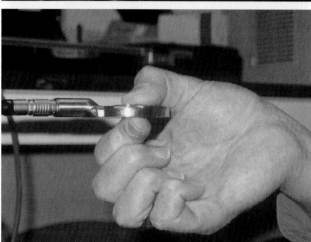

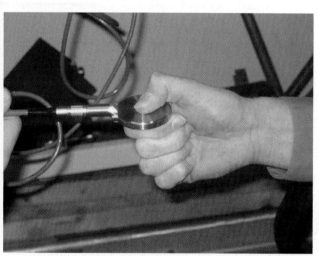

6

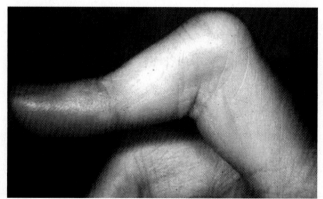

FIG. 6-45 Boutonniere deformity. (From Dell PC, Sforzo CR: Ulnar intrinsic anatomy and dysfunction, *J Hand Ther* 18[2]:198-207, 2005.)

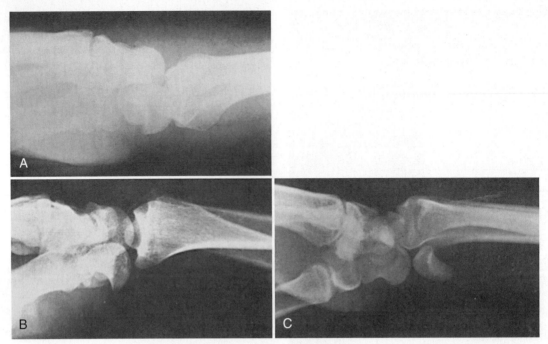

FIG. 6-46 Volar carpal dislocation. A volar dislocation of the carpus on the radius produces the duck bill wrist deformity and risks rupture of the extensor tendons. In a patient with a carpal dislocation, the initial lateral radiograph may depict a configuration at any point in the spectrum of injury. **A,** Dorsal perilunate dislocation. **B,** An intermediate state. **C,** Volar lunate dislocation (duck bill deformity). (From Browner BD: *Skeletal trauma: basic science, management, and reconstruction,* Philadelphia, ed 3, 2003, Saunders.)

PROCEDURE

- The examiner gives mild-to-moderate lateral compression of the lower ends of the radius and ulna (Fig. 6-47).
- This compression causes acute forearm, wrist, and hand pain (Fig. 6-48).
- The test is significant for rheumatoid arthritis.

Next Steps/Procedures
Clinical laboratory and diagnostic imaging

CLINICAL PEARL

The bracelet test can be similar to a manual tourniquet test. The examiner must carefully compress osseous structures and must avoid occluding arterial structures.

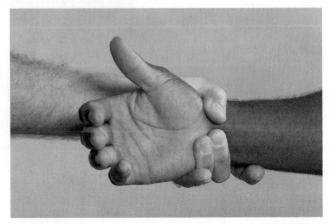

FIG. 6-47 The patient is seated with the elbow flexed. The examiner grasps the affected wrist, applying lateral compression to the distal radius and ulna. This action may cause acute pain that indicates rheumatoid arthritis of the wrist.

FIG. 6-48 While the examiner applies the lateral compression, the patient attempts to make a fist. This action, which will intensify the pain, will detect and localize the structures more involved in the arthritic degeneration.

BUNNEL-LITTLER TEST

Assessment for Interphalangeal Capsular Contractures

Comment

OA is a common abnormality that affects the hands. This type of arthritis attacks the DIP joints, where bony enlargement occurs. Sometimes, acute Heberden nodes occur, characterized by erythematous periarticular inflammation. Osseous hypertrophy of the PIP joints is characteristic of Bouchard nodes. Heberden and Bouchard nodes may affect one or all of the fingers, but the effects are usually symmetric (Fig. 6-49).

> Heberden arthritis has an exceptional position among the various types of primary OA of the hand. The peculiar predilection for the DIP joints facilitates diagnosis and differentiation from inflammatory arthropathies. Heberden nodes are a characteristic sign. Both osteophytes in Heberden arthritis and hyaluronic acid cysts, which are observed in young patients, are described as Heberden nodes (Irlenbusch, Schaller, 2006).

Except for the thumb, the MCP joints are not involved. Rheumatoid arthritis usually involves the ulnar aspect of the hand, and OA typically involves the radial aspect. The first carpometacarpal (CMC) joint is one of the joints most commonly involved. The wrists are usually spared, except for some volar swelling that occurs when an associated carpel tunnel syndrome exists. Contrary to what is widely believed, the erythrocyte sedimentation rate is sometimes slightly elevated. Other than that, systemic manifestations are lacking. Deformities such as ankylosis of the DIP joints, flexion contractures of the PIP joints, and unstable sublux-

ation of the first MCP or CMC joints are common (Fig. 6-50). Lateral deviations at both the DIP and PIP joints, particularly when radiad at one digit and ulnad at another, are more suggestive of OA than they are of rheumatoid arthritis. Although extensive deformations may occur, disability is usually not great. Diagnostic images will show characteristic subchondral sclerosis, marginal spur formation, joint space narrowing, and cystic changes at the involved joint.

With a pathologic condition such as arthritis, an inflammatory lesion is usually found in the muscles, the cell elements of which include lymphocytes, plasma cells, epithelioid cells, and, occasionally, mononuclear, eosinophile, and polymorphonuclear cells. These cells usually have a nodular arrangement in the tissue but are occasionally scattered. Muscles demonstrate degeneration as evidenced by enlargement, increase in number, and vacuolization of the nuclei. Muscle fibers shrink and break into small elements. Many of the fibers are replaced by fatty and fibrous connective tissue. The blood vessels thicken with collagen and periadventitial or paraadventitial round-cell infiltration. These changes involve the extensor mechanism, subcutaneous tissue, joint capsule, connective tissue septa, and the intrinsic muscles. The PIP joints usually demonstrate limitation of motion; thus the patient cannot oppose the fingertip to the thumb tip. When the patient tries to grasp an object with the fingers, the thumb opposes the PIP joint. This pressure will eventually lead to a thumb that pushes the fingers in an ulnar direction (Fig. 6-51).

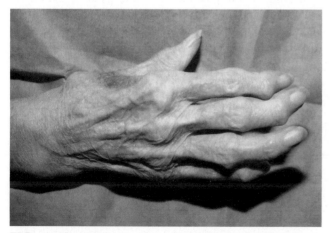

FIG. 6-49 Arthritic nodes of Heberden and Bouchard. (From Delcambre B, Bera-Louville A, Guyot-Drouot M-H: Arthrose des doigts et rhizarthrose, *Revue du Rhumatisme* 68[4]:339-347, 2001.)

ORTHOPEDIC GAMUT 6-11

STAGES OF BASAL JOINT THUMB ARTHRITIS, BASED ON RADIOLOGIC APPEARANCE

- Stage 1: Articular contours are normal.
  - Patient exhibits slight widening of joint space caused by effusion or ligamentous laxity.
- Stage 2: Slight narrowing of the trapeziometacarpal joint with minimal sclerosis of the subchondral bone.
  - Scaphotrapeziotrapezoid joint is unaffected.
  - Joint debris is less than 2 mm.
- Stage 3: Marked narrowing of the trapeziometacarpal joint.
  - Scaphotrapeziotrapezoid joint are not affected.
  - Joint debris is more than 2 mm.
- Stage 4: Identical to stage 3 but with involvement of the scaphotrapeziotrapezoid joint.

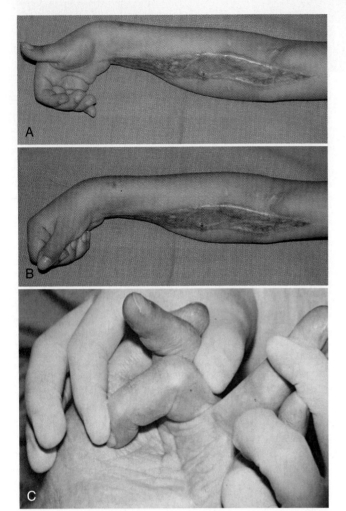

FIG. 6-50 A 5-year-old boy who sustained a Gartland Type III supracondylar humerus fracture with an ipsilateral distal radius fracture. He was treated with closed reduction and percutaneous pinning of the humerus and casting of the radius. Six hours later, the patient developed signs of compartment syndrome and was returned immediately to the operating room, where a fasciotomy was performed. Exploration of the brachial artery demonstrated a severely contused brachial artery with thrombosis. An interpositional vein graft was used to reconstruct the brachial artery. Despite early intervention, the patient developed a moderate-type Volkmann ischemic contracture. After 9 months of occupational therapy and splinting, he was left with residual contracture. **A,** Preoperative extension. **B,** Preoperative flexion. (Adapted from Stevanovic M, Sharpe F. Management of established Volkmann's contracture of the forearm in children, *Hand Clin* 2006;22 [1]:99–111.) **C,** Intrinsic contracture and Volkmann contracture of the forearm secondary to axillary artery disruption. (From Cooney WP, Linscheid RL, Dobyns JH: *The wrist diagnosis and operative treatment,* vol 1–2, St Louis, 1998, Mosby.)

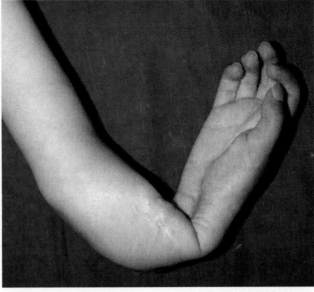

FIG. 6-51 Late sequelae of severe type Volkmann ischemic contracture. (From Stevanovic M, Sharpe F: Management of established Volkmann's contracture of the forearm in children, *Hand Clin* 2006;22[1]: 99–111.)

For thumb involvement, the *Swanson grind test* may be used to confirm the diagnosis (pain on circular movements of the thumb metacarpal with axial compression). The pain presentation needs to be differentiated from de Quervain tenosynovitis, in which the pain and tenderness are located more proximally over the radial styloid.

Exactly why OA affects the basal joint of the thumb is poorly understood. Stability of the saddle-shaped joint surfaces is provided by small ligaments. Instability of this joint leading to excessive movements may result in OA (Eaton, Glickel, 1987).

PROCEDURE

- The examiner slightly extends the MCP joint while moving the PIP joint into flexion (Figs. 6-52 and 6-53).
- A PIP joint that cannot be flexed indicates a tight intrinsic muscle or contracture of the joint capsule, which is a positive finding (Fig. 6-54).
- This joint will not flex fully if the capsule is tight (Fig. 6-55).

Next Steps/Procedures
Cascade sign, test for tight retinacular ligaments, clinical laboratory tests, and diagnostic imaging

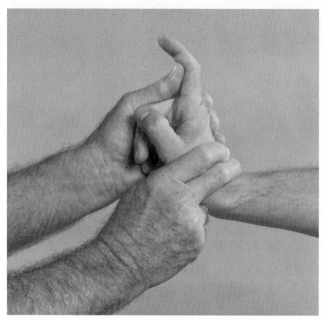

FIG. 6-52 The patient is seated with the elbow flexed and the forearm pronated. The examiner slightly extends the MCP joint of the digit under examination.

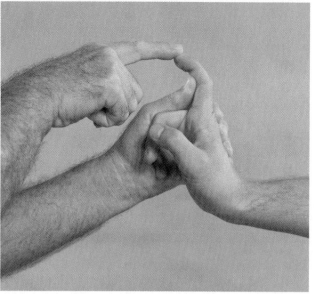

FIG. 6-53 After extending the MCP joint, the examiner tries to move the PIP joint into flexion. The test is positive if the PIP joint cannot be flexed, indicating tight intrinsic musculature or contracture of the joint capsule.

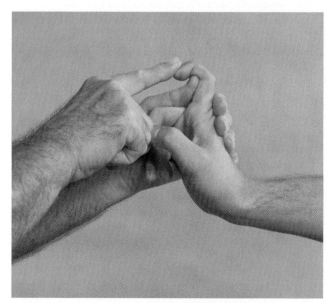

FIG. 6-54 From the position attained in Figure 6-53, the examiner then slightly extends the PIP joint of the digit and tries to move the DIP joint into flexion.

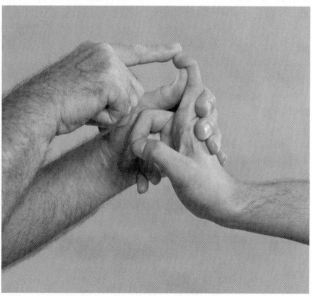

FIG. 6-55 The test is positive if the DIP joint cannot be flexed, which indicates tight intrinsic musculature or contracture of the joint capsule.

Assessment for Carpal Fracture or Sprain

Comment

Because a sprain is a ligament injury, by definition, it is uncommon in the wrist. Most of the so-called sprains that are commonly diagnosed are not sprains at all; rather, they are strains of tendon attachments or osseous injuries. The ligaments of the wrist permit a large amount of motion in the radiocarpal joint but very little motion in the intercarpal joints. The massive ligaments on the volar aspect of the wrist are so strong that a hyperextension injury is more likely to produce an incomplete fracture of the carpal bones, a contusion of the articular surfaces, or possibly a chondral fracture rather than a tearing of the ligaments. With hyperextension, slipping of one row of carpals on the other may actually occur. This slipping permits damage to the dorsal carpal ligaments. However, demonstrating this action is rather difficult. Suffice to say that, with the common dorsiflexion injury of the wrist, the damage is usually on the dorsal aspect. Therefore, the examiner should be wary of the diagnosis of sprain of the wrist with a common dorsiflexion injury. During dorsiflexion of the wrist, pain is more common over the back of the wrist and forearm than over the front. However, stress on the ligament would appear to have been on the volar side. If tenderness is felt over the carpus, a complete X-ray study should be made, and the carpal bones should be studied closely regarding their position and condition.

Fractures of the scaphoid are the most common fractures occurring in the wrist joint. These injuries are also prone to complications, most notably non-union, malunion, and late degenerative changes. Although scaphoid fracture is still predominately a fracture seen in men, it is not uncommon in active women (Fig. 6-56). The most common fracture line is through the scaphoid midpoint. The scaphoid takes a good deal of stress at the wrist, whether it is in dorsiflexion or palmar flexion, because of its position bridging the two rows of carpals, leading to bone bruise complaints.

A *bone bruise* is a term used to describe the finding on magnetic resonance imaging (MRI) of marrow edema (increased signal intensity on T2 weighting), representing capillary damage causing edema and hemorrhage. When bone bruising is associated with disruption of the overlying cortical bone, a fracture is considered to be present. In the absence of a fracture, a bone bruise of the scaphoid is a benign injury with predictable recovery over time and is unlikely to result in long-term morbidity (La Hei et al, in press).

Subluxation and dislocation may accompany ligament injury and may have peculiar characteristics when they occur in the wrist. Dislocation of the radiocarpal joint is extremely uncommon, even though it occurs as the result of violent action. A complete carpal dislocation is also uncommon and is obviously a serious injury. Both conditions are accompanied by deformity and disability, are readily diagnosed, and usually receive effective treatment. Diagnosing the exact dislocation through the carpus is difficult, but a complete X-ray examination of both the normal and injured wrist in several positions will reduce the margin of error. Being diagnosed early is particularly important for these conditions because, as with most dislocations, the longer the dislocation remains unreduced, the greater the likelihood is that it will recur and permanent residual impairment will result.

The outer layer of the deep fascia of the dorsum of the hand is continuous with the antebrachial fascia. The deep fascia is modified over the wrist to form the dorsal carpal ligament. On either side of the hand, the deep fascia becomes fused with the second and fifth metacarpals, with the inner layer forming a compartment through which the extensor tendons can move freely. Distally, the deep fascia fuses with the capsules of the MCP joints and adjacent periosteum. The inner layers invest the underlying carpal and metacarpal bones and interosseous muscles.

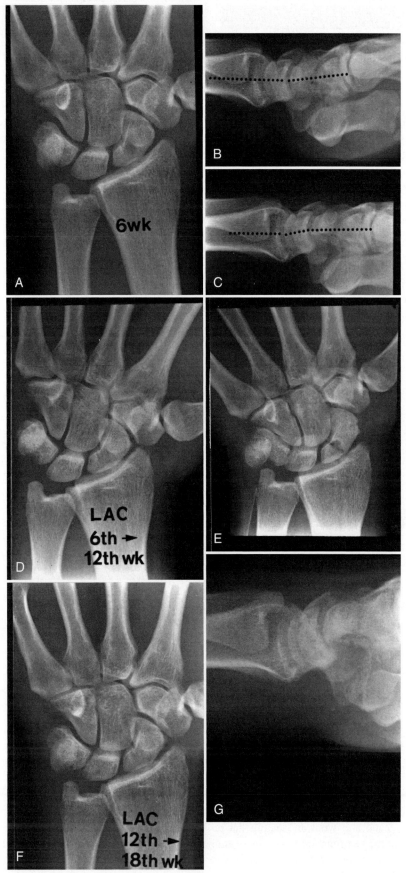

FIG. 6-56 Sprain of wrist. Initial radiograph was negative. **A-G,** Course of healing over 18 weeks. (From Cooney WP, Linscheid RL, Dobyns JH: *The wrist diagnosis and operative treatment,* vol 1-2, St Louis, 1998, Mosby.)

PROCEDURE

- While fixing the other fingers to the examination table, the examiner applies pressure to the dorsum of the digit being examined.
- The patient attempts to lift or extend the finger off the table (Fig. 6-57).
- The sign is present if this action causes pain at the dorsum of the wrist.
- The presence of this sign indicates carpal fracture or sprain.

Next Steps/Procedures

Finsterer sign, Maisonneuve sign, Finkelstein test, and diagnostic imaging

CLINICAL PEARL

Carpal lift is accomplished when the finger is extended against resistance. The earliest sign of carpal fracture or degeneration, before using imaging, is the pain elicited with this test. With a carpal fracture, the carpal lift activity shifts bony fragments and produces the corresponding discomfort.

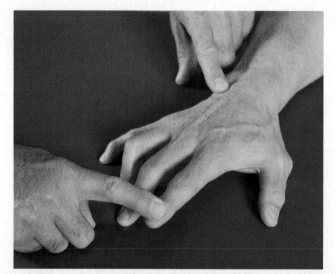

FIG. 6-57 The patient is seated with the elbow flexed. The arm is pronated, and the affected hand and wrist are resting flat on the examining table. While fixing the other fingers to the examination table, the examiner applies pressure to the dorsum of the digit under examination. The patient attempts to lift or extend the finger from the table. The sign is present if this action causes pain at the dorsum of the wrist. Such pain indicates carpal fracture or sprain. The pain may be emanating from the proximal or distal row of carpals or from the base of a metacarpal. The examiner should test each digit.

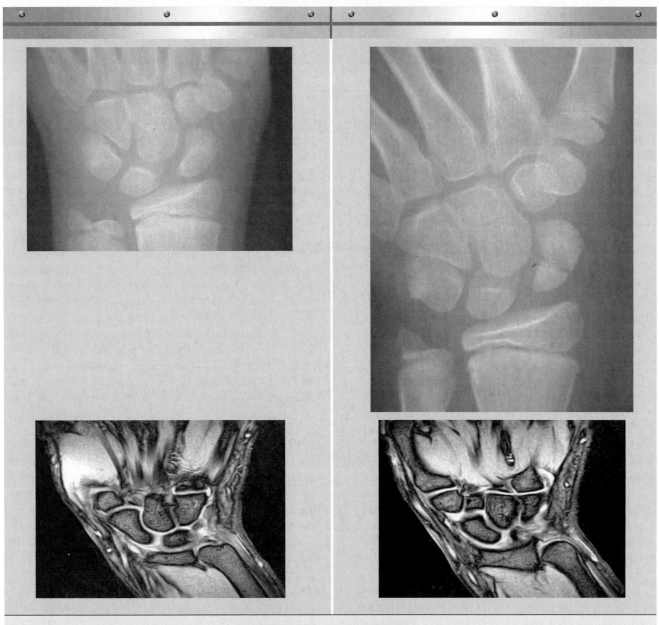

6

AT THE VIEWBOX

A young patient presenting with a history of a fall on an outstretched hand. There is pain in the anatomic snuffbox and positive orthopedic tests for scaphoid fracture. Initial radiographs are negative for fracture, with a wide appearance of the scapholunate joint space. In an adult, a scapholunate joint space exceeding 2.0 mm is indicative of scapholunate ligament tear, but this may be normal in a child, since the carpal bones are not fully ossified. Comparison to the opposite side and MRI would help to distinguish between normal variation and scapholunate ligament tear producing scapholunate dissociation. Note the negative ulnar variance (developmentally short ulna), which has been associated with increased incidence of avascular necrosis of the lunate, ulnar impingement syndrome and tears of the triangular fibrocartilage complex. **(A)** MRI would further assess. CT could be utilized to assess for scaphoid fracture when radiographs are negative, but with strong clinical suspicion for fracture. Repeat radiography was performed two weeks later due to

ongoing pain in the anatomic snuffbox. **(B)** The fracture of the scaphoid waist is now obvious. More subtle is evidence of increased density of the proximal pole of the scaphoid, suggesting avascular necrosis (Preiser disease). A high degree of clinical suspicion for scaphoid fracture warrants imaging beyond a standard radiographic study of the wrist. A dedicated scaphoid view with angulation of the X-ray beam through the waist of the scaphoid is often helpful. Advanced imaging is most sensitive and CT, MRI or radionuclide imaging may be used to avoid the common complications of fracture non-union and avascular necrosis. In some cases, a cast is applied when clinical findings strongly suggest scaphoid fracture, even when imaging findings are inconclusive or negative for fracture. In another patient with a fall on an outstretched hand, MRI demonstrates scapholunate ligament tear, with widened scapholunate joint. **(C)** The intercarpal joint spaces are normally uniform. (From the teaching file of Timothy Mick, DC, DACBR.)

Assessment for Internal Derangement of Carpometacarpal Articulations and Internal Derangement of Phalanges

Comment

Intra-articular fractures of the second through fifth metacarpal bases (**Bennett Fracture**) are uncommon injuries but may be underreported and underdiagnosed. Failure to properly diagnose and treat these fractures can lead to debilitating complications such as weakness of grip strength and of wrist extension, decreased range of motion, degenerative osteoarthritis, tendon rupture, unstable carpal boss, and poor appearance. These injuries usually occur because of forced flexion of the wrist with simultaneous extension of the arm, as occurs with a punch or a fall . . . These fractures are relatively stable because of the associated strength provided by the dorsal and palmar carpometacarpal ligaments and the interosseous ligaments. However, the stability provided by these ligaments decreases sequentially in a radial-to-ulnar direction, and much more motion exists at the fourth and fifth carpometacarpal joints than at the second and third carpometacarpal joints. The increased mobility at the fourth and fifth carpometacarpal joints leads to increased fracture instability at the fourth and fifth metacarpal bases. Also, tendon insertions of the extensor carpi radialis longus, extensor carpi radialis brevis, and the extensor carpi ulnaris can lead to avulsion fractures of the second, third, and fifth metacarpals, respectively, which may prove difficult to appreciate on plain radiographs. (Bushnell et al, 2008)

In the normal wrist and hand, the digits are medially deviated slightly in relation to the carpal bones. In addition, the metacarpals are at an angle to each other. These positions increase the dexterity of the hand and oblique flexion of the medial four digits and contribute to deformities seen in conditions such as rheumatoid arthritis and phalangeal fractures.

Treatment of fractures of the proximal phalanx is difficult because of the necessity of restoring alignment (Fig. 6-58). Fractures of the base are often angulated volarly because of the pull of the intrinsic muscles. The degree of angulation is difficult to visualize by lateral radiograph because the proximal phalanges of the uninjured fingers are superimposed on the film. An oblique radiograph is helpful, but it may fail to show the true severity of the angulation.

Volar angulation of the fracture is often noticed by a depression on the dorsal aspect of the bone, which can be palpated as the examiner's finger moves across the MCP joint and along the dorsal aspect of the phalanx.

Rheumatoid arthritis is a connective-tissue disease characterized by chronic inflammatory changes in the synovial membranes and other structures and by migratory swelling and stiffness of the joints in the early stage. Rheumatoid arthritis is also characterized by a variable degree of deformity, ankylosis, and invalidism in its late stage.

Although the cause of rheumatoid arthritis remains unclear, a slight familial tendency has been demonstrated. Hypotheses of the etiologic factors have included infection, abnormality of peripheral circulation, endocrine imbalance, metabolic disturbance, allergic phenomenon, faulty adaptation to physical or psychologic stress, and many other concepts. Evidence suggests that infection by slow viruses or organisms of the *Mycoplasma* species may play a role, but proof is lacking. The autoimmune mechanisms may be the underlying cause, and proteolytic enzymes released from disrupted lysosomes within the joint may play a part in the chronic synovial inflammation and the destruction of articular cartilage.

Rheumatoid arthritis is currently regarded as one of a group of connective-tissue diseases that exhibit somewhat similar clinical and pathologic changes. Other members of the group include systemic lupus erythematosus, polyarteritis nodosa, dermatomyositis, progressive systemic sclerosis, and rheumatic fever.

In the hand and wrist, the lesions of rheumatoid arthritis are characteristic and progressively disabling. The thumb is often drawn into adduction, the fingers deviate toward the ulnar side, and individual digits may develop grotesque deformities and severe restriction of function (Fig. 6-59). Arthritic destruction at the wrist may result in dorsal subluxation of the distal end of the ulna, medial subluxation of the carpus on the radius, and radial deviation of the hand. The inflammatory synovial reaction damages the joints and involves the tendon sheaths and tendon in producing a variety of deformities.

The available tests for demonstrating the action of flexor digitorum superficialis can be used on one finger at a time. The cascade sign can test all the four flexor digitorum superficialis tendons simultaneously (Fig. 6-60). It correlates fully with the standard test on middle and ring fingers and with the pulp-to-pulp forced pinch test with the thumb on index fingers. The cascade sign is more accurate than the standard test in detecting the presence of the flexor digitorum superficialis action on the little finger.

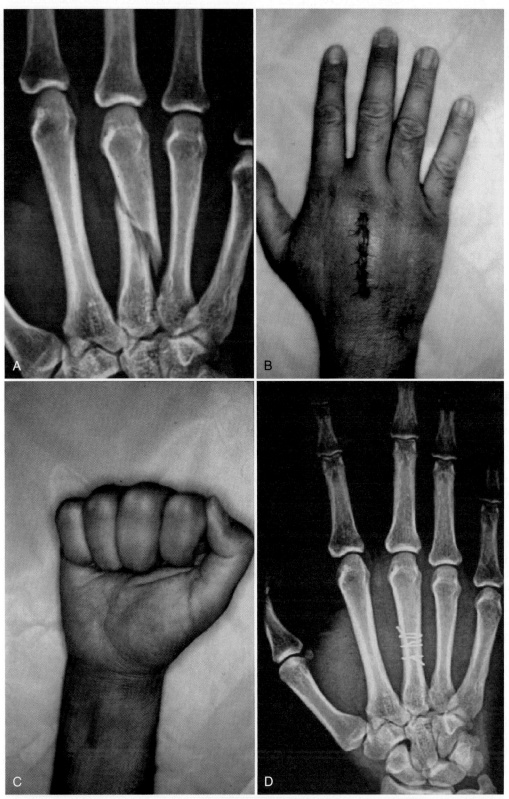

FIG. 6-58 A spiral mid-shaft metacarpal fracture (with scissoring of the finger) treated by open reduction and internal fixation using three cerclage wires. **A,** Preoperative X-ray; **B and C,** demonstration that full range of motion is obtained without formal physiotherapy consultation at 2 weeks after surgery (before removal of sutures); **D,** the healed fracture at 9 weeks. (From Al-Qattan MM, Al-Lazzam A: Long oblique/spiral mid-shaft metacarpal fractures of the fingers: treatment with cerclage wire fixation and immediate post-operative finger mobilisation in a wrist splint, *J Hand Surg Eur Vol* 2007;32[6]:637–640.)

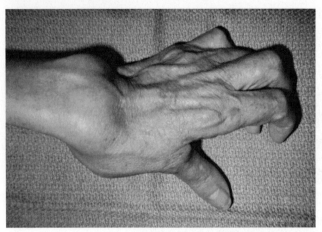

FIG. 6-59 55-year-old female—rheumatoid arthritis for 28 years (left hand). The photo shows hand deformity and contractures caused by rheumatoid arthritis. The patient has had no hand surgery. (From Cooney WP, Linscheid RL, Dobyns JH: *The wrist diagnosis and operative treatment*, vol 1-2, St Louis, 1998, Mosby.)

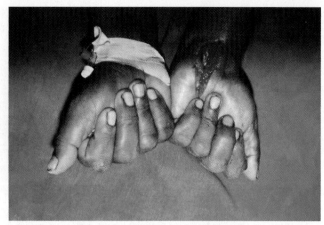

FIG. 6-60 The uninjured right hand demonstrates action of all the tendons; the injured left hand demonstrates the absence of function of the flexor digitorum superficialis tendons of the middle and little fingers caused by cut injury. (From Mishra S: A new test for demonstrating the action of flexor digitorum superficialis (FDS) tendon, *J Plast Reconst Aesthet Surg* 59[12]:1342-1344, 2006.)

PROCEDURE

- The patient is seated, elbow flexed, and forearm supinated. The patient flexes the fingers at the MCP and PIP joints, as if the hand is gripping a golf club. A complete fist should not be made (Fig. 6-61).
- In the normal hand, the longitudinal axis of the four fingers converges over or near the scaphoid tubercle (Fig. 6-62).
- The sign is present if any of the fingers are askew, which indicates internal derangement of the metacarpals or carpals or both (Fig. 6-63).

Next Steps/Procedures

Bunnel-Littler test, test for tight retinacular ligaments, clinical laboratory, and diagnostic imaging

CLINICAL PEARL

A faulty cascade of the fingers, indicating internal derangement of the wrist and hand, is an impediment of the hand grasp in daily activities. Patients usually have adopted accommodating grips. Pain or grip weakness is what precipitates the need for professional care.

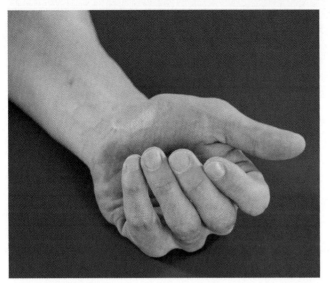

FIG. 6-61 The patient is seated with the elbow flexed and the forearm supinated. The patient flexes the fingers at the MCP and PIP joints, as if the hand is gripping a golf club. A complete fist should not be made.

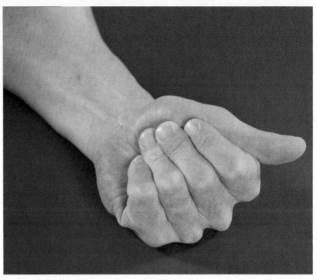

FIG. 6-62 In the normal hand, the longitudinal axis of the four fingers converges over or near the scaphoid tubercle.

6

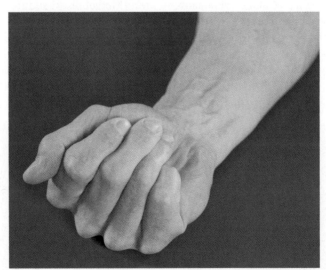

FIG. 6-63 The sign is present if any of the fingers are askew, which indicates internal derangement of the metacarpals or carpals or both.

DELLON MOVING TWO-POINT DISCRIMINATION TEST

Assessment for Dermatome Sensory Disturbances

Comment

Sensation is the acceptance and activation of impulses in the afferents of the nervous system. The four primary modes of sensation are determined by the peripheral terminal endings of the sensory axons. These modes are the mechanoreceptors (touch-pressure), nociceptors (pain), and thermoreceptors (cold and warmth). Determination of the electrical conduction velocity of sensory nerves is the only objective way to measure sensation.

Sensibility is the cutaneous appreciation and precise interpretation of sensation. For example, two-point discrimination is a judgment, not a primary sensation. No correlation exists between sensory nerve conduction velocity and two-point discrimination values after repair of peripheral nerves.

Atrophy of the opponens muscle is a finding in advanced carpal tunnel syndrome (CTS) (Fig. 6-64,*A*). Opponens muscle weakness alone can be an earlier finding in CTS but is difficult to identify. To test for motor weakness associated with CTS, the clinician should examine only the opponens muscle. To perform this test, the patient is asked to place the back of the hands on a table and point the thumb tip at the ceiling (Fig. 6-64,*B*). The examiner then attempts to flatten the thumb on the table with two fingers. Most people with normal opponens power are able to prevent the force of the examiner's two fingers from flattening the thumb to the table.

Normal cutaneous sensation provides normal-quality sensibility that has been termed *tactile gnosia*. All current testing to examine the degree of loss of sensibility is related to cutaneous touch-pressure sensation. The sensation of touch is mediated through myelinated axons that are termed *quickly adapting* and *slowly adapting* in relation to their peripheral receptors. Touch-pressure can be divided into moving touch and constant (static) pressure, in relation to the receptors that are stimulated. Moving touch can be demonstrated with a 30-cycles-per-second (cps) tuning fork for flutter, which will affect the Meissner corpuscles, or a 256-cps tuning fork for vibration, which will affect the Pacini corpuscles. Static pressure, which will affect the Merkel discs, is evaluated by the Weber two-point discrimination test (Merkel discs) and the *von Frey test*.

Detection of grid patterns by the fingers is best for longitudinal, then oblique, and, last, horizontal orientations. The anisotropy is caused by the number of cortical neurons tuned to a stimulus orientation. The *2-point* threshold on the arm

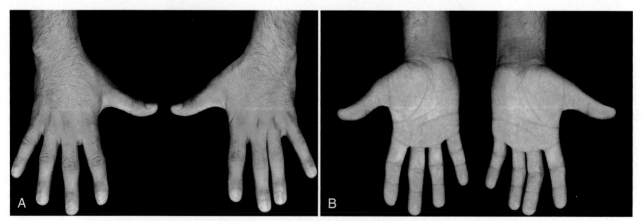

FIG. 6-64 A twenty-eight-year-old male sustained an industrial injury while operating a roller machine used to compress plastic material into plates. On the 21st day post-injury, small muscles of his left hand (dorsal interossi, hypothenar and thener muscles) appeared wasted in comparison with the right hand (**A** and **B**), and his hand function was significantly restricted. There is clawing of the little and ring fingers. Worsening pins and needles in all four fingers was noted together with positive Wartenberg and Froment signs. Both Phalen and Tinel tests were positive. (From Dakhil-Jerew F, Ikram MS, Schreuder F: Delayed onset ulnar nerve palsy and carpal tunnel syndrome following blunt injury to the wrist, *Injury Extra* In Press.)

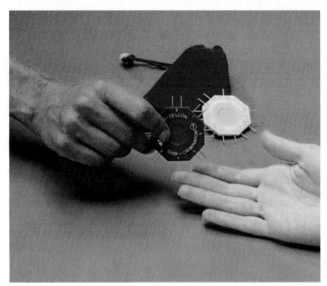

FIG. 6-65 Two-point discriminator diagnostic instrument tests both static and moving one- and two-point discrimination. Two plastic disks, each containing a series of metal rods, spaced at varying intervals from 1 to 25 mm. Useful for measuring the innervation density of any surface area after nerve injury and repair and for testing areas of skin before and after skin grafts. (Photo from Benefitsnow Ltd Unit 4 17d Riverway Newport, Isle of Wight, PO30 5UX www.benefitsnowshop.co.uk)

ORTHOPEDIC GAMUT 6-12

TWO-POINT DISCRIMINATION

The normal threshold for two-point discrimination distance for the volar surface of the hand varies according to the zone being tested:

1. Between the fingertip and the DIP joint, two-point discrimination is normal from 3 to 5 mm, diminished if 6 to 10 mm, and absent if greater than 10 mm.
2. Between the DIP joint and the PIP joint, normal is 3 to 6 mm, diminished is 7 to 10 mm, and absent is greater than 10 mm.
3. Between the PIP joint and the finger web, normal is 4 to 7 mm, diminished is 9 to 10 mm, and absent is greater than 10 mm.
4. Between the web and the distal palmar crease, normal is 5 to 8 mm, diminished is 9 to 20 mm, and absent is greater than 20 mm.
5. Between the distal crease and the central palm, normal is 6 to 9 mm, diminished is 10 to 20 mm, and absent is greater than 20 mm.
6. At the base of the palm and wrist, normal is 7 to 10 mm, diminished is 11 to 20 mm, and absent is greater than 20 mm.
7. The threshold for the dorsal surface is higher in all zones: normal is 7 to 12 mm, diminished is 13 to 20 mm, and absent is greater than 20 mm.
8. Below the elbow but above the wrist, normal is 40 to 50 mm, diminished is between 55 and 80 mm, and absent is greater than 80 mm.
9. Above the elbow, normal is 65 to 75 mm, diminished is between 80 and 100 mm, and absent is greater than 100 mm.

---

is lower for horizontal than it is for longitudinal orientations, which is explained by elongated *sensory circles*—areas of skin served by single nerve fibers. The elongation follows the axis of the main sensory nerves (longitudinal in the arm). Horizontal acuity is finer because the stimulus interval covers more separate fibers (Ross, 1999).

Moving touch is evaluated by the moving two-point discrimination test or using the ridge sensimeter (Fig. 6-65). Functional tests, such as a picking-up test or coin test, evaluate both receptor populations. The tests are subjective and related to factors other than sensation, such as comprehension, motor strength, and coordination or concentration.

The testing instrument can be a **Boley gauge,** a blunt-eye caliper, or a paper clip. Testing is begun distally and proceeds proximally. The points of the caliper are set at 10 mm and are brought progressively closer together after each accurate response is obtained. The pressure from the testing instrument should not produce an ischemic area on the skin. When the two points are applied, they make contact simultaneously, and the line between the points is in the longitudinal axis of the finger. The patient closes the eyes for this test and indicates immediately if one or two points are felt.

From 3 to 5 seconds should be allowed between applications of the points. A series of one or two points is applied with varied sequence in each finger zone, and the procedure is performed three times. If the patient does not report two of the three correctly, the result is considered a failure at that distance. If the patient correctly identifies the number of points applied, the testing distance is decreased by 5 mm. The test has 10 applications of two points and 10 applications of one point, both of which occur randomly. The total incorrect one-point applications are subtracted from the total of correct two-point applications. (A score of 5 or more is considered passing.)

Abnormal skin texture, such as heavy scales or calluses, has a marked influence on the test results. Testing can be performed in the presence of edema or infection, but the results demonstrate the sensibilities present, which may not reflect the true status of the nerve.

PROCEDURE

- Two blunt points are moved proximally and distally in the long axis of the digit (Fig. 6-66).
- One or two points of the Boley gauge are randomly used.
- The distance between the two points is decreased until the two points can no longer be distinguished (Fig. 6-67).
- The object is to determine whether the patient can discriminate between being touched with one or two points and the minimal distance at which two points touching the skin are recognized.
- Several areas on the uninvolved hand should be checked because some patients have congenitally abnormal two-point discrimination.

Next Steps/Procedures

Interphalangeal neuroma testing, shrivel test, Weber two-point discrimination test, and electrodiagnosis

CLINICAL PEARL

Janet test can be performed simultaneously with Dellon test. If the patient's responses are bizarre and do not follow anatomic distributions, psychogenic anesthesia is suspected. The patient is instructed to say *yes* when the stimulus is felt and *no* when the stimulus is not felt. The patient will say *no* if functional anesthesia exists.

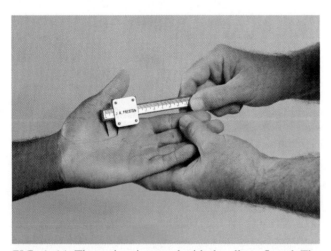

FIG. 6-66 The patient is seated with the elbow flexed. The hand is supinated and is resting on the examining table. The Boley gauge is set at 10 mm of distance or greater. The gauge is applied to the proximal axis of the digit under investigation. The two points must make contact simultaneously and with equal pressure. The patient's eyes should be closed.

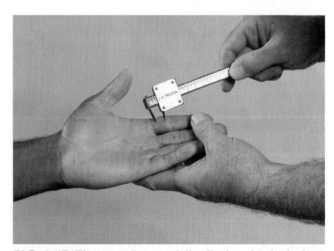

FIG. 6-67 The gauge is moved distally, keeping in the long axis of the finger. The gauge distance is decreased in increments of 5 mm. The test is positive for loss of sensibility if the gauge cannot be perceived as two points at the expected threshold distances for the area tested.

FINKELSTEIN TEST

Assessment for de Quervain Disease (Hoffman Disease, Tenosynovitis of the Thumb)

Comment

Stenosing tenosynovitis of the tendon sheath of the abductor pollicis longus and the extensor pollicis brevis was first clearly recognized by Fritz de Quervain (1895). In this process, an additional etiologic agent may be the presence of accessory tendons in the sheath.

As the tendons to the thumb cross over the lower end of the radius on its radial aspect, they pass through tunnels of grooves on the lower end of the radius (Fig. 6-68). A fibrous retinaculum forms the roof of these tunnels. In particular, the long abductor and short extensor of the thumb pass directly over the styloid process of the radius. Multiple tendons of the abductor may pass through the same sheath, which is subcutaneous. Tenosynovitis in this area is common, usually as a result of overuse of the wrist and thumb. These tendons slide through the tunnel not only during movements of the thumb, but also during movements of the wrist while the thumb is fixed. As the condition progresses, the tendons swell, the sheath thickens, and a situation arises that is analogous to trigger finger. While one tendon slides through the

groove, another one hangs and doubles up. In the early stages, the tendon may then slip through the constriction with a palpable click.

de Quervain disease (Hoffman disease) usually affects women between the ages of 30 and 60 years. This disease is usually the result of repetitive thumb abduction or extension or of ulnar wrist deviation. It is more common in repetitive activities such as keyboarding, filing, carpentry, assembly-line work, and golfing. Pain, tenderness, and swelling over the first dorsal compartment, increased with thumb motion, dominate the physical findings. Palpable crepitus is occasionally present over the compartment. Affected individuals develop bilateral involvement 30% of the time.

Lymphedema of the arm after axillary lymph node dissection for primary breast cancer is a common disorder. Its incidence has been estimated to vary between 6% and 30% in survivors of breast carcinoma; it is also associated with radiation therapy to the axillary lymph nodes. Lymphedema may occur at any time after axillary lymph node dissection or radiation or both. The incidence of lymphedema increases over time. The pathophysiologic mechanism of de Quervain tenosynovitis in patients with lymphedema and cancer is unclear.

Although de Quervain tenosynovitis is generally considered an overuse disorder, patients with lymphedema and cancer often have diminished use of the involved extremity because of its bulk, fear of injury, or superimposed brachial plexopathy (Fig. 6-69). Furthermore, patients with lymph-

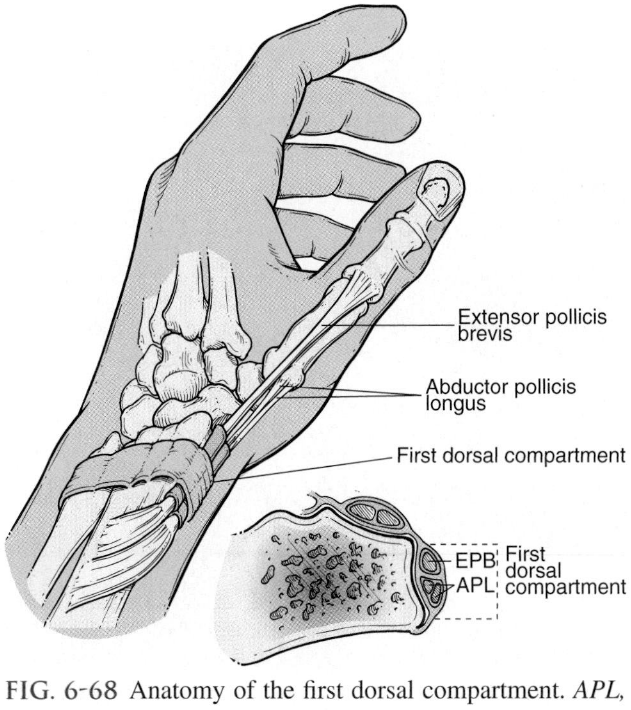

FIG. 6-68 Anatomy of the first dorsal compartment. *APL,* Abductor pollicis longus; *EPB,* extensor pollicis brevis. (From Cooney WP, Linscheid RL, Dobyns JH: *The wrist diagnosis and operative treatment,* vol 1-2, St Louis, 1998, Mosby.)

Extensor pollicis brevis

Abductor pollicis longus

First dorsal compartment

EPB First dorsal APL compartment

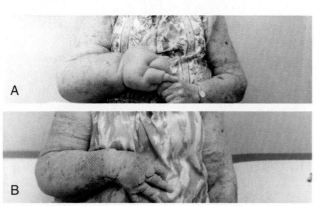

FIG. 6-69 **A,** Before treatment, an 84-year-old woman with severe, elephantitic lymphedema of her right upper extremity for 20 years, secondary to surgery and radiation treatment for breast cancer 30 years ago. **B,** After 20 complete decongestive therapy treatments, she has achieved a 77% reduction in the lymphedema in her right upper extremity and has begun to use her right hand functionally again. (From Goodman C: *Pathology: implications for the physical therapist,* ed 3. St Louis, 2009, Saunders.)

edema are generally counseled to avoid activities that might exacerbate the edema. Tonometry and perometry help define the dimensions of the brawny lymphedema (Figs. 6-70 and 6-71). This regime includes avoidance of excessive exertion while performing mopping, scrubbing, and many other precipitants.

In a patient who is compliant with these general lymphedema recommendations, overuse may not be the sole explanation for de Quervain tenosynovitis. Such patients might be at increased risk for developing de Quervain tenosynovitis with minimal repetitive trauma as a result of their overlying lymphedema (Lin, Stubblefield, 2003).

Differential diagnosis of de Quervain includes entrapment of the superficial branch of the radial nerve, arthrosis of the thumb axis and surrounding joints, and intersection syndrome.

de Quervain disease must be differentiated from intersection syndrome. Although this condition is generally thought to be the result of friction between the abductor pollicis longus and extensor pollicis brevis muscle bellies and the radial wrist extensors, it is tenosynovitis of the second dorsal compartment. Pain and swelling approximately 4 cm proximal to the wrist joint is characteristic of this problem (Ankarath, 2006).

During the early stage of de Quervain disease, use of the wrist is increasingly painful. Swelling appears over the styloid of the radius. This tissue feels very firm and tender when palpated. The tendon sheath is tender and often swollen (Fig. 6-72).

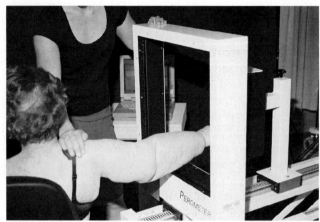

FIG. 6-71 Perometry is rapidly becoming the gold standard for the measurement of changes in circumference and volume of affected limbs. Perometry measures the circumference and volume at 3.7-mm intervals by opto-electronic means. (From Harris R, Piller N: Three case studies indicating the effectiveness of manual lymph drainage on patients with primary and secondary lymphedema using objective measuring tools, *J Bodywork Move Ther* 7[4]:213-221, 2003.)

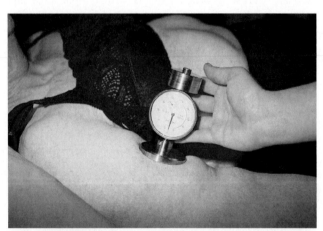

FIG. 6-70 Tonometry is use a means to detect fibrotic induration in the tissues. Resistance to compression, which relates the extent of induration, is measured by placing the weight-based tonometer over the mid point of a lymphatic region. A measurement is taken of the depth that the plunger penetrates after a period of 2 seconds. All tonometry points for the patient are on the forearm, upper arm, anterior and posterior thorax. The lymphedematous and contralateral normal limbs are always compared. (From Harris R, Piller N: Three case studies indicating the effectiveness of manual lymph drainage on patients with primary and secondary lymphedema using objective measuring tools, *J Bodywork Move Ther* 7[4]:213-221, 2003.)

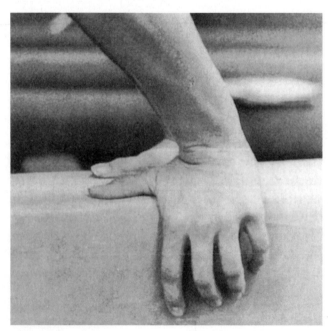

FIG. 6-72 Position of hand on beam that causes symptoms of both ulnar sprains and radial tendonitis (de Quervain tenosynovitis). (From Nicholas JA, Hershman EB: *The upper extremity in sports medicine*, ed 2, St Louis, 1995, Mosby.)

PROCEDURE

- The patient makes a fist with the thumb inside the fingers. The examiner deviates the wrist in an ulnar direction (Figs. 6-73 and 6-74).
- If this action produces pain over the abductor pollicis longus and the extensor pollicis brevis tendons at the wrist, the test is positive (Fig. 6-75).
- Pain indicates tenosynovitis in these two tendons.

Next Steps/Procedures
Carpal lift sign, Finsterer sign, Maisonneuve sign, clinical laboratory testing, and diagnostic imaging

CLINICAL PEARL

Finkelstein test produces an exquisitely painful response in a patient with stenosing tenosynovitis. Initially, determining the severity of the condition is somewhat easier when the patient actively tucks the thumb in, then deviating the hand and wrist in an ulnar direction. Depending on the response this produces, the passive test can then be performed. The pain elicited by this test is discrete and can be long lasting once excited.

6

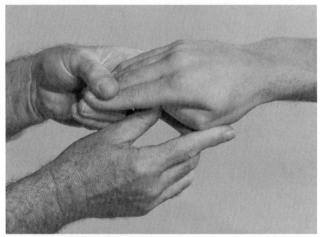

FIG. 6-73 The patient is seated with the elbow flexed and the forearm pronated. The examiner tucks the affected thumb into the palm of the patient's hand.

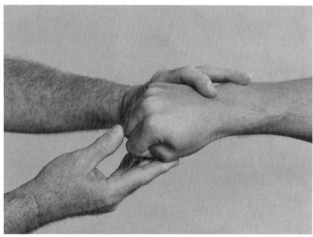

FIG. 6-74 The patient makes a fist over the thumb, and the examiner helps maintain the fist.

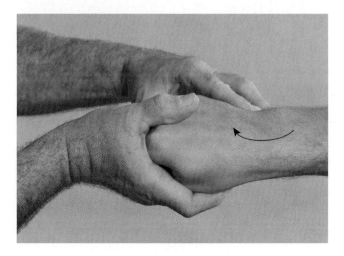

FIG. 6-75 The examiner moves the hand and wrist into sharp ulnar deviation. Pain elicited at the abductor pollicis longus and the extensor pollicis brevis tendons indicates stenosing tenosynovitis.

Assessment for Lunate Carpal Septic Necrosis

Comment

After trauma, whether severe or trivial, the carpal bones may undergo aseptic necrosis. However, in many cases, no history of trauma is obtainable. Most commonly the semilunar bone is affected (Kienböck disease), less often the scaphoid bone is affected (Preiser disease), and rarely are the other hand bones affected (Fig. 6-76). The amount of aseptic necrosis varies in degree. Regardless, the necrotic trabeculae are slowly resorbed and replaced by creeping substitution.

Resorption is often incomplete, and cystlike areas form that are filled with fibrous tissue or amorphous debris. The articular cartilage degenerates and is replaced by fibrocartilage. The carpal bones become irregular, and the inevitable result is degenerative arthritis of the entire wrist joint.

Radiographic evaluation of the carpus is accomplished with a wrist series, which includes a neutral PA and neutral lateral. The series is completed with pronated PA views of the wrist in radial and ulnar deviation, along with an AP grip or clenched fist view.

The cause of Kienböck disease is unknown but is thought to be related to antecedent trauma, with microfracture perhaps disrupting the vascular supply to the lunate.

Kienböck theorized that lunate malacia was the result of a traumatic disruption of the blood supply to the lunate and subsequent disturbance of the bony nutrition. The cause of lunatomalacia has remained a source of controversy. Theories regarding the mechanism for the development of osteo-necrosis of the lunate include primary compression fracture, traumatic disruption of the extraosseous blood supply of the lunate, repetitive loading of the lunate, and emboli. Up to 26% of the time, only a single volar or dorsal blood supply to the lunate exists. Possibly this singularity of blood supply may lead to lunate necrosis (Lamas et al, 2007).

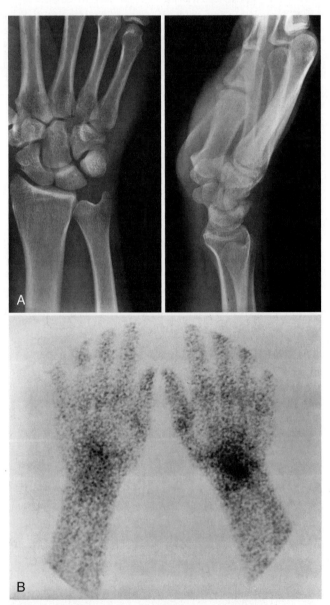

FIG. 6-76 Stage 1 Kienböck disease. **A,** Normal appearance of radiographs of the wrist. **B,** Increased uptake at the lunate level on the bone scan. (Modified from Cooney WP, Linscheid RL, Dobyns JH: *The wrist diagnosis and operative treatment,* vol 1-2, St Louis, 1998, Mosby.)

ORTHOPEDIC GAMUT 6-13
KIENBÖCK DISEASE

Kienböck disease staging:
- Stage I: No changes in plain-film radiographs, but MRI will show deceased signal within the lunate.
- Stage II: Increased density of the lunate in plain-film radiographs. Height of lunate is maintained with no collapse.
- Stage IIIa: Collapse of lunate with loss of carpal height is present, but the scapholunate relationship is maintained.
- Stage IIIb: Collapse of the lunate and loss of carpal height is associated with rotary subluxation of the scaphoid.
- Stage IV: Generalized degenerative arthritis of the carpus is associated with fixed rotary subluxation of the scaphoid.

The scaphoid articulates with five bones is predominately covered by articular cartilage and is the most commonly fractured carpal bone. Blood supply to the proximal pole may be tenuous, with approximately one third of scaphoids having one or no vascular foramina proximal to the scaphoid waist (mid portion). As a result, proximal fractures require longer periods of immobilization for union, with avascular necrosis of the proximal pole seen in 30% of mid-third fractures and almost 100% of proximal pole fractures.

Symptoms that occur even before roentgenographic evidence appears include wrist pain that radiates up the forearm, tenderness over the affected bone, swelling of the wrist, and limitation of motion, usually dorsiflexion. By passively dorsiflexing either the long finger, if the semilunar bone is involved, or the thumb and index finger, if the scaphoid bone is involved, pain is reproduced.

A prominent feature of Kienböck disease is its insidious onset, which often occurs without known prior injury. A considerable difference of opinion has been raised about the events leading up to this initial complex of findings. Of the possibilities, the occurrence of a simple transverse fracture, resulting from a single episode of trauma; numerous compression fractures, resulting from repeated compression strains; and lunate or perilunate dislocation, leading to avascular necrosis in anatomically at-risk individuals, are the most popular. These theories have not been supported by well-conceived studies. On the other hand, clearly, once the process of lunate necrosis has begun, a consistent and progressive sequence of events follows.

PROCEDURE

- The sign is present when grasping an object hard, clenching the hand, or making a fist fails to show the normal prominence of the third metacarpal on the dorsal surface and when percussion of the third metacarpal elicits tenderness just distal to the center of the wrist joint (Figs. 6-77 and 6-78).
- The test is significant for Kienböck disease (aseptic necrosis of the lunate).

Next Steps/Procedures
Carpal lift sign, Maisonneuve sign, Finkelstein test, and diagnostic imaging

6

CLINICAL PEARL

For this sign, all the metacarpal heads are percussed. This gross, low-frequency vibration will localize any cortical defect. In addition, an important point to remember is that ganglions are the most common soft-tissue swellings of the wrist region. They are usually outpouchings of the capsule from the carpal joints, but they may also arise in relation to the tendons. The most common site of origin is from the scapholunate joint. In nearly every instance, a connection to the underlying joint or tendon sheath exists. Patients often have a painless swelling but, in some cases may, complain only of wrist pain, with no visible swelling. This scenario is particularly likely in early stages when the ganglion is small and not visible.

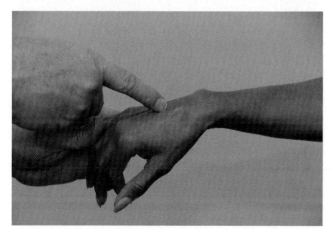

FIG. 6-77 The patient is seated with the elbow flexed and the arm pronated. The examiner locates the proximal head of the third metacarpal. This area may be a site of discomfort and abnormal bony contour.

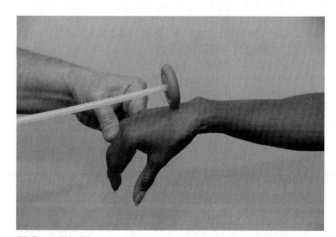

FIG. 6-78 The examiner percusses the proximal head of the third metacarpal with a reflex hammer or tuning fork. Pain elicited distal to the center of the wrist indicates Kienböck disease (aseptic necrosis of the carpal lunate).

ALSO KNOWN AS FROMENT SIGN

Assessment for Ulnar Nerve Palsy

Comment

Testing the function of the median and ulnar nerves is the important first step in evaluating injuries of the volar aspect of the wrist.

Neuralgic amyotrophy, a disorder with many synonyms, is believed to be an inflammatory disease that afflicts the brachial plexus or one or more peripheral nerves in the shoulder girdle or upper extremity. It is a rare disorder with an estimated annual incidence of 1.64 cases per 100,000 population, affecting adults most often and peaking during their 20 s. Men are affected twice as often as women. Neuralgic amyotrophy is usually unilateral, but it is sometimes bilateral and asymmetric; it is rarely recurrent. Most cases have no specific precipitating factors, but some follow upper respiratory tract infection, vaccination, childbirth, and surgical procedures.

As the name implies, neuralgic amyotrophy is characterized by painful weakness of the upper limb. An abrupt onset of deep, boring shoulder pain occurs, which is severe, worse during the night, and maximal during the first few days of illness. Many patients visit the emergency room for pain control. Typically, the patient notices upper limb weakness during the first week, as the pain starts to subside. Sensory loss is usually mild but may be more prominent in severe cases. Deep-tendon reflexes are depressed or absent if the appropriate muscles are weakened significantly.

The anterior interosseous nerve is a purely motor branch of the median nerve. Entrapment may result from compression by aberrant or accessory muscles, by fibrous bands beneath the pronator teres, or by pressure from an enlarged bicipital muscle.

Because no sensory fibers are in the anterior interosseus nerve, the patient has no sensory complaints and experiences only motor weakness. The typical pattern is loss of distal flexion of the thumb and index finger, giving a characteristic pinch sign (Figs. 6-79 and 6-80). The pronator quadratus is tested with the elbow fully flexed.

Severance of the median nerve at the wrist results in the inability to oppose the thumb and anesthesia of the volar surface of the thumb, the index finger, and the long, radial half of the ring finger. When this severance occurs, sensation is the most important function lost. In adults, the recovery of sensation is rarely complete after repair of the median nerve. Although a casual examination may show that the patient appreciates pinprick and light touch in a normal manner, a thorough examination reveals loss or diminution

of two-point discrimination. The patient thereby loses a measure of tactile gnosia, which is essential for rapid and precise manipulation of small objects and for the tactile differentiation of objects.

Severance of the ulnar nerve at the wrist results in the loss of function of the dorsal and volar interossei, the adductor pollicis, the hypothenar muscles, and the lumbricales to the ring and little fingers. The patient exhibits anesthesia over the volar surface of the little finger and over the ulnar half of the volar surface of the ring finger. The key function lost is the use of the adductor pollicis and the first dorsal interosseous. The adductor is essential for strong pinching

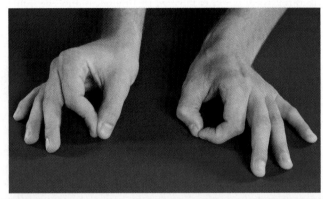

FIG. 6-79 Anterior interosseous nerve paralysis (right hand).

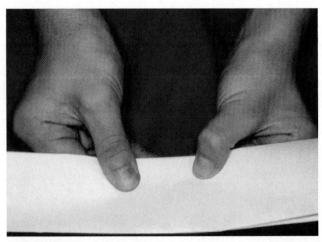

FIG. 6-80 Positive Froment sign with typical atrophy of the first dorsal interosseous muscle of the left hand. (From Jeon I-H et al: Tardy ulnar nerve palsy in cubitus varus deformity associated with ulnar nerve dislocation in adults, *J Shoulder Elbow Surg* 15[4]:474-478, 2006.)

by the thumb. The first dorsal interosseous stabilizes the index finger against the thumb during pinching. The strength of the ulnar-innervated intrinsic muscles fails to return to functional levels in 75% of all ulnar nerve injuries in adults.

Compression in Guyon canal is a rare cause of ulnar nerve palsy and is in many cases associated with certain occupations (i.e., prolonged bicycling, known as *cyclist's palsy*). Dependent on the location of the compression, different patterns of sensory and motor disturbances can be distinguished. The combination of ulnar and median nerve palsy has been described in persons engaged in long-distance cycling but not in other sports (Paul et al, 2007).

PROCEDURE

- The patient grasps a piece of paper between any two fingers (Fig. 6-81).
- Failure to maintain the grip when the paper is pulled away indicates ulnar nerve paralysis (Fig. 6-82).
- This result indicates a positive test.
- The test indicates ulnar nerve paralysis.

Next Steps/Procedures
Pinch grip test, Wartenberg sign, and electrodiagnosis

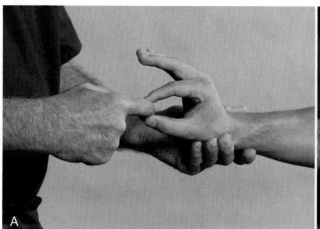

FIG. 6-81 The patient's elbow is flexed, and the forearm is pronated. The patient abducts the fingers from each other. The examiner places a sheet of paper between any two fingers, and the patient adducts the fingers, gripping the paper. Failure to maintain this grip as the examiner tugs on the paper suggests ulnar nerve paralysis.

CLINICAL PEARL

A change from a tip-to-tip pinch grip position to a pulp-to-pulp position is the earliest sign of ulnar entrapment (anterior interosseous nerve lesions must be differentiated). An electromyogram requires more gross muscle deficiency for conclusive findings, and the nerve conduction velocity may be equivocal in the early stages of nerve degeneration.

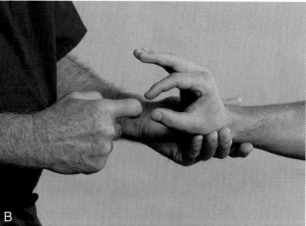

FIG. 6-82 In a modification of the Froment paper test, the patient adducts and flexes the tip of the finger to the tip of the thumb. The examiner tries to pull the digits apart. Failure of the fingers to maintain sufficient strength to resist this motion suggests ulnar nerve paralysis. (Anterior interosseous nerve lesions must be differentiated by electromyogram.)

Assessment for Interdigital Neuroma

Comment

Neuromas can form at the cut end of an injured nerve. A neuroma in continuity may develop along the pathway of an injured nerve. Neurofibroma is a nerve tumor arising from the Schwann cells and fibrocytes. This tumor is usually intertwined with the nerve fascicles, and complete removal requires a segmental resection of the nerve and reconstruction with a nerve graft (Fig. 6-83). Neurofibrolipoma is a benign nerve tumor with elements of fibrous and lipomatous hyperplasia. Similar to neurofibroma, neurofibrolipoma tends to be intimately associated with nerve, and removal requires segmental nerve resection.

When stimulated, the neuromas may cause exquisite discomfort in the extremity, which usually consists of a pins-and-needles sensation or a shooting pain that radiates from a localized area. The pain may sometime become so severe and diffuse that it spreads up the entire extremity. This spread of pain from a neuroma to the point at which it involves the entire extremity may be the result of the fiber interaction in injured nerves. Alternatively, painful nerve impulses stimulate or excite the internuncial pool of the spinal cord so much that normal impulses reaching this area from the periphery are interpreted as painful.

Patients with pain in the thumb or finger tips may have a glomus tumor. In histopathologically proven glomus tumors, neuroma and hemangioma have been found to coexist. Symptoms of glomus tumors are chronic, averaging 1.9 years in duration. Cold-sensitivity and Hildreth tests have sensitivities of 100% and 77.4%, respectively, and specificity of 100%. Hildreth test, which is based on the relief of pain by inflating a tourniquet applied proximally on the arm, is virtually pathognomonic of a glomus tumor. Love pin test has a sensitivity of 100%.

> Eliciting pain by applying precise pressure with the tip of a pencil or pin (Love test) helps locate the lesion. Love and Hildreth tests demonstrate 78% accuracy, whereas the cold-sensitivity test is 100% accurate (Bhaskaranand, Navadgi, 2002).

> Cold sensitivity is associated with vasomotor phenomena, and in some instances a bluish discoloration can be seen beneath the nail immediately overlying the lesion. Pain is consistently elicited by applying pressure or tapping the pulp of the finger. Remarkably, the pain is always localized in the pulp, even in cases in which tumors are paraungual or subungual. This phenomenon is probably the result of the transmission of pressure during grip (Carroll, Berman, 1972).

Such painful neuromas are often confused with the phantom limb syndrome, which does not imply that the phantom limb syndrome is caused by a painful neuroma. The point is that the painful neuroma excites and stimulates certain areas of the central nervous system to the extent that the phantom sensation becomes painful.

Painful neuromas should not be confused with causalgia. Pain produced by neuromas should not be called *minor causalgia* because doing so only adds to the confusion.

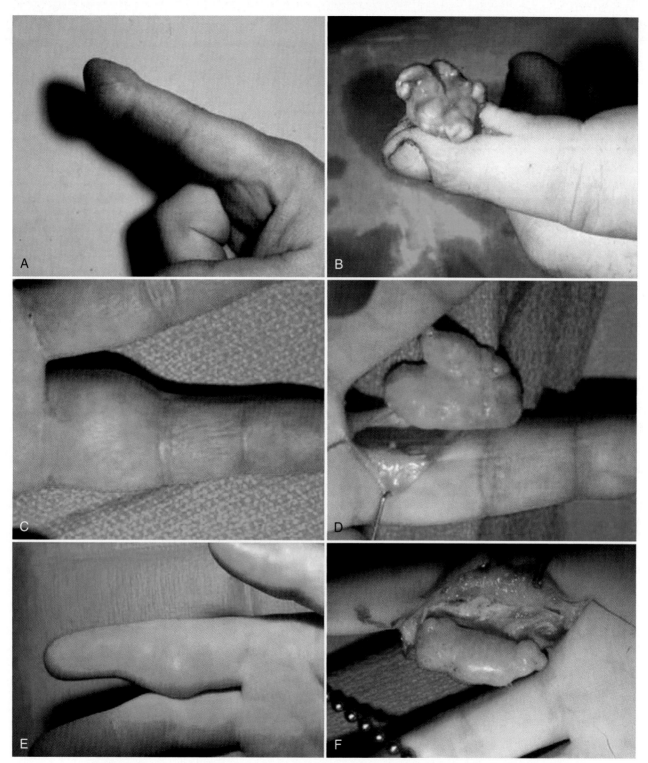

FIG. 6-83 **A** and **B,** Giant-cell tumour of the tendon sheath affecting distal phalanx of the index finger; preoperative and intraoperative views. **C** and **D,** Lipoma of proximal phalanx of the small finger; preoperative and intraoperative views. **E** and **F,** Schwannoma involving ulnar digital nerve of the index finger; preoperative and intraoperative views.

(From Hsu CS, Hentz VR, Yao J: Tumours of the hand, *Lancet Oncol* 2007;8[2]:157–166.)

PROCEDURE

- Neuromas should be carefully sought out by examining the area using a slender instrument for palpating, such as the blunt end of a reflex hammer (Fig. 6-84).
- A localized spot in a scar will cause severe pain and is associated with paresthesia.
- The neuroma itself may be felt as a discrete mass.

Next Steps/Procedures

Dellon moving two-point discrimination test, shrivel test, Weber two-point discrimination test, and electrodiagnosis

CLINICAL PEARL

Although neuromas in continuity develop more frequently in the lower extremity and near amputations, they do develop elsewhere. Neuromas in continuity are observed at the bifurcation of nerve branches near the base of digits and may result from the chronic mechanical irritation caused by malalignment of the digit structures.

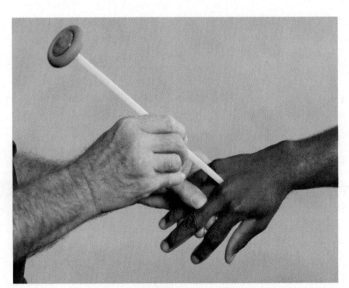

FIG. 6-84 The patient's forearm is pronated. The MCP interdigital tissues are probed with the blunt end of a reflex hammer. If a neuroma is present, severe pain and paresthesia will be elicited. The neuroma may be palpated as a discrete mass.

Assessment for Colles Fracture

Comment

A fracture through the flared distal metaphysis of the radius, also known as *Colles fracture,* is a common fracture in adults older than age 50. This type of fracture occurs more often in women than in men and has the same age and sex incidence as fractures of the neck of the femur. Both fractures occur through bone that has become markedly weakened by a combination of senile and postmenopausal osteoporosis.

> Distal radius (Colles) fractures are a common injury in older women and generally result from a fall onto an outstretched hand. Although not life-threatening, these fractures cause significant impairment and are frequently associated with complications after healing, such as decreased grip strength and range of motion, wrist instability, contractures, CTS, and OA. Because Colles fractures usually occur during impact from a fall from standing height or lower and are considered low-energy fractures, diminished bone quality (i.e., osteopenia or osteoporosis) has been implicated as a risk factor for sustaining these and hip fractures (Troy, Grabiner, in press).

The incidence of Colles fracture is particularly high when walking conditions are slippery because the typical mechanism of injury is as follows: The patient either slips or trips, and in an attempt to break the fall, the patient lands on the open hand with the forearm pronated. This pressure breaks the wrist. Therefore the forces that fracture the distal end of the radius involve not only dorsiflexion and radial deviation, but also supination, all of which account for the typical fracture deformity.

The fracture pattern is constant, the main fracture line being transverse within the distal 2 cm of the radius. Radiographs in traction after closed reduction are helpful in determining the severity of injury and potential for instability.

Unstable injuries are often the result of cortical comminution (dorsal with Colles fracture, volar in Smith fracture) (Fig. 6-85). Impact forces at the time of injury may compress trabecular bone, especially in older individuals with osteopenia.

Even though only two major fragments exist, comminution of the thin cortex is common, especially in the osteo-

---

ORTHOPEDIC GAMUT 6-14
COLLES FRACTURE

Poor results from Colles fracture secondary to:
1. Residual dorsal tilt more than 20 degrees (normal, 11 to 12 degrees of volar tilt)
2. Radial inclination more than 10 degrees (normal, 22 to 23 degrees)
3. Articular incongruity more than 2 mm
4. Radial translation more than 2 mm

---

porotic bone of older adults. The ulnar styloid is often avulsed. The distal end of an intact radius extends beyond the distal end of the ulna. The joint surface is angulated 15 degrees toward the anterior (palmar) aspect of the wrist. After a Colles fracture, these relationships are reversed, and some degree of subluxation of the distal radioulnar joint is always present.

The clinical deformity, often called a *dinner fork* deformity, is typical. In addition to the swelling, an obvious jog can be found just proximal to the wrist resulting from the posterior displacement and posterior tilt of the distal radial fragment. The hand is radially deviated, and although it is often less obvious clinically, the wrist appears supinated in relation to the forearm.

Two main types of Colles fractures can be identified. The stable type of fracture produces one main transverse fracture line with little cortical comminution. The unstable type exhibits gross comminution, particularly of the dorsal cortex, and marked crushing of the cancellous bone (Fig. 6-86). The intact periosteal hinge is on the dorsal aspect of the fracture in both types.

Median nerve injury occurring coincident with a Colles fracture (laceration or contusion) is rare but should be considered when the fracture is compound. Most early-median nerve problems are related to the progressive edema and hematoma that follow injury and to the reduction of the fracture. During the healing phase, exuberant fracture callus, especially in the presence of persistent bony deformity, can result in median nerve symptoms. The residual scarring and thickening that follow healing can eventually result in CTS or tardy median nerve palsy at a much later date.

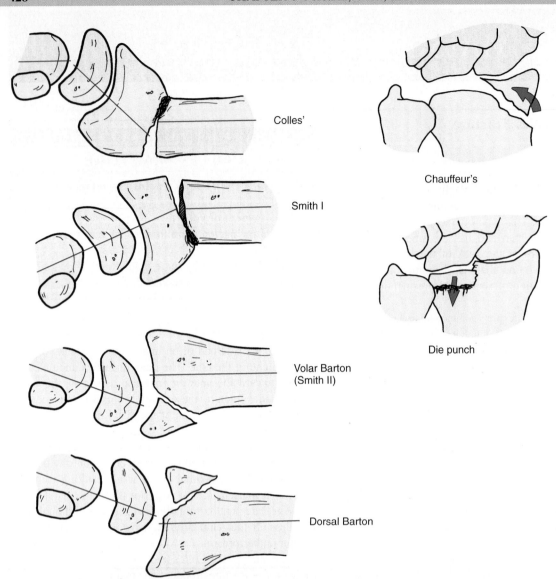

Colles'

Smith I

Volar Barton
(Smith II)

Dorsal Barton

Chauffeur's

Die punch

FIG. 6-85 Distal radius fracture classification. (From Bucholz RW: *Orthopaedic decision making,* ed 2, St Louis, 1996, Mosby.)

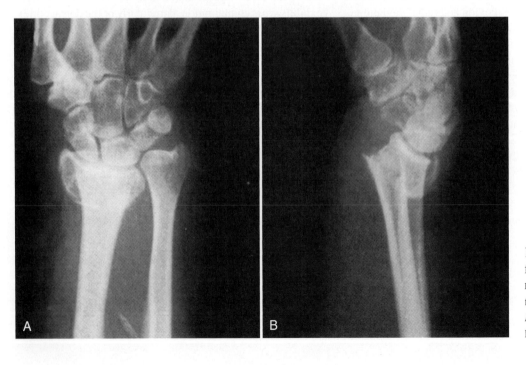

FIG. 6-86 Typical Colles fracture with dorsal and radial displacement. (Modified from Mercier LR, Pettid FJ: *Practical orthopedics,* ed 4, St Louis, 1995, Mosby.)

PROCEDURE

- A positive Maisonneuve sign is characterized by marked hyperextensibility (dorsiflexion) of the hand (Fig. 6-87).
- The sign is present in Colles fracture.

Next Steps/Procedures
Carpal lift sign, Finsterer sign, Finkelstein test, and diagnostic imaging

CLINICAL PEARL

Maisonneuve sign remains a finding long after the fracture healing process is completed. A marked hyperextension of the wrist, with or without complaint, warrants imaging.

6

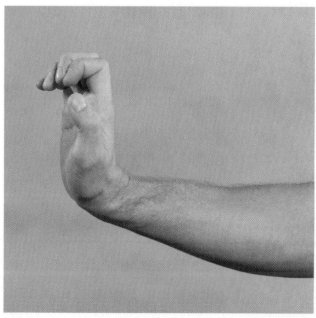

FIG. 6-87 The patient's arm is pronated with the elbow flexed. The hand and wrist are actively dorsiflexed. The sign is present if marked hyperextension of the wrist is apparent. The sign is present in Colles fracture.

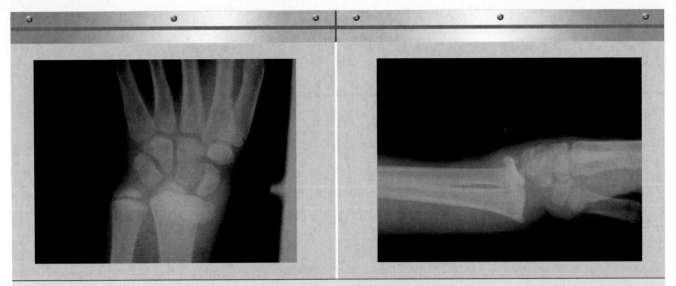

AT THE VIEWBOX

Adolescent male who fell on an outstretched hand. The markedly displaced fracture represents a variant of a Colles fracture (more common in adults, especially osteoporotic females). There was typical associated "silver fork" deformity. This is a Salter-Harris type 1 fracture with marked dorsal displacement of the distal radial epiphysis. Note the marked dorsal displacement of the carpus, along with the fracture. Physeal fractures such as this may result in premature and asymmetric physeal fusion, with associated deformities. Closed reduction and casting resulted in a favorable outcome in this case. (From the teaching file of Timothy Mick, DC, DACBR)

PHALEN SIGN

ALSO KNOWN AS PRAYER SIGN

Assessment for Carpal Tunnel Syndrome (Median Nerve Palsy)

Comment

In the distal forearm, the median and ulnar nerves are surrounded by soft tissues and untethered by bone or dense ligamentous tissues. Distal to the sublimis muscle belly, the median nerve lies just beneath the fascia and is protected only by the palmaris longus tendon. Within the carpal tunnel, the median nerve is in the most volar layer of structures and is easily compressed by the volar carpal ligament. The four unyielding walls of the carpal tunnel fix the volume of the tunnel and guarantee compression of the contained structures if edema or bone fragments occupy part of the available space.

The median nerve may be compressed in the carpal tunnel, producing CTS. Pain is usually felt over the median nerve distribution. As the disease progresses, a definite pattern of hypesthesia or anesthesia will appear over this area. Opposition of the thumb may disappear before definite sensory changes in the hand are noted (Fig. 6-88). The large fibers (motor) in the nerves are damaged more than the smaller fibers (sensory) in such types of indirect trauma. Percussion of the median nerve at the flexor crease of the wrist may produce paresthesia along the median nerve. As the disease further progresses, the pain may reach the forearm and even the shoulder. The symptoms may be more prominent at night.

The symptoms are aggravated by temporarily occluding the circulation of the arm above the elbow. A partially injured nerve is more susceptible to ischemia than is a normal one. Therefore paresthesia and numbness will appear first along the median nerve distribution rather than in the ulnar nerve.

Several provocative signs for CTS have been discovered and are extremely useful in diagnosing the condition. The nerve is located just ulnar to the palmaris longus tendon. Tinel's sign demonstrates irritability of a nerve, as evidenced by direct tapping with a reflex hammer or finger directly on the median nerve. If struck vigorously, any peripheral nerve responds by sending electric shock sensations in the distribution of the nerve. In CTS, tapping the median nerve at the wrist causes tingling or paresthesias (or both) in part, or all, of the distribution in the hand. Occasionally, an electric shock sensation also is transmitted proximally toward the elbow or shoulder.

The carpal tunnel is a semi-rigid conduit that contains the median nerve and the nine digital flexor tendons. The boundaries of the tunnel are, dorsally, the extrinsic palmar wrist ligaments covering the carpal bones and, on the palmar side, the transverse carpal ligament. Although not technically a closed compartment, the carpal tunnel functions as a confined area with little free space. Any process that either increases the volume of its contents or reduces its capacity leads to compression of the median nerve. "Even a slight swelling of the synovial sheath of the flexor tendons," Phalen wrote, "may be sufficient to force the median nerve up against the firm inelastic transverse carpal ligament, causing motor and sensory changes" (Sternbach, 1999).

Phalen test (Fig. 6-89,*B*) is performed by asking the patient to maximally palmar flex the wrist for 60 seconds. The test is considered positive if paresthesias occurs in the median nerve distribution of the hand. Modifications of this test include placing the hand in maximal dorsiflexion with the fingers extended *(reverse Phalen)* (Fig. 6-89,*C*) or holding the fingers flexed *(Berger test),* which may crowd the lumbrical muscles into the tunnel of Guyon.

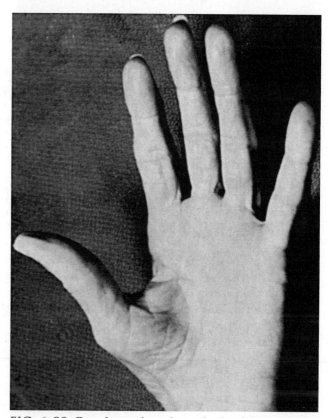

FIG. 6-88 Carpal tunnel syndrome in the right hand. The thenar eminence has atrophied as a result of compression of the medial nerve. (From Parsons M, Johnson M: *Diagnosis in color neurology,* St Louis, 2001, Mosby.)

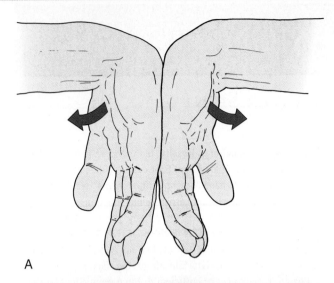

A

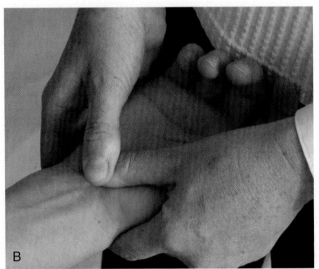

B

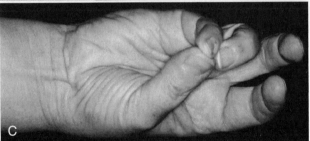

C

The carpal compression test is preferred as the most accurate provocative sign in CTS. The patient opposes the thumb to the small finger and flexes the wrist (Fig. 6-89,A). The examiner's thumb firmly compresses the area between the two tendons, indenting the skin 4 to 5 mm. In CTS, paresthesias in the median nerve distribution occur within 60 seconds. Paresthesias within 15 seconds or less indicate more advanced disease.

PROCEDURE

- The patient's wrists are flexed maximally. The position is held for up to 1 minute as the dorsums are pushed together (Fig. 6-90).
- Tingling sensations that radiate into the thumb, the index finger, and the middle and lateral half of the ring finger are a positive sign.
- A positive sign indicates CTS caused by median nerve compression (Fig. 6-91).

Next Steps/Procedures
Tinel sign at the wrist, wringing test, electrodiagnosis, and diagnostic imaging (MRI)

CLINICAL PEARL

Phalen sign duplicates the wrist flexion-extension maneuvers that irritate the median nerve. The presence of Phalen sign is a good indicator that wrist splints will be useful in the management of CTS. As a screening test, a reverse Phalen maneuver can be performed. The patient is asked to press the hands together in the vertical plane and raise the elbows until they are horizontal. Loss of any dorsiflexion should be obvious. The most common cause of lost dorsiflexion is stiffness after a Colles fracture.

FIG. 6-89 **A,** A positive test is indicated by tingling in the thumb, index finger, and middle and lateral half of the ring finger and is indicative of carpal tunnel syndrome caused by pressure on the median nerve. (From Magee DJ: *Orthopedic physical assessment,* ed 5, St Louis, 2008, Saunders.) **B,** Carpal compression test. Production of the patient's symptoms is considered to be a positive test for carpal tunnel syndrome. This test is a modification of the reverse Phalen test. (From Magee DJ: *Orthopedic Physical Assessment,* ed 5, St Louis, 2008, Saunders.) **C,** Reverse Phalen test. (From Cooney WP, Linscheid RL, Dobyns JH: *The wrist diagnosis and operative treatment,* vol 1-2, St Louis, 1998, Mosby.)

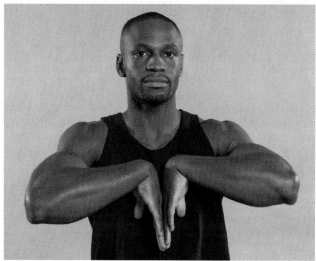

FIG. 6-90 The patient is seated with both elbows flexed and the arms pronated. The wrists are flexed, and the dorsal surfaces of the hands are approximated to each other. The position is maintained for at least 60 seconds. In addition, the elbows can be dropped slightly to increase the wrist flexion angle. Median nerve paresthesia indicates CTS. In the flexed wrist position, the syndrome is caused by neural ischemia.

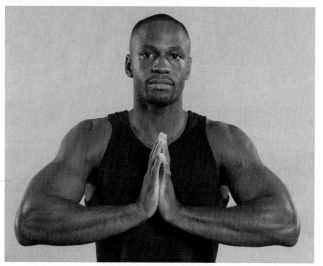

FIG. 6-91 A reversed position for this test is with the patient's wrists extended and the palms of the hands approximated to each other. The patient maintains this position for at least 60 seconds. Median nerve paresthesia indicates CTS caused by neural stretch and compression by surrounding tissues.

6

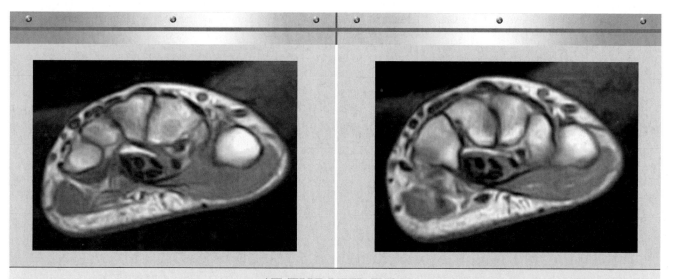

AT THE VIEWBOX

Adult female with symptoms of carpal tunnel syndrome. Axial MR images demonstrate the normal low signal (black) band of the flexor retinaculum (arrow) defining the palmar aspect of the carpal tunnel. This contains the black flexor tendons, the median nerve (asterisk) with its intermediate signal (gray) and fat, dorsally, which has high signal (white) on these T2-weighted images. There is no obvious imaging abnormality of the median nerve, which is often the case. A diagnosis of carpal tunnel syndrome is most often established primarily on the basis of clinical findings and, in some cases, electrodiagnostic studies including nerve conduction tests. MRI signs of median nerve compression may include flattening or other deformation and, in some cases, signal alteration. Masses or other causes of median nerve compression may also be identified on MRI. (From the teaching file of Timothy Mick, DC, DACBR)

Assessment for Anterior Interosseous Nerve Syndrome

Comment

Anterior interosseous nerve syndrome (Kiloh-Nevin syndrome) is the triad of weakness of the flexor pollicis longus, the flexor digitorum profundus of the index finger, and the pronator quadratus. It is a manifestation of neuropathy affecting either the anterior interosseous nerve itself (anterior interosseous neuropathy) or its fascicles more proximally within the median nerve or brachial plexus (pseudo–anterior interosseous neuropathy) (Chin, Meals, 2001).

In anterior interosseous nerve syndrome, the pronator quadratus is nonfunctioning. Pronation is accomplished entirely by the pronator teres, and selective pronation tests are positive in varying degrees. The pronator teres muscle is strongest while the elbow joint is in extension and weaker while the elbow is flexed to 145 degrees. The patient pronates the arm against resistance if the pronator quadratus is nonfunctioning. The patient will have more pronation power while the arm is extended, when the pronator teres is at its maximal advantage, than while the elbow is flexed, when the pronator quadratus contributes its force in pronation (Fig. 6-92).

After supplying the pronator teres, flexor carpi radialis, palmaris longus, and flexor digitorum sublimis muscles, the median nerve divides into two branches. The main trunk continues into the hand, and the anterior interosseous branch supplies the flexor pollicis longus, the flexor digitorum profundus to the index and middle fingers, and the pronator quadratus. Compression of the anterior interosseous branch of the median nerve in the forearm, usually secondary to anomalous muscle and tendon origins, produces the anterior interosseous syndrome.

The ligament of Struthers is a fibrous band of tissue that runs between the supracondylar process, which is a bony spur on the shaft of the distal humerus, and the medial epicondyle. The supracondylar process is not required for the presence of the ligament. The median nerve (anterior interosseous nerve) passes under this ligament, often along with the brachial artery or one of its branches. The ligament is present in approximately 1% to 2% of the population; the associated bony spur from which the ligament originates may be pal-

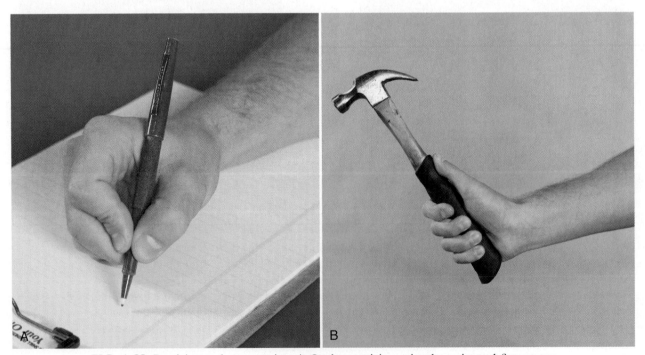

FIG. 6-92 Precision and power grips. **A,** In the precision grip, the wrist and fingers are flexed by the larger muscles, and the intrinsic hand muscles make small incremental movements of the fingers. **B,** The power grip involves the long flexor tendons and the palmar muscles, and the object is to create a rigid grip on the object being held.

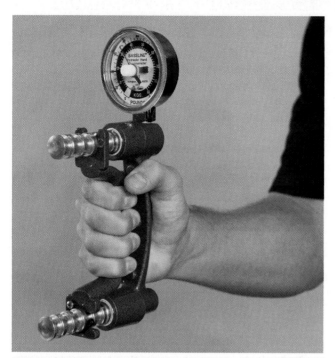

FIG. 6-93 The Jamar Hand Dynamometer for screening of grip strength and initial and ongoing evaluation of patients with hand trauma and dysfunction. The dual-scale readout displays isometric grip force from 0 to 200 lbs and adjusts to five grip positions, from $1\frac{3}{8}$ inches to $3\frac{3}{8}$ inches, in half-inch increments.

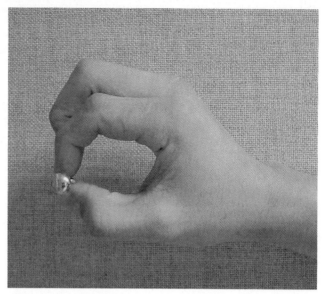

FIG. 6-94 Opposition occurs between the thumb and index finger and is used for picking up small objects. A tip prehension is used to hold a small a sharp object, such as a nail or a piece of page. (Courtesy of Jae Kun Shim, PhD.)

6

ORTHOPEDIC GAMUT 6-15
STAGES OF HAND GRASP

Hand grasp consists of three stages:
1. Opening of the hand
2. Closing of the digits to grasp an object
3. Regulating the force of pressure

ORTHOPEDIC GAMUT 6-16
DIVISIONS OF HAND GRASP

Hand grasp is divided into two types:
1. Power
2. Precision

---

pated in thin patients. Entrapment of the median nerve by the ligament of Struthers is probably the rarest of the proximal median nerve entrapment syndromes. Most patients who have this anomaly are asymptomatic, and the spur, when present, is detected incidentally by radiograph (Gross, Tolomeo, 1999).

The characteristic physical finding of this compression is paralysis of the muscles that this section of the nerve supplies. The Jamar® hydraulic hand dynamometer provides an accurate and reliable method of measuring grip strength (Fig. 6-93). The adjustable handle allows an accurate evaluation of overall hand strength. Grip strength is altered by the size of the objects being grasped; therefore readings should be taken in all five grip spans. Measuring grip strength requires that the arm be held at the side. The elbow should be flexed at 90 degrees with the wrist held in a neutral position. The patient is instructed to apply a grip force smoothly without rapid wrenching or jerking motions. The examiner should ensure that substitute patterns are not used. Initially, the right and left hand should be tested alternately. The noninvolved extremity may be used for comparison.

During physical examination, the examiner may note a weakness of grip and a characteristic pinch grip in which the index finger is extended at the DIP joint with hyperflexion of the PIP joint. The MCP joint of the thumb has increased

flexion, and the IP joint is hyperextended. Thenar muscle function and sensory function in the median nerve distribution are normal.

Various injuries to the hand and wrist can interfere with the worker's ability to perform activities requiring grip.

Grip depends on skeletal mobility, joint integrity, and a combination of contraction and relaxation of the intrinsic and the extrinsic muscle groups.

The intrinsic muscles play an important role in required finger motion. Precision grip is required in grasping a smaller object or a ball (Figs. 6-94 to 6-96).

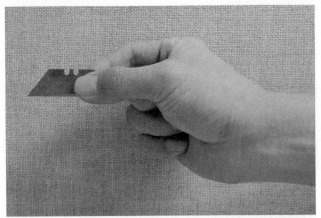

FIG. 6-95 Three-point prehension is used to grasp and stabilize large objects most commonly during functional activity. A palmar prehension is used for a thin and relatively thick object. (Courtesy of Jae Kun Shim, PhD.)

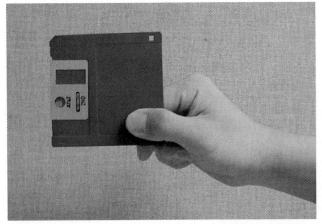

FIG. 6-96 Lateral or key pinch. The most powerful form of pinch. A lateral prehension is used for a thin and flat object. (Courtesy of Jae Kun Shim, PhD.)

PROCEDURE

- The patient pinches the tips of the index finger and thumb together in tip-to-tip pinch (Fig. 6-97).
- If the patient is unable to pinch tip to tip and has a pulp-to-pulp pinch of the index finger and thumb, the sign for anterior interosseous nerve syndrome is positive (Fig. 6-98).
- This sign may indicate entrapment of the anterior interosseous nerve (Figs. 6-99 and 6-100).

Next Steps/Procedures

Froment paper sign, Wartenberg sign, and electrodiagnosis

CLINICAL PEARL

Even minor irritation of the anterior interosseous nerve produces this sign. The inability to pinch grip tip to tip influences the patient's ability to pick up small objects, which is the dysfunction that usually causes the patient to seek professional care.

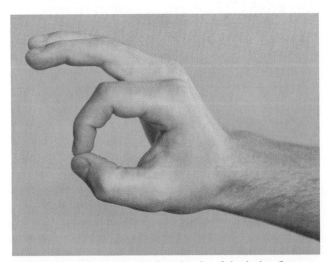

FIG. 6-97 The patient pinches the tip of the index finger to the tip of the thumb in tip-to-tip pinch.

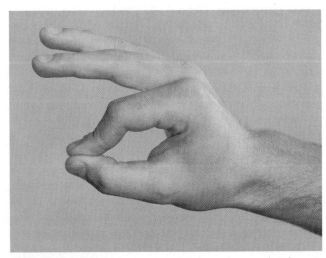

FIG. 6-98 If the grip is tip to pulp or pulp to pulp, the test is positive. A positive test indicates involvement of the anterior interosseous nerve.

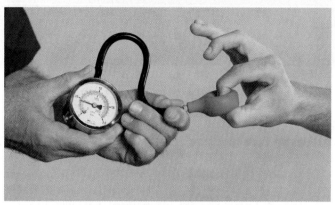

FIG. 6-99 The pinch grip also can be determined with pinch dynamometers. Again, the normal grip is tip to tip. The grip strength of each digit is recorded.

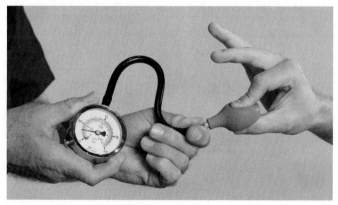

FIG. 6-100 The abnormal grip is tip to pulp or pulp to pulp, both of which produce a corresponding loss of pinch-grip strength.

6

SHRIVEL TEST

ALSO KNOWN AS O'RIAIN SIGN

Assessment for Peripheral Nerve Denervation

Comment

Wrinkling of fingertips after prolonged immersion in water is a well-known and common phenomenon. However, the exact mechanism remains obscure. As early as 1935, investigators found that the skin in the median nerve distribution failed to wrinkle in patients with median nerve palsy.

> The wrinkling test has been employed as a bedside test for assessing sympathetic nerve function. Experts agree that intact sympathetic nerves are required for wrinkling, but other factors such as temperature, fluid tonicity and pH, and the thickness of stratum corneum may also influence this process. Use of the wrinkling test is limited by the time taken for wrinkling to occur. If the onset of wrinkling could be hastened, the test would probably be more widely used (Tsai, Kirkham, 2005).

O'Riain recorded a common but unappreciated observation: *The skin of denervated fingers does not wrinkle or shrivel as normal skin does when immersed in warm water.* This objective test can be performed without the patient's concentration or cooperation and is particularly indicated for use with small children. Shriveling of the skin returns progressively with recovery of nerve function. O'Riain recommends immersion in water at approximately 40°C for 30 minutes. Smooth skin indicates a loss of sensibility. The patient may have already noticed this phenomenon with routine bathing.

PROCEDURE

- The affected fingers are placed in warm (40°C) water for approximately 30 minutes (Fig. 6-101).
- The fingers are removed from the water, and skin wrinkling is observed, especially over the finger pulp (Fig. 6-102).
- Normal fingers wrinkle; denervated fingers do not.
- O'Riain sign is valid only in the first 90 to 120 days after injury, consistent with reactions of degeneration.

Next Steps/Procedures

Dellon moving two-point discrimination test, interphalangeal neuroma test, Weber two-point discrimination test, and electrodiagnosis

CLINICAL PEARL

Muscle wasting in CTS is a good illustration of the trophic relationship that exists between striated muscle and the nerves that innervate them. When the nerve input to such a muscle is interrupted, the muscle wastes away, loses its strength, and eventually becomes much reduced in size. Even when the nerve-muscle relationship remains intact, if physiologic transmission of impulses is blocked, the muscle similarly wastes away. Smooth muscle is innervated by autonomic nerves, but no such trophic relationship exists in the case of smooth muscle.

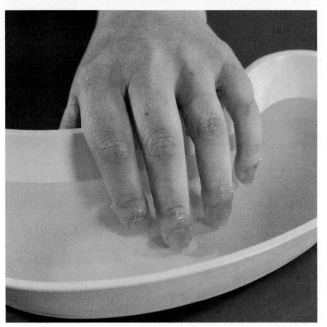

FIG. 6-101 The patient's fingers are immersed in warm (40° C) water for approximately 30 minutes.

6

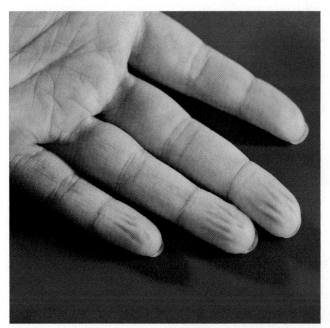

FIG. 6-102 After the patient removes the digits from the water, skin wrinkling is noted. If the skin of the pulp of a finger is not wrinkled, the test is positive. A positive shrivel test indicates denervation of that area. This sign usually is not elicited beyond 90 to 120 days after injury.

TEST FOR TIGHT RETINACULAR LIGAMENTS

Assessment for Fixation of Phalangeal Retinacular Ligaments

Comment

A study of the structure and function of the dorsal aponeurosis is essential for understanding the forces that are active during flexion and extension of the finger. The dorsal aponeurosis is the main structural basis for the integration and coordination of the extensor and intrinsic muscles.

An important portion of the terminal tendon is the retinacular ligament. This ligament consists of two parts: a transverse layer that is spread over both lateral tendons and a very slender but strong band that merges with the most lateral fibers of the terminal tendon. The first or broad thin ligament passes proximally across the PIP joint. Some of the ligament's fibers reach as far as the flexor tendon sheath over the first phalanx, to which they adhere. The fibers of the second or oblique ligament pass underneath the transverse part of the retinacular ligament and insert into the lateral border of the first phalanx. Therefore the lateral aspect of the PIP joint is crossed by two structures: the lateral tendon and the retinacular ligament. At the level of the PIP joint, the dorsal aponeurosis forms a hood that is drawn over the joint, further reinforcing the joint at its sides. Tight intrinsic ligaments limit PIP joint flexion, commonly found in trauma and is often associated with rheumatoid arthritis (Fig. 6-103).

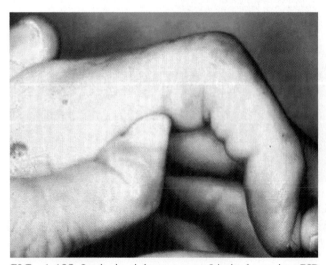

FIG. 6-103 Intrinsic tightness test. Limited passive PIP joint flexion with passive MCP joint hyperextension. (From Dell PC, Sforzo CR: Ulnar intrinsic anatomy and dysfunction, *J Hand Ther* 18[2]:198-207, 2005.)

Tight intrinsics limit PIP joint flexion, but patients often also have complaints of pain with digital flexion. Intrinsic tightness commonly occurs after trauma and can be associated with rheumatoid arthritis. Because the intrinsics flex the MCP and extend the IP joints, the test for intrinsic tightness is to maintain the MCP joint in extension and passively flex the PIP joint. Normally, passive PIP joint flexion is full, independent of MCP joint position. When the intrinsics are tight, passive flexion of the PIP joint is limited when the MCP joint is extended. This test is valid if only passive motion of both MCP and PIP joints is full. In rheumatoid disease, in which the patient may have ulnar deviation of the fingers, the ulnar deviation has decompressed tight intrinsics. Hence digital alignment needs to be corrected before an accurate assessment of intrinsic tightness. The oblique retinacular ligament (Landsmeer ligament), if contracted, will limit simultaneous PIP and DIP joint flexion. The test for oblique retinacular ligament tightness is similar to intrinsic tightness, except it is one joint more distally. The PIP joint is maintained in extension, and the DIP joint is passively flexed. With tightness of the ligament, passive flexion of the DIP joint is incomplete with the PIP joint held extended. Commonly, this circumstance occurs after trauma or edema of the finger (Dell, Sforzo, 2005).

The position of the lateral tendon and the retinacular ligament is important, especially the oblique part of the ligament in relation to the axis of motion of the PIP joint. In the fully extended joint, the lateral tendon passes dorsally, and the oblique band passes ventrally to the axis. This relationship changes as the joint is flexed until both structures become displaced ventrally. Disruption of the terminal extensor mechanism at the DIP joint produces an extensor lag at that joint. This lesion, the mallet finger, which has also been called a *baseball* finger, is incurred when an object, often a ball, strikes the tip of the extended finger, forcing it suddenly into flexion (Fig. 6-104). This activity tears the extensor mechanism from the base of the distal phalanx. The tendon may be just stretched or attenuated, or it may be torn completely from the bone, resulting in a soft-tissue mallet finger. If the deformity is associated with a fracture in which a fragment of bone comes off from the dorsum of the distal phalanx with the tendon, a mallet fracture is present (Fig. 6-105).

Erythema may be detected over the dorsum of the joint and some pain with the injury, but the patience may experience remarkably few symptoms. Inability to extend the distal phalanx actively is present to a varying degree. The exact amount of extension loss can be better estimated when the distal phalanx is compared with an adjacent normal

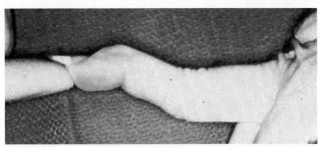

FIG. 6-104 Swan neck deformity. (From Dell PC, Sforzo CR: Ulnar intrinsic anatomy and dysfunction, *J Hand Ther* 18[2]:198-207, 2005.)

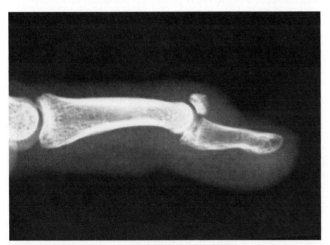

FIG. 6-105 Wehbe and Schnieder classification Type IIB, displaced large fragment, mallet fracture with subluxation. (From Teoh LC, Lee JYL: Mallet fractures: a novel approach to internal fixation using a hook plate, *J Hand Surg J Br Soc Surg Hand* 32[1]:24–30, 2007.)

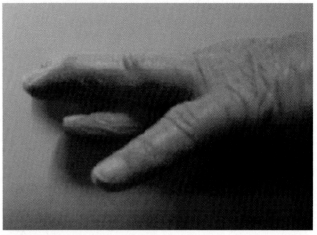

FIG. 6-106 Patient with displaced distal phalanx greater than 1/3 articular surface who was unable to undergo surgery for medical reasons and developed a significant lag post splint period. (From Thomas C: Moon socks for mallets, *J Hand Ther* 19[3]:365–367, 2006.)

6

finger because many patients normally hyperextend at the DIP joint (Fig. 6-106).

Mallet injuries are avulsions of the terminal extensor tendon, from the base of the distal phalanx, with or without a bony fragment. The disruption of the terminal extensor mechanism results in a characteristic flexion deformity of the DIP joint. These injuries are commonly encountered in ball-related sports injuries from axial loading or a forceful flexion of the extended digit. Inadequate treatment can result in extensor lag, significant swan neck deformity and early osteoarthritic changes (Teoh, Lee, 2007).

On the dorsal side of the second phalanx, a triangular lamina of connective tissue that joins the two lateral tendons with each other prevents both tendons from sliding off the base of the second phalanx. According to Bunnell, a fascial sheet extending from the lateral band to the collateral ligament and to the base of the second phalanx causes the volar shift of the lateral bands during flexion.

The term *no man's land* (NML) to describe flexor tendon lacerations within the digital sheath has been attributed to Bunnell. "Primary suture of the flexor tendon between the distal crease in the palm and the middle crease in the finger (no man's land) . . . In the zone between the distal crease in the palm and middle crease of a finger (no man's land), the juncture of a tendon always adheres after secondary repair." NML refers to the area of the hand where the flexor digitorum superficialis and the flexor digitorum profundus change their position relative to one another while passing through a synovial sheath with minimal tolerance, approximately from the distal palmar crease to the midportion of the middle phalanx. The 2 tendons have a large amplitude, the loss of which (e.g., from dense scar) will result in marked diminution of either finger flexion or extension or both. (Newmeyer and Manske, 2004) (Fig. 6-107)

Zone classification of injuries to the flexor tendons

Zone I contains flexor digitorum profundus only, and is from its insertion to the insertion of flexor digitorum superficialis.

Zone II (once known as 'no-man's land') is from the insertion of flexor digitorum superficialis to the proximal edge of the A1 pulley.

Zone III is in the palm from the proximal end of A1 to the distal edge of carpal tunnel, and contains the origin of the lumbrical muscles.

Zone IV is within the carpal tunnel.

Zone V is proximal to the carpal tunnel in the forearm.

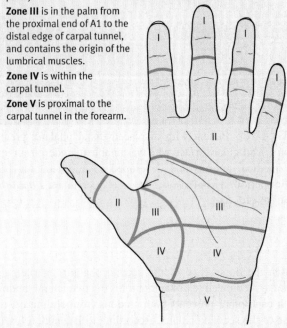

FIG. 6-107 Zone classification of injuries to hand flexor tendons. (From WilsonJones N, Laing H: Acute injuries to the flexor and extensor tendons of the hand, *Surgery (Oxford)* 24(12):441-445, 2006.

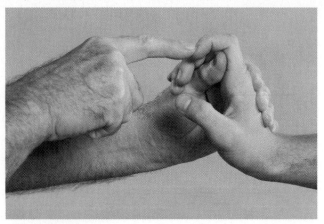

FIG. 6-108 The patient's elbow is flexed, and the forearm is pronated. The examiner fixes the PIP joint in the neutral position. The examiner tries to flex the DIP joint. If the joint does not flex, the collateral ligaments and the joint capsule are tight. If the joint flexes freely, the collateral ligaments are tight, and the joint capsule is normal.

PROCEDURE

- The PIP joint is placed in a neutral position as the DIP joint is flexed passively (Fig. 6-108).
- If the DIP joint does not flex, the ligaments or capsule are tight or contracted.
- If the PIP joint flexes easily, the retinacular ligaments are tight, but the capsule is normal.

Next Steps/Procedures

Bunnel-Littler test, cascade sign, clinical laboratory testing, and diagnostic imaging

ORTHOPEDIC GAMUT 6-17

PROXIMAL INTERPHALANGEAL DISLOCATIONS

Acute dorsal proximal interphalangeal dislocation categories:

I.   Hyperextension: joint surfaces in contact
II. Dorsal dislocation: with dorsal dislocation of the middle phalanx on the proximal phalanx (bayonet)
III. Proximal dislocation: fracture of the volar base of the middle phalanx

CLINICAL PEARL

Rupture of the ulnar collateral ligament of the metacarpophalangeal joint of the thumb is an injury frequently encountered by the emergency physician. The mechanism of injury is usually a fall onto the abducted thumb. The setting is frequently one of athletic endeavor, especially skiing, in which this is the most commonly encountered upper extremity injury. The physical findings typical of collateral ligament rupture may easily be overlooked on casual examination. When not appropriately managed, the injury may result in chronic pain, weakness, and joint instability. The eponym "gamekeeper thumb" derives from a report of similar injuries described as occurring in a series of British gamekeepers.

TINEL SIGN AT THE WRIST

ALSO KNOWN AS FORMICATION SIGN, DISTAL TINGLING ON PERCUSSION (DTP) SIGN, AND HOFFMAN-TINEL SIGN

Assessment for Peripheral Neuropathy in Median or Ulnar Nerve Distribution

Comment

Pressure applied to an injured nerve trunk often produces a tingling sensation that is transmitted to the periphery of the nerve and localized to a precise cutaneous region. Pain is a sign of nerve irritation; tingling is a sign of regeneration. More precisely, tingling reveals the presence of regenerating axons.

The point of nerve irritation is present as a localized pain that is felt at the point where pressure is applied. If this pain extends along the nerve trunk, it is most intense at the point of pressure. This type of pain is associated with pain produced by pressure of the muscles, and the muscular pain is most often more pronounced than the pain along the nerve trunk.

Although ulnar neuropathy at or distal to the wrist has been well characterized in the literature, it is not as common as other mononeuropathies, such as median mononeuropathy at the wrist. In addition, with common entrapments at the cubital tunnel and above the elbow, additional opportunities exist for electrodiagnostic confusion. Patients with traumatic causes of ulnar neuropathy of the wrist tend to have motor symptoms. Patients with cumulative stress tend to have no symptoms or sensory symptoms only. This circumstance is paralleled in the physical examination in which most patients with cumulative trauma have a normal examination, whereas patients with traumatic etiologies have weakness. Electromyography confirms these changes by noting sensory and motor-evoked amplitude changes in patients with traumatic ulnar neuropathy of the wrist. Those from cumulative stress or with sensory signs have only more variable electrodiagnostic findings without motor changes (Chiodo, Chadd, 2007).

Although the tingling of regeneration is not a painful sensation, it is a vaguely disagreeable feeling. The patient may compare the sensation with that of an electric shock. This sensation may be felt at the point of compression but is most commonly felt in the skin along the corresponding nerve distribution. The patient does not experience pain in the muscles adjacent to the nerve where tingling is found.

The two types of sensation, pain and tingling, produced by pressure on the nerve are easily differentiated in all cases. The two sensations rarely exist simultaneously in the same nerve or, more exactly, at the same point during examination of a nerve. The sensations may follow one another along the

---

ORTHOPEDIC GAMUT 6-18

FIVE PATTERNS OF ULNAR NEUROPATHY DEPENDING ON THE SITE OF THE LESION

- Type I lesion
  - Either outside or just within the proximal end of Guyon's canal.
  - Affects the mixed ulnar nerve.
  - All of the hand intrinsic muscles and sensation of the medial 1.5 digits are affected.
  - Dorsal ulnar cutaneous sensory branch distribution is spared.
- Type II lesion
  - Located within Guyon's canal and affects only the superficial sensory branch.
  - Creates a pure sensory neuropathy of the medial 1.5 digits.
- Type III lesion
  - Involves the deep motor branch distal to its bifurcation from the superficial sensory nerve but proximal to the motor branch to the hypothenar compartment.
  - Results in a pure motor neuropathy affecting all the hand intrinsics including the hypothenar muscles.
- Type IV lesion
  - Occurs on the deep motor branch distal to the hypothenar branch; preserves hypothenar function.
  - Affect other ulnar-innervated hand intrinsics.
- Type V lesion
  - Occurs just proximal to the branches supplying the first dorsal interosseous and adductor pollicis muscles; results in decreased activity of these muscle groups only.

---

same nerve trunk. The two different signs produced by pressure applied to the nerve are similar to the symptoms that are revealed by examination of the skin sensation. Regeneration of the nerve is manifested by paresthesia of a more constant type, such as that associated with hypoesthesia produced by touch, by puncture, and especially by slight friction of the skin.

However, in all cases, pain indicates irritation of the axons, and tingling indicates their regeneration. These situations are much easier to differentiate than the signs of cutaneous sensibility. The symptoms of neural compression are also more constant and appear much earlier. They furnish more precise, more localized, and more important information.

Specific pain symptoms differ between patients with peripheral neuropathic pain and those with nonneuropathic inflammatory and musculoskeletal pain. Specifically, patients with neuropathic pain report significantly more intense hot, cold, sensitive, itchy, and surface pain and significantly less intense dull and deep pain than patients with nonneuropathic pain.

In total nerve interruption along the course of the nerve trunk, a definite zone can be found where pressure produces tingling in the cutaneous distribution of the nerve. This zone of tingling is not extended; it does not exceed 2 or 3 cm. This zone indicates that, at this precise point, the suddenly interrupted axons have undergone local degeneration.

With complete interruptions of the nerve produced by very tight entrapment, the same characteristics of fixation, prominence, and precise limitation are found, but the zone of tingling is more extended.

In certain instances the examiner might find along the course of the same nerve two different sites of tingling corresponding to two different lesion levels.

Incomplete interruption of a nerve or, more exactly, lesions permitting the passage of regenerating axons, are characterized by progressive extension of the tingling. The same progressive extension of the tingling zone is found in incomplete interruption with nerve irritability.

Tingling induced by pressure of the nerve does not appear before the fourth or even the sixth week after trauma. The tingling disappears as soon as the nerve returns to its normal structure and the newly formed axons become mature. After 8 or 10 months, the tingling stops. Tingling may be absent in certain rare cases.

The first clinical manifestation of regeneration of a nerve is that paresthesia occurs while the nerve is being percussed. As this task is performed, beginning distally and proceeding proximally, a point will be reached at which the patient feels a tingling or buzzing sensation accompanied by radiation of sensation down to the involved area. The advancing edge of this sensitive area in the nerve is measured at monthly intervals using some bony prominence as a guide. The steady progress of this sensation down the nerve is a rough test of recovery (Figs. 6-109 and 6-110).

A sign found commonly in CTS, called the *volar hot dog*, is a firm hot dog-type swelling at the wrist. This sausage-shaped structure (1 cm wide and 2.5 cm long) is located on the ulnar side of the palmaris longus tendon (Fig. 6-111) and extends proximally from the wrist crease.

Although CTS is diagnosed based on the patient's history and clinical examination, imaging and electrodiagnostic studies may be useful in confirming the diagnostic impression.

The most important electrodiagnostic study is the measurement of sensory nerve conduction velocity across the carpal tunnel. A slowed conduction velocity, along with prolongation of distal motor latency, lends support to the diagnosis of CTS.

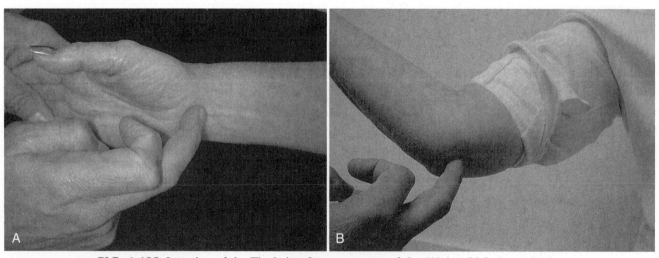

FIG. 6-109 Location of the Tinel sign for entrapment of the (**A**) brachial plexus in the thoracic inlet and the (**B**) radial nerve in the radial tunnel. (From Dellon AL, Shookster LA, Chistopher T et al: Diagnosis of compressive neuropathies in patients with fibromyalgia, *J Hand Surg* 28[6]:894-897, 2003.)

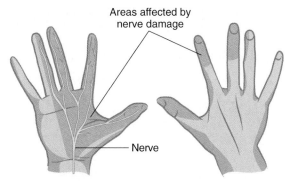

Areas affected by nerve damage

Nerve

FIG. 6-110 The classic symptoms of carpal tunnel syndrome are pain, numbness, and tingling in the distribution of the median nerve, although numbness in all fingers may be a more common presentation. Symptoms are usually worse at night and can awaken patients from sleep. To relieve the symptoms, patients often "flick" their wrist as if shaking down a thermometer (flick sign). (From Beare PG, Myers JL: *Adult health nursing*, ed 3, St. Louis 1998, Mosby.) (In: *Mosby's dictionary of medicine, nursing, and health professions*, ed 7, St. Louis, 2006, Mosby.)

6

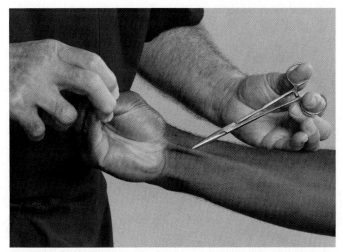

FIG. 6-111 Palmaris longus tendon. The hemostat tip identifies the tissue of the palmaris longus tendon, a major landmark in carpal canal compression syndromes.

PROCEDURE

- The carpal tunnel is percussed at the wrist (Fig. 6-112).
- Tingling in the thumb, index finger, forefinger, and the middle and lateral half of the ring finger is a positive finding.
- Tingling and paresthesia must be felt distal to the point of percussion for a positive finding.
- The test can demonstrate the rate of regeneration of the sensory fibers.
- The most distal point of the abnormal sensation represents the distal limit of nerve regeneration.

Next Steps/Procedures

Phalen sign, Wartenberg sign, electrodiagnosis, and diagnostic imaging (MRI)

CLINICAL PEARL

Tinel sign is extremely useful in identifying (1) the most proximal point of nerve regeneration or (2) the most distal point of nerve degeneration. These points are one and the same. Tinel sign is most evidenced at the Valleix points (tender points) along the course of the peripheral nerve (as in a neuralgia or neuritis). The examiner also may slide the tip of the index finger across the palm, noting frictional resistance and temperature. Increased thenar resistance from lack of sweating and temperature rise (vasodilation) may occur with median involvement.

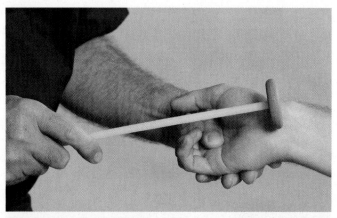

FIG. 6-112 The patient's elbow is flexed and the forearm supinated. The wrist and hand are slightly dorsiflexed by the examiner. The examiner percusses the volar surface of the wrist over the carpal tunnel with a reflex hammer or tuning fork. Tingling felt along the median nerve distribution and distal to the point of percussion indicates regeneration of the nerve. Pain felt after the same distribution, above and below the point of percussion, indicates neural inflammation and degeneration. Percussion at the tunnel of Guyon reveals the condition of the ulnar nerve as it passes into the hand.

Assessment for Neural Irritability as a Result of Posterior Interosseous or Median Nerve Compression

Comment

Nerve compressions are often caused by mechanical or dynamic compression of a nerve segment, and they occur more frequently in the upper limb than in the lower limb. The nerve compressions are localized to regions where the nerves pass through the anatomically narrow tunnels. The nerve may be damaged by localized pressure or inflammation caused by surrounding tissue (Oberlin et al, 2006).

Ganglion cyst compression of nerves in the forearm can result in pain, decreased motor function, and decreased sensation. Radial nerve compression, in particular, can occur anywhere along the course of the nerve, with the antecubital fossa and proximal forearm being the most common sites of origination. The posterior interosseous and sensory branches of the radial nerve can be compressed, resulting in decreased supination and decreased sensation with lateral elbow pain, respectively. Posterior interosseous nerve compression affects the dominant arm twice as often as the nondominant arm. Men are twice as often affected as women. Most reported cases in the literature demonstrate progressive weakness over several days to weeks (Ly et al, 2005).

Ganglion cysts can arise where damage and inflammation of tendon and ligamentous structures are found. They are formed when joint fluid extrudes through a defect in the joint capsule (Carlson, Logigian, 1999).

Lipomas are usually subcutaneous and asymptomatic. Rarely, they can occur in a deeper soft-tissue plane exerting pressure on adjacent nerves. When adjacent to the neck of the radius, it can cause **posterior interosseous nerve compression** (Ganapathy et al, 2006).

Significant diminution of blood flow to individual digits or to an entire hand results in pale nail beds, slow capillary recovery after skin compression, diminished bleeding after skin puncture, lowering of the skin temperature, and pain of varying intensity. Symptoms and signs of pain, pulselessness, pallor, paresthesia, and paralysis indicate arterial insufficiency or inadequate capillary perfusion (Table 6-5). The coexistence of pallor with cyanosis and rubor is consistent with vasoconstriction and subsequent vasodilation. This sign may occur in the presence of posterior interosseous nerve compression (Fig. 6-113).

Pallor and a significant drop in skin temperature will cause pain that is moderately severe and described as a deep, dull, aching sensation. As the ischemia state persists, pain becomes more intense.

The term *Raynaud disease* is used to describe vasospasm without an underlying primary disease. If vasospasm is associated with a known connective-tissue disease, Raynaud phenomenon is implied. Recognition of Raynaud syndrome and the patient's response to this condition is important in explaining pain and cold tolerance associated with a known pathologic condition. When the symptoms of pain occur in a digit of the hand or on the entire extremity, the existence of adequate blood flow in the large and small vessels must be determined.

Most cold tests in the medical literature are either complex and expensive or unreliable for routine clinical use. Cold-induced postischemic reactive hyperemia seen in Raynaud phenomenon of the hand is demonstrated by immersing the hand in a stirred water bath at $13°\,C$, and ischemia is induced by placing an inflatable tourniquet around a finger for 5 minutes. Afterward the tourniquet is deflated while the hand remained in the cold water bath. The temperature of the finger with the deflated tourniquet is compared with that of an adjacent finger serving as control.

Hyperemia is established by the increase in differential temperature between these two fingers after tourniquet release minus the difference in temperature existing before deflating the tourniquet, with a normal lower limit of $0.7°\,C$ for hyperemia. This simple and inexpensive cold test can reliably diagnose Raynaud phenomenon.

In patients known to have a nerve lesion, such as ulnar nerve compression at the elbow, posterior interosseous nerve compression in the supinator muscle, or median nerve compression at the wrist, diminished blood flow will cause abnormal sensory changes to occur earlier than would happen in the normal patient. Motor weakness occurs more quickly when partial or complete ischemia occurs.

Various conditions, such as atherosclerotic stenosis, thromboembolism, or compression of major arteries in the thoracic outlet, cause pain, claudication, paresthesia, and intermittent episodes of pallor. The lesions may be partial or complete, and the clinical symptoms vary according to the degree of ischemia (Figs. 6-114 and 6-115).

ORTHOPEDIC GAMUT 6-19

TWO TYPES OF POSSIBLE GANGLION CYST

- Type I
  - An expanding cyst in the nerve trunk leaving the epineurium intact
- Type II
  - An expanding cyst that penetrates the epineurium

TABLE 6-5

BLOND McINDOE COLD INTOLERANCE SYMPTOM SEVERITY (CISS) QUESTIONNAIRE

Question	Score
1. Which of the following symptoms of cold intolerance do you experience in your injured limb on *exposure to cold?* Please give each symptom a score between 0 and 10, where 0 = no symptoms at all and 10 = the most severe symptoms imaginable. *Pain, numbness, stiffness, weakness, aching, swelling, skin color change (white/bluish white/blue)*	Not scored
2. How often do you experience these symptoms? (Please check.)	
Continuously, all the time	10
Several times a day	8
Once a day	6
Once a week	4
Once a month or less	2
3. When you develop cold induced symptoms on your return to a warm environment are the symptoms relieved? (Please check.)	
Within a few minutes	2
Within 30 minutes	6
After more than 30 minutes	10
4. What do you do to ease or prevent your symptoms occurring? (Please check.)	
Take no special action	0
Keep hand in pocket	2
Wear gloves in cold weather	4
Wear gloves all the time	6
Avoid cold weather; stay indoors	8
Other (Please specify.)	10
5. How much does cold bother your injured hand in the following situations? (Please score 0-10.)	
Holding a glass of ice water	10
Holding a frozen package from the freezer	10
Washing in cold water	10
When you get out of a hot bath or shower with air at room temperature	10
During cold wintry weather	10
6. Please state how each of the following activities have been affected as a consequence of cold induced symptoms in your injured hand and score each. (Please score 0-4.)	
Domestic chores	0 1 2 3 4
Hobbies and interests	0 1 2 3 4
Dressing and undressing	0 1 2 3 4
Tying your shoe-laces	0 1 2 3 4
Your job	0 1 2 3 4

The scores given in question #1 do not count; with an overall minimal score of 4 and a maximal score of 100, a score of 30 is the cut-off point for abnormal cold intolerance. Numbness is the most frequent cold-induced symptom present in 80% of the time. Other symptoms of frequency are stiffness (77%), weakness (72%), aching (67%), pain (63%), skin color change (50%) and swelling (33%).

From Irwin MS et al: Cold intolerance following peripheral nerve injury. Natural history and factors predicting severity of symptoms, *J Hand Surg* 22B(3):308-316, 1997.

Acute occlusion of the ulnar artery is associated with unrelenting pain, pallor, and, later, rubor and cyanosis. Cold tolerance is diminished, and intrinsic muscle weakness occurs.

Obliteration of the brachial artery because of trauma causes the occurrence of an anterior compartment compression of the forearm muscles, vessels, and nerve and causes pallor of the hand, diminished pulse volume, and severe pain. The effect of diminished arterial inflow and lessened venous outflow on pain has been calibrated by analyzing the effects of traumatic lesions at various levels of the extremity. Decompression of a tight compartment anterior to the elbow and in the forearm will diminish pain almost immediately. Elimination of nerve compression syndromes at the wrist and elbow will provide measurable relief of pain.

Causalgia is a mixed nerve lesion with accompanying or secondary vascular insufficiency. Sympathetic dystrophy is a part of the spectrum that may occur, although no particular nerve injury is demonstrated. Median nerve distributions are commonly present, but the ulnar nerve is rarely involved. However, a vasospastic element can be found that occurs secondary to a major or minor insult of the extremity or an adjacent organ.

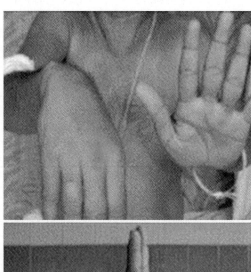
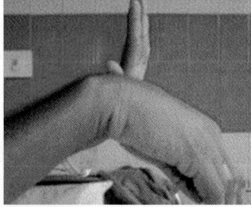

FIG. 6-113 A 54-year-old diabetic man with a swelling in the right forearm of 12 years' duration. Progressive weakness of the right hand of 3 months' duration. Finger extensors paralyzed (0/5 power). Extensor carpi radialis longus weak (power 3/5). No sensory deficit. (From Ganapathy K, Winston T, Seshadri V: Posterior interosseous nerve palsy due to intermuscular lipoma, *Surg Neurol* 65[5]:495-496, 2006.)

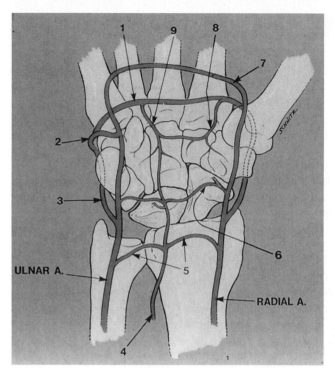

FIG. 6-114 The two main arteries of the forearm anastomose to form two primary vascular arches in the palm. Most frequently, the ulnar artery will chiefly supply the superficial palmar arch, and the radial artery will chiefly contribute to the deep palmar arch. *1*, deep palmar arch; *2*, branch of ulnar artery to deep arch; *3*, medial branch of ulnar artery; *4*, palmar branch of intermediate artery; *5*, palmar radiocarpal arch; *6*, palmar intercarpal arch; *7*, superior palmar arch; *8*, radial rec. artery; *9*, ulnar rec. artery. (From DeLee: *DeLee and Drez's orthopaedic sports medicine*, ed 2, St Louis, 2003 Saunders.)

Carpal tunnel: palmar view

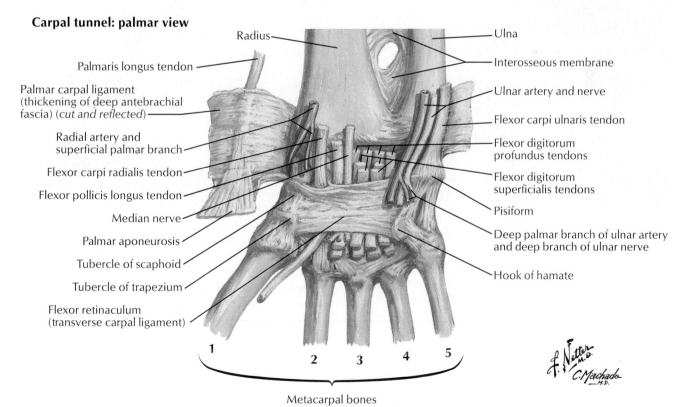

FIG. 6-115 Vascular supply to the wrist. Note the relationship of the wrist ligaments to the neurovascular supply to the wrist. (From Netter: *Atlas of human anatomy*, ed 4, St Louis, 2004, Mosby.)

PROCEDURE

- Application of a pneumatic tourniquet to a normal extremity with pressure elevated to 20 mm Hg above the patient's resting diastolic blood pressure will obliterate arterial inflow and venous outflow, slow motor nerve conduction, decrease sensory conduction, and cause severe pain in the hand and forearm, all of which occur at the site of tourniquet compression (Fig. 6-116).
- Anoxia and nerve compression occur simultaneously, and muscle weakness is evident within 3 to 5 minutes.
- Digital paresthesia occurs, and sensation diminishes gradually to anesthesia in approximately 30 minutes.
- These painful sensations are a combination of muscle and nerve ischemia and nerve compression.
- The appearance of symptoms at less than 20 mm Hg above the patient's resting diastolic blood pressure, or sooner than 3 to 5 minutes, is a positive test result.
- A positive test indicates neural instability as a result of posterior interosseous nerve or median nerve compression syndromes (Fig. 6-117).

Next Steps/Procedures
Allen test and vascular assessment

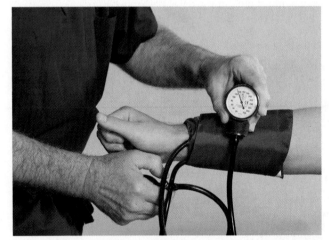

FIG. 6-116 The patient's elbow is flexed, and the arm is supinated and resting on the examination table. A blood pressure cuff is applied to the forearm at a spot above the area of complaint. The cuff is inflated to 20 mm Hg above the patient's resting diastolic blood pressure. Pressure may be increased to reach blanching of the distal extremity. Arm and hand pain, paresthesia, and muscle weakness appearing in less than 5 minutes indicate arterial insufficiency.

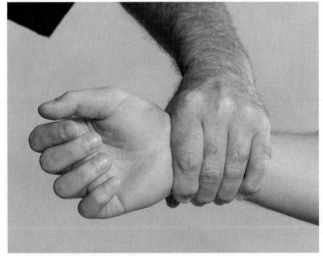

FIG. 6-117 A modified tourniquet test is performed with the examiner occluding the circulation of the extremity manually instead of using a blood pressure cuff. The same principles apply, but this modification does not rely on the accuracy of the pressure to establish occlusion of the arteries.

Assessment for Ulnar Palsy

Comment

The ulnar nerve descends from the medial cord of the brachial plexus on the medial side of the arm and pierces the medial intramuscular septum. The nerve continues in a groove behind the medial humeral epicondyle into the forearm. A branch to the flexor carpi ulnaris is given off in the region of the elbow and, distal to this, a branch to the medial half of the flexor digitorum profundus. The nerve trunk enters the forearm posteriorly between the two heads of the flexor carpi ulnaris. The nerve is constricted by a fibrous band between the muscle and the ulna, and here is the location where the nerve trunk is vulnerable to compression. The nerve, which lies to the medial side of the ulnar artery in the distal half of the forearm and proximal to the wrist, emerges from under the flexor carpi ulnaris to enter the canal of Guyon, the roof of which is the volar carpal ligament. From here, the nerve passes between the pisiform and hamate bones, and at this point the nerve divides into a deep motor branch to the ulnar innervated intrinsic muscles and a superficial sensory branch. The latter supplies both the dorsal and the volar aspects of the ulnar side of the hand, as well as all of the small fingers and the ulnar half of the ring finger. The deep motor branch swings across the mid palm, dorsal to the flexor tendons, as it gives off branches to the palmaris brevis and the three hypothenar muscles: the abductor, opponens, and flexor digiti quinti. The nerve then supplies the four dorsal and three volar interossei, the lumbricales of the small and ring fingers, the adductor pollicis, and the deep head of the flexor pollicis brevis. Proximal to the wrist, the palmar and dorsal cutaneous nerves of the hand are given off.

Anomalous innervation patterns can occur in the normally innervated ulnar muscles. A forearm ulnar-median communication pattern known as the *Martin-Gruber anastomosis* occurs in 17% of the population. Most commonly (60%), connections involve motor branches from the median nerve to the ulnar nerve to innervate *median* muscles. Palmar communications also exist and are called *Riche-Cannieu anastomoses*. The first dorsal interosseous, third and fourth lumbricals, and adductor pollicis have all been described as having dual innervation. Thus all of these variations have an affect on the observed functional deficit that is encountered in patients with ulnar nerve lesions (Dell, Sforzo, 2005).

The ulnar nerve is the most commonly injured nerve of the upper extremity. Open wounds, especially at the wrist, are the most common cause of injury, but compression or irritation of the nerve at either the wrist or the elbow can occur. The major functional loss in low median nerve palsy is a sensory loss. Loss of ulnar nerve function, as with radial nerve function, is a motor loss. Anesthesia in the ulnar distribution of the hand, at its worst, is an inconvenience, but loss of all the interossei and the adductor pollicis interferes seriously with the strength and effectiveness of the patient's grasp.

Cubitus valgus deformity is a well-described complication of a lateral condyle fracture, which is frequently associated with *tardy ulnar nerve palsy*. However, cubitus varus after a pediatric supracondylar fracture of the humerus is usually considered only as a cosmetic deformity and not a functional problem. Recently, though, functional problems of posterolateral instability or tardy ulnar nerve palsy have been reported. Causative factors such as instability of the nerve, internal rotation deformity, and snapping of triceps have been described in the literature (Jeon et al, 2006).

Ulnar clawhand *(main en griffe)* is caused primarily by loss of the interossei, the major function of which is to flex the MCP joints (Fig. 6-118). With the loss of the interossei, the action of the extrinsic finger extensors is unopposed, and a hyperextension deformity of the MCP joints begins. As the volar capsule of these joints stretches, the deformity, which may be barely present in the recently injured extremity, progresses. Lumbricales one and two are most commonly median innervated. Therefore the index and middle fingers usually do not develop the deformity. The interossei and lumbricales also act as IP joint extensors, and with their paralysis, these joints are held in flexion by the now unopposed flexor digitorum profundi and flexor digitorum sublimis. These flexors are overactive in their attempt to com-

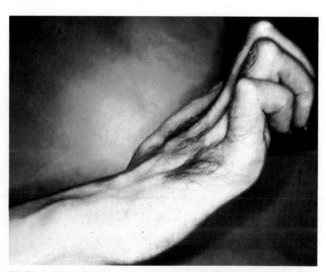

FIG. 6-118 Claw hand associated with ulnar nerve palsy.
(From Dell PC, Sforzo CR: Ulnar intrinsic anatomy and dysfunction, *J Hand Ther* 18[2]:198-207, 2005.)

pensate for the lack of the interossei as MCP flexors. Thus a vicious cycle is started. The more the patient attempts to correct the deformity actively, the more exaggerated it will become. The degree of clawing is usually less apparent in the high ulnar palsy than when the ulnar half of the flexor digitorum profundus is spared.

Workers involved in activities that require repetitive forearm rotation along with ulnar deviation of the wrist can develop a branch of the radial nerve that was originally described in nonathletes by Wartenberg (Fig. 6-119). This condition, the persistent abduction of the little finger, is also seen in workers who wear equipment that encompasses the wrist. Anatomically, the radial sensory nerve is located in a subcutaneous position between the extensor carpi radialis longus and the brachioradialis at the junction of the mid and distal thirds of the forearm. The fascia at this point of transition sends fibers from the musculotendinous area of the brachioradialis to the extensor carpi radialis longus. These fibers create a relatively unyielding bridge under the nerve, which is the most common location of entrapment.

The patient experiences pain and numbness over the dorsoradial aspect of the hand and thumb. Pertinent physical findings include Tinel sign over the nerve and exacerbation of symptoms with wrist flexion and ulnar deviation. Most obvious in the ulnar clawhand is the apparent deformity of clawing, which is a loss of the transverse arch of the hand, and visible atrophy of the interossei, particularly the first dorsal interosseous muscle mass (Fig. 6-120). Hypothenar atrophy also occurs.

The next most apparent condition is the clumsy grip and the marked weakness of grasp. Normal grip strength in the male adult is approximately 90 pounds and is 53 pounds for female adults. In the ulnar-palsied hand, the grip strength will be only one fourth to one third of that. This weakness is the one most responsible for gross dysfunction of the hand, such as the loss of the ability to grasp a shovel or a suitcase handle.

More disabling for fine sophisticated use of the hand is the interference with normal pinch or prehension. The average strength of pinch in the male adult is 20 to 25 pounds, but with ulnar palsy, the strength is only 10% to 20% of that. This loss in strength is the result of paralysis of the adductor pollicis, one half of the flexor pollicis brevis, and the first dorsal interosseous muscles. The paralysis of these muscles leads not only to weakness, but also to gross deformity of pinch, characterized by hyperextension of the thumb MCP joint and hyperflexion of the thumb IP joint. A good test of adductor pollicis and first dorsal interosseous

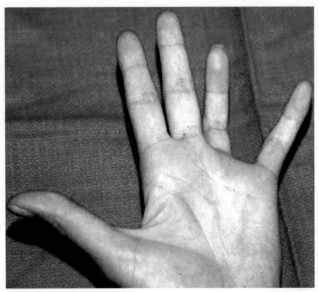

FIG. 6-119 Wartenberg sign. (From Dell PC, Sforzo CR: Ulnar intrinsic anatomy and dysfunction, *J Hand Ther* 18[2]:198-207, 2005.)

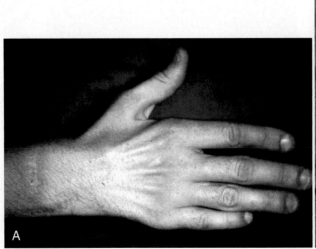
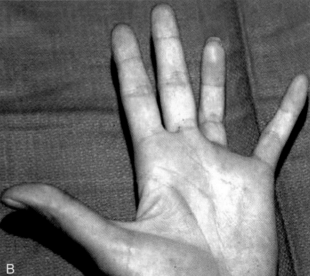

FIG. 6-120 **A,** Intrinsic atrophy from ulnar nerve palsy. **B,** Wartenberg sign. (From Dell PC, Sforzo CR: Ulnar intrinsic anatomy and dysfunction, *J Hand Ther* 2005;18[2]:198–207.)

function is to observe the position of the fingers for pinch and test the muscle strength of each digit. Palpation of the first dorsal interosseous muscle on the radial side of the second metacarpal and the adductor pollicis is deep in the thumb web. This action can be accomplished while the patient attempts maximal strength of pinch.

The ulnar pinch deformity represents a reversal of the normal longitudinal arch of the first metacarpal and thumb, the integrity of which depends on the presence of the adductor pollicis and normal MCP flexion. Many variations of classic ulnar-palsied pinch are possible and are caused by variations in median and ulnar innervation of the intrinsics, whether the patient has loose or tight joints.

Ulnar palsy is usually caused by trauma of the ulnar nerve as it passes behind the medial humeral epicondyle. The most common causes are old fractures of the elbow and arthritis. Paresthesia or hypesthesia develops in the ulnar nerve distribution with increasing weakness of the intrinsic muscles. Percussion of the nerve in the epicondylar groove will produce paresthesia along its course.

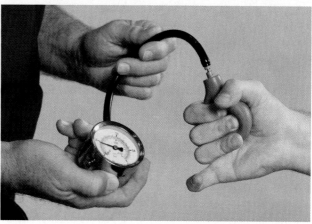

FIG. 6-121 The patient grasps a dynamometer for grip-strength testing. The sign is present if the fifth digit remains abducted and does not contribute to the grip strength. The presence of the sign indicates ulnar nerve paralysis.

PROCEDURE

- The patient performs a hard grasp strength test with a dynamometer.
- The examiner observes the position and function of the digits in the action.
- If the position of abduction is assumed by the little finger, the sign is present (Fig. 6-121).
- The sign is present in ulnar palsy.

Next Steps/Procedures
Froment paper sign, pinch grip test, and electrodiagnosis

Assessment for Diminished Peripheral Nerve Sensibility

Comment

The human nervous system is bombarded simultaneously by a multitude of stimuli. The afferent input is limited by the inconstant threshold of the peripheral nerve endings and the specialized receptor organs associated with them. Sensation is the acceptance and activation of impulses in the afferent nerve fibers of the nervous system.

The brain receives and elaborates a continuously changing flood of sensations. Varied sensations are synthesized into three-dimensional experiences. Central neural mechanisms, such as memory storage and introspection, influence the conscious perception of the external and internal environment. Sensibility is the conscious appreciation and interpretation of the stimulus that produced sensation. Tactile discrimination requires interpretation by the cerebral cortex.

Stereognosis is the ability to recognize objects by touching and manipulating them. Stereognosis should be tested with universally familiar objects, such as a key, safety pin, or coin (Fig. 6-122).

In graphesthesia, the patient identifies letters or numbers written on the palm with a blunt point. The patient who does not have graphesthesia can correctly identify the letters or numbers inscribed (Fig. 6-123).

To test for extinction, the examiner should touch the same areas on both sides of the body simultaneously. Failure of the patient to perceive touch on one side is called the *extinction phenomenon.* Normally, sensation is perceived on both sides (Figs. 6-124 and 6-125).

Position sense *(kinesthetic sensation)* is facilitated by proprioceptive receptors in the muscles, tendons, and joints. Perception of the position, orientation, and motion of limbs and body parts is obtained from kinesthetic sensations. A sensory unit is a single first-order afferent neuron, including all peripheral and central branches.

Cold intolerance is defined as abnormal pain, with or without discoloration, numbness and weakness, or stiffness of the hand and fingers after exposure to mild to severe cold. Although this condition is a frequent sequel of upper extremity trauma, the incidence is particularly high after upper extremity nerve injury. In the majority of peripheral nerve–injured patients, cold intolerance is the most bothersome,

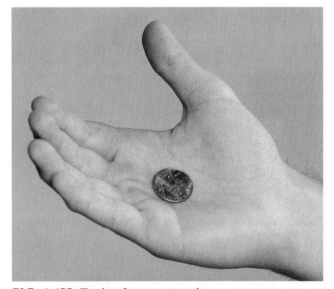

FIG. 6-122 Testing for stereognosis.

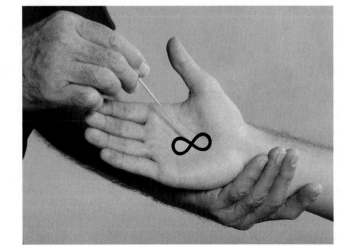

FIG. 6-123 Testing for graphesthesia.

ORTHOPEDIC GAMUT 6-20
TACTILE DISCRIMINATION

Four types of tactile discrimination are:
1. Stereognosis
2. Graphesthesia
3. Extinction
4. Two-point discrimination

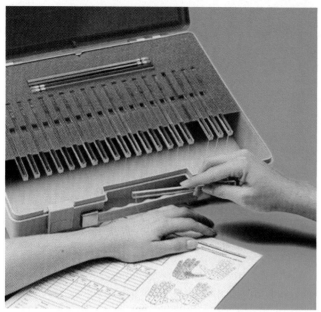

FIG. 6-124 The use of the Rolyan Semmes-Weinstein monofilaments has been found through repeated testing to be an extremely accurate method of measuring cutaneous sensibility. This test measures both diminishing and returning sensation. (Photo from Benefitsnow Ltd Unit 4 17d Riverway Newport, Isle of Wight, PO30 5UX www.benefitsnowshop.co.uk.)

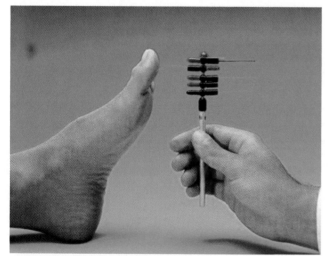

FIG. 6-125 Weinstein Enhanced Sensory Test (WEST) for the Hand and Foot uses five monofilaments to measure skin sensitivity and determine peripheral nerve involvement. WEST for the Hand and Foot provides reliable test results with textured, round monofilament tips. Two or more filaments can be in position for testing. (Photo from Benefitsnow Ltd Unit 4 17d Riverway Newport, Isle of Wight, PO30 5UX www.benefitsnowshop.co.uk.)

ORTHOPEDIC GAMUT 6-21

QUALITIES OF SENSIBILITY

Five elementary qualities of sensibility evoked by stimulation via:
1. Touch-pressure
2. Warmth
3. Coldness
4. Pain
5. Movement and position

ORTHOPEDIC GAMUT 6-22

NEURAL SENSORY UNIT

Factors influencing the neural sensory unit:
1. The diameter of the first-order afferent neuron
2. The properties of the sensory receptors
3. The size and population of the receptive field
4. The threshold for the entire sensory unit

TABLE 6-6

IMAI CLASSIFICATION OF SENSORY RECOVERY

Quality of Sensation (Range 1-5)	Filament Marking
1. Normal	2.83
2. Diminished light touch	3.61
3. Diminished protective sensation	4.31
4. Loss of protective sensation	4.56
5. Anesthetic	6.10

From Imai H, Tajima T, Natsuma Y: Interpretation of cutaneous pressure threshold (Semmes-Weinstein monofilament measurement) following median nerve repair and sensory reeducation in the adult, *Microsurgery* 10(2):142-144, 1989.

prolonged, and disabling symptom, affecting both work and leisure activities (Ruijs et al, in press).

Ten zones in the hand are tested, six in the territory of the median nerve and four in the territory of the ulnar nerve. The scores are interpreted as suggested by Imai and colleagues (Table 6-6). A score of 6.10 is interpreted as having no sensation.

PROCEDURE

- The test should be demonstrated while the patient is watching the procedure. The patient then closes the eyes.
- Several areas on the uninvolved hand are checked because some patients have congenitally abnormal two-point discrimination.
- The testing instrument can be a Boley gauge, a blunt-eye caliper, or an ordinary paper clip (Fig. 6-126).
- Testing is begun distally and proceeds proximally (Fig. 6-127).
- The points of the caliper are set at 10 mm and are brought together progressively as accurate responses are obtained (Fig. 6-128).
- The pressure from the testing instrument should not produce an ischemic area on the skin.
- When two points are applied, they make contact simultaneously.
- The patient indicates immediately if one or two points are felt.
- An interval of 3 to 5 seconds should be allowed between applications of the points.
- A series of one or two points is applied with varied sequence in each finger zone.
- The procedure is performed three times; if the patient does not record two of the three points correctly, the result is considered a failure at that test distance.
- If the patient correctly identifies the number of points applied, the testing distance is decreased in varying increments.
- The test has 10 applications of two points and 10 applications of one point at random.
- The total incorrect one-point applications are subtracted from the total of correct two-point applications.
- A score of 5 or more is considered passing.

Abnormal skin texture, such as heavy scales or calluses, has a marked influence on the test results. Testing can be performed in the presence of edema or infection, but the results demonstrate the sensibilities present, which may not reflect the true status of the nerve.

Next Steps/Procedures

Dellon moving two-point discrimination test, interphalangeal neuroma test, shrivel test, and electrodiagnosis

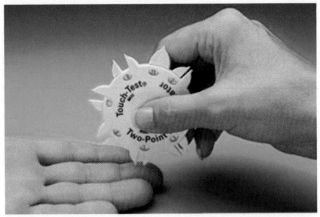

FIG. 6-126 Two-point discriminator, consisting of two rotating, plastic disks that are joined together. Tests static and moving two-point discrimination of fingers, toes or sensory flaps. Ideal for testing after nerve repair, grafts, and innervated tissue transfer for desensitization or to deter the level of impairment. Rounded tips are spaced at standard testing intervals from 1 to 15 mm apart; 20- and 25-mm spacing are also available. (Photo from Benefitsnow Ltd Unit 4 17d Riverway Newport, Isle of Wight, PO30 5UX www.benefitsnowshop. co.uk.)

CLINICAL PEARL

As with Dellon moving two-point discrimination test, bizarre responses are reasons for suspicion as to the origin of the symptoms. *Janet test* can help identify psychogenic anesthesia.

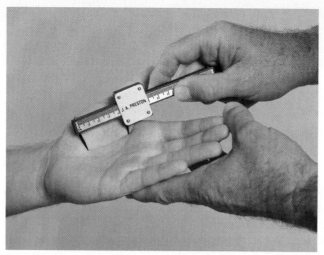

FIG. 6-127 The patient is seated with the elbow flexed. The arm is supinated and resting on the examination table. The hand is relaxed. The Boley gauge is set for 10 mm or more distance. The contact points are made randomly, beginning at the distal portions of the hand. The contacts must touch simultaneously and with equal pressure. The patient's eyes are closed.

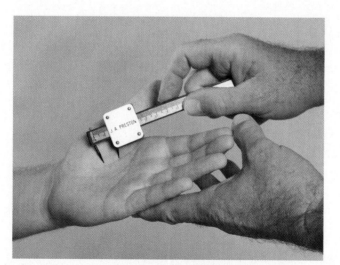

FIG. 6-128 As the testing progresses, the gauge contacts are reset closer together in 5-mm increments. If the patient cannot detect the points in two out of three attempts, the test is positive. A positive test indicates diminished sensibility for the area tested, according to established norms.

WRINGING TEST

Assessment for Elbow, Wrist, or Hand Derangement

Comment

The median nerve enters the hand through the carpal tunnel, a bony trough covered with a stout fibrous roof called the *flexor retinaculum,* which it shares with nine tendons, each covered with two layers of synovium. The carpal tunnel is a defined space with rigid and semirigid circumferential boundaries. The tube of space making up the carpal tunnel provides a channel for passage of all the flexor tendons of the thumb and digits from the forearm to the hand. The median nerve also passes through this space, completing the contents of the carpal canal. In addition to providing a protected passageway for these vital structures into the hand,

the transverse carpal ligament functions as a pulley to increase the power of the flexor tendons. The underlying bones form the floor of the carpal canal and are somewhat more distal (Fig. 6-129).

The tissue has no room to expand, and any swelling of the tendons or the synovium around them compresses the median nerve.

The palmaris longus muscle has a common area of origin with the flexor digitorum superficialis muscle, the flexor carpi ulnaris muscle, and the flexor carpi radialis muscle, which is the medial epicondyle of the humerus. It is located just under the skin, the subcutaneous fat, and the forearm's fascia, superficial to the flexor digitorum superficialis muscle and between the flexor carpi ulnaris and flexor carpi radialis muscle. The palmaris longus muscle runs downwards and outwards. It is muscular up to the forearm's middle, where

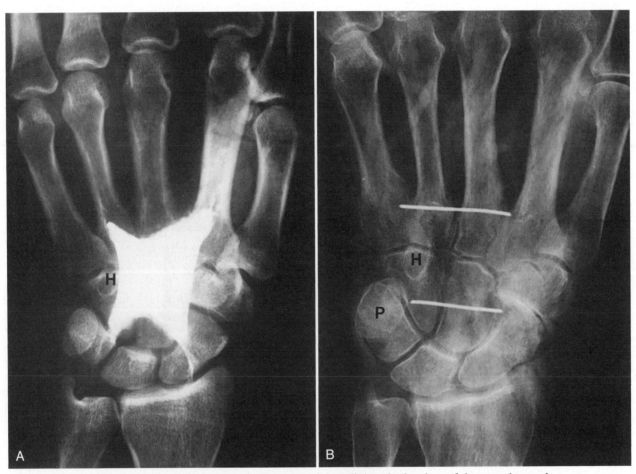

FIG. 6-129 **A,** Radiographic contrast material outlining the borders of the carpal tunnel. **B,** Lines representing border of carpal tunnel superimposed on radiograph. (From Cooney WP, Linscheid RL, Dobyns JH: *The wrist diagnosis and operative treatment,* vol 1-2, St Louis, 1998, Mosby.)

it is toggled into a thin and broad tendon that is inserted into the flexor retinaculum and the palmar aponeurosis (Natsis et al, 2007).

The palmaris longus muscle, tendinous in its upper part and muscular in its lower part, is termed a *reversed palmaris longus*. A three-headed palmaris longus muscle may be a source of edema and pain in the wrist.

The most common overall cause of CTS is fluid retention, the most common cause of which is pregnancy. However, overuse of the tendons from repeated forceful movements of the wrist, either at work or recreation, is probably the most common cause of CTS referred to orthopedic and neurosurgical clinics. Any condition that causes synovial thickening, including rheumatoid arthritis and Colles fracture, can also be responsible.

Median nerve compression causes paresthesia in the median nerve distribution, which is the front of the thumb, index finger, middle finger, and the radial half of the ring finger. The palm is not involved because the palmar branch of the median nerve arises above the wrist.

The symptoms are worse at night, and the patient will wake and fling the hand up and down to try and relieve the symptoms. In time, the paresthesia is replaced by pain, which can be felt as far up as the elbow, and eventually by numbness in the median distribution.

Most patients notice the little finger is not affected, and those who report that all the fingers are involved should be treated with suspicion.

The differential diagnosis includes peripheral neuropathy, mononeuritis, cervical spondylosis, and tumors of the thoracic outlet that involve the brachial plexus, but these are often forgotten because CTS is such a common condition. If any doubt exists, the diagnosis can be confirmed by nerve conduction studies.

PROCEDURE

- The patient, using both hands, wrings a towel (Fig. 6-130).
- Paresthesia in the hand indicates CTS.
- Pain elicited at the elbow indicates epicondylitis.
- Wrist discomfort indicates arthropathy or carpal derangement.

Next Steps/Procedures

Phalen sign, electrodiagnosis, diagnostic imaging, and further testing based on the area of localized complaint

CLINICAL PEARL

The wringing test is useful to determine the area for primary investigation. The patient may also be asked to hold both wrists in a fully flexed position for 1 to 2 minutes. The appearance or exacerbation of paresthesia suggests CTS. This test is the most sensitive clinical test for CTS. Advanced CTS can produce thenar atrophy and distal phalangeal acroasphyxia. The wringing test is particularly useful in eliciting responses in more subtle afflictions of the median nerve.

6

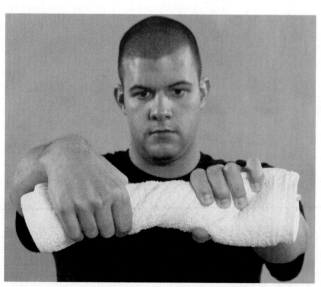

FIG. 6-130 The patient, using both hands, wrings a towel. Maximal effort is applied. The test will localize the discomfort to the primary site of origin. If the test elicits pain at the elbow, epicondylitis is indicated. If the discomfort is felt at the wrist, arthropathy or carpal derangement is indicated. Paresthesia in the hand suggests CTS.

CRITICAL THINKING

1. Name the tendons involved in de Quervain tendinopathy (first compartment tendinopathy).
2. The second area of the wrist that is clinically significant is on the dorsal side over the tubercle of the radius, or Lister tubercle. Name three tunnels of the wrist that transverse the area of Lister tubercle.
3. What is a cystic mass that arises on the ulnar side of the radial tubercle?
4. Name the structures that lie within the carpal tunnel.
5. Describe the two physical signs that are helpful in determining CTS.
6. Which muscles are affected by the anterior interosseous nerve palsy?
7. How does one physically test for compression of the pronator teres between the superficial and deep heads?
8. What is a boxer knuckle?
9. List the contents of the carpal tunnel.
10. What is Guyon canal?
11. What are the borders of the *anatomic snuffbox?*
12. What is Allen test?
13. Where is the *no man's land* of the hand?
14. What structure is involved in Dupuytren contracture?
15. Where do most wrist ganglia originate?
16. What is a boxer fracture?
17. How can rotational malalignment be evaluated?
18. What is a Bennett fracture?
19. What is a gamekeeper thumb?
20. Which carpal bone is fractured most often?
21. Fractures at which location in the scaphoid have the lowest rate of healing?
22. What is a Colles fracture?
23. What other connective tissue disorders are associated with Dupuytren disease?
24. What are Heberden nodes?
25. What is caput ulna syndrome?
26. What is the role of trauma in the etiology of Kienböck disease?
27. What are the criteria for making the diagnosis of Kienböck disease?
28. What is the most commonly encountered compressive neuropathy of the upper extremity?
29. What are the most common causes of CTS?
30. Name the provocative test used to substantiate the diagnosis of CTS.
31. What is de Quervain disease?
32. How is de Quervain disease diagnosed?
33. When injury occurs to the carpal system of the wrist, what are the four determining factors?
34. The carpal bones form a volar concave arch or carpal tunnel. What forms the roof of the carpal tunnel?
35. The carpal tunnel contains what nerve?
36. What are the four carpal bones making up the floor or volar concave arch of the carpal tunnel?
37. The ulnar tunnel, or *tunnel of Guyon,* contains what structures?
38. Acute pain in the *anatomical snuffbox* is suggestive of injury to which carpal bone?
39. What are the potential serious consequences of misdiagnosis, delay in treatment, or an undesirable outcome from treatment of this injury?
40. The *Terry Thomas sign* is classic for injury to what ligament? What two carpal bones are involved?
41. What is the normal gap between the bones that is considered normal?
42. What X-ray view accentuates this gap?
43. What is the most common cause of scapholunate advance collapse?
44. What are other causes?
45. What is one of the most serious complications that can occur after an injury to the wrist?
46. What patient reaction would you expect with RSD-CRPS to your examination of the wrist?
47. What would you expect to see on observation and examination of the wrist in this patient?
48. What is the classic plain-film imaging presentation?
49. OA in the hands results in a progressive loss of articular cartilage resulting in new bone formation at the joint surfaces and the subchondral area. Where are Heberden and Bouchard nodes located?
50. Name four findings in the wrist and hand that are suggestive of rheumatoid arthritis.
51. The most common fracture occurring in the wrist is to which bone?
52. Which muscle of the hand atrophies in advanced CTS?
53. Stenosing (de Quervain) tenosynovitis is diagnosed with which examination test or procedure?
54. What two tendons are inflamed with this condition?
55. What is the common cause of this condition?
56. What sex and age range does this affect primarily?
57. What findings are present with a positive Phalen test?
58. How long must the patient hold the test position to determine if the test is positive or negative?
59. What carpal tunnel test is the most accurate provocative sign in CTS?
60. Weakness of the flexor pollicis longus, the flexor digitorum profundus of the index finger, and the pronator quadratus constitute a triad of findings consistent with what syndrome?
61. How is Raynaud disease characterized?
62. What is the most commonly injured nerve in the upper extremity?
63. What is the most common cause of ulnar palsy?
64. What area of the hand does median nerve compression causes paresthesias?

BIBLIOGRAPHY

Abrams WB, Berkow R: *The Merck manual of geriatrics,* Rahway, NJ, 1990, Merck Sharp & Dohme Research Laboratories.

Adams JC, Hamblen DL: *Outline of orthopaedics,* ed 11, Edinburgh, 1990, Churchill Livingstone.

Agee JM et al: Endoscopic release of the carpal tunnel: a randomized prospective multicenter study, *J Hand Surg* 17A:987, 1992.

Akbas M, Yegin A, Karsli B: 778 reflex sympathetic dystrophy in a 10 year old pediatric, *Eur J Pain* 10(suppl 1):S202-S203, 2006.

Alario AJ: *Practical guide to the care of the pediatric patient,* St Louis, 1997, Mosby.

Amadio PC: The Mayo Clinic and carpal tunnel syndrome, *Mayo Clin Proc* 67:42, 1992.

American Board of Chiropractic Orthopedists: *Proceedings 1997,* New Orleans, 1997, American Board of Chiropractic Orthopedists.

American Medical Association: *Guides to the evaluation of permanent impairment,* ed 4, Chicago, 1993, The Association.

American Medical Association: *How to use guides to the evaluation of permanent impairment,* ed 4, Falmouth, Conn, 1993, SEAK.

American Society for Surgery of the Hand: *The hand examination and diagnosis,* Aurora, Colo, 1978.

Anderson B, Kayes S: Treatment of flexor tenosynovitis of the hand trigger finger with corticosteroids: a prospective study of the response to local injection, *Arch Intern Med* 151:153, 1991.

Ankarath S: Chronic wrist pain: diagnosis and management, *Curr Orthop* 20(2):141-151, 2006.

Apley AG, Solomon L: *Concise system of orthopaedics and fractures,* London, 1988, Butterworth-Heinemann.

Arner M, Jonsson K, Aspenberg P: Complete palmar dislocation of the lunate in rheumatoid arthritis: avascularity without avascular changes, *J Hand Surg* 21(3):384-387, 1996.

Aulicino P: Neurovascular injuries in the hands of athletes, *Hand Clin* 6:455, 1990.

Baird KS, Crossan JF, Ralston SH: Abnormal growth factor and cytokine expression in Dupuytren's contracture, *J Clin Pathol* 46:425, 1993.

Baird KS et al: T-cell-mediated response in Dupuytren's disease, *Lancet* 341:1622, 1993.

Barkauskas VH et al: *Health & physical assessment,* ed 2, St Louis, 1998, Mosby.

Beckenbaugh RD et al: Kienböck's disease: the natural history of Kienböck's disease and consideration of lunate fractures, *Clin Orthop* 149:98, 1980.

Beekman RA et al: Extensor mechanism slide for the treatment of proximal interphalangeal joint extension lag: an anatomic study, *J Hand Surg* 29(6):1063-1068, 2004.

Bell JA: Sensibility evaluation. In Hunter JM, et al, editors: *Rehabilitation of the hand,* St Louis, 1978, Mosby.

Belsole RJ et al: Computed analyses of the pathomechanics of scaphoid waist nonunions, *J Hand Surg* 16A:899, 1991.

Berger RA: Endoscopic carpal tunnel release, a current perspective, *Hand Clin* 10:625, 1994.

Berthelot J-M: Current management of reflex sympathetic dystrophy syndrome (complex regional pain syndrome type I), *Joint Bone Spine* 73(5):495-499, 2006.

Birchard D, Pichora D: Experimental corrective scaphoid osteotomy for scaphoid malunion with abnormal wrist mechanics, *J Hand Surg* 15A:863, 1990.

Bourne G: *The structure and function of nervous tissue,* New York, 1968, Academic Press.

Braithwaite IJ, Jones WA: Scapho-lunate dissociation occurring with scaphoid fracture, *J Hand Surg* 17B:286, 1992.

Brashear HR Jr, Raney RB: *Shands' handbook of orthopaedic surgery,* St Louis, 1978, Mosby.

Brondum V, Larsen CF, Skov O: Fracture of carpal scaphoid: frequency and distribution in a well-defined population, *Eur J Radiol* 15:118, 1992.

Brooks M, Evans R, Fairclough J: *Sports injuries,* ed 2, London, 1992, Gower Medical.

Brotzman SB: *Clinical orthopaedic rehabilitation,* St Louis, 1996, Mosby.

Brown DE, Neumann RD: *Orthopedic secrets,* Philadelphia, 1995, Hanley & Belfus.

Brown M: The well elderly. In Guccione A, editor: *Geriatric physical therapy,* St Louis, 1993, Mosby.

Brown MG, Keyser B, Roghtnberg ES: Endoscopic carpal tunnel release, *J Hand Surg* 17A:1009, 1992.

Brown RA et al: Carpal tunnel release: a prospective, randomized assessment of open and endoscopic methods, *J Bone Joint Surg* 75A:1265, 1993.

Buchler U: *Wrist instability,* St Louis, 1996, Mosby.

Bucholz RW: *Orthopaedic decision making,* ed 2, St Louis, 1996, Mosby.

Bunnell S: Surgery of the rheumatic hand, *J Bone Joint Surg* 27:759, 1955.

Burton RI: Extensor tendons-late reconstruction. In Green DP, editor: *Operative hand surgery,* ed 3, New York, 1993, Churchill Livingstone.

Cahalan T et al: Biomechanics of the golf swing in players with pathologic conditions of the forearm, wrist, and hand, *Am J Sports Med* 19:288, 1991.

Cailliet R: *Hand pain and impairment,* ed 2, Philadelphia, 1975, FA Davis.

Cambridge CA: Range of motion measurements of the hand. In Hunter JM et al, editors: *Rehabilitation of the hand,* ed 3, St Louis, 1990, Mosby.

Canale ST: *Campbell's operative orthopaedics,* vol 1-4, ed 9, St Louis, 1998, Mosby.

Canoso JJ: Bursitis, tenosynovitis, ganglions, and painful lesions of the wrist, elbow and hand, *Curr Opin Rheumatol* 2:276, 1990.

Cardon LJ, Toh S, Tsubo K: Traumatic boutonniere deformity of the thumb, *J Hand Surg* 25(5):505-508, 2000.

Chen Y-G et al: Innervation of the metacarpophalangeal and interphalangeal joints: a microanatomic and histologic study of the nerve endings, *J Hand Surg* 25(1):128-133, 2000.

Chiodo A, Chadd E: Ulnar neuropathy at or distal to the wrist: traumatic versus cumulative stress cases, *Arch Phys Med Rehabil* 88(4):504-512, 2007.

Christiansen TG et al: Diagnostic value of ultrasound in scaphoid fractures, *Injury* 22:397, 1991.

Chusid JG, McDonald JJ: *Correlative neuroanatomy and functional neurology,* Los Altos, Calif, 1962, Lange Medical.

Cipriano JJ: *Photographic manual of regional orthopaedic and neurological test,* ed 3, Baltimore, 1997, Williams & Wilkins.

Cobb TK et al: Anatomy of the flexor retinaculum, *J Hand Surg* 18A:91, 1993.

Cohn RE: *Impairment rating examination and disability evaluation,* ed 3, Wilkesboro, NC, 1994, R Ernest Cohn.

Collo MC et al: Evaluating arthritic complaints, *Nurse Pract* 15:9, 1991.

Compson JP, Waterman JK, Spencer JD: Dorsal avulsion fractures of the scaphoid: diagnostic implications and applied anatomy, *J Hand Surg* 18B:58, 1993.

Cooney WP III, Dobyns JH, Linscheid RL: Complications of Colles' fracture, *J Bone Joint Surg* 62A:613, 1980.

Cooney WP III, Linscheid RL, Dobyns JH: External pin fixation for unstable Colles' fracture, *J Bone Joint Surg* 61A:840, 1979.

Cooney WP III, Linscheid RL, Dobyns JH: *The wrist diagnosis and operative treatment,* vol 1-2, St Louis, 1998, Mosby.

Cooney WP, Dobyns JH, Linscheid RL: Arthroscopy of the wrist: anatomy and classification of carpal instability, *Arthroscopy* 6(2):133-140, 1990.

Copeland SA et al: *Joint stiffness of the upper limb,* St Louis, 1997, Mosby.

Dambro MR, Griffith JA: *Griffith's 5 minute clinical consult,* Baltimore, 1997, Williams & Wilkins.

D'Ambrogio KJ, Roth GB: *Positional release therapy assessment & treatment of musculoskeletal dysfunction,* St Louis, 1997, Mosby.

D'Ambrosia RD: *Musculoskeletal disorders regional examination and differential diagnosis,* Philadelphia, 1977, JB Lippincott.

Dandy DJ: *Essential orthopaedics and trauma,* Edinburgh, 1989, Churchill Livingstone.

De Smet L: Avascular necrosis of multiple carpal bones: a case report, *Annales de Chirurgie de la Main* 18(3):202-204, 1999.

De Smet L: The distal radioulnar joint in rheumatoid arthritis, *Int Congr Ser* 129:63-68, 2006.

Dellon AL, Curtis RM, Edgerton MT: Evaluating recovery of sensation in the hand following nerve injury, *Johns Hopkins Med J* 130:235, 1972.

Dellon AL, Curtis RM, Edgerton MT: Reeducation of sensation in the hand after nerve injury and repair, *Plast Reconstr Surg* 53:297, 1974.

Dellon AL et al: Diagnosis of compressive neuropathies in patients with fibromyalgia, *J Hand Surg* 28(6):894-897, 2003.

Deltoff MN, Kogon PL: *The portable skeletal x-ray library,* St Louis, 1998, Mosby.

Demeter SL, Anderson GBJ, Smith GM: *Disability evaluation,* St Louis, 1996, Mosby.

Deshpande JK, Tobias JD: *The pediatric pain handbook,* St Louis, 1996, Mosby.

Dettenmeier PA: *Radiographic assessment for nurses,* St Louis, 1995, Mosby.

Dias J, Buch K: Palmar wrist ganglion: does intervention improve outcome? A prospective study of the natural history and patient-reported treatment outcomes, *J Hand Surg* 28(2):172-176, 2003.

Dias JJ et al: Suspected scaphoid fractures, the value of radiographs, *J Bone Joint Surg* 72B:98, 1990.

Dilley DF, Tonkin MA: Acute calcific tendinitis in the hand and wrist, *J Hand Surg* 16B:215, 1991.

Dimitriou CG, Chalidis B, Pournaras J: Bilateral volar lunate dislocation, *J Hand Surg* (in press, corrected proof).

Doherty M, Doherty J: *Clinical examination in rheumatology,* London, 1992, Wolfe.

Doherty M, George E: *Self-assessment picture tests in rheumatology,* London, 1995, Mosby-Wolfe.

Doherty M: *Color atlas and text of osteoarthritis,* London, 1994, Wolfe.

Doyle JR: Extensor tendons-acute injuries. In Green DP, editor: *Operative hand surgery,* ed 3, New York, 1993, Churchill Livingstone.

Dray GJ, Eaton RG: Dislocation and ligament injuries in the digits. In Green DP, editor: *Operative hand surgery,* ed 3, New York, 1993, Churchill-Livingstone.

Duchenne GB: *Physiology of motion (translated by Emanuel B. Kaplan),* Philadelphia, 1975, WB Saunders.

Dworkin RH et al: Symptom profiles differ in patients with neuropathic versus non-neuropathic pain, *J Pain* 8(2):118-126, 2007.

Elster AD: *Questions and answers in magnetic resonance imaging,* St Louis, 1994, Mosby.

Epstein O et al: *Clinical examination,* ed 2, London, 1997, Mosby.

Evangelisti S, Realve VF: Fibroma of tendon sheath as a cause of carpal tunnel syndrome, *J Hand Surg* 17A:1026, 1992.

Feldmann E: *Current diagnosis in neurology,* St Louis, 1994, Mosby.

Ferezy JS: *The chiropractic neurological examination,* Gaithersburg, Md, 1992, Aspen.

Finkelstein H: Stenosing tendovaginitis at the radial styloid process, *J Bone Joint Surg* 12:509, 1930.

Finneson BE: *Diagnosis and management of pain syndromes,* Philadelphia, 1969, WB Saunders.

Flatt AE: *The care of minor hand injuries,* St Louis, 1972, Mosby.

Frank ED, et al: *Merrill's atlas of radiographic positioning and procedures,* ed 11, St Louis, 2007, Mosby.

Frykman G: Fracture of the distal radius including sequelae-shoulder-hand-finger syndrome, disturbance in the distal radioulnar joint and impairment of nerve function: a clinical and experimental study, *Acta Orthop Scand Suppl* 108:1, 1967.

Frykman GK: *The orthopedic clinics of North America,* vol 12(2), Philadelphia, April 1981 and April 1984, WB Saunders.

Gabel G, Bishop AT, Wood MB: Flexor carpi radialis tendinitis. part II: results of operative treatment, *J Bone Joint Surg* 76A:1015, 1994.

Ganz PA: The quality of life after breast cancer. Solving the problem of lymphedema, *N Engl J Med* 340(5):383-385, 1999.

Garcia JH: *Neuropathology the diagnostic approach,* St Louis, 1997, Mosby.

Gelberman RH et al: The vascularity of the lunate bone and Kienböck's disease, *J Hand Surg* 5A:272, 1980.

Goldie BS: *Orthopaedic diagnosis and management: a guide to the care of orthopaedic patients,* ed 2, Oxford, UK, 1998, ISIS Medical Media.

Goldner JL et al: Metacarpophalangeal joint arthroplasty with silicone-Dacron prosthesis, Niebauer type, six and a half years experience, *J Bone Joint Surg* 2:200, 1977.

Goldner JL: Volkmann's ischemic contracture. In Flynn JE, editor: *Hand surgery,* ed 2, Baltimore, 1975, Williams & Wilkins.

Gordon M: *Nursing diagnosis: process and application,* ed 3, St Louis, 1994, Mosby.

Green DP: Carpal dislocations and instabilities. In Green DP, editor: *Operative hand surgery,* ed 3, New York, 1993, Churchill-Livingstone.

Greenstein GM: *Clinical assessment of neuromusculoskeletal disorders,* St Louis, 1997, Mosby.

Grossman ZD et al: *Cost-effective diagnostic imaging: the clinician's guide,* ed 3, St Louis, 1995, Mosby.

Grundberg AB, Reagan DS: Pathologic anatomy of the forearm: intersection syndrome, *J Hand Surg* 10(2):299-302, 1985.

Guimberteau JC, Panconi B: Recalcitrant non-union of the scaphoid treated with a vascularized bone graft based on the ulnar artery, *J Bone Joint Surg* 72A:88, 1990.

Hammer WI: *Functional soft tissue examination and treatment by manual methods: the extremities,* Gaithersburg, Md, 1991, Aspen.

Harris R, Piller N: Three case studies indicating the effectiveness of manual lymph drainage on patients with primary and secondary lymphedema using objective measuring tools, *J Bodywork Move Ther* 7(4):213-221, 2003.

Hartley A: *Practical joint assessment upper quadrant,* ed 2, St Louis, 1995, Mosby.

Harvey FJ, Harvey PM, Horsely MW: De Quervain's disease: surgical or nonsurgical treatment, *J Hand Surg* 15A:83, 1990.

Hawkins RJ: *An organized approach to musculoskeletal examination and history taking,* St Louis, 1995, Mosby.

Hinkle CZ: *Fundamentals of anatomy & movement a workbook and guide,* St Louis, 1997, Mosby.

Hoppenfeld S: *Physical examination of the spine and extremities,* New York, 1976, Appleton-Century-Crofts.

Hori Y, Tamai S, Okuda H: Blood vessel transplantation to bone, *J Hand Surg* 4(1):23-33, 1979.

Hornberger JP: *Exercise physiology therapeutic exercise,* Sarasota, Fla, 1991, Joseph P Hornberger.

Hunter JM: Recurrent carpal tunnel syndrome, epineural fibrous fixation, and traction neuropathy, *Hand Clin* 7:491, 1991.

Imaeda T et al: Magnetic resonance imaging in scaphoid fractures, *J Hand Surg* 17B:20, 1992.

Johnson MK: *The hand book,* Springfield, Ill, 1973, Charles C Thomas.

Jonsson K: Nonunion of a fractured scaphoid tubercle, *J Hand Surg* 15A:283, 1990.

Jupiter JB: Current concepts review: fractures of the distal end of the radius, *J Bone Joint Surg* 73A:461, 1991.

Kanner R: *Pain management secrets,* Philadelphia, 1997, Hanley & Belfus.

Kasdan ML: *Occupational hand & upper extremity injuries & diseases,* ed 2, Philadelphia, 1998, Hanley & Belfus.

Katirji B: *Electromyography in clinical practice: a case study approach,* St Louis, 1998, Mosby.

Katz WA: *Rheumatic diseases diagnosis and management,* Philadelphia, 1977, JB Lippincott.

Keats TE: *Atlas of roentgenographic measurement,* ed 6, St Louis, 1990, Mosby.

Kendall HO, Kendall FP, Wadsworth GE: *Muscle testing and function,* ed 2, Baltimore, 1971, Williams & Wilkins.

Kerluke L, McCabe SJ: Nonunion of the scaphoid: a critical analysis of recent natural history studies, *J Hand Surg* 18A:1, 1993.

Kerr CD, Sybert DR, Albarracin NS: An analysis of flexor synovium in idiopathic carpal tunnel syndrome: report of 625 cases, *J Hand Surg* 17A:1028, 1992.

Kiebhaber TR, Stern P: Upper extremity tendinitis and overuse syndrome in the athlete, *Clin Sports Med* 11:39, 1992.

Klippel JH, Dieppe PA: *Rheumatology,* vol 1-2, ed 2, London, 1998, Mosby.

Kloth LC, McCulloch JM, Feedar JA: *Wound healing: alternatives in management,* Philadelphia, 1990, FA Davis.

Koenigsberg R: *Churchill's illustrated medical dictionary,* New York, 1989, Churchill Livingstone.

Kraemer BA, Young BL, Arfken S: Stenosing flexor tenosynovitis, *South Med J* 83:806, 1990.

Lamas C et al: The anatomy and vascularity of the lunate: considerations applied to Kienböck's disease, *Chirurgie de la Main* 26(1):13-20, 2007.

Landsmeer JMF: *Atlas of anatomy of the hand,* Edinburgh, 1976, Churchill Livingstone.

Larsen CF, Brondum V, Skov O: Epidemiology of scaphoid fractures in Odense, Denmark, *Acta Orthop Scand* 63:216, 1992.

Lavy CBD, Barrett DS: *Questions and answers on Apley's concise system of orthopaedics and fractures,* Oxford, UK, 1991, Butterworth-Heinemann.

Lee MLH: The intraosseous arterial pattern of the carpal lunate bone and its relation to avascular necrosis, *Acta Orthop Scand* 33:43, 1963.

Lefevre-Colau MM et al: Reliability, validity, and responsiveness of the modified kapandji index for assessment of functional mobility of the rheumatoid hand, *Arch Phys Med Rehabil* 84(7):1032-1038, 2003.

Leibovitz A et al: Edema of the paretic hand in elderly post-stroke nursing patients, *Arch Gerontol Geriatr* 44(1):37-42, 2007.

Lerner AJ: *The little black book of neurology,* ed 3, St Louis, 1995, Mosby.

Leslie BM, Ericson WB Jr, Morehead JR: Incidence of a septum within the first dorsal compartment of the wrist, *J Hand Surg* 15A:88, 1990.

Lewis CB, Knortz KA: *Orthopedic assessment and treatment of the geriatric patient,* St Louis, 1993, Mosby.

Lewis MH: Median nerve decompression after Colles' fracture, *J Bone Joint Surg* 60B:195, 1978.

Lin JT, Stubblefield MD: De Quervain's tenosynovitis in patients with lymphedema: a report of 2 cases with management approach, *Arch Phys Med Rehabil* 84(10):1554-1557, 2003.

Lindstrom G, Nystrom A: Incidence of post-traumatic arthrosis after primary healing of scaphoid fractures: a clinical and radiological study, *J Hand Surg* 15B:11, 1990.

Lindstrom G, Nystrom A: Natural history of scaphoid non-union, with special reference to "asymptomatic" cases, *J Hand Surg* 17B:697, 1992.

Linscheid RL, Dobyns JH: Rheumatoid arthritis of the wrist, *Ortho Clin North Am* 2:649, 1971.

Linscheid RL et al: Instability patterns of the wrist, *J Hand Surg* 8A:682, 1983.

Linscheid RL et al: Traumatic instability of the wrist, *J Bone Joint Surg* 54A:1612, 1972.

Lister G: *The hand: diagnosis and indications,* Edinburgh, 1977, Churchill Livingstone.

Lluch AL: Thickening of the synovium of the digital flexor tendons: cause or consequence of the carpal tunnel syndrome? *J Hand Surg* 17B:209, 1992.

Lynch AC, Lipscomb PR: The carpal-tunnel syndrome and Colles' fractures, *JAMA* 185:363, 1963.

Magee DJ: *Orthopedic physical assessment,* ed 3, Philadelphia, 1997, WB Saunders.

Malone TR, McPoil TG, Nitz AJ: *Orthopedic and sports physical therapy,* ed 3, St Louis, 1997, Mosby.

Mannerfelt L et al: Rupture of the extensor pollicis longus tendon after Colles' fracture and by rheumatoid arthritis, *J Hand Surg* 15B:49, 1990.

Marchiori DM: *Clinical imaging with skeletal, chest, and abdomen pattern differentials,* St Louis, 1999, Mosby.

Maritz NGJ et al: The rheumatoid wrist in black south African patients, *J Hand Surg* 28(4):373-375, 2003.

Martin JH: *Neuroanatomy text and atlas,* ed 2, Stamford, Conn, 1996, Appleton & Lange.

Mathers LH et al: *Clinical anatomy principles,* St Louis, 1996, Mosby.

Mayfield JK et al: Biomechanical properties of human carpal ligaments, *Orthop Trans* 3:143, 1979.

Mayfield JK, Johnson RP, Kilcoyne RF: Carpal dislocations: pathomechanics and progressive perilunar instability, *J Hand Surg* 5:226, 1980.

Mayfield JK: Mechanism of carpal injuries, *Clin Orthop* 149:45, 1980.

Mayo Clinic: *Clinical examinations in neurology,* ed 3, Philadelphia, 1971, WB Saunders.

Mazion JM: *Illustrated manual of neurological reflexes/signs/tests, part I, Orthopedic signs/tests/maneuvers for office procedure, part II,* Orlando, Fla, 1980, Daniels Publishing.

McCarty DJ, Koopman WJ, editors: *Arthritis and allied conditions,* ed 12, Philadelphia, 1993, Lea & Febiger.

McLain RF, Steyer CM: Tendon ruptures with scaphoid nonunion, a case report, *Clin Orthop* 255:117, 1990.

McNurty RY et al: Kinematics of the wrist, II, clinical applications, *J Bone Joint Surg* 600:955, 1978.

McRae R: *Clinical orthopaedic examination,* ed 3, Edinburgh, 1990, Churchill Livingstone.

Medical Economics Books: *Patient care flow chart manual,* ed 3, Oradell, NJ, 1982, Medical Economics Books.

Mellion MB: *Office sports medicine,* ed 2, St Louis, 1996, Mosby.

Mellion MB: *Sports medicine secrets,* Philadelphia, 1994, Hanley & Belfus.

Mennell JM: *The musculoskeletal system differential diagnosis from symptoms and physical signs,* Gaithersburg, Md, 1992, Aspen.

Mercier LR, Pettid FJ: *Practical orthopedics,* ed 4, St Louis, 1995, Mosby.

Millender LH, Nalebuff EA, Feldon PG: Rheumatoid arthritis, In Green D, editor: *Operative hand surgery,* New York, 1982, Churchill Livingstone.

Minamikawa Y et al: de Quervain's syndrome: surgical and anatomical studies of the fibroosseous canal, *Orthopedics* 14:545, 1991.

Mino DE, Palmer AK, Levinsohn EM: The role of radiography and computerized tomography in the diagnosis of subluxation and dislocation of the distal radioulnar joint, *J Hand Surg* 8A:23, 1983.

Mishra S: A new test for demonstrating the action of flexor digitorum superficialis (FDS) tendon, *J Plast Reconst Aesthet Surg* 59(12):1342-1344, 2006.

Moberg E: Criticism and study of methods for examining sensibility of the hand, *Neurology* 12:8, 1962.

Moberg E: Relation of touch and deep sensation to hand reconstruction, *Am J Surg* 109:353, 1965.

Mody BS et al: Nonunion of fractures of the scaphoid tuberosity, *J Bone Joint Surg* 75B:423, 1993.

Moldaver J: Tinel's sign: its characteristics and significance, *J Bone Joint Surg* 60A:412, 1978.

Moran SL et al: The use of the 4 + 5 extensor compartmental vascularized bone graft for the treatment of Kienböck's disease, *J Hand Surg* 30(1):50-58, 2005.

6

Mosby-Year Book, Inc: *Expert 10-minute physical examination,* St Louis, 1997, Mosby-Year Book.

Mourad LA: *Orthopedic disorders,* St Louis, 1991, Mosby.

Mulliken JB: Cutaneous vascular anomalies. In McCarthy JG, editor: *Plastic surgery. Vol 5, tumors of the head and neck and skin,* Philadelphia, 1990, WB Saunders.

Naidu SH, Heppenstall RB: Compartment syndrome of the forearm and hand, *Hand Clin* 10:13, 1994.

Nakamura P, Imaeda T, Miura T: Scaphoid malunion, *J Bone Joint Surg* 73B:134, 1991.

Nakamura R et al: Analysis of scaphoid fracture displacement by three-dimensional computed tomography, *J Hand Surg* 16A:485, 1991.

Nakamura R et al: Scaphoid non-union with D.I.S.I. deformity, a survey of clinical cases with special reference to ligamentous injury, *J Hand Surg* 16B:156, 1991.

Nettina SM: *The Lippincott manual of nursing practice,* ed 6, Philadelphia, 1996, JB Lippincott.

Newton RW: *Color atlas of pediatric neurology,* St Louis, 1995, Mosby-Wolfe.

Nicholas JA, Hershman EB: *The upper extremity in sports medicine,* ed 2, St Louis, 1995, Mosby.

Nolan WV III et al: Results of treatment of severe carpal tunnel syndrome, *J Hand Surg* 17A:1020, 1992.

Nordin M, Anderson GBJ, Pope MH: *Musculoskeletal disorders in the workplace: principles and practice,* St Louis, 1997, Mosby.

Oaklander AL et al: Evidence of focal small-fiber axonal degeneration in complex regional pain syndrome-I (reflex sympathetic dystrophy), *Pain* 120(3):235-243, 2006.

O'Donoghue DH: *Treatment of injuries to athletes,* ed 3, Philadelphia, 1976, WB Saunders.

Oka Y, Umeda K, Ikeda M: Cyst-like lesions of the lunate resembling Kienböck's disease: a case report, *J Hand Surg* 26(1):130-134, 2001.

Olson WH et al: *Handbook of symptom-oriented neurology,* ed 2, St Louis, 1994, Mosby.

Omer GE Jr et al: The neurovascular cutaneous island pedicles for deficient median nerve sensibility: new technique and results of serial functional tests, *J Bone Joint Surg* 52A:1181, 1970.

Omer GE Jr, Vogel JA: Determination of physiological length of a reconstructed muscle tendon unit through muscle stimulation, *J Bone Joint Surg* 47A:304, 1965.

Omer GE Jr: Evaluation and reconstruction of the forearm and hand after acute traumatic peripheral nerve injuries, *J Bone Joint Surg* 50A:1454, 1968.

Omer GE Jr: Sensation and sensibility in the upper extremity, *Clin Orthop* 104:30, 1974.

Omer GE, Spinner M: *Management of peripheral nerve problems,* Philadelphia, 1980, WB Saunders.

O'Riain S. New and simple test of nerve function in hand, *BMJ* 3(5881):615-616, 1973.

O'Riain S: Shrivel test: a new and simple test of nerve function in the hand, *BMJ* 3:615, 1973.

O'Young B, Young MA, Stiens SA: *PM&R secrets,* Philadelphia, 1997, Hanley & Belfus.

Pagnanelli DM, Barrer SJ: Bilateral carpal tunnel release at one operation: report of 228 patients, *Neurosurgery* 31:1030, 1992.

Pahle JA, Raunio P: The influence of wrist position on finger deviation in the rheumatoid hand: a clinical and radiological study, *J Bone Joint Surg* 51B:664, 1969.

Palmer AK, Glisson RR, Werner FW: Ulnar variance determination, *J Hand Surg* 7:376, 1982.

Palmer AK, Livensohn EM, Kuzma GR: Arthrography of the wrist, *J Hand Surg* 8:15, 1983.

Palmer AK: Fractures of the distal radius. In Green DP, editor: *Operative hand surgery,* ed 2, New York, 1993, Churchill Livingstone.

Palmer DH et al: Endoscopic carpal tunnel release, *Arthroscopy* 9:498, 1993.

Pap G et al: Evaluation of wrist and hand handicap and postoperative outcome in rheumatoid arthritis, *Hand Clin* 19(3):471-481, 2003.

Patten J: *Neurological differential diagnosis,* ed 2, London, 1996, Springer.

Pecina MM, Krmpotic-Nemanic J, Markiewitz AD: *Tunnel syndromes,* Boca Raton, Fla, 1991, CRC Press.

Pegoli L et al: The ishiguro extension block technique for the treatment of mallet finger fracture: indications and clinical results, *J Hand Surg* 28(1):15-17, 2003.

Perleik PC, Guilford WB: Magnetic resonance imaging to assess vascularity of scaphoid nonunions, *J Hand Surg* 16A:479, 1991.

Petrek JA, Heelan MC: Incidence of breast carcinoma-related lymphedema, *Cancer* 83(12 suppl II):2776-2781, 1998.

Phalen GS: The carpal-tunnel syndrome: seventeen years' experience in diagnosis and treatment of six hundred fifty-four hands, *J Bone Joint Surg* 48A:211, 1966.

Pheasant S: *Ergonomics, work and health,* Gaithersburg, Md, 1991, Aspen.

Pitner MA: Pathophysiology of overuse injuries in the hand and wrist, *Hand Clin* 6:355, 1990.

Porter JN: Raynaud's syndrome. In Sabiston DC Jr, editor: *Davis Christopher textbook of surgery,* Philadelphia, 1977, WB Saunders.

Protas JM, Jackson WT: Evaluating carpal instabilities with fluoroscopy, *AJR Am J Roentgenol* 135:137, 1980.

Resnick D, Niwayama G: *Diagnosis of bone and joint disorders,* Philadelphia, 1981, WB Saunders.

Royle SG: Compartment syndrome following forearm fracture in children, *Injury* 21:73, 1990.

Saidoff DC, McDonough AL: *Critical pathways in therapeutic intervention,* St Louis, 1997, Mosby.

Sampson SP, Wisch D, Badalamente MA: Complications of conservative and surgical treatment of de Quervain's disease and trigger fingers, *Hand Clin* 10:73, 1994.

Scheck M: Long-term follow up of treatment of comminuted fractures of the distal end of the radius by transfixation with Kirschner wires and cast, *J Bone Joint Surg* 44A:337, 1962.

Schiltenwolf M, Martini AK, Mau H: Measurement of intraosseous pressure in lunate necrosis, *J Hand Surg* 19(suppl 1):28-29, 1994.

Schumacher HR, Klippel JH, Koopman WJ: *Primer on the rheumatic diseases,* ed 10, Atlanta, 1993, Arthritis Foundation.

Sennwald G: *The wrist,* New York, 1990, Springer-Verlag.

Shankman GA: *Fundamental orthopedic management for the physical therapist assistant,* St Louis, 1997, Mosby.

Silver D: Circulatory problems of the upper extremity. In Sabiston DC Jr, editor: *Davis Christopher textbook of surgery,* Philadelphia, 1985, WB Saunders.

Skoff HD: "Postpartum/newborn" de Quervain's tenosynovitis of the wrist, *Am J Orthop* 30(5):428-430, 2001.

Smith KL, Harvey FJ, Stalley PD: Nonunion of a pathologic juvenile scaphoid fracture after osteomyelitis, *J Hand Surg* 16A:493, 1991.

Southmayd WW, Millender LH, Nalebuff EA: Rupture of the flexor tendons in the index finger after Colles' fracture case report, *J Bone Joint Surg* 57A:562, 1975.

Specht NT, Russo RD: *Practical guide to diagnostic imaging,* St Louis, 1998, Mosby.

Spencer PS: The traumatic neuroma and proximal stump, *Bull Hosp Joint Dis Orthop Inst* 35:85, 1974.

Spinner M: *Injuries of the major branches of peripheral nerves of the forearm,* Philadelphia, 1972, WB Saunders.

Stern PJ: Tendinitis, overuse syndromes, and tendon injuries, *Hand Clin* 6:467, 1990.

Stewart DL, Abeln SH: *Documenting functional outcomes in physical therapy,* St Louis, 1993, Mosby.

Stoller DW: *Magnetic resonance imaging in orthopaedics & sports medicine,* Philadelphia, 1993, JB Lippincott.

Strunk J et al: Three-dimensional Doppler sonographic vascular imaging in regions with increased MR enhancement in inflamed wrists of patients with rheumatoid arthritis, *Joint Bone Spine* 73(5):518-522, 2006.

Sugden P et al: Dermal dendrocytes in Dupuytren's disease: a link between the skin and pathogenesis? *J Hand Surg* 18B:662, 1993.

Sunderland S: *Nerves and nerve injuries,* Baltimore, 1968, Williams & Wilkins.

Sutton D, Young JWR: *A concise textbook of clinical imaging,* ed 2, St Louis, 1995, Mosby.

Swanson AB et al: Pathogenesis of rheumatoid deformities in the hand. In Cruess RL, Mitchell NS, editors: *Surgery of rheumatoid arthritis,* Philadelphia, 1971, JB Lippincott.

Swanson AB: Disabling arthritis at the base of the thumb: treatment by resection of the trapezium and flexible (silicone) implant arthroplasty, *J Bone Joint Surg* 54(3):456-471, 1972.

Taleisnik J: The ligaments of the wrist, *J Hand Surg* 1(2):110-118, 1976.

Taleisnik J: Rheumatoid arthritis of the wrist. In Strickland JW, Steichen JB, editors: *Difficult problems in hand surgery,* St Louis, 1982, Mosby.

Taleisnik J: The ligaments of the wrist, *J Hand Surg* 1A:110, 1976.

Tan JC, Horn SE: *Practical manual of physical medicine and rehabilitation,* St Louis, 1998, Mosby.

Taybi H, Lachman RS: *Radiology of syndromes, metabolic disorders, and skeletal dysplasias,* ed 4, St Louis, 1996, Mosby.

Thibodeau GA, Patton KT: *Anatomy & physiology,* ed 3, St Louis, 1996, Mosby.

Thibodeau GA, Patton KT: *Pocket reference to accompany anatomy & physiology,* ed 3, St Louis, 1996, Mosby.

Thompson JM: *Clinical outlines for health assessment,* St Louis, 1997, Mosby.

Thompson JS, Phelph TH: Repetitive strain injuries, how to deal with the epidemic of the 1990's, *Postgrad Med* 88:143, 1990.

Thorson E, Szabo RM: Common tendinitis problems in the hand and forearm, *Orthop Clin North Am* 23:65, 1992.

Tiel-van Buul MM et al: Radiography and scintigraphy of suspected scaphoid fracture, a long-term study in 160 patients, *J Bone Joint Surg* 75B:61, 1993.

Tiel-van Buul MM et al: Radiography of the carpal scaphoid, experimental evaluation of "the carpal box" and first clinical results, *Invest Radiol* 27:954, 1992.

Tinel J: *Nerve wounds: symptomatology of peripheral nerve lesions caused by war wounds (translated by F Rothwell; edited by CA Joll),* New York, 1918, William Wood.

Toghill PJ: *Examining patients: an introduction to clinical medicine,* London, 1990, Edward Arnold.

Tollison CD, Satterthwaite JR, Tollison JW: *Handbook of pain management,* ed 2, Baltimore, 1994, Williams & Wilkins.

Torg JS, Shepard RJ: *Current therapy in sports medicine,* ed 3, St Louis, 1995, Mosby.

Trumble TE, Benirschke SK, Vedder NB: Ipsilateral fractures of the scaphoid and radius, *J Hand Surg* 18A:8, 1993.

Tubiana R: *The hand,* Philadelphia, 1981, WB Saunders.

Turek SL: *Orthopaedics principles and their application,* ed 3, Philadelphia, 1977, JB Lippincott.

Turkcapar N et al: Late onset rheumatoid arthritis: clinical and laboratory comparisons with younger onset patients, *Arch Gerontol Geriatr* 42(2):225-231, 2006.

Urbaniak JR: Complication of treatment of carpal tunnel syndrome. In Gelberman RH, editor: *Operative nerve repair and reconstruction,* vol 2, Philadelphia, 1991, JB Lippincott.

US Preventative Services Task Force: *Guide to clinical preventive services,* ed 2, Alexandria, Va, 1996, International Medical Publishing.

Van Holsbeeck M, Introcaso JH: *Musculoskeletal ultrasound,* St Louis, 1991, Mosby.

Vance RM, Gelberman RH: Acute ulnar neuropathy with fractures at the wrist, *J Bone Joint Surg* 60A:962, 1978.

Vayssairat M et al: A new cold test for the diagnosis of Raynaud's phenomenon, *Ann Vasc Surg* 1(4):474-478, 1987.

Vidal MA et al: Preiser's disease, *Ann Chir Main Memb Super* 10:227, 1991.

Voche P, Merle M. Wartenberg's sign: a new method of surgical correction, *J Hand Surg* 20(1):49-52, 1995.

von Prince K, Butler B: Measuring sensory function of the hand in peripheral nerve injuries, *Am J Occup Ther* 21:385, 1967.

von Prince K: Occupational therapy's interest in function following peripheral nerve injury, *Med Bull US Army, Europe* 23:143, 1966.

Wakefield TS, Frank RG: *The clinicians guide to neuro musculoskeletal practice,* Abbotsford, Wisc, 1995, Allied Health of Wisconsin, S.C.

Warwick R, Williams PL: *Gray's anatomy,* Philadelphia, 1973, WB Saunders.

Watson HK, Ashmead D IV, Makhlouf MV: Examination of scaphoid, *J Hand Surg (Am)* 13(5):657-660, 1988.

Wavreille G et al: Anatomical bases of the second toe composite dorsal flap for simultaneous skin defect coverage and tendinous reconstruction of the dorsal aspect of the fingers, *J Plast Reconst Aesthet Surg* (in press, corrected proof).

Wehbe MA, Schneider LH: Mallet fractures, *J Bone Joint Surg* 66(5):658-669, 1984.

Weineck J: *Functional anatomy in sports,* ed 2, St Louis, 1990, Mosby.

Weinstein S: Tactile sensitivity of the phalanges, *Percept Mot Skills* 14:351, 1962.

Weinstein SL, Buckwalter JA: *Turek's orthopaedics principles and their application,* ed 5, Philadelphia, 1994, JB Lippincott.

Weiss AP, Steichen JB: Synovial sarcoma causing carpal tunnel syndrome, *J Hand Surg* 17A:1024, 1992.

Weiss A-PC, Akelman E, Tabatabai M: Treatment of de Quervain's disease, *J Hand Surg* 19A:595, 1994.

Werner JL, Omer GE Jr: Evaluating cutaneous pressure sensation of the hand, *Am J Occup Ther* 24:247, 1970.

Williams TM et al: Verification of the pressure provocative test in carpal tunnel syndrome, *Ann Plast Surg* 19:8, 1992.

Windsor RE, Lox DM: *Soft tissue injuries: diagnosis and treatment,* Philadelphia, 1998, Hanley & Belfus.

Witczak JW, Masear VR, Meyer RD: Triggering of the thumb with de Quervain's stenosing tendovaginitis, *J Hand Surg* 15A:265, 1990.

Witt J, Pess G, Gelberman RH: Treatment of de Quervain's tenosynovitis: a prospect study of the results of injection of steroids and immobilization in a splint, *J Bone Joint Surg* 73A:219, 1991.

Wu WC, Wong TC, Yip TH: Chronic finger joint instability reconstructed with bone-ligament-bone graft from the iliac crest, *J Hand Surg* 29(5):494-501, 2004.

Wynn-Parry CB: *Rehabilitation of the hand,* ed 3, London, 1973, Butterworth.

Xiao Y, Zhang G, Zuo X: Diagnostic value of high-resolution ultrasonography for imaging of the knee, elbow and wrist joints in rheumatoid arthritis, *Ultrasound Med Biol* 32(5, suppl 1):P253-P268, 2006.

Yacoe ME et al: Dupuytren's contracture: MR imaging findings and correlation between MR signal intensity and cellularity of lesions, *AJR Am J Roentgenol* 160:813, 1993.

Yazaki N et al: Bilateral Kienböck's disease, *J Hand Surg* 30(2):133-136, 2005.

Yosipovitch G et al: Trigger finger in young patients with insulin dependent diabetes, *J Rheumatol* 17:951, 1990.

Younger CP, DeFiore JC: Rupture of the flexor tendons to the fingers after a Colles' fracture: a case report, *J Bone Joint Surg* 59A:828, 1977.

Zangger P et al: Assessing damage in individual joints in rheumatoid arthritis: a new method based on the Larsen system, *Joint Bone Spine* 71(5):389-396, 2004.

Zoega H: Fracture of the lower end of the radius with ulnar nerve palsy, *J Bone Joint Surg* 48V:514, 1966.

6

CITATIONS

Ankarath S: Chronic wrist pain: diagnosis and management, *Curr Orthop* 20(2):141-151, 2006.

Bhaskaranand K, Navadgi BC: Glomus tumour of the hand, *J Hand Surg* 27(3):229-231, 2002.

Bushnell BD et al: Management of intra-articular metacarpal base fractures of the second through fifth metacarpals, *J Hand Surg* 33(4):573-583, 2008.

Carlson N, Logigian EL: Radial neuropathy, *Neurol Clin* 17(3):499-523, 1999.

Carroll RE, Berman AT: Glomus tumors of the hand: review of the literature and report on twenty-eight cases, *J Bone Joint Surg* 54(4):691-703, 1972.

Chin DHCL, Meals RA: Anterior interosseous nerve syndrome, *J Am Soc Surg Hand* 1(4):249-257, 2001.

Chiodo A, Chadd E: Ulnar neuropathy at or distal to the wrist: traumatic versus cumulative stress cases, *Arch Phys Med Rehabil* 88(4):504-512, 2007.

Dell PC, Sforzo CR: Ulnar intrinsic anatomy and dysfunction, *J Hand Ther* 18(2):198-207, 2005.

Eaton RG, Glickel SZ: Trapeziometacarpal osteoarthritis: staging as a rationale for treatment, *Hand Clin* 3:455-469, 1987.

Ganapathy K, Winston T, Seshadri V: Posterior interosseous nerve palsy due to intermuscular lipoma, *Surg Neurol* 65(5):495-496, 2006.

Gelberman RH, Menon J: The vascularity of the scaphoid bone, *J Hand Surg* 5(5):508-513, 1980.

Gross PT, Tolomeo EA: Proximal median neuropathies, *Neurol Clin* 17(3):425-445, 1999.

Hoii E G-EM et al: A kinematic study of luno-triquetral dissociations, *J Hand Surg* 16A:355-362, 1991.

Imai H, Tajima T, Natsuma Y: Interpretation of cutaneous pressure threshold (Semmes-Weinstein monofilament measurement) following median nerve repair and sensory reeducation in the adult, *Microsurgery* 10(2):142-144, 1989.

Irlenbusch U, Schaller T: Investigations in generalized osteoarthritis. Part 1: genetic study of Heberden's nodes, *Osteoarthr Cartil* 14(5):423-427, 2006.

Jeon I-H et al: Tardy ulnar nerve palsy in cubitus varus deformity associated with ulnar nerve dislocation in adults, *J Shoulder Elbow Surg* 15(4):474-478, 2006.

La Hei N et al: Scaphoid bone bruising—probably not the precursor of asymptomatic non-union of the scaphoid. *J Hand Surg* (in press, corrected proof).

Lamas C et al: The anatomy and vascularity of the lunate: considerations applied to Kienböck's disease, *Chirurgie de la Main* 26(1):13-20, 2007.

Lin JT, Stubblefield MD: de Quervain's tenosynovitis in patients with lymphedema: a report of 2 cases with management approach, *Arch Phys Med Rehabil* 84(10):1554-1557, 2003.

Ly JQ et al: MRI diagnosis of occult ganglion compression of the posterior interosseous nerve and associated supinator muscle pathology, *Clin Imaging* 29(5):362-363, 2005.

Manning DC: Reflex sympathetic dystrophy, sympathetically maintained pain, and complex regional pain syndrome: diagnoses of inclusion, exclusion, or confusion? *J Hand Ther* 13(4):260-268, 2000.

Mazet RHM Jr: Conservative treatment of old fractures of the carpal scaphoid, *J Trauma* 1:115-127, 1961.

Merritt WH: The challenge to manage reflex sympathetic dystrophy/complex regional pain syndrome, *Clin Plast Surg* 32(4):575-604, 2005.

Natsis K et al: Three-headed reversed palmaris longus muscle and its clinical significance, *Ann Anat Anatomischer Anzeiger* 189(1):97-101, 2007.

Newmeyer WL, Manske PR: No man's land revisited: the primary flexor tendon repair controversy, *J Hand Surg* 29(1): 1-5, 2004; with quote from Bunnell S: *Surgery of the hand*, ed 3, Philadelphia, 1956, JB Lippincott.

Oberlin C et al: Hourglass-like constriction of the axillary nerve: report of two patients, *J Hand Surg* 31(7):1100-1104, 2006.

Paul F et al: Combined ulnar nerve palsy in Guyon's canal and distal median nerve irritation following excessive canoeing, *Clin Neurophysiol* 118(4):e81-e82, 2007.

Reagan DS, Linscheid RL, Dobyns JH: Lunotriquetral sprains, *J Hand Surg* 9(4):502-514, 1984.

Ross HE: Tactile sensory anisotropy: Weber's contribution. *J Exp Psychol Hum Percept Perform* 25(4):1159-1161, 1999.

Ruijs AC et al: Cold intolerance following median and ulnar nerve injuries: prognosis and predictors, *J Hand Surg Eur Vol* (in press, corrected proof).

Sternbach G: The carpal tunnel syndrome, *J Emerg Med* 17(3):519-523, 1999.

Teoh LC, Lee JYL: Mallet fractures: a novel approach to internal fixation using a hook plate, *J Hand Surg* 32(1):24-30, 2007.

Troy KL, Grabiner MD: Off-axis loads cause failure of the distal radius at lower magnitudes than axial loads: a finite element analysis, *J Biomech* (in press, corrected proof).

Tsai N, Kirkham S: Fingertip skin wrinkling—the effect of varying tonicity, *J Hand Surg* 30(3):273-275, 2005.

Weber ER, Chao EY: An experimental approach to the mechanism of scaphoid waist fractures, *J Hand Surg* 3(2):142-148, 1978.

CHAPTER SEVEN

THORACIC SPINE

AXIOMS IN ASSESSING THE THORACIC SPINE

- The thoracic spine requires evaluation in isolation and in combination with the cervical and lumbar spine.
- Thoracic pain can be perplexing and difficult to diagnose.
- The most commonly involved spinal area is the transitional thoracolumbar junction.

INTRODUCTION

Thoracic spinal pain and dysfunction present a particularly challenging clinical dilemma. Thoracic spinal pain may arise from somatic and visceral origins. Pain felt along the thoracic spine may arise from the ribs, the abdomen, or the vertebral column.

The thoracic spine is the part of the vertebral column that is most rigid because of the rib cage. The rib cage, in turn, provides protection for the heart and lungs.

Thoracic pain can occur as a referred visceral symptom, radiating from the chest and abdomen. The pain may also appear as a symptom of musculoskeletal origin. Sudden pain in the thoracic region occurs less often than in the more mobile cervical and lumbar spines.

The structure of the thorax as a whole is such that overall motion of this portion of the spine is limited.

Added to the bony and discal stabilizing influences of the thoracic spine are the muscles supporting the spinal column.

ORTHOPEDIC GAMUT 7-1
THORACIC AREA PAIN

Diagnostic keys for thoracic area pain include the following:
1. Identify postural strain syndromes.
2. Identify radicular syndromes.
3. Always check for myelopathy.

ORTHOPEDIC GAMUT 7-2
MECHANICAL SPINAL SYNDROME CLASSIFICATIONS

1. Posture syndrome. Pain arises as a result of mechanical deformation of normal soft tissues from prolonged end-range loading of periarticular structures.
2. Dysfunction syndrome. Pain occurs as a result of mechanical deformation of structurally impaired tissues (scarred, adhered, or adaptively shortened tissue).
3. Derangement syndrome. Pain occurs as a result of a disturbance in the normal resting position of the affected joint surfaces.
4. Other. Patient exhibits signs and symptoms of other known abnormality (i.e., spinal stenosis, hip disorders, sacroiliac disorders, low back pain in pregnancy, zygapophyseal disorders, spondylolysis and spondylolisthesis, and postsurgical problems).

Adapted from Hefford C: McKenzie classification of mechanical spinal pain: profile of syndromes and directions of preference, *Man Ther* 13(1): 75-81, 2008.

The thoracic spinal column serves as the attachment for many of the muscles of the trunk, shoulder, and arm.

Among these muscles are the trapezius and latissimus dorsi. The deeper muscles of the trunk include the levator scapulae, rhomboid major, and rhomboid minor. Still deeper are the sacrospinalis muscle groups, which include the spinalis dorsi, longissimus dorsi, and the iliocostalis lumborum.

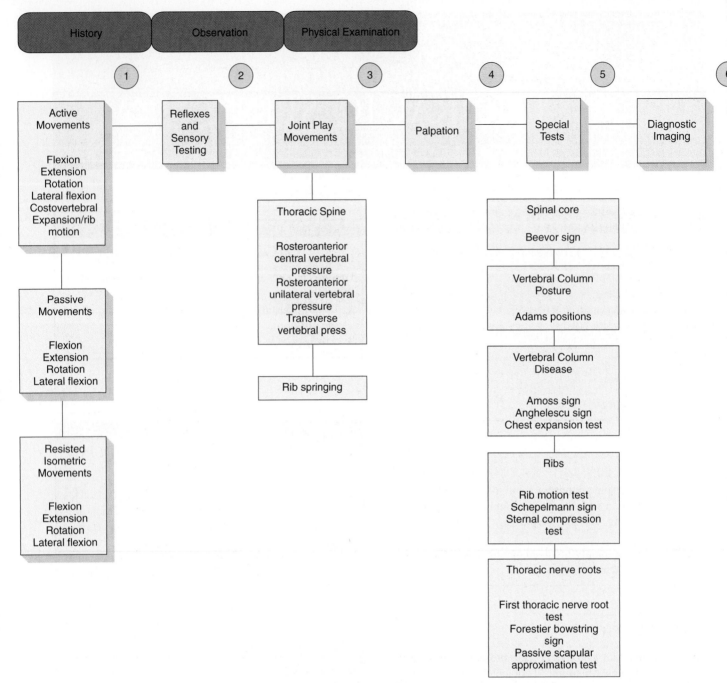

FIG. 7-1 Thoracic spine assessment.

During an examination of the thorax and thoracic spine, the assessment is primarily of the thoracic spine. The examination is extensive. Without a history of specific trauma or injury to the thoracic spine, the examiner must be prepared to assess the other implicated tissues. For problems superior to the thoracic spine, a thorough examination of the cervical spine and upper limb is a part of the examination scheme. If a problem exists inferior to the thoracic spine, the examination of the lumbar spine and lower limb is completed.

The shape of the spine and its structural relationship to the shoulder girdle, thorax, and pelvis should be assessed.

The normal spinal curvatures are concave at the cervical area, convex at the thoracic area, and concave at the lumbar area. Any differences in heights of the shoulders and the iliac crests should be noted. Unusual heights of the iliac crests suggest uneven leg lengths. Variations in spinal curvature may indicate a structural problem. Scoliosis is a deformity of the spine that appears as a lateral deviation (Fig. 7-2). The normal anteroposterior curve needs to be assessed as well (Fig. 7-3, *A*). Kyphosis is a flexion deformity (Fig. 7-3, *B*). When the angle of the defect is sharp, the apex is called a *gibbus*. Lordosis (swayback) is an extension deviation of the spine, commonly in the lumbar area (Fig. 7-3, *C*).

TABLE 7-1

THORACIC SPINE CROSS-REFERENCE TABLE BY ASSESSMENT PROCEDURE

Thoracic Spine Test/Sign	Scoliosis	Ankylosing Spondylitis	Intervertebral Disc Syndrome	Sprain	Tuberculosis	Myelopathy	T1-T2 Nerve Root	Rib Injury	Intercostal Syndrome	Fracture	Strain	Fibrositis
Adams positions	•											
Amoss sign		•	•	•								
Anghelescu sign					•							
Beevor sign						•						
Chest expansion test		•										
First thoracic nerve root test							•					
Forestier bowstring sign		•										
Passive scapular approximation test							•					
Rib motion test		•						•	•			
Schepelmann sign								•	•			
Spinal percussion test			•	•						•	•	
Sponge test												•
Sternal compression test								•				

7

TABLE 7-2

THORACIC SPINE CROSS-REFERENCE TABLE BY SYNDROME OR TISSUE

Ankylosing spondylitis	Amoss sign
	Chest expansion test
	Forestier bowstring sign
	Rib motion test
Fibrositis	Sponge test
Fracture	Spinal percussion test
Intercostal syndrome	Rib motion test
	Schepelmann sign
Intervertebral disc syndrome	Amoss sign
	Spinal percussion test
Myelopathy	Beevor sign
Rib injury	Rib motion test
	Schepelmann sign
	Sternal compression test
Scoliosis	Adams positions
Sprain	Amoss sign
	Spinal percussion test
Strain	Spinal percussion test
T1–T2 nerve root	First thoracic nerve root test
	Passive scapular approximation test
Tuberculosis	Anghelescu sign

ORTHOPEDIC GAMUT 7-3

THORACIC SPINE

Stabilizing influences for the thoracic spine include the following:

- The first element is the vertebral articular process. The interlocking arrangement of the thoracic facets prevents anterior displacement of the vertebra and forms the imbrication of the thoracic spine.
- The second primary stabilizing influence of the thoracic spine is the vertebral body. At the posterior of the vertebral bodies, the height of the body is greater than in the anterior. This circumstance contributes to the thoracic spine kyphosis.
- The third stabilizing influence is the structure of the ribs and their attachments to the spine. The ribs help stiffen the thoracic spine.
- The fourth primary stabilizing influence for the thoracic spine is the structure of the intervertebral disc. The thoracic spine intervertebral discs are more narrow and thin than in the cervical or lumbar spines. They are also less elastic than all the other disc tissues of the spine.

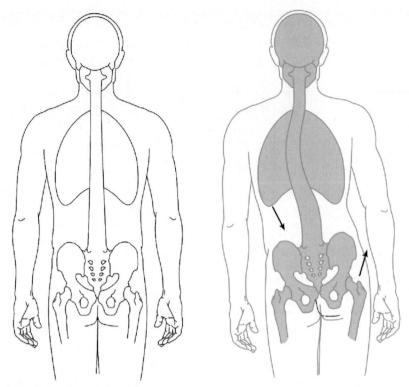

FIG. 7-2 Deformity of the spine. (From Barkauskas VH et al: *Health & physical assessment,* ed 2, St Louis, 1998, Mosby.)

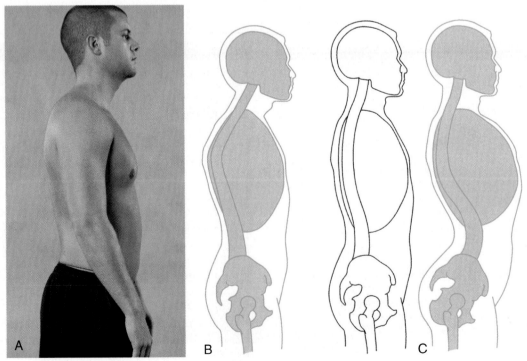

FIG. 7-3 **A,** Normal curvature of the spine. **B,** Kyphosis. **C,** Lordosis and extension deformity of the spine. (From Barkauskas VH et al: *Health & physical assessment,* ed 2, St Louis, 1998, Mosby.)

ESSENTIAL ANATOMY

The thoracic spine consists of 12 thoracic vertebrae. They are characterized by down-swept spines, prominent transverse processes, and heart-shaped bodies, and they are unique in articulating with the normal 12 pairs of ribs. Ribs 1 to 10 articulate both with the vertebral body and with its transverse process. Ribs 11 and 12 articulate only with the vertebral body and are not jointed to the transverse processes on these vertebrae. The thoracic spine and the ribs are intimately related to many neural, vascular, and visceral structures (Figs. 7-4 and 7-5). Each intercostal nerve (and the subcostal and upper two lumbar nerves) sends a white ramus communicans to the sympathetic ganglion of the same level. Each intercostal nerve provides sensory, motor (somatic motor), and sympathetic (visceral motor to blood vessels and sweat glands) innervation to the thoracic or abdominal wall.

ESSENTIAL MOTION ASSESSMENT

The facets of the thoracic vertebrae are oriented 60 degrees to the horizontal plane. These facets are more vertically oriented than the articular processes of the cervical region. This vertical orientation dramatically limits forward flexion (Fig. 7-6). Extension is limited by the inferior articular processes contacting the laminae of the vertebrae below and by contact between adjacent spinous processes. Rotation is the dominant movement in the thoracic region.

ESSENTIAL MUSCLE FUNCTION ASSESSMENT

In addition to the bony and discal stabilizing influences of the thoracic spine are muscles that support the spinal column. The thoracic spinal column serves as the attachment for many of the muscles of the trunk, shoulder, and arm.

FIG. 7-4 Relationship of the vertebrae and the ribs to the vessels and nerves of the thorax. (From Cramer GD, Darby SA: *Basic and clinical anatomy of the spine, spinal cord, and ANS,* St Louis, 1995, Mosby.)

ORTHOPEDIC GAMUT 7-4

THORACOLUMBAR SPINE

To assess range of motion of the thoracolumbar spine, the patient is directed to do the following:

1. Slowly bend forward at the waist and try to touch the toes (while observed for scoliosis) (Figs. 7-7 and 7-8).
2. Bend back as far as possible (hyperextending the spine) (Fig. 7-9).
3. Bend to the right and left side as far as possible (lateral bending with the pelvis stabilized) (Fig. 7-10).
4. Turn to the right and left in a circular motion (with the pelvis stabilized) (Figs. 7-11 and 7-12).

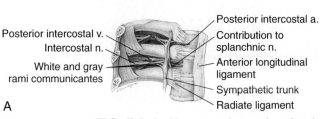
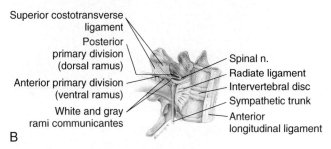

FIG. 7-5 **A,** Nerves and vessels related to three adjacent vertebrae and the ribs that articulate with them. **B,** Close-up of the nerves associated with a single thoracic motion segment. (From Cramer GD, Darby SA: *Basic and clinical anatomy of the spine, spinal cord, and ANS,* St Louis, 1995, Mosby.)

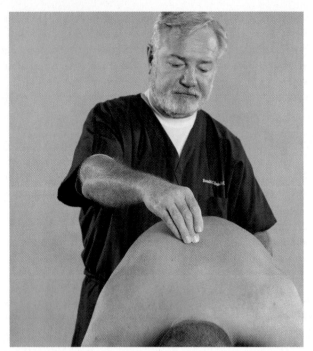

FIG. 7-6 Palpation of the spinal processes as the patient bends forward.

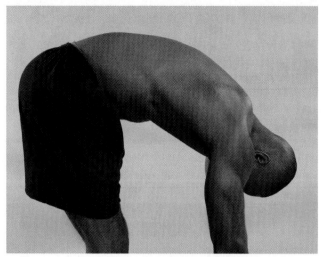

FIG. 7-7 Flexion range of motion in the thoracic spine is 20 to 45 degrees. In an indirect measurement of the thoracic range of motion, the length of the spine from the C7 spinous process to the T12 spinous process is measured. The patient bends forward, and the spine is again measured. A minimum of a 2.7-cm difference is considered normal. A measurement from the C7 spinous process to S1 can also be made. The spine is measured a second time with the patient bending. A minimum of a 10-cm difference is normal. Alternatively, the patient bends forward attempting to touch the toes. The patient tries to keep the knees straight. The distance from the patient's fingertips to the floor is assessed.

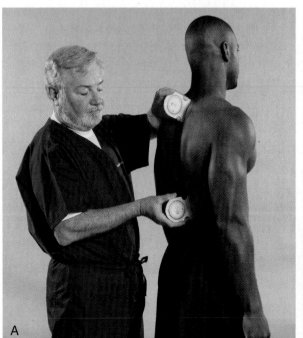

A

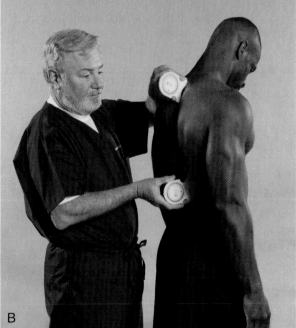

B

FIG. 7-8 For testing flexion with an inclinometer, the patient is seated or standing. One inclinometer is placed in the sagittal plane at the T1 level and the other at the T12 level, also in the sagittal plane (**A**). Both instruments are zeroed. If seated, the patient places the hands on the hips, and if standing, the patient crosses the arms in front of the chest. The thoracic spine is flexed forward so as not to involve lumbar spine motion (**B**). Both instrument readings are recorded. The T12 value is subtracted from the T1 value to arrive at the thoracic flexion angle. Retained flexion of the thoracic spine of 30 degrees or less is an impairment of the thoracic spine in the activities of daily living.

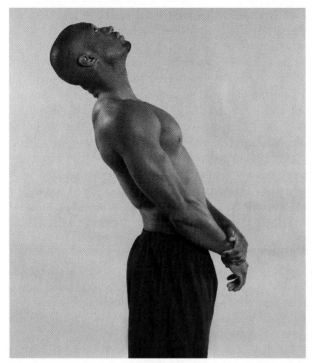

FIG. 7-9 Extension in the thoracic spine is normally 25 to 35 degrees. The distance between C7 and T12 spinous processes is determined with a tape measure. A minimum of a 2.5-cm difference in tape measure length between standing and extension is normal.

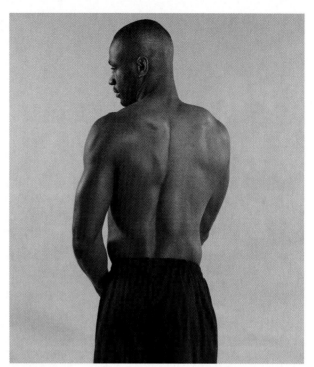

FIG. 7-11 Rotation in the thoracic spine is approximately 35 to 50 degrees. The patient rotates to the right or left. The examiner assesses the amount of rotation, comparing both ways.

7

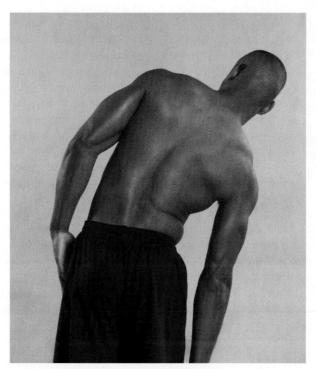

FIG. 7-10 Lateral flexion is approximately 20 to 40 degrees to the right and left. For accuracy of movement, the patient runs a hand down the side of the leg, without bending forward or backward. The distance from the fingertips to the floor is measured. The measurements are compared bilaterally. The distances should be equal.

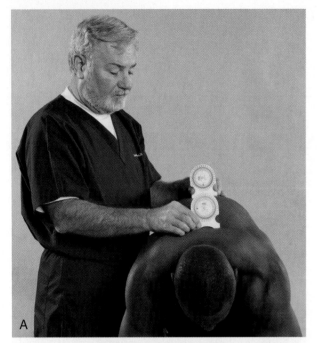

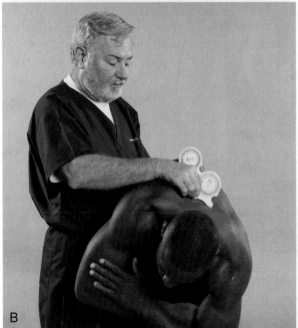

FIG. 7-12 When an inclinometer is used to assess thoracic spinal rotation, the patient is standing. The patient is flexed forward. The patient may brace the position with the arms. One inclinometer is placed at the T1 level in the coronal plane and the other at the T12 level, also in the coronal plane (**A**). Both instruments are zeroed. The patient rotates to one side and the angles indicated on both instruments are recorded (**B**). The T12 measurement is subtracted from the T1 measurement to arrive at the thoracic rotation angle. The measurements are repeated for rotation to the opposite side. Retained active rotation of the thoracic spine of 20 degrees or less is an impairment of the function of the thoracic spine in the activities of daily living.

Among these muscles are the trapezius and latissimus dorsi. The deeper muscles of the trunk include the levator scapulae, rhomboid major, and rhomboid minor. Still deeper are the sacrospinalis muscle groups, which include the spinalis dorsi, longissimus dorsi, and iliocostalis lumborum.

The trapezius muscle attaches to the spinous processes from the upper cervical to the lower thoracic spine. In the lower part, the muscle overlaps the long attachment of the latissimus dorsi muscle.

The latissimus dorsi muscle attaches to the spinous processes, beginning in the mid thoracic region, and extends to the pelvis. The trapezius and latissimus dorsi are the two most superficial muscles of the back. In addition to movement, these muscles also serve to enclose the deeper muscle layers.

The deeper muscles are broad and flat and are not as frequently subjected to injury. These muscles are the levator scapulae, rhomboid major, and rhomboid minor. They lie under the trapezius, in the upper portion of the dorsal spine. The muscles extend down toward the level of the upper limit of the latissimus dorsi.

Still deeper are the muscles that run from the spine to the pelvis and form the sacrospinalis group. This group is a combination of many muscles, the course of which parallels the spinal column. The sacrospinalis group of muscles includes the spinalis dorsi, longissimus dorsi, and iliocostalis lumborum.

The sacrospinalis group fills the sulcus between the spinous processes, the bodies of the vertebrae, and the arc of the ribs. This group of muscles interdigitates in such a manner that each muscle supports the others. These muscles make up the lumbar mass of muscles that extends from the occiput to the sacrum and laterally to the spinous processes.

These muscles have multiple actions depending on the relationship between them. One muscle may serve to stabilize the spine while another muscle member moves.

The back extensors are the most important of all the trunk muscles. Several reasons exist as to why abdominal muscles are discussed in detail in literature and back extensors have little emphasis. Weakness of the lower back musculature is seldom encountered except in paralytic cases. The incidence among nonparalytic or so-called *normal* individuals is probably less than 1%.

On the other hand, abdominal muscle weakness is commonly encountered. Parts of the abdominal muscles can be tested separately, but the back extensors can be tested only as a group.

During the trunk extension test, the latissimus dorsi, quadratus lumborum, and trapezius assist back extensors. The head and neck extensor muscles and the hip extensors should be tested before the back extensors are tested (Fig. 7-13).

ESSENTIAL IMAGING

Several radiographic views have been frequently described to evaluate the osseous and soft-tissue anatomy of the thoracic spine. Frontal (anteroposterior [AP]) (Figs. 7-14 and 7-15), lateral (left) (Figs. 7-16 to 7-18), and *swimmer's* views (Figs. 7-19 to 7-24) are the standard evaluation projections (Fig. 7-25).

Although plain-film radiographs are generally unreliable in the early detection and assessment of osteoporosis, plain-film findings of osteoporosis can be a helpful adjunct to the diagnosis. The trabecular bone becomes sparse, resulting in overall reduction in bone density. Nontraumatic compression deformities are a sure sign that bone density is compromised.

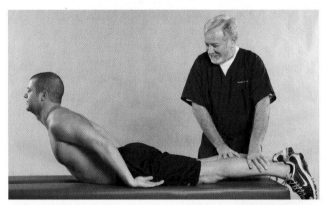

FIG. 7-13 The patient is prone. The hip extensors must be given fixation of the pelvis to the thighs, and the examiner must stabilize the legs firmly on the examining table. The patient then attempts trunk extension. The ability to complete spine extension and hold against strong pressure with hands clasped behind the head is normal. The ability to perform this only with the hands behind the back is good. If performed only with the hands clasped behind the back, the ability to lift the thorax so that the xiphoid process of the sternum is raised slightly from the table is fair. When marked weakness is present, such weakness usually extends throughout the back. If cervical extensors can lift the head, a head-raising movement can furnish slight resistance against other back extensors. When the lower back is strong and the upper back is weak, an attempt to raise the thorax will result in the back extensors extending the lower back by anteriorly tilting the pelvis, but the thorax will not be lifted from the table.

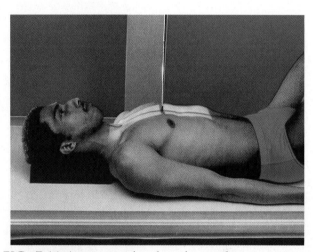

FIG. 7-14 Anteroposterior thoracic vertebrae. (From Frank ED, et al: *Merrill's atlas of radiographic positioning and procedures,* vol 1-3, ed 11, St Louis, 2007, Mosby.)

7

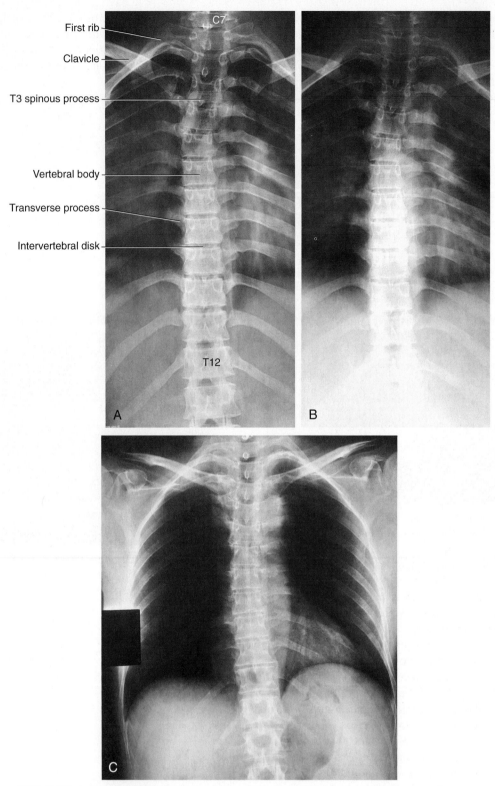

First rib

Clavicle

T3 spinous process

Vertebral body

Transverse process

Intervertebral disk

C7

T12

A

B

C

FIG. 7-15 Anteroposterior thoracic views of the thorax. (From Frank ED et al: *Merrill's atlas of radiographic positioning and procedures,* vol 1-3, ed 11, St Louis, 2007, Mosby.)

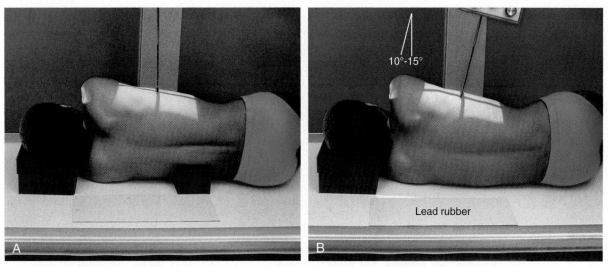

FIG. 7-16 Recumbent lateral thoracic spine. (From Frank ED et al: *Merrill's atlas of radiographic positioning and procedures,* vol 1-3, ed 11, St Louis, 2007, Mosby.)

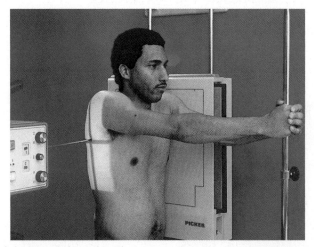

FIG. 7-17 Upright lateral thoracic spine. (From Frank ED et al: *Merrill's atlas of radiographic positioning and procedures,* vol 1-3, ed 11, St Louis, 2007, Mosby.)

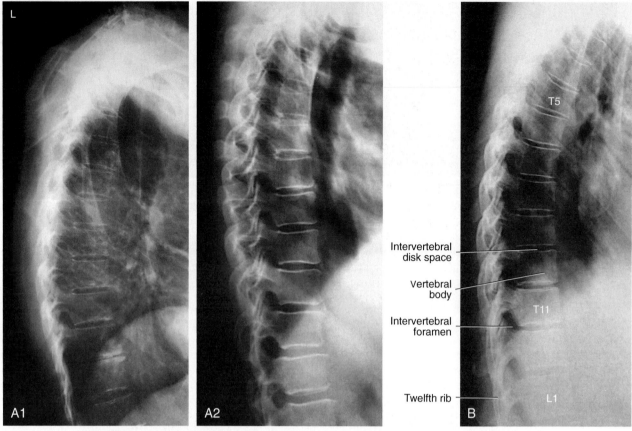

FIG. 7-18 Lateral thoracic spine. (From Frank ED et al: *Merrill's atlas of radiographic positioning and procedures,* vol 1-3, ed 11, St Louis, 2007, Mosby.)

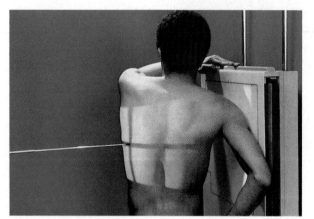

FIG. 7-19 Posteroanterior oblique zygapophyseal joints (Z-joints). (From Frank ED et al: *Merrill's atlas of radiographic positioning and procedures,* vol 1-3, ed 11, St Louis, 2007, Mosby.)

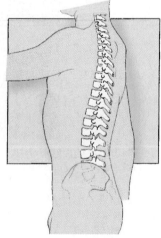

FIG. 7-20 Posteroanterior oblique Z-joints, right anterior oblique for joints closest to film. (From Frank ED et al: *Merrill's atlas of radiographic positioning and procedures,* vol 1-3, ed 11, St Louis, 2007, Mosby.)

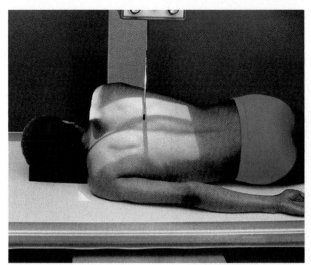

FIG. 7-21 Posteroanterior oblique Z-joints, left anterior oblique for joints closest to film. (From Frank ED et al: *Merrill's atlas of radiographic positioning and procedures,* vol 1-3, ed 11, St Louis, 2007, Mosby.)

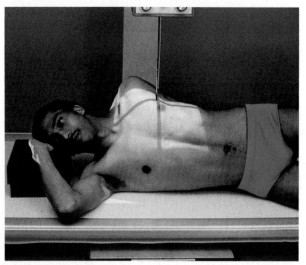

FIG. 7-22 Anteroposterior oblique Z-joints, right posterior oblique for joints farthest from film. (From Frank ED et al: *Merrill's atlas of radiographic positioning and procedures,* vol 1-3, St Louis, 2007, Mosby.)

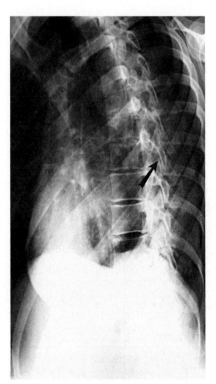

FIG. 7-23 Upright posteroanterior oblique Z-joints. (From Frank ED et al: *Merrill's atlas of radiographic positioning and procedures,* vol 1-3, ed 11, St Louis, 2007, Mosby.)

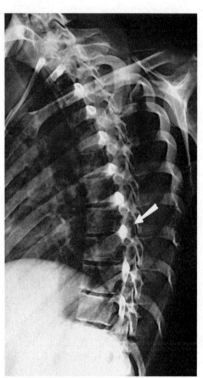

FIG. 7-24 Recumbent anteroposterior oblique Z-joints. (From Frank ED et al: *Merrill's atlas of radiographic positioning and procedures,* vol 1-3, ed 11, St Louis, 2007, Mosby.)

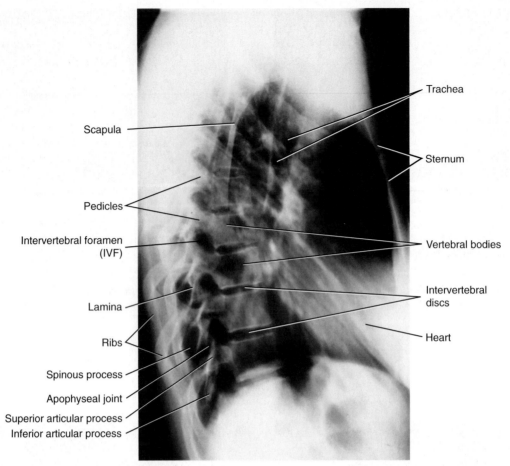

Scapula

Trachea

Sternum

Pedicles

Intervertebral foramen
(IVF)

Vertebral bodies

Intervertebral
discs

Lamina

Ribs

Heart

Spinous process

Apophyseal joint

Superior articular process

Inferior articular process

FIG. 7-25 Lateral radiographic view of the thoracic spine and ribs. (From Greenstein GM: *Clinical assessment of neuromusculoskeletal disorders,* St Louis, 1997, Mosby.)

ORTHOPEDIC GAMUT 7-5

VERTEBRAL COMPRESSION DEFORMITIES

Compression deformities of vertebrae may take several shapes:

1. An isolated central end-plate impression may be present.
2. Biconcave end-plate deformities may be present.
3. The segment may lose anterior vertebral body height with maintenance of the end-plate integrity.
4. The segment may demonstrate loss of anterior and posterior vertebral body height.
5. Fractures of the ribs are quite common.

Assessment for Pathologic or Structural Scoliosis

Comment

The spinal column centers the mass of the torso and head in a line along the vertical axis that falls through the pelvis. Disturbances of the spine, such as the curvatures associated with scoliosis, may significantly alter the normal balance and coordination of the spine (Table 7-3).

Scoliosis, or lateral curvature of the spine, may be idiopathic, congenital, or neuromuscular in origin. Idiopathic scoliosis is responsible for 85% to 95% of all cases of scoliosis. Infantile idiopathic scoliosis spans the ages of 0 to 3 years.

Infantile scoliosis is unique in many ways. It is more commonly seen in boys and usually produces a curve convex to the left; the curve is generally located in the thoracic and thoracolumbar regions. Most curves develop within the first 6 months of life. The frequently resolving thoracic and thoracolumbar curves account for 85% of all infantile curves, whereas double structural curves with a thoracic component tend to be progressive, leading to severe deformities. Also observed is that right-sided thoracic curves in girls have a worse prognosis. Associated anomalies often include plagio-

cephaly (cranial molding), bat-ear deformity, congenital muscular torticollis, and developmental hip dysplasia (Dobbs, Weinstein, 1999).

Juvenile idiopathic scoliosis occurs in patients ages 4 to 10 years, and adolescent idiopathic scoliosis occurs in patients older than 10 years (Fig. 7-26).

Juvenile idiopathic scoliosis is defined by detection of the scoliosis deformity in patients between 4 and 10 years of age; it represents 12% to 21% of patients with idiopathic scoliosis. The cause remains unknown and may differ depending on age of presentation. Because juvenile and adolescent scoliosis appear to be more closely related to each other than to infantile scoliosis, theories regarding the cause of adolescent scoliosis also may be applicable to juvenile scoliosis. A variety of neuromuscular theories has been offered, ranging from proposed posterior column spinal cord dysfunction to central nervous system processing abnormalities. A neurohormonal theory also has been advanced suggesting a pineal gland abnormality resulting in deficiency of certain neurotransmitters. In addition, several reports have been published of an increased familial occurrence of juvenile idiopathic scoliosis, similar to that reported in adolescent idiopathic scoliosis (Dobbs, Weinstein, 1999).

A slight lateral curve with the convexity on the same side as handedness (i.e., convexity to the left in left-handed indi-

TABLE 7-3

THORACIC SPINE SYNDROMES

	Sprain or Strain	Vertebral Subluxation	Scoliosis	Scheuermann's Disease
Physical examination findings	Palpable tenderness over intervertebral joint Supraspinous ligament tenderness Pain on twisting, cervical flexion, or extreme extension Paraspinal myospasm or hypertonicity	Pain over spinous process or supraspinous ligament Flexion or extension fixation; malposition Loss of normal springy end-feel Alteration of normal muscle or joint physiologic response	Structural deformity, such as hip or pelvis unleveling, leg length discrepancy, posterior scapula, high shoulder Muscular asymmetry and unilateral hypertonicity Lateral curvature of spine Chronologic age versus skeletal maturity	Kyphotic deformity of dorsal spine Rigid musculature of thoracic spine Discomfort of back in growing children and adolescents Tight anterior shoulder girdle and thorax
X-ray findings	Usually unremarkable	Normal Need to rule out concomitant mechanical factors that can delay recovery	Lateral deviation of spine (D1 to S1 view)	End-plate irregularity, abnormal vertebral ossification patterns, anterior plate or body deformity, involvement of three or more vertebral bodies More than 40-45 degrees of kyphosis

Modified from Brier SR: *Primary care orthopedics*, St Louis, 1999, Mosby.

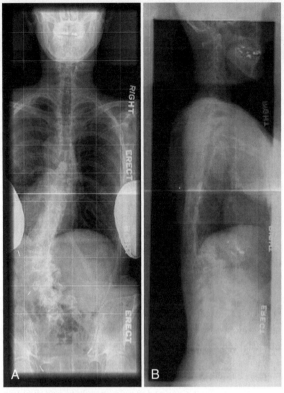

FIG. 7-26 Scoliosis. (From Brier SR: *Primary care orthopedics,* St Louis, Mosby, 1999.)

ORTHOPEDIC GAMUT 7-6

SCOLIOSIS

Scoliosis predictive indexing:

1. Curves less than 20 degrees will improve spontaneously more than 50% of the time.
2. No accurate method is available to help predict which curves will improve or worsen.
3. In curves of less than 30 degrees, 20% will progress.
4. Progression is more common in young children, at the beginning of their growth spurt.
5. The larger the curve at detection, the greater the chance of progression.
6. Curves in female patients and double curves in male or female patients are more likely to progress.
7. Scoliosis is more common in female patients than in male patients (idiopathic); 9 : 1 ratio.

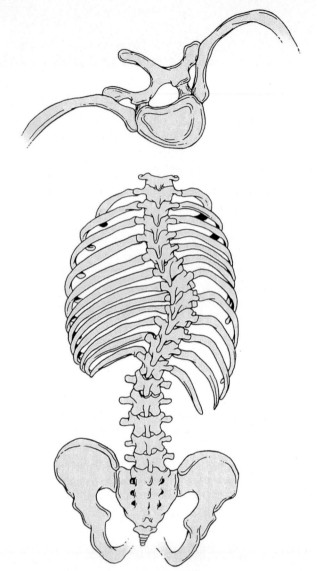

FIG. 7-27 Posterior view of a scoliotic spine. (From Cramer GD, Darby SA: *Basic and clinical anatomy of the spine, spinal cord, and ANS,* St Louis, 1995, Mosby.)

---

viduals) is normally found in the upper thoracic region (Fig. 7-27). The diagnosis is usually made on routine physical examination. Attention should be focused on the problem in all children, but especially in those between the ages of 10 and 14 years, when spinal growth is most rapid (Fig. 7-28). The diagnosis is confirmed by a standing plain-film study of the spine (Fig. 7-29). Pathologic anomalies at birth are responsible for scoliosis in some individuals. The problem usually results from a *failure of formation* (Fig. 7-30).

Scoliosis is also classified as either structural or nonstructural. Structural curves are fixed and nonflexible and fail to correct with side bending. Nonstructural curves, on the other hand, are flexible and readily correct with side bending. The Lenke Classification System helps examiners develop a more complete picture of the patient's condition by understanding the scoliosis as multidimensional and considering it from more than one view. The Lenke classification method also gives more detailed shorthand for communicating about scoliosis in professional settings, using a widely understood set of criteria (Table 7-4).

Side-bending radiographs have been the gold standard technique by which spinal flexibility is assessed. In the Lenke Classification System for adolescent idiopathic scoliosis

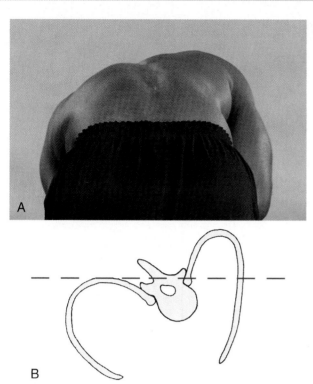

FIG. 7-28 **A,** Scoliosis with rib prominence from vertebral rotation is best exhibited on forward bending. **B,** Cross-section of the chest showing rib distortion from vertebral rotation. (From Mercier LR, Pettid FJ: *Practical orthopedics,* ed 4, St Louis, 1995, Mosby.)

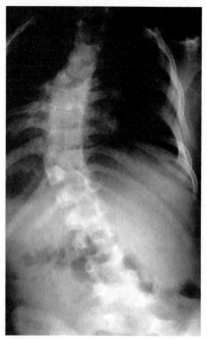

FIG. 7-30 Thoracolumbar curve with hemivertebra. (From Brier SR: *Primary care orthopedics,* St Louis, Mosby, 1999.)

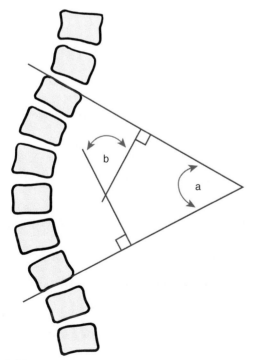

FIG. 7-29 Cobb method of measuring the severity of a curve. (From Mercier LR, Pettid FJ: *Practical orthopedics,* ed 4, St Louis, 1995, Mosby.)

(AIS), a residual side-bending curve equal to or more than 25 degrees indicates that a minor curve is structural, but inherent variability exists in the subjective nature of the procedure. Because a supine X-ray is not effort or technician dependent, it will be more reliable and reproducible. The supine x-ray provides a consistent, nonsubjective, single x-ray assessment of curve flexibility in the preoperative evaluation of AIS and predicts structural curve accurately. Supine curves less than 40 degrees in the thoracolumbar-lumbar region, and less than 30 degrees in the main thoracic or proximal thoracic regions can be considered nonstructural minor curves (Cheh et al, 2006).

Curvature of the spine in the AP direction in which the convexity is directed posteriorly is termed *kyphosis.* This curvature exists in the normal spine at the thoracic and sacral regions. Disease of the discs and vertebral bodies is the most common cause. Congenital kyphosis is rare and usually is secondary to a localized malformation of the spine.

Senile kyphosis is relatively common in the elderly patient and may be symptomatic (Fig. 7-31).

Scheuermann kyphosis is a fixed kyphosis that develops near the time of puberty. The origin of Scheuermann kyphosis is unknown, but the deformity is caused by typical wedging abnormalities in the dorsal and dorsolumbar spine that result in a decrease in the anterior height of the vertebrae. Mild forms may clinically resemble postural round back. Wedging of the vertebrae, irregularity of the end plates and typical Schmorl nodules are seen on the lateral view, usually between T2 and T12 (Fig. 7-32). Synostoses and osteophyte formation are not uncommon in adults. *Gibbus* refers to a focal flexion deformity (Fig. 7-33).

7

TABLE 7-4

LENKE SCOLIOSIS CLASSIFICATION

Curve Type (1-6)

Lumbar Spine Modifier	Type 1 (Main Thoracic)	Type 2 (Double Thoracic)	Type 3 (Double Major)	Type 4 (Triple Major)	Type 5 (TL/L)	Type 6 (TL/L-MT)
A	1A°	2A°	3A°	4A°		
B	1B°	2B°	3B°	4B°		
C	1C°	2C°	3C°	4C°	5C°	6C°
Possible sagittal structural criteria (To determine specific curve type)	Normal	PT Kyphosis	TL Kyphosis	PT and TL Kyphosis	Normal	TL Kyphosis

°T5-12 sagittal alignment modifier:-, N, or +
−: <10°
N: 10-40°
+: >40°

The Lenke Classification System is simple, accurate, and easy to reproduce and communicate between health care providers. It relies on measurements taken from standard radiographs (x-rays). In this method, the examiner evaluates x-rays of the patient from the front, the side, and in bending positions. Each scoliosis curve is then classified in three steps by the region of the spine, the degree or angle of the curve, and the relationship of the side-to-side curve to the sagittal plane. For example, many scoliosis curves affect the presence or absence of kyphosis, which is the outward or convex curve normally found in the upper back. In addition, each aspect of the curve is evaluated for its relative stiffness or flexibility.

From Dr. Lawrence Lenke, Washington University School of Medicine, St. Louis, Missouri. Available at: www.spinal-deformity-surgeon.com.

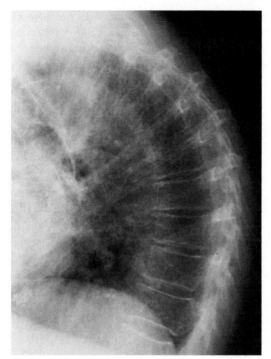

FIG. 7-31 Senile kyphosis. (From Mercier LR, Pettid FJ: *Practical orthopedics,* ed 4, St Louis, 1995, Mosby.)

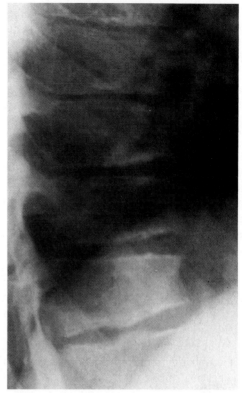

FIG. 7-32 Scheuermann disease. (From Mercier LR, Pettid FJ: *Practical orthopedics,* ed 4, St Louis, 1995, Mosby.)

7

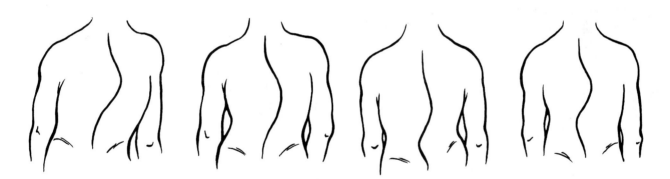

Right thoracic
curve

Right thoracic
lumbar curve

Left lumbar
curve

Right thoracic and
left lumbar curve
(double major curve)

FIG. 7-33 Examples of scoliosis curve patterns. (From Barkauskas VH, et al: *Health and physical assessment,* ed 2, St Louis, 1998, Mosby.)

Few conditions produce decreased kyphosis. The lordotic interscapular thoracic spine (Pottenger saucering) involves the T2 to T6 vertebrae. This type of flattened thoracic spine may have its beginning in the juvenile years, ages 2 through 5. The cause of this flattened spine may be a congenital fixation of the thoracic spine.

The examiner should also be aware that if a thoracolumbar kyphosis exists, the kyphosis is caused by a postural deficit resulting from poor postural habits. This cause of kyphosis is most prevalent in adolescents. A patient with this condition is not round-shouldered, rather round-backed. The classification for thoracolumbar kyphosis is round back type I or type II. Type I results from postural habitus and type II from structural abnormalities. Among causes for thoracolumbar kyphosis are juvenile osteochondrosis (Scheuermann disease) and vertebra plana (Calvé disease).

The lower the thoracolumbar kyphosis occurs in the thoracic spine, the more it is a fixed and unyielding kyphosis. The patient may have normal and supple flexion in the areas of the spine above the thoracolumbar kyphosis.

Concerning the thoracic kyphosis, the examiner must observe for gibbus deformity. The gibbus deformity is associated with spinal tuberculosis and involves only two or three vertebral elements. The gibbus is a short, sharply angled, and acute kyphosis. This deformity may also be observed in significant compression fracture of one or more thoracic vertebrae.

Often, with the dramatic and adverse changes of thoracic kyphosis, a parallel development of lateral curvature (scoliosis) is present.

The presence of scoliosis needs to be determined. Nonstructural scoliosis is associated with poor postural habits. When the patient with nonstructural or postural scoliosis assumes proper standing or seated attitudes, the scoliosis disappears. Poor posture, hysteria, nerve root irritation, inflammation in the spine area, leg length discrepancy, or hip contracture can cause nonstructural scoliosis.

An idiopathic structural scoliosis does not have any specific cause. Structural changes may result from a congenital problem, such as wedge vertebrae, hemivertebrae, or failure of segmentation. The increase or decrease of kyphosis in a juvenile will alert the examiner to other postural deficits that may indicate the onset of scoliosis.

Senile scoliosis is the result of spinal column changes associated with aging of the adult thoracic spine. A scoliotic curve develops but does not have all the characteristics demonstrable in adolescent scoliosis. On a more thorough examination, senile scoliosis might actually be mild or moderate adolescent structural scoliosis that was previously undetected. Changes or increases in curvature usually result from the effects of gravity or injury to the thoracic spine. These patients are often experiencing thoracic pain and are surprised to learn that scoliosis exists.

Once scoliosis is identified, the degree of curvature has to be determined. Accurate techniques of measurement must be used. Once a particular method of curvature measurement is established, all further studies must be measured in the same way.

PROCEDURE

- If the patient has an S or C scoliosis, the curvature may straighten when the spine flexes forward.
- A curvature that does straighten is a negative sign, indicating functional scoliosis.
- A positive sign occurs when the scoliosis does not improve after flexing forward.
- A positive sign is evidence of pathologic or structural scoliosis, and it indicates an altered morphologic abnormality, a pathologic condition, trauma, and subluxation.
- A posterior Adams position requires the examiner to be behind the patient (Figs. 7-34 and 7-35).
- An anterior Adams position requires the examiner to be in front of the patient (Fig. 7-36).

Next Steps/Procedures
Postural assessment and diagnostic imaging

CLINICAL PEARL

When the scoliotic curvature disappears in the Adams position, the curves are mild to moderate, or less than 25 degrees. These curves have more of a functional component than a structural component and are amenable to conservative management.

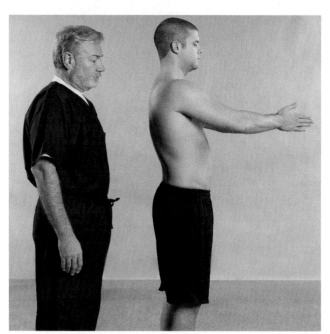

FIG. 7-34 The patient is standing. The examiner notes any spinal asymmetry, scapular winging, chest rotational deformity, and so forth.

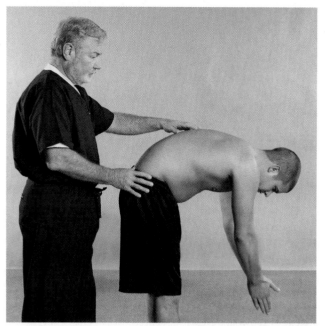

FIG. 7-35 For posterior Adams position, the patient flexes forward at the waist. The arms are allowed to hang toward the floor, and the hands are placed together in a prayer position. The examiner, who is posterior to the patient, observes the patient's thoracolumbar spine for deformity, which includes persistent scoliotic curvature, rib humping, and muscular atrophy.

7

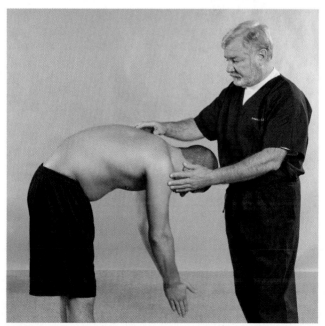

FIG. 7-36 In anterior Adams position, the patient assumes the Adams position by flexing the spine at the waist and flexing the cervical spine. The examiner, who is anterior to the patient, observes for upper thoracic scoliosis defects.

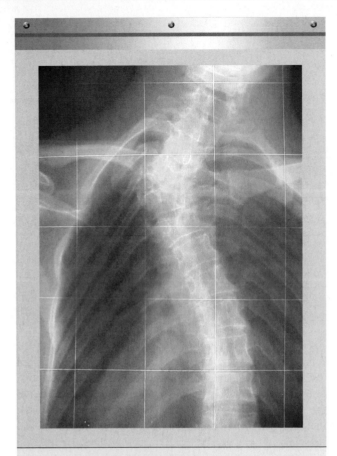

AT THE VIEWBOX

This type of angular, short radius scoliosis in the upper thoracic spine, indicates an underlying segmentation anomaly such as lateral hemivertebra. Structural scolioses do not reduce on flexion. The compensatory right mid to lower thoracic scoliosis is typically flexible ("functional"). The complex segmentation anomalies warrant follow-up with MRI to assess for associated anomalies of the spinal cord. (From the teaching file of Timothy Mick, DC, DACBR)

Assessment for Ankylosing Spondylitis, Severe Sprain, and Intervertebral Disc Syndrome

Comment

The early erosive sclerotic changes of bone adjacent to the sacroiliac joints in ankylosing spondylitis are well recognized. Less well recognized is the fact that similar erosive sclerotic changes may on occasion involve the intervertebral disc and adjacent bone, producing a lesion termed *spondylodiscitis*.

The radiographic appearance of spondylodiscitis is fairly typical (Fig. 7-37). Erosion of the subchondral bony plates widens the disc space. The surrounding bone becomes sclerotic and radiodense. Either erosion or sclerosis may be more prominent. The reported incidence of spondylodiscitis is 5% to 6% (Fig. 7-38). It occurs most frequently in the lower thoracic spine.

Nontuberculous discitis and spondylodiscitis may be either nonspecific (nonpyogenic, traumatic) or infectious (mainly bacterial). In this latter instance, primary focus may be detected (ear, throat). The commonest causal agents are *Staphylococcus, Streptococcus,* and *Coxiella.* Sometimes the organism is not cultured. The spine is involved by infectious organisms through hematogenous spread or from a contaminated contiguous source. Spine infection represents approximately 2% to 4% of all osteomyelitis cases. The diagnosis is often delayed, and the mean age at diagnosis is 7.5 years. Three clinical forms according to age have been identified. In patients 1 year of age or younger, a serious form with septicemia is observed. The infantile form (1 to 4 years) is associated with stiff gait and limping. After 4 years of age, spondylodiscitis is associated with back pain and has a benign course, more so in the younger child. In addition, symptoms may include fever, malaise, weight loss, bone pain, irritability, and a refusal to walk (Khoury et al, 2006).

Ankylosing spondylitis (AS), an ascending disease, affects the thoracic region after the lumbar. Patients with this condition experience back pain, but the anterolateral chest pain and the limited chest expansion bother them the most. In some patients, these symptoms may occur rather early in the life of the disease, but they usually become bothersome after 6 years of illness. Chest pain, which usually occurs during inspiration, and limited chest expansion are caused primarily by involvement of costovertebral and manubriosternal joints, as well as the costochondral junctions and the clavicular joints. The girdle-like restriction may cause a sense of anxiety and dyspnea, particularly during exertion. However, respiratory problems are surprisingly uncommon, although restricted ventilatory volumes are detected by pulmonary function studies (Table 7-5). Of course, should concomitant disease result in impaired diaphragmatic breathing, a problem is likely to develop.

Tenderness is elicited over the manubriosternal joint, the costochondral junctions, and the entire dorsal spine. With more advanced disease, a dorsal kyphosis is evident, and the thoracic cage remains in the expiratory position. Chest expansion, normally no less than 1 inch in female patients and 1.5 inches in male patients, may be diminished by 50%

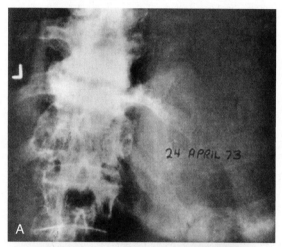
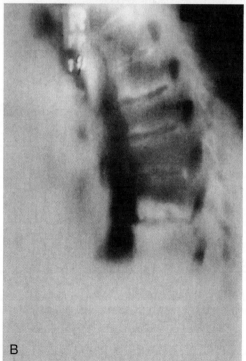

FIG. 7-37 Ankylosing spondylitis with discitis. (From Watkins RG: *The spine in sports,* St Louis, 1996, Mosby.)

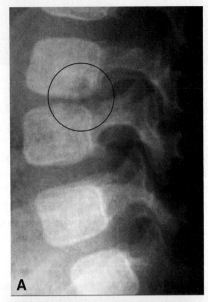

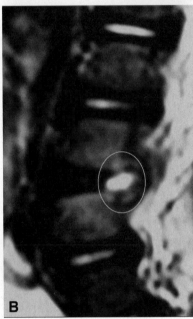

FIG. 7-38 Bacterial spondylodiscitis in a 18-month-old child with fever and irritation. Lateral spine radiograph shows narrowing of the L3–L4 disc space with lucencies at both endplates *(circle)*. (Adapted From Khoury NJ et al: Imaging of back pain in children and adolescents, *Cur Probl Diagn Radiol* 35[6]:224-244, 2006.)

or more. A football abdomen, a spherical protrusion, may result from abdominal breathing.

The posture of the *hang-dog* cervical spine, dorsal kyphosis with the chest cage fixed in expiration, straightening of the lumbar spine, marked flexion contractures of the hips

TABLE 7-5

MODIFIED NEW YORK CRITERIA FOR ANKYLOSING SPONDYLITIS DIAGNOSIS

Clinical criteria	Low back pain and stiffness for more than 3 months that improves with exercise but is not relieved by rest
	Limitation of motion of the lumbar spine both the sagittal and the frontal planes
	Limitation of chest expansion relative to normal values corrected for age and sex
Radiological criterion	Sacroiliitis grade 2 bilaterally or sacroiliitis grade 3-4 unilaterally

Adapted from Moll JMH: New criteria for the diagnosis of ankylosing spondylitis, *Scand J Rheum* 16(suppl 65):12-24, 1987.

and knees, and a gaze that is fixed on the floor are highly characteristic of the terminal stage of AS and should offer no problems with diagnosis.

AS may be primarily or secondarily associated with a variety of conditions. Most of these disorders follow manifestation of spondylitis, but some may precede the actual onset of musculoskeletal symptoms by several months and occasionally by years. In some instances, these allied conditions may overlap one another. Aortitis may be found both in idiopathic AS and in Reiter syndrome. Heel pain is common to psoriatic arthritis, Reiter syndrome, and enteropathic arthropathy, with and without an associated inflammation of the spine. The detection of human leukocyte antigen (HLA)-B27 antigen, not only in AS, but also in Reiter disease and psoriatic arthritis, creates an even closer relationship between these conditions.

PROCEDURE

- The recumbent patient places the hands far behind the body and tries to arise from the supine position to the seated position.
- The patient can also be in a side-lying position (Fig. 7-39).
- The examiner should note the patient's position of comfort and any spinal complaints that the patient presents.
- The patient arises from the side-lying position to a sitting position (Fig. 7-40).
- The sign is present when either action elicits a localized thoracic or thoracolumbar spinal pain.
- The sign suggests AS, severe sprain, or intervertebral disc syndrome.

Next Steps/Procedures

Chest expansion test, Forestier bowstring sign, clinical laboratory testing, and diagnostic imaging

CLINICAL PEARL

The patient sometimes defers to a side-lying posture when trying to stand after lying supine. This action represents Amoss sign. Amoss sign may not produce pain, but it reveals stiffness and lack of mobility and is still useful for detecting chronic spondylitis, which, at the least, requires imaging of the thoracolumbar spine.

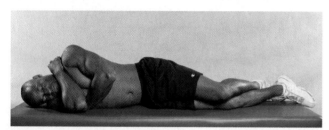

FIG. 7-39 The patient is in a side-lying position on the examining table. The examiner notes the position of comfort and any spinal complaints that the patient expresses.

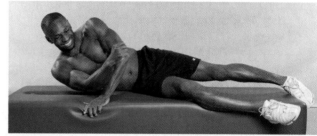

FIG. 7-40 The patient arises from the side-lying position to a seated position. The sign is present when this action elicits a localized thoracic or thoracolumbar spinal pain. The sign suggests ankylosing spondylitis, severe sprain, or intervertebral disc syndrome.

7

Assessment for Tuberculosis of the Vertebrae and Other Destructive Processes of the Spine

Comment

Spinal infections are rare, constituting only 2% to 4% of all cases of osteomyelitis. Patients with vertebral osteomyelitis often have few systemic symptoms, such as fever or sepsis, and may have normal white blood cell counts; therefore delay in diagnosis is not uncommon (Fig. 7-41). A high index of suspicion is necessary to diagnose spinal infections accurately in the early stages.

Tuberculosis (TB) is a major cause of morbidity and mortality. The World Health Organization (WHO) has noted that the global incidence of TB is increasing by 0.4% per annum. For example, in South Africa the prevalence has increased from 190 in 100,000 in 1980 to 339 in 100,000 in 2001. The human immunodeficiency virus (HIV) contributes to the increased disease burden of TB. Central nervous system TB accounts for approximately 5% of all extrapulmonary TB, and tuberculous meningitis (TBM) is the most serious complication. Without treatment, most patients die, and any delay in treatment results in significant morbidity. The mortality rates vary from 7% to 45% (Bhigjee et al, in press).

With tuberculous spondylitis, any single vertebra or several vertebrae may be involved. The disease most often involves the lower thoracic and the lumbar spine. The infection starts in the cancellous bone area of the vertebral body. Most commonly, an exudative reaction with marked hyperemia produces severe generalized osteoporosis. The body softens and easily yields to compression forces. In the

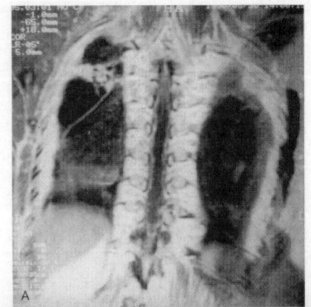
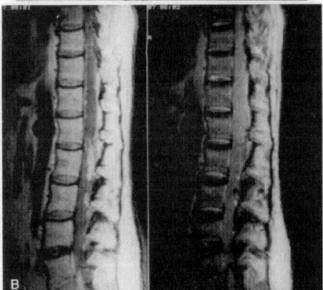

FIG. 7-41 Syringomyelia complicating tuberculous meningitis 17 years after the initial infection. **A,** Coronal T1-weighted magnetic resonance image showing extensive residual tuberculous lung involvement and a syringomyelic cavity extending along the dorsolumbar spinal cord. **B,** Sagittal T1 *(right)* and T2 *(left)* image showing the same cavity with residual inflammatory nodules mainly at middle dorsal level. (From Garcia-Monco JC: Central nervous system tuberculosis, *Neurol Clin* 17[4]:737-759, 1999.)

ORTHOPEDIC GAMUT 7-7

SIGNS AND SYMPTOMS OF TUBERCULOUS MENINGITIS

- **Fever**
  - Headache
  - Meningismus
  - Abnormal mental status
  - Vomiting
  - Malaise–anorexia
  - Papilledema
  - Cranial-nerve palsies
  - Hemiparesis, hemiplegia
  - Seizures
  - Hydrocephalus (computed tomographic scan)

Adapted from Garcia-Monco JC: Central nervous system tuberculosis, *Neurol Clin* 17(4):737-759, 1999.

thoracic spine, normal kyphotic curve increases the pressure on the vertebrae anteriorly, and anterior wedging is severe. An angular kyphosis results if the vertebral body is crushed.

The infection advances and destroys the epiphyseal cortex, the intervertebral disc, and the adjacent vertebrae. The infective exudate may spread anteriorly beneath the anterior longitudinal ligament to reach the neighboring vertebrae.

Infection of the posterior bony arch and the transverse processes is unusual. More commonly, granulation tissue develops and compresses the spinal cord and the nerve roots. Pressure on nerve structures is more likely in the thoracic spine, where the caliber of the spinal canal is small. Sequestra and bone fragments do not often extrude into the canal, limited by the strong posterior longitudinal ligament.

The most common vertebral infection is an exudative type that constitutes a severe hypergic reaction. This circumstance causes an extreme degree of osteoporosis that spreads rapidly. Abscess formation is common, and constitutional symptoms are pronounced.

PROCEDURE

- Anghelescu sign is used for identifying TB of the vertebrae or other destructive processes of the spine.
- In the supine position, the patient places weight on the head and heels while lifting the body upward (Fig. 7-42).
- Inability to hyperextend the spine indicates a disease process (Fig. 7-43).

Next Steps/Procedures

Chest expansion test, Forestier bowstring sign, clinical laboratory testing, and diagnostic imaging

---

ORTHOPEDIC GAMUT 7-8

PROBLEMS IN CONFIRMING THE CLINICAL SUSPICION OF TUBERCULOSIS MENINGITIS

- Approximately 45% of patients will have chest radiographic evidence of past or present TB, and approximately 50% will have a positive tuberculin test.
- Typical routine cerebrospinal fluid (CSF) profile demonstrates a lymphocyte predominant pleocytosis, a raised protein, and a low glucose; TBM can be excluded on the absence of these parameters alone.
- The CSF may be acellular in as many as 3% to 6% of HIV-negative patients. The CFS may be acellular in as many as 16% of HIV-positive patients.
- HIV-negative patients may have a neutrophilic predominance in 20% to 25% of cases.
- The protein level may be normal in approximately 6% of patients with HIV, the glucose level may be normal in approximately 25% of HIV-negative patients.
- The protein and glucose figures are increased in HIV-positive patients.
- Smears of the CSF, although diagnostic, are positive in only 5% to 20% of cases.
- Culture, though the gold standard, is positive in approximately 40% of cases. Cultures and may take up to 6 weeks to return a positive result.

Adapted From Garcia-Monco JC: Central nervous system tuberculosis, *Neurol Clin* 17(4):737-759, 1999.

7

CLINICAL PEARL

When testing for Anghelescu sign, the loss of the ability to achieve a near opisthotonos posture is significant. Although the true opisthotonos posture involves the cervical spine, very few patients normally have enough strength in the neck to accomplish this task.

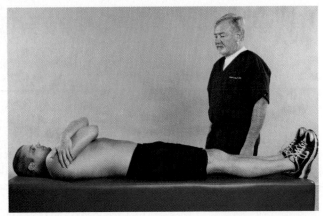

FIG. 7-42 The patient is supine on the examining table. The examiner observes for postural symmetry and notes any positions of antalgia.

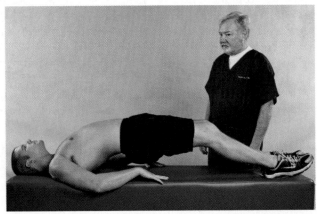

FIG. 7-43 From the supine position, the patient attempts to extend the thoracic spine sufficiently to raise it from the table. Without a thoracic spinal abnormality, the patient will be able to rest the weight of the body on the heels and the shoulders (a near opisthotonos posture). This position cannot be achieved in tuberculous spondylitis.

BEEVOR SIGN

Assessment for Myelopathy Associated with the T10 Spinal Level

Comment

Probably the most important diagnosis to make in thoracic and thoracic-radiating pain is that of a thoracic disc herniation.

The incidence of symptomatic thoracic disc herniation has been reported to be 1 in 1 million per year. More than 70% of the thoracic disc herniations are asymptomatic. In addition, the symptoms and signs are usually slowly progressive and not closely related with the localization, level, composition, and size of the herniated disc. The clinical presentation of this uncommon disorder is often atypical. Most patients have either pain in the chest wall, usually in the distribution of a thoracic nerve root, or thoracic myelopathy involving the lower extremities. However, on rare occasions, localization of the pain from a symptomatic thoracic disc herniation may be unclear, and the character of the pain may sometimes mimic cardiopulmonary, gastrointestinal, or genitourinary disorders or may even suggest a psychiatric disease (Ozturk et al, 2006).

Pressure on or damage to the spinal cord carries the grave risk of permanent cord injury. A thoracic disc herniation can result in paraplegia, with weakness and numbness in the legs and complete loss of bowel, bladder, sexual, and leg function. Up to 50% of patients with thoracic disc herniation can have significant spinal cord injury.

Thoracic disc herniation may produce a great variety of symptoms. In the lower thoracic spine, a flaccid neurologic loss may occur rather than the spastic presentation of an upper thoracic disc herniation, and it often mimics lumbar spine disease. Lower herniated thoracic disc may produce signs and symptoms of neurogenic claudication or sciatica. Upper thoracic disc herniations at T1–T2 or T2–T3 may cause a cervical spine problem, with pain radiating to the medial aspect of the arm, hand, and shoulder, with possible intrinsic hand weakness or Horner syndrome or both.

Within the thoracic spine is an overlap of dermatomes. The dermatomes follow the ribs, and the absence of only one dermatome may lead to no loss in sensation at all.

Absence of the abdominal reflexes may be an early sign of corticospinal disease, which is a common sign of multiple sclerosis but is by no means pathognomonic of this disease. When the abdominal reflexes are absent, hyperreflexia of the lower extremities and the Babinski sign are present.

The T5 segment is at the level of the nipple, T10 at the umbilicus, and T12 at the groin.

The motor and sensory roots become progressively longer as they proceed from their respective cord segments to their points of exit.

Acute postinfectious polyneuropathy (Guillain-Barré syndrome), an acute idiopathic polyneuritis, is a disease of unknown origin characterized by rapid onset of ascending weakness with associated sensory disturbance. All races, all age groups, and both sexes are susceptible to this disease. Peripheral nerve demyelination and often a mononuclear inflammatory reaction characterize the pathologic picture. Numerous theories have been suggested as to causation of this disease. One theory is that the disease results from an autoimmune reaction against a peripheral nerve antigen, specifically myelin. Other theories postulate that the disease is secondary to a bacterial, viral, or neurotoxic substance. Approximately one half of the cases of acute postinfectious polyneuropathy will occur after an upper respiratory or gastrointestinal infection.

ORTHOPEDIC GAMUT 7-9

GUILLAIN-BARRÉ SYNDROME DISABILITY SCORE

The Guillain-Barré syndrome (GBS) disability score is a widely accepted scoring system to assess the functional status of patients with GBS in which scores range from 0 (normal) to 6 (dead).

- Poor outcome is a GBS disability score at 6 months of 3 or more, which corresponds with the inability to walk 10 m independently
- Fairly good outcome is defined as a GBS disability score at 6 months of 2 or less.
- The endpoint is at 6 months because most of the recovery process has occurred by this time in select patients who do recover.
- The GBS index:
  0 A healthy state
  1 Minor symptoms and capable of running
  2 Able to walk 10 m or more without assistance but unable to run
  3 Able to walk 10 m across an open space with help
  4 Bedridden or chair bound
  5 Requiring assisted ventilation for at least part of the day
  6 Dead

Adapted from van Koningsveld R et al: A clinical prognostic scoring system for Guillain-Barré syndrome, *Lancet Neurol* 6(7):589-594, 2007.

ORTHOPEDIC GAMUT 7-10

MEDICAL RESEARCH COUNCIL SUM SCORE

1. The Medical Research Council (MRC) sum score is the sum of the scores of six muscle groups, which include shoulder abductors, elbow flexors, wrist extensors, hip flexors, knee extensors, and foot dorsiflexors, bilaterally. Scores range from 60 (normal) to 0 (quadriplegic).

2. The MRC score of an individual muscle group ranges from 0 to 5:

   0 No visible contraction

   1 Visible contraction without movement of the limb

   2 Active movement of the limb, but not against gravity

   3 Active movement against gravity over (almost) the full range

   4 Active movement against gravity and resistance

   5 Normal power

Adapted from van Koningsveld R et al: A clinical prognostic scoring system for Guillain-Barré syndrome, *Lancet Neurol* 6(7):589-594, 2007.

The typical medical history includes an acute upper respiratory illness followed by a few days of pins-and-needles paresthesia, followed by lower extremity weakness, which is characteristically a symmetrically ascending motor weakness accompanied by minimal sensory changes and intact sphincter control. Aching or tenderness may be present, but neither symptom is a prominent feature. A minority of patients exhibits profound sensory losses. Temporary bowel or bladder paralysis may occur but occurs in a lesser degree than the lower extremity paralysis. The disease may ascend to involve the bulbar muscles, resulting in respiratory paralysis and death. The course of the disease ranges from several days to a week. If the patient survives the first 2 weeks, the prognosis is good. Motor power returns gradually over the course of a year.

The Guillain-Barré syndrome disability score is probably the easiest to apply in clinical practice, although the Medical Research Council sum score might be more accurate. Moreover, a variable measured at 1 week supplies information in an early phase of the disease and therefore might be more helpful in early decision making concerning therapeutic intervention (van Koningsveld et al, in press).

PROCEDURE

- Beevor sign, although not an abdominal reflex, is seen during an examination.
- In this test, the recumbent patient lifts the head off the examining table (Figs. 7-44 and 7-45).
- Normally, the upper and lower abdominal muscles contract equally and the umbilicus does not move or drift.
- When the lower abdominal muscles alone are weakened, the umbilicus will be drawn upward by the contraction of the intact upper musculature (Figs. 7-46 and 7-47).
- This effect is associated with a spinal cord lesion at the T10 level.

Next Steps/Procedures

Sensory assessment, reflex testing, electrodiagnosis, and diagnostic imaging (magnetic resonance imaging)

CLINICAL PEARL

In the presence of prolonged illness followed by lower extremity paresthesia (regardless of how minor), this test needs to be performed. Beevor sign affords an early, noninvasive indicator of the existence of thoracic spinal cord myelopathy.

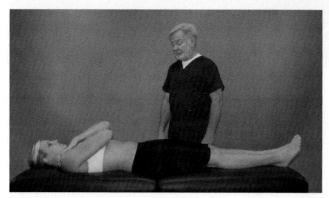

FIG. 7-44 The patient is supine on the examining table. The abdominal muscles are palpated and the position of the umbilicus established.

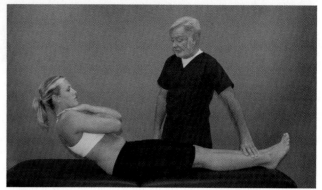

FIG. 7-45 The examiner fixes the patient's legs to the table with mild downward pressure. The patient performs a partial sit-up with the arms folded across the chest. The examiner notes any drift of the umbilicus. During a sit-up, the uppermost fibers of the abdominal musculature are primarily the ones tested. Drift occurs toward the stronger or uninvolved musculature. Cephalad drift implicates lower thoracic spine involvement. Caudad drift implicates upper thoracic spine involvement but not above T7.

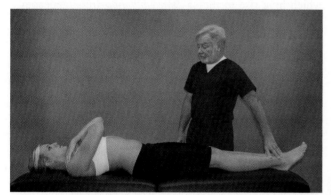

FIG. 7-46 If extensive abdominal muscle weakness or paresis exists, the back will arch from the table as the patient attempts the partial sit-up. The thorax may pull away from the pelvis until it is firmly fixed by extension of the thoracic spine. The arching of the back stretches the abdominal muscles, and they may appear firm under tension. The examiner needs to be careful to avoid mistaking this tautness for firmness resulting from actual contraction of the muscles.

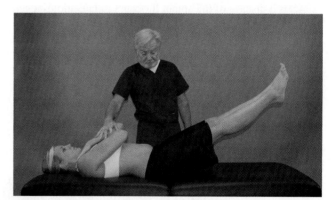

FIG. 7-47 As an alternative, the patient can perform a partial bilateral leg lift to test the abdominal musculature. In this procedure, the examiner can apply a mild downward pressure to the patient's thorax, fixing it to the examining table for stability. Umbilical drift is noted. Leg lifting tests primarily the lowermost fibers of the abdominal musculature.

Assessment for Spinal Ankylosis

Comment

Children breathe abdominally. Women perform upper thoracic breathing. Men are both upper and lower thoracic breathers. In elderly adults, the breathing is in the lower thoracic and abdominal regions. Chest wall movement that occurs during breathing displaces the pleural surfaces, thorax musculature, nerves, and ribs. Breathing and coughing accentuate pain if any of these structures is injured.

In pectus carinatum (pigeon chest), the sternum projects more anterior and inferior. This deformity increases the AP dimension of the chest and can impair ventilation volume.

In pectus excavatum (funnel chest), the sternum is displaced posteriorly by an overgrowth of the ribs. The AP dimension of the chest is decreased. The heart is displaced or compressed.

In barrel chest, often associated with emphysema, the sternum projects anterior and superior, and the AP chest diameter is increased.

AS is a disease of the spine. It occurs in late adolescence or early adulthood and is characterized pathologically by progressive inflammation of the spine, sacroiliac joints, and the larger joints of the extremities—particularly the hips, knees, and shoulders—leading to fibrous or bony ankylosis and deformity.

AS starts insidiously in a young adult. Symptoms at first are vague and poorly localized. Aching and stiffness around both sacroiliac joints occur as a morning backache that subsides with activity but returns after sitting in one position for prolonged periods. The pain and stiffness become progressively worse and spread slowly, within 6 months to a year, to the rest of the spine. Limitation of motion appears first in the lower spine but is finally notable throughout the spine. Chest expansion is restricted because of disease of the costovertebral joints.

Rigidity of the rib cage has been accepted as an important sign of AS for centuries. Pulmonary function tests typically show mild restrictive respiratory pattern. These observations are considered depending on inflammation of the costovertebral joints, resulting in reduction in rib cage mobility (Ragnarsdottir, Geirsson, Gudbjornsson, in press).

The early roentgenographic features usually are those of bilateral sacroiliitis. Eventually, complete fusion of the sacroiliac and hip joints may occur as healing takes place after the inflammation. As the disease progresses, calcifications of the anulus fibrosis and paravertebral ligaments develop, which give rise to the so-called *bamboo-spine* appearance characteristic of AS (Fig. 7-48). The HLA-B27 antigen is important in the diagnosis of AS. This antigen occurs in nearly 100% of Caucasian patients with AS.

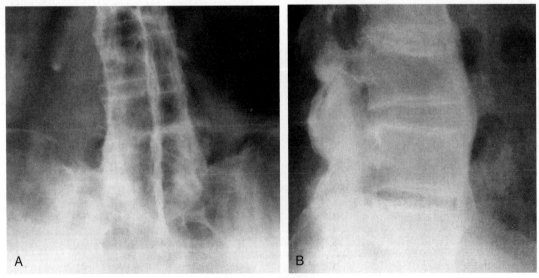

FIG. 7-48 Ankylosing spondylitis. **A,** Anteroposterior view. **B,** Lateral view. (From Mercier LR, Pettid FJ: *Practical orthopedics,* ed 4, St Louis, 1995, Mosby.)

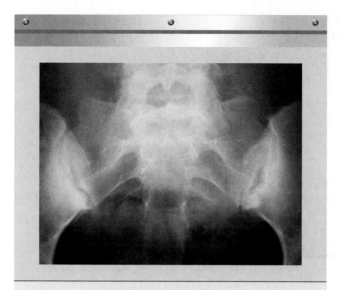

AT THE VIEWBOX

A 34-year-old female with chronic Crohn disease, and a family history of rheumatoid arthritis. Chronic left sacroiliac pain, with exacerbations several times per year. Note the bilateral, symmetric ill-defined joint margins, attended by reactive sclerosis and apparent joint space widening ("pseudo widening"). Seronegative spondyloarthropathies, especially ankylosing spondylitis, tend to affect the sacroiliac joints initially, but spinal involvement may predominate. Clinical findings of bilateral, symmetric joint pain and stiffness, especially of the sacroiliac joints, along with tenderness over entheses (ligament and tendon insertions on bone) may indicate seronegative spondyloarthropathy (SSA), especially ankylosing spondylitis. Diminished chest expansion is a later clinical finding, which may show associated imaging abnormality of the costovertebral and costotransverse joints. Chronic colitis should always raise the question of ankylosing spondylitis. (From the teaching file of Timothy Mick, DC, DACBR)

PROCEDURE

- The chest diameter is measured at the level of the fourth intercostal space.
- The measurement is taken as the patient exhales maximally (Fig. 7-49).
- A second measurement is made as the patient inhales deeply (Fig. 7-50).
- The normal difference between inspiration and expiration is 5.75 to 7.62 cm (1.5 to 3 inches).

Next Steps/Procedures

Amoss sign, Forestier bowstring sign, clinical laboratory testing, range-of-motion testing, spirometer testing, and diagnostic imaging of the pelvis and sacroiliac joints.

CLINICAL PEARL

Chest expansion measurements are sensitive indicators of early involvement of the costovertebral joints in ankylosing spondylitis. The chest expansion test is often positive before the patient realizes a change in chest comfort.

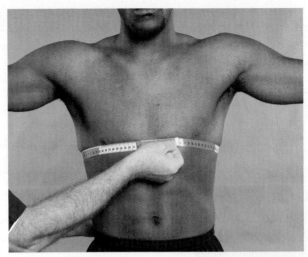

FIG. 7-49 The patient is standing with the arms elevated to 90 degrees. The examiner places a tape measure around the patient's chest at any of the following points: (1) at the fourth intercostal space, (2) at the axillary level, (3) at the level of the nipples, or (4) at the T10 rib level. The patient exhales maximally, and the chest diameter is measured.

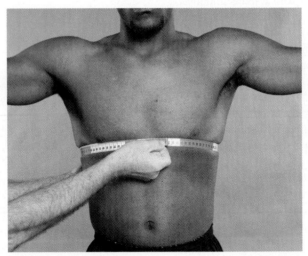

FIG. 7-50 The patient inhales deeply, and a second measurement is made. The normal difference between inspiration and expiration is 5.75 to 7.62 cm (1.5 to 3 inches). Decreases, in the absence of trauma, suggest ankylosing spondylitis.

Assessment for First or Second Thoracic Nerve Root Involvement

Comment

Herniations of the thoracic intervertebral disks can mimic a myriad of medical conditions and have been misdiagnosed as cardiac, abdominal, gastrointestinal, neoplastic and demyelinating diseases, to name a few. Thoracic disk herniation is a relatively uncommon occurrence. Estimates suggest that only 4% to 5% of all disk herniations take place in the thoracic region. Although uncommon, this condition poses a significant problem because it is often misdiagnosed and can be the cause of severe morbidity. Despite the diagnostic challenge caused by this condition, certain signs and symptoms are suggestive of the diagnosis. Back pain of gradual onset is generally reported along with some degree of myelopathy or sensory disturbance (Linscott, Heyborne, 2007).

Thoracic disc herniations are rare, seen in less than 0.3% of the population, and affect both men and women equally from the fourth through the sixth decades of life. The most common segments affected are between the T9 and T12 vertebrae.

Central disc prolapse generally produces symptoms of spastic paraparesis, increased deep-tendon reflexes, and a positive Babinski response. However, lateral thoracic disc protrusions produce signs more consistent with nerve root compression.

Compression of the spinal cord usually results in paresthesias (pins and needles) that are bilateral and disregard segmentation of the body. Other associated neural structures, compressed simultaneously, cause pain that follows dermatome patterns.

At the point of emergence from the dura, a dural sleeve invests the nerve root. Pressure on the dural sleeve produces discomfort. Pain occurs in all or any part of the dermatome. Paresthesia, a compression phenomenon, occurs at the distal end of the dermatome. Paresthesia often conspicuously occupies an area supplied by multiple nerve roots. The paresthesia has no edge or depth, and numbness displaces paresthesia. Pressure on a nerve root causes analgesia. Minimal pressure evokes paresthesia.

Weakness results from compression of the nerve root within the parenchyma. Weakness is discernible during resisted movements.

In compression of a nerve root, pressure on the surrounding dural sleeve, at the transverse process, will cause pain. Impaired conduction along a nerve leads to muscle weakness, manifested during resisted movements. Paresthesia rather than numbness represents a release phenomenon. The lesion always lies proximal to the upper edge of the paresthetic area.

In compression of a peripheral nerve or cutaneous nerve, numbness, rather than paresthesia, occupies the cutaneous area supplied by the nerve. The edge is well defined, and toward the center of the area, full anesthesia is often demonstrable.

The dura mater does not conform to the rules of segmental reference. The dura mater descends from the foramen magnum of the skull to the inferior edge of the first or second sacral vertebra. The dura mater keeps the spinal cord buffered in cerebrospinal fluid. From the dura mater protrude 30 pairs of nerve roots covered by the dural sheath.

Compression or stretching of the dura mater causes extra segmentally referred pain. The dura mater is adjacent to the intervertebral discs and vulnerable to posterior pressure exerted by the posterior longitudinal ligament.

Dura mater pain often pervades many dermatomes simultaneously. This pain is a common cause of scapular pain, and the symptoms are usually central or unilateral. Pressure on the dura mater at thoracic levels may radiate pain to the base of the neck, and this pain may also radiate to the posterior or anterior aspect of the trunk. The pain will spread over many dermatomes simultaneously. The symptoms are usually central or unilateral.

Pressure on the dura mater at lumbar levels may cause pain that reaches the lower thorax in the posterior, the lower abdomen, the upper buttocks, the sacrum, and the coccyx. Again, many dermatomes may be occupied simultaneously.

Pain perceived elsewhere in places other than its true site is referred pain. Nearly all pain is referred. The examiner's task is to determine the origin of the pain.

The sensory cortex determines the site where symptoms are referred. The sensory cortex attributes the impulses it receives to the appropriate areas of the body. With stimuli to the skin, the sensory cortex achieves a high degree of accuracy. Over time, a stimulus reaching certain cells in the

---

ORTHOPEDIC GAMUT 7-11

NERVOUS SYSTEM

The four components of the nervous system that refer pain or discomfort follow:

1. The spinal cord
2. The dural sleeve of a nerve root
3. The nerve trunk
4. A peripheral or cutaneous nerve

ORTHOPEDIC GAMUT 7-12

COMMON HISTORICAL AND PHYSICAL FINDINGS IN THORACIC INTERVERTEBRAL DISK HERNIATION

Historical findings
- Pain
- Back pain
- Pain not in back
- Paresthesias
- Numbness
- Tingling
- Weakness
  - Lower extremities
  - Upper extremities
- Bowel/bladder involvement

Physical findings
- Weakness—lower extremities
- Localized spine tenderness
- Sensation abnormalities
- Reflex abnormalities

Adapted from Linscott MS, Heyborne R: Thoracic intervertebral disk herniation: a commonly missed diagnosis, *J Emerg Med* 32(3):235-238, 2007.

cortex is interpreted as damage in a specific area of the skin.

The same cortical cells receive a painful stimulus arising from a deep-seated structure. The sensory cortex interprets this new impulse based on experience. Pain is referred to the area of skin served by those particular cortical cells.

The area of skin associated with sensory cells is the dermatome. The dermatome corresponds to the embryologic neural segment from which the structure was derived. Thus the sensory cortex will refer a pain in tissue of T5 segmental origin to the T5 dermatome and from the T8 structure to the T8 dermatome.

The 40 dermatome segments of a 1-month-old fetus are distributed horizontally. At this stage, the dermatomes are superimposed directly over the segments from which they are derived. The growth of the four limbs draws the dermatomes down the arms and the legs. However, in the trunk, the original arrangement of circular dermatome bands remains intact.

PROCEDURE

- Pain from stretching the first thoracic nerve root via the ulnar nerve identifies the T1 or T2 roots.
- Disc lesions at either level are rarities and are not accompanied by easily identifiable neurologic signs.
- If weakness is present, the possibility of serious disease should be considered.

ORTHOPEDIC GAMUT 7-13

PAIN REFERRAL

Pain referral rules are as follows:
1. Pain refers segmentally. A T5 tissue refers pain to the T5 dermatome. Pain can occupy all or any part of the dermatome. If the patient describes symptoms straddling more than one dermatome, or if the pain migrates from one dermatome to another, four possibilities arise: (a) The patient is describing a nonorganic pain; (b) the lesion itself is shifting, which often happens with vertebral element displacements; (c) the lesion is spreading, as in metastasis; or (d) the pain stems from a tissue that cannot refer pain segmentally. An exception of importance is the dura mater, which refers pain extrasegmentally.
2. Pain refers distally. The source of symptoms is sought locally or proximally.
3. Referred pain does not cross the midline. A T5 left rib will not cause discomfort on the right side of the body. A pain felt centrally must originate from a central structure. Pain that cannot be accounted for by a unilateral structure must be sought centrally. A pain alternating from one side of the body to the other must have a central source. This central source must be able to shift from one side to the other, such as during an intervertebral disc displacement.
4. The extent of pain reference is controlled. The referred pain is controlled by the size of the dermatome and the position in the dermatome of the tissue lesion. A large dermatome permits greater reference than a small one. A lesion in the proximal part of the dermatome refers pain farther than a lesion in the distal part.
5. The more intense the pain is, the greater the number will be of cortical cells excited. The spread to adjacent cells in the sensory cortex is interpreted as an enlargement of the painful area.
6. The deeper a soft-tissue lesion lies, the larger the reference to be expected. However, bone lesions produce minimal pain radiation.

- The affected arm is abducted to 90 degrees. The elbow is flexed with the pronated forearm to 90 degrees (Figs. 7-51 to 7-53).
- The patient places the hand behind the neck (Fig. 7-54).
- The ulnar nerve and the T1 nerve root are stretched.
- A positive test is indicated by scapular pain on the ipsilateral side.

Next Steps/Procedures

Cervical range of motion, thoracic spinal range of motion, reflex testing, sensory assessment, electrodiagnosis, Roos test, and diagnostic imaging

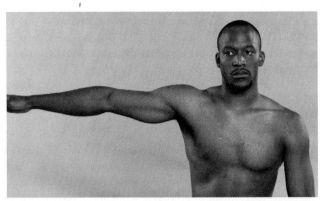

FIG. 7-51 The patient is seated and abducts the shoulder to 90 degrees. The arm is pronated.

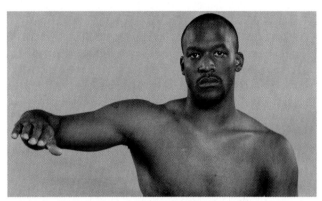

FIG. 7-52 The elbow is flexed to 90 degrees.

7

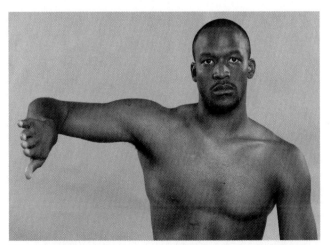

FIG. 7-53 The forearm is pronated fully to a 90-degree position, which should not be uncomfortable at this point.

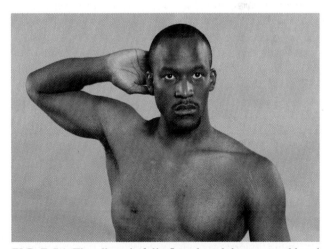

FIG. 7-54 The elbow is fully flexed, and the pronated hand is placed behind the head. Pain elicited in the scapular region suggests T1 nerve root involvement.

Assessment for Ankylosing Spondylitis

Comment

AS is viewed as the archetypal spondyloarthritis, its hallmark being inflammation of the axial skeleton (i.e., the spine and sacroiliac joints). AS is the second most common inflammatory joint disease after rheumatoid arthritis, with a prevalence ranging across studies from 0.1% to 0.9%. Nevertheless, the diagnosis is often made late, with an estimated time from symptom onset to diagnosis ranging from 5 to 8 years. Factors that contribute to delay the diagnosis include the insidious and nonspecific nature of the initial symptoms, delayed development of radiographic changes (sacroiliitis and syndesmophytes), absence in many patients of laboratory evidence of inflammation and, until recently, restricted therapeutic armamentarium consisting solely of nonsteroidal antiinflammatory drugs (Pavy et al, in press).

A well-recognized fact is that severe flexion deformities of the spine may occur in patients with AS.

Vertebral fractures are the hallmark of osteoporosis and are associated with significant physical impairments. One such impairment is increased thoracic kyphosis, which is itself associated with increased spinal loading, back extensor muscle weakness, limitations in functional activities, and increased risk of further fracture. The relationship between vertebral fracture and thoracic kyphosis is recognized in the literature, with agreement that greater numbers of vertebral fractures are associated with increases in thoracic kyphosis (Greig et al, in press).

AS is an inflammation of the joints of the spine that often results in bony ankylosis. The process is chronic, usually low grade, and begins mainly in young men. Early symptoms include pain and stiffness of the back; later, disability occurs because of the so-called *poker spine.*

On one hand, AS is a disease of the cartilaginous and fibrocartilaginous joints of the spine. On the other hand, the disease affects the diarthrodial articulations, such as the sacroiliac joint, the hips, and the shoulders. AS is primarily an axial disease. However, in approximately 35% of the patients, peripheral involvement of the hands, knees, ankles, and other joints does occur and is sometimes the first manifestation of the disease. However, rarely does peripheral arthritis result in significant deformity. All axial joints, including the manubriosternal, costovertebral, and symphysis pubis, may be affected.

Although AS is an entity distinct from rheumatoid arthritis, the early pathologic changes are similar. As is the case with rheumatoid arthritis, AS is a synovial disease characterized grossly by proliferative granulation tissue, adhesions of the joint, and probably a greater tendency for fibrous and bony ankylosis. The earliest findings of the disease are found in the sacroiliac joint and typify those also seen in the apoph-

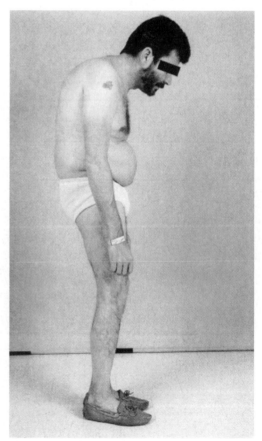

FIG. 7-55 Ankylosing spondylitis. (From Watkins RG: *The spine in sports,* St Louis, 1996, Mosby.)

ORTHOPEDIC GAMUT 7-14
THORACIC KYPHOSIS

Patients with thoracic kyphosis are classified into the following two groups:

1. Patients in the first group exhibit a major increase in thoracic kyphosis, with an associated loss of lumbar lordosis and a rigid spine. With sufficient extension of the lumbar spine, compensation can be achieved for the thoracic kyphosis, allowing a horizontal gaze and erect posture (Fig. 7-55).
2. Patients in the second group have thoracic kyphotic deformity but maintain a normal or even increased (compensatory) cervical and lumbar lordosis.

yseal joints of the lumbar, dorsal, and cervical spine, as well as the shoulders, hips, costovertebral, manubriosternal, and symphysis pubis articulations. Joint spaces are initially widened because of proliferative synovitis that gives way to erosive changes of the articular margins, narrowing, and then fusion.

The area may contain no semblance of a joint. The histologic counterpart of these findings is synovial membrane thickening with plasma cell and lymphocyte infiltration that are arranged in nests surrounding the smaller synovial blood vessels. Foci of chronic inflammation may also be found in adjacent bone, usually independent of the synovial process.

Most of the patient's discomfort and disability are caused by involvement of the dorsolumbar spine, albeit the sacroiliacs are concomitantly affected. Muscle pains, initially diffuse, may become increasingly concentrated in the dorsolumbar region. Stiffness is profound at times. Bending, lifting, and turning become formidable chores. Examination usually shows mild to severe direct tenderness of the dorsolumbar apophyseal joints, marked paravertebral muscle spasm, straightening of the lumbar spine, and sometimes an ironed-out appearance caused by muscle atrophy. Limitation of motion can be marked even if symptoms are minimal or absent.

The normal arching of the spine during flexion is lost, but this feature may not be fully appreciated because of the compensatory flexion at the hips (Fig. 7-56). Lateral flexion of the dorsolumbar spine cannot be disguised so well; it is sometimes lost. Minor limitations of motion can be confirmed by marking a point 10 cm above the L5 process and measuring the linear distance between the L5 spinous process and this point during flexion and extension. The distance should normally increase by 5 cm (2 inches) or more *(Schober test)*. Spondylitis of the dorsolumbar area, even if a fixed ankylosis ensues, does not usually pose a serious threat of disability.

Patients who seek help because of the apparent spinal deformity may have their main deformity in the hip joints, the lumbar spine, or the thoracic spine, or it may be primarily cervical in situation (Fig. 7-57). The most reliable measure of trunk deformity is the chin-brow to vertical angle. This is a measure of the angle formed by a line from the brow to the chin through the vertical, when the patient stands with the hips and knees extended, and the neck in its neutral or fixed position (Fig. 7-58).

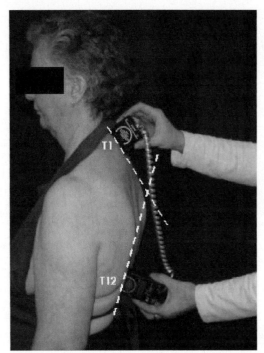

FIG. 7-56 Thoracic kyphosis measured using a dual inclinometer (The Dualer Electric Inclinometer, J. Tech, 1992, North American Fork, Utah). Spinous processes of T1 and T12 are used as landmarks for positioning the inclinometer sensors. The angle of the intersection of the dashed lines demonstrates the angle of thoracic kyphosis. (From Greig AM et al: Postural taping decreases thoracic kyphosis but does not influence trunk muscle electromyographic activity or balance in women with osteoporosis, *Man Ther* 13(3):249-257, 2008.)

7

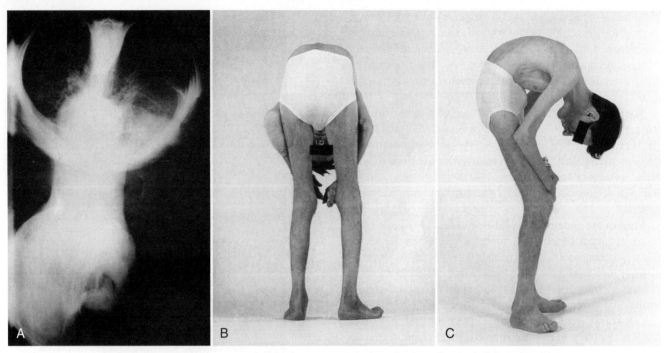

FIG. 7-57 Ankylosing spondylitis demonstrating complexity of spinal deformity. (From Watkins RG: *The spine in sports,* St Louis, 1996, Mosby.)

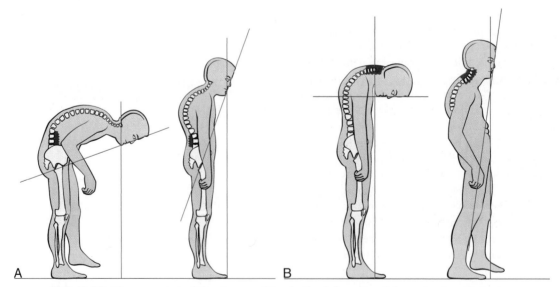

FIG. 7-58 Measurement of the degree of kyphotic deformity of the spine in ankylosing spondylitis using the chin-to-vertical angle. *(From Watkins RG: The spine in sports, St Louis, 1996, Mosby.)*

PROCEDURE

- The standing patient performs side bending and reveals ipsilateral tightening and contracture of the paraspinal musculature (Figs. 7-59 and 7-60).
- Normally, the contralateral musculature demonstrates tightening (Fig. 7-61).
- The test is significant for AS.

Next Steps/Procedures

Amoss sign, Anghelescu sign, chest expansion test, clinical laboratory testing, and diagnostic imaging

CLINICAL PEARL

Although the presence of Forestier bowstring sign suggests spondylitis, this test also indicates strain and intervertebral disc involvement. Any loss of symmetric motion must be examined further.

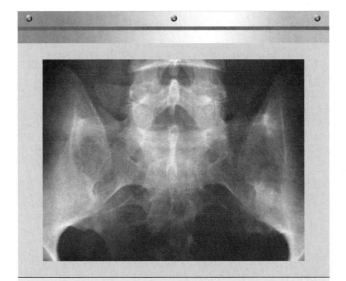

AT THE VIEWBOX

More advanced sacroiliitis from ankylosing spondylitis has produced bilateral, symmetric sacroiliac joint fusion. Note the "star sign" resulting from ankylosis across the superior sacroiliac joints. (From the teaching file of Timothy Mick, DC, DACBR)

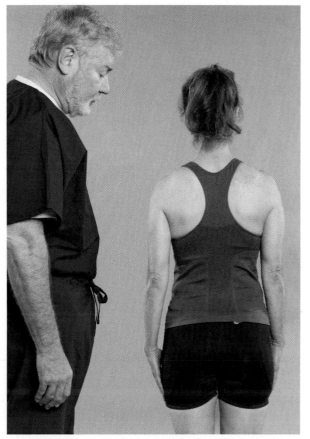

FIG. 7-59 The patient is standing with the arms at the sides. The examiner notes any loss of symmetry of the spinal musculature and notes the posture.

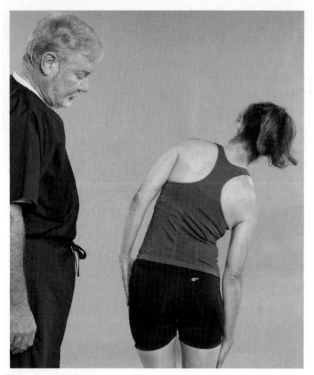

FIG. 7-60 The patient flexes the thoracic spine laterally. The sign is present when tightening or contracture of the musculature occurs on the same side as flexion, which suggests ankylosing spondylitis.

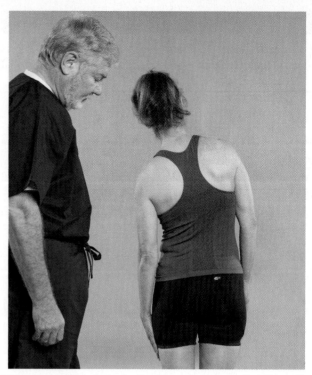

FIG. 7-61 The lateral flexion is compared bilaterally. Motion toward the opposite side is expected to produce normal tightening on the contralateral side. Overall, this tightening represents asymmetric motion of the thoracic spine.

PASSIVE SCAPULAR APPROXIMATION TEST

Assessment for T1 or T2 Nerve Root Problem

Comment

The scapular reflex is a contraction of the scapular muscles on stimulation of the interscapular region. This reflex demonstrates the integrity of the cord between the upper two or three dorsal and lower two or three cervical nerves. However, only a third of the patients exhibit a good reflex response. The examiner should observe the quality of the skin's vascular response after the reflex stimulus. Each side should be equally hyperemic.

The dorsal (erector spinae) reflex is a local contraction of the erector spinae musculature that follows stimulation of the skin along the border of the muscle. This reflex demonstrates integrity of the dorsal region of the cord.

These reflexes are carried out by stimulating the respective area with a Wartenberg pinwheel or a reflex hammer. Reflexes are examined bilaterally.

In acute intervertebral disc herniation, sequestered disc fragments are forced into the spinal canal. Although compression of the theca may be slight, impingement of the anterior median longitudinal artery, an end artery, produces ischemia of the spinal cord over several segments.

The critical zone of the spinal cord is that portion of the cord that lies within the area of the spinal canal extending from the vertebral segments T4 to T9. This portion of the spinal canal is the narrowest zone of the canal and corresponds to that part of the cord possessing the least amount of vascular supply. Therefore the spinal cord may be compromised by two factors: compression and interruption of the vascular supply. Ischemia produces edema and central necrosis of the cord.

> Because it courses along the midaxillary line of the lateral chest wall, the long thoracic nerve may be injured in traction, blunt trauma, penetrating trauma, or surgery (i.e., first rib resection, transaxillary sympathectomy, thoracotomy) that damages this area, resulting in an ipsilateral winged scapula in which the medial border and inferior angle of the scapula pull away from the posterior thoracic wall when the arm is raised. Dysfunction of the anterior serratus muscle from the long thoracic nerve is the most common cause of scapular winging. Functional loss will include the inability to pull and lift heavy objects and to perform tasks that involve reaching objects at a higher level of the shoulders (Krasna, Forti, 2006).

Injury to the long thoracic nerve often occurs along with sprain or other injury at the base of the neck. The long thoracic nerve comes directly off the nerve roots and does not participate in the brachial plexus. The nerve passes down and supplies the various striations of the serratus anterior (Fig. 7-62). Bruising or damage to this nerve may occur and pass unrecognized until distressing winging of the scapula is noted. The cause of this winging may be a sharp blow at the base of the neck that laterally impinges the nerve against the lower cervical vertebrae. Because the long thoracic nerve is primarily a motor nerve, usually little pain or discomfort is noted to guide the examiner. The patient may exhibit weakness or complete paralysis of the nerve, resulting in loss of fixation of the scapula to the chest wall.

PROCEDURE

- The examiner passively approximates the patient's scapulae (Fig. 7-63).
- Ipsilateral T1 or T2 nerve root problem is indicated by scapular pain (Fig. 7-64).

Next Steps/Procedures

First thoracic nerve root test, Roos test, electrodiagnosis, and diagnostic imaging

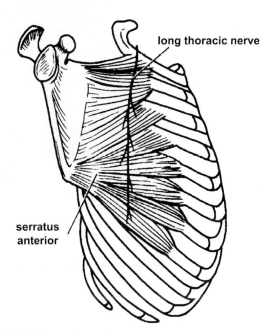

FIG. 7-62 Long thoracic nerve and serratus anterior muscle. (From Krasna MJ, Forti G: Nerve injury: injury to the recurrent laryngeal, phrenic, vagus, long thoracic, and sympathetic nerves during thoracic surgery, *Thorac Surg Clin* 16[3]:267-275, 2006.)

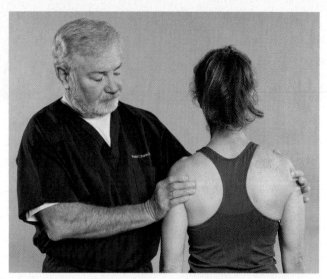

FIG. 7-63 The patient is standing, with the arms at the sides. The examiner observes for thoracic spinal symmetry and posture.

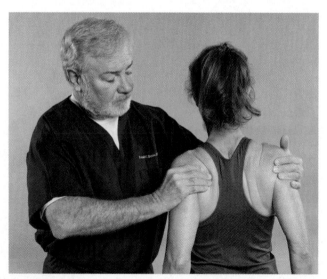

FIG. 7-64 The examiner approximates the scapulae by pulling the shoulder tips backward. Pain in the scapular area indicates a T1 or T2 nerve root involvement.

Assessment for Hypermobile or Hypomobile Costal Structures

Comment

The costocorporeal articulation is a joint between the head of a rib and the adjoining typical thoracic vertebrae. The ligaments of the costotransverse articulation include the articular capsule, costotransverse ligament (both described previously), superior costotransverse ligament, and lateral costotransverse ligament.

The costovertebral joints are synovial joints that are found between the ribs and the vertebral body (Fig. 7-65). The 24 joints are divided into two parts. Ribs 1, 10, 11, and 12 form joints with a single vertebra. Ribs 2 through 9 have an intraarticular ligament. The intraarticular ligament divides the joint into two parts; therefore each rib forms a joint with two adjacent vertebrae. Ribs 2 through 9 also articulate with the intervening intervertebral disc.

The costotransverse joints are synovial joints found between the ribs and the transverse processes of the vertebrae for ribs 1 through 10. Ribs 11 and 12 do not form a joint with the transverse processes; therefore this joint does not exist at these two levels.

The costochondral joints are formed between the ribs and the costal cartilage. The sternocostal joints are found between the costal cartilage and the sternum. The costochondral joints of ribs 2 through 6 are synovial. The first rib costal cartilage is united with the sternum by a synchondrosis and is not synovial. Ribs form joints with an adjacent rib or

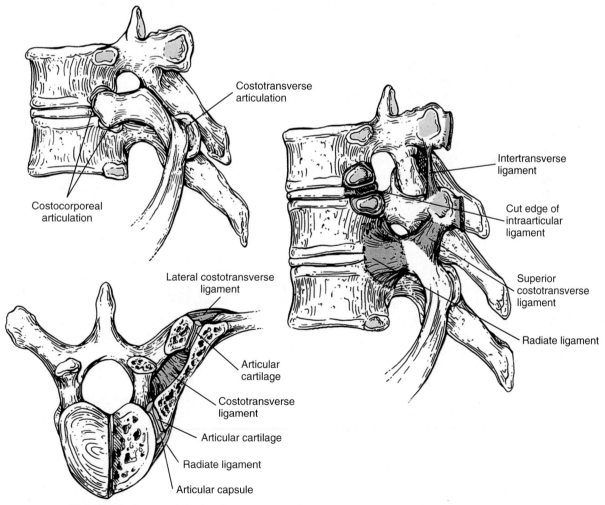

FIG. 7-65 Costovertebral articulations. **A,** Bony costocorporeal and costotransverse articulations. **B,** Ligamentous attachments of these joints. **C,** Superior view. (From Cramer GD, Darby SA: *Basic and clinical anatomy of the spine, spinal cord, and ANS,* St Louis, 1995, Mosby.)

511

costal cartilage. At each of these articulations, a synovial interchondral joint exists.

The ribs help stiffen the thoracic spine. The ribs articulate with the demifacets on vertebrae T2 to T9. For T1 and T10 vertebrae, a complete facet for ribs 1 and 10 exists, respectively. The first rib forms a joint with T1 only, the second rib with T1 and T2, and so on.

Ribs 1 through 7 articulate with the sternum directly and are classified as true ribs. Ribs 8, 9, and 10 join with the costocartilage of the rib above and are classified as false ribs. Ribs 11 and 12 are classified as floating ribs because they do not attach to the sternum or costal cartilages at their distal ends.

Ribs 11 and 12 form joints only with the bodies of T11 and T12 vertebrae. These ribs do not have a joint with the transverse processes of the vertebrae or with the costocartilage of the rib above. The ribs are held by ligaments to the body of the vertebrae and to the transverse processes of the same vertebrae. Some of these ligaments also bind the ribs to the vertebrae above.

At the top of the rib cage, the ribs are horizontal. As the rib cage descends, the ribs become more and more oblique. Rib 12 is more vertical than horizontal. During inspiration, the ribs are pulled up and forward. The first six ribs increase the AP dimension of the chest, mainly by rotating around their long axes. Downward rotation of the rib neck is associated with depression of the chest. Upward rotation of the same portion of the ribs is associated with chest elevation. Collectively, these motions are known as the *pump handle action.* These movements are accompanied by elevation of the manubrium and sternum, superior and anterior.

Ribs 7 through 10 mainly increase lateral, or transverse, dimension. The ribs move superiorly, posteriorly, and medially to increase the infrasternal angle, or inferiorly, anteriorly, and laterally to decrease the angle. These movements are known as the *bucket handle action.*

Ribs 8 through 12 move laterally in a caliper action that increases the lateral dimension.

The ribs are elastic in children but become increasingly brittle with age. Rib hyperostosis is seen with the seronegative spondyloarthropathies (Fig. 7-66). In the anterior half of the chest, the ribs are subcutaneous. In the posterior half, the ribs are covered by muscles.

Rib hyperostosis can be observed in patients with diffuse idiopathic skeletal hyperostosis (DISH), AS, psoriasis, and quadriplegia. According to Huang and colleagues, the frequency of rib hyperostosis was significantly higher in DISH (21.6%), AS (10.3%), and quadriplegia (6.6%) than in the healthy control group (0.5%). In their study, the main radiographic features were a short segment of cortical thickening and sclerosis, which predominated in the medial aspect of the posterior portion of the rib. The resulting radiographic

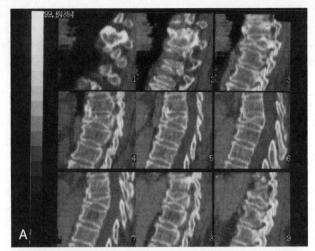
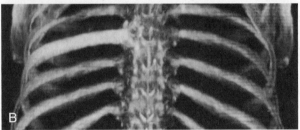

FIG. 7-66 Rib hyperostosis (isolated). (Adapted From Arslan G et al: Single rib sclerosis as a sequel of compression fracture of adjacent vertebra and costovertebral joint ankylosis, *Eur J Radiol Extra* 51[1]:43-46, 2004.)

features simulated the appearance of Paget disease. Osseous excrescences of adjacent costovertebral articulations were significantly related to the rib hyperostosis, seen in 73% of instances of rib involvement. In most of the patients, sclerosis can be observed in one level, but two- or three-level sclerosis can also be seen. Rib sclerosis is significantly related to exuberant bony excrescences of the adjacent costovertebral articulations, and rib sclerosis is caused by hypomobility of costovertebral joints in the setting of bony outgrowths and ankylosis (Arslan et al, 2004).

PROCEDURE

- As the supine patient inhales and exhales, the AP movement of the ribs is palpated (Fig. 7-67).
- Restriction in motion is noted.
- Rib abnormalities during exhalation suggest an elevated rib (lowest rib).
- Rib abnormalities during inhalation suggest a depressed rib (uppermost rib).

Next Steps/Procedures
Chest expansion test, sternal compression test, and diagnostic imaging

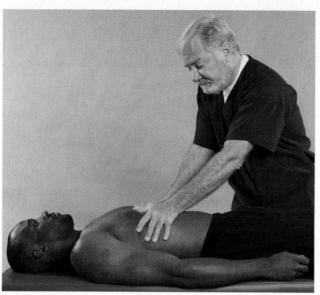

FIG. 7-67 With the patient supine, the examiner's hands are placed over the chest. The examiner feels for the anteroposterior movement of the ribs as the patient inhales and exhales. Any restriction or difference in motion is noted. Rib abnormalities during exhalation suggest an elevated rib. Rib abnormalities during inhalation suggest a depressed rib. A depressed rib is usually the uppermost rib. An elevated rib is usually the lowest rib.

7

Assessment for Costal and Intercostal Tissue Integrity

Comment

Any fixation or aberrant movement of the costovertebral articulations, or ribs, can have an impact on the synovial joints of the dorsal spine. The examiner rarely finds concomitant loss of joint play at the rib angle and corresponding vertebral motor unit. Experts have suggested that the rib cage may act as a splint to the thoracic spine. This splinting effect may prevent stresses placed directly on the mid spine. In addition, it may be one of the reasons that thoracic disc herniations are less common. The fully developed ribs protect the underlying thoracic viscera while simultaneously providing attachment sites for a wide variety of muscles (Table 7-6).

Because a multitude of muscles attach to the chest, almost any manifestation of strain may occur. Strain may be caused by violent exertion or by overstretching of the muscles. The symptoms depend entirely on the area involved. In the long muscles of the back of the thorax, this condition may be indistinguishable from or may be a part of a lumbar strain. In the front of the chest, the strain may involve the muscles of the abdominal wall, where the muscles attach to the lower ribs. Strain also may involve the intercostal muscles, although this involvement is uncommon because the muscles are well protected by other muscle structures. These muscles do not act forcibly enough to rupture their fibers. A strain is much more likely to involve an area connecting to the chest

than the chest itself, particularly the scapular muscles. Strain of the rhomboids will occur either at the scapular attachment or along the spine much more often than at the costal attachment.

Similarly, the serrati may be more likely to get injured in their substance than in their costal origins. Thorough analysis of the active motion that causes pain will usually determine the proper muscle group.

Strain of the muscle at its attachment to the rib is likely to be more painful than it is disabling. However, considerable attendant muscle spasms may occur that will splint the chest and interfere with deep breathing, occasionally marking intercostal nerve injury as well. These spasms may actually prevent certain types of activity. A strain of the abdominal recti attached to the lower ribs may interdict undertaking of certain sports, such as rowing or wrestling, in which forcible use of the abdominal muscles is required. Similarly, a spasm of the shoulder muscles may interdict throwing.

The incidence of postthoracotomy pain is 80% at 3 months, 75% at 6 months, and 61% at 1 year after surgery. Pain is severe in 3% to 5% of patients and interferes with quality of life. Characterized by incisional pain with radiation along the distribution of intercostal nerves, it may be predicted by poor postoperative analgesia. The etiology of intercostal nerve damage may be the result of focal nerve injury or ischemia related to rib retraction. Minimally invasive procedures, such as video-assisted thoracoscopic surgery (VATS), may be associated with a reduced incidence of postthoracotomy pain. When occurring after the resolution of postoperative pain, other causes, such as recurrent intrathoracic disease, require consideration. When established, intercostal neuralgia is often refractory to treatment and results in significant morbidity (Brewer, 2003).

Chronic abdominal pain of uncertain etiology is a common clinical problem that often leads to many diagnostic evaluations and treatment interventions and sometimes multiple surgeries. Numerous reports emphasize that patients with pain originating in the structures of the abdominal wall are frequently misdiagnosed and treated as suffering from visceral pain. In 1919, Cyriax reported conditions simulating referred visceral pain from somatic structures by causing intercostal nerve irritation. Three years later, Janowski pointed out that symptoms attributed to visceral disease could arise from the abdominal wall. In 1926, Carnett, a surgeon, published the seminal article recognizing the syndrome that he believed was caused by intercostal neuralgia. A 1991 editorial in *The Lancet* and other reports emphasize that the lack of physician awareness of abdominal wall pain is economically costly. Hershfield reported that 100 patients ultimately diagnosed as having abdominal wall pain had previously had 418 diagnostic procedures. In another study,

TABLE 7-6

THORACIC CAGE ARCHITECTURE

Region	Tissues
Superiorly	Sternocleidomastoid, sternohyoid, sternothyroid, and anterior, middle, and posterior scalene muscles
Anteriorly	Pectoralis major and minor muscles, mammary glands
Posteriorly	Serratus posterior superior and inferior, and deep back muscles; trapezius, rhomboid minor and major, scapula, and all muscles related to it reset against the thoracic cage
Laterally	Serratus anterior muscles
Inferiorly	Abdominal muscles attaching to thoracic cage (i.e., rectus abdominis, external and internal abdominal oblique, transverses abdominis)

From Cramer GD, Darby SA: *Basic and clinical anatomy of the spine, spinal cord, and ANS,* ed 2, St Louis, 2005, Mosby.

30 patients with chronic abdominal pain, subsequently found to be from the abdominal wall, had earlier undergone 67 diagnostic procedures, including four laparoscopies. The conservatively estimated average cost was $1269 (1993 dollars) per patient, not taking into account the costs of blood or urine tests, office or emergency department visits, and lost pay. In both studies, all procedures were exclusionary, and none pointed to the diagnosis or management. In 2001, Thompson and colleagues (C. Thompson, Pennsylvania State College of Medicine, personal communication, June 15, 2001) estimated an average cost of $6727 per patient for previous diagnostic testing and hospital charges for 16 patients ultimately diagnosed as having *abdominal wall syndrome*. (Srinivasan, Greenbaum, 2002).

PROCEDURE

- Schepelmann sign identifies rib integrity (Fig. 7-68).
- The patient raises the arms while standing and then bends laterally.
- Pain created on the concave side is caused by intercostal neuritis (Fig. 7-69)
- If pain is created on the convex side, the diagnosis is intercostal myofascitis (Fig. 7-70).
- Intercostal myofascitis must be differentiated from the fibrous inflammation of pleurisy.

Next Steps/Procedures

Rib motion testing, chest expansion test, Amoss sign, Forestier bowstring sign, sternal compression test, and diagnostic imaging.

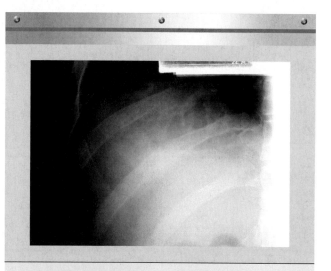

AT THE VIEWBOX

There is a subtle, nondisplaced oblique fracture of the ninth posterior rib. Rib fractures and other rib, costal cartilage, costovertebral and sternocostal injuries are often diagnosed largely on clinical findings. Imaging studies may provide confirmation of fracture and may help to assess for complications, such as pneumothorax. However, negative or equivocal radiographs certainly do not exclude non-displaced rib fractures. Advanced imaging such as radionuclide imaging or CT may be used to more definitively assess for rib fracture. (From the teaching file of Timothy Mick, DC, DACBR)

CLINICAL PEARL

Schepelmann test provides an efficient method for localizing rib injury. The patient moves actively and can limit the motion according to the pain.

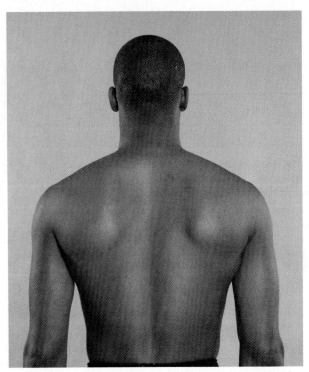

FIG. 7-68 The patient is standing, and the spinal contours are noted.

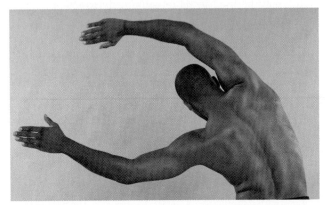

FIG. 7-69 The patient fully abducts the shoulders, bringing the hands overhead. The patient flexes the thoracic spine laterally. Pain elicited on the side of flexion (concave) indicates intercostal neuritis. Pain elicited on the convex side indicates intercostal myofascitis.

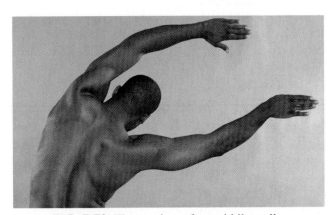

FIG. 7-70 The test is performed bilaterally.

Assessment for Spinal Osseous and Paraspinal Soft-Tissue Integrity

Comment

Several mechanisms of injury to the thoracic spine can lead to a sprain or strain disability. Flexion and extension loading in a ballistic fashion can damage the joints and paravertebral soft tissues of the thoracic spine. Lifting can also injure the mid spine if the weight is too heavy or the mechanics are incorrect. Excessive contraction and rotation can place undue strain on the facet joints and erector muscles of the spine.

Multiple-level spinal fractures, which may be contiguous or separated, are estimated to occur in 3% to 5% of patients with spinal fractures (Fig. 7-71). Multiple noncontiguous spinal fractures rarely occur without injury to the spinal cord. Three patterns of injury have been identified (Fig. 7-72).

Patients with multiple-level, noncontiguous fractures usually have a disproportionate number of primary vertebral injuries in the middle and upper thoracic spine.

In thoracolumbar spine injuries, a three-column concept of spinal injury exists (Fig. 7-73). The anterior column contains the anterior longitudinal ligament, the anterior half of

---

ORTHOPEDIC GAMUT 7-15

MULTIPLE-LEVEL SPINAL FRACTURES

Three patterns of injury in multiple-level spinal fractures are:

Pattern A: The primary lesion occurs between C5 and C7, with secondary injuries at T12 or the lumbar spine

Pattern B: The primary injury occurs at T2 and T4, with secondary injuries in the cervical spine

Pattern C: The primary injury occurs between T12 and L2, with secondary injuries from L4 to L5

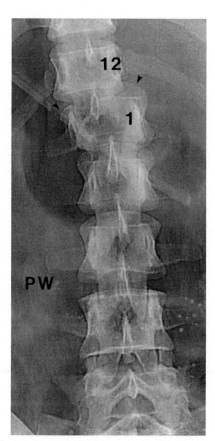

FIG. 7-71 Anteroposterior view of the thoracolumbar spine shows noncontiguous translation injury at T12–L1 level. (From Canale ST: *Campbell's operative orthopaedics,* vol 1-4, ed 9, St Louis, 1998, Mosby.)

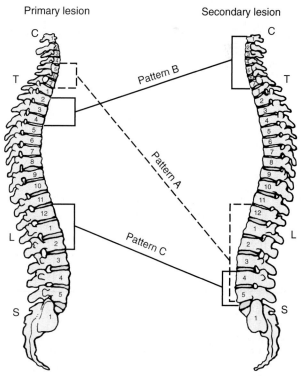

FIG. 7-72 Three patterns of multiple level injury. (From Canale ST: *Campbell's operative orthopaedics,* vol 1-4, ed 9, St Louis, 1998, Mosby.)

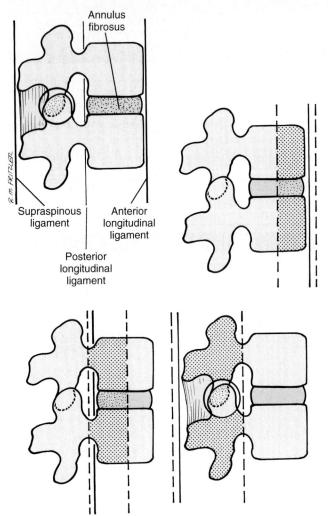

FIG. 7-73 Three-column classification of spinal instability. (From Canale ST: *Campbell's operative orthopaedics,* vol 1-4, ed 9, St Louis, 1998, Mosby.)

THORACOLUMBAR FRACTURES

Thoracolumbar fracture classifications (based on three-column concepts) follow:

- Wedge compression fractures cause isolated failure of the anterior column and result from forward flexion.
- In stable burst fractures, the anterior and middle columns fail because of a compressive load.
- In unstable burst fractures, the anterior and middle columns fail in compression, and the posterior column is disrupted.
- Chance fractures are horizontal avulsion injuries of the vertebral bodies caused by flexion about an axis anterior to the anterior longitudinal ligament.
- In flexion distraction injuries, the flexion axis is posterior to the anterior longitudinal ligament. The anterior column fails in compression, and the middle and posterior columns fail in tension.
- Translational injuries are characterized by malalignment of the neural canal, which has been totally disrupted. Usually, all three columns have failed in shear.

the vertebral body, and the anterior portion of the annulus fibrosus. The middle column consists of the posterior longitudinal ligament, the posterior half of the vertebral body, and the posterior aspect of the annulus fibrosus. The posterior column includes the neural arch, the ligamentum flavum, the facet capsules, and the interspinous ligaments.

The incidence of fractures of the spine is significantly increased because of osteoporosis in the later years of life. Even after relatively minor trauma, compression fractures with vertebral collapse are common in older people. After age 70 in the asymptomatic population, the incidence of such fractures is 20%.

Fracture risk increases with age, prior fracture at any site and decreasing bone mineral density (BMD). The risk of recurrent fracture is highest in the first 2 years after a fracture (12%), and especially in the first year. Early diagnosis and treatment of osteoporosis immediately after fracture is therefore vital. Effective, easy-to-use medication may reduce fracture risk by one half if BMD *T*-score at or below −2.5, WHO threshold value for osteoporosis (Blonk et al, 2007).

In the aging spine, the cause of such fractures may be spontaneous and obscure without a major traumatic event. The fractures may occur because of sneezing, raising windows, or lifting weights. The patient can experience severe pain in the spine, although absence of discomfort is common. Minor falls may also produce such fractures. In addition to having back pain, these patients may have local tenderness and may be reluctant to move while in bed to avoid further pain. Some patients have root pain, and a very small minority has injury to the spinal cord. Approximately 15% of such patients may develop paralytic ileus, particularly in association with fractures of T12 and L1. Experts generally consider that retroperitoneal hemorrhage is the underlying factor in the production of the ileus either by the size of the hemorrhage or by irritation of the celiac plexus.

Osteoporosis is the most commonly seen metabolic disease in the United States (Fig.7-74). It is almost universally found in elderly adults and, as with atherosclerosis, develops slowly over many years. The two most common types of osteoporosis are postmenopausal and *age associated* (sometimes called *senile*). The age-associated form is seen equally in men and women. The postmenopausal type is the most common symptomatic form of osteoporosis. This disorder becomes increasingly more common with age, usually developing within 15 to 20 years after menopause. Estimates indicate that 1.5 million fractures occur yearly because of osteoporosis. The disorder is less common in African Americans and more common in Caucasians and Asians. Spontaneous fractures, vertebral collapse, and osteo-

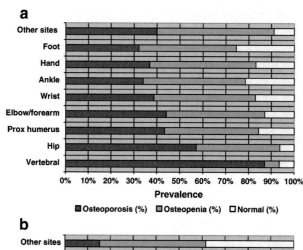

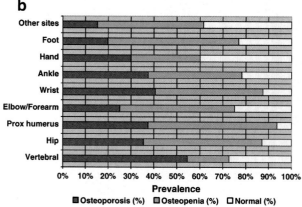

FIG. 7-74 **A,** Osteoporosis, osteopenia, and normal bone density in female fracture patients (*N* = 804) according to WHO criteria. **B,** Osteoporosis, osteopenia and normal bone density in male fracture patients (*N* = 254) according to WHO criteria. (From Blonk MC et al: The fracture and osteoporosis clinic: 1-year results and 3-month compliance, *Bone* 40[6]:1643-649, 2007.)

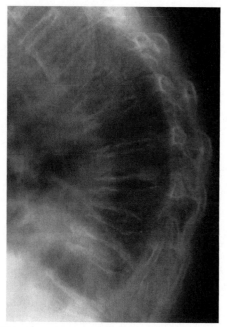

FIG. 7-75 Osteoporosis. Multiple compression fractures are present. (From Mercier LR, Pettid FJ: *Practical orthopedics,* ed 4, St Louis, 1995, Mosby.)

porosis are often discovered as incidental findings on roentgenograms (Fig. 7-75).

Several methods are currently available for evaluating bone status. Standard radiography is useful for identifying fractures, but fails to detect osteoporosis in its initial stage. Dual-energy X-ray absorptiometry (DXA) is the most widely known and employed method to detect BMD (in g/cm^2). Quantitative computed tomography (QCT) assists in evaluating the trabecular portion and is the only method that expresses bone density as a volumetric unit. Last, quantitative ultrasound techniques (QUS) seem to be correlated not only to the mineral content, but also to some qualitative properties of bone (Camozzi et al, in press).

PROCEDURE

- While the patient is seated or standing and the thoracic spine is slightly flexed, the examiner percusses the spinous processes and the associated musculature of each of the thoracic vertebrae with a neurologic reflex hammer.
- Evidence of localized pain indicates a possible fractured vertebra.
- Evidence of radicular pain indicates a possible disc lesion.
- Because of the nonspecific nature of this test, other conditions also will elicit a positive pain response.
- If a ligamentous sprain exists, percussion of the spinous processes will elicit pain (Fig. 7-76).
- Percussion of the paraspinal musculature will elicit a positive sign for strain (Fig. 7-77).

Next Steps/Procedures
Soto-Hall sign, Dejerine sign, Valsalva maneuver, Lhermitte sign, and diagnostic imaging

CLINICAL PEARL

When soft-tissue percussion reproduces the complaint, the examiner may expect the same phenomenon from applications of ultrasound to the tissue. The uses of such therapies may be delayed until the soft tissue is no longer reactive to percussion.

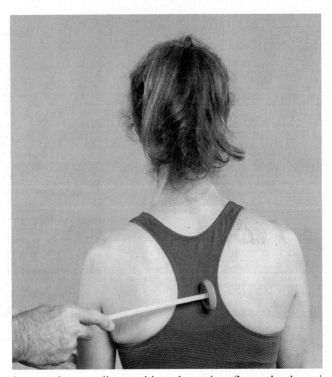

FIG. 7-76 In the seated or standing position, the patient flexes the thoracic spine, exposing the spinous processes as much as possible. The examiner percusses the spinous processes of each vertebra. Localized pain is evidence of a fracture or severe sprain. Radiating pain suggests intervertebral disc syndrome.

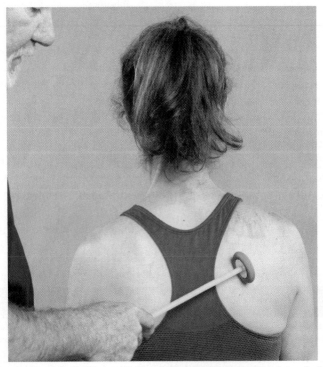

FIG. 7-77 The paravertebral tissues are percussed. Pain elicited in the soft tissues suggests muscular strain and highly sensitive myofascial trigger points.

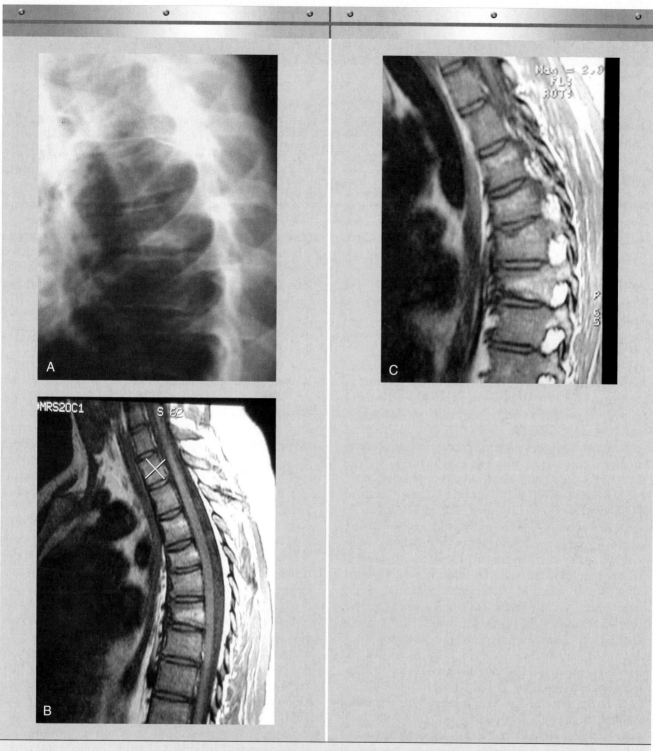

AT THE VIEWBOX

19-year-old male with upper thoracic and cervical spine pain since motor vehicle accident two months ago. Patient was examined and released from the emergency room without X-rays. He presented to a chiropractic physician, who obtained thoracic spine radiographs. The lateral view demonstrates a compression fracture of T6. **A,** MRI was obtained, to help exclude extension of the fracture into the middle or posterior columns and to exclude other radiographically occult lesions, such as associated disc herniation. This demonstrates four consecutive subacute compression fractures, including the one at T6 visible on plain films. **B** and **C,** A careful clinical examination, to include spinal percussion, led to obtaining the appropriate imaging to diagnose these fractures. (From the teaching file of Timothy Mick, DC, DACBR)

Assessment for Acute Inflammatory Lesions of the Spine

Comment

Minor injuries of the soft tissue result from mild overuse or overstretching. Severe thoracic soft-tissue injuries are characterized by traumatic effusion, pain, and loss of function. Traumatic effusion consists of four types of physiologic tissue reactions.

Tissue tearing or crushing with rupture of the blood vessels causes bleeding into the tissue. The capillaries are constricted in the injury area or site. Resultant clotting seals the damaged vessels. Fibroblasts begin the repair process, and lymphatic drainage takes place.

Local inflammation causes the undamaged capillaries to dilate and become more permeable, allowing inflammatory exudates to form. The exudates stimulate fibroblast repair and white blood cell activity with resultant local heat, redness, swelling, and pain.

Formation of tissue thickening or tissue adhesions from the blood and exudates occur, especially if any of the lymphatics are damaged or if the circulation is impaired.

If a thoracic spinal joint is involved in the soft-tissue injury, synovial effusion may result. With muscle strain, the interstitial exudates and fluids gel when the muscle is at rest. The patient experiences a stiffening of the muscle on resting the injured part. This stiffening is followed by the onset of a cramp or spasm of the injured muscle, and associated pain and ache occur in the part. This pain is completely relieved by movement. As the exudates are forced out of the tissue, through mechanical action of muscle contraction, the part is no longer stiff or sore. However, after excessive movement, the strained muscle fibers are once again aggravated and become uncomfortable. The patient is forced to rest the part, and the cycle begins again.

Myofascial fibrositis, an inflammatory nonsuppurative condition affecting the interstitial tissues of the body, is an established clinical syndrome. Previous terms applied to this condition often caused confusion. These terms are *nonarticular rheumatism, fibromyositis, myositis,* and *muscular rheumatism.* Other commonly used terms include *wry neck* and *lumbago.*

Primary myofascial fibrositis occurs independent of pathologic causes elsewhere in the body. Secondary myofascial fibrositis is myofascial inflammation that is secondary to the development of another pathologic condition and is associated with conditions such as rheumatoid arthritis, osteoarthritis, hypertrophic or degenerative arthritis, spondylosis, septic foci, rheumatic fever, diabetes, and influenza.

Secondary myofascial fibrositis may also be the residual effect of traumatic injuries.

When the tissues involved fail to heal completely after injury, the condition of myofascial inflammation is called a *residual* complication.

Older patients who develop clinical cases of myofascial fibrositis experience a gradual onset of their symptoms (senile myofascial fibrositis). The etiology of this type of myofascial fibrositis is one that is mixed and complex and is probably associated with a combination of factors that include endocrine imbalances, dietary deficiencies, and degenerative tissue changes.

Normal fibrous tissue is made up of bands of collagen, fibroblasts, elastic tissue fibrils, fluid spaces, reticuloendothelial cells, capillaries, and nerves.

The inflammatory reaction of these tissues includes the swelling and fragmentation of the bands of collagen and the proliferation of fibroblasts. If the fibroblasts proliferate, the proliferation causes contractures and blocks the free flow of tissue fluids. This blockage results in difficulty moving the joints and produces pressure on the vessels and nerves in the immediate vicinity. Although small nodules form, they are often too small to be palpated. The nodules are discovered because of tenderness produced by pressure or other means.

The onset of the clinical symptoms may be sudden or insidious. The limitation of joint movement in acute cases is caused by muscle spasm. In chronic cases, the spasm may be mixed with contractures. Post inertial dyskinesia, which is the *gelling* stiffness that results from movement of a part that has been rested, is a consistent complaint.

Swelling of the tissues is sometimes found by the examiner. However, the swelling sensation is often subjective. The nodules that have been described are located by palpation, especially when the nodules form over a firm undersurface, such as bone. By carefully searching the area, the examiner can discern acutely tender areas of myofascial fibrositis, which are called *trigger points.*

Sensitive areas in the soft tissues throughout the body have been described for years. Pressure on these areas causes local and referred pain into distal areas of the body. These tender areas are often identified as symptoms of the following conditions: myofascial pain syndrome, myalgia, myositis, fibrositis, fibromyositis, fibromyalgia fascitis, myofascitis, muscular rheumatism, strain, and sprain.

The small hypersensitive area that makes up a trigger site may be stimulated by pressure, goading, needling, excessive heat, local icing, and motion.

Trigger points are characterized as hard nodules of fibrous connective tissue that surrounds sparse muscle fibers. Infiltrations of lymphocytes also occur. Trigger points may be worsened by stress, infection, or metabolic upset.

Myofascial fibrositis is classified as acute, subacute, or chronic, depending on the pain, pressure sensitivity, reflex spasm, swelling, impaired mobility, and increased temperature in the area.

Diagnostic criteria for myofascial fibrositis include exquisite pain and tenderness, circumscribed painful tissue hardening, and pressure on the trigger point, which causes pain referral.

Predisposing factors for myofascial fibrositis include chronic muscular strain, repeated excessive muscular activity and direct trauma, chilling of fatigued muscles, arthritis, nerve root injury, and psychogenic anxiety.

The cardinal symptom of fibromyalgia is diffuse, chronic pain. The pain often begins in one location, particularly the neck and shoulders but then becomes more generalized. Generally, patients state that "it hurts all over" and have difficulty locating the site of pain arising from articular or nonarticular tissues. Patients often describe the muscle pain as burning, radiating, or gnawing and the intensity of the pain as modest or severe but varying greatly. Most patients also report profound fatigue. Headaches, either tension or more typical migraine headaches and symptoms suggestive

---

ORTHOPEDIC GAMUT 7-17

FIBROMYALGIA TENDER POINT EXAMINATION PROTOCOL

The examiner surveys 18 standard points and three control points. The purpose of the control points is to assess the patient's baseline pain perception.

Palpation Technique
- Patient should wear a standard examination gown.
- Survey sites are first located visually and then with light palpation.
- Pressure is applied with the dominant thumb pad perpendicular to each survey site.
- Each site is pressed for a total of 4 seconds only once to prevent sensitization that may occur with repeated palpation.
- The force is increased by 1 kg per second until 4 kg pressure is achieved.
- Whitening of the examiner's nail bed usually occurs when applying 4 kg force.
- Examiners can learn the approximate feel of 4 kg force by using a dolorimeter or by using the thumb to counterbalance the 4-kg weight on a standard scale.

Patient Instruction
- "Please say *yes* or *no* if you feel any pain when a specific point is pressed."
- When the patient responds *yes* to indicate pain, the examiner should assess pain severity by asking for a numeric pain intensity rating: on a scale from 0 to 10, where 0 is no pain, and 10 is the worst pain ever experienced.
- By mid test, the patient is reminded of the meaning of the pain intensity range.

Tender Point Locations for Testing
- Seated
  - Mid-forehead (control)
  - Occiput: suboccipital muscle insertions

- Trapezius: midpoint of upper border
- Supraspinatus: above medial border of scapular spine
- Gluteal: upper outer quadrant of buttocks
- Low cervical: anterior aspect of the intertransverse space of C5–C7
- Second rib: second costochondral junction
- Lateral epicondyle: 2 cm distal to epicondyle
- Dorsum right forearm (control): junction of proximal two thirds and distal one third
- Left thumbnail (control):
- Side lying
  - Greater trochanter: posterior to trochanteric prominences
- Supine, feet slightly apart
  - Knee: medial fat pad proximal to the joint line

Number of positive survey sites: _____ Sum of survey site scores (SS): _____	
Number of positive control sites: _____ Sum of control site scores (CS): _____	
FMS Intensity Score (SS/18): _____ Control Intensity Score (CS/3): _____	
FMS? Widespread pain for more than 3 months: _____ Yes _____ No	
Eleven or more positive survey sites: _____ Yes _____No	
If answer to both questions is yes, patient fits FMS criteria.	

Adapted from Sinclair JD, Startz TW, Turk DC: The manual tender point survey. Pittsburgh, 1997, University of Pittsburgh Medical Center, Center of Continuing Education in the Health Sciences.
Okifuji A, Turk DC, Sinclair JD, et al: A standardized manual tender point survey. I. Development and determination of a threshold point for the identification of positive tender points in fibromyalgia syndrome, *J Rheumatol* 24:377-383, 1997.

of irritable bowel syndrome are present in more than 50% of patients. True Raynaud phenomenon or a Raynaud-like excess sensitivity to cold has also been commonly reported.

Patients with fibromyalgia are hypersensitive to heat, cold, and cutaneous electric, intramuscular electric, sural nerve electric (to assess nociceptive spinal reflex), ischemic, and intramuscular hypertonic saline. Furthermore, allodynia to warmth, cold, and pressure has been documented. Temporal summation has been demonstrated by using heat and cold and intramuscular electric stimuli. Sensitivity to noise, as often complained by patients with fibromyalgia syndrome, has been demonstrated in a human pain laboratory by using a noise generator (Yunus, 2007).

Patients invariably complain of muscle weakness; however, formal muscle testing does not reveal significant weakness, provided the pain does not prevent the patient from achieving maximal effort. The only reliable finding on examination is the presence of multiple tender points (Fig.

7-78). Nine pairs of tender points should be examined routinely. Patients with fewer than 11 tender points certainly can be diagnosed with fibromyalgia provided other symptoms and signs are present.

Other common findings on examination include muscle *spasm* or taut bands of muscle, sometimes called nodules by patients; skin sensitivity, in the form of skin roll tenderness of dermatographism (Fig. 7-79); or purplish mottling of the skin, especially of the legs after exposure to the cold. Myofascial pain syndromes also overlap with fibromyalgia (Table 7-7). The relationship of trigger points and tender points is not clear. The location of the trigger point is deep within the muscle belly. Trigger points result in decreased muscle stretch and pain with contraction. A *twitch response* (or jump sign), pathognomonic of an active trigger point, is a visible or palpable contraction of the muscle produced by a rapid snap of the examining finger on the taut band of muscle, or by stroking the skin with a blunt instrument. A characteristic referred pain pattern is present (Fig. 7-80).

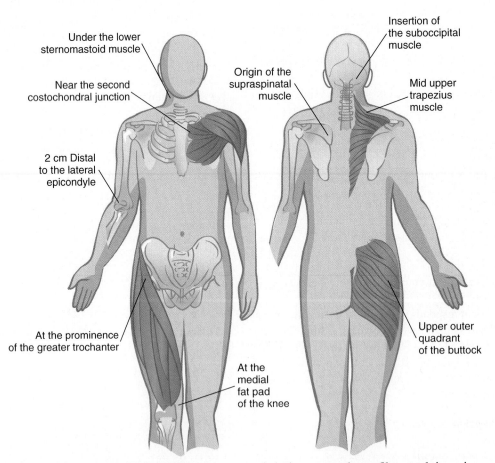

FIG. 7-78 American Pain Society–recommended sites to evaluate fibromyalgia pain.

(From American Pain Society: *Guidelines for the management of fibromyalgia syndrome pain in adults and children,* Copyright © 2005 by American Pain Society; all rights reserved.)

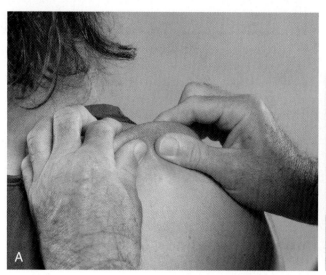 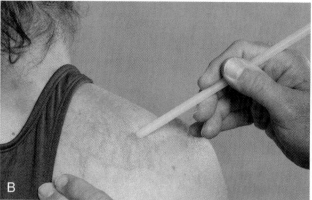

FIG. 7-79 Skin-rolling tenderness (**A**) and reactive hyperemia (**B**).

FIG. 7-80 **A,** The tender point location of fibromyalgia. The nine paired tender points recommended by the 1990 American College of Rheumatology Criteria Committee for establishing a diagnosis of fibromyalgia are (1) insertion of the nuchal muscles into the occiput; (2) upper border of the trapezius, midportion; (3) muscle attachments to the upper medial border of the scapula; (4) anterior aspects of the C5, C7 intertransverse spaces; (5) second rib space approximately 3 cm lateral to the sternal border; (6) muscle attachments to the lateral epicondyle, approximately 2 cm below the bony prominence; (7) upper outer quadrant of gluteal muscles; (8) muscle attachments just posterior to the greater trochanter; and (9) medial fat pad of the knee proximal to the joint line. A total of 11 or more tender points in conjunction with a history of widespread pain is characteristic of the fibromyalgia syndrome. (From Bradley WG: *Neurology in clinical practice,* ed 5, New York, 2008, Butterworth-Heinemann.) **B,** Overlap between syndromes with unexplained etiologies such as fibromyalgia, chronic fatigue syndrome (CFS), irritable bowel syndrome, temporomandibular disorder, and multiple chemical sensitivity. (From Harris ED: *Kelley's textbook of rheumatology,* ed 7, Philadelphia, 2005, WB Saunders.)

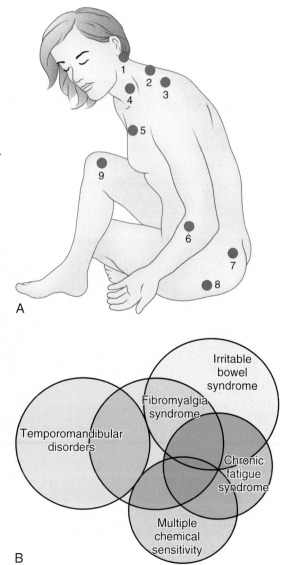

TABLE 7-7

MISDIAGNOSES THAT MAY BE GIVEN TO PATIENTS WHO EVENTUALLY ARE FOUND TO HAVE THE FIBROMYALGIA SYNDROME

Alzheimer disease
Depression
Early spondyloarthropathy
Hypochondriasis
Hypothyroidism
Inflammatory bowel disease
Inflammatory myopathy
Interstitial cystitis
Malingering
Menière–Age disease
Metabolic myopathy
Multiple sclerosis
Neuropathy
Polymyalgia rheumatica
Sciatica
Somatoform pain disorder
Systemic lupus erythematosus/rheumatoid arthritis

From Kelley WN et al: *Textbook of rheumatology,* ed 5, Philadelphia, 1997, WB Saunders.

PROCEDURE

- A hot moist sponge is passed up and down the spine several times (Figs. 7-81 and 7-82).
- If any lesion of the spine is present, pain is felt as the sponge passes over the lesion.
- The test is positive for acute inflammatory lesions of the spine.

Next Steps/Procedures

Palpation, thoracic spinal range of motion, and thoracic spinal muscle testing

CLINICAL PEARL

As with spinal percussion, the focal areas of tenderness found with the sponge test may be hypersensitive to mechanical stimulation. This sensitivity represents spasmophilia and must be absent before aggressive physical therapy can begin.

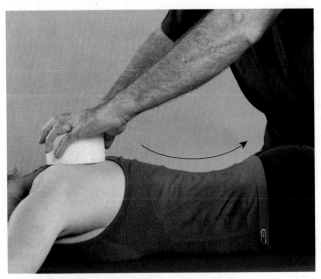

FIG. 7-81 The patient is prone. The examiner notes spinal symmetry and any muscular induration. A hot sponge is placed at the superior aspect of the thoracic spine.

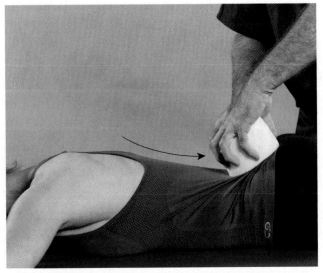

FIG. 7-82 The sponge is passed down the spinal column to the lumbosacral area. This action is repeated several times. Pain is felt in locally inflamed areas as the sponge passes over them. This pain indicates local acute inflammation.

STERNAL COMPRESSION TEST

Assessment for Costal Structure Fracture

Comment

The participation of women in sports has steadily increased over recent decades because of the implementation of Title IX. As participation increases, so does physical stress placed on the musculoskeletal system of the female athlete. Chest wall pain is a common symptom in athletes. Costochondritis is typically associated with pain on the anterior chest wall of the costochondral or costosternal joints. This condition is more common in women and associated with physical stresses experienced in athletics. Costochondritis is typically a benign and self-limiting condition. However, other more ominous conditions such as *Escherichia coli* infection in the cartilage, intravenous drug abuse, primary tumors, and rheumatologic disorders are reported to be an associated cause of symptoms (Aspegren, Hyde, Miller, 2007).

Also known as *Tietze syndrome*, costochondritis is an inflammation of the rib cartilage at the costosternal junction. The differential diagnosis includes angina pectoris, intercostal strain and neuralgia, rib subluxation, and, in cases of substantial trauma, rib fracture. The patient with costochondritis complains of point tenderness over one or two rib heads or costal junctions lateral to the sternum (Table 7-8). Symptoms are most commonly localized to the second, third, or fourth costochondral junctions (Fig. 7-83). Abduction of the arm reproduces the patient's pain, which may radiate down the arm. Acute inflammation causes discomfort or pain on deep inspiration as the rib cage expands. Bogginess or swelling over the costal cartilage is possible but does not always occur.

Fractures of the ribs are common, and they usually are caused by a direct blow from a blunt object. In this instance, a fracture of one rib or, at most, two ribs is likely. Forceful compression of the chest in one of its diameters may produce single or multiple fractures. In the first instance, the patient will relate a history of a blow to the chest that may have been forceful enough to knock the wind out of the person and cause severe localized pain. As the patient tries to breathe deeply, severe pain occurs. Muscle spasm splints the chest and prevents deep breathing. The result is rapid, shallow respiration caused by the combination of air hunger and pain during inspiration. In the second instance, the patient may relate a history of being crushed in a pileup or of falling forcibly onto a side with an object between the chest and the ground. Here again, the patient will experience labored breathing accompanied by severe pain. Thorough examination at the time of injury will elicit tenderness directly over the rib or ribs, and pain occurs in this same area during deep breathing. Although direct pressure on the involved rib is avoided, compression of the chest will cause pain. If the sixth rib is broken at the anterior axillary line, pressure made directly backward on the sternum will cause pain in the area of the fracture, and deep inspiration will be painful. Any attempt at coughing or sneezing is disastrous. A patient who tries to do so will grab the chest and attempt to restrict the motion manually.

A palpable defect in the rib maybe found if the fracture is complete, and crepitus might be elicited. Manipulation to elicit such an effect is not justifiable. Fracture can be differentiated from a simple contusion because contusion does not usually cause pain during motion of the rib.

Physical examination findings for costochondritis typically include anterior chest wall tenderness that is localized to the costochondral junction of one or more ribs but does not include swelling, heat, or erythema. The second through fifth costal cartilage areas are most commonly involved. Associated restriction of corresponding costovertebral and costotransverse joints may be discovered on joint play assessment, such as by motion palpation (Aspegren, Hyde, Miller, 2007; Humphreys, Delahaye, Peterson, 2004; Pringle, 2004).

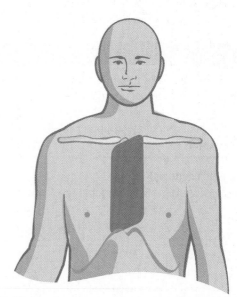

FIG. 7-83 Tenderness localized over the costochondral joints may be the only clinical finding in costochondritis, whereas Tietze syndrome may be associated with swelling, heat, and erythema. (Adapted from Ian Rabey M: Costochondritis: are the symptoms and signs due to neurogenic inflammation? Two cases that responded to manual therapy directed towards posterior spinal structures, *Man Ther* 13[1]:82-86, 2008.)

TABLE 7-8

THORAX AND RIB SYNDROMES

	Costochondritis (Tietze Syndrome)	Intercostal Strain	Intercostal Neuralgia	Costovertebral Syndrome	Pectoralis Strain
Physical examination findings	Painful arm abduction Palpable tenderness at costosternal junction Commonly at second to fourth rib cartilage Normal results on cardiac examination Exacerbation of pain on stretching of pectoralis muscle	Palpable tenderness at rib interspace Splinting or spasm of affected intercostal muscle Reproduction of pain at deep inspiration with arms overhead	Painful rib interspace Possible strain of intercostal muscle Referral of pain from anterior to posterior or vice versa Exacerbation of pain with deep inspiration or spinal rotation Need to rule out infection (e.g., herpes zoster) and organic disease	Tenderness over rib angle or head Fixation of costovertebral articulation Inferoanterior subluxation of corresponding dorsal vertebral level Muscle guarding, spasm over affected rib cage Palpable spinal rotation or cervicodorsal fixation Referral to anterior thorax possible	Pain on examination at pectoralis muscle, either proximally or distally Swelling or bogginess of muscle belly Discomfort on abduction of arm Ecchymosis at injury site possible Pain reproduced by adduction against resistance Need to rule out costochondral injury, avulsion of pectoralis tendon at proximal humerus
X-ray findings	Usually normal Need to rule out rib fracture in cases of blunt trauma	Not applicable	Only needed for suspected organic disease or rib trauma	Not applicable	Not applicable unless rupture or avulsion is suspected

Adapted from Brier SR: *Primary care orthopedics,* St Louis, 1999, Mosby.

PROCEDURE

- While the patient is in the supine position, the examiner exerts downward pressure on the patient's sternum (Fig. 7-84).
- Localized pain at the lateral border of the ribs indicates a rib fracture.

Next Steps/Procedures

Chest expansion test, Schepelmann test, and diagnostic imaging

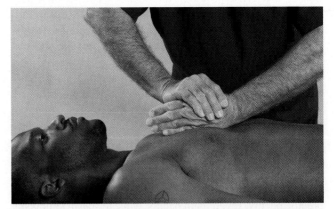

FIG. 7-84 The patient is supine, with the arms at the sides or crossed low over the abdomen. The examiner places the ulnar aspect of one hand in the vertical axis of the sternum. The other hand is placed on top of it. The examiner exerts a downward pressure on the sternum. Localized pain in the ribs indicates fracture.

CRITICAL THINKING

1. List the seronegative spondyloarthropathies.
2. List the common features of the seronegative spondyloarthropathies.
3. List the three basic types of spinal deformity.
4. List the common classifications of scoliosis.
5. List other disease processes in which scoliosis and kyphosis are also seen.
6. What is the prevalence of AIS?
7. Describe the physical examination for a patient with scoliosis.
8. What is Adams position?
9. What is infantile and juvenile idiopathic scoliosis?
10. What is kyphosis?
11. What is the prevalence of Scheuermann disease?
12. What are the three columns of the spine?
13. Describe a compression fracture.
14. What is a burst fracture?
15. What is a flexion-distraction injury?
16. What are the stabilizing influences for the thoracic spine?
17. What is the Lenke Classification System for scoliosis, and why is it important?
18. What axioms need to be understood to manage or co-manage patients with scoliosis successfully?
19. What does the modified New York criteria for the diagnosis of ankylosing spondylitis include?
20. The detection of HLA-B27 antigen is not only a marker for ankylosing spondylitis, but also for what other arthritic conditions?
21. The incidence of symptomatic thoracic disc herniation is thought to be approximately 1 in 1 million. When present, the clinical presentation is often atypical. What are some of the symptoms that can be noted with this type of lesion?
22. Ankylosing spondylitis generally starts insidiously in a young adult. The symptoms are initially vague and poorly localized. Why does reduced chest expansion accompany this condition?
23. Where is the correct location to measure chest inspiration and expiration?
24. What is chest expansion in the female and male patient that suggests ankylosing spondylitis?
25. Dysfunction of the serratus muscle will include the inability to pull and lift heavy objects and perform tasks that involve reaching objects at a higher level than the shoulders. Scapular winging will occur with dysfunction of this muscle. Injury to which nerve is the most common cause of scapular winging? What is the nerve involved and nerve root level?
26. What test is performed to determine intercostal muscle strain or myofascitis versus intercostal neuritis? How is the test performed?
27. What finding determines if the patient has intercostal myofascitis or neuritis?
28. Physical examination findings in costochondritis typically include anterior chest wall tenderness. What costal cartilages are the most commonly involved?

7

BIBLIOGRAPHY

Abrams WB, Berkow R: *The Merck manual of geriatrics,* Rahway, NJ, 1990, Merck Sharp & Dohme Research Laboratories.

Adams JC, Hamblen DL: *Outline of orthopaedics,* ed 11, Edinburgh, 1990, Churchill Livingstone.

Adams RD, Victor M: *Principles of neurology,* ed 3, New York, 1985, McGraw-Hill.

Alario AJ: *Practical guide to the care of the pediatric patient,* St Louis, 1997, Mosby.

American Medical Association: *Guides to the evaluation of permanent impairment,* ed 4, Chicago, 1993, The Association.

American Medical Association: *How to use guides to the evaluation of permanent impairment,* ed 4, Falmouth, Conn, 1993, SEAK.

American Orthopaedic Association: *Manual of orthopaedic surgery,* Chicago, 1972, The Association.

Aminoff MJ: *Electrodiagnosis in clinical neurology,* ed 2, New York, 1986, Churchill Livingstone.

Anderson PA et al: Flexion distraction and chance injuries to the thoracolumbar spine, *J Orthop Trauma* 5:153, 1991.

Ansel BM: Rheumatic disorders in childhood, *Clin Rheum Dis* 2:303, 1976.

Apley AG, Solomon L: *Concise system of orthopaedics and fractures,* London, 1988, Butterworth-Heinemann.

Appelrouth D, Gottlieb NL: Pulmonary manifestations of ankylosing spondylitis, *J Rheumatol* 2:446, 1975.

Asbury AK, McKhann GM, McDonald WI: *Disease of the nervous system,* Philadelphia, 1986, WB Saunders.

Avioli LV: Osteoporosis, pathogenesis and therapy. In Avioli LV, Vrane SM, editors: *Metabolic bone disease,* New York, 1977, Academic Press.

Avioli LV: Senile and post-menopausal osteoporosis, *Adv Intern Med* 21:391, 1976.

Avioli LV: Significance of osteoporosis: a growing national health care problem, *Orthop Rev* 21:1126, 1992.

Baker AB, Joynt RJ: *Clinical neurology,* New York, 1985, Harper & Row.

Barkauskas VH et al: *Health & physical assessment,* ed 2, St Louis, 1998, Mosby.

Bauer DC et al: Factors associated with appendicular bone mass in older women, *Ann Intern Med* 118:657, 1993.

Beetham WP et al: *Physical examination of the joints,* Philadelphia, 1965, WB Saunders.

Bennett RM et al: A multidisciplinary approach to fibromyalgia treatment, *J Musculoskel Med* 8:21, 1991.

Benson MKD, Byrnes DP: The clinical syndromes and surgical treatment of thoracic intervertebral disc prolapse, *J Bone Joint Surg* 57B:471, 1975.

Berg EE: The sternal-rib complex: a possible fourth column in thoracic spine fractures, *Spine* 18:1916, 1993.

Bernat JL: A dangerous backache, *Hosp Pract (Off Ed)* 12:36, 1977.

Blount WP, Moe JH: *The Milwaukee brace,* Baltimore, 1973, Williams & Wilkins.

Boden SD et al: *The aging spine: essentials of pathophysiology, diagnosis and treatment,* Philadelphia, 1991, WB Saunders.

Bodley R: Imaging in chronic spinal cord injury—indications and benefits, *Eur J Radiol* 42(2):135-153, 2002.

Bogduk N, Twomey LT: *Clinical anatomy of the lumbar spine,* ed 2, New York, 1991, Churchill Livingstone.

Bogduk N, Valencia F: Innervation and pain patterns of the thoracic spine. In Grant R, editor: *Physical therapy of the cervical and thoracic spine,* ed 2, New York, 1994, Churchill Livingstone.

Bondilla KK: Back pain: osteoarthritis, *J Am Geriatr Soc* 25:62, 1977.

Bordurant FJ et al: Acute spinal cord injury: a study using physical examination and magnetic resonance imaging, *Spine* 15:161, 1990.

Bourdillon JR: *Spinal manipulation,* ed 3, New York, 1982, Appleton-Century-Crofts.

Bradford DS et al: Scheuermann's kyphosis and roundback deformity: results of Milwaukee brace treatment, *J Bone Joint Surg* 56A:740, 1974.

Bradford DS et al: Scheuermann's kyphosis: results of surgical treatment by posterior spine arthrodesis in 22 patients, *J Bone Joint Surg* 57A:439, 1975.

Bradford DS: Juvenile kyphosis, *Clin Orthop* 128:45, 1977.

Brashear HR, Raney RB: *Shand's handbook of orthopaedic surgery,* St Louis, 1978, Mosby.

Brier SR: *Primary care orthopedics,* St Louis, 1999, Mosby.

Brooks M, Evans R, Fairclough J: *Sports injuries,* ed 2, London, 1992, Gower Medical.

Brotzman SB: *Clinical orthopaedic rehabilitation,* St Louis, 1996, Mosby.

Brown CW et al: The natural history of thoracic disc herniation, *Spine* 17:597, 1992.

Brown DE, Neumann RD: *Orthopedic secrets,* Philadelphia, 1995, Hanley & Belfus.

Brown MD: Diagnosis of pain syndromes of the spine, *Orthop Clin North Am* 6:233, 1975.

Bucholz RW: *Orthopaedic decision making,* ed 2, St Louis, 1996, Mosby.

Buckwalter J: Spine update: aging and degeneration of the human intervertebral disc, *Spine* 20:1307, 1995.

Bunnell WP: Treatment of idiopathic scoliosis, *Orthop Clin North Am* 10:813, 1979.

Cailliet R: *Scoliosis: diagnosis and management,* Philadelphia, 1975, FA Davis.

Canale ST: *Campbell's operative orthopaedics,* vol 1-4, ed 9, St Louis, 1998, Mosby.

Carman DL et al: Measurement of scoliosis and kyphosis radiographs, intraobserver and interobserver variation, *J Bone Joint Surg* 72A:328, 1990.

Castro FP: Adolescent idiopathic scoliosis, bracing, and the Hueter-Volkmann principle, *Spine J* 3(3):180-185, 2003.

Cipriano JJ: *Photographic manual of regional orthopaedic and neurological test,* ed 3, Baltimore, 1997, Williams & Wilkins.

Cohn RE: *Impairment rating examination and disability evaluation,* ed 3, Wilkesboro, NC, 1994, R Ernest Cohn.

Cramer GD, Darby SA: *Basic and clinical anatomy of the spine, spinal cord, and ANS,* St Louis, 1995, Mosby.

Croft P, Schollum J, Silman A: Population study of tender point counts and pain as evidence of fibromyalgia, *Br Med J* 309:696, 1994.

Crosby EC, Humphrey T, Lauer EW: *Correlative anatomy of the nervous system,* New York, 1962, Macmillan.

Cyriax J: *Textbook of orthopaedic medicine, vol 1: diagnosis of soft tissue lesions,* London, 1982, Bailliere Tindall.

Cyriax JH, Cyriax PJ: *Illustrated manual of orthopaedic medicine,* London, 1983, CM Publications.

Daffner RH et al: The radiology assessment of post-traumatic vertebral stability, *Skeletal Radiol* 19:103, 1990.

Dambro MR, Griffith JA: *Griffith's 5 minute clinical consult,* Baltimore, 1997, Williams & Wilkins.

D'Ambrogio KJ, Roth GB: *Positional release therapy assessment & treatment of musculoskeletal dysfunction,* St Louis, 1997, Mosby.

D'Ambrosia RD: *Musculoskeletal disorders: regional examination and differential diagnosis,* Philadelphia, 1977, JB Lippincott.

Dandy DJ: *Essential orthopaedics and trauma,* Edinburgh, 1989, Churchill Livingstone.

Dawson DM, Hallett M, Millender LH: *Entrapment neuropathies,* Boston, 1983, Little, Brown.

DeJong RN: *The neurologic examination,* ed 4, New York, 1978, Harper & Row.

Deltoff MN, Kogon PL: *The portable skeletal x-ray library,* St Louis, 1998, Mosby.

Demeter SL, Andersson GBJ, Smith GM: *Disability evaluation,* St Louis, 1996, Mosby.

Deshpande JK, Tobias JD: *The pediatric pain handbook,* St Louis, 1996, Mosby.

Dettenmeier PA: *Radiographic assessment for nurses,* St Louis, 1995, Mosby.

Dickson RA: Conservative treatment for idiopathic scoliosis, *J Bone Joint Surg* 67B:176, 1985.

Doherty M, Doherty J: *Clinical examination in rheumatology,* London, 1992, Wolfe.

Doherty M, George E: *Self-assessment picture tests in rheumatology,* London, 1995, Mosby-Wolfe.

Doherty M: *Color atlas and text of osteoarthritis,* London, 1994, Wolfe.

Elattrache N, Fadale PD, Fu F: Thoracic spine fracture in a football player, *Am J Sports Med* 21:157, 1984.

Elster AD: *Questions and answers in magnetic resonance imaging,* St Louis, 1994, Mosby.

Engelman EG, Engleman EP: Ankylosing spondylitis: recent advances in diagnosis and treatment, *Med Clin North Am* 61:347, 1977.

Epstein O et al: *Clinical examination,* ed 2, London, 1997, Mosby.

Feldmann E: *Current diagnosis in neurology,* St Louis, 1994, Mosby.

Ferezy JS: *The chiropractic neurological examination,* Gaithersburg, Md, 1992, Aspen.

Ferris B, Edgar M, Leyshon A: Screening for scoliosis, *Acta Orthop Scand* 59:417, 1988.

Fokkema DS et al: Different breathing patterns in healthy and asthmatic children: responses to an arithmetic task, *Respir Med* 2006; 100 (1):148-156.

Frank ED et al: *Merrill's atlas of radiographic positioning and procedures,* vol 1-3, ed 11, St Louis, 2007, Mosby.

Froissart A, Pagnoux C, Cherin P: Lymph node paradoxical enlargement during treatment for tuberculous spondylodiscitis (Pott's disease), *Joint Bone Spine* 74(3):292-295, 2007.

Garcia F, Florez MT, Conejero JA: A butterfly vertebra or a wedge fracture? *Int Orthop* 17:7, 1993.

Garcia JH: *Neuropathology: the diagnostic approach,* St Louis, 1997, Mosby.

Gartland JJ: *Fundamentals of orthopaedics,* London, 1968, E & S Livingstone.

Gavin TM, Shurr DG, Patwardhan AG: Orthotic treatment for spinal disorders. In Weinstein SL, editor: *The pediatric spine,* New York, 1993, Raven.

Gertzbein SD: Spine update: classification of thoracic and lumbar fractures, *Spine* 19:626, 1994.

Goldenberg DL: Fatigue in rheumatic disease, *Bull Rheum Dis* 44:4, 1995.

Goldie BS: *Orthopaedic diagnosis and management: a guide to the care of orthopaedic patients,* ed 2, Oxford, UK, 1998, ISIS Medical Media.

Goldstein LA, Waugh TR: Classification and terminology of scoliosis, *Clin Orthop* 93:10, 1973.

Goshi K et al: Thoracic scoliosis fusion in adolescent and adult idiopathic scoliosis using posterior translational corrective techniques (Isola): is maximum correction of the thoracic curve detrimental to the unfused lumbar curve? *Spine J* 4(2):192-201, 2004.

Greenspan A, Montesano P: *Imaging of the spine in clinical practice,* London, 1993, Wolfe.

Greenstein GM: *Clinical assessment of neuromusculoskeletal disorders,* St Louis, 1997, Mosby.

Gregersen GG, Lucas DB: An in vivo study of the axial rotation of the human thoracolumbar spine, *J Bone Joint Surg* 49A:247, 1967.

Grieve GP: *Common vertebral joint problems,* New York, 1981, Churchill Livingstone.

Grootboom MJ, Govender S: Acute injuries of the upper dorsal spine, *Injury* 24:389, 1993.

Grossman ZD et al: *Cost-effective diagnostic imaging: the clinician's guide,* ed 3, St Louis, 1995, Mosby.

Hamilton MG, Thomas HG: Intradural herniation of a thoracic disc presenting as flaccid paraplegic: case report, *Neurosurgery* 27:482, 1990.

Harvey J, Tanner S: Low back pain in young athletes: a practical approach, *Sports Med* 12:394, 1991.

Harvey MA, James B: *Differential diagnosis,* Philadelphia, 1972, WB Saunders.

Hawkins RJ: *An organized approach to musculoskeletal examination and history taking,* St Louis, 1995, Mosby.

Heim HA: Scoliosis, *Clin Symp* 25:1, 1973.

Hinkle CZ: *Fundamentals of anatomy & movement: a workbook and guide,* St Louis, 1997, Mosby.

Hollingshead WH, Jenkins DR: *Functional anatomy of the limbs and back,* Philadelphia, 1981, WB Saunders.

Hornberger JP: *Exercise physiology: therapeutic exercise,* Sarasota, Fla, 1991, Joseph P Hornberger.

James JP: The etiology of scoliosis, *J Bone Joint Surg* 52B:410, 1970.

Jones DH, Kilgour RD, Comtois AS: Test-retest reliability of pressure pain threshold measurements of the upper limb and torso in young healthy women, *J Pain* (in press, corrected proof).

Judge RD, Zuidema GD, Fitzgerald FT: *Clinical diagnosis: a physiologic approach,* Boston, 1982, Little, Brown.

Kanner R: *Pain management secrets,* Philadelphia, 1997, Hanley & Belfus.

Kapandji IA: *The physiology of the joints: the trunk and vertebral column,* vol 3, New York, 1974, Churchill Livingstone.

Katirji B: *Electromyography in clinical practice: a case study approach,* St Louis, 1998, Mosby.

Katz WA: *Rheumatic diseases: diagnosis and management,* Philadelphia, 1977, JB Lippincott.

Keats TE, Lusted LB: *Atlas of roentgenographic measurements,* ed 6, St Louis, 1990, Mosby.

Keim HA: *The adolescent spine,* New York, 1982, Springer-Verlag.

Kelley WN et al: *Textbook of rheumatology,* vol 1, ed 4, Philadelphia, 1993, Saunders.

Kendall HO, Kendall FP, Wadsworth GE: *Muscle testing and function,* ed 2, Baltimore, 1971, Williams & Wilkins.

Kimura J: *Electrodiagnosis in disease of nerve and muscle: principles and practice,* Philadelphia, 1983, FA Davis.

Klippel JH, Dieppe PA: *Rheumatology,* vol 1-2, ed 2, London, 1998, Mosby.

Koenigsberg R: *Churchill's illustrated medical dictionary,* New York, 1989, Churchill Livingstone.

Korovessis P, Sidiropoulos P, Dimas A: Complete fracture-dislocation of the thoracic spine without neurologic deficit: case report, *J Trauma* 36:122, 1994.

Kostuik JP: Adult scoliosis. In Weinstein J, Wiesel SW, editors: *The lumbar spine,* Philadelphia, 1990, WB Saunders.

Krupp MA, Chatton MJ: *Current diagnosis and treatment,* Los Altos, Calif, 1972, Lange Medical.

Kuklo T, Lehman R, Lenke L: Select poster presentations: preoperative and postoperative computer tomography evaluation of structures at risk with anterior spinal fusion, *Spine J* 2(5, suppl 1):110-111, 2002.

Lavy CBD, Barrett DS: *Questions and answers on Apley's concise system of orthopaedics and fractures,* Oxford, UK, 1991, Butterworth-Heinemann.

Lenke LG et al: Modern anterior scoliosis surgery, St Louis, 2004, Quality Medical Publishing.

Lenke LG et al: Selection of the lowest instrumented vertebra in thoracic adolescent idiopathic scoliosis Lenke type 1 and 2 following segmental posterior spinal fusion, *Spine J* 4(5, suppl 1):474-475, 2004.

Lerner AJ: *The little black book of neurology,* ed 3, St Louis, 1995, Mosby.

Levene DL: *Chest pain: an integrated diagnostic approach,* Philadelphia, 1977, Lea & Febiger.

Lewis CB, Knortz KA: *Orthopedic assessment and treatment of the geriatric patient,* St Louis, 1993, Mosby.

Lonstein JE, Winter RB: Milwaukee brace treatment of adolescent idiopathic scoliosis—review of 1020 patients, *J Bone Joint Surg* 76A:1207, 1994.

7

MacConaill MA, Basmajian JV: *Muscles and movements: a basis for human kinesiology,* Baltimore, 1969, Williams & Wilkins.

Macnab I: *Backache,* Baltimore, 1977, Williams & Wilkins.

Magee DJ: *Orthopedic physical assessment,* ed 3, Philadelphia, 1997, WB Saunders.

Maguire MF et al: A study exploring the role of intercostal nerve damage in chronic pain after thoracic surgery, *Eur J Cardiothorac Surg* 29(6):873-879, 2006.

Maigne JY, Maigne R, Guerin-Surville H: Upper thoracic dorsal rami: anatomic study of their medial cutaneous branches, *Surg Radiol Anat* 13:190, 1991.

Maigne R: *Orthopaedic medicine: a new approach to vertebral manipulation,* Springfield, Ill, 1972, Charles C Thomas.

Maitland GD: *Vertebral manipulation,* London, 1973, Butterworths.

Malone TR, McPoil TG, Nitz AJ: *Orthopedic and sports physical therapy,* ed 3, St Louis, 1997, Mosby.

Manniche C et al: Clinical trial of intensive muscle training for chronic low back pain, *Lancet* 24:1473, 1988.

Marchiori DM: *Clinical imaging with skeletal, chest, and abdomen pattern differentials,* St Louis, 1999, Mosby.

Marrero GH: Juvenile kyphosis, *Spine State Art Rev* 4:173, 1990.

Martin JH: *Neuroanatomy text and atlas,* ed 2, Stamford, Conn, 1996, Appleton & Lange.

Mather's LH et al: *Clinical anatomy principles,* St Louis, 1996, Mosby.

Mazion JM: *Illustrated manual of neurological reflexes/signs/tests, part I, orthopedic signs/tests/maneuvers for office procedure, part II,* Orlando, Fla, 1980, Daniels Publishing.

McGoey BV et al: Effect of weight loss on musculoskeletal pain in the morbidly obese, *J Bone Joint Surg* 72B:322, 1990.

McKenzie RA: *The lumbar spine: mechanical diagnosis and therapy,* Wikanae, New Zealand, 1981, Spinal Publications.

McRae R: *Clinical orthopaedic examination,* ed 3, Edinburgh, 1990, Churchill Livingstone.

Medical Economics Books: *Patient care flow chart manual,* ed 3, Oradell, NJ, 1982, Medical Economics Books.

Mellion MB: *Office sports medicine,* ed 2, St Louis, 1996, Mosby.

Mellion MB: *Sports medicine secrets,* Philadelphia, 1994, Hanley & Belfus.

Mengel MB, Schwiebert LP: *Ambulatory medicine: the primary care of families,* ed 2, Stamford, Conn, 1996, Appleton & Lange.

Mennell JM: *The musculoskeletal system differential diagnosis from symptoms and physical signs,* Gaithersburg, Md, 1992, Aspen.

Mercier LR, Pettid FJ: *Practical orthopedics,* ed 4, St Louis, 1995, Mosby.

Modic MT, Masaryk TJ, Ross JS: *Magnetic resonance imaging of the spine,* ed 2, St Louis, 1994, Mosby.

Moe JH, Kettleson DN: Idiopathic scoliosis, *J Bone Joint Surg* 52A:1509, 1970.

Moe JH et al: *Scoliosis and other spinal deformities,* Philadelphia, 1978, WB Saunders.

Moldofsky H: Chronobiological influences on fibromyalgia syndrome: theoretical and therapeutic implications, *Baillieres Clin Rheumatol* 8:801, 1994.

Moll JH, Wright V: Measurement of spinal movement. In Jayson M, editor: *Lumbar spine and back pain,* New York, 1976, Grune & Stratton.

Moll JMH, Wright V: An objective clinical study of chest expansion, *Ann Rheum Dis* 31:1, 1972.

Montgomery SP, Erwin WE: Scheuermann's kyphosis: long-term results of Milwaukee brace treatment, *Spine* 6:5, 1981.

Moore KL: *Clinically oriented anatomy,* ed 3, Baltimore, 1992, Williams & Wilkins.

Morrisey RT et al: Measurement of Cobb angle on radiographs of patients who have scoliosis, evaluation of intrinsic error, *J Bone Joint Surg* 72A:320, 1990.

Mosby-Year Book, Inc: *Expert 10-minute physical examination,* St Louis, 1997, Mosby-Year Book.

Nash CL, Moe JH: A study of vertebral rotation, *J Bone Joint Surg* 52A:223, 1969.

Nash CL: Scoliosis bracing, *J Bone Joint Surg* 62A:848, 1980.

Netter F: *The Ciba collection of medical illustration, vol 8: the musculoskeletal system,* Summitt, NJ, 1990, Ciba Geigy.

Nettina SM: *The Lippincott manual of nursing practice,* ed 6, Philadelphia, 1996, Lippincott.

Newton RW: *Color atlas of pediatric neurology,* St Louis, 1995, Mosby-Wolfe.

Noonan KJ et al: Use of the Milwaukee brace for progressive idiopathic scoliosis, *J Bone Joint Surg* 78A:557, 1996.

Nordin M, Andersson GBJ, Pope MH: *Musculoskeletal disorders in the workplace: principles and practice,* St Louis, 1997, Mosby.

O'Connor MI, Carrier BI: Metastatic disease of the spine, *Orthopedics* 15:611, 1992.

O'Donoghue DH: *Treatment of injuries to athletes,* ed 4, Philadelphia, 1984, WB Saunders.

Olson WH et al: *Handbook of symptom-oriented neurology,* ed 2, St Louis, 1994, Mosby.

Omer GE, Spinner M: *Management of peripheral nerve problems,* Philadelphia, 1980, WB Saunders.

O'Young B, Young MA, Stiens SA: *PM&R secrets,* Philadelphia, 1997, Hanley & Belfus.

Panjabi MM et al: Thoracolumbar burst fracture: a biomechanical investigation of its multidirectional flexibility, *Spine* 19:578, 1994.

Panjabi MM, White AA: *Clinical biomechanics of the spine,* ed 2, Philadelphia, 1990, JB Lippincott.

Panjabi MM: The stabilizing system of the spine, part II, neutral zone and instability hypothesis, *J Spinal Disord* 5:390, 1992.

Papaioannu T, Stokes I, Kenwright J: Scoliosis associated with limb length inequality, *J Bone Joint Surg* 64A:59, 1982.

Papakonstantinou DK et al: Unilateral pulmonary oedema due to lung re-expansion following pleurocentesis for spontaneous pneumothorax. The role of non-invasive continuous positive airway pressure ventilation, *Int J Cardiol* 114(3):398-400, 2007.

Patten J: *Neurological differential diagnosis,* ed 2, London, 1996, Springer.

Pheasant S: *Ergonomics, work and health,* Gaithersburg, Md, 1991, Aspen.

Pope MH, Frymoyer JW, Krag MH: Diagnosing instability, *Clin Orthop* 279:60, 1992.

Prescott E et al: Fibromyalgia in the adult Danish population. I: a prevalence study, *Scand J Rheumatol* 22:233, 1993.

Puno R et al: Treatment recommendations for idiopathic scoliosis: an assessment of the Lenke classification, *Spine J* 2(5, suppl 1):61, 2002.

Puno R et al: A comparison of the King and the Lenke classification systems of adolescent idiopathic scoliosis, *Spine J* 2(5, suppl 1):60-61, 2002.

Qin C, Farber JP, Foreman RD: Gastrocardiac afferent convergence in upper thoracic spinal neurons: a central mechanism of postprandial angina pectoris, *J Pain* (in press, corrected proof).

Rachlin ES: *Myofascial pain and fibromyalgia trigger point management,* St Louis, 1994, Mosby.

Ramsey RG: *Neuroradiology,* Philadelphia, 1987, WB Saunders.

Resnick NW, Greenspan SL: Senile osteoporosis reconsidered, *JAMA* 261:1025, 1989.

Riggs BL, Melton LJ III: *Osteoporosis: etiology, diagnosis and management,* New York, 1988, Raven.

Rodnitzky RL: *Van Allen's pictorial manual of neurologic tests,* St Louis, 1988, Mosby.

Rolak LA: *Neurology secrets,* ed 2, Philadelphia, 1998, Hanley & Belfus.

Rose KA, Kim WS: The effect of chiropractic care for a 30-year-old male with advanced ankylosing spondylitis: a time series case report, *J Manipulative Physiol Ther* 26(8):524-532, 2003.

Rothman RH, Simeone FA: *The spine,* Philadelphia, 1982, WB Saunders.

Rowland LP: *Merritt's textbook of neurology,* ed 7, Philadelphia, 1984, Lea & Febiger.

Ruge D, Wiltse LL: *Spinal disorders: diagnosis and treatment,* Philadelphia, 1977, Lea & Febiger.

Rumball K, Jarvis J: Seat-belt injuries of the spine in young children, *J Bone Joint Surg* 74B:572, 1992.

Sacsh BL et al: Primary osseous neoplasms of the thoracic and lumbar spine, *Orthop Trans* 8:422, 1984.

Saidoff DC, McDonough AL: *Critical pathways in therapeutic intervention,* St Louis, 1997, Mosby.

Saito Y et al: Facioscapulohumeral muscular dystrophy with severe mental retardation and epilepsy, *Brain Dev* 29(4):231-233, 2007.

Schumacher HR, Klippel JH, Koopman WJ: *Primer on the rheumatic diseases,* ed 10, Atlanta, 1993, Arthritis Foundation.

Seror P: The long thoracic nerve conduction study revisited in 2006, *Clin Neurophysiol* 117(11):2446-2450, 2006.

Shankman GA: *Fundamental orthopedic management for the physical therapist assistant,* St Louis, 1997, Mosby.

Shehata SMK, Shabaan BS: Diaphragmatic injuries in children after blunt abdominal trauma, *J Pediatr Surg* 41(10):1727-1731, 2006.

Simmons EH, Bernstein AJ: Fractures of the spine in ankylosing spondylitis. In Floman Y, Farcy JP, Argenson C, editors: *Thoracolumbar spine fractures,* New York, 1993, Raven.

Simmons EH, Graziano GP, Heffner R Jr: Muscle disease as a cause of kyphotic deformity in ankylosing spondylitis, *Spine* 16:5351, 1991.

Simmons EH: Kyphotic deformity of the spine in ankylosing spondylitis, *Clin Orthop* 128:65, 1977.

Simons GW, Sty JR, Storkshak RJ: Retroperitoneal and retrofascial abscesses, *J Bone Joint Surg* 65A:1041, 1983.

Sledge CB, Poss R: *The year book of orthopedics 1997,* St Louis, 1997, Mosby.

Spapen HD et al: The straight back syndrome, *Neth J Med* 36:29, 1990.

Specht NT, Russo RD: *Practical guide to diagnostic imaging,* St Louis, 1998, Mosby.

Spivak JM, Vaccaro AR, Cotler JM: Thoracolumbar spine trauma, I, evaluation and classification, *J Am Acad Orthop Surg* 3:345, 1995.

Starlanyl D, Copeland ME: *Fibromyalgia & chronic myofascial pain syndrome: a survival manual,* Oakland, Calif, 1996, New Harbinger.

Stewart DL, Abeln SH: *Documenting functional outcomes in physical therapy,* St Louis, 1993, Mosby.

Stillerman C, Weiss M: Management of thoracic disc disease, *Clin Neurosurg* 38:325, 1992.

Stoller DW: *Magnetic resonance imaging in orthopaedics & sports medicine,* Philadelphia, 1993, JB Lippincott.

Sunderland S: *Nerves and nerve injuries,* ed 2, New York, 1979, Churchill Livingstone.

Sutton D, Young JWR: *A concise textbook of clinical imaging,* ed 2, St Louis, 1995, Mosby.

Tan JC, Horn SE: *Practical manual of physical medicine and rehabilitation,* St Louis, 1998, Mosby.

Taybi H, Lachman RS: *Radiology of syndromes, metabolic disorders, and skeletal dysplasias,* ed 4, St Louis, 1996, Mosby.

Thibodeau GA, Patton KT: *Anatomy & physiology,* ed 3, St Louis, 1996, Mosby.

Thibodeau GA, Patton KT: *Pocket reference to accompany anatomy & physiology,* ed 3, St Louis, 1996, Mosby.

Thompson JM: *Clinical outlines for health assessment,* St Louis, 1997, Mosby.

Toghill PJ: *Examining patients: an introduction to clinical medicine,* London, 1990, Edward Arnold.

Tollison CD, Satterthwaite JR, Tollison JW: *Handbook of pain management,* ed 2, Baltimore, 1994, Williams & Wilkins.

Torg JS, Shepard RJ: *Current therapy in sports medicine,* ed 3, St Louis, 1995, Mosby.

Tsou PM, Yau A, Hodgson AR: Embryogenesis and prenatal development of congenital vertebral anomalies and their classification, *Clin Orthop* 152:211, 1980.

Tsou PM: Embryology of congenital kyphosis, *Clin Orthop* 128:18, 1977.

Turek SL: *Orthopaedics principles and their application,* ed 3, Philadelphia, 1977, JB Lippincott.

Turk DC et al: Effects of type of symptom onset on psychological distress and disability in fibromyalgia syndrome patients, *Pain* 68(2-3):423-430, 1996.

Turner PG, Green JH, Galasko CS: Back pain in childhood, *Spine* 14:812, 1989.

Van Holsbeeck M, Introcaso JH: *Musculoskeletal ultrasound,* St Louis, 1991, Mosby.

Veeming A et al: The posterior layer of the thoracolumbar fascia, its function in load transfer from spine to legs, *Spine* 20:753, 1995.

Vernon L, Dooley J, Acusta A: Upper lumbar and thoracic disc pathology: a magnetic resonance imaging analysis, *J Neuromuscoskeletal Syst* 59:63, 1993.

Wakefield TS, Frank RG: *The clinician's guide to neuro musculoskeletal practice,* Abbotsford, Wisc, 1995, Allied Health of Wisconsin, S.C.

Wang Z et al: Treatment of spinal tuberculosis with ultrashort-course chemotherapy in conjunction with partial excision of pathologic vertebrae, *Spine J* (in press, corrected proof).

Watkins RG: *The spine in sports,* St Louis, 1996, Mosby.

Wedgewood RJ, Schaller JG: The pediatric arthritides, *Hosp Pract (Off Ed)* 12:83, 1977.

Weineck J: *Functional anatomy in sports,* ed 2, St Louis, 1990, Mosby.

Weinerman SA, Bockman RS: Medical therapy of osteoporosis, *Orthop Clin North Am* 21:109, 1990.

Weinstein SL, Buckwalter JA: *Turek's orthopaedics principles and their application,* ed 5, Philadelphia, 1994, JB Lippincott.

Weinstein SL: Adolescent idiopathic scoliosis: prevalence and natural history, *Am Acad Orthop Surg Lect* 38:115, 1989.

White AA: Kinematics of the normal spine as related to scoliosis, *J Biomech* 4:405, 1971.

White AH, Schofferman JA: *Spine care,* vol 1-2, St Louis, 1995, Mosby.

White AW, Panjabi MM: *Clinical biomechanics of the spine,* Philadelphia, 1990, JB Lippincott.

White KP et al: Fibromyalgia in rheumatology practice: a survey of Canadian rheumatologists, *J Rheumatol* 22:722, 1995.

White KP, Nielson WR: Cognitive behavioral treatment of fibromyalgia syndrome: a follow-up assessment, *J Rheumatol* 22:717, 1995.

Whiteside TE: Traumatic kyphosis of the thoracolumbar spine, *Clin Orthop* 128:78, 1977.

Whitmore I, Willan PLT: *Multiple choice questions in human anatomy,* London, 1995, Mosby.

Wiles P, Sweetnam R: *Essentials of orthopaedics,* London, 1965, JA Churchill.

Williams P, Warwick R: *Gray's anatomy,* ed 36, Philadelphia, 1980, WB Saunders.

Windsor RE, Lox DM: *Soft tissue injuries: diagnosis and treatment,* Philadelphia, 1998, Hanley & Belfus.

Wolfe F et al: The prevalence and characteristics of fibromyalgia in the general population, *Arthritis Rheum* 38:19, 1995.

Wyke B: Morphological and functional features of the innervation of the costovertebral joints, *Folia Morphol* 23:296, 1975.

Yokoyama T et al: Neurological findings for screening thoracic myelopathy *Spine J* 4(5, suppl 1):S30, 2004.

Zatouroff M: *Diagnosis in color: physical signs in general medicine,* ed 2, London, 1996, Mosby-Wolfe.

Zitelli BJ, Davis HW: *Atlas of pediatric physical diagnosis,* ed 2, London, 1992, Wolfe.

7

CITATIONS

Arslan G et al: Single rib sclerosis as a sequel of compression fracture of adjacent vertebra and costovertebral joint ankylosis, *Eur J Radiol Extra* 51(1):43-46, 2004.

Aspegren D, Hyde T, Miller M: Conservative treatment of a female collegiate volleyball player with costochondritis, *J Manipulative Physiol Ther* 30(4):321-325, 2007.

Bhigjee AI et al: Diagnosis of tuberculous meningitis: clinical and laboratory parameters, *Int J Infect Dis* (in press, corrected proof).

Blonk MC et al: The fracture and osteoporosis clinic: 1-year results and 3-month compliance. *Bone* 40(6):1643-1649, 2007.

Brewer R: Diabetic thoracic radiculopathy: an unusual cause of post-thoracotomy pain, *Pain* 103(1-2):221-223, 2003.

Camozzi V et al: Quantitative bone ultrasound at phalanges and calcaneus in osteoporotic postmenopausal women: influence of age and measurement site, *Ultrasound Med Biol* (in press, corrected proof).

Cheh G et al: Use of a supine radiograph to accurately predict structural curve in operative adolescent idiopathic scoliosis, *Spine J* 6(5, suppl 1):67S-68S, 2006.

D'Arcy Y, McCarberg BH: New fibromyalgia pain management recommendations, *J Nurs Pract* 1(4):218-225, 2005.

Dobbs MB, Weinstein SL: Infantile and juvenile scoliosis, *Orthop Clin North Am* 30(3):331-341, 1999.

Greig AM et al: Postural taping decreases thoracic kyphosis but does not influence trunk muscle electromyographic activity or balance in women with osteoporosis, *Man Ther* (in press, corrected proof).

Humphreys B, Delahaye M, Peterson C: An investigation into the validity of cervical spine motion palpation using subjects with congenital block vertebrae as a 'gold standard', *BMC Musculoskeletal Disord* 5(1):19, 2004.

Ian Rabey M: Costochondritis: are the symptoms and signs due to neurogenic inflammation? Two cases that responded to manual therapy directed towards posterior spinal structures, *Man Ther* (in press, corrected proof).

Khoury NJ et al: Imaging of back pain in children and adolescents, *Curr Probl Diagn Radiol* 35(6):224-244, 2006.

Krasna MJ, Forti G: Nerve injury: injury to the recurrent laryngeal, phrenic, vagus, long thoracic, and sympathetic nerves during thoracic surgery, *Thorac Surg Clin* 16(3):267-275, 2006.

Linscott MS, Heyborne R: Thoracic intervertebral disk herniation: a commonly missed diagnosis, *J Emerg Med* 32(3):235-238, 2007.

Ozturk C et al: Far lateral thoracic disc herniation presenting with flank pain, *Spine J* 6(2):201-203, 2006.

Pavy S et al: Imaging for the diagnosis and follow-up of ankylosing spondylitis: development of recommendations for clinical practice based on published evidence and expert opinion, *Joint Bone Spine* (in press, uncorrected proof).

Pringle RK: Guidance hypothesis with verbal feedback in learning a palpation skill, *J Manipulative Physiol Ther* 27(1):36-42, 2004.

Ragnarsdottir M, Geirsson AJ, Gudbjornsson B: Rib cage motion in ankylosing spondylitis patients: a pilot study, *Spine J* (in press, corrected proof).

Srinivasan R, Greenbaum DS: Chronic abdominal wall pain: a frequently overlooked problem: Practical approach to diagnosis and management, *Am J Gastroenterol* 97(4):824-830, 2002.

van Koningsveld R et al: A clinical prognostic scoring system for Guillain-Barré syndrome, *Lancet Neurol* (in press, corrected proof).

Yunus MB: Fibromyalgia and overlapping disorders: the unifying concept of central sensitivity syndromes, *Semin Arthritis Rheum* 36(6):339-356, 2007.

LUMBAR SPINE

AXIOMS IN ASSESSING THE LUMBAR SPINE

- Low back pain is common from the second decade of life on.
- Intervertebral disc disease and disc herniation are most prominent in the third and fourth decades of life.
- Low back and posterior thigh pain arises from many areas of the spine, including the facet joints, longitudinal ligaments, and the periosteum of the vertebrae.
- Radicular pain often extends below the knee in the affected dermatome.

INTRODUCTION

As many as 90% of patients with back pain have a mechanical reason for their pain. Mechanical low back pain may be defined as pain secondary to overuse of a normal anatomic structure or pain secondary to trauma or deformity of an anatomic structure. The age of a patient is helpful in determining the potential cause of back pain. In considering spondyloarthropathies, clinical characteristics help in differentiating the diseases belonging in this group (Table 8-3 and Table 8-4). The sex of the patient may also help select potential causes of low back pain. Certain disorders occur more often in men, whereas others are associated more commonly with women. Other disorders occur equally in both sexes (Table 8-5).

> Despite considerable research efforts, chronic low back pain (cLBP) remains a poorly understood condition, causing substantial disability, work absenteeism, and high health care costs. Although statistics have shown that many patients with an episode of acute low back pain improve clinically without specific treatment, less clear is why others progress to develop recurrent or chronic symptoms. A generally recognized fact is that cLBP is a dynamic, fluctuating condition with multifactorial etiology and complex pathogenesis. Historically, mechanistic models for cLBP have tended to focus on musculoskeletal tissues, on the nervous system, or on behavior (Langevin, Sherman, 2007).

Other than the common cold, back pain is the most prevalent human affliction. As stated earlier, most patients have a mechanical cause (muscle strain or annular tear) for their

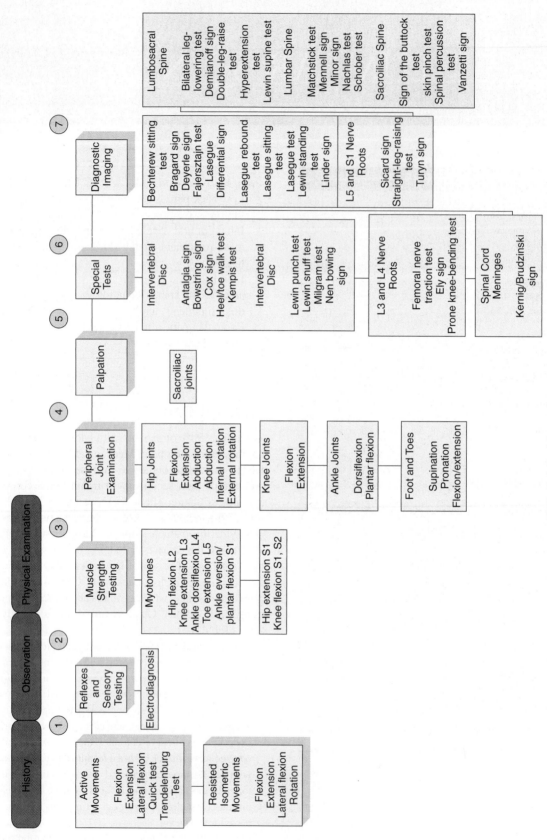

FIG. 8-1 Lumbar spine assessment.

TABLE 8-1

LUMBAR SPINE CROSS-REFERENCE TABLE BY ASSESSMENT PROCEDURE

DISEASE ASSESSED

Test/Sign	Intervertebral Disc Syndrome	Sciatica	Intervertebral Foramen Encroachment	Dural Adhesions	Subluxation	Mechanical Lower Back	Cord Tumor	Spinal Neuropathy	Sprain	Hip Lesion	Femoral Nerve	L2-L3-L4	Meningitis	Sacroiliac Lesion	Hamstring Spasm	Myofascitis	Denervation	Fracture	Lower Extremity Joints
Antalgia sign	•																		
Bechterew sitting test	•	•	•	•	•														
Bilateral leg-lowering test	•		•			•													
Bowstring sign								•											
Bragard sign	•	•					•	•											
Cox sign	•																		
Demianoff sign						•													
Deyerle sign		•																	
Double-leg-raise test	•					•			•										
Ely sign								•		•	•								
Fajersztajn test	•			•															
Femoral nerve traction test								•			•	•							
Heel/toe walk test	•	•						•											
Hyperextension test											•	•							
Kemp test	•					•		•											
Kernig/Brudzinski sign													•						
Lasègue differential sign								•											
Lasègue rebound test	•																		
Lasègue sitting test		•						•											
Lasègue test	•	•	•	•		•	•							•					
Lewin punch test	•																		
Lewin snuff test	•	•																	
Lewin standing test		•													•				
Lewin supine test	•	•												•		•			
Linder sign																			
Matchstick test	•																•		
Mennell sign														•					
Milgram test	•						•												
Minor sign	•													•				•	
Nachlas test					•	•								•					
Neri sign	•					•								•					
Prone knee-bending test											•	•							
Quick test																			•
Schober test						•													
Sicard sign		•						•											
Sign of the buttock						•				•									
Skin pinch test	•					•										•	•		
Spinal percussion test	•					•		•										•	
Straight-leg-raising test	•			•			•												
Turyn sign		•																	
Vanzetti sign		•																	

TABLE 8-2

LUMBAR SPINE CROSS-REFERENCE TABLE BY SYNDROME OR TISSUE

Cord tumor	Bragard sign	Mechanical lower back	Bilateral leg-lowering test
	Lasègue test		Demianoff sign
	Milgram test		Double-leg-raise test
	Straight-leg-raising test		Kemp test
Denervation	Matchstick test		Lasègue test
	Skin pinch test		Nachlas test
Dural adhesions	Bechterew sitting test		Neri sign
	Fajersztajn test		Schober test
	Lasègue test		Sign of the buttock
	Straight-leg-raising test		Skin pinch test
Femoral nerve	Ely sign		Spinal percussion test
	Femoral nerve traction test	Meningitis	Kernig/Brudzinski sign
	Hyperextension test	Myofascitis	Lewin supine test
	Prone knee-bending test		Skin pinch test
Fracture	Minor sign	Sacroiliac lesion	Lasègue test
	Spinal percussion test		Lewin supine test
Hamstring spasm	Lewin standing test		Mennell sign
Hip lesion	Ely sign		Minor sign
	Sign of the buttock		Nachlas test
Intervertebral disc syndrome	Antalgia sign		Neri sign
	Bechterew sitting test	Sciatica	Bechterew sitting test
	Bilateral leg-lowering test		Bragard sign
	Bragard sign		Deyerle sign
	Cox sign		Fajersztajn test
	Double-leg-raise test		Heel/toe walk test
	Fajersztajn test		Lasègue sitting test
	Heel/toe walk test		Lasègue test
	Kemp test		Lewin snuff test
	Lasègue rebound test		Lewin standing test
	Lasègue test		Lewin supine test
	Lewin punch test		Sicard sign
	Lewin snuff test		Turyn sign
	Lewin supine test		Vanzetti sign
	Matchstick test	Spinal neuropathy	Bowstring sign
	Milgram test		Bragard sign
	Minor sign		Ely sign
	Neri sign		Femoral nerve traction test
	Skin pinch test		Heel/toe walk test
	Spinal percussion test		Kemp test
	Straight-leg-raising test		Lasègue differential sign
Intervertebral foramen encroachment	Bechterew sitting test		Lasègue sitting test
	Bilateral leg-lowering test		Sicard sign
	Lasègue test	Sprain	Double leg-raise test
L2–L3–L4	Femoral nerve traction test		Spinal percussion test
	Hyperextension test	Subluxation	Bechterew sitting test
	Prone knee-bending test		Nachlas test
Lower extremity joints	Quick test		

back pain and do not have an underlying, serious, systemic medical illness.

Even if treatment involves only a localized part of the lumbar spine, in each case, the lumbar spine has to be considered as a functional unit consisting of bones, ligaments, intervertebral discs, muscles, and all other soft tissues. Because of their central location, spinal elements represent the focal point for the equilibrium of the body. Because of the many connections and relations, spinal changes influence some organs directly, and the functional equilibrium of the spine depends on the efficient performance of other organs.

The spine contributes to many mutual relationships within the total body. With its equilibrium (statics), the spine exerts

TABLE 8-3

CLINICAL CHARACTERISTICS OF SPONDYLOARTHROPATHIES

- Typical pattern of peripheral arthritis: predominantly of lower limb, asymmetric
- Tendency to radiographic sacroiliitis
- Absence of rheumatoid factor
- Absence of subcutaneous nodules and other extraarticular features of rheumatoid arthritis
- Overlapping extraarticular features characteristic of the group (e.g., anterior uveitis)
- Significant familial aggregation
- Association with HLA-B27

HLA, Human leukocyte antigen.
Adapted From Kelley WN et al: *Textbook of rheumatology*, ed 5, Philadelphia, 1997, WB Saunders.

TABLE 8-4

DISEASES BELONGING TO THE SPONDYLOARTHROPATHIES

- Ankylosing spondylitis
- Reiter syndrome, reactive arthritis
- Arthropathy of inflammatory bowel disease (Crohn disease, ulcerative colitis)
- Psoriatic arthritis
- Undifferentiated spondyloarthropathies
- Juvenile chronic arthritis: juvenile-onset ankylosing spondylitis

Adapted From Kelley WN et al: *Textbook of rheumatology*, ed 5, Philadelphia, 1997, WB Saunders.

TABLE 8-5

GENDER PREVALENCE IN LOW BACK PAIN

Male predominance	Spondyloarthropathies
	Vertebral osteomyelitis
	Benign and malignant neoplasms
	Paget disease
	Retroperitoneal fibrosis
	Peptic ulcer disease
	Work-related mechanical disorders
Female predominance	Polymyalgia rheumatica
	Fibromyalgia
	Osteoporosis
	Parathyroid disease

Data from Klippel JH, Dieppe PA: *Rheumatology*, vol 1-2, ed 2, London, 1998, Mosby.

influences and receives forces (dynamics), all of which are interwoven with the far-reaching chain of motion (kinetics). In addition, the spine is able to exercise considerable influence on neighboring structures, as well as on remote organs. This influence is its action on nerves and blood vessels. To a considerable degree, this complicated system depends on the metabolism, the mineral metabolism of the bones, and the nutrition of the bradytrophic ligamentous and disc tissues. Improper function of the endocrine glands also affects the spine.

During fetal development, the spine may be exposed to many influences, such as drug-induced malformations, lack of oxygen, and radiation.

Embryologic studies have shown that the ossification pattern of vertebral bodies and arches follows a definite sequence, namely, regular bidirectional proximodistal progression for the bodies, starting from T10-L1 and regularly progressing both cephalad (quickly) and to the sacral region (slowly), and craniocaudal progression for the arches starting from the first cervical vertebrae. Neural arch ossification starts at the base of the transverse process and proceeds anteriorly into the pedicles and posteriorly into the laminae. In addition, craniocaudal extension into the articular processes and lateral extension into the transverse process occur. Ossification progress in the laminae occurs first cephalad and then caudally, as the fetus matures (Vignolo et al, 2005).

Occupational and daily-living stresses, as well as traumatic influences, may combine to have an unfavorable effect when coupled with the aging process, which has a marked effect on the disc apparatus and the bony substance. More resources for the diagnosis and treatment of spinal diseases are available today than previously.

Degeneration of posture during early years, lack of exercise, physical weakness, and degenerative changes in later life have taken on a serious social significance for the cultures of industrialized nations.

The spine is an intricate and interesting mechanical structure. The spine's functions are mechanical, and it is well suited for serving its basic mechanical roles. The materials used to execute the design are appropriate for enhancing these functions. The spine must transfer loads from the trunk to the pelvis, must allow for physiologic motion, and must protect the spinal cord from damage. When a proper appreciation of normal anatomy and mechanics has been gained, the pathophysiologic features of the diseased or deformed spine become clear.

The lumbar spine is designed to withstand loading and to provide truncal mobility. The primary plane of motion is during flexion-extension, although axial rotation at the L5 level is significant. This rotation in the lower lumbar spine is particularly important, considering that the annulus fails and tears with torsional forces. Coupling in the lumbar spine is the opposite of cervical and thoracic spine coupling. The spinous processes move toward the concavity of the curve in physiologic lateral flexion.

Optimal spinal mobility in relation to age is difficult to pin down. The only generalization that can be made is that spinal mobility is probably greatest during adolescence and early adulthood. This tendency is significant when planning treatment and in determining prognoses.

The anatomic structures of the lumbosacral spine receive specific types of sensory innervation that are associated with distinct qualities of pain (Table 8-6).

TABLE 8-6

SUMMARY OF THE CHARACTERISTICS OF LOW BACK PAIN OF VARIOUS ORIGINS

Source of Pain	Distribution	Nature	Aggravating Factors	Neurologic Changes
Spinal pain	Sclerotomal Local	Sharp Dull	Motion	None
Discogenic pain	Sclerotomal	Deep, aching	Increased intradiscal pressure (e.g., bending, sitting, Valsalva maneuver)	None
Nerve root pain	Radicular	Paresthesias Numbness	Root stretching	Present
Multiple lumbar spinal stenosis pain	Radicular Sclerotomal	Paresthesias Spinal claudication pattern	Lumbar extension Walking	Present
Referred visceral pain	Dermatomal	Deep, aching	Related to affected organ	None

From Kelley WN et al: *Textbook of rheumatology,* ed 5, Philadelphia, 1997, WB Saunders.

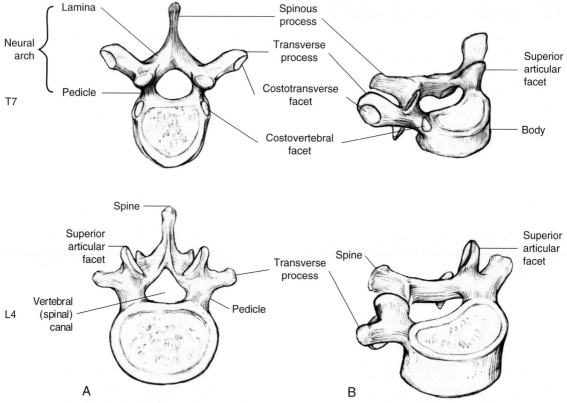

FIG. 8-2 Representative vertebrae. **A,** Superoinferior view. **B,** Right anterior oblique views. (From Mathers LH et al: *Clinical anatomy principles,* St Louis, 1996, Mosby.)

ESSENTIAL ANATOMY

The lumbar spine consists of five lumbar vertebrae, numbered L1 to L5, followed by five fused sacral bodies that form the sacrum and the coccyx. The alignment of the lumbar spine generally has a lordotic contour. The normal lordosis is 30 to 50 degrees (apex L3) in a standing person.

Lumbar vertebrae are specialized for weight bearing and strength. They have strong, thick bodies (Fig. 8-2) and stout spines and transverse processes to which attach several large paravertebral muscles (Fig. 8-3). The anterior longitudinal ligament extends from the sacrum to the inferior surface of the occipital bone.

The intrinsic musculature of the back is innervated by the posterior primary rami of segmental spinal nerves (Fig. 8-4). These nerves also innervate the skin and subcutaneous tissues overlying the intrinsic muscles of the back, the vertebral column, and the meninges.

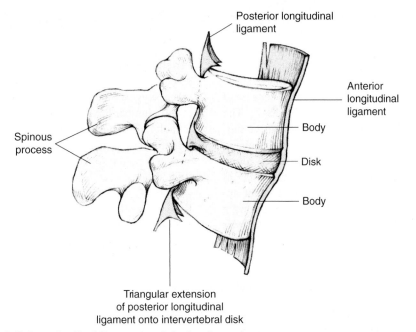

FIG. 8-3 Longitudinal ligaments of the lumbar spine. (From Mathers LH et al: *Clinical anatomy principles,* St Louis, 1996, Mosby.)

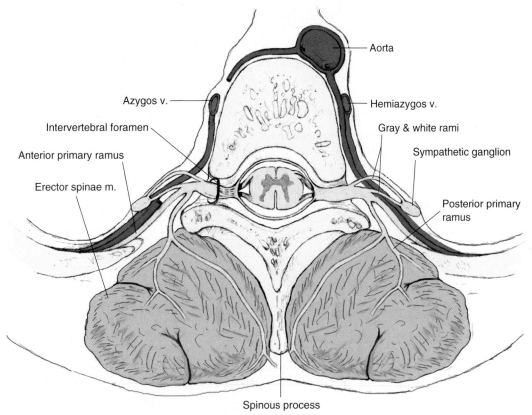

FIG. 8-4 Spinal cord and the intercostal space. (From Mathers LH et al: *Clinical anatomy principles,* St Louis, 1996, Mosby.)

Within the intervertebral foramina, the ventral and dorsal roots of each segment unite to form a true spinal nerve (Fig. 8-5). Spinal nerves represent all of the axons leaving and entering the spinal cord at that level (Fig. 8-6).

Below L2, the vertebral canal contains the many nerve roots that make up the cauda equina (so named because it resembles the many hairs in a horse's tail) (Fig. 8-7). The systematic dermatome pattern is evident as consecutive segments in order from proximal to distal along the cephalic border of the limb and then from distal to proximal along the caudal border of the limb (Fig. 8-8). The posterior margin of the annulus and the posterior longitudinal ligament are supplied by the sinuvertebral nerve, which is formed by a branch of the ventral rami (somatic) and a branch of the gray ramus communicans (autonomic) (Fig. 8-9).

ESSENTIAL MOTION ASSESSMENT

Range-of-motion findings are most helpful in pinpointing a vertebral structure that may be compromised in the lumbar spine. Pain at an early point in the extension of the lumbar spine suggests an inflamed posterior joint or pars disease. Painful lumbar flexion in the early-to-middle range connotes a faulty disc mechanism or muscular stain. Because the terminal range of flexion causes the facet joint capsule to stretch, a pain response at this point may indicate a posterior joint sprain.

Patients with acute spasm or significant trauma often have multidirectional complaints and severe limitation of motion in all planes. Therefore, range-of-motion testing may be initially inconclusive as to the severity of the injury.

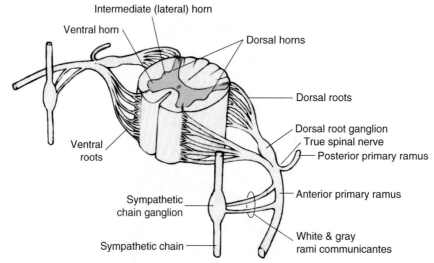

FIG. 8-5 Spinal cord and sympathetic chain. (From Mathers LH et al: *Clinical anatomy principles,* St Louis, 1996, Mosby.)

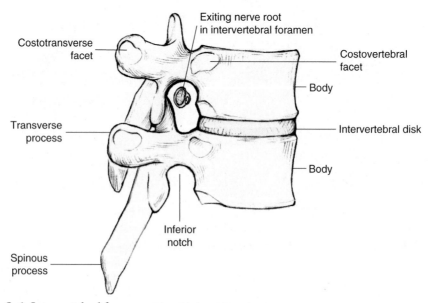

FIG. 8-6 Intervertebral foramen. (From Mathers LH et al: *Clinical anatomy principles,* St Louis, 1996, Mosby.)

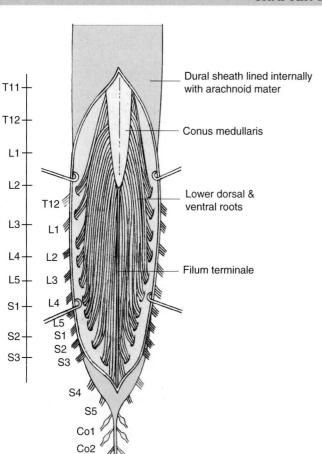

T11
T12
L1
L2
L3
L4
L5
S1
S2
S3

T12
L1
L2
L3
L4
L5
S1
S2
S3

S4
S5
Co1
Co2
Co3

Dural sheath lined internally
with arachnoid mater

Conus medullaris

Lower dorsal &
ventral roots

Filum terminale

FIG. 8-7 Cauda equina. (From Mathers LH et al: *Clinical anatomy principles,* St Louis, 1996, Mosby.)

8

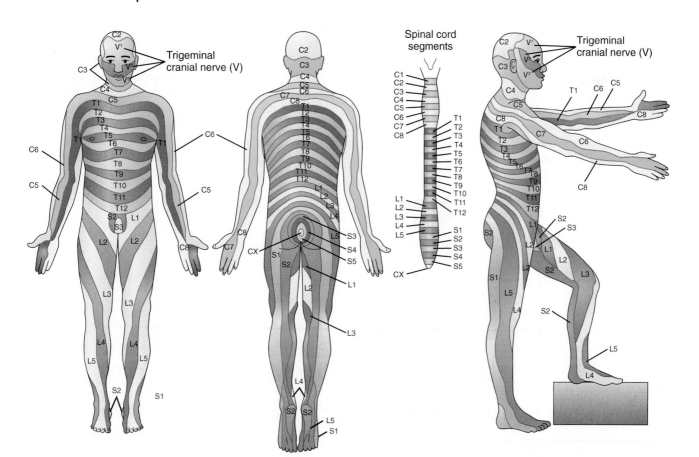

FIG. 8-8 Dermatomes. Segmental dermatome distribution of spinal nerves to the front, back, and side of the body. *C,* Cervical segments; *CX,* coccygeal segment; *L,* lumbar segments; *S,* sacral segments; *T,* thoracic segments. (From Thibodeau GA, Patton KT: *Structure and function of the body,* St Louis, 1997, Mosby.)

To assess the contribution made to flexion by the lumbar spine, the examiner should mark the spine at the lumbosacral junction and then 10 cm above and 5 cm below this point. On forward flexion, the distance between the two upper marks should increase by approximately 4 cm, the distance between the lower two remaining unaltered (Figs. 8-10 to 8-13).

ESSENTIAL MUSCLE FUNCTION ASSESSMENT

The erector spinae consist of a minor portion (the spinalis) and two major portions (the longissimus and iliocostalis).

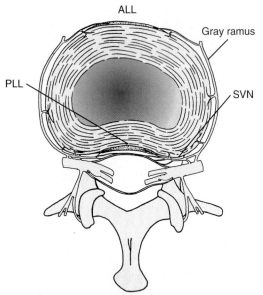

FIG. 8-9 Nerve supply of the lumbar intervertebral disc. *ALL,* Anterior longitudinal ligaments; *PLL,* posterior longitudinal ligaments; *SVN,* sinuvertebral nerves. (From Nicholas JA, Hershman EB: *The lower extremity & spine in sports medicine,* vol 1-2, ed 2, St Louis, 1995, Mosby.)

The spinalis connects spinous processes, and the longissimus and iliocostalis connect homologous portions of the costal and transverse elements of the lumbar, thoracic, and cervical vertebrae and skull (Fig. 8-14).

Useful in screening is muscle testing of the legs, which measures strength on a 5-point scale for extension and flexion (knee), abduction and adduction (hip), and eversion and inversion, as well as dorsiflexion and plantar flexion (foot) (Table 8-7).

For patients in whom the objective findings do not match the subjective complaints, close observation helps identify the inconsistencies (Table 8-8). A finding of three or more of the five signs of the Waddell index is clinically significant. Isolated positive signs are ignored.

The most superficial layer of tissue, below the subcutaneous layer, contains the thoracolumbar fascia. This tissue attaches medially to the thoracic spinous processes and inferiorly to the iliac crest and lateral crest of the sacrum. Laterally, the tissue serves as the origin of the latissimus dorsi and transversus abdominis muscles. Superiorly, the tissue attaches to the angles of the ribs in the thoracic region. Below the fascia lie the superficial multisegmental muscles, collectively named the erector spinae muscles. Their origin is a thick tendon attached to the posterior aspect of the sacrum, iliac crest, lumbar spinous processes, and supraspinous ligament. The muscle fibers split into three columns at the level of the lumbar spine: the lateral iliocostalis, the intermediate longissimus, and the more medial spinalis. The action of this group of muscle is to extend the spine. With unilateral action, the muscle group flexes the spine to one side.

Deep to the erector spinae lie the transversospinal muscles, including the multifidus and rotators. The multifidus originates at the posterior surface of the sacrum, the aponeurosis of the sacrospinalis, the posterior-superior iliac spine, and the posterior sacroiliac ligament. The multifidus inserts two to four segments above its origin into the spinous processes. The multifidus extends the spine and rotates it toward the opposite side. The rotators have similar attach-

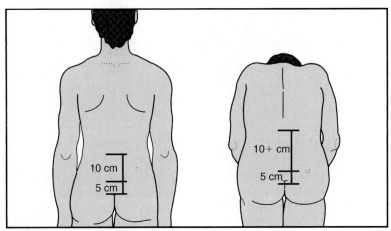

FIG. 8-10 Measuring lumbar flexion. (From Epstein O et al: *Clinical examination,* ed 2, London, 1997, Mosby.)

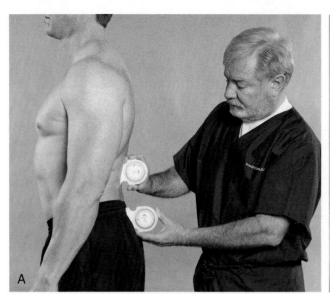
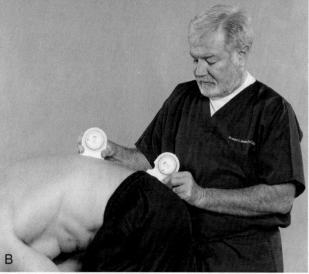

FIG. 8-11 For flexion, 80 degrees of movement is normal. Movement must occur from the lumbar spine and not the hips or thoracic spine. The distance that the patient is able to bend forward is compared with the straight-leg-raising tests. When using an inclinometer to measure the lumbar flexion range of motion, the patient is standing. One inclinometer is placed over the T12 spinous process in the sagittal plane. The second inclinometer is placed at the level of the sacrum, also in the sagittal plane (**A**). Both inclinometers are zeroed at these positions. The patient flexes forward, and the angle of both inclinometers is recorded (**B**). The sacral inclination is subtracted from the T12 inclination to obtain the lumbar flexion angle. Flexion movement of 60 degrees or less is an impairment to the lumbar spine in the activities of daily living.

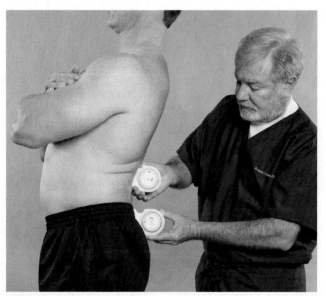

FIG. 8-12 Extension is limited to 35 degrees in the lumbar spine. Extension, as measured with an inclinometer, is performed with the patient standing. One inclinometer is placed over the T12 spinous process in the sagittal plane. The second inclinometer is placed at the sacrum, also in the sagittal plane. Both instruments are zeroed in this position. The patient extends the lumbar spine, and the angles of both instruments are recorded. The sacral inclination angle is subtracted from the T12 inclination angle to obtain the lumbar extension angle. Lumbar extension range of motion that is 20 degrees or less is an impairment to the lumbar spine in the activities of daily living.

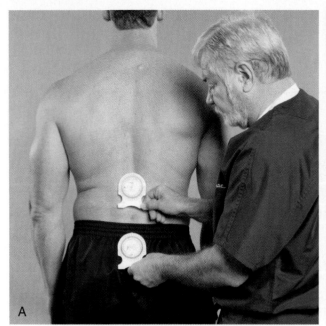
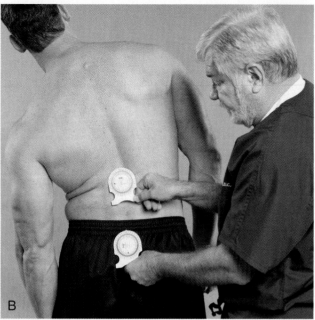

FIG. 8-13 Lateral flexion is approximately 25 degrees in the lumbar spine. The patient slides a hand down the side of the leg. The patient cannot bend forward or backward during the movement. The movement is compared with the opposite side. To use an inclinometer to measure the lateral lumbar flexion, the patient is standing and the lumbar spine is in neutral position. One inclinometer is placed at the T12 spinous process, in the coronal plane. The second inclinometer is placed at the superior aspect of the sacrum in the coronal plane. Both instruments are zeroed to this position (**A**). The patient laterally flexes the lumbar spine to one side, and the inclinations of both instruments are recorded (**B**). The sacral angle is subtracted from the T12 angle to obtain the lumbar lateral flexion angle. The procedure is repeated for the range of motion to the opposite side. Lateral flexion of 20 degrees or less to either side is an impairment of the lumbar spine in the activities of daily living.

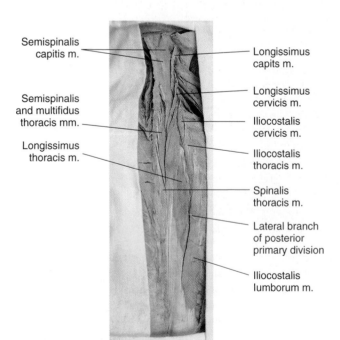

FIG. 8-14 Fifth layer of back muscles of the right side.
(From Cramer GD, Darby SA: *Basic and clinical anatomy of the spine, spinal cord, and ANS,* St Louis, 1995, Mosby.)

Labels (left):
Semispinalis capitis m.
Semispinalis and multifidus thoracis mm.
Longissimus thoracis m.

Labels (right):
Longissimus capits m.
Longissimus cervicis m.
Iliocostalis cervicis m.
Iliocostalis thoracis m.
Spinalis thoracis m.
Lateral branch of posterior primary division
Iliocostalis lumborum m.

ORTHOPEDIC GAMUT 8-1

LOWER EXTREMITY MUSCULATURE

Sequential innervation lower extremity musculature:
1. L2 and L3 supply hip flexion
2. L4 and L5 hip extension
3. L3 and L4 supply knee extension
4. L5 and S1 knee flexion
5. L4 and L5 supply ankle dorsiflexion
6. S1 and S2 ankle plantar flexion
7. L4 supplies ankle inversion
8. L5 and S1 supply ankle eversion

TABLE 8-7

LUMBAR RADICULAR SYNDROMES

Disc Level	Any Central Disc Herniation	L5/S1	L4/L5	L3/L4
Nerve root involved	Cauda equina (L4/L5 > L5/S1)	S1	L5	L4
Pain referral pattern	Perineum	Unilateral	Unilateral	Unilateral
	Low back	Low back	Low back	Low back
	Buttocks	Buttocks	Buttocks	Buttocks
	Either or both legs	Posterior leg	Lateral leg and thigh	Posterolateral leg
Motor deficit	Unilateral or bilateral leg weakness	Unilateral weakness; plantar flexion of foot; difficulty with toe walking	Unilateral weakness; dorsiflexion of foot; difficulty with heel walking	Unilateral quadriceps weakness
Sensory deficit	Perineum/buttocks, low back, thighs, legs, feet	Lateral foot, posterolateral calf	Lateral calf; between the first and second toes	Knee distal, anterior thigh
Reflexes compromised	Ankle jerk	Ankle jerk	0	Knee jerk

From Demeter SL, Andersson GBJ, Smith GM: *Disability evaluation,* St Louis, 1996, Mosby.

TABLE 8-8

NONORGANIC PHYSICAL SIGNS INDICATING ILLNESS BEHAVIOR

	Physical Disease/Normal Illness Behavior	Abnormal Illness Behavior
Symptoms		
Pain	Anatomic distribution	Whole leg pain
		Tailbone pain
Numbness	Dermatomal	Whole leg numbness
Weakness	Myotomal	Whole leg giving away
Time pattern	Varies with time and activity	Never free of pain
Response to treatment	Variable benefit	Intolerance of treatments
		Emergency admissions to hospital
Signs		
Tenderness	Anatomic distribution	Superficial
		Widespread nonanatomic
Axial loading	No lumbar pain	Lumbar pain
Simulated rotation	No lumbar pain	Lumbar pain
Straight leg raising	Limited on distraction	Improves with distraction
Sensory	Dermatomal	Regional
Motor	Myotomal	Regional, jerky, giving way

From Demeter SL, Andersson GBJ, Smith GM: *Disability evaluation,* St Louis, 1996, Mosby.

ments and action, but they ascend only one or two segments. Additional deep muscles include the interspinalis, which connects pairs of adjacent lumbar spinous processes, and the intertransversarii (medial, dorsal lateral, and ventral lateral groups), which connect pairs of adjacent transverse process. These muscles extend and bend the column to the same side, respectively.

The forward and lateral flexor muscles of the lumbar spine are located anterior and lateral to the vertebral bodies and transverse processes. The iliopsoas consists of two separate muscular heads: the iliacus and psoas major. The origins of the psoas major arise from the intervertebral disc by five slips, each of which start from adjacent upper and lower margins of two vertebrae, and membranous arches that emanate from the bodies of the four upper lumbar vertebrae. These arches permit the lumbar arteries and veins and the sympathetic rami communicantes to pass beneath them.

The iliacus arises from the iliac fossa and joins the psoas under the inguinal ligament. The iliacus then crosses the hip joint capsule and inserts into the lesser trochanter of the femur. These muscles flex the lumbar spine and bend it toward the same side. The quadratus lumborum, which lies lateral to the vertebral column, arises from the posterior part of the iliac crest and iliolumbar ligament and inserts into the twelfth rib and the tips of the transverse processes of the upper four lumbar vertebrae. This muscle fixes the diaphragm during inspiration and bends the trunk toward the same side when it acts alone (Figs. 8-15 to 8-17).

ESSENTIAL IMAGING

A variety of radiographic views can be taken when the lumbosacral region is evaluated. The standard views consist of the anteroposterior (AP), lateral (Figs. 8-18 and 8-19),

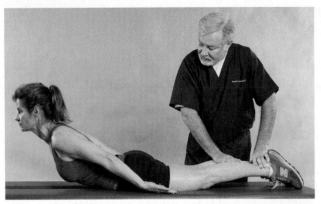

FIG. 8-15 During trunk extension, back extensors are assisted by the latissimus dorsi, quadratus lumborum, and trapezius. The patient is lying prone on the examination table. Hip extensors must give fixation of the pelvis to the thighs, and the examiner must stabilize the legs firmly on the table. The patient then extends the trunk.

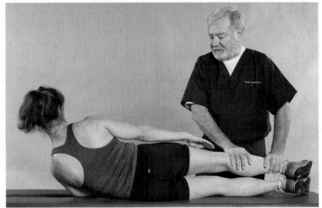

FIG. 8-16 Lateral flexion of the trunk requires a combination of lateral flexion and hip abduction. The patient is side lying, with the head, upper trunk, pelvis, and lower extremities in a straight line. The top arm is extended down along the side. The patient is not allowed to hold on to the pelvis and attempt to pull up with the hand. The under arm is forward, across the chest. This position rules out assistance by pushing up with the elbow. The legs must be held down by the examiner to counterbalance the weight of the trunk. During the test, the patient laterally flexes the trunk away from the examination table.

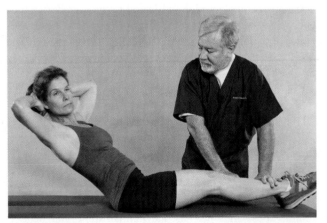

FIG. 8-17 Raising the trunk obliquely forward combines trunk flexion and rotation. It is accomplished by the combined actions of the external oblique on one side, the internal oblique on the opposite side, and the rectus abdominis. The patient is supine on the examination table, and the legs are supported by the examiner. The patient clasps the hands behind the head. The patient flexes, rotates the trunk, and holds the position.

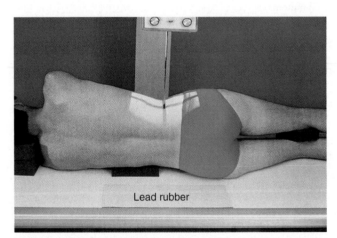

Lead rubber

FIG. 8-18 Lateral lumbar spine positioning, recumbent. (From Frank ED et al: *Merrill's atlas of radiographic positioning and procedures,* ed 11, St Louis, 2007, Mosby.)

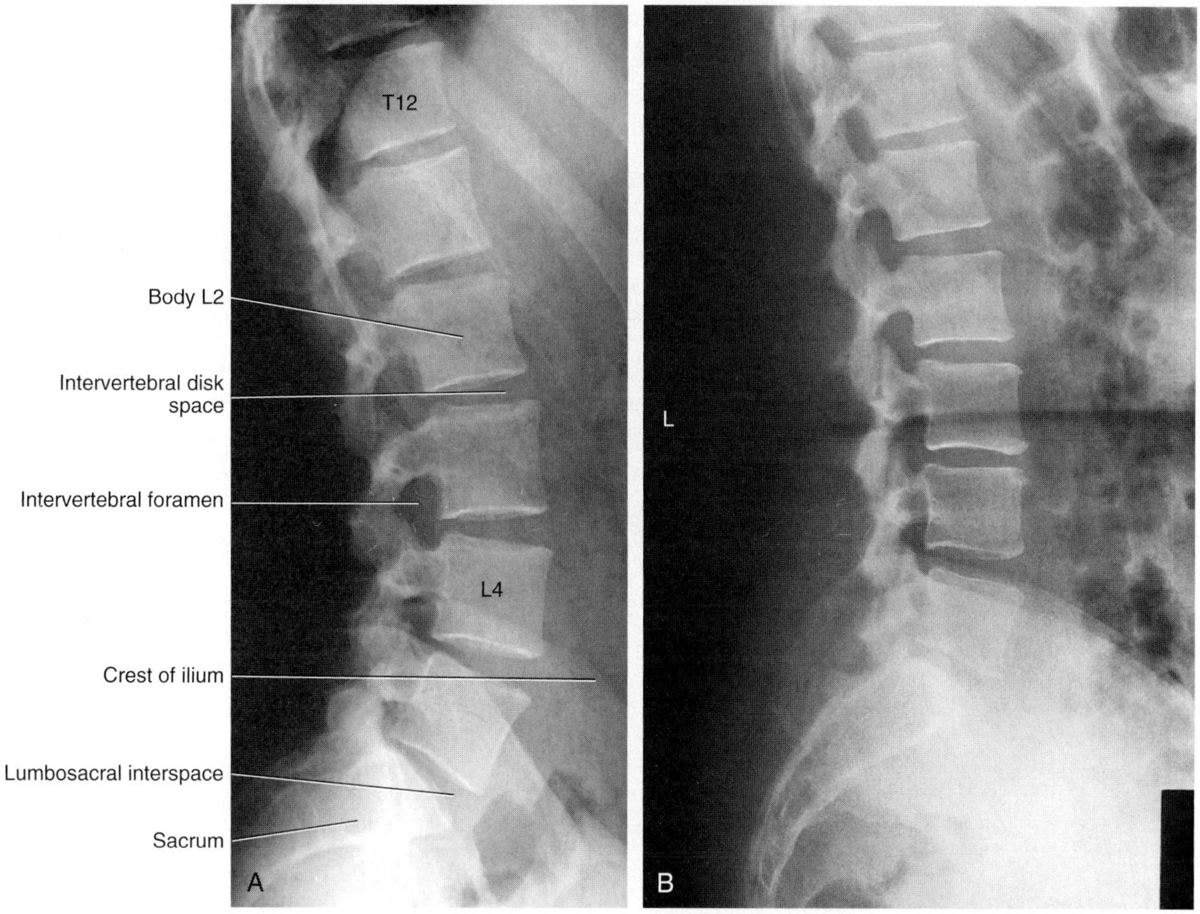
T12
Body L2
Intervertebral disk space
Intervertebral foramen
L4
Crest of ilium
Lumbosacral interspace
Sacrum
A
L
B

FIG. 8-19 Lateral lumbar spine. (From Frank ED et al: *Merrill's atlas of radiographic positioning and procedures,* ed 11, St Louis, 2007, Mosby.)

8

oblique (Figs. 8-20 to 8-22), and either a frontal or a lateral lumbosacral spot (Figs. 8-23 and 8-24).

The AP projection has generally been used for recumbent examinations. This position places the lumbar spine fully arched by extension of the lower limbs. The extended limb position accentuates the lordotic curve, which increases the angle between the vertebral bodies and the divergent rays, with resultant distortion of the bodies, as well as poor delineation of the intervertebral disc spaces (Figs. 8-25 and 8-26). The lordotic curve can be reduced and the intervertebral disc spaces clearly delineated in the AP projection simply by flexing the hips and knees enough to place the back in firm contact with the table (Figs. 8-27 to 8-29).

Bone scintigraphy is of limited utility in patients with low back pain (Fig. 8-30).

Computed tomography (CT) is useful for evaluating abnormalities of the lumbosacral spine, where the spatial anatomy is complex (Fig. 8-31). CT can visualize cortical bone destruction, calcified tumor matrix, and soft-tissue extension of tumors affecting the spine and is superior to magnetic resonance imaging (MRI) in this regard (Fig. 8-32). MRI is an excellent technique to view the spinal

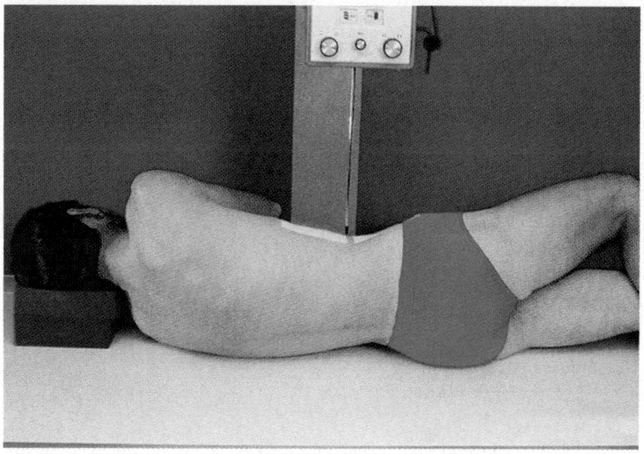

FIG. 8-20 Anteroposterior oblique lumbar spine positioning, recumbent. (From Frank ED et al: *Merrill's atlas of radiographic positioning and procedures,* ed 11, St Louis, 2007, Mosby.)

cord. MRI identifies syringomyelia, atrophy, cord infarction, cord injury, multiple sclerosis, and intramedullary tumors (Fig. 8-33). MRI can identify the vertebral bodies in which bone marrow has been replaced with tumor (Fig. 8-34).

Text continued on p. 556

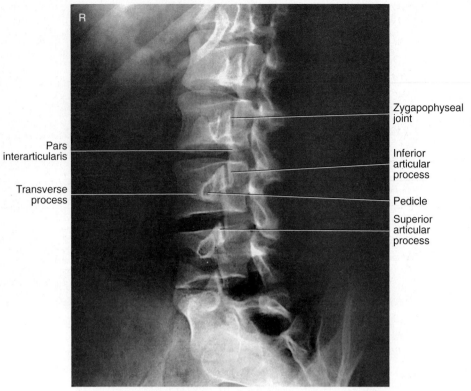

Zygapophyseal joint

Inferior articular process

Pedicle

Superior articular process

Pars interarticularis

Transverse process

FIG. 8-21 Anteroposterior oblique lumbar spine, right posterior oblique. (From Frank ED et al: *Merrill's atlas of radiographic positioning and procedures*, ed 11, St Louis, 2007, Mosby.)

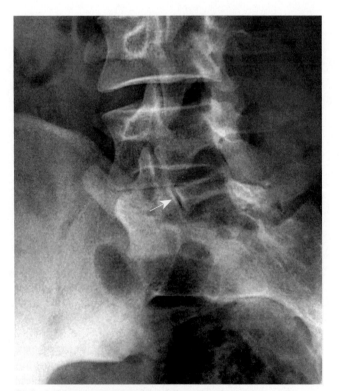

FIG. 8-22 Anteroposterior oblique lumbar spine, right posterior oblique. (From Frank ED et al: *Merrill's atlas of radiographic positioning and procedures*, ed 11, St Louis, 2007, Mosby.)

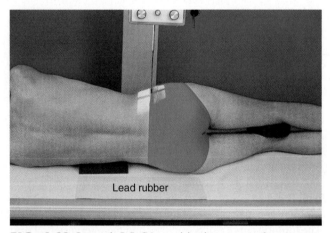

Lead rubber

FIG. 8-23 Lateral L5–S1 positioning, recumbent. (From Frank ED et al: *Merrill's atlas of roentgenographic positioning and procedures*, ed 11, St Louis, 2007, Mosby.)

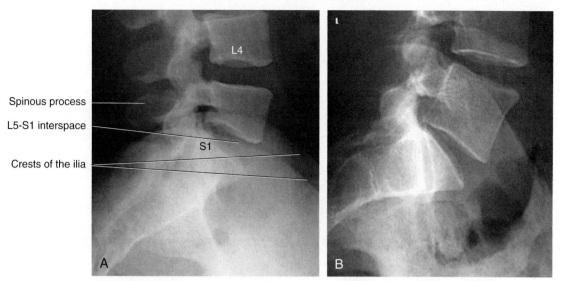

Spinous process

L5-S1 interspace

Crests of the ilia

FIG. 8-24 Lateral L5–S1. (From Frank ED et al: *Merrill's atlas of radiographic positioning and procedures,* ed 11, St Louis, 2007, Mosby.)

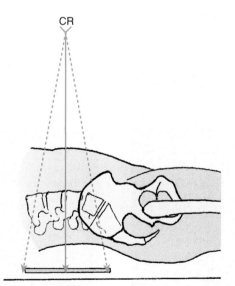

FIG. 8-25 Lumbar spine positioning demonstrating intervertebral disc spaces and diverging central ray are not parallel. (From Frank ED et al: *Merrill's atlas of radiographic positioning and procedures,* ed 11, St Louis, 2007, Mosby.)

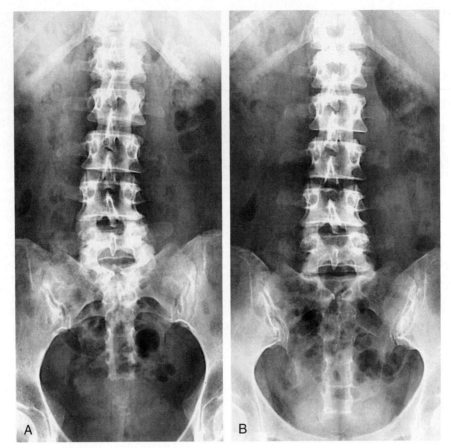

FIG. 8-26 Anteroposterior lumbar spine. (From Frank ED et al: *Merrill's atlas of radiographic positioning and procedures,* ed 11, St Louis, 2007, Mosby.)

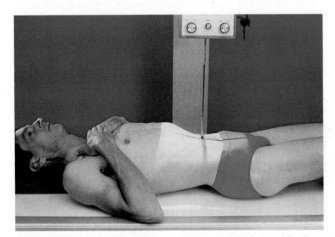

FIG. 8-27 Anteroposterior lumbar spine positioning, recumbent with the limbs extended, creating increased lordotic curve. (From Frank ED et al: *Merrill's atlas of radiographic positioning and procedures,* ed 11, St Louis, 2007, Mosby.)

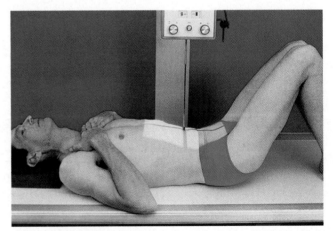

FIG. 8-28 Anteroposterior lumbar spine positioning, recumbent with limbs flexed, decreasing lordotic curve. (From Frank ED et al: *Merrill's atlas of radiographic positioning and procedures,* ed 11, St Louis, 2007, Mosby.)

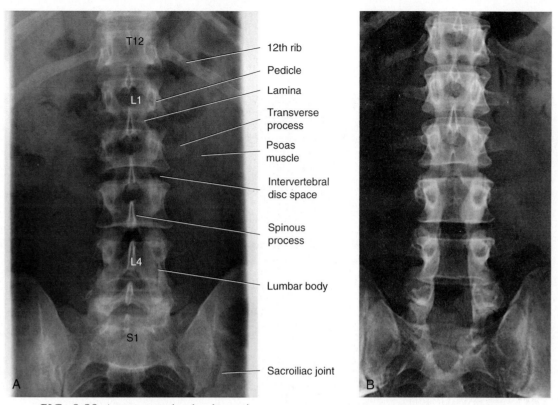

FIG. 8-29 Anteroposterior lumbar spine. (From Frank ED et al: *Merrill's atlas of radiographic positioning and procedures,* ed 11, St Louis, 2007, Mosby.)

8

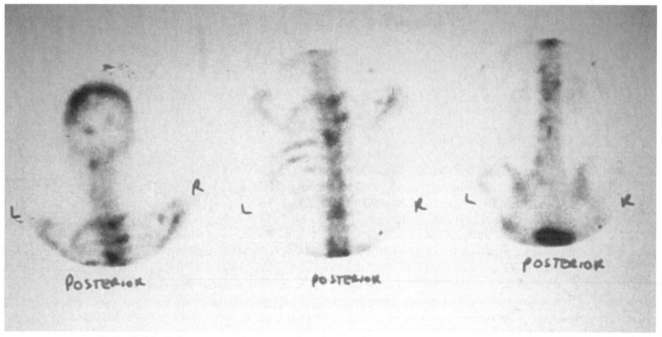

FIG. 8-30 A bone scan demonstrating the random uptake of radioisotope. Note the absence of uptake symmetry and variation of sizes of the foci throughout the skeleton. (From Deltoff MN, Kogon PL: *The portable skeletal x-ray library,* St Louis, 1998, Mosby.)

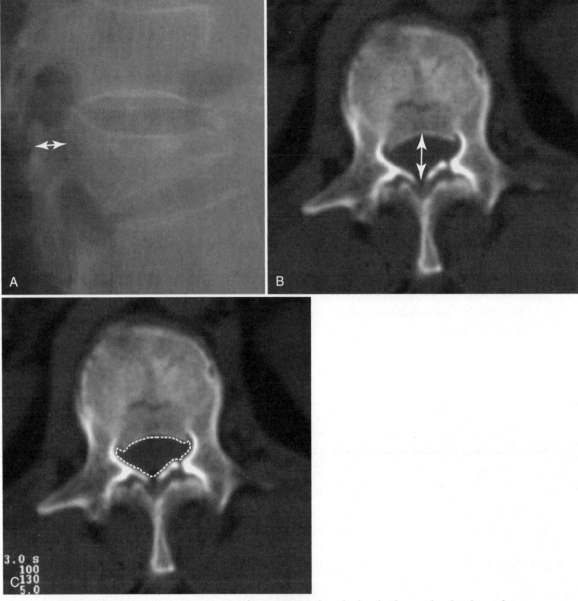

FIG. 8-31 Measurement methods of percent canal occlusion in thoracolumbar burst fractures. **A,** Ratio 1 for measurement of sagittal diameter of spinal canal on plain radiographs. **B,** Ratio 2 for measurement of sagittal diameter of spinal canal on axial CT scans. The sagittal diameter is defined as the distance between the anterior and posterior margins of the canal at the midline. **C,** Ratio 3 for measurement of cross-sectional area of spinal canal on axial CT scans. The canal area defined as an area enclosed by the inner bony margins of spinal canal. (From Dai L-Y, Wang X-Y, Jiang L-S: Evaluation of traumatic spinal canal stenosis in thoracolumbar burst fractures: A comparison of three methods for measuring the percent canal occlusion, *Europ J Radiol* In Press.)

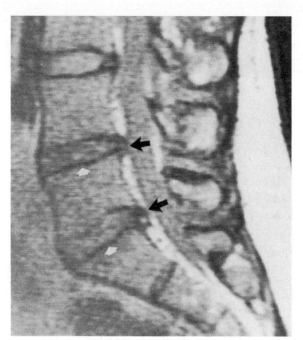

FIG. 8-32 On a T1-weighted sagittal image, abnormal findings include posterior disc protrusion *(black arrows)* and decreased signal intensity is the nucleus pulposus *(white arrows)* at L4–L5, L5–S1. (From Sartoris DJ: *Musculoskeletal imaging: the requisites*, St Louis, 1996, Mosby.)

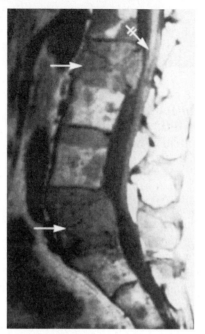

FIG. 8-34 T1-weighted magnetic resonance imaging scan reveals mild effacement of the thecal sac *(crossed arrow)* and multiple hypointense regions where normal hyperintense marrow has been replaced by tumor tissue *(arrows)*. This feature is particularly the case at L5, which appears homogeneously hypointense. (From Marchiori DM: *Clinical imaging with skeletal, chest, and abdomen pattern differentials,* St Louis, 1999, Mosby.)

8

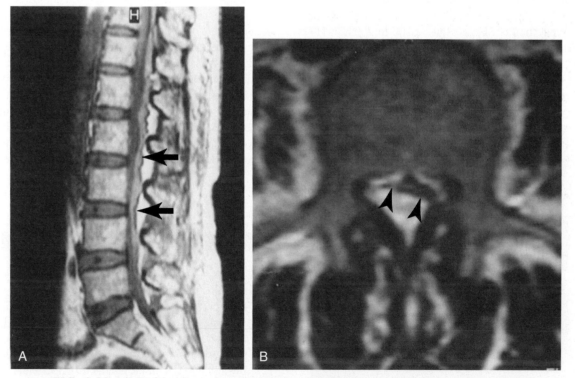

FIG. 8-33 MRI of lumbar spine. Sagittal T1 WI **(A)** showed the lumbar extension of acute spinal epidural hematoma (ASEDH) mass *(arrows)* along the entire lumbar spinal canal. Transverse T2 WI **(B)** at the level of L4 demonstrated severe dural sac compression *(arrowheads)*. (From Firat AK, Firat MM, Akmangit I et al: Acute epidural hematoma involving entire thoracic and lumbar spine, *Eur J Radiol Ex* 59[1]:7-10, 2006.)

Assessment for Posterolateral, Posteromedial, and Posterocentral Intervertebral Disc Protrusion

Comment

Small disc lesions can cause significant spinal impairment. Central lesions may cause thecal sac displacement or lumbar spinal canal compromise (Fig. 8-35).

Two major types of low back abnormalities center on the intervertebral disc: acute impairment from herniated discs and chronic impairment from degenerative disc disease (Table 8-9).

When applying compression and axial rotation, the **posterolateral** inner annular zones of the intervertebral disc show high stress peaks and centripetal pressure gradients. Asymmetrical loads (rotation) combined with postural changes in the sagittal plane increase these effects and may be responsible for a chronic mechanical overload of these regions (Steffen et al, 1998).

The usual pressure in the nucleus pulposus is 30 pounds per square inch (psi). This pressure is 30% to 40% less in the standing position than in the seated position and is 50% less in the reclining position than in the seated position. Cerebrospinal fluid (CSF) pressure is 100 to 200 mm H_2O in the recumbent position and 400 mm H_2O in the seated posture.

Two anatomically different types of lumbar disc herniation (LDH), contained and noncontained, have been recognized. In the contained type, the outer layer of the annulus fibrosus is intact and the herniated nucleus pulposus is not in direct contact with epidural tissue; in the noncontained type, the herniated nucleus pulposus is in direct contact with epidural tissue (Nakagawa et al, 2007).

A disc may protrude lateral to a nerve root, medial to a nerve root, under a nerve root, or central to the nerve root.

Approximately 95% or more of the lumbar lesions occur at either the L4–L5 or the L5–S1 disc level. The L4–L5 disc usually compresses the L5 nerve root, resulting in pain sensations down the lower extremity in the L5 dermatome. The L5–S1 disc usually compresses the first sacral nerve root, resulting in pain distribution down the S1 dermatome. Of these patients, 60% will have an antalgic lean. Two factors are important: the side of sciatic pain distribution and the side of antalgic inclination. By evaluating the antalgic posture, the examiner may determine whether the problem is a medial, central, or lateral disc protrusion.

A well-known problem related to intervertebral discs is the advent of degenerative discs. A loss of proteoglycan, and hence water and thus disc height and stiffness, occurs with aging and is one of the first changes seen in disc degeneration. Degenerated discs become dehydrated and disorganized; stress peaks occur and appear associated with pain in some instances. Degenerative disc disease results in biochemical changes; the amount of type-I collagen increases at the expense of type-II collagen, and the content in water and proteoglycans decreases. In contrast to the expected appearance of degenerated discs, which become dehydrated, hydrated intervertebral disc herniations are sometimes encountered in radiologic practice. In these cases,

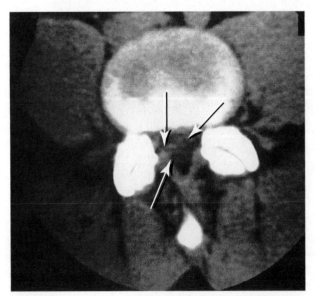

FIG. 8-35 Computed tomographic scan demonstrating a large right paracentral herniated disc at the L4–L5 level. (From Brier SR: *Primary care orthopedics,* St Louis, 1999, Mosby.)

ORTHOPEDIC GAMUT 8-2

DISC INJURIES

Definitions of disc injuries are as follows:

1. Disc protrusion is present when nuclear material does not extend beyond the annulus in a contained herniated nucleus pulposus.
2. Disc extrusion is a focal herniation contained by the posterior longitudinal ligament that extends into the spinal canal.
3. Sequestered disc is a free fragment that has broken off or through the annular peripheral fibers in the vertebral canal (prolapsed).

TABLE 8-9

LUMBAR DISC SYNDROMES

	Lumbar Herniated Nucleus Pulposus	Degenerative Disc Disease

Physical examination findings	Back or leg pain
	Sciatic nerve tension signs:
	    Positive SLR less than 60 degrees
	    Positive Bragard sign
	    Positive bowstring test
	    Positive Bechterew test
	    Painful arc of lumbar flexion, extension, or both
	True nerve root signs:
	    Radiculopathy
	    Motor or sensory deficit
	    Paresthesias
	    Diminished or absent deep-tendon reflexes
	    Possible antalgia, muscle spasm, instability
		Morning stiffness
		Lumbopelvic hypomobility
		Pain in lumbar flexion
		History consistent with spinal degeneration

X-ray findings	Need to rule out organic abnormality Hypolordosis secondary to muscle spasm Possible loss of intervertebral disc height Possible diagnosis of degenerative arthritis	Radiologic signs in acute exacerbation Spur formation Loss of intervertebral disc height Discogenic spondylosis Compatible findings on CT or MRI scans

CT, Computed tomography; *MRI,* magnetic resonance imaging.
Adapted from Brier SR: *Primary care orthopedics,* St Louis, 1999, Mosby.

the presence of hydrated discs may indicate another pathophysiologic basis rather than the well-known degenerative changes related to senility and wear and tear (Rasekhi et al, 2006).

> Proprioceptive input from the muscles of the legs and trunk plays an important role in maintaining postural stability, suggesting that sensory deficits from either location might result in instability. Postural instability has been observed in patients with low back pain, as well as in elderly persons. Patients with low back pain have also been attributed reduced lumbosacral proprioception, which might be a causative factor in their instability (Brumagne, Cordo, Verschueren, 2004).

PROCEDURE

- When the disc protrudes lateral to the nerve root, the patient assumes an antalgic lean away from the side of the disc lesion or pain (Fig. 8-36).
- When the disc protrudes medial to the nerve root, the patient assumes an antalgic lean into the side of the disc lesion or pain (Fig. 8-37).
- With a central disc lesion, the patient assumes a flexed posture of the lumbar spine, with or without leaning to either side (Fig. 8-38).
- With protrusion under the nerve root, the patient may not lean at all.

Next Steps/Procedures

Bowstring sign, Cox sign, heel/toe walk test, Kemp test, Lewin punch test, Lewin snuff test, Milgram test, and Neri sign

CLINICAL PEARL

I f the antalgia is not readily apparent in a static posture, it will appear with forward flexion of the trunk. If a disc protrusion exists, even in the mildest degree, trunk flexion exerts enough pressure to irritate the inflamed muscle or to stretch neural structures over the bulging disc. The antalgia is evident at this point. Patients with low back pain might stiffen the trunk and pelvis and hyperextend the knees in an effort to decrease the number of degrees of freedom.

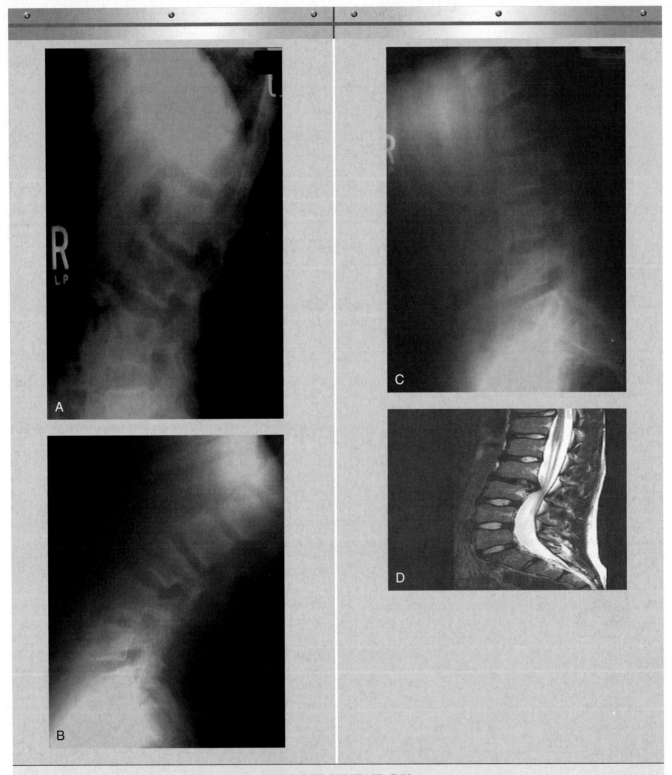

AT THE VIEWBOX

16-year-old male with moderate generalized back pain and stiffness, including extreme muscle guarding. No report of trauma, but the patient is active in sports. Neutral lateral lumbar spine radiograph (**A**) demonstrates retrolisthesis subluxation of L2, measuring one centimeter, which increases minimally on extension (**B**) and decreases markedly on flexion. **C,** There is also increased flexion-exten-sion focally at L2 on L3. These findings indicate motion segment instability at L2–3. The patient was referred for MRI, which demonstrates a large central disc herniation at L2–3. **D,** There is associated avulsive injury of the ring apophysis at the posterosuperior vertebral body margin of L3, a variant of a posterior limbus bone. (From the teaching file of Timothy Mick, DC, DACBR)

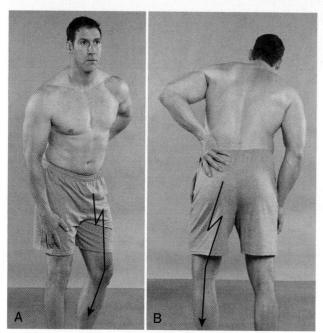

FIG. 8-36 When the disc protrudes lateral to the nerve root, the patient assumes an antalgic lean away from the side of the disc lesion or pain. In this illustration, the patient is experiencing left leg sciatica.

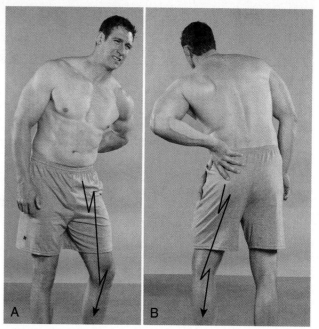

FIG. 8-37 When the disc protrudes medial to the nerve root, the patient assumes an antalgic lean into the side of the disc lesion or pain. In this illustration, the patient is experiencing left leg sciatica.

8

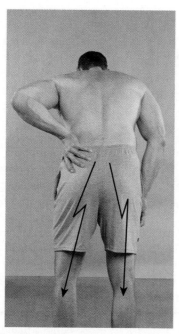

FIG. 8-38 With a central disc lesion, the patient assumes a flexed posture of the lumbar spine, with or without leaning to either side.

Assessment for Sciatica, Intervertebral Disc Lesion, Vertebral Exostoses, Dural Sleeve Adhesions, Muscular Spasm, or Vertebral Subluxation

Comment

The dura mater of the lumbar spine has a series of attachments to neighboring vertebrae and ligaments. These attachments are found at each segmental level and are usually found in the region of the intervertebral disc. They have been known as the *dural attachment complex* or *Hoffmann ligaments* (also known as the *dorsolateral dural ligaments of Hofmann*).

The neural elements pass over an intervertebral disc before exiting through an intervertebral foramen (IVF) (Fig. 8-39).

A typical lumbar IVF (Fig. 8-40) is sometimes described as having the shape of an inverted teardrop or an inverted pear.

Compression, or entrapment, of neural elements as they pass through the nerve root canal or the IVF can occur. Causes of such compression include degenerative changes of the superior articular facets and posterior vertebral bodies,

intervertebral disc protrusion, and pressure from the superior pedicle of the IVF.

Strong ligamental attachments absorb the craniocaudal tractive forces, and the transverse fibers are important to the transversal pressure of the spinal nerves. However, many theories have been suggested about the clinical role of the epidural ligaments. They would play an important mechanical part in low back pain and radiculopathy. The rather impressive investigation by Kuslich and colleagues seems to confirm indirectly the important part the epidural ligaments are playing. The stimulus of a swollen or compressed nerve root or both, responsible for sciatic pain, might be the result of to its fixation by an epidural ligament. Furthermore, the origin of low back pain can sometimes be partially explained by traction transmitted via the ligament of Trolard to the posterior longitudinal ligament and the annulus fibrosus, respectively, the dura mater, all these structures being well innervated by the sinuvertebral nerve and consequently extremely sensitive to pain (van Dun, Girardin, 2006).

Lumbar disc protrusions are a common cause of lower back pain with sciatica. This protrusion usually occurs against a background of degenerative joint disease. The disc protrusion of a young adult is likely to be traumatic and should not be classified as osteoarthritis.

The precipitating trauma of an intervertebral disc syndrome is usually slight. The annulus fibrosus ruptures posteriorly, and a fragment of the nucleus is extruded into the vertebral canal. In other instances, a frank prolapse of the nucleus pulposus may occur through the tear. If concomitant rupture of the posterior longitudinal ligament occurs, the protrusion may be in the midline posteriorly, which is instead of a usual posterolateral position. The fibrocartilage or nucleus pulposus may impinge on the related nerve root and compress it against the lamina and ligamentum flavum.

Because the rupture is usually to one side of the midline, only one nerve root is affected in its extrathecal course. Because the roots of the cauda equina run vertically within the theca, one or more of these passing caudal nerves may also be compressed. If the rupture is in the midline, roots on both sides may be involved. If it is large enough, the protrusion also may compress the cauda equina. Most disc lesions are at the L4–L5 or L5–S1 level. Only here can a disc lesion produce the syndrome of lower backache with sciatica. Unlike the situation in the cervical spine, cord compression is not a feature of lumbar disc lesions because the spinal cord ends opposite the lower border of L1. However, cauda equina compression can occur at these levels.

The apophyseal joints are usually involved pari passu with disc degeneration. They are also part of the pattern of joint involvement in multiple osteoarthritis and are likely to contribute to the patient's symptoms.

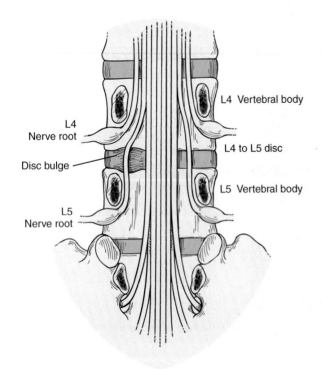

FIG. 8-39 Lumbar intervertebral discs and the exiting nerve roots. (From Greenstein GM: *Clinical assessment of neuromusculoskeletal disorders*, St Louis, 1997, Mosby.)

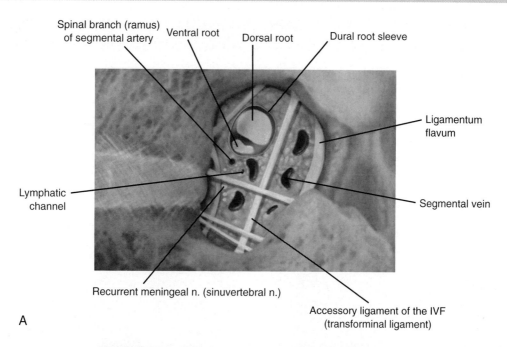

Spinal branch (ramus) of segmental artery — Ventral root — Dorsal root — Dural root sleeve

Ligamentum flavum

Lymphatic channel

Segmental vein

Recurrent meningeal n. (sinuvertebral n.)

Accessory ligament of the IVF (transforminal ligament)

A

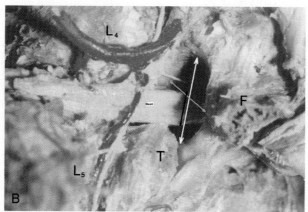

FIG. 8-40 **A,** The lumbar intervertebral foramen (IVF). (From Greestein GM: *Clinical assessment of neuromusculoskeletal disorders*, St Louis, 1997, Mosby.) **B,** Lumbar intervertebral foramen and lumbar root. L4 indicates fourth lumbar vertebrae; L5, fifth lumbar vertebrae; F, facet; T, transverse process; white arrow, sagittal diameter; blue arrow, transverse diameter; black arrow, root diameter. (From Torun F, Dolgun H, Tuna H, et al: Morphometric analysis of the roots and neural foramina of the lumbar vertebrae, *Surg Neurol* 66[2]:148-151, 2006.)

Pain is aggravated by movement of the spine, such as rolling over in bed, and by any maneuver that causes elevation of the CSF pressure within the theca. Pain is more constantly aggravated by maneuvers that stretch the sciatic nerve. Forward flexion of the lumbar spine or straight leg raising with the patient supine produces pain. The back usually is held rigid, and movements are limited by muscle spasm, which results in antalgia to one side or the other and flattening of the lumbar lordosis. Forward flexion is more limited than lateral flexion.

- The examiner restricts the patient's attempts at hip flexion with downward pressure on the thigh (Fig. 8-43).
- This extension is followed by an attempt to extend both legs.
- The test is positive if backache or sciatic pain is increased or if the maneuver is impossible.
- In disc involvement, extending both legs will usually increase the spinal and sciatic discomfort.
- A positive test indicates sciatica, a disc lesion, exostoses, adhesions, spasm, or subluxation.

Next Steps/Procedures

Bragard sign, Deyerle sign, Fajersztajn test, Lasègue differential sign, Lasègue rebound test, Lasègue sitting test, Lasègue test, Lewin standing test, Lindner sign, Sicard sign, straight-leg-raising test, and Turyn sign

PROCEDURE

- While in a seated position, the patient attempts to extend each leg one at a time (Figs. 8-41 and 8-42).

CLINICAL PEARL

Simple flattening or even reversing the lumbar curve is often not associated with radicular pain. The pain is localized in the lower lumbar spine, and any movement of the spine accentuates the pain. In these instances, the prime pathologic feature is sprain of an intervertebral joint rather than root irritation.

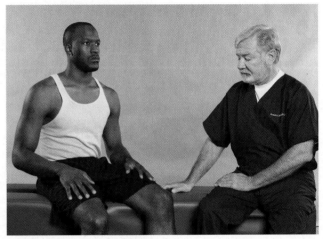

FIG. 8-41 The patient is in the seated position.

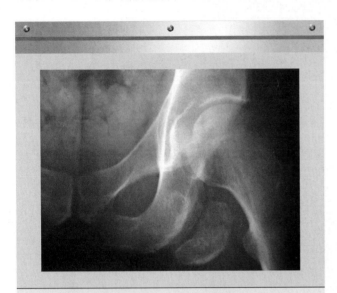

AT THE VIEWBOX

31-year-old male with left sciatica. No report of trauma. Lumbar spine imaging was unremarkable. Left hip radiograph demonstrates a "rider's bone," a hypertrophied, ununited avulsion fracture of the ischial tuberosity apophysis. This was related to a "hamstring pull" from sports activity in adolescence, recalled by the patient upon directed questioning. Though sciatica most often originates from lumbar spine abnormality, such as disc herniation, compromise of the sciatic nerve anywhere along its course may produce sciatica. Sciatica, with negative lumbar spine imaging should raise the question of a less common peripheral lesion of the sciatic nerve, such as a compressive lesion or neural tumor and directed imaging along the course of the sciatic nerve may be necessary. MRI of the pelvis and leg will directly assess the sciatic nerve. (From the teaching file of Timothy Mick, DC, DACBR)

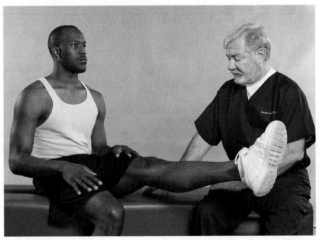

FIG. 8-42 The patient attempts to extend each leg one at a time.

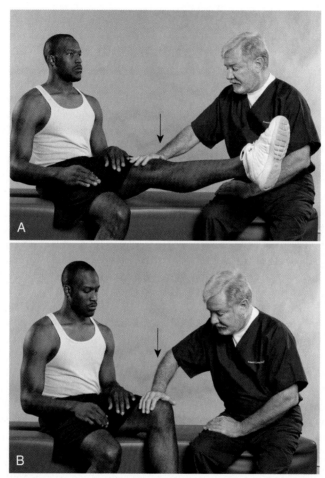

FIG. 8-43 The examiner resists the patient's attempts at hip flexion with downward pressure on the thigh. The test is positive if the maneuver increases backache or sciatic pain or if the maneuver is impossible. Unilateral leg testing is followed by the patient's attempt to extend both legs simultaneously. With disc involvement, extending both legs will usually increase the spinal and sciatic discomfort. A positive test suggests sciatica, disc lesion, exostoses, adhesions, spasm, or subluxation.

Assessment for Mechanical Lumbosacral Lesion, Intervertebral Disc Lesion, or Vertebral Exostoses

Comment

The lumbar zygapophyseal joints (Z-joints) are complex synovial joints that are oriented in the vertical plane (Fig. 8-44).

During rotation of the lumbar region, distraction, or gapping, occurs between adjacent lumbar articular facets on the side of rotation. An articular capsule covers the posterior aspect of each lumbar Z-joint. Effusion within the Z-joint may enter the superior recess, and as little as 0.5 mL of effusion may cause the superior recess of the capsule to enter the anteriorly located IVF. Such a protrusion of the Z-joint is known as a *synovial cyst* (Fig. 8-45).

> Intraspinal cysts (juxtafacet cysts, juxtaarticular cysts) in the immediate vicinity of the lumbar Z-joints are generally accepted as representing either true synovial cysts or ganglion cysts. The cysts are most common at the L4-L5 level (50% to 75% of reported cases) but are also seen at other lumbar and cervical levels. The diagnosis of Z-joint–induced radicular pain is based on correlation of an appropriate history with imaging studies. The patient usually has a history of slowly progressive or intermittent radicular pain, commonly neuroclaudicatory in nature. Coupled with imaging documentation of a cyst at a level that correlates with the patient's symptoms, the examiner can be relatively certain of the diagnosis. Imaging studies that document the presence of a cyst include myelography, Z-joint arthrography, CT, and MRI (Sabers et al, 2005).

Degenerative changes of the Z-joints often accompany aging. Such changes include an inflammatory reaction at the synovial lining of the Z-joint, changes of the articular cartilage, loose bodies in the Z-joint, and laxity of the joint capsule.

Degeneration of the disc leads to increased rotational instability of the Z-joints, resulting in further degeneration of these structures.

Osteophytes (bony spurs) often develop with age on the superior and inferior articular processes. This abnormality often occurs on the periphery of the Z-joint along the attachment sites of the ligamentum flavum or the articular capsule.

> Juxtafacet cysts (JFCs), histologically divided into ganglion and synovial cysts, are a rare pathologic condition of the lumbar spine. They originate from the facet joint and are usually characterized by intraspinal extradural masses, which compress nerve root and dural sac from posterolaterally. Posteromedial JFCs, anterolateral JFCs with contact to the posterior longitudinal ligament, and foraminal or extra-foraminal JFCs are an exceptional finding. A JFC, which arises intraspinally and extends through the neural foramen to become an extraspinal lesion compressing the upper nerve root, is a unique phenomenon (Oertel et al, 2006).

As the legs are raised or lowered, they exert a strong, downward pull on the pelvis. This pull is in opposition to the upward pull of the abdominal muscles. If the patient can tilt the pelvis posteriorly to flex the spine and hold the low back flat on an examining table as the legs are raised or lowered, the abdominal muscles must act to hold that position.

If the abdominal muscles are weak and the hip flexor muscles are strong, the back cannot be held flat while the legs are raised or lowered. The lower back will appear hyperextended as the legs are raised, and the abdominal muscles will be put on stretch.

The actions of various segments of the abdominal muscles are so closely allied with and interdependent on other parts that no specific functions can be ascribed to any single segment.

From a mechanical standpoint, the pelvis can be tilted toward the posterior rib cage by an upward pull on the pubis, by a downward pull on the ischium, and by an oblique pull from the anterior iliac crest. The muscle or muscle fibers that lie in these lines of pull are the rectus abdominis, the hip extensors, and the lateral fibers of the external oblique. These muscles act to tilt the pelvis posteriorly, whether the subject is standing or lying supine. During double leg raising from a supine position, the hip extensors cease to assist actively in tilting the pelvis posteriorly. The rectus abdominis and the external oblique muscles assume the major roles if an effort is made to flex the lumbar spine and keep the lower back flat on the examination table while the thoracic spine remains extended. Without the resistance of the lower extremities, the pelvis can be tilted posteriorly by the external oblique without assistance from the rectus abdominis. Against resistance, as occurs during double leg raising, the rectus abdominis must come into strong action.

The abdominal muscles elongate, and the back starts to arch if the patient's strength is not sufficient to maintain the pelvis in posterior tilt.

At the initiation of double leg raising or leg lowering, the thorax will show a tendency for the ribs to pull inward, decreasing the infrasternal angle. This movement is compatible with the line of pull and the action of the external oblique.

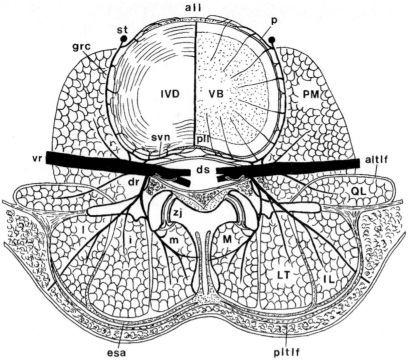

FIG. 8-44 Innervation of the lumbar motion segment showing the vertebral body (VB) on the right and the intervertebral disc (IVD) on the left. *ds*, dural sac; *zj*, zygapophyseal joint; *pll*, posterior longitudinal ligament; *all*, anterior longitudinal ligament; *vr*, ventral ramus; *dr*, dorsal ramus; m, medial branch; *svn*, sinuvertebral nerve; *grc*, gray ramus communications; *st*, sympathetic trunk.

8

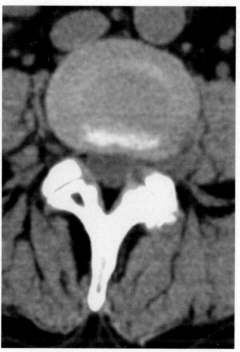

FIG. 8-45 Preoperative non–contrast-enhanced axial CT scan at segment L3–L4 showing a left-sided soft tissue density mass located both pan- and extra-foraminally, causing nerve root compression with an associated intraspinal extradural cystic lesion adjacent to the facet joint. (Adapted from Oertel MF, Ryang YM, Gilsbach JM, et al: Lumbar foraminal and far lateral Juxtafacet cyst of intraspinal origin, *Surg Neurol* 66[2]:197-199, 2006.)

PROCEDURE

- The patient lowers the straightened legs from a 90-degree angle to a 45-degree angle (Figs. 8-46 and 8-47).
- The test is positive if the legs drop or if the move produces pain.
- A positive test indicates lumbosacral involvement, disc lesions, or exostoses.

Next Steps/Procedures

Demianoff sign, double leg-raise test, hyperflexion test, Lewin supine test, matchstick test, Mennell sign, Minor sign, Nachlas test, Quick test, Schober test, sign of the buttock, skin pinch test, spinal percussion test, and Vanzetti sign

CLINICAL PEARL

Because of the presence of the nociceptive nerve ending within the annulus fibrosus of the disc, annular tears can cause pain in the lower back, buttocks, sacroiliac region, and lower extremity. This pain can occur without nerve compression by a disc protrusion. Disc protrusion that does not compress the nerve root can cause an inflammatory response and secondary radiculitis by chemically induced inflammatory neural pain.

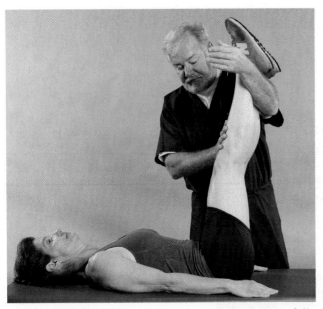

FIG. 8-46 The patient is supine with both legs fully extended. The examiner lifts both legs, simultaneously, to a near 90-degree, hip-flexion angle.

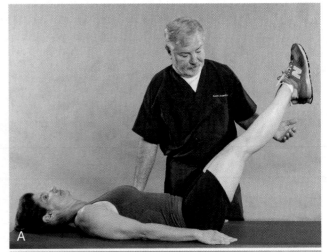

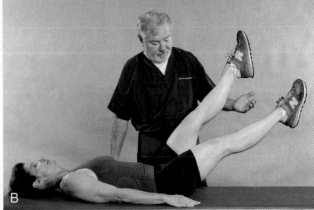

FIG. 8-47 From this elevated leg position, the patient is instructed to lower the legs from a 90-degree angle to a 45-degree angle. The test is positive if the legs drop or if lower back pain is produced. A positive test suggests lumbosacral involvement, disc lesions, or exostoses.

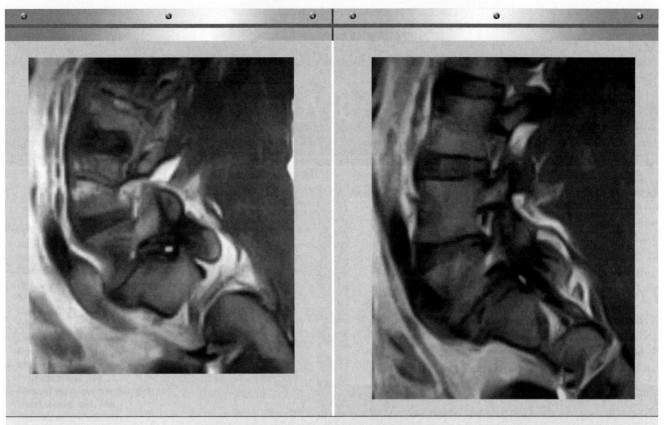

AT THE VIEWBOX

8

This patient with L5 lower extremity radiculopathy has high grade nerve root canal stenosis due to combined L5 spondylolytic spondylolisthesis and disc bulge into the foraminal zone. T1 weighted MR images through the intervertebral foramina show marked effacement of the normal perineural fat, surrounding the exiting L5 nerve root at the L5–S1 level, with compression of the L5 nerve root. **A** and **B,** At L3–4 and L4–5, the normal exiting L3 and L4 nerve roots are well seen as oval low signal foci, surrounded by the normal high signal perineural fat. (From the teaching file of Timothy Mick, DC, DACBR)

BOWSTRING SIGN

Assessment for Lumbar Nerve Root Compression

Comment

Lower back pain is often associated with sciatica and can be elicited in the posterior part of a degenerated disc because the posterior longitudinal ligament in this region contains sensory nerve fibers. However, lower back pain is not the direct result of nerve root compression.

> The lumbosacral nerve roots are often involved in disease processes and injuries such as disc herniation, spinal stenosis, tumor and vertebral fracture. General consensus asserts that the genesis of radiculopathy associated with the pathologic conditions of the spine may result from mechanical compression of the nerve root. This factor may change the intraradicular circulation and produce nerve fiber dysfunction. The mechanical compression may also lead to a series of intraneurial tissue reactions, including edema formation, demyelination, and fibrosis (Kobayashi, Yoshizawa, Yamada, 2004a).

Disc degeneration does not elicit a referred radiating pain that can be confused with the pain of lumbosacral nerve root compression. Lower back pain is present in most cases of sciatica and often appears earlier than does the radiating pain. In some cases, the pain has its onset with the onset of the radiating pain. The lower back pain is not as important in the diagnosis as the levels and sites of nerve root compression.

In adults, the cord ends near the caudal end of the first lumbar vertebra. In its caudal extension, the dural sac encloses the lumbosacral nerve roots. At each segment, a pair of nerve roots, symmetrically enclosed by dural nerve root sleeves, leaves the dural sac and departs from the spinal canal through the IVF at that level. In the lower lumbar region, the point of departure of the nerve roots from the dural sac is more cranial than the point at which the nerve roots depart from the spinal canal through their respective IVF. The difference in height amounts to approximately one segment.

All of the lower sacral nerve roots depart from the tapering end cone of the dural sac, which is caudal to the level of the L5 disc. This end cone varies in how far it reaches into the sacral canal. The levels at which the lower sacral nerve roots depart from the dural sac are different in individual cases.

The neurologic symptoms caused by disc protrusions bulging from different lumbar discs depend on the nerve root that is closest to the site of the disc protrusion, making it the first one compressed. At their point of departure from the dural sac, the nerve roots are firmly fixed to the dural sac and cannot at this point be easily pushed aside by disc protrusions. This firmness contributes to the occurrence of typical nerve root syndromes caused by disc protrusions located near the point from which the nerve roots depart.

ORTHOPEDIC GAMUT 8-3
LUMBOSACRAL NERVE ROOTS

After leaving the dural sac, the lumbosacral nerve roots run caudally and laterally in the direction of departure from the spinal canal:

1. The fourth lumbar root (L4) leaves the dural sac slightly caudal of the intervertebral disc between the third and fourth lumbar vertebrae (third lumbar disc).
2. The fifth lumbar root (L5) leaves the dural sac near the level of the fourth lumbar disc.
3. The first sacral root (S1) leaves the dural sac medial of S1 and slightly below the level of the L5 disc.

ORTHOPEDIC GAMUT 8-4
WALLERIAN DEGENERATION SEQUENCE

- When axonal continuity is disrupted by mechanical compression or nerve trunk ischemia:
  - Axons distal to the stump divide finely and begin to degenerate.
  - At the same time, the myelin sheaths that have lost axons begin to break down.
- Wallerian degeneration occurs peripheral to the site of compression in the anterior root and central to this site (i.e., toward the spinal cord) in the posterior root when the cauda equina or nerve root is compressed by a herniated intervertebral disc or spinal canal stenosis.
- Nerve roots have a regenerative capacity similar to that of peripheral nerves.
- While regeneration of the anterior root approximates that of peripheral nerves, recovery of sensation presents problems in the posterior root because degeneration extends into the spinal cord.

PROCEDURE

- With the patient in the supine position, the examiner moves the patient's leg until it is above the examiner's shoulder.
- At this point, firm pressure should be exerted on the hamstring muscles (Fig. 8-48).
- If pain is not elicited, pressure is applied to the popliteal fossa.
- Pain in the lumbar region or radiculopathy is a positive sign for nerve root compression.

Next Steps/Procedures

Antalgia sign, Cox sign, heel/toe walk test, Kemp test, Lewin punch test, Lewin snuff test, Milgram test, and Neri sign

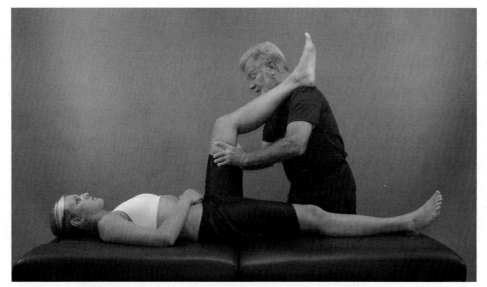

FIG. 8-48 The patient is in the supine position with both legs fully extended. The examiner places the patient's affected leg atop a shoulder. The examiner exerts firm pressure near the insertion of the hamstring muscles. If this maneuver is painful, firm pressure is applied to the popliteal fossa. Pain in the lumbar region or radiculopathy is a positive sign for nerve root compression. This is followed by a confirmation maneuver in attempting to pull the patient's knee into *full* extension, usually exacerbating the radicular complaint.

CLINICAL PEARL

Nerve roots must change their lengths depending on the degree of flexion, extension, lateral flexion, and rotation of the lumbar spine. Lumbar nerve roots that are limited in motion by fibrosis of either intraspinal or extraspinal origin will create traction on the nerve root complex, causing ischemia and secondary neural dysfunction.

BRAGARD SIGN

Assessment for Sciatic Neuritis, Spinal Cord Tumor, Intervertebral Disc Lesions, and Spinal Nerve Irritation

Comment

An intervertebral disc typically consists of a nucleus pulposus surrounded by an annulus fibrosus, both sandwiched between superior and inferior vertebral end-plates (Fig. 8-49). The nucleus pulposus of a lumbar intervertebral disc consists of a central core of a well-hydrated proteoglycan matrix surrounded by fibrocartilage. The annulus fibrosus consists of 10 to 12 concentric lamellae of collagen fibers. In any given lamella, the collagen fibers run in parallel at an angle of approximately 65 degrees to the vertical, but the direction of this angle alternates in successive layers.

Pain in the segmental distribution of a root is the hallmark of root compression syndrome. Pain in the spine and restriction of spinal movement are common and are the result of local involvement of the sensitive tissues and the root.

Herniated disc, metastatic malignancy, primary neoplasm, recent trauma, or inflammation may be responsible.

Signs of nerve trunk hypersensitivity, such as spontaneous activity and mechanosensitive responses to pressure at the site of injury, can develop in injured afferents after a neuroma or a chronic constriction injury. Responses to stretch can also develop in A-fibers in a neuroma. However, for many patients with widespread painful conditions, a nerve lesion is not apparent on clinical examination. Researchers have suggested that, in these patients, pain can occur after relatively minor nerve damage and that inflammation of the nerve trunk alone may play a major role in symptom production (Dilley, Lynn, Pang, 2005).

Pain that radiates down the leg follows the primary anterior division of the nerve and may be localized by the patient anywhere in the distribution of the root. This root pain is aggravated by spinal movement, local pressure over the nerve, or straining of the nerve. Pressure over the muscle in the area of pain usually produces discomfort.

Paresthesia in root distribution is common and is usually experienced distally in the foot. This paresthesia may be

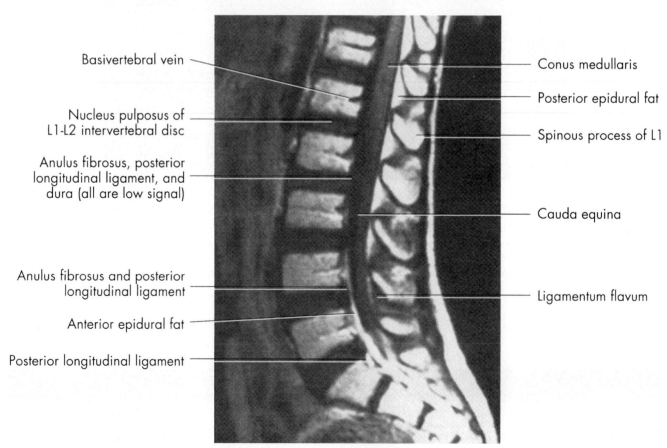

FIG. 8-49 (From Enzmann DR, De La Paz PL, Rubin JB: *Magnetic resonance of the spine*, St Louis, 1990, Mosby.)

aggravated or relieved by the same factors that influence the pain, but the paresthesia is constant.

Weakness and atrophy in the corresponding myotonic distribution result from prolonged or severe root compression, and stretch reflexes, with arcs that are largely or entirely incorporated in the involved root, will be diminished or lost.

Suspicion of a single nerve root compression syndrome should be prompted by the combination of a history of pain and the presence of paresthesia in the appropriate distribution of one nerve root only. Findings necessary to confirm the diagnosis are those that relate spinal movement to the radiating pain, those that demonstrate muscular weakness and tenderness in the myotome, and those that localize sensory and reflex deficits to the dermatome and myotome.

A herniated intervertebral disc produces a persistent, unilateral, isolated syndrome. Bilateral and multiple nerve root involvement can be caused by extensive degenerative joint disease. When nerve root involvement is progressive and acute or subacute, metastatic malignancy or inflammation is suggested.

Nerve root compression may herald an intraspinal mass that later will impinge on the spinal cord or cauda equina. The examiner must always look closely for motor, sensory, and reflex changes below the affected root because these changes may indicate involvement of the cord or cauda equina.

A herniated intervertebral disc is the most common cause of frank root compression syndromes affecting the extremities.

> The nerve root compression that occurs in lumbar disc herniation and lumbar canal stenosis often results in a range of symptoms, including low back pain, sciatic pain, and sensory disturbances and muscle weakness in the legs. In experimental studies, many acute subacute and chronic nerve root compression models have been created and have been studied pathologically and electrophysiologically. The results obtained so far suggest that impaired intraradicular blood flow and nerve fiber deformation are implicated in the appearance of radicular symptoms associated with nerve root compression. However, few studies have examined the effect of lumbar nerve root compression on axonal flow in the nerve fibers deformation caused by compression. Apparently, various neurotransmitters produced by the primary sensory neurons in the dorsal root ganglion and transported to the spinal dorsal horn by axonal flow in the central branches of the dorsal root neurons are implicated in the development of radicular pain and sensory disturbance associated with nerve root compression (Kobayashi, Yoshizawa, Yamada, 2004b).

PROCEDURE

- If the Lasègue test or the straight-leg-raising test is positive, the leg is lowered below the point of discomfort, and the foot is sharply dorsiflexed (Fig. 8-50).
- The sign is present if pain is increased.
- The presence of the sign is a finding associated with sciatic neuritis, spinal cord tumors, intervertebral disc lesions, and spinal nerve irritations.

Next Steps/Procedures
Bechterew sitting test, Deyerle sign, Fajersztajn test, Lasègue differential sign, Lasègue rebound test, Lasègue sitting test, Lasègue test, Lewin standing test, Lindner sign, Sicard sign, straight-leg-raising test, and Turyn sign

CLINICAL PEARL

Either the *Bragard sign* or the *Hyndman sign* (for neck flexion movement) must be accomplished as a finishing maneuver in any positive straight-leg-raising test. Pain that increases during neck flexion, ankle dorsiflexion, or both indicates an inflamed nerve root. Pain that does not increase with these maneuvers may indicate a problem in the hamstring area or in the lumbosacral or sacroiliac joints.

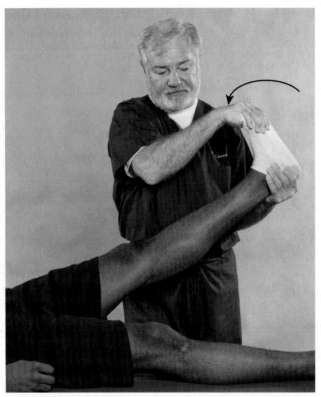

FIG. 8-50 If a straight-leg-raising test is positive, the affected leg is lowered just below
the angle of pain production and is held by the examiner. The foot is sharply dorsiflexed
by the examiner. The sign is present if the pain is duplicated or increased. The presence
of the sign indicates sciatic neuritis, spinal cord tumors, intervertebral disc lesions, and
spinal nerve irritations.

Assessment for Prolapse of Intervertebral Disc Nucleus

Comment

The lumbar discs become thinner during the day because they carry the load of the torso *(relaxation)*. They usually regain their shape within 5 hours of sleep *(creep)*. The disc bulging of intervertebral discs is a direct parameter of the outer annular strain distribution and is an indirect parameter of the internal stress of the disc. Disc bulging is known to be sometimes a few tenths of a millimeter.

> Static lumbar flexion develops creep in the lumbar visco-elastic structures. The musculature, however, compensates for the decreased capacity of the viscoelastic tissues to generate passive forces by initiating and maintaining active force in the necessary periods. This further confirms the neurologic synergy between ligaments and muscles in the control of movement and preservation of skeletal stability. Creep of viscoelastic tissues seems to be associated with microdamage to the collagen structure (Solomonow et al, 2003).

During the active hours, the discs require movement to maintain proper hydration. In fact, decreased movement and decreased axial loading have been strongly associated with disc degeneration. Significant hyperexcitability of the multifidus muscles develop in the resting period after the static lumbar flexion, peaking between the sixth and seventh hours of rest. Full recovery of muscular hyperexcitability and creep may take up to 48 hours. Overall, a transient neuro-muscular disorder is elicited after 20 minutes of static lumbar flexion.

Several maneuvers tighten the sciatic nerve and compress an inflamed nerve root against a herniated lumbar disc (Fig. 8-51). With the straight-leg-raising tests, the L5 and S1 nerve roots move several millimeters at the level of the foramen. The L4 nerve root moves a smaller distance, and the proximal roots show little motion. The straight-leg-raising tests are most important and valuable for detecting lesions of the L5 and S1 nerve roots. Young patients with herniated discs have marked propensities for positive straight-leg-raising tests. Although the test itself is not pathognomonic, a negative test rules out the possibility of a herniated disc. After age 30, a negative straight-leg-raising test no longer precludes this diagnosis. Lumbosacral transistional vertebrae complicates this further (Table 8-10).

The straight-leg-raising tests are performed while the patient is supine. The examiner raises the affected leg slowly. Only when leg pain or radicular symptoms are reproduced is the straight-leg-raising test considered positive. Back pain alone is not a positive finding for straight leg raising.

Many variations of the straight-leg-raising test have been developed. Contralateral straight leg raising is performed in a way similar to the straight-leg-raising test except that, with the former test, the examiner raises the unaffected leg. If this movement reproduces the patient's sciatica in the affected extremity, the test is positive. This result suggests a herniated disc and is an indication that the prolapse, although it may be large, is medial to the nerve root in the axilla.

When the roots of the femoral nerve are involved, they are tensed, not by the straight-leg-raising test but by the reverse of straight leg raising, such as hip extension and knee flexion.

From a morphologic perspective, peripheral nerves are naturally structured to withstand mild levels of stretch. The tortuous pattern of axonal elements and surrounding axo-lemma offer a protective mechanism against stretch injuries. Previously, several studies have been conducted in an attempt to define tensile loads that translate into measurable anatomic damage. However, a reasonable assumption is that functional damage may occur before any permanent morphologic change (Li et al, 2006).

For nearly a century, the clinical significance of lumbosacral transitional vertebra (LSTV) has been debated. In 1917, Bertolotti described the association between low back pain and assimilation of the L5 vertebrae into the sacrum, sometimes called Bertolotti syndrome. This association has been disputed, and Tini and colleagues, in a series of 4000 individuals, demonstrated no relationship between low backache and the presence of a LSTV. However, other studies

---

TABLE 8-10

CASTELLVI CLASSIFICATION OF LUMBOSACRAL TRANSITIONAL VERTEBRA (FIG. 8-53)

- Type I: dysplastic transverse process
  - Type Ia (unilateral) height >19 mm
  - Type Ib (bilateral) height >19 mm
  - Type I is not considered a true lumbosacral transitional vertebra because no articulation with the sacrum is present
- Type II: incomplete lumbarization/sacralization
  - Type IIa enlarged transverse process with unilateral pseudoarthrosis with the adjacent sacral ala
  - Type IIb enlarged transverse process with bilateral pseudoarthrosis with the adjacent sacral ala
- Type III Complete lumbarization/sacralization
  - Type IIIa enlarged transverse process that has unilateral complete fusion with the adjacent sacral ala
  - Type IIIb enlarged transverse process that has bilateral complete fusion with the adjacent sacral ala
- Type IV: mixed (type IIa on one side and type IIIa on the other)

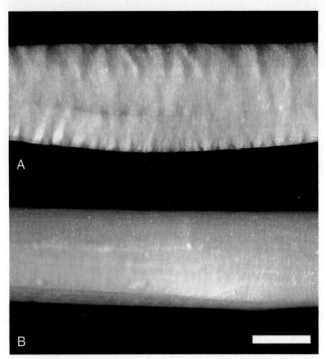

FIG. 8-51 Upper picture, nerve tissue at rest (retracted) length. The vertical light and dark bands are an optical phenomena (bands of Fontana) caused by the microscopic undulations of the nerve architecture. Lower picture, during stretch, the axonal undulations straighten and the vertical bands of Fontana disappear. On release of stretch, the bands are restored as the nerve rebounds to initial length. (Adapted from Li J, Shi R: A device for the electrophysiological recording of peripheral nerves in response to stretch, *J Neurosci Methods* 154(1-2):102-108, 2006.)

have shown a larger than expected proportion of patients with LSTV among those being imaged for back pain or surgery for a prolapsed disc. Type-II LSTVs (pseudarthroses) appear to be related to pain in some series. Large series have shown no difference in the incidence of spondylolysis or spondylolisthesis between patients with LSTVs and controls. However, the degree of slip in patients with lytic spondylolisthesis is greater at L4-L5 above an L5 transition than at L5-S1 above an S1 transition, which is postulated to be caused by the restraining action of the iliolumbar ligament, which stabilizes the L5 vertebra (Hughes, Saifuddin, 2004).

In general, the intervertebral discs of the lumbar region are the thickest of the spine (Fig. 8-53).

PROCEDURE

- Cox sign occurs during straight leg raising when the pelvis rises from the table instead of the hip flexing (Figs. 8-54 and 8-55).
- Cox sign is present when patients have a prolapse of the nucleus into the IVF.

Next Steps/Procedures
Antalgia sign, bowstring sign, heel/toe walk test, Kemp test, Lewin punch test, Lewin snuff test, Milgram test, and Neri sign

CLINICAL PEARL

Cox sign is a consistent finding associated with disc prolapse. The sign is often overlooked in the patient's pain presentation. A false-negative test result may occur if the examiner does not observe the movements of the buttocks on the affected side. The sign is present the moment hip flexion motion is locked and the buttock rises from the examination table.

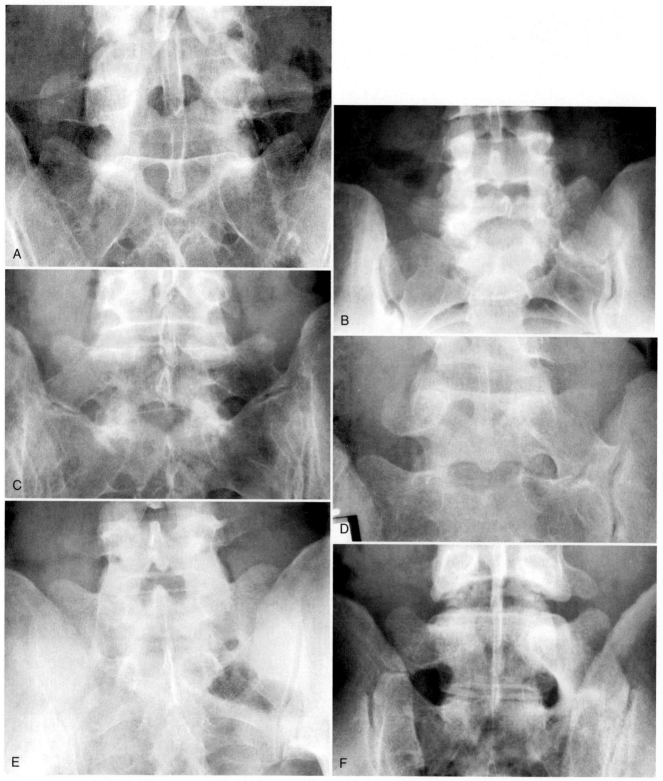

FIG. 8-52 **(A)** Type 1b lumbosacral transitional vertebra with bilaterally enlarged L5 transverse processes but no articulation with the sacrum. **(B)** Type 2a lumbosacral transitional vertebra with unilateral pseudarthrosis. **(C)** Type 2b lumbosacral transitional vertebra with bilateral pseudarthroses. **(D)** Type 3a lumbosacral transitional vertebra with unilateral fusion of the enlarged transverse process to the sacral ala. **(E)** Type 3b lumbosacral transitional vertebra with bilateral fusion. **(F)** Type 4 lumbosacral transitional vertebra appearance with fusion on the left side and a pseudarthrosis on the right. (Adapted from Hughes RJ, Saifuddin A: Imaging of lumbosacral transitional vertebrae, *Clin Radiol* 59[11]:984-991, 2004.)

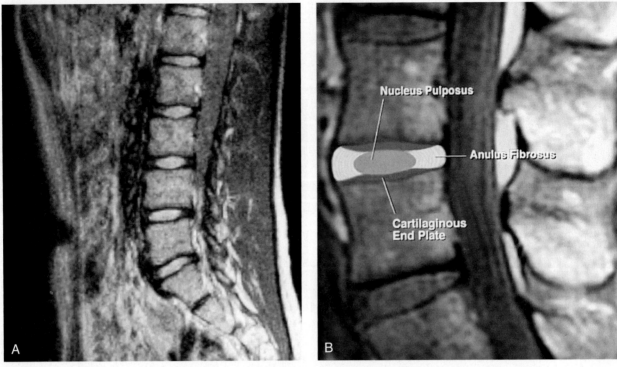

FIG. 8-53 Midsagittal magnetic resonance imaging scan of the lumbar spine. (From Greenstein GM: *Clinical assessment of neuromusculoskelatal disorders*, St. Louis, 1997, Mosby.)

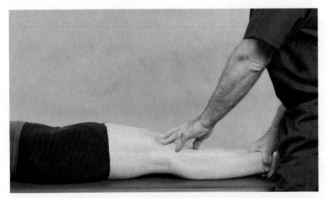

FIG. 8-54 The patient is supine with the legs fully extended. The examiner places one hand under the ankle of the patient's affected leg and the other hand on the patient's knee.

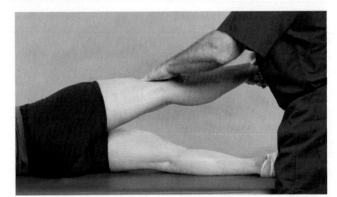

FIG. 8-55 The examiner performs a straight-leg-raising test on the affected leg. Cox sign is present if, during the straight leg raising, the pelvis rises from the table rather than the hip flexing. The sign is present in patients with prolapse of the nucleus into the intervertebral foramen.

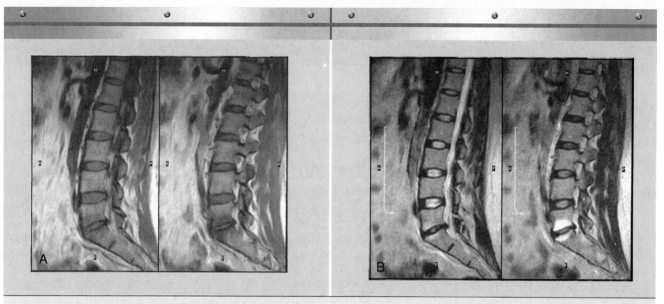

AT THE VIEWBOX

In patients with mechanical back pain from segmental instability and in other cases of discopathy, MRI may demonstrate fibrovascular subchondral marrow changes, with a bone marrow edema pattern. There is diminished T1 (**A**) and increased T2 signal (**B**). These have been described as Modic type 1 changes, which may convert to fibrofatty marrow changes (Modic type 2), which show increased signal on both T1 and T2-weighted images. These marrow signal changes are not seen on X-rays. Modic type 3 changes show low signal on both T1 and T2 weighted images, corresponding to reactive sclerosis, which may be seen on radiographs. (From the teaching file of Timothy Mick, DC, DACBR)

8

Assessment for Spasm of the Sacrolumbalis (Iliocostalis Lumborum) Musculature

Comment

Back strain can be defined as nonradiating lower back pain associated with mechanical stress to the lumbosacral spine. The exact number of patients with back strain is difficult to determine. Most patients with back pain (90%) have it for a mechanical reason. Of patients with mechanical lower back pain, back strain may account for 60% to 70%.

> After several decades of research, the cause of low back pain (LBP) is still a controversial issue. However, the degeneration of trunk extensor muscles (decrease of mass, alteration of fiber characteristics) after a first episode of LBP is proposed as a potential cause of the recurrence of LBP. Furthermore, poor back extensor muscle endurance is a predictor of first-time occurrence of LBP (Lariviere et al, 2002).

The cause of back strain is not always clear, but it may be related to muscular strain secondary to either a specific traumatic episode or a continuous mechanical stress. The lumbosacral spine has two major biomechanical functions. The first function is to support the upper body in a balanced, upright position while allowing the second function—locomotion. In a static, upright position, maintenance of erect posture is achieved through a balance among the expansile pressure of the intervertebral discs, the stretch placed on the anterior and posterior longitudinal and facet joint ligaments, and the sustained involuntary tone of the surrounding lumbosacral and abdominal muscles. The balance of the spine is also related to the reciprocal physiologic curves in the cervical, thoracic, and lumbosacral areas of the vertebral column. The balance in curvature results in an individual's posture. Proper alignment is also influenced by structures in the pelvis and lower extremities, including the hip joint capsule and the hamstring and gluteus maximus muscles.

Movement of the lumbar spine is associated with a lumbar pelvic rhythm that results in the simultaneous reversal of the lumbar lordosis and rotation of the hips. During flexion and extension of the lumbar spine, tension is produced in the paraspinous, hamstring, and gluteal muscles; the fascia that surrounds the muscles; and the ligaments that support the vertebral bodies and discs. In addition to the normal stresses placed on these structures during lowering and rising of the torso, the stresses on these anatomic structures are increased to an even greater degree when an individual must lift a heavy object. During lateral flexion, paraspinous muscle activity increases on both sides of the spine, but it increases primarily on the side toward the lateral flexion. During axial rotation of the spine, the erector spinae muscles on the ipsi-lateral side and the rotator and multifidus muscles on the contralateral side are active. Lateral flexion is accomplished by contraction of the abdominal wall oblique muscles with the ipsilateral quadratus lumborum and psoas major muscles.

Spinal infections involving the vertebrae and the intervertebral discs, usually known as *disc space infections* because of the characteristic radiographic appearance, are rare causes of LBP (Fig 8-56). When present and in the early stages, spinal infection may be confused with back strain.

> In most patients with disk space infection, the clinical and imaging study findings suggest the diagnosis before microbiologic confirmation is obtained. Nevertheless, the broad range of organisms potentially responsible for discitis and the risk of severe complications warrants investigations aimed at recovering the causative organism and testing its susceptibility to antibiotics. Microbiologic studies remain negative in 8% to 30% of patients with typical features of pyogenic discitis and no evidence of parasitic or fungal infection (Gillard et al, 2005).

Although a number of serious conditions, including benign and malignant tumors, Paget disease, vascular disease, infections, and fractures, cause discomfort in the lower back, most patients who experience LBP do not have underlying medical disease. The history of a previous infection, and in particular a urinary tract infection with abdominal symptoms, suggests the possibility of disc space infection. Pyogenic infections of the lower spine is usually characterized by persistent increasing pain. Pyrexia, local tenderness, muscle spasm, constitutional symptoms, and neurologic deficits may or may not be present. Pain radiating to the abdomen or both legs and the presence of abdominal discomfort and symptoms may confuse the diagnosis.

The early diagnosis of a disc space infection requires a high level of clinical suspicion. Any patient in whom this possibility is considered should have blood cultures, urine cultures, a complete blood count, erythrocyte sedimentation

---

ORTHOPEDIC GAMUT 8-5

COMMON INFECTIVE ORGANISMS IN DISCITIS

- *Neisseria gonorrhoeae*
- *Neisseria meningitidis*
- *Listeria monocytogenes*
- *Mycoplasma*
- *Ureaplasma urealyticum*

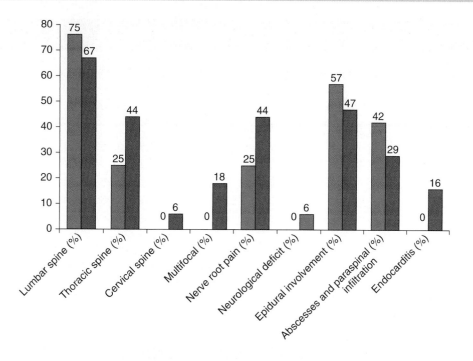

■ Negative microbiology (n = 8)   ■ Positive microbiology (n = 18)

FIG. 8-56 Prevalence of symptoms (back pain and neurological manifestations), vertebral levels with discitis, soft tissue involvement, and endocarditis in the patients with and without microbiological documentation of pyogenic discitis. (From Gillard J, Boutoille D, Varin S et al. Suspected disk space infection with negative microbiological tests–report of eight cases and comparison with documented pyogenic discitis, *Jt Bone Spine* 72(2):156-162, 2005.)

8

ORTHOPEDIC GAMUT 8-6
DISC SPACE INFECTION

The radiographic evidence of established disc space infection includes:

1. Symmetric destruction of adjacent end-plate surfaces of two vertebrae
2. Loss of disc height
3. Reactive new bone formation
4. Sclerosis of bone end-plates, with or without evidence of bone destruction or bone formation
5. Soft-tissue abscesses
6. Kyphosis or subluxation after previous significant bone destruction

rate, and AP and lateral radiographs of the spine. The radiographs may show evidence of soft-tissue expansion around the disc height. A bone scan may be helpful, showing a localized hot spot before radiographic change, and spinal MRI may show the abscess and disc space changes in the

early stage of evolution. In addition, CT scans, as carried out in the case, may help delineate the anatomic changes.

PROCEDURE

- While the patient is in the supine position, the examiner performs a straight-leg-raising test with either leg.
- The sign is present when this action produces a pain in the lumbar region.
- This pain prevents the patient from raising the leg high enough to form an angle between the examination table and the leg of 15 degrees or more (Fig. 8-57).
- The sign differentiates pain that originates in the sacrolumbalis muscles from lumbar pain of any other origin.
- A positive test demonstrates that the pain is caused by the stretching of the sacrolumbalis (iliocostalis lumborum).

Next Steps/Procedures
Bilateral leg-lowering test, double leg-raising test, hyperextension test, Lewin supine test, matchstick test, Mennell sign, Minor sign, Nachlas test, Quick test, Schober test, sign of the buttock, skin pinch test, spinal percussion test, and Vanzetti sign

CLINICAL PEARL

D emianoff sign is clearly separate from Cox sign. Demianoff sign involves production of lower back pain, which prevents further raising of the leg. Sciatica is absent. Cox sign is present when the pelvis is locked, which prevents further elevation of the leg because of increasing sciatica.

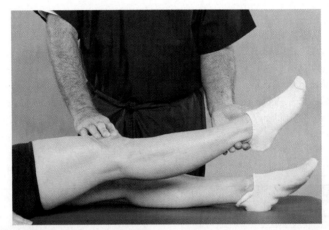

FIG. 8-57 The patient is in a supine position. The examiner performs a straight-leg-raising test on the affected leg. The sign is present when this action produces a pain in the lumbar region. The pain prevents the examiner from raising the patient's leg high enough to form an angle of 15 degrees or more with the examination table. When the sign is present, it demonstrates that pain occurs because of the stretching of the sacrolumbalis (iliocostalis lumborum) musculature.

Assessment for Sciatic Nerve Irritation

Comment

Patients with acute LBP often complain of pain that radiates from the low back into the posterior thigh.

Patients with lesions compressing the L2 and L3 nerve roots may experience pain on the medial and lateral portions of the posterior thigh.

Meralgia paresthetica, originally known as Bernhardt-Roth syndrome, was first described by Bernhardt and Roth in 1895. The term was coined from the Greek words *meros,* meaning thigh, and *algos,* meaning pain. By definition, meralgia paresthetica is a syndrome of pain or dysesthesia or both in the anterolateral thigh. The most common causes are entrapment or neurinoma formation of the lateral femoral cutaneous nerve (LFCN). Pathogenetic factors are manifold, including anatomic variations either of the nerve itself or of its course at the anterior-superior iliac spine (Trummer et al, 2000).

Meralgia-like symptoms caused by a disc herniation at L1–L2 or L2–L3 is grouped with other misleading symptoms of disc herniation in the upper lumbar spine such as isolated sciatica or abdominogenital pain. Meralgia itself can mimic the symptoms of a nerve root compression, explained by the origin of the LFCN from the nerve roots at L2 and L3.

Occasionally, L4 lesions may also cause similar symptoms and signs. The phase of degeneration or spondylosis often determines the level of intervention (Table 8-11).

The pain pattern that is associated with nerve root irritation resulting from a movable lamina arch or neural arch (spondylolisthesis) resembles the pain caused by compression of the nerve root by an intervertebral disc or by compression of the nerve root by other mechanical means. Pain usually occurs when the spine is extended or when the spinous process is compressed or manipulated, causing secondary irritation of the dura. Pain may radiate along the course of the femoral or sciatic nerve, depending on the site of the bone abnormality.

Degenerative arthritis in the hip or alteration of the hip joint capsule or of the surrounding osseous structures may cause pain anteriorly, laterally, and posteriorly in the groin. Pain radiation may be associated with this through the LFCN, through the obturator nerve along the medial aspect of the thigh, or through branches of the sciatic nerve along the posterior thigh.

Destructive lesions of the sacrum, pelvis, pubis, or ischium cause pain along the femoral, obturator, or sciatic nerves. The onset of this pain may be vague and gradual, and the distribution of the pain may be deep, with few cutaneous changes. The radiculopathy may resemble a primary nerve root irritation.

TABLE 8-11

OVERVIEW OF SCHEME OF TREATMENT RELATIVE TO THE PHASE OF SPONDYLOSIS

Phase	Lesion	Treatment
Dysfunction	Facet joint	Mobilization, manipulation, injection
	Sacroiliac joint	Mobilization, manipulation, injection
	Myofascial syndromes	Contraction stretching, injection
	Disc herniation	Epidural injection, discectomy
Unstable	Disc herniation	Epidural injection, discectomy
	Segmental instability	Injection, fusion
	Lateral stenosis	Nerve root block, decompression, fusion
	Central stenosis	Epidural injection, decompression, fusion
	Degenerative olisthesis	Epidural injection, decompression, fusion
	Isthmic olisthesis	Epidural injection, decompression, fusion
Stabilization	Disc herniation	Epidural injection, discectomy
	Lateral stenosis	Nerve root block, decompression
	Central stenosis	Epidural injection, decompression
	Degenerative olisthesis	Epidural injection, decompression, rarely fusion
	Isthmic olisthesis	Epidural injection, decompression, rarely fusion

From Kirkaldy WH: *Managing low back pain,* ed 4, Philadelphia 1999, Churchill Livingstone.

Postoperative neuropathy is a known complication of major pelvic oncologic surgery. Although rare, obturator nerve injury complicating pelvic lymph node dissection has been noted in several case reports. This nerve originates from L2-L3 and innervates the medial thigh adductor muscles: gracilis, pectineus, adductor longus, adductor brevis, adductor magnus, and obturator internus. The nerve enters the pelvic cavity after piercing the medial border of the psoas muscle. It is located along the retroperitoneum within the obturator fossa. Finally, the nerve leaves the pelvis through the obturator foramen. Different types of lesions have been identified. Neurapraxia is a simple neuronal contusion. A more severe lesion is axonotmesis with degeneration of the distal elements. Neurotmesis is the most severe lesion that is induced by a complete section of the nerve. In cases of injury, the patient will have adductor weakness with or without associated sensory loss over the medial thigh. Severity and duration of the symptoms are determined by the severity of the initial nerve lesion (Rafii, Querleu, 2006).

PROCEDURE

- While the patient is seated, the affected leg is passively extended at the knee until pain is reproduced (Fig. 8-58).
- The knee is then slightly flexed while strong pressure is applied by the examiner into the popliteal fossa (Fig. 8-59).
- The sign is present if this pressure increases radicular symptoms.
- The sign demonstrates irritation of the sciatic nerve above the knee.
- This irritation is caused by stretching the nerve over an abnormal mechanical obstruction.

Next Steps/Procedures

Bechterew sitting test, Bragard sign, Fajersztajn test, Lasègue differential sign, Lasègue rebound test, Lasègue sitting test, Lasègue test, Lewin standing test, Lindner sign, Sicard sign, straight-leg-raising test, and Turyn sign

CLINICAL PEARL

Deyerle sign is a variation of the Lasègue sitting test. The sign demonstrates the effects of inflammation or partial denervation (neural compression) in the sciatic distribution. The pain response may be caused by myalgic hyperalgesia as a response to denervation hypersensitivity.

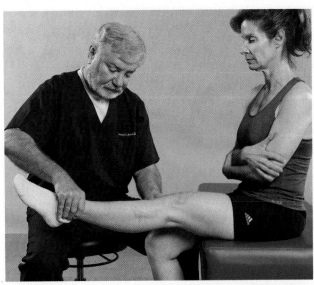

FIG. 8-58 The patient is seated. The examiner extends the patient's affected leg to the point at which pain is reproduced.

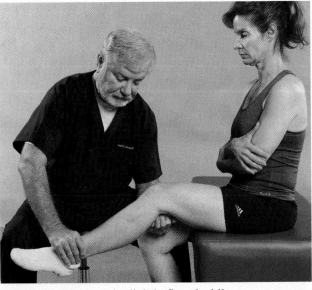

FIG. 8-59 The knee is slightly flexed while strong pressure into the popliteal fossa is applied by the examiner. The sign is present if radicular symptoms are increased.

DOUBLE-LEG-RAISE TEST

ALSO KNOWN AS BILATERAL STRAIGHT-LEG-RAISING TEST

Assessment for Lumbosacral Joint Involvement

Comment

Sprain is common in the mobile lumbar spine, which has many ligaments giving support to the various joints. The supraspinous ligament, which extends along the tips of the spinous processes, is particularly susceptible. A sprain involving this ligament can be diagnosed by tenderness over the ligament or over the tip of the spinous process, where the ligament attaches. Active contraction of the muscles to pull the spine into hyperextension is pain free, as is passive extension. Active flexion of the back, which occurs during an attempt to sit up from the supine position, is pain free until tension is put on the spinous process by forcing the head toward the knees. Passive hyperflexion of the spine will cause pain.

Injury to other ligaments of the back is much more difficult to diagnose. The interspinous ligament is rarely damaged because it has elastic fibers and is not readily overstretched. However, the articular ligaments around the apophyseal joints are commonly damaged, as are the anterior spinal and the lateral spinal ligaments. Whether the ligamentum flavum is damaged by hyperflexion is problematic because it is also an elastic structure and will probably allow as much motion without damage as the range of flexion of the back will permit. Diagnosis of these sprains depends on whether tests that bring stress on certain areas are used. With a sprain, passive movements that put stress on the involved ligament will cause pain. For example, sprain of the capsule on the left will cause pain during lateral flexion to the right or during flexion of the trunk.

Persistent LBP without nerve root tension signs should signal the possibility of a stress reaction or fracture of the pars interarticularis.

Spondylolysis appearing between ages 6 and 7 is caused by a fatigue fracture of the pars interarticularis and is seldom caused by one acute, traumatic event.

Patients with an impending or existing pars fractures complain of LBP. Young patients often report that they have been playing a sport, even though they had a backache and some spasm, and that they noted a sudden worsening of symptoms after a specific traumatic episode.

The facet joints and the supraspinous ligament play a crucial role in the stability of the lumbosacral junction whereas the interspinous, and yellow ligaments play a minor role at this level. In case of lumbosacral dislocation (LD), soft-tissue disruption involves not only the posterior ligament complex, but also the posterior longitudinal ligament and the annulus fibrosus. The mechanism of injury is complex and a subject of controversy. Watson-Jones was the first to hypothesize that dislocations were caused by a hyperextension force. Roaf suggested that hyperflexion, axial rotation, and compression forces were responsible for LD. Denis described a type-C fracture-dislocation corresponding to a flexion distraction injury and consisting of bilateral facet dislocation. Conditions required are as follows: A high-velocity impact is directly applied below the level of the lumbosacral junction or indirectly when the pelvis is locked. Then, the trunk describes a flexion motion and is projected forward, providing the distractive component (Roche et al, 1998).

Affected patients often complain of chronic, dull, aching, or cramping pain in the low back. The pain may be unilateral or bilateral, usually *along the belt line*. The ache is usually constant and worsens with rotation or hyperextension of the low back. In most instances, no radicular findings or true sciatic tension signs are present. The range of motion, although painful, is usually full. Palpable, paraspinal spasms and hamstring tightness may be present. Commonly, having the patient stand on one leg and bend backward (*Jackson test*) reproduces and accentuates the pain if a fatigue fracture is present (Fig. 8-60). In the presence of a unilateral defect, hyperextension while standing on the ipsilateral leg will worsen the pain on the side of the defect.

PROCEDURE

- While the patient is supine, the examiner performs a straight-leg-raising test on each of the patient's lower extremities, noting the angle at which the pain is produced.
- Next, both lower limbs are raised together (Fig. 8-61).
- If pain is produced at an earlier angle by raising both legs together, the test is positive (Fig. 8-62).
- In the presence of disc disease with resulting vertebral instability, the double-leg-raising movement will cause pain in the lumbar area.
- The test is specific and highly accurate for lumbosacral joint involvement.

Next Steps/Procedures
Bilateral leg-lowering test, Demianoff sign, hyperextension test, Lewin supine test, matchstick test, Mennell sign, Minor sign, Nachlas test, Quick test, Schober test, sign of the buttock, skin pinch test, spinal percussion test, and Vanzetti sign

CLINICAL PEARL

Atypical cases of disc prolapse are common. A definite history of injury or strain is often lacking. The pain may begin gradually rather than suddenly, and the symptoms may be confined to the back and never radiate down the leg. On the other hand, the pain is sometimes felt predominantly in the limb and is scarcely perceptible in the back.

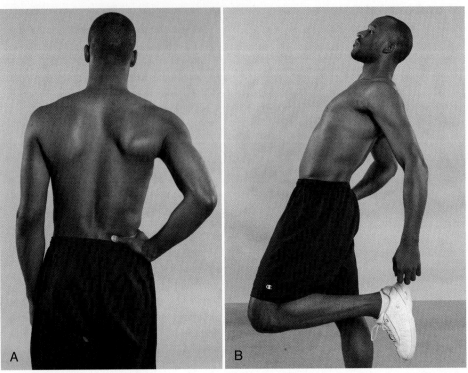

A   B

FIG. 8-60 Jackson one-legged hyperextension test. The patient stands on one leg and hyperextends the back. Back pain will be reproduced on the symptomatic side if an impending pars fracture exists.

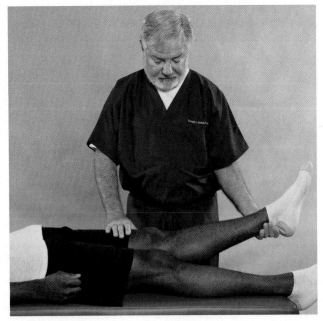

FIG. 8-61 The patient is supine with both legs fully extended. The examiner performs a straight-leg-raising test on each of the lower extremities and notes the angle at which the pain is produced. The examiner then raises both lower limbs together.

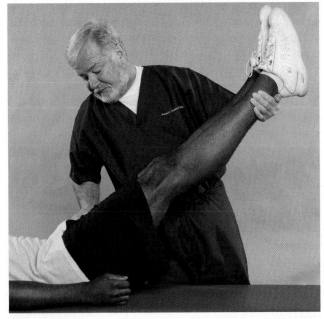

FIG. 8-62 If raising both legs together produces pain at an earlier angle than raising each leg singly, then the sign is positive. The test is specific and highly accurate for lumbosacral joint involvement.

ELY HEEL-TO-BUTTOCK TEST

Assessment for Lumbar Radicular or Femoral Nerve Inflammation

Comment

The size of the lumbar vertebral canal ranges from 12 to 20 mm in its AP dimension at the mid sagittal plane and 18 to 27 mm in its transverse diameter. Stenosis has been defined as a narrowing below the lowest value of the range of normal (Table 8-12).

The dura mater of the lumbar spine has a series of attachments to neighboring vertebrae and ligaments. They have been called the *dural attachment complex* or *Hoffmann ligaments* (Fig. 8-63). Narrowing of the vertebral canal (spinal canal) is most often known as *spinal canal stenosis*. Lumbar spinal canal stenosis affects the nerves of the cauda equina or the dorsal and ventral roots as they leave the vertebral canal and enter IVFs. The exiting nerve roots travel through the more narrow, lateral aspect of the vertebral canal, known as the *lateral recess*, before entering the IVF. As the roots pass through this region of the vertebral canal, pressure may

TABLE 8-12	
DIMENSIONS OF THE LUMBAR VERTEBRAL FORAMINA (VERTEBRAL CANAL)*	
Dimension	**Size (Range)[†]**
Anteroposterior (in midsagittal plane)	12–20 mm
Transverse (interpedicular distance)	18–27 mm

*Dimensions below the lowest value indicate spinal (vertebral) canal stenosis. A typical vertebral foramen is rather triangular (trefoil) in shape. However, the upper lumbar vertebral foramina are more rounded than the lower lumbar foramina. L1 is the most rounded, and each succeeding lumbar vertebra becomes increasingly triangular, with L5 the most dramatically trefoil of all.

[†]Dimensions of lumbar vertebral foramina are usually smaller than those of the cervical region but larger than those of the thoracic region.

From Cramer GD, Darby SA: *Basic and clinical anatomy of the spine, spinal cord, and ANS,* St Louis, 1995, Mosby.

From Dommisse GF, Louw JA: Anatomy of the lumbar spine. In Floman Y, editor: *Disorders of the lumbar spine,* Rockville, Md, and Tel Aviv, Israel, 1990, Aspen and Freund Publishing House.

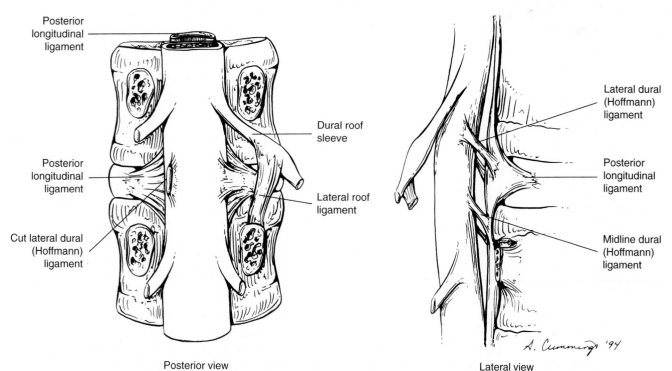

Posterior longitudinal ligament

Posterior longitudinal ligament

Cut lateral dural (Hoffmann) ligament

Dural roof sleeve

Lateral roof ligament

Lateral dural (Hoffmann) ligament

Posterior longitudinal ligament

Midline dural (Hoffmann) ligament

Posterior view

Lateral view

FIG. 8-63 Attachments of the dura mater to surrounding structures. (From Cramer GD, Darby SA: *Basic and clinical anatomy of the spine, spinal cord, and ANS,* St Louis, 1995, Mosby.)

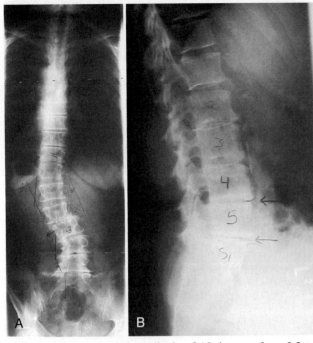

FIG. 8-64 Left lumbar scoliosis of 18 degrees from L2 to L4, with right L3 radiculopathy. (From Jabri RS, Hepler M, Benzon HT: Overview of low back pain disorders. In Benzon HT, Raja SN, Molloy RE, et al: *Essentials of pain medicine and regional anesthesia,* ed 2, Philadephia, 2005, Elsevier.)

ORTHOPEDIC GAMUT 8-7

MODIFIED ARNOLD INTERNATIONAL CLASSIFICATION OF LUMBAR SPINAL STENOSIS AND NERVE ROOT ENTRAPMENT SYNDROMES

- Congenital stenosis
  - Idiopathic
  - Achondroplastic
- Acquired stenosis
  - Degenerative
  - Combined
  - Spondylolisthetic, spondylolytic
  - Iatrogenic
  - Posttraumatic
  - Paget disease
  - Fluorosis
- Degenerative lumbar spinal stenosis with scoliosis

In degenerative lumbar spinal stenosis with scoliosis, nerve root compression is almost always seen on the concave side of the scoliosis, and L4 and L5 nerve roots are the most often involved (Fig 8-64).

---

be placed on them. This condition is known as *lateral recess stenosis.*

In sequestration of nuclear tissue adjacent to or under a nerve, adhesions may form within and without the nerve root sheath, binding the root firmly to the floor of the spinal canal. During movements of the trunk and legs, the nerve roots are no longer freely movable or capable of moving in and out of the intervertebral foramina without tension. When fixed to the floor of the spinal canal or within the foramina, the nerve roots are subjected to abnormal tension during movement of the trunk and legs, particularly movements that require the extended leg to flex at the hip. Tension on the nerve roots causes radicular pain.

The condition is characterized by the localization of the pain in the dermatome supplied by the affected nerve root. The pain, although often widely distributed throughout the dermatome, is occasionally limited to a small area within it. Although dermatomal in distribution, nerve root pain in the leg seldom extends beyond the ankle. However, any associated dermatomal paresthesia or dysesthesia is usually most prominent distally and may be described in the foot.

Pain is present in the spinal column and is temporarily associated with pain in the leg or paresthesia or both.

Root pain often is produced or aggravated by coughing, sneezing, and straining (e.g., during defecation) or by any other measures that suddenly increase intrathoracic and intraabdominal pressure. Such increases in pressure block venous flow from the epidural space through the intervertebral veins. Because the intervertebral veins do not contain valves, such increases in pressure may also permit a return of blood with consequent distension of the veins in the epidural space. This condition in turn forces the dura, which envelops the nerve roots, toward the spinal cord. Because the nerve roots are affixed to the spinal cord proximally and peripherally at the IVF, the displacement of the dura results in stretching of the involved nerve root. This stretching results in pain if the root is diseased. In addition, distension of the intervertebral vein may result in direct compression of the nerve root.

Root pain may awaken the patient at night after several hours of sleep and may be relieved 15 to 30 minutes after the patient assumes an upright position. The patient may learn to prevent the pain by sleeping in a chair. However, in contrast to peripheral neuritis, the position is the important determining factor. If the patient lies down in a similar position during the day, the pain occurs as it does at night. This feature of root pain has its basis in the lengthening of the spinal column that takes place when the horizontal position is assumed and the shortening that takes place when the patient is in the upright position. Because the length of the spinal cord remains the same regardless of the position assumed by the patient, the lengthening of the spinal column results in a tensing of, or traction on, the nerve roots that emerge from the lumbar and sacral segments of the cord. From these segments, the roots course downward and outward to emerge from their respective intervertebral foramina.

ORTHOPEDIC GAMUT 8-8

COMPLEX REGIONAL PAIN SYNDROME DIAGNOSTIC CRITERIA (INTERNATIONAL ASSOCIATION FOR THE STUDY OF PAIN)

1. Complex regional pain syndrome type I (CRPS-I) is a syndrome that develops after an initiating noxious event.
2. Spontaneous pain or allodynia/hyperalgesia occurs, is not limited to the territory of a single peripheral nerve, and is disproportionate to the inciting event.
3. Evidence exists or has existed of edema, skin blood flow abnormality, or abnormal sudomotor activity in the region of the pain since the inciting event.
4. This diagnosis is excluded by the existence of conditions that would otherwise account for the degree of pain and dysfunction.
5. For the diagnosis of CRPS-I, criteria 2 through 4 must be fulfilled.

Complex regional pain syndrome type II (CRPS-II) develops after tissue trauma, displaying clinical signs and symptoms reminiscent of those induced by the injury itself; however, more pronounced and long lasting. Nevertheless a detailed knowledge of physiologic tissue response to trauma is mandatory to differentiate clearly the physiologic trauma reaction from a possible pathologic response, as it is seen in CRPS-I. Recent animal models employing tissue trauma in order to imitate human CRPS-I substantiate the idea of CRPS-I being an abnormal posttraumatic inflammatory reaction (Gradl et al, 2006).

CRPS-I is characterized by a variety of sensory and autonomic disturbances of an extremity, usually as a consequence of trauma. Clinical evaluation and diagnosis of CRPS-I is based on clinical assessment of signs and symptoms, according to predetermined sets of diagnostic criteria (Perez et al, in press).

PROCEDURE

- The patient is prone, with the toes hanging over the edge of the table and legs relaxed.
- One or the other heel is approximated to the opposite buttock (Figs. 8-65 and 8-66).
- After flexion of the knee, the thigh is hyperextended.
- With any significant hip lesion, performing this test will normally be impossible.
- With irritation of the iliopsoas muscle or its sheath, extending the thigh to any normal degree will be impossible.
- This test will aggravate inflammation of the lumbar nerve roots and will be accompanied by production of femoral radicular pain.
- The test will also stretch lumbar nerve root adhesions, which will be accompanied by upper lumbar discomfort.

Next Steps/Procedures

Femoral nerve traction test and prone knee-bending test

CLINICAL PEARL

In the uncommon cases of high lumbar and mid lumbar disc prolapse, the pain radiates toward the groin and front of the thigh rather than to the back of the thigh and leg.

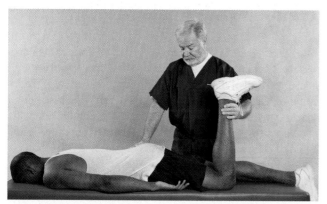

FIG. 8-65 The patient is prone. The legs are fully extended, with the toes hanging over the edge of the table. The examiner flexes the knee of the affected leg to 90 degrees.

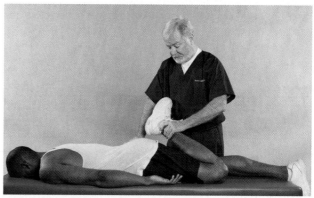

FIG. 8-66 The heel of the affected leg is approximated to the opposite buttock. After flexion of the knee, the thigh can be hyperextended. With irritation of the iliopsoas muscle or its sheath, extending the thigh to any degree will be impossible. Pain in the anterior thigh is a positive finding and indicates inflammation of the lumbar nerve roots.

FAJERSZTAJN TEST

ALSO KNOWN AS WELL-LEG-RAISING TEST OF FAJERSZTAJN, PROSTRATE LEG-RAISING TEST, SCIATIC PHENOMENON, AND CROSS-OVER SIGN

Assessment for Lumbar Nerve Root Lesion Caused by Intervertebral Disc Syndrome or Dural Sleeve Adhesion

Comment

Although clearly evident in most advanced imaging tests, spinal stenosis is the cause of many cases of low back problems that are refractory to conservative treatment. Lumbar stenosis can occur at the central spinal canal or at the peripheral canal where the nerve root exits (Fig. 8-67). Two major conditions, both of which compromise the vertebral canal and its neural contents, contribute to lumbar stenosis: facet disease and discogenic spondylosis. Degenerative arthritis of the facets has the potential to cause stenosis by encroaching on the lateral recess of the spinal canal.

Patients with discogenic spondylosis develop multidirectional pain in addition to flexion discomfort.

Patients with central lumbar canal stenosis exhibit neurogenic claudication with pain on walking and feel as if their legs *give way*. Temperature changes and weakness of the legs are common. Night pain and sciatic tension signs are equally common.

Patients with lateral lumbar canal stenosis have nerve root entrapment. Pain occurs intermittently over years, with exacerbations. Pain may be referred to the hips, buttocks, or posterior thigh (**pseudoradiculopathy**) (Fig. 8-69). Pain is rarely referred to the foot or toes. Sensory changes at the calf are common.

ORTHOPEDIC GAMUT 8-9
LUMBAR CENTRAL CANAL STENOSIS

Structural causes for lumbar central canal stenosis are as follows:

1. *Osseous:* inferior facet arthrosis
2. *Discogenic:* central disc herniation
3. *Ligamentous:* ligamentum flavum buckling in degenerative spinal disease (Fig. 8-68)

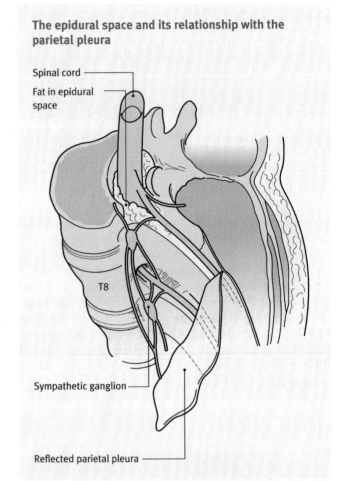

The epidural space and its relationship with the parietal pleura

Spinal cord
Fat in epidural space
T8
Sympathetic ganglion
Reflected parietal pleura

FIG. 8-67 Each spinal nerve, as it passes through its intervertebral foramen into the paravertebral space, carries with it an extension of the extradural fat. The paravertebral spaces communicate with each other contralaterally via the epidural space. This communication between the epidural and the paravertebral space explains the negative pressure in the epidural space. The paravertebral spaces in the thoracic region are separated from the negative pressure of the pleural space only by the parietal pleura; pressure changes in the pleural cavity are transmitted to the paravertebral, and thence to the epidural space. Thus, deep inspiration will increase the negative epidural pressure, and coughing will produce a positive pressure (Valsalva Maneuver; Dejerine Triad). (Adapted from Ellis H: The anatomy of the epidural space, *Anaesthesia Intensive Care* 7[11]:402-404, 2006.)

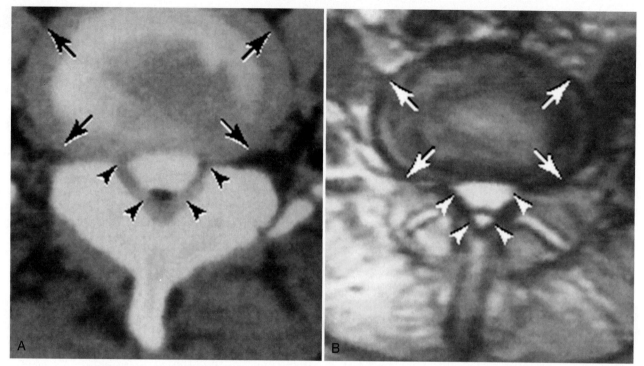

FIG. 8-68 Central canal stenosis attributable to a diffusely bulging disc and hypertrophy of the ligamentum flavum. **A,** Axial computed tomography. **B,** Magnetic resonance imaging. (From Brier SR: *Primary care orthopedics,* St Louis, 1999, Mosby.)

8

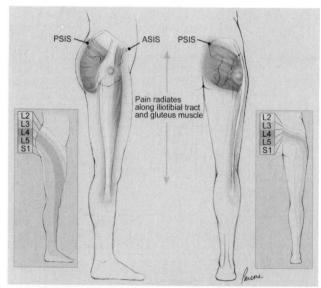

FIG. 8-69 Inflammation of the bursa may cause irritation and radiation of pain distally along the entire iliotibial tract and proximally along the fibers of the tensor fasciae lata and gluteus maximus toward the anterior and posterior superior iliac spines (ASIS and PSIS, respectively) of the pelvis. (Adapted from Tortolani PJ, Carbone JJ, Quartararo LG: Greater trochanteric pain syndrome in patients referred to orthopedic spine specialists, *Spine J* 2[4]:251-254, 2002.)

Limitation of motion is usually noted during the symptomatic phase of disc disease. The range of motion should be noted not only in flexion and extension, but also in rotation. The examiner must not equate flexion of the hips with flexion of the lumbar spine, and attention should be directed to whether reversal of the normal lumbar lordosis occurs. Even in patients who have only sciatica, marked restriction of motion may be present in the lumbar spine.

When acute sciatica is present, the patient usually lists away from the side of the sciatica, producing the sciatic scoliosis. When the disc herniation is lateral to the nerve root, the patient will incline away from the side of the irritated nerve root in an attempt to draw the nerve root away from the disc fragment. On the contrary, when the herniation is in an axillary position medial to the nerve root, the patient will list toward the side of the lesion to decompress the nerve root.

Pseudoradiculopathy, that is, radiation of pain along the iliotibial tract that mimics true nerve root irritation, may complicate the diagnosis of greater trochanteric pain syndrome (GTPS). Although anatomic overlap of the iliotibial tract is present (particularly L2, L3, and L4 dermatomes), radiation of pain in GTPS does not extend distal to the proximal tibia (at the insertion of the iliotibial tract at Gerdy tubercle). In contrast, patients with true nerve root irritation experience pain extending into the lower leg and foot. Moreover, on physical examination, patients with nerve root irritation do not exhibit a positive *jump* sign secondary to thumb pressure over the most prominent ridge of the greater trochanter. Other physical examination features (e.g., pain on resisted leg abduction or pain at the extreme of thigh external rotation and abduction) should be specifically investigated (Tortolani, Carbone, Quartararo, 2002).

When performing a unilateral straight-leg raising test, 80 to 90 degrees of hip flexion is normal. If one leg is lifted and the patient complains of pain on the opposite side, a space-occupying lesion (herniated disc) is indicated. This finding indicates a rather large intervertebral disc protrusion, usually medial to the nerve root. The test causes stretching of the ipsilateral, as well as the contralateral nerve root, pulling laterally on the dural sac.

PROCEDURE

- Straight-leg-raising and dorsiflexion of the foot are performed on the asymptomatic side of a sciatic patient (Figs. 8-70 and 8-71).
- When this test causes pain on the symptomatic side, Fajersztajn sign is present.
- The sign indicates sciatic nerve root involvement, such as a disc syndrome or dural root sleeve adhesions.

Next Steps/Procedures
Bechterew sitting test, Bragard sign, Deyerle sign, Lasègue differential sign, Lasègue rebound test, Lasègue sitting test, Lasègue test, Lewin standing test, Lindner sign, Sicard sign, straight-leg-raising test, and Turyn sign

CLINICAL PEARL

Several factors my produce pain in the back or lower extremities. Some of these causes are (1) tumors of the spinal cord or cauda equina, (2) tumors of the spinal column, (3) tuberculosis of the spine, (4) osteoarthritis, (5) tumors of the ilium or sacrum, (6) spondylolisthesis, (7) prolapsed intervertebral disc, (8) ankylosing spondylitis, (9) vascular occlusion, (10) intrapelvic mass, and (11) arthritis of the hip. All of these possible causes must be considered in differential diagnosis.

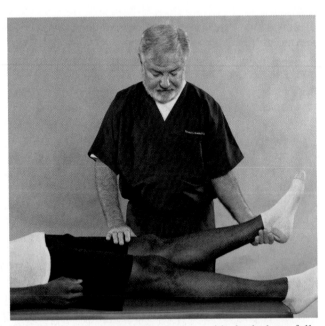

FIG. 8-70 The patient is supine with both legs fully extended. The examiner performs a straight-leg-raising test on the patient's unaffected leg.

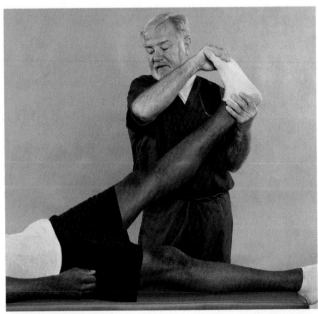

FIG. 8-71 The leg is lowered to a point just below that which produces sciatic symptoms in the affected leg. The examiner sharply dorsiflexes the patient's foot (Bragard's sign). If this maneuver causes pain on the symptomatic side, the test is positive. A positive test indicates sciatic nerve root involvement, such as medial disc protrusion syndrome or dural root sleeve adhesions.

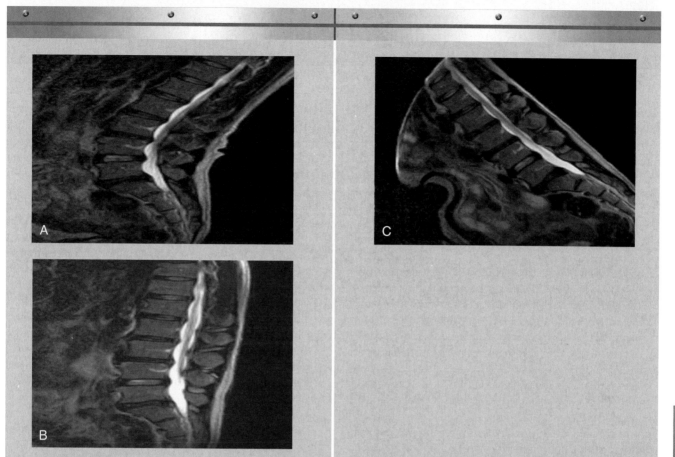

AT THE VIEWBOX

The most comprehensive study for the assessment of low back and leg pain, especially when position dependent, is upright MRI, with flexion-extension images. Note the difference in appearance of the L5–S1 disc herniation between the upright neutral sagittal, extension and flexion images. As may be suspected, disc lesions, especially bulges and protruded herniations (contained herniations) are often most prominent on extension images (**A**), less prominent on neutral images (**B**), and even less conspicuous or not visualized at all on flexion images. (**C**) Note the variation in the appearance of the L5–S1 disc herniation. There are also disc bulges more diffusely in the lumbar spine. (From the teaching file of Timothy Mick, DC, DACBR)

8

Assessment for Mid-lumbar Nerve Root Involvement (L2, L3, and L4)

Comment

Redundant nerve roots refers to roots of the cauda equina that bend (undulate within the vertebral canal) or buckle during their course through the cauda equina. Degenerative spinal stenosis is thought to be the usual cause of this condition (Fig. 8-72).

> This disorder (degenerative spinal stenosis) mainly affects men. The clinical history ranges from months to decades. The illness often starts with LBP or sciatica or both. Motor and sensory impairment of the legs dominate the further course of the disease. Serpentine filling defects in the column of contrast area characteristic (but inconstant) feature on myelograms (Pau et al, 1981).

The vertebral column decreases in superior-to-inferior length with age (an average of 14 mm). Shortening of the vertebral canal forces the roots of the cauda equina to become redundant. The pressure from compressive elements over time results in friction neuritis. Friction neuritis results in the large redundant roots. With walking and extension, increased pressure is placed on the nerve roots (Fig. 8-73), which causes ischemia of the neural elements. Nerve root ischemia results in the signs and symptoms of neurogenic claudication pain. Weakness in the lower extremities during standing and walking is often associated with spinal stenosis and redundant nerve roots. These changes are often permanent.

> The effect on the lumbar spine of axial compression has concentrated on the assessment of changes in dural sac cross-sectional area (DCSA). Willen and colleagues assessed the effects of axial compression in three patient groups, those with cLBP, neurogenic claudication, or sciatica. They determined the additional valuable information obtained on compression studies. This information was defined as a greater than 15 mm^2 reduction in DCSA to levels below 75 mm^2 (the borderline DCSA, below which spinal stenosis is considered to be present based on intradural pressure measurements), accentuation of disc herniation, lateral recess or foraminal stenosis or the development of an intraspinal synovial cyst (Saifuddin, Blease, MacSweeney, 2003).

When a herniated annulus fibrosus compresses a nerve root, the irritation produces pain and motor and sensory loss of the lower extremities. As the nerve root becomes irritated, it becomes inflamed and even more sensitive to pressures. The patient will notice a lancinating pain that begins in the thigh and progresses distally in a pattern typical of a dermatome. The onset of pain may be gradual or extremely sudden and may be associated with a popping or tearing in the spine. This pain may represent the extrusion of disc material against the nerve root. When this circumstance occurs, the back pain often resolves, and the patient is left with the radicular symptoms.

The disc rupture is usually lateral to the nerve root, and the patient lists or leans away from the side of the sciatica to release the pressure. Occasionally, the disc presents medially or in the axilla of the nerve root, and the patient will list toward the side of the sciatica. The pain is increased by any maneuver that suddenly increases intraspinal pressures, such as a Valsalva maneuver or the triad of Dejerine (coughing, sneezing, or bearing down with defecation). The pain may be so severe as to paralyze the patient in a fixed position.

In rare instances, the major presenting symptom is motor weakness, particularly if the L4 or L5 nerve is affected. Weakness of the quadriceps with later buckling of the knee (L4) or a complete foot drop (L5), without pain, may present a confusing picture.

A large, midline disc herniation can compress several nerve roots of the cauda equina and can mimic an intraspinal tumor. Usually, lower back and perineal symptoms predominate, with radicular symptoms being masked. Difficulty with urination, such as frequency or overflow incontinence, may develop early. In male patients, a recent history of sexual impotence may be elicited. The patients experience pain down the posterior thighs to the soles of the feet accompanied by weakness of the legs and feet. L2, L3, and L4 radiculopathies are less common than the L5 and S1 radiculopathies, probably because of their relatively short course within the cauda equina, which makes them less susceptible to compression (Table 8-13).

ORTHOPEDIC GAMUT 8-10

UPPER LUMBAR RADICULOPATHY

The electrophysiologic confirmation of an upper lumbar radiculopathy is challenging for the following reasons:

1. The exact compressed root is difficult to identify among upper lumbar roots because of the limited number of muscles innervated by the roots (Fig. 8-74).
2. The myotomal representation of these roots occurs in proximally situated muscles, mostly above the knee (except for the tibialis anterior).
3. A lack of available sensory nerve action potential exists for confirming that the upper lumbar lesion is preganglionic.

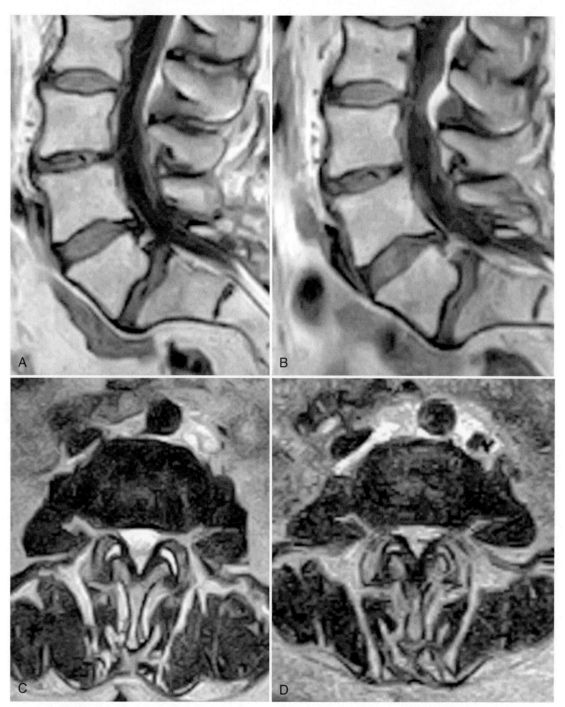

FIG. 8-72 Change in lumbar spine central canal dimensions, with and without axial loading. **A,** Sagittal T1-weighted spin-echo sequence without axial loading. A moderate degree of central stenosis is demonstrated at the L2–L3 level but cerebrospinal fluid (CSF) is still identified ventral to the cauda equina. **B,** Sagittal T1-weighted spin-echo sequence with axial loading. Critical stenosis has developed at L2–L3, mainly as a result of posterior impression on the theca from the fat pad. **C,** Axial T2-weighted fast spin-echo sequence without axial loading. Plentiful CSF is seen ventral to the cauda equina. **D,** Axial T2-weighted spin-echo sequence with axial loading. At this point, complete loss occurs of CSF around the cauda equina, indicating the presence of occult central canal stenosis.

(From Saifuddin A, Blease S, MacSweeney E: Axial loaded MRI of the lumbar spine, *Clin Radiol* 58[9]:661-671, 2003.)

TABLE 8-13

DIFFERENTIAL ELECTRODIAGNOSIS OF UPPER LUMBAR RADICULOPATHY (FIG. 8-74)

	Femoral Neuropathy	**Lumbar Plexopathy**	**Lumbar Radiculopathy**
Thigh adductors	Normal	Denervation	Denervation
Tibialis anterior	Normal	Denervation*	Denervation*
Saphenous SNAP†	Low or absent‡	Low or absent‡	Normal
Paraspinal fibrillations	Absent	Absent	Usually present

SNAP, Sensory nerve action potential.
*Abnormal in L4 radiculopathy/plexopathy only.
†May be technically difficult, particularly in the elderly patients or if leg edema is present.
‡Normal in purely demyelinating lesions.
From Katirji B: *Electromyography in clinical practice: a case study approach,* St Louis, 1998, Mosby.

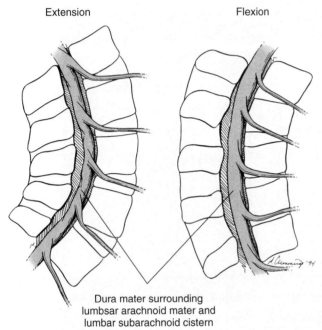

Extension   Flexion

Dura mater surrounding
lumbsar arachnoid mater and
lumbar subarachnoid cistern

FIG. 8-73 Changes that occur within the lumbar vertebral canal during flexion and extension. (From Cramer GD, Darby SA: *Basic and clinical anatomy of the spine, spinal cord, and ANS,* St Louis, 1995, Mosby.)

Separating upper lumbar radiculopathies from lumbar plexopathy is sometimes difficult, especially in chronic situations in which fibrillation potentials are less common in the paraspinal muscles. This difficultly is most relevant in diabetic patients in whom diabetic amyotrophy (diabetic proximal neuropathy) also is in question.

PROCEDURE

- The side-lying patient slightly flexes the hip and knee on the unaffected side (Fig. 8-75).
- With neck slightly flexed, the patient's back is straight (not hyperextended).
- The affected limb is extended at the hip 15 degrees.
- The affected knee is flexed, stretching the femoral nerve (Fig. 8-76).
- If the test is positive, pain radiates into the anterior thigh.

Next Steps/Procedures
Ely sign and prone knee-bending test

CLINICAL PEARL

Upper lumbar disc disturbances may cause weakness of the quadriceps muscle and a diminished or absent patellar reflex. The straight-leg-raising tests and signs may be negative. Pinwheel examination usually reveals hyperesthesia or hypoesthesia of the L4 dermatome.

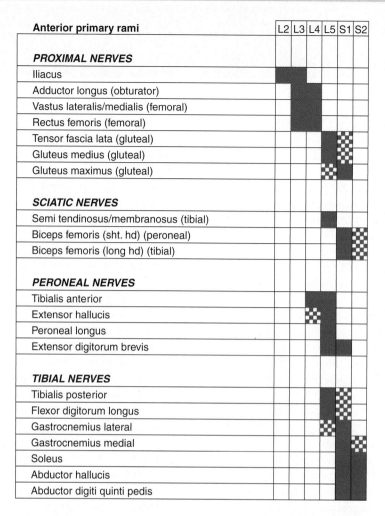

Anterior primary rami	L2	L3	L4	L5	S1	S2
PROXIMAL NERVES						
Iliacus		■	■			
Adductor longus (obturator)		■	■			
Vastus lateralis/medialis (femoral)		■	■			
Rectus femoris (femoral)		■	■			
Tensor fascia lata (gluteal)				■	▦	
Gluteus medius (gluteal)				■	▦	
Gluteus maximus (gluteal)				▦	■	
SCIATIC NERVES						
Semi tendinosus/membranosus (tibial)				■	■	
Biceps femoris (sht. hd) (peroneal)					■	▦
Biceps femoris (long hd) (tibial)					■	▦
PERONEAL NERVES						
Tibialis anterior			■	■		
Extensor hallucis			▦	■		
Peroneal longus				■	■	
Extensor digitorum brevis				■	■	
TIBIAL NERVES						
Tibialis posterior				■	▦	
Flexor digitorum longus				■	▦	
Gastrocnemius lateral				▦	■	
Gastrocnemius medial					■	▦
Soleus					■	■
Abductor hallucis					■	■
Abductor digiti quinti pedis					■	■

Posterior primary rami	L2	L3	L4	L5	S1	S2
Lumbar paraspinals	■	■	■	■	■	
High sacral paraspinals				■	■	■

FIG. 8-74 Chart of lower extremity muscles useful in the electromyographic recognition of lumbosacral radiculopathy. (From Brown WF, Bolton CF: *Clinical electromyography,* ed 2, Philadelphia, 1993, Butterworth-Heinemann.)

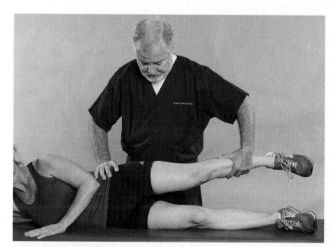

FIG. 8-75 The patient lies on the unaffected leg and slightly flexes the hip and knee. The patient straightens the back and flexes the neck. The affected leg is extended at the hip approximately 15 degrees.

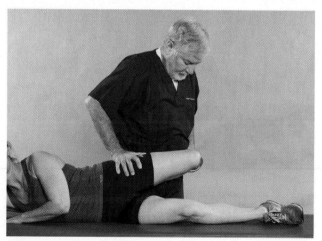

FIG. 8-76 The affected knee is flexed. This stretches the femoral nerve. The test is positive if pain radiates down the anterior thigh. A positive test indicates a radiculopathy that involves L2, L3, and L4.

8

Assessment for L5 or S1 Nerve Root Motor Deficiency

Comment

Muscle weakness, atrophy, or the inability to perform functional testing maneuvers all suggest the presence of nerve root compression that is more significant than the alteration of sensation (Table 8-14).

When lower-extremity weakness is apparent, atrophy may signify a lower motor neuron lesion or muscular disorder. However, disuse of a muscle from any cause—whether pain, immobilization, or paralysis of central origin—will result in some loss of muscle mass. The quadriceps are prone to disuse atrophy, which happens quite rapidly.

The patient who can hop well does not have a serious weakness of the gastrocnemius, which is a strong muscle and is difficult to evaluate through direct testing. The examiner observes the patient walk on the toes, during which the patient's body weight is completely supported on one foot and then the other. If weakness exists, the heel will drop while the patient is walking. The contours of the musculature may demonstrate atrophy or hypertrophy. A patient who has had a stroke and who has a moderate degree of spasticity and increased tone in antigravity muscles may still be able to rise on the toes. When weakness is evident while attempting this maneuver, the disorder is usually a primary lesion of the nerve root, peripheral nerve, or muscle.

Having the patient walk on the heels is an especially valuable screening test because dorsiflexion of the ankles and toes is weakened in many muscular and neural disorders. If necessary, the examiner may help the patient maintain balance in this maneuver. A healthy patient can hold the foot and toes anteriorly off the floor while strongly dorsiflexing the great toe during walking on the heels. If the patient can perform this action, foot drop does not exist. However, the patient might still have minor weakness of the muscles of the anterior compartment, and these areas should be tested directly. Foot drop may be of either central or peripheral origin. Severe foot drop of peripheral origin is clearly revealed by the abnormal nature of the gait and by an observable loss of dorsiflexion of the ankle and toes. If foot drop of a peripheral origin (lower motor neuron) has been present for several weeks, shrinkage and softness of the anterior compartment also will be apparent.

Piriformis syndrome is defined by a loose cluster of symptoms arising from the entrapment of the sciatic nerve passing the sciatic notch, and it may lead to buttock or hamstring pain. Causes for anatomic abnormalities of the piriformis muscle and the sciatic nerve may result in irritation of the sciatic nerve by the piriformis muscle. Clinically, piriformis syndrome often mimics sciatica caused by the spine. Although some available evaluation methods, including imaging studies of piriformis syndrome as shown by Rossi and Filler and colleagues, have greatly enhanced diagnostic specificity and sensitivity to anatomic abnormalities, elec-

TABLE 8-14

SPECIFIC DORSOLUMBAR RADICULOPATHY PATTERNS

Nerve	HNP	Foramen	Muscle	Reflex	Sensation
T10					Umbilicus
T12					Pubis
L1	T12–L1	L1–L2			Upper anterior thigh
L2	L1–L2	L2–L3			Mid anterior thigh
L3	L2–L3	L3–L4	Quadriceps femoris		Lower anterior thigh
L4	L3–L4	L4–L5	Quadriceps femoris Anterior tibial	Patella	Anterior thigh Medial leg Foot (occasionally)
L5	L4–L5	L5–S1	Anterior tibial EHL	Posterior tibial	Lateral leg Dorsum of foot Big toe
S1	L5–S1	Heel raise Peroneal		Achilles tendon	Posterior leg Sole of foot Lateral foot Little toe

EHL, Extensor hallicis longus; *HNP,* herniated nucleus pulposus.
Adapted from Brier SR: *Primary care orthopedics,* St Louis, 1999, Mosby.

TABLE 8-15

ELECTROPHYSIOLOGIC DIFFERENCES BETWEEN L5 RADICULOPATHY AND PERONEAL NEUROPATHY

	L5 Radiculopathy	Peroneal Neuropathy
Nerve Conduction Studies		
Peroneal CMAP, recording extensor digitorum brevis	Normal or low amplitude	Conduction block at fibular head, low amplitude, or both
Peroneal CMAP, recording tibialis anterior	Normal or low amplitude	Conduction block at fibular head, low amplitude, or both
Superficial peroneal SNAP	Normal	Low or absent; normal in deep peroneal or purely demyelinating lesions
Needle EMG		
Tibialis anterior	Abnormal	Abnormal
Extensor digitorum brevis	Abnormal	Abnormal
Extensor hallucis	Abnormal	Abnormal
Peroneus longus	Abnormal	Abnormal; normal in selective deep peroneal lesions
Tibialis posterior	Abnormal	Normal
Flexor digitorum longus	Abnormal	Normal
Gluteus medius	May be normal	Normal
Tensor fasciae latae	May be normal	Normal
Lumbar paraspinals	May be normal	Normal

CMAP, Compound muscle action potential; *EMG*, electromyography; *SNAP*, sensory nerve action potential.
From Katirji B: *Electromyography in clinical practice: a case study approach*, St Louis, 1998, Mosby.

ORTHOPEDIC GAMUT 8-11

ANATOMIC RELATIONS BETWEEN THE SCIATIC NERVE AND THE PIRIFORMIS MUSCLE

- Both peroneal and tibial components of sciatic nerve pass inferior to the piriformis muscle.
- Tibial component of the sciatic nerve passes inferior to the piriformis muscle; the common peroneal nerve passes through the muscle.

trodiagnostic tools to examine functional entrapment of the sciatic nerve at the crossing level of piriformis muscle are still limited. In the previous study by Fishman and Zybert, the H-reflex was used to evaluate patients with piriformis syndrome. Their study showed that H-reflex was normal at rest, but latencies in the FAIR position (hip flexion, adduction, and internal rotation) were delayed (Chang et al, 2006).

The sciatic nerve seems to be compressed from the above piriformis muscle but less entrapped through the muscle.

When the leg is shaken, such as during the test for alternating motion rate, the foot will be unstable and flop about. The foot is less floppy with central disorders (upper motor neuron lesions) and may be fixed in plantar flexion. When dorsiflexion of the ankles and toes is weak, the toes of the spastic leg are dragged during walking. Before the examiner

concludes that weakness of dorsiflexion exists, the foot should be passively dorsiflexed to be certain that previous weakness, now healed, did not permanently shorten the gastrocnemius. Patients with severe L5 radiculopathy, in whom significant motor axon loss has occurred, sometimes have foot drop (Table 8-15).

PROCEDURE

- The examiner observes the patient walking on the toes, which requires each foot, one at a time, to support the patient's body weight completely (Fig. 8-77).
- If weakness exists, the heel will drop while the patient is walking.
- The contours of the musculature may demonstrate atrophy or hypertrophy.
- Having the patient walk on the heels is an especially valuable screening test because many muscular and neural disorders result in weakened dorsiflexion of the ankles and toes (Fig. 8-78).
- The patient may need help maintaining balance during this maneuver.
- The normal patient can hold the foot and toes anteriorly off the floor while strongly dorsiflexing the great toe during walking on the heels.
- If the patient can perform this maneuver, foot drop does not exist.

Next Steps/Procedures

Antalgia sign, bowstring sign, Cox sign, Kemp test, Lewin punch test, Lewin snuff test, Milgram test, and Neri sign

CLINICAL PEARL

The inability to walk on the toes indicates an L5–S1 disc problem based on weakness of the calf muscles supplied by the tibial nerve. The inability to walk on the heels indicates an L4–L5 disc problem based on weakness of the anterior leg muscles supplied by the common peroneal nerve.

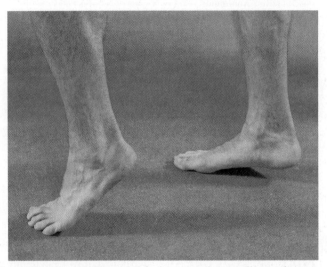

FIG. 8-77 The patient is standing and is instructed to walk on the toes. Weakness is evident if the heel drops while walking.

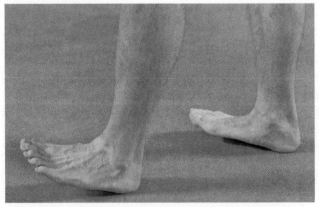

FIG. 8-78 The patient then walks on the heels. If necessary, the examiner may help the patient maintain balance during this maneuver. If the patient cannot walk on the heels, foot drop exists.

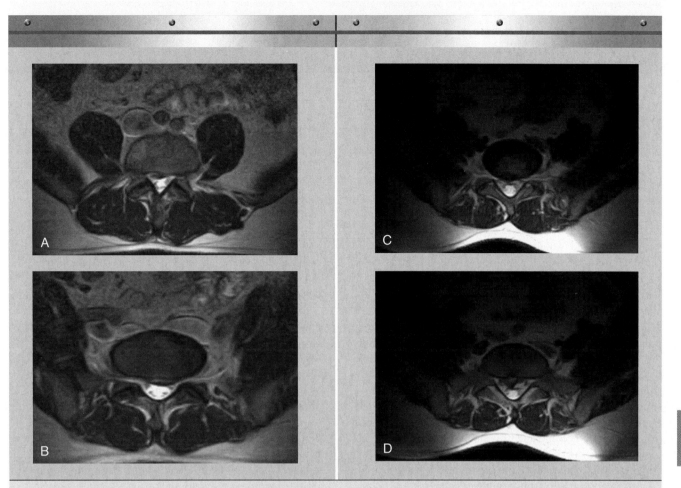

AT THE VIEWBOX

Axial MR images are essential for localizing disc herniations in a coronal plane and for assessing associated neural impingement due to central canal and/or nerve root canal compromise. This patient had bilateral lower extremity radiculopathy due to right L4–5 (A) and left L5–S1 (B) disc herniations, impinging upon the traversing right L5 and left S1 nerve roots, respectively. Unfortunately, the clinical-imaging correlation is not as straightforward in every case. Another patient had left sciatica, following an S1 distribution, yet the large, extruded disc herniation is eccentric to the right, without obvious impingement upon the traversing right S1 nerve root. (C and D) This type of case is challenging and frustrating to the patient, doctors, and other interested parties. (From the teaching file of Timothy Mick, DC, DACBR)

8

Assessment for L3 and L4 Nerve Root Inflammation

Comment

Spondylolisthesis in the adult, with the exception of traumatic and pathologic spondylolisthesis, is typically associated with a long history of back pain that may be punctuated with waxing and waning symptoms. An association with acute neurologic loss is unusual for spondylolisthesis in the adult. A more common scenario is the onset of intermittent radicular or neurogenic claudicatory-type symptoms that slowly become a more prominent part of the patient's history. Traumatic spondylolisthesis is caused most typically by a fall from a height. Generally, the fractures are not simply through the pars interarticularis, as is seen in isthmic spondylolisthesis, but may include the facets, the pedicles, the pars interarticularis, or any combination. Degenerative spondylolisthesis is based on the advancement of the degenerative cascade with disc degeneration and facet degeneration over time, accompanied by incompetence of the facet joint and anterior listhesis of the proximal on the distal vertebra. This abnormality most commonly occurs at the L4–L5 level (Fig. 8-79) and to a lesser degree at L3–L4 and L5–S1. Isthmic spondylolisthesis (Fig. 8-80) occurs in two varieties: subtype A, a lytic pars defect, and subtype B, an elongation of the pars interarticularis. The elongation occurs with repetitive stress fractures and healing over time. Pathologic fractures consist of a defect in the posterior arch because of abnormalities of the bone itself, either underlying metabolic bone disease or neoplasia.

Congenital spondylolisthesis consists of structural anomalies of the lumbosacral junction resulting in inadequate mechanical support to prevent forward slippage of L5 on S1 (Fig. 8-81).

During the third through the fifth decades of life, changes that occur in the lumbar spine can be quite pronounced, with the first manifestations of aging reflected in the intervertebral disc. One of three different phenomena can produce biochemical changes: degeneration of the annulus with disc nuclear herniation through posterolateral annular rents, nuclear degeneration with intact annulus, or simultaneous degeneration of both the annulus and the nucleus.

The biomechanical insufficiency of the involved disc compels the posterior elements, or the facets and capsules, to assume a more compressive, tensile, and shear load, resulting in capsular strain, hypermobility, and articular cartilage degeneration. The hypermobility can produce traction spurs. The ligamentum flavum also will be compelled to assume more tensile loads while becoming redundant as the total spine length decreases with disc degeneration. The vertebrae themselves tend toward a lowering and broadening in the superior, inferior, and midbody transverse breadth, a total change that, in static terms, begins to acutely or insidiously affect the neural elements.

If a disc lesion occurs in a spinal canal that is small, compression of the neural elements will result, and the patient will experience symptoms. In pure terms, this situation can be considered as a relative spinal stenosis. The stenosis occurs secondarily to the herniated nucleus pulposus occupying space in a small spinal canal. On the other hand, a similarly sized disc herniation in a large spinal canal

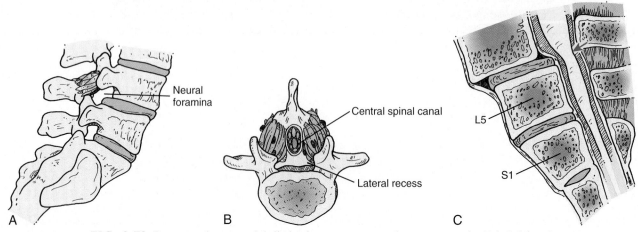

FIG. 8-79 Degenerative spondylolisthesis most commonly occurs at the L4–L5 level.
(From Bucholz RW: *Orthopaedic decision making,* ed 2, St Louis, 1996, Mosby.)

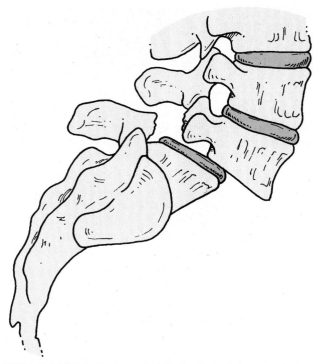

FIG. 8-80 Isthmic spondylolisthesis. (From Bucholz RW: *Orthopaedic decision making*, ed 2, St Louis, 1996, Mosby.)

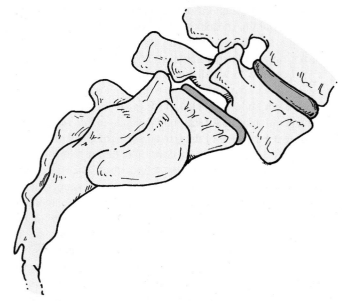

FIG. 8-81 Congenital spondylolisthesis caused by inadequate development of the L5–S1 facet complexes. (From Bucholz RW: *Orthopaedic decision making*, ed 2, St Louis, 1996, Mosby.)

8

ORTHOPEDIC GAMUT 8-12

MODIFIED WILTSE CLASSIFICATION OF LUMBAR SPONDYLOLISTHESIS ETIOLOGY

- Type 1, dysplastic (congenital) spondylolisthesis (congenital dysplasia of articular processes)
  - Type 1a. The articular processes of L5 and S1 are dysplastic, having a horizontal rather than coronal orientation.
  - Type 1b. The orientation of the facet joints is sagittal and the facets are malformed, allowing spondylolisthesis to occur typically in adult life.
  - Type 1c includes other congenital malformations of the lumbar spine that permit spondylolisthesis.
- Type 2, isthmic (lytic) spondylolisthesis (This type occurs in the presence of bilateral pars defects, which can result from a variety of causes.)
  - Type 2a. Lytic defects arise in the pars because of congenital weakness in the bone or repeated mechanical strain or both.
  - Type 2b. The elongated pars is a true stress fracture of the pars.
  - Type 2c. The pars fractures under acute trauma in cases that show complex fractures of the spine. Acute isolated pars fracture is exceedingly rare.
- Type 3, degenerative spondylolisthesis (This type is the most common cause of lumbar spondylolisthesis in patients older than 50 years. The neural arch is intact and the slip occurs because of degenerative changes in the facet joints with associated disc degeneration.)
- Type 4, traumatic spondylolisthesis (This type is rare and results from fractures or dislocations involving any part of the neural arch except the pars interarticularis, for example the pedicle or the facet joints. It is almost always secondary to severe trauma.)
- Type 5, pathological spondylolisthesis (This type can be divided into two types.)
  - Type 5a can occur when a generalized bone disease weakens the spine (e.g., Paget disease, osteoporosis, osteogenesis imperfecta, achondroplasia, arthrogryposis, osteopetrosis).
  - Type 5b can occur when a focal disease process weakens the pars interarticularis, resulting in pathologic fracture and spondylolisthesis (e.g., syphilis, tuberculosis, and neoplastic processes).
- Type 6, iatrogenic spondylolisthesis (This type can follow spinal decompression performed for spinal stenosis, laminectomy for disc removal, or any other spine surgery in which decompressing the spinal canal is necessary.)

will cause no symptoms because the neural elements have enough room to escape the pressure.

Thus, symptoms in persons of this age group are a result of not only a disc herniation itself but also the size of the spinal canal with which the individual is born.

Patients in the fifth decade of life and older can exhibit the hypermobile end-stage changes of the aging process. Degeneration of both facet joints and the intervertebral disc leads to a narrowing of the spinal canal. The canal is rimmed by large osteophytes, which develop to diminish the load on the now incompetent intervertebral disc. The facets are hypertrophic and deformed by the osteophytic spurs that are encased within the thickened joint capsule. The ligamentum flavum becomes redundant, and in combination with the changes just mentioned, the spinal canal and foramina are affected. Changes in the lumbar spinal canal occur to some degree in all active people as they age. However, not everyone suffers from significant impairment. The symptoms a person will have depend on the original size of the spinal canal. If the individual's spinal canal is small, the changes that are caused by aging and that occur in the disc and facet joints will lead to an absolute spinal stenosis with compression of the neural elements. If the spinal canal is large, the normal changes of aging will lead to a relative spinal stenosis with no neural compression (Fig 8-82).

> Numerous papers report that adjacent segment disease occurs after fusion surgery in the lumbar spine. The incidence of adjacent segment disease after lumbar fusion surgery ranges from 25% to 40%. The belief is that the disease is related to increased biomechanical stress on the motion segment adjacent to the fused area. Biomechanical studies have shown that the mobility and the intradiscal pressure of the adjacent disc are increased after spinal fusion. By using roentgen stereophotogrammetric analysis in humans, Axelsson and colleagues found that fusion of the lumbosacral segment can alter the kinematics of the adjacent segment, redistributing the mobility toward relative hypermobility in the juxtafused segment (Kawaguchi et al, 2007).

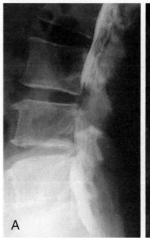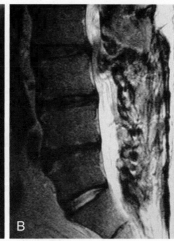

FIG. 8-82 Postoperative MRI at 11 years after L3–L5 laminoplasty. Spinal stenosis, demonstrating remarkable posterior indentation of the dura mater. (Adapted From Kawaguchi Y, Ishihara H, Kanamori M, et al: Adjacent segment disease following expansive lumbar laminoplasty, *Spine J* 7[3]:273-279, 2007.)

PROCEDURE

- The patient is prone, and the legs are fully extended (Fig. 8-83).
- The examiner anchors the patient's lumbosacral spine with one hand.
- With the other hand, the examiner slowly extends the hip of the patient's affected leg (Fig. 8-84).
- The test is positive if the patient experiences radiating pain in the anterior thigh.
- A positive test indicates inflammation of the L3 and L4 nerve roots.

Next Steps/Procedures

Bilateral leg-lowering test, Demianoff sign, double-leg-raise test, Lewin supine test, matchstick test, Mennell sign, Minor sign, Nachlas test, Quick test, Schober test, sign of the buttock, skin pinch test, spinal percussion test, and Vanzetti sign

CLINICAL PEARL

Five criteria have been established for diagnosis of sciatica caused by a herniated intervertebral disc. (1) Leg pain is the dominant symptom when compared with back pain, and it affects only one leg and follows a typical sciatic or femoral nerve distribution. (2) Paresthesia is localized to a dermatomal distribution. (3) Straight leg raising is reduced to 50% of what is considered normal, and pain is elicited in the symptomatic leg when the unaffected leg is elevated. This pain radiates proximally or distally with digital pressure on the tibial nerve in the popliteal fossa. (4) Two of four neurologic signs (atrophy, motor weakness, diminished sensory appreciation, and diminution of reflex activity) are present. (5) A contrast study or other diagnostic imaging is positive and corresponds to the clinical level.

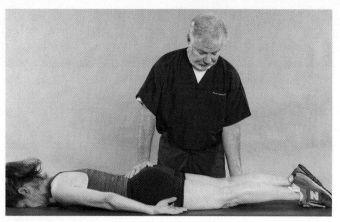

FIG. 8-83 The patient is prone, and the legs are fully extended. The examiner anchors the patient's lumbosacral spine with one hand.

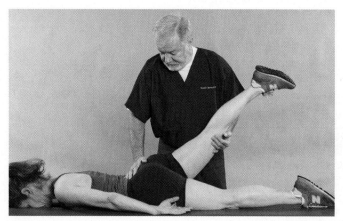

FIG. 8-84 With the other hand, the examiner slowly extends the hip of the patient's affected leg. The test is positive if the patient experiences radiating pain in the anterior thigh. A positive test indicates inflammation of the L3 and L4 nerve roots.

Assessment for Intervertebral Nerve Root Encroachment, Muscular Strain, Ligamentous Sprain, or Pericapsular Inflammation

Comment

Idiopathic LBP has confounded health care practitioners for decades. Although many advances have been made in the understanding of the biomechanics of the *lumbar* spine over the last 25 years, the cellular and neural mechanisms that lead to *facet* pain are not well understood. (Cavanaugh et al, 1996)

Patients with chronic facet syndrome develop adhesions of the synovial joint, which is innervated by the primary dorsal rami. When facet disease is advanced, bony encroachment on a susceptible spinal canal can occur (Fig. 8-85). Lateral mass stenosis and neuroforaminal impingement can produce symptoms commonly seen in patients with lumbar stenosis.

Disc prolapse occurs in three stages, and it occurs only if the disc has deteriorated as a result of repeated microtrauma and if the annulus fibers have started to degenerate.

The hernia causes acute pain, which is felt in the lower back. This occurrence corresponds to the initial phase of the

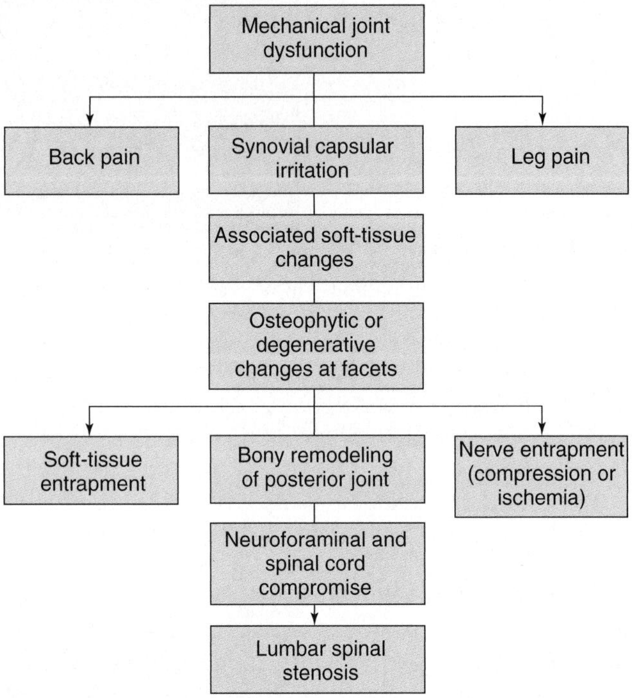

FIG. 8-85 Pathogenesis of the lumbosacral Z-joints. (From Brier SR: *Primary care orthopedics,* St Louis, 1999, Mosby.)

ORTHOPEDIC GAMUT 8-13

MECHANISMS OF LUMBAR FACET PAIN

1. The facet joint can carry a significant amount of the total compressive load on the spine when the human spine is hyperextended.
2. Extensive stretch of the human facet joint capsule occurs when the spine is in the physiologic range of extreme extension.
3. An extensive distribution of small nerve fibers and free and encapsulated nerve endings exists in the lumbar facet joint capsule, including nerves containing substance P, a putative neuromodulator of pain.
4. Low- and high-threshold mechanoreceptors fire when the facet joint capsule is stretched or is subject to localized compressive forces.
5. Sensitization and excitation of nerves in facet joint and surrounding muscle occur when the joint is inflamed or exposed to certain chemicals that are released during injury and inflammation.
6. Marked reduction in nerve activity occurs in facet tissue injected with hydrocortisone and lidocaine.

ORTHOPEDIC GAMUT 8-14

DISC PROLAPSE

Disc prolapse usually follows lifting or twisting while the trunk is in flexion:

1. During the first stage, trunk flexion flattens the discs anteriorly and opens out the intervertebral space posteriorly.
2. During the second stage, as soon as the weight is lifted, the increased axial compression force crushes the whole disc and violently drives the nuclear substance posteriorly until it reaches the deep surface of the posterior longitudinal ligament.
3. During the third stage, when the trunk is nearly straight, the path taken by the herniating mass is closed by the pressure of the vertebral plateaus, and a hernia remains trapped under the posterior longitudinal ligament.

lumbar sciatica complex. This initial acute lower back pain can regress spontaneously or with treatment, but as a result of repeated trauma, the herniation grows in size and protrudes more and more into the vertebral canal. Once this protrusion occurs, the herniation meets with a nerve root, often one of the roots of the sciatic nerve. In fact, the herniation progressively pushes on the nerve root until the latter is jammed against the posterior wall of the IVF. The posterior wall is formed by the joint between the articular processes, its anterior capsular ligament, and the lateral border of the ligamentum flavum. The compressed nerve root causes pain in the spinal segment that corresponds to the root and, finally, impairs reflexes and creates motor disturbances, such as those that occur in sciatica with paralysis (Fig. 8-86).

The clinical picture depends on the spinal level of disc prolapse and nerve root compression.

If prolapse occurs at L4–L5, the root of L5 is compressed, and pain is felt in the posterolateral aspect of the thigh, the knee, the lateral border of the calf, the lateral border of the instep of the foot, and the dorsal surface of the foot to the great toe. If the prolapse lies at L5–S1, S1 is compressed, and pain is referred to the posterior aspect of the thigh, knee, and calf, as well as the heel and the lateral border of the foot to the fifth toe. However, this correlation of clinical picture and lesion level is not absolute. A herniation at L4–L5 may lie closer to the midline and compress L5 and S1 simultaneously, or even occasionally, S1 alone. Surgical exploration at L5–S1, performed on the strength of the S1 root pain, may fail to recognize that this lesion lies one level above.

PROCEDURE

- While in a seated position, the patient is supported by the examiner, who reaches around the patient's shoulders and upper chest from behind (Fig. 8-87).
- The patient is directed to lean forward to one side and then around until the patient is eventually bending obliquely backward (Figs. 8-88 and 8-89).
- The maneuver is similar to that used for cervical compression.
- If this compression causes or aggravates a pattern of radicular pain in the thigh and leg, the sign is positive and indicates nerve root compression.
- Local back pain should be noted, but it does not constitute a positive test.
- However, local back pain may indicate a strain or sprain and thus be present when the patient leans obliquely forward or at any point in motion.
- Because elderly adults are less prone to an actual herniation of a disc because of lessened elasticity involved in the aging process, other reasons for nerve root compression are usually the cause.
- Degenerative joint disease, exostoses, inflammatory or fibrotic residues, narrowing from disc degeneration, and tumors must all be considered.
- This test must elicit a more positive finding when the patient is standing than when sitting (Figs. 8-90 and 8-91).

Next Steps/Procedures
Antalgia sign, bowstring sign, Cox sign, heel/toe walk test, Lewin punch test, Lewin snuff test, Milgram test, and Neri sign

CLINICAL PEARL

Kemp test can be performed when the patient is either standing or sitting. Sitting increases intradiscal pressure and therefore maximizes stress on the disc. Standing increases weight bearing and maximizes stress to the facets. The test should be performed in both positions.

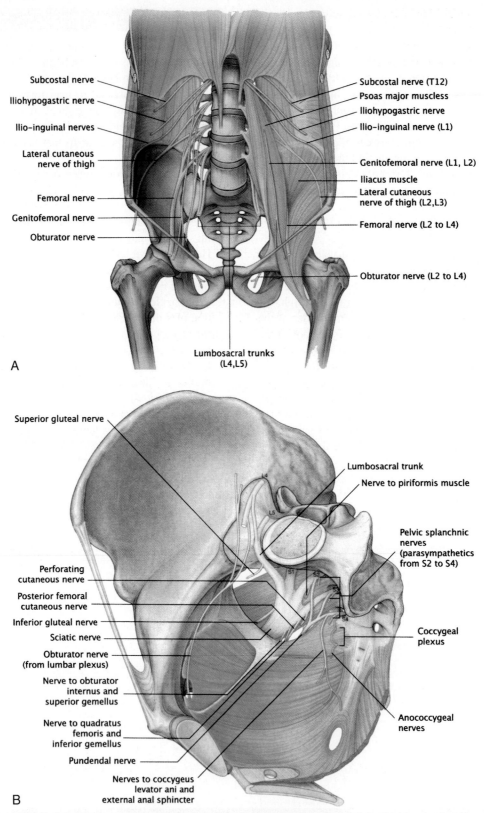

FIG. 8-86 Lumbosacral plexus subdivided functionally and anatomically into the lumbar and sacral plexus. The lumbar plexus is formed from the anterior rami of the T12–L5 nerve roots and the sacral plexus represents the union of the lumbosacral trunk and the anterior rami of the S1–5 nerve roots. (From Planner AC, Donaghy M, Moore NR: Causes of lumbosacral plexopathy, *Clin Radiol* 61(12):987-995, 2006.)

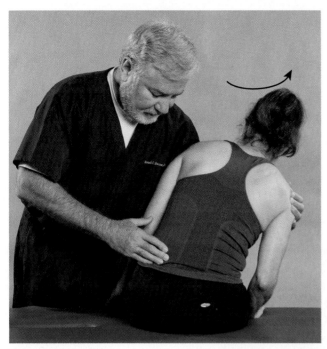

FIG. 8-87 While in a seated position, the patient is supported by the examiner, who reaches around the patient's shoulders and upper chest from behind. The patient is directed to lean obliquely forward and away from the affected side.

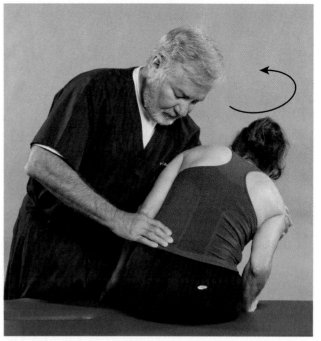

FIG. 8-88 The examiner actively rotates the patient's trunk from the original position and circumducts the trunk toward the affected side.

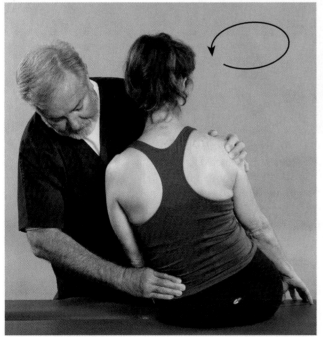

FIG. 8-89 Circumduction of the trunk toward the affected side occurs to the point at which the spine is posterolaterally extended. If this compression causes or aggravates a pattern of radicular pain in the thigh and leg, the test is positive and indicates nerve root compression. Local pain should be noted, but it does not constitute a positive test. Degenerative joint disease, exostoses, inflammatory or fibrotic residues, narrowing from disc degeneration, and tumors must be evaluated.

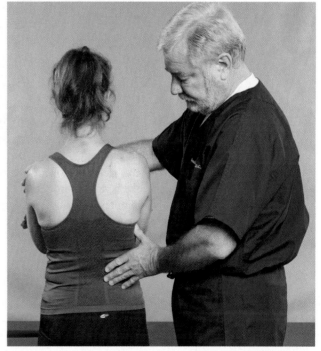

FIG. 8-90 An alternative is to have the patient assume a standing position. The examiner anchors the pelvis on the patient's affected side with one hand. With the other hand, the examiner grasps the patient's opposite shoulder.

8

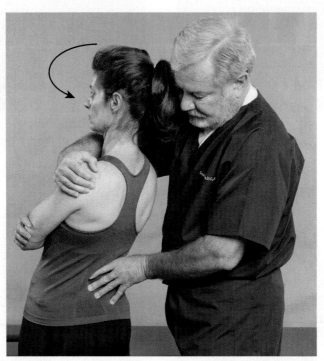

FIG. 8-91 While fixing the pelvis, the examiner firmly moves the patient's opposite shoulder obliquely backward toward the affected side. This maneuver rotates the trunk, extends it, and exerts downward pressure over the affected lumbosacral area. The test is positive if this compression causes or aggravates a pattern of radicular pain in the thigh and leg. A positive test indicates nerve root compression. In the standing position, the test must elicit a more positive finding than is elicited in the seated position.

KERNIG/BRUDZINSKI SIGN

Assessment for Meningeal Irritation or Inflammation

Comment

Meningitis is the most common central nervous system (CNS) infection caused by viruses, and viral meningitis is a far more common condition than bacterial or fungal meningitis. Approximately 10,000 to 15,000 cases of lymphocytic or presumed viral meningitis are reported each year, with an incidence of 5 to 10 cases per 100,000 individuals. Unreported cases, however, may be as much as 10-fold higher. CSF pleocytosis has also been reported in random individuals infected with measles, mumps, and human immunodefi- ciency virus, and similar asymptomatic CNS involvement probably occurs with other viral agents as well. Although viral meningitis may affect all age groups, it is predominantly a disease of childhood (Greenlee, Michael, Robert, 2003).

With treatment, the fatality rate of *adult bacterial meningitis* is usually less than 10%, but severe neurologic sequelae are possible. The two leading causes of these sequelae in the adult are pneumococci *(Streptococcus pneumoniae)* and meningococci *(Neisseria meningitidis)*.

Pneumococcal meningitis is usually preceded by pneumonia and is often associated with alcoholism, debilitation, and old age. This type of meningitis usually occurs sporadically, except in developing countries.

ORTHOPEDIC GAMUT 8-15

MENINGEAL PATHOGENS AND ASSOCIATED OR PREDISPOSING CONDITIONS*

Organism	Associated Factors/Condition	Organism	Associated Factors/Condition
Streptococcus pneumoniae	Pneumonia	*Staphylococcus*	CSF shunt
	Otitis media		Ommaya reservoir
	Acute sinusitis		Lumbar puncture
	Diabetes		Infective endocarditis
	Splenectomy		Parameningeal infection
	Hypogammaglobulinemia		(empyema, epidural abscess,
	Head trauma		osteomyelitis)
	CSF rhinorrhea	*Streptococcus agalactiae*	Neonates, elderly adults
	Neonates, elderly adults		Diabetes
	Alcoholism, cirrhosis, peritonitis		Alcoholism
Neisseria meningitidis	College dormitory living		Acquired immunodeficiency
	Exposure in an endemic area		syndrome
	Complement deficiencies	*Haemophilus influenzae* type b	Age over 60
	Splenectomy		Otitis media
	Hypogammaglobulinemia		Sinusitis
Listeria monocytogenes	Immunosuppressive therapy		CSF leak
	Organ transplantation		Immunodeficiency
	Pregnancy		Diabetes
	Diabetes		Alcoholism
	Alcoholism		
	Neonates, elderly adults		
Enteric gram-negative bacilli	Diabetes		
	Cirrhosis, alcoholism		
	Craniotomy		
	Head trauma		

CSF, Cerebral spinal fluid.

*Meningeal pathogens and associated or predisposing conditions adapted from Roos KL: Bacterial meningitis. *Curr Treat Options Neurol* 1(2):147-156, 1999.

Meningococcal meningitis occurs in epidemics (serogroup A or C) in the pediatric age group and may be acquired by susceptible adults.

Meningitis caused by gram-negative enteric bacteria is always a disease of the hospitalized or nursing home patient and often follows bacteremia from other foci, such as cellulitis or urinary tract infection.

The possibility of bacterial meningitis must be considered in any patient with fever and even minimal mental or neurologic symptoms.

Whenever the diagnosis is suspected, a referral for lumbar puncture must be accomplished immediately and bacterial cultures obtained. When the cerebrospinal fluid is abnormal, tuberculous and fungal cultures should be obtained.

Prognosis depends on the interval between the onset of the illness and the institution of therapy.

If severe backache, stiff neck, and the Kernig/Brudzinski sign are absent but mental symptoms are prominent, and the cerebrospinal fluid shows normal sugar, a low number of cells, or a mononuclear pleocytosis (lymphocytosis), then encephalitis must be suspected. Patients with herpes simplex encephalitis classically exhibit an acute onset of mental and behavioral symptoms and often with an amnestic syndrome. The patients may have lateralized findings, such as hemiparesis or aphasia.

Onset of viral meningitis may occur following a symptomatic, systemic illness or as an isolated event after inapparent systemic infection. Patients complain of headache, photophobia, and, in many instances, symptomatic neck stiffness or back pain. Significant alteration of consciousness is far less common than in bacterial meningitis but does occasionally occur. Seizures or focal neurologic signs are unusual and raise concerns about concomitant viral encephalitis or infection caused by some other process, such as brain abscess. Patients are usually uncomfortable but do not appear severely ill. Physical examination may reveal evidence of systemic illness, including rash, lymphadenopathy, pharyngitis, or splenomegaly, depending on the infectious agent. Neurologic examination will reveal nuchal rigidity. The patient may be unable to touch chin to chest. Resistance to passive neck flexion and Kernig sign or Brudzinski sign or both may be present but are inconsistent, and both signs may be absent in milder cases. A useful test of nuchal rigidity is to ask the patient to touch forehead to knee; this test will often be positive when all other tests of meningeal irritation are questionable or absent (Greenlee et al, 2003).

PROCEDURE

- For the Brudzinski part of the sign, the patient is in the supine position, and the examiner passively flexes the patient's head (Fig. 8-92).
- The sign is present if flexion of both knees occurs (Fig. 8-93).
- The sign is often accompanied by flexion of both hips and is present with meningitis.
- For the Kernig part of the sign, the patient is supine.
- The examiner flexes the patient's hip and knee of either leg to 90 degrees (Fig. 8-94).
- The examiner attempts to completely extend the patient's leg (Fig. 8-95).
- If this maneuver causes pain, the sign is present.
- The sign is often accompanied by involuntary flexion of the opposite knee and hip and is present in meningitis.

Next Steps/Procedure
Cerebrospinal fluid examination

CLINICAL PEARL

After myelographic examination, a percentage of patients experience general malaise, headache, nausea, pain, and stiffness for a week or longer, and the symptoms are strikingly aggravated by the erect position or activity. These conditions may be signs of arachnoiditis. Subarachnoid fibrosis typically affects the lowermost segment of the thecal sac. This whole process represents meningismus or the apparent irritation of the spinal cord in which the symptoms simulate meningitis. However, no actual infectious agent—such as bacteria, fungi, or viruses—can be found.

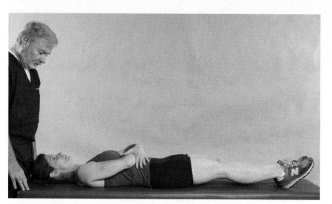

FIG. 8-92 For the Brudzinski sign, the patient is in the supine position.

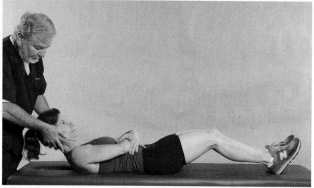

FIG. 8-93 The patient's head is passively flexed by the examiner. The sign is present if flexion of both knees occurs. The sign is often accompanied by flexion of both hips. The sign is present in meningitis.

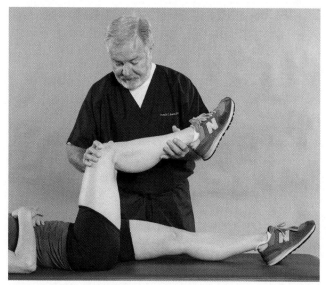

FIG. 8-94 For Kernig sign, the patient is supine. The examiner flexes the patient's hip and knee of either leg to 90 degrees.

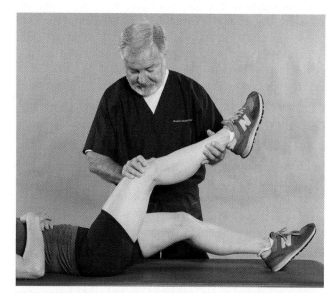

FIG. 8-95 The examiner attempts to extend the leg completely. If pain prevents this extension, the sign is present. The sign is often accompanied by involuntary flexion of the opposite knee and hip. The sign is present in meningitis.

8

Assessment for Intervertebral Radiculopathy Versus Hip Joint Disease

Comment

Pain that radiates distally at the extremities is clinically divided into radicular and pseudoradicular syndromes. Radicular pain is defined as a pain that radiates below the knee, whereas pseudoradicular pain does not cross this border. The rationale behind this distinction stems from the hypothesis that pain from local proximal disorders that do not affect any nerves or nerve roots, that is, facet joint affection, piriformis syndrome, might be perceived in proximal dermatomes within the thigh (referred pain, head zones), whereas pain from disorders associated with nerve root compression is often felt in distal dermatomes below the knee (projected pain). This distinction is thought to be clinically relevant because a projected pain always involves a damage or irritation of peripheral nerves or nerve roots (i.e., it has a neuropathic component), whereas referred pain occurs without nerve involvement and might therefore be purely nociceptive (Freynhagen et al, in press).

Osteoarthritis (OA) of the hip and knee are prevalent musculoskeletal complaints worldwide, affecting 7.5% to 50% of the population older than 65 years. Patients with OA experience increasing pain and progressive loss of function,

---

ORTHOPEDIC GAMUT 8-16

MODIFIED ALTMAN CLASSIFICATION OF HIP OSTEOARTHRITIS

Different classification systems have been described using as criteria the direction of migration of the femoral head and the evolution of the destructive changes within the joint. The two main types of head migration are as follows:

- The superior migration (or eccentric) may be superolateral or superomedial. The differential diagnosis of the superior migration pattern of the hip includes the calcium pyrophosphate dihydrate crystal deposition disease and the osteonecrosis, both of which might be complicated by secondary degenerative changes.
- The medial migration (concentric) is also known as axial or global. The concentric loss of articular cartilage poses diagnostic difficulties because it should be differentiated from infectious arthritis and rheumatoid arthritis.

---

particularly in walking and stair climbing (Kapstad et al, 2007).

The symptoms in OA are usually unilateral and asymmetric at early stage. In late stages multiple joints may be involved. Patients usually show symptoms of OA after middle age, although in some forms of secondary OA (e.g., congenital hip displacement/dislocation) symptoms start earlier. Pain is the usual presenting symptom. Initially pain is worsened by activity and relieved by rest, but eventually rest and night pain develop. Typically, the symptoms of hip OA follow an intermittent course, with periods of remission sometimes lasting for months. Pain arising in the hip joint is felt in the groin, down the front of the thigh and, sometimes, in the knee; occasionally, knee pain is the only symptom. Pain at the back of the hip is seldom from the joint; it usually derives from the lumbar spine. Limp is a common symptom and it may be caused by a change in limb length, weakness of the hip abductors or joint instability. Decreased range of motion and crepitus are also common. Stiffness, deformity, leg length discrepancy and Trendelenburg sign are late symptoms, associated with pelvic obliquity. Restriction of walking distance, difficulty in climbing stairs, and progressive inability to perform everyday tasks or enjoy recreation may eventually drive the patient to seek help. The eccentric type of idiopathic OA is more painful and has poor prognosis as a result of rapid deterioration. The concentric type has a better prognosis and is better tolerated by patients (Karachalios, Karantanas, Malizos, 2007).

The intervertebral disc is the source of most LBP. Of disc lesions in the lumbar spine, 95% occur at the fourth and fifth spaces. With normal aging and repetitive trauma, progressive degeneration of the nucleus pulposus occurs. Protrusion of nuclear material usually occurs in the area of greatest weakness at the posterolateral aspect of the disc (Fig. 8-96).

Examination often reveals restriction of low back motion. Bending toward the affected side typically exacerbates the pain. Variable degrees of local tenderness and muscle guarding are present. In an attempt to relieve tension on the nerve root, the patient may list or bend away from the painful side and stand with the affected hip and knee slightly flexed. A characteristic clinical picture may be present, depending on the level of nerve root involvement (Table 8-16).

With lower lumbar compression, attempted forward bending is limited by pain and inflexibility of the lumbar spine, and percussion by a fist or reflex hammer over the lower segments may aggravate the complaint in the thigh or leg (*doorbell sign*). The motor deficits that ensue from paresis of these roots are most apparent below the knee. Seldom is weakness of the calf so severe that the patient cannot walk on the toes, but atrophy of the gastrocnemius

TABLE 8-16

LUMBAR DISC SYNDROME PATTERNS

Level	Pain	Sensory	Motor Weakness Atrophy	Reflex
L3–L4 (L4 root)	Low back, posterolateral aspect of thigh, across patella, anteromedial aspect of leg	Anterior aspect of knee, anteromedial aspect of leg	Quadriceps (knee extension)	Knee jerk
L4–L5 (L5 root)	Lateral, posterolateral aspect of thigh, leg	Lateral aspect of leg, dorsum of foot, first web space, great toe	Great toe extension, ankle dorsiflexion, heel walking difficult (foot drop may occur)	Minor (posterior tibial jerk depressed)
L5–S1 (S1 root)	Posterolateral aspect of thigh, leg, heel	Posterior aspect of calf, heel, lateral aspect of foot (three toes)	Calf, plantar flexion of foot, great toe; toe walking weak	Ankle jerk
Cauda equina syndrome (massive midline protrusion)	Low back, thigh, legs; often bilateral	Thighs, legs, feet, perineum; often bilateral	Variable; may be bowel, bladder incontinence	Ankle jerk (may be bilateral)

Adapted from Mercier LR, Pettid FJ: *Practical orthopedics,* ed 4, St Louis, 1995, Mosby.

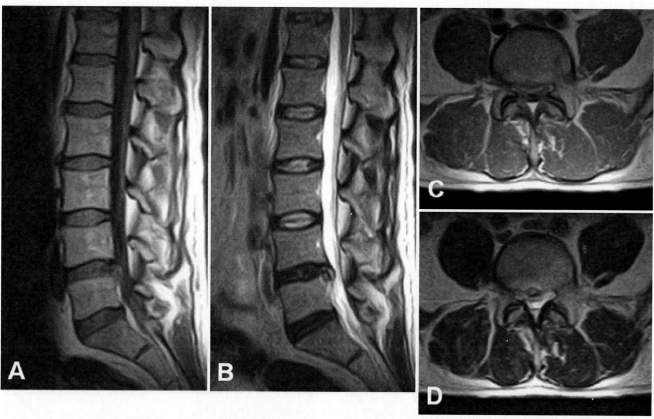

FIG. 8-96 Examples of magnetic resonance images. Sagittal (**A** and **B**) and axial (**C** and **D**) T1- and T2-weighted magnetic resonance images of a 44-year-old man. Right subarticular extrusion is seen at the L4–L5 level with compromise of the right L5 nerve root.

(From Jensen TS, Albert HB, Sorensen JS, et al: Magnetic resonance imaging findings as predictors of clinical outcome in patients with sciatica receiving active conservative treatment, *J Manip Physiol Ther* 30(2):98-108, 2007.)

8

may be noted. Heel walking is especially revealing. Severe foot drop is unlikely, but toe drop is common with some atrophy of the anterior compartment. Nevertheless, dorsiflexion of the foot and toes should be tested directly for minor weakness. The straight-leg-raising test often demonstrates marked limitation in range of thigh flexion on the painful side. Squeeze tenderness of the calf is common. The ankle jerk reflex is a stretch reflex of the gastrocnemiussoleus. It is commonly diminished or absent when S1 root impingement occurs but may be normal in L5 root syndromes.

Neoplasms or inflammation of the spine or cauda equina may produce a syndrome similar to that produced by compression of the lower lumbar root, as may a retroperitoneal tumor and invasive neoplasm in the pelvis.

PROCEDURE

- If the examiner flexes the hip of a patient with sciatica while the knee is extended and this movement elicits pain (Fig. 8-97) but flexing the thigh on the pelvis while the knee is flexed produces no sciatic pain, the sign is present (Fig. 8-98).
- This sign rules out hip joint disease.

Next Steps/Procedures
Bechterew sitting test, Bragard sign, Deyerle sign, Fajersztajn test, Lasègue rebound test, Lasègue sitting test, Lasègue test, Lewin standing test, Lindner sign, Sicard sign, straight-leg-raising test, and Turyn sign

CLINICAL PEARL

Lasègue described how painful sciatica is for patients when the sciatic nerve is stretched by extending the knee while the hip is flexed. He also described the pain relief that occurs when the knee was then flexed. This reaction is the classic leg-raising sign. Variations of this sign, with interpretations of its meaning, lend much more knowledge to the examining physician than merely noting at what degree of leg raise the patient experiences either back pain, leg pain, or both.

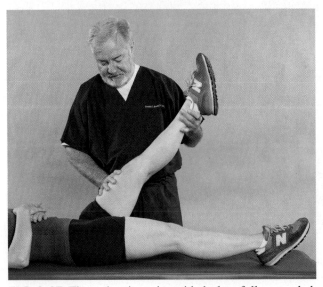

FIG. 8-97 The patient is supine with the legs fully extended. The examiner performs a straight-leg-raising test on the affected leg and notes the angle at which sciatic pain is produced.

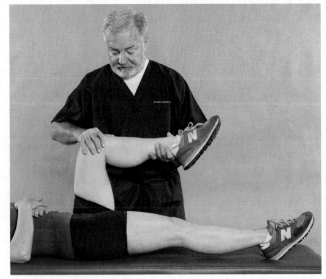

FIG. 8-98 The examiner flexes the thigh and the knee, relieving the stretch on the sciatic nerve. The sign is present if the pain is relieved. The presence of the sign indicates neural pain rather than hip articular pain.

Assessment for Intervertebral Nerve Root Lesion, Piriformis Muscular Spasm, Ischiotrochanteric Groove Adhesion, or Intervertebral Disc Syndrome

Comment

Patients with chronic postural or mechanical problems in the lumbar spine or individuals who are vulnerable to repetitive injury may develop a chronic lumbar strain.

Hip flexion with rotation causes pain in an individual with this problem because it stretches the piriformis muscle, thereby compromising or irritating the sciatic nerve. Activities that externally rotate the thigh can strain the piriformis muscle and can refer pain to the buttocks; toward the hip, posterior thigh, and calf; and even to the sole of the foot, on occasion, as in typical cases of *sciatica* in radiculopathies.

Spasm of the posterior trunk muscles, sometimes accompanied by functional scoliosis and often by pain, usually indicates an underlying strain of the posterior joints, disc, or both. Unilateral spasm suggests a unilateral posterior joint strain. Lesions involving both disc and posterior joints are often accompanied by spasm of the spinal flexors, producing a straight or slightly kyphotic lumbar spine. Psoas spasm produces flexion deformity at the hip, and this may be missed at the initial examination. Spasm of the piriformis muscle, a common cause of buttock pain, can be diagnosed by palpation medial to the lower part of the neck of the femur.

In piriformis syndrome, the piriformis muscle spasms and places pressure on the sciatic nerve, causing pain in the buttock, which can radiate along the back of the leg to the posterior aspect of the knee. Some investigators consider piriformis syndrome to be a form of myofascial pain syndrome. Clinical history and physical examination are the mainstay in the diagnosis of piriformis syndrome. Physical examination findings in piriformis syndrome include local-ized tenderness to palpation, pain with straight leg raise, pain on forced internal rotation of the extended thigh (positive Freiberg test), pain with resisted abduction/external rotation (positive Pace test), and pain radiating to the posterior thigh. The clinician must have a high index of suspicion for this syndrome because laboratory and routine radiology studies are usually normal. However, when the diagnosis is unclear, electromyography can detect myopathic and neuropathic changes, whereas CT and MRI can be helpful in differentiating muscle infection, soft-tissue inflammation, and spine disease (Vallejo et al, 2004)

Sciatic nerve entrapment usually occurs at the sciatic notch as the nerve exits from the pelvis. The nerve is compressed against the bony edge as it traverses the belly of the piriformis muscle. The syndrome is characterized by pain that is behind the greater trochanter and is referred down the thigh, the outer side of the leg, and the sole of the foot. Diagnostic findings include a positive Lasègue test, hypoesthesia of the lateral half of the sole of the foot, and pain behind the greater trochanter when the hip and knee joints are flexed to a right angle and the thigh is forced into adduction and internal rotation.

Pain during hip movement is emphasized as the diagnostic feature that differentiates sciatica because of a disc (when only straight leg raising is painful) from peripheral entrapment of the nerve as it traverses the sciatic notch. When the nerve is stretched by straight leg raising, pain is aggravated by internal rotation and relieved by external rotation.

ORTHOPEDIC GAMUT 8-17

CAUSES AND PREDILECTION FOR PIRIFORMIS SYNDROME

- The female-to-male predominance is 6:1.
- The most common cause of piriformis syndrome is trauma to the pelvis or buttock (50%).
- However, the trauma is usually not dramatic and may occur several months before initial symptoms.
- Prolonged sitting, although uncommon, has been recognized as a cause of piriformis syndrome.

ORTHOPEDIC GAMUT 8-18

DISC HERNIATION VERSUS OTHER CAUSES OF BACK PAIN

The following elements apply when early disc herniation is difficult to differentiate from other causes of back pain:

1. Plain-film roentgenograms are indicated within 2 to 4 weeks of onset.
2. Electromyography, computed tomography (CT), magnetic resonance imaging (MRI), or myelography confirm the diagnosis (Fig. 8-99).
3. Electromyography (EMG), CT, and MRI are not usually indicated for at least 4 to 6 weeks from onset.
4. EMG, CT (if surgical intervention is being contemplated), or MRI is indicated if other more serious spinal disease is suspected.
5. Discography is considered to be of only limited value.

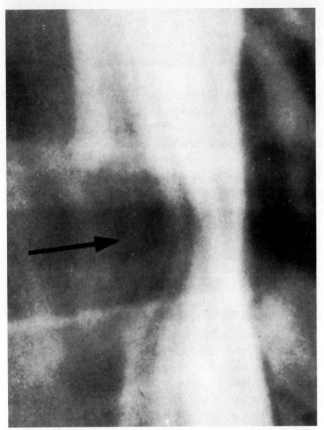

FIG. 8-99 Abnormal myelogram revealing a large extradural defect in the dye column that is consistent with disc herniation. (From Mercier LR, Pettid FJ: *Practical orthopedics,* ed 4, St Louis, 1995, Mosby.)

Sensory changes, when present, are below the buttock and in the sole of the foot. Pressure on the nerve roots by a disc may involve the peroneal distribution above the ankle and the buttock itself. The condition is not common and may coexist with a prolapsed disc. The diagnosis of nerve entrapment is often missed initially and recognized only when sciatica persists after excision of the disc.

PROCEDURE

- To continue a differential after the straight-leg-raising test, the examiner fixes the patient's pelvis on the same side by pressing heavily with a hand on the region of the ipsilateral anterosuperior iliac spine and repeats this straight-leg-raising test (Fig. 8-100).
- Any undue pain experienced by the patient is associated with sciatic involvement resulting from a nerve root disorder, piriform spasm, or ischiotrochanteric groove adhesions (Fig. 8-101).
- Differentiation of piriformis spasm from other causes can be accomplished by reproducing the pain during internal rotation of the femur when it is at a lower level than the original point of pain.
- After a positive Lasègue test, the examiner may permit the leg to drop to the examination table without warning the patient (Fig. 8-102).
- If this Lasègue rebound test causes a marked increase in the back pain, sciatic neuralgia, and muscle spasm, then disc involvement is suspected.

Next Steps/Procedures

Bechterew sitting test, Bragard sign, Deyerle sign, Fajersztajn sign, Lasègue differential sign, Lasègue sitting test, Lasègue test, Lewin standing test, Lindner sign, Sicard sign, straight-leg-raising test, and Turyn sign

CLINICAL PEARL

The relationship of the lumbar roots and the lumbar discs is of major clinical importance. A massive posterior extrusion of one of the lumbar discs may severely injure the cauda equina (both intrathecal and extrathecal roots). Although these lesions are rare, they do occur. In these instances, the size and shape of the spinal canal and the size of the extruded mass are major factors in the severity of the clinical syndrome.

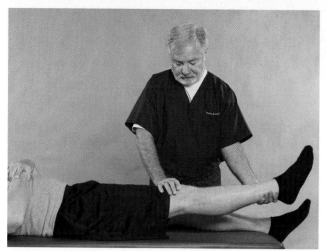

FIG. 8-100 The patient is in a supine position with both legs fully extended. The examiner performs a straight-leg-raising test on the affected leg.

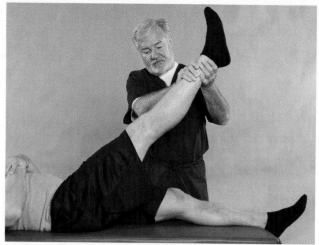

FIG. 8-101 The leg is elevated to the point at which pain is produced.

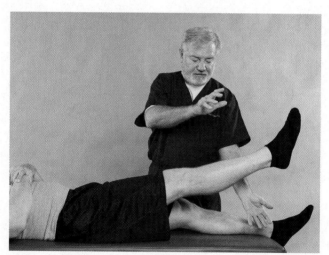

FIG. 8-102 Without warning, the examiner removes support from the elevated leg, allowing it to drop to the examination table. If the test causes marked increase in back pain, sciatic neuralgia, and muscle spasm, the test is positive. A positive test indicates disc involvement.

8

Assessment for Sciatic Nerve Inflammation

Comment

The lumbar spinal canal is bounded anteriorly by lumbar discs, vertebrae bodies, and the posterior longitudinal ligament; laterally by the lamina and facet joints; and posteriorly by the ligamentum flavum (Fig. 8-103).

The epidemiologic mechanism of lumbar spinal stenosis is unclear. The prevalence of narrowing of the lumbar spinal canal rises with increasing age. Midsagittal narrowing to less than 12 mm has been proposed as being probably pathologic and less than 10 mm unequivocally pathologic. Clinical recognition of the syndrome is very much age related, with few cases diagnosed in patients younger than 50 years.

The most characteristic symptom is neurogenic claudication. *Neurogenic claudication* is any discomfort that occurs in the buttock, thigh, or leg on standing or walking that is relieved by rest. Neurogenic claudication is not produced by peripheral vascular insufficiency.

Patients with neurogenic claudication primarily complain of pain radiating down the legs, as well as weakness, numbness, and tingling in the lower extremities. Given that pain is such a dominant component of neurogenic claudication, this syndrome must be distinguished from vascular claudication, which can be associated with similar complaints in a similar subset of patients. Vascular claudication differs from neurogenic claudication in several ways. Neurogenic claudication occurs with little or no exercise and, in some cases, with just standing. In contrast, vascular claudication typically requires some exertion on the part of the patient to

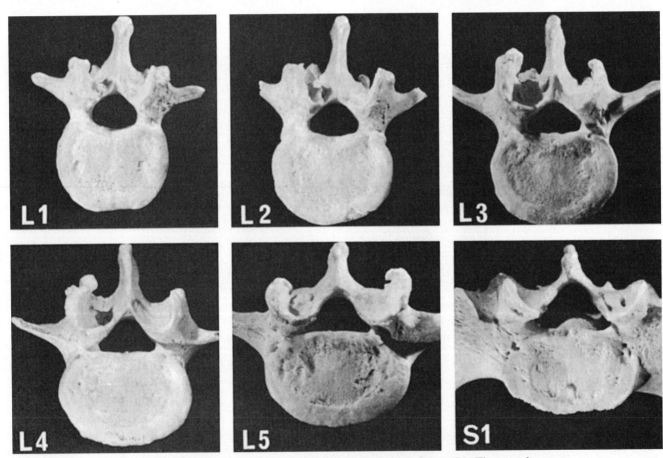

FIG. 8-103 The changing shape of the spinal canal from L1 to S1. The vertebrae are viewed from above. From L1 to S1, the spinal canal changes from an oval on its side to a more trefoil shape as the posterior wall of the vertebrae changes from concave to convex and the pedicles grow shorter and broader, migrate more laterally, and project more posterolaterally. (From Kirkaldy WH: *Managing low back pain*, ed 4, Philadelphia, 1999, Churchill Livingstone.)

ORTHOPEDIC GAMUT 8-19

ETIOLOGY OF NEUROGENIC CLAUDICATION PAIN

- Direct compressive forces on the nerves, particularly in the lateral recesses and foramina of the lumbar spinal canal, where the nerves exit
- Compromised blood supply to the nerve root as a result of the compression, leading to nerve pain similar to the muscular pain of vascular claudication
- Lack of nerve root nutrition resulting from stenosis-induced stagnation of cerebrospinal fluid

ORTHOPEDIC GAMUT 8-20

LUMBAR CANAL STENOSIS

Electromyographic (EMG) findings in lumbar canal stenosis include the following:

1. An entirely normal EMG
2. Absent H-reflex only, unilaterally or bilaterally
3. Denervation in a single root distribution (single radiculopathy), unilaterally or bilaterally and asymmetrically
4. Occurrence of bilateral and asymmetric lumbosacral radiculopathies, affecting the L5, S1, and S2 roots (the most common EMG finding associated with lumbar canal stenosis) (Table 8-17)

ORTHOPEDIC GAMUT 8-21

LUMBOSACRAL RADICULOPATHY

Electromyographic (EMG) limitations in lumbosacral radiculopathy are as follows:

1. If the dorsal root is the only root compressed, and if the ventral root is normal, then the EMG examination is normal. This scenario occurs in a significant number of patients whose symptoms are limited to pain or paresthesia or both. Thus a normal EMG does not exclude root compression.
2. Fibrillation potentials can be absent from the paraspinal muscles, particularly in chronic radiculopathies. This circumstance is likely caused by reinnervation. In contrast, fibrillation potentials can be present in the paraspinal muscles after lumbar laminectomy because of denervation during surgical exposure.
3. The lower-extremity sensory nerve action potentials (SNAPs) often are unevocable bilaterally in elderly patients. When this circumstance occurs, differentiating a preganglionic lesion (i.e., lumbosacral radiculopathy) from a postganglionic lesion (i.e., lumbosacral plexopathy) is often difficult, unless fibrillation potentials are evident in the paraspinal muscles.
4. No SNAPs have been devised to assess the L2 or L3 fibers up to the dorsal root ganglion, and the saphenous SNAP is not technically reliable (especially in elderly and obese patients) to assess the L4 fibers. Thus, separating an upper lumbar radiculopathy (especially L2 and L3) from lumbar plexopathy is often difficult unless fibrillations are present in the paraspinal muscles.

8

stress the blood supply to the musculature of the lower extremities. One of the key differences between the conditions is that standing and resting fail to relieve leg pain in neurogenic claudicators, whereas cessation of activity, regardless of posture or position, relieves the pain in the vascular group. Furthermore, the character of the pain may be described differently, with vascular claudication manifesting as a dull ache in a calf muscle, for example, whereas neurogenic claudication may describe more of a radicular pain radiating from the back or buttocks down the leg and into the calf or foot (Gerber et al, 2003).

Sciatica resulting from lumbar spinal stenosis is distinct from the sciatica that typically follows herniation of the nucleus pulposus. Objective neurologic signs are often absent. Restriction of straight leg raising (*Lasègue test*) is present in only 10% of cases of sciatica resulting from lumbar spinal stenosis. Deep-tendon reflexes at the ankle are absent in 40%, deep-tendon reflexes at the knee are absent in 10%, and a small percentage have sensory loss or weakness. A condition identical to meralgia paresthetica can be produced by stenosis at the upper lumbar levels.

Restless leg syndrome (RLS) produces a predominantly nocturnal discomfort that profoundly disturbs sleep and is relieved only by moving the legs either in bed or forcing the patient to arise and walk around to settle the discomfort. The cause of this condition is uncertain, but it has been attributed to lumbar spinal stenosis syndrome.

RLS is a sensorimotor disorder typically characterized by an uncomfortable feeling in the legs that leads to an urge to move. A recent large multinational survey in the primary care population indicated that RLS is a common cause of sleep disruption that remains undiagnosed in the primary care setting. The same survey reported that physicians often gave a wide range of diagnoses for RLS symptoms, including varicose veins or venous problems, back or spinal problems, neuropathy, and depression. In fact, only approximately 25% of patients with RLS symptoms were appropriately diagnosed (Allen, Earley, 2001).

Traumatic lumbar intervertebral disc prolapse is found in young adults who are most often men and usually employed in work that involves the lifting of heavy weights. Furniture movers, dockers, miners, truck drivers (who have to load

TABLE 8-17

ELECTROPHYSIOLOGIC DIFFERENTIATION OF CHRONIC S1/S2 RADICULOPATHY

	Chronic S1/S2 Radiculopathy	Tarsal Tunnel Syndrome	Peripheral Polyneuropathy
Nerve Conduction Studies			
Sural sensory study*	Normal	Normal	Usually abnormal
Peroneal motor study	Normal or low amplitude	Normal	Low amplitude, or slow latency, or both
Tibial motor study	Normal or low amplitude	Low amplitude, or slow	Low amplitude, or slow latency, or both
Motor conduction velocities	Normal or slowed	latency, or both	Slowed
Plantar studies*	Norma	Normal	Slow latencies or absent
H-reflex*	Abnormal	Slow latencies or absent	Abnormal
Upper extremity conductions	Normal	Normal	Can be abnormal
		Normal	
Needle EMG			
AH/ADQP	Denervated	Denervated	Denervated
EDB†	Denervated	Normal	Denervated
Medial gastrocnemius	Denervated	Normal	Denervated
Tibialis anterior	Normal	Normal	Denervated
Paraspinal muscles	Normal or fibs	Normal	Normal or fibrillations
Symmetry of findings (when bilateral)	Asymmetric	Asymmetric	Symmetric

ADQP, Abductor digiti quinti pedis; *AH,* abductor hallucis; *EDB,* extensor digitorum brevis; *EMG,* electromyography.
*Commonly absent in asymptomatic elderly subjects.
†May be denervated, selectively, in healthy subjects.
From Katirji B: *Electromyography in clinical practice: a case study approach,* St Louis, 1998, Mosby.

ORTHOPEDIC GAMUT 8-22

DISTINGUISHING FEATURES OF RESTLESS LEGS SYNDROME

- Onset at rest, restless leg syndrome is unrelated to body position or other activity and occurs when resting or lying down.
- The patient has an internal urge to move a body part, usually the limbs (not a spontaneous general body movement).
- Focal akathisia is relieved immediately (at least partially) by movement of the affected limb.
- Relief with movement persists as long as the limb is being moved.
- Symptoms may reoccur as soon as movement ceases.
- Usually, a time of day exists when symptoms are not present or are less severe, typically a circadian pattern when symptoms appear at the end of the day or at bedtime.
- No signs of disease are found in the affected limbs.

ORTHOPEDIC GAMUT 8-23

DIFFERENTIAL DIAGNOSIS FOR RESTLESS LEG SYNDROME*

- Neuropathic pain syndromes
- Peripheral neuropathy
- Arthritis
- Nocturnal leg cramps
- Restless insomnia
- Painful legs and moving toes
- Vascular insufficiencies
- Drug-induced akathisia

*Adapted from Allen RP, Earley CJ: Restless legs syndrome: a review of clinical and pathophysiologic features, *J Clin Neurophysiol* 18(2):128-147, 2001.

---

their own trucks), and medical and nursing workers are particularly vulnerable.

The patient develops acute pain in the back immediately after lifting a weight or unexpectedly bearing a heavy load, such as when the worker slips or helpers release their grip prematurely. The sudden force is taken by the flexed and rotated spine. The patient develops immediate, midline lumbar pain that is severe enough to stop motion. The patient is afraid to move and feels as if the back is locked by the pain.

The pain may extend into the leg in the sciatic distribution, and loss of nerve root function may occur. The pain is severe enough to drive the sufferer to bed after the first attack. Recumbency relieves the symptoms.

ORTHOPEDIC GAMUT 8-24

DIAGNOSTIC CRITERIA OF RESTLESS LEG SYNDROME*

Essential criteria:

1. Urge to move legs is usually accompanied or caused by uncomfortable or unpleasant sensations in the legs.
2. Urge to move or unpleasant sensation begins or worsens during periods of rest or inactivity.
3. Urge to move or unpleasant sensation is partially or totally relieved by movement as long as activity continues.
4. Urge to move or unpleasant sensation is worse in the evening or at night than during the day, or the urge occurs only during the evening or at night.

Supportive clinical features:

1. Positive family history
2. Response to dopaminergic therapy (>90%)
3. Periodic limb movements (during wakefulness or sleep)

Associated features:

1. Natural clinical course
2. Sleep disturbance
3. Medical or physical evaluation is generally normal

*Adapted from Ilen RP, Earley CJ: Restless legs syndrome: a review of clinical and pathophysiologic features, *J Clin Neurophysiol* 18(2):128-147, 2001.

PROCEDURE

- The patient is seated upright on the edge of a table with the legs dangling (Fig. 8-104).
- The examiner faces the patient and extends the patient's leg at the knee.
- The lower extremity from the hip to the foot is made parallel with the floor (Fig. 8-105).
- When radiculoneuropathy is not present, the patient should not experience discomfort from this action.
- Initially, the significance of the test is the same as the Lasègue test.
- However, the modification of performing the straight leg raise while the patient is in the seated position provides several advantages.
- In the supine position, straight leg raising may be difficult because the patient may squirm and shift the pelvis, making the leg abduct and rotate.
- The apprehensive patient may attempt to ward off anticipated pain and make the test positive sooner than is warranted.
- When the test is performed in the seated position, the patient faces the examiner, feels more secure and at ease, and is less likely to even know the part is being tested.
- The test has excellent objective values when the examiner is able to determine immediately the slightest attempt on the part of the patient to withdraw by leaning back from the induced pain.

Next Steps/Procedures

Bechterew sitting test, Bragard sign, Deyerle sign, Fajersztajn test, Lasègue differential sign, Lasègue rebound test, Lasègue test, Lewin standing test, Lindner sign, Sicard sign, straight-leg-raising test, and Turyn sign

8

CLINICAL PEARL

By raising the patient's foot, the examiner has performed a modified straight-leg-raising test. Because the thigh is already flexed to 90 degrees in this position, straightening the knee to the horizontal places stretching forces on the nerve roots. The results of this seated tension should correspond to the results obtained from the tests performed in the supine position.

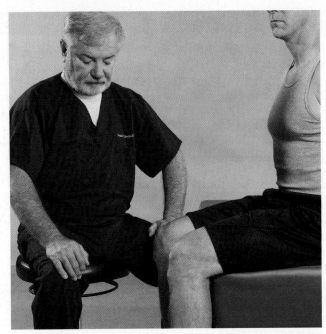

FIG. 8-104 The patient is seated with the legs hanging over the edge of the examination table.

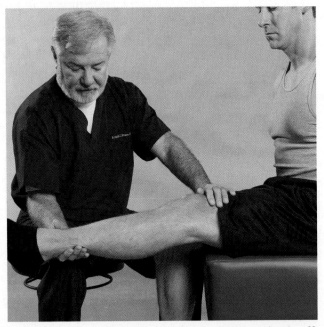

FIG. 8-105 The examiner faces the patient and extends the patient's affected leg at the knee. The lower extremity, from the hip to the foot, is brought up until parallel with the floor. Pain in the sciatic distribution is a positive finding. A positive test indicates radiculoneuropathy.

LASÈGUE TEST

ALSO KNOWN AS LASÈGUE SIGN

Assessment for Sciatica Resulting from Lumbosacral or Sacroiliac Lesions, Lumbar Subluxation Syndrome, Intervertebral Disc Lesion, Spondylolisthesis, Dural Sleeve Adhesions, or Intervertebral Foramen Occlusion (Encroachment)

Comment

A high percentage of adults older than 40 have degenerative disc disease at one or more levels on roentgenographic examination (Fig. 8-106). Significant thinning of the disc accompanied by osteophyte formation is often present. Degenerative changes in the adjacent facet joints and surrounding soft tissues often lead to intermittent LBP and even nerve root irritation.

A positive Lasègue test is the pain induced by stretching the sciatic nerve or one of its roots. The sign is elicited by gradual and slow extension of the knee of the elevated lower limb, which is performed while the patient is supine. The pain that is induced is similar to that felt spontaneously by the patient.

Every **nerve** must have the capacity to adapt to different positions by passive movement relative to the surrounding tissue. This capacity is provided by a gliding apparatus around the **nerve trunk.** The interfascicular epineurium provides another level of gliding that allows the fascicles to glide against one another. The clinical significance of the gliding apparatus in the context of external and internal neurolysis and nerve repair is discussed. An explanation is offered for the occurrence of the so-called meander-like deformity of fascicles, seen in nerve entrapment syndromes (Millesi, Zoch, Rath, 1990).

The nerve root glides freely through the IVF and during extension of the knee. The nerve roots are pulled out of the foramen for several millimeters at the L5 level.

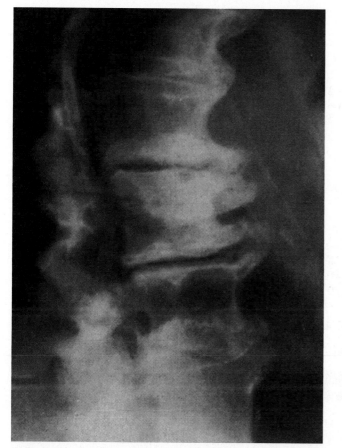

FIG. 8-106 Chronic degenerative disc disease. (From Mercier LR, Pettid FJ: *Practical orthopedics,* ed 4, St Louis, 1995, Mosby.)

ORTHOPEDIC GAMUT 8-25
LASÈGUE TEST

Interpretations of the Lasègue test:
1. When the patient is supine and the lower limbs are resting on the examination table, the sciatic nerve and its roots are under no tension.
2. When the lower limb is raised while the knees are flexed, the sciatic nerve and its roots are still under no tension.
3. If the knee is extended while the leg is elevated, the sciatic nerve, which must cover a longer distance, is subjected to increasing tension. In the normal patient, the nerve roots slide freely through the intervertebral foramen, and no pain results. When the lower limb is nearly vertical for people with diminished flexibility, pain is felt on the posterior aspect of the thigh as a result of stretching the hamstrings. However, this pain does not constitute a positive Lasègue sign.
4. When one nerve root is trapped in the foramen or when the root must cover a longer distance because of a prolapsed disc, any stretching of the nerve will become painful with moderate elevation of the lower limb. This result constitutes a positive Lasègue sign, which is evident before 60 degrees of flexion is attained. Pain may be elicited at 10, 15, or 20 degrees of flexion, which allows a rough quantification of the severity of the lesion.

ORTHOPEDIC GAMUT 8-26

PRECAUTIONS FOR LASÈGUE TEST

Two precautions to observe in performing Lasègue test:

1. The examiner must always elicit the Lasègue sign cautiously and stop when the patient feels pain.
2. The examiner must never attempt to elicit the Lasègue sign when the patient is under general anesthesia because the protective pain reflex is absent. The reflex can occur when the patient is being placed prone on an operating table and the hips are allowed to flex while the knees are extended. Hip flexion must always be associated with knee flexion, which relaxes the sciatic nerve and the trapped root.

One point deserves emphasis. During extension of the knee while the leg is elevated, the force of the traction on the nerve roots can reach 3 kg. The resistance to traction of the nerve roots is 3.2 kg.

If a root is trapped or shortened by a prolapsed disc, any rough manipulation of the leg can cause rupture of some axons and may result in paralysis. This condition is usually short lived, but it may occasionally take a long time to disappear.

PROCEDURE

- The patient lies supine with legs extended.
- The examiner places one hand under the ankle of the patient's affected leg and the other hand on the knee and flexes the thigh on the pelvis while the knee is flexed (Fig. 8-107).
- The examiner then slowly extends the patient's knee while the leg is elevated (Fig. 8-108).
- If this maneuver is markedly limited because of pain, the test is positive and suggests sciatica from lumbosacral or sacroiliac lesions, subluxation syndrome, disc lesions, spondylolisthesis, adhesions, or IVF occlusion.

Next Steps/Procedures

Bechterew test, Bragard sign, Deyerle sign, Fajersztajn test, Lasègue differential sign, Lasègue rebound test, Lasègue sitting test, Lewin standing test, Lindner sign, Sicard sign, straight-leg-raising test, and Turyn sign

---

CLINICAL PEARL

Whenever the presence of the Lasègue sign is questionable, the examiner should combine this test with flexion of the cervical spine *(Lindner sign)*. This combination places the greatest pull and stretch on the nerve roots behind the intervertebral discs and often elicits pain.

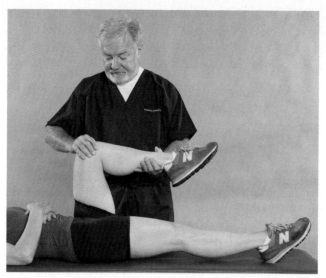

FIG. 8-107 The patient is supine, with both legs fully extended. The examiner places one hand under the ankle of the affected leg and the other hand at the knee. The hip and knee are both flexed to 90 degrees. The nerve roots are under no tension, and pain should not be elicited.

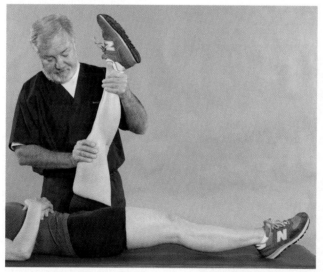

FIG. 8-108 The patient's knee is extended by the examiner. If this maneuver is limited by pain, the Lasègue test is positive. The positive test suggests sciatica from lumbosacral or sacroiliac lesions, subluxation syndrome, disc lesions, spondylolisthesis, adhesions, or interventricular foramen occlusion.

Assessment for Generalized Spinal Lesion or Intervertebral Disc Protrusion

Comment

A defect in the pars interarticularis with no forward displacement is termed *spondylolysis*. Defects can be dysplastic, isthmic, degenerative, traumatic, or pathologic. In Western world cultures, spondylolysis is believed to occur in approximately 6% of the population, with 80% to 90% of these defects occurring at the L5 level. Lumbosacral spine films with additional oblique views help the examiner investigate or confirm defects of the pars interarticularis (Fig. 8-109).

Upright posture and ambulation appear to have a role in its development because no known cases in nonambulatory patients have been found. Spondylolysis in newborns is virtually nonexistent, whereas its incidence by age 6 years is approximately 5%, close to that seen in the general population. Repetitive loading appears to be a likely contributing cause. The fact that hyperlordosis, such as seen in Scheuer-mann kyphosis, as well as sports such as diving, weight lifting, wrestling, and gymnastics, are associated with higher incidences of spondylolysis is well described. This theory is supported by biomechanical and structural studies. An increased familial incidence, as well as an association of spondylolysis and spina bifida occulta, appears to exist. This association may suggest a dysplastic component to the cause of spondylolysis. Certain populations also demonstrate a higher incidence of spondylolysis, including Alaskans (40% by adulthood) and Eskimos (13% in young patients and 54% of adults). Although spondylolysis has been reported to be more common in men than women, progression is more likely in women than men. This condition also has a lower incidence in African Americans than in Caucasians (Smith, Hu, 1999).

The symptomatic patient has LBP, which may radiate into the buttocks or leg. Early extension of the lumbar spine causes pain over the affected vertebra. Having the patient stand on the ipsilateral leg and extend the spine (*Jackson test*) is a unilateral weight-bearing posture in extension that usually evokes pain over the defect or fracture.

When compressed axially, the substance of the nucleus pulposus can stream out in various directions. If the annulus is still strong, the increase in pressure within the disc can cause the vertebral plateaus to give way. This circumstance corresponds to intravertebral prolapse.

The annulus fibers begin to degenerate after 25 years of age, allowing the tearing of fibers within each of its layers. Therefore, under axial stress, the nuclear material can stream out through the torn annulus. This streaming of nuclear material can be concentric but is more often radial.

Anterior prolapse is the rarest. Posterior prolapse is the most common, especially posterolateral prolapse. Thus, when the disc is crushed, part of the nuclear substance may stream out anteriorly, but it more often streams out posteriorly and can thus reach the posterior edge of the disc to touch the posterior longitudinal ligament. At first, the streamer, which is still attached to the nucleus, gets trapped under the posterior longitudinal ligament. When this event happens, bringing the streamer back into its fibrous casing is still possible by using vertebral traction. Very often, the streamer breaks through the posterior longitudinal ligament and may lie within the vertebral canal, which produces the so-called *free type* of disc prolapse. In other cases, the nuclear streamer is trapped under the posterior longitudinal ligament and gets nipped off by the annulus fibers, which precludes any restoration to normal because the fibers snap back into position. In some cases, the streamer, after reaching the deep aspect of the posterior longitudinal ligament, slides either superiorly or inferiorly. This situation is a case of subligamentous prolapse.

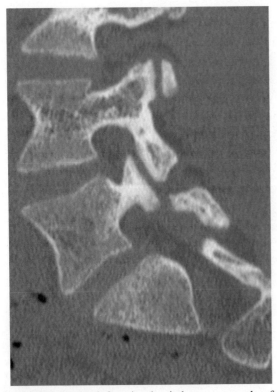

FIG. 8-109 Bony defect in the isthmus or neck of the Scottie dog in oblique view of spondylosis. (From Brier SR: *Primary care orthopedics*, St Louis, 1999, Mosby.)

Only when the herniating nucleus presses against the deep surface of the posterior longitudinal ligament can the nerve endings of the ligament be stretched, which causes LBP. Finally, compression of the nerve roots by the herniating disc causes nerve root pain, or sciatica.

PROCEDURE

- Punching the buttock produces a referred pain in the back.
- While the patient is standing, the examiner punches the side of the patient's buttock with the lesion (Fig. 8-110).
- If this punch elicits pain, the test is positive.
- Punching the opposite buttock should not elicit pain.
- The test is significant for a spinal lesion, usually involving a protruded disc.

Next Steps/Procedures
Antalgia sign, bowstring sign, Cox sign, heel/toe walk test, Kemp test, Lewin snuff test, Milgram test, and Neri sign

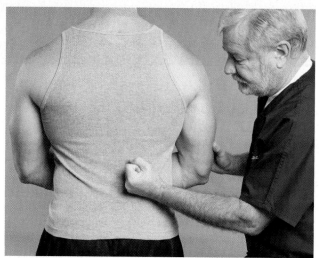

FIG. 8-110 While the patient is standing, the examiner firmly percusses the patient's buttock on the affected side. If the *punch* produces a referred pain in the back, the test is positive. Punching the opposite buttock does not produce pain. The positive test indicates a spinal lesion, usually a protruded disc.

8

CLINICAL PEARL

The sneeze produces a sudden Valsalva maneuver. If the examiner assumes that motion of an irritated nerve root over a disc bulge is one of the causes of pain, any production of a Valsalva effect abruptly increases the patient's pain as the defect appears and disappears and thereby moves the nerve root over the disc.

Assessment for Intervertebral Disc Rupture or Space-Occupying Mass

Comment

Tumors of the spinal canal are traditionally categorized as to location as follows: intramedullary, intradural, extramedullary, and extradural. With the exception of the rare primary bone tumor, MRI is the method of choice in evaluation of tumors of the spinal column. In intramedullary spinal cord lesions, myelography and CT myelography may demonstrate cord enlargement or contour irregularities. Intradural extramedullary tumors and extradural tumors are more completely demonstrated on MRI than on CT (Fig. 8-111 and Fig. 8-112).

Angiolipomas are benign tumors of mature adipose tissue containing abnormal vascular elements. They generally occur in the subcutaneous tissue of trunk and limbs. Spinal locations are rare, estimated to account for between 0.004% and 1.2% of all spinal axis tumors and 2% to 3% of extradural spinal tumors. Angiolipomas can be further categorized into two subtypes: noninfiltrating and infiltrating. The noninfiltrating type is more common and is usually well encapsulated. The infiltrating ones are rare, and partially or entirely unencapsulated, ill-defined, and infiltrate the surrounding tissues, especially the bone (Guzey et al, in press).

The most common extradural or bony neoplastic disease of the spine is metastatic disease, commonly involving bone marrow because of its rich vascularity. The lumbar spine is most commonly affected, followed by the thoracic and cervical spine. The most common primary tumors are breast, prostate, and lung.

Primary spinal tumors are relatively rare in children. They represent approximately 5% to 10% of CNS tumors within the pediatric age group. They are also relatively infrequent; the possibility of a spinal tumor as the cause of a child's complaints is often not considered until the clinical manifestations have progressed significantly (Loh et al, 2005).

In children, tumors of the spine are less common relative to intracranial tumors than in adults. The most common clinical presentation is limb weakness, which is usually spastic, but may be flaccid if the conus medullaris or the cauda equina is involved. The next most frequent symptom is back pain. The diagnosis of a spinal tumor in a child may be delayed by not in attention to these complaints. The incidence of neurologic findings varies in most series.

The intervertebral discs are not solid lumps of inert gristle, as patients often think, but rather are living structures that flatten during the day and reexpand at night. The discs consist of a firm nucleus pulposus surrounded by the annulus fibrosus, a ring of fibrocartilage, and fibrous tissue that links two vertebrae together. The disc is a symphysis between each pair of vertebrae and, with the two posterior facet joints, allows movement between the vertebrae.

The tension within the disc is maintained by fluid imbibition at the cellular level. If imbibition fails, the pressure within the disc falls, and the disc collapses. Increased movement occurs between the adjacent vertebrae, and the annulus fibrosus is exposed to increased stress. This condition is accompanied by vague LBP.

As the degeneration proceeds, the annulus fibrosus softens, and the degenerative disc bulges the annular ligament backward, usually just lateral to the midline. If this bulge occurs in a tight spinal canal opposite a nerve root, the function of the root is affected.

Of all lumbar disc protrusions, 90% involve the lowest two spaces, L4–L5 or L5–S1. Lesions that press on the L5 nerve root cause altered sensibility on the outer side of the calf and weakness of the peronei and ankle extensors, whereas those lesions affecting the S1 nerve root produce altered sensibility on the foot or back of the calf, weak ankle flexors, and a depressed ankle jerk. The resting muscle tone of the glutei, hamstrings, calf muscles, and other posterior muscle groups also may be reduced, and these muscles may atrophy.

Unless neurologic symptoms and signs below the knee are present, the patient probably does not have a true prolapsed intervertebral disc. If the disc presses on a nerve root, the postural reflexes work to diminish the pressure on the root. The spine is held curved to produce a sciatic scoliosis, and straight leg raising, which stretches the nerve, is restricted by pain.

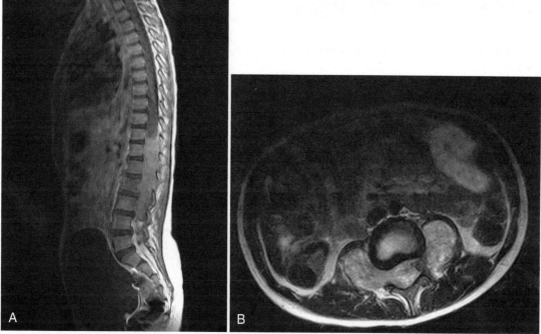

FIG. 8-111 A 4-year-old girl presented with a 3-month history of limping after a fall, back pain, and progressive left lower extremity pain that later became bilateral. She developed constipation and difficulty urinating over a few days, and finally inability to stand up or walk. Spinal magnetic resonance imaging. (A) Sagittal post-contrast T1-weighted image reveals abnormal marrow signal including L1–L3 vertebral bodies, and a soft tissue mass filling the spinal canal. (B) Axial T$_2$-weighted image at the level of L2/3 disc space reveals tumor extension through the neural foramina. (From Song X, Choi J, Rao C, et al: Primary ewing sarcoma of lumbar spine with massive intraspinal extension, *Ped Neurol* 38(1):58-60, 2008.)

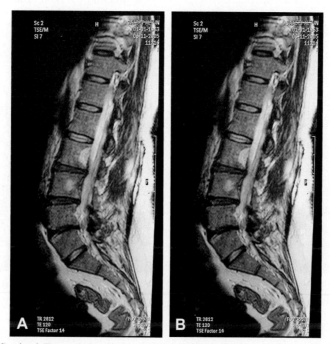

FIG. 8-112 Sagittal T1-weighted (A) and T2-weighted (B) magnetic resonance images demonstrates a spinal posteriorly located extradural tumor extending into the L2 and L3 vertebral bodies. (Adapted from Guzey FK, Bas NS, Ozkan N, et al: Lumbar extradural infiltrating angiolipoma: a case report and review of 17 previously reported cases with infiltrating spinal angiolipomas, *Spine J* 7[6]:739-744, 2007.)

PROCEDURE

- An aromatic substance is introduced, and the patient is instructed to sniff it up the nostril so as to induce sneezing (Fig. 8-113).
- The test is positive when sneezing elicits an exacerbation of well-localized spinal and radicular pain (Fig. 8-114).
- The test is significant for intervertebral disc rupture.

Next Steps/Procedures
Antalgia sign, bowstring sign, Cox sign, heel/toe walk test, Kemp test, Lewin punch test, Milgram test, and Neri sign

CLINICAL PEARL

In some instances of an acute attack, even light fist percussion over the lumbar spine in the midline will produce such severe accentuation of the local and radiating pain that the patient's knees may buckle. Some evidence of a vasovagal response may be found. In patients with spondylolysis or spondylolisthesis, hamstring tightness and the classic Phalen-Dickson sign—a knee-flexed, hip-flexed gait—may be demonstrated, regardless of degree of slippage. The mechanism for hamstring tightness is unclear, but it may be caused by nerve root irritation from the instability. For higher degrees of slip, the sacrum becomes more vertical so that the pelvis is more flexed and the hips cannot hyperextend enough to maintain upright posture. Therefore the patient must flex the knees to stand upright.

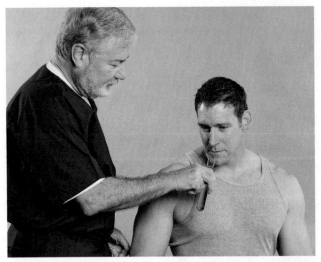

FIG. 8-113 The patient is introduced to a pungent, aromatic substance and instructed to inhale it through a nostril to induce sneezing or coughing.

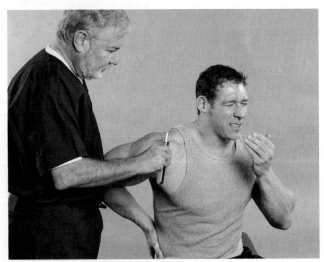

FIG. 8-114 The test is positive when sneezing or coughing elicits an exacerbation of well-localized spinal and radicular pain. The positive test indicates intervertebral disc rupture.

Assessment for Unilateral or Bilateral Hamstring Spasm

Comment

Rupture of a muscle is felt as a tearing sensation. Swelling and tenderness at the site of the rupture follow within hours, and bruising appears approximately 24 hours later. The bruising, which is caused by bleeding from the ends of the ruptured muscle, can be dramatic and even alarming.

During examination, a defect can be felt in the muscle belly, and the belly becomes prominent as the muscle contracts. The swelling can occasionally be mistaken for a soft-tissue mass. The rectus femoris and hamstrings are the muscles most often affected.

A hematoma in a muscle is a serious lesion that is sometimes called a *charley horse*. The lesion usually follows direct trauma or, more rarely, a tear of the central fibers of the muscle.

As the blood in the hematoma becomes organized, it interferes with normal muscle function. In some patients, the hematoma becomes ossified, which restricts muscle movement severely.

Muscle intolerance to exercise may result from different processes. Diagnosis involves confirming first the source of pain then potential pathologic myalgia. Delayed-onset muscle soreness (DOMS), commonly termed *tiredness,* occurs frequently in sports. DOMS usually develops 12 to 48 hours after intensive or unusual eccentric muscle action. Symptoms usually involve the quadriceps muscle group but may also affect the hamstring and triceps surae groups. The muscles are sensitive to palpation, contraction, and passive stretch. Acidosis, muscle spasm, and microlesions in both connective and muscle tissues may explain the symptoms. However, inflammation appears to be the most common explanation. Interestingly, strong evidence exists that the progression of the exercise-induced muscle injury proceeds no further in the absence of inflammation. Even though unpleasant, DOMS should not be considered as an indicator of muscle damage but rather a sign of the regenerative process, which is well known to contribute to the increased muscle mass. DOMS can be associated with decreased proprioception and range of motion, as well as maximal force and activation. DOMS disappears 2 to 10 days before complete functional recovery. This painless period is ripe for additional joint injuries (Coudreuse, Dupont, Nicol, 2004).

If a child has tight hamstrings that prevent flexion of the trunk or hip, spondylolisthesis should be suspected. Radiographs of the lumbosacral spine are essential in any child with tight hamstrings or calf muscles.

The sciatic nerve is considered to supply the posterior aspect of the hip and thigh.

The innervation to the short muscles of the hip and thigh (the obturator, sciatic, and sacral plexuses) also supplies the sensory branches from the hip joint capsule. The cutaneous branches around the hip originate at a higher level than the motor and capsular nerves. The LFCN that covers the anterolateral thigh is L2. The anterior of the thigh is covered by the continuation of the femoral nerve by L2 to L4, the upper portion of the thigh is covered by the iliohypogastric, and the buttocks are covered by the posterior primary division of T12 to L3 (Fig 8-115). Superficial cutaneous abnormality is referred from higher spinal levels.

Disorders of the iliohypogastric nerve are rare. The nerve may be involved in lower abdominal wall entrapment as a mononeuropathy by a suture or healing scar, resulting in severe disability. In addition, the nerve may be entrapped in a cartilaginous tunnel as it crosses over the iliac crest or damaged from retroperitoneal disease, surgical procedures involving abdominal wall incisions (e.g., appendectomy), inguinal hernia repair, cesarean section, nephrectomy or endoscopy, and from possible microtraumata caused by friction from belts and tight clothing pressing directly on the iliac crest. Lesions of the lateral cutaneous branch result in sensory loss or pain over the superolateral gluteal region.

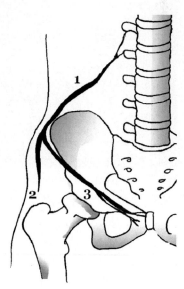

FIG. 8-115 Anatomy of the iliohypogastric nerve. 1 = Intra-abdominal course of the iliohypogastric nerve; 2 = Lateral cutaneous branch; 3 = Anterior cutaneous branch. (From Rabie M, Drory VE: A test for the evaluation of the lateral cutaneous branch of the iliohypogastric nerve using somatosensory evoked potentials, *J Neurolog Sci* 238(1-2):59-63, 2005.)

The anterior cutaneous branch causes a much more common clinical problem of lower abdominal pain and paresthesia on the involved side, radiating to the lower back (Rabie, Drory, 2005).

PROCEDURE

- The patient is standing.
- From behind, the examiner stabilizes the patient's pelvis with one hand while sharply pulling the knee on that side into extension (Figs. 8-116 and 8-117).
- The examiner then repeats this move on the opposite side and braces a shoulder against the patient's sacrum and sharply pulls both of the patient's knees into extension.
- The test is positive when pulling one or both knees into extension elicits pain that is followed by one or both knees snapping back into flexion.
- This positive finding represents unilateral or bilateral hamstring spasm.

Next Steps/Procedures

Bechterew sitting test, Bragard sign, Deyerle sign, Fajersztajn test, Lasègue differential sign, Lasègue rebound test, Lasègue sitting test, Lasègue test, Lindner sign, Sicard sign, straight-leg-raising test, and Turyn sign

CLINICAL PEARL

Tight or contracted hamstrings pull eccentrically on the pelvis. The patient with suspected tight hamstring disorder can be examined in the supine position. Keeping the hips and buttocks in contact with the table, straight-leg-raising is performed bilaterally. The comparison will indicate any hamstring contracture or tightness.

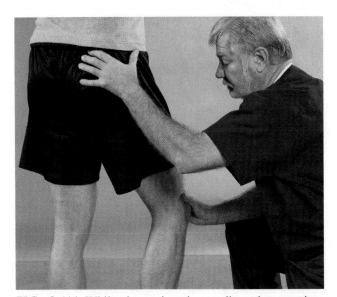

FIG. 8-116 While the patient is standing, the examiner stabilizes the patient's pelvis on the affected side with one hand.

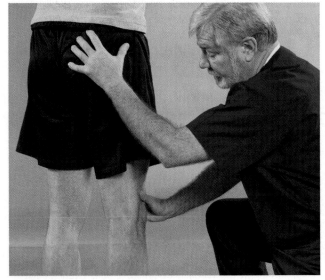

FIG. 8-117 The examiner then sharply pulls the knee of the patient's affected leg into extension. This maneuver is repeated on the unaffected side. Next, the examiner braces a shoulder against the patient's sacrum and pulls both knees sharply into extension. The test is positive if pulling the knee into extension causes pain and is followed by a snapping back, of either knee, into flexion. This positive finding represents unilateral or bilateral hamstring spasm, as seen in sciatic radiculopathy.

LEWIN SUPINE TEST

Assessment for Lumbar Arthritis, Lumbar Fibrosis, Spondylosis, Sacroiliac or Lumbosacral Arthrosis, or Sciatica

Comment

The cervical spine is frequently affected by rheumatoid arthritis (RA), and surgical treatment is sometimes required. The reported frequency of cervical involvement in RA varies from 25% to 90%, depending on diagnostic criteria. Furthermore, numerous reports have been published on surgical treatment for RA-related cervical disorders such as anterior atlantoaxial subluxation, vertical subluxation of the atlas, and subaxial subluxation. On the other hand, thoracic or lumbar involvement is rarely treated surgically, and little attention has been paid to this area clinically. Helliwell and colleagues reported that chronic back pain lasting more than 3 months occurred in 33% of patients with RA. Lawrence and colleagues, in a series involving patients with RA ages 55 to 64 years, found lumbar RA lesions in 5% of men and 3% of women (Sakai et al, in press).

Approximation of the spinous processes (kissing spines) and the development of a bursa between them have been indicated as a cause of LBP after hyperextension injuries. *Sprung back* is a term describing rupture of the supraspinous ligament after a sudden flexion strain applied to the spine with the pelvis fixed, as in falling on the buttocks with the legs outstretched (Fig. 8-118).

Normally, on flexion of the spine, the discal borders of the vertebral bodies become parallel above the level of L5. This extent is the maximal movement permitted. In the stage of segmental instability, excessive degrees of extension and flexion are permitted, and a certain amount of backward and forward gliding movement also occurs (Fig. 8-119). This abnormal type of movement can be shown clinically by roentgenograms taken with the patient holding the spine in full extension and in full flexion. Two radiologic changes are indicative of instability: the Knutsson phenomenon (vacuum sign) of gas in the disc and the *traction spur* (Fig. 8-120).

Lumbar spondylosis is a condition characterized by progressive degeneration of the intervertebral discs leading to changes of the adjacent vertebrae and ligaments and to OA.

Most patients with lumbar spondylosis are older than those with primary disc lesions. A chief symptom is LBP, which is often described as both generalized and specific aching, involving certain areas of point tenderness. Activity increases the discomfort, and rest eases it. Sciatic pain is rare. When present, sciatic pain is generalized, it involves

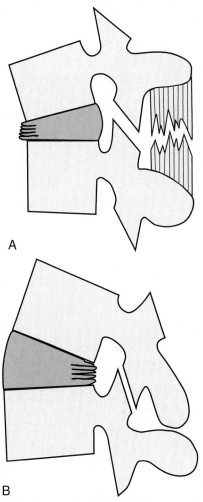

A

B

FIG. 8-118 **A,** Sprung back. **B,** Kissing spines. (From Torg JS, Shephard RJ: *Current therapy in sports medicine,* ed 3, St Louis, 1995, Mosby.)

ORTHOPEDIC GAMUT 8-27
DISC DEGENERATION

Observations in disc degeneration:
1. Disc degeneration may occur and may remain asymptomatic.
2. Disc degeneration may be associated with changes within the disc itself, which may produce pain.
3. Disc degeneration may give rise to mechanical instability that renders the spine vulnerable to trauma.

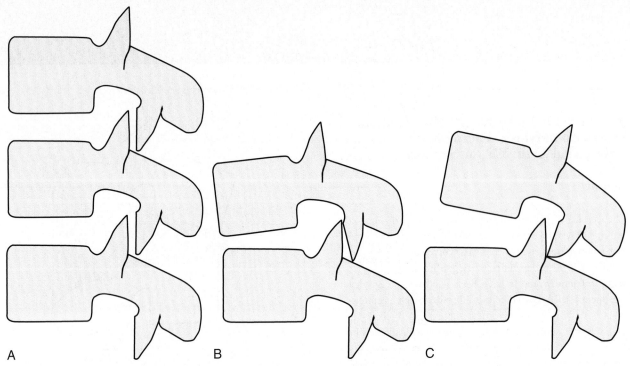

FIG. 8-119 Facet degeneration patterns. (From Torg JS, Shephard RJ: *Current therapy in sports medicine,* ed 3, St Louis, 1995, Mosby.)

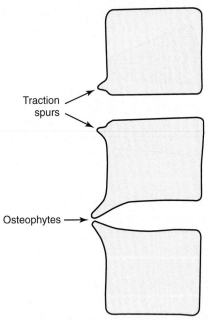

Traction spurs

Osteophytes

FIG. 8-120 The traction spur projects horizontally from the vertebral body approximately 1 mm away from the discal border. (From Torg JS, Shephard RJ: *Current therapy in sports medicine,* ed 3, St Louis, 1995, Mosby.)

one or both lower extremities, and it often reflects root compression at several levels.

Examination reveals moderate paraspinal muscle spasm in the lumbar region, with some limitation of the lumbar spine mobility in most movements. Extension is usually a bit more restricted than flexion. Some flattening of the normal lumbar lordosis is observed. A moderate paraspinal muscle spasm usually is present. Straight leg raising is not as painful with spondylosis as with a herniated lumbar disc. Deep-tendon reflex changes are elicited but are somewhat vague, which reflects nerve root compression at several levels.

The patient with lumbar spondylosis and a stenotic canal has a long history of intermittent LBP that is often related to specific positions and activities. The patient is often unable to sleep in a prone position, which tends to increase the lumbar lordosis. The patient is forced to sleep on a side with the hips and knees flexed to maintain a strong lumbar flexion.

With lumbar spondylosis accompanied by a stenotic lumbar spinal canal, the physical examination is unrevealing despite intermittent symptoms that are often severe. Flexion and straight leg raising are often performed without difficulty. Severe pain during lumbar extension may be the only positive result. RA must be included in the differential diagnoses (Tables 8-18 and 8-19).

Loss of periarticular bone is one of the classification criteria for RA, and it occurs early during the course of the disease. RA itself may contribute to bone loss, but generalized bone loss is multifactorial. Functional impairment and the duration of the illness have a negative effect on bone mineral density (BMD) in both axial and peripheral bone. Disease activity seems to be more prominently associated with functional capacity in early RA, while in later stages joint damage contributes more to incapacitation (Hamalainen et al, in press).

TABLE 8-18

THE LARSEN AND THE MODIFIED LARSEN RHEUMATOID ARTHRITIS GRADING SYSTEM

	Larsen system	Modified Larsen system Erosions		Joint space narrowing (JSN)
Grade 0	Intact bony outlines and normal joint space	Definitely no erosions "There is no doubt that there is no damage at all"	And/or	Definitely no JSN "There is no doubt that there is no damage at all"
Grade 1	Erosion less than 1 mm in diameter or joint space narrowing	Possible erosions "I am not sure whether what I am seeing is an erosion, and I could not assign this finding to either grade 0 or grade 2"	And/or	Possible JSN "I am not sure whether JSN is present even if I compare with neighboring joints and I could not assign this finding to either grade 0 or grade 2"
Grade 2	One or several small erosions	Definite, but moderate, erosions "I am sure that some damage is present, but I had to look extensively to come to this conclusion; it is definitely not striking"	And/or	Definite, but moderate, JSN "I am sure that some damage is present, but I had to look extensively to come to this conclusion; it is definitely not striking"
Grade 3	Marked erosions	Striking erosions, bony outlines at joint line more than 50% preserved. Damage is gross, visible at first glance, even from some distance. Definitely more than what grade 2 would be, but the joint line is intact"	And/or	Striking JSN, but both subchondral bony outlines still separated Damage is gross, visible at first glance, even from some distance. Definitely more than what grade 2 would be"
Grade 4	Severe erosions: there is usually no joint space left; the original bony outlines have been partly preserved	Severe erosions, bony outlines at joint lines less than 50% preserved. The joint appears completely destroyed, but a portion of the joint line is still intact	And/or	Complete JSN, subchondral bony outlines in contact
Grade 5	Mutilating changes: the bony outlines have been completely destroyed	Complete disorganization of the joint, bony outlines destroyed	And/or	Complete disorganization of the joint, bony outlines destroyed

The following joints are graded: five metacarpophalangeal joints, the interphalangeal joint of the thumb, four proximal interphalangeal joints, and four quadrants of the wrist on both sides, to give a total of 28 joints or sectors.

Either erosions or joint space narrowing must be present to assign to more than grade 1. If both are present, the worse finding is taken into account. Any amount of erosion or JSN associated with dislocation of the joint = grade 5. (Adapted from Zangger P, Kachura JR, Bombardier C et al: Assessing damage in individual joints in rheumatoid arthritis: a new method based on the Larsen system, *J Bone Spine* 71 (5):389-396, 2004.)

PROCEDURE

- While the patient is supine, the examiner supports the patient's legs on the table (Fig. 8-121).
- The patient is directed to sit up without using the hands (Fig. 8-122).
- The test is positive if the patient is unable to perform this action.
- A positive test is often associated with lumbar arthritis, lumbar fibrosis, degenerative disc thinning with protrusion, sacroiliac or lumbosacral arthritis, and sciatica.
- The patient is often able to localize the site of the complaint.

Next Steps/Procedures
Bilateral leg-lowering test, Demianoff sign, double leg-raise test, hyperextension test, matchstick test, Mennell sign, Minor sign, Nachlas test, Quick test, Schober test, sign of the buttock, skin pinch test, spinal percussion test, and Vanzetti sign

CLINICAL PEARL

The security and comfort of the back depend not only on the lumbar muscles and ligaments, but also on the strength of the abdominal wall and prevertebral muscles. The abdomen should be palpated to determine whether divarication of the rectus abdominis muscle is present. The clinical test for diagnosis of rectus divarication involves instructing the supine patient to raise the head from the examination table. The examining hand can easily feel the gap between the contracted pillars of the rectus, and the fingers will sink into the soft abdominal wall. The width of the gap may vary from 1 cm to a hand's breadth.

TABLE 8-19

LUMBAR SPINAL RHEUMATOID ARTHRITIS LESION GRADES

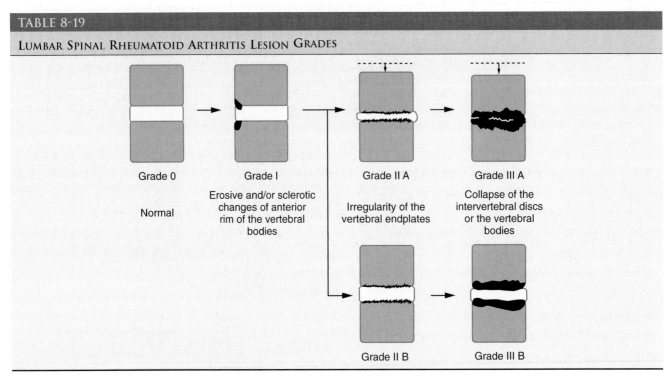

Grades II and III are further divided into two types. Type A includes grade IIA (presence of disc narrowing) and grade IIIA (disc space collapsed and vertebral bodies fused), and type B includes grade IIB (absence of disc narrowing) and grade IIIB (vertebral body collapsed but intervertebral disc remains or appears ballooned).

From Sakai T et al: Radiological features of lumbar spinal lesions in patients with rheumatoid arthritis with special reference to the changes around intervertebral discs, *Spine J* 8[4]:605-611, 2008.)

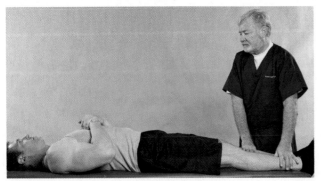

FIG. 8-121 The patient is supine, with both legs fully extended. The examiner firmly applies downward pressure to the patient's legs.

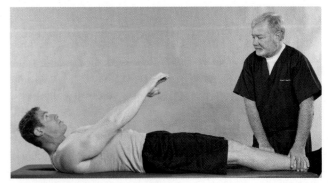

FIG. 8-122 The patient is directed to sit up without using the hands. The test is positive if the patient is unable to perform this action. A positive test indicates lumbar arthritis, lumbar fibrosis, a degenerative disc with protrusion, sacroiliac or lumbosacral arthritis, or sciatica. The patient is often able to localize the site or origin of the pain.

LINDNER SIGN

Assessment for Lumbar Nerve Root Irritation or Inflammation

Comment

Before the development of signs and symptoms compatible with a diagnosis of a herniated lumbar disc, most patients have previously experienced LBP and other symptoms, which in retrospect can be related to the ensuing disc syndrome. In many instances, the preexisting LBP is not severe and does not cause impairment. When the back pain becomes associated with pain radiating down the course of the sciatic nerve, the possibility of lumbar disc disease should be seriously considered. Position is usually a factor in intensifying or decreasing the pain.

Most patients report that weight bearing, prolonged standing, walking, and sometimes sitting aggravate the pain. Resting in bed eases the pain. Symptoms may be aggravated by coughing, sneezing, or straining at the stool. Physical activity aggravates the pain, particularly flexion activities or postures.

Spinal nerve roots are subjected to tensile strains in various traumatic, as well as pathologic conditions. In clinical situations, spinal nerve roots may be subjected to tension during disk protrusion, disk herniation, foraminal stenosis, and nerve root avulsion injuries that lead to the development of edema and demyelination, subsequently causing radicular pain, paresthesias, numbness, and loss of motor control. Several surgical diseases of the spinal column have also been known to cause tension on the spinal nerve roots. Congenital abnormalities such as spina bifida occulta have been known to induce traction on the spinal nerve roots and the spinal cord. Additionally, intradural spinal tumors may induce stretch on the spinal nerve roots on one or both sides, often causing bilateral hyperesthesias. These and various other conditions of the spine induce tension on the nerve roots at low strain rates (Singh, Lu, Chen, 2006).

Whenever the straight-leg-raising test produces a questionable result of pain, it should be combined with flexion of the cervical spine (Lindner's sign). This combination places pull and stretch on the nerve roots behind the intervertebral disc and often elicits pain. The simultaneous flexion of the neck and elevation of the contralateral leg can produce pain in the ipsilateral sciatic notch in patients with either free fragments or herniated discs. Raising the contralateral leg alone might not elicit pain in either leg.

The various nerve roots, when compressed by the protruding disc, produce characteristic signs and symptoms. Nerve roots, similar to other viscoelastic materials, are strain rate dependent and exhibit higher tensile stress at higher strain rates.

ORTHOPEDIC GAMUT 8-28

UNILATERAL DISC HERNIATION BETWEEN L3 AND L4

Unilateral disc herniation between L3 and L4 usually compresses the fourth lumbar root as it crosses the disc before exiting at the L4 intervertebral foramen with the following results:

1. Pain may be localized around the medial side of the leg.
2. Numbness may be present over the anteromedial aspect of the leg.
3. The quadriceps and hip adductor group, both innervated from L2, L3 and L4, may be weak and, in extended ruptures, atrophic.
4. Reflex testing may reveal a diminished or absent patellar tendon reflex (L2, L3, and L4) or tibialis anterior tendon reflex (L4).
5. Sensory testing may show diminished sensibility over the L4 dermatome, the isolated portion of which is the medial leg, and the autonomous zone, which is at the level of the medial malleolus.

ORTHOPEDIC GAMUT 8-29

UNILATERAL DISC HERNIATION BETWEEN L4 AND L5

Unilateral disc herniation between L4 and L5 results in compression of the fifth lumbar root with the following results:

1. Fifth lumbar root radiculopathy should produce pain in the dermatomal pattern.
2. Numbness, when present, follows the L5 dermatome along the anterolateral aspect of the leg and the dorsum of the foot, including the great toe.
3. The autonomous zone for this nerve is the first web of the foot and the dorsum of the third toe. Weakness may involve the extensor hallucis longus (L5), gluteus medius (L5), or extensor digitorum longus and brevis (L5).
4. Reflex change is not usually found.
5. A diminished tibialis posterior reflex is possible but difficult to elicit.

ORTHOPEDIC GAMUT 8-30

UNILATERAL DISC HERNIATION BETWEEN L5 AND S1

In a unilateral disc herniation between L5 and S1, the findings of an S1 radiculopathy are noted as follows:

1. Pain and numbness involve the dermatome of S1.
2. The S1 dermatome includes the lateral malleolus and the lateral and plantar surface of the foot, occasionally including the heel.
3. Numbness is present over the lateral aspect of the leg and, more important, over the lateral aspect of the foot, including the lateral three toes.
4. The autonomous zone for this root is the dorsum of the fifth toe.
5. Weakness may be demonstrated in the peroneus longus and brevis (S1), gastrocnemius-soleus (S1), or gluteus maximus (S1).
6. In general, weakness is not a usual finding in S1 radiculopathy.
7. Occasionally, mild weakness may be demonstrated by asymmetrical fatigue with exercise of these motor groups.
8. The ankle jerk usually is reduced or absent.

PROCEDURE

- Passive flexion of the patient's head onto the chest can be accomplished in a supine, seated, or standing position (Figs. 8-123 and 8-124).
- If pain occurs in the lumbar spine and along the sciatic nerve distribution, the test is positive and, according to Lindner, is an indication of root sciatica (Figs. 8-125 and 8-126).

Next Steps/Procedures

Bechterew sitting test, Bragard sign, Deyerle sign, Fajersztajn test, Lasègue differential sign, Lasègue rebound test, Lasègue sitting test, Lasègue test, Lewin standing test, Sicard sign, straight-leg-raising test, and Turyn sign

CLINICAL PEARL

Flexion of the head to the chest increases the traction of the nerve root against the disc bulge. When the disc is a contained disc, in which the annulus is not ruptured, the flexion or maintenance of a flexed position of the trunk obliterates the disc bulge. Motion of an irritated nerve root over a bulging disc is often the source of the patient's back and leg pain. Relief of pain with trunk flexion occurs only because the disc bulge has disappeared.

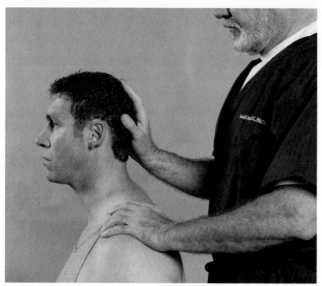

FIG. 8-123 The patient is seated with the arms in a comfortable position.

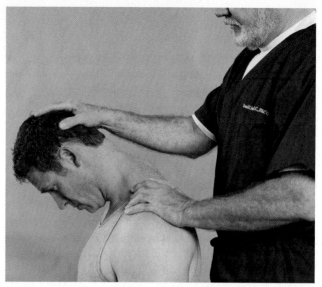

FIG. 8-124 The examiner passively flexes the patient's head onto the chest. If pain occurs in the lumbar spine and the sciatic nerve distribution, the test is positive. A positive test is an indication of root sciatica.

8

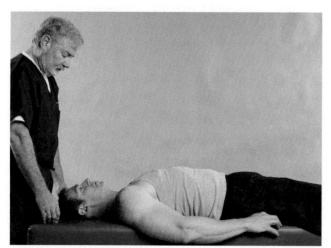

FIG. 8-125 A supine version of this test can also be performed.

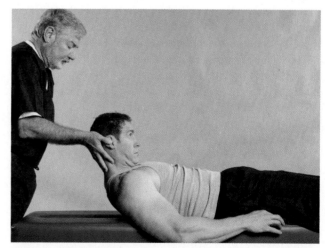

FIG. 8-126 For the supine version, the head is passively flexed toward the chest. If pain occurs in the lumbar spine and the sciatic nerve distribution, the test is positive. A positive test is an indication of root sciatica. This result should be differentiated from Brudzinski sign and the Soto-Hall maneuver. These tests are similar but have slightly different significance.

Assessment for Denervation Hypersensitivity

Comment

Many cases of acute LBP that are not correctly identified evolve into a chronic spinal problem with significant disability at the muscular level (Table 8-20). Patients with muscular dysfunction of the lumbar spine can have varying types of clinical findings and case histories.

The sensory distribution of each nerve root, or dermatome, varies from person to person, and overlap is often present. A *dermatome* is the area of skin supplied by a single nerve root.

The examiner must also be aware of the sensory, motor, and sympathetic distribution of peripheral nerves to be able to differentiate between lesions of the nerve roots and peripheral nerves.

Pressure on a peripheral nerve resulting in a neurapraxia leads to temporary nonfunctioning of the nerve. This type of injury is associated with primarily motor involvement. Pressure on a nerve root leads to a loss of tone and muscle mass. Spinal nerve roots have a poorly developed epineurium and lack a perineurium, which makes the nerve root more susceptible to compressive forces, tensile deformations, chemical irritants (e.g., alcohol, lead, arsenic), or metabolic abnormalities. For example, diabetes may cause a metabolic peripheral neuropathy of one or more nerves.

In peripheral nerves, the epineurium consists of a loose areolar connective tissue matrix surrounding the nerve fiber that allows changes in growth length of the bundled nerve fibers (funiculi) without allowing the bundles to be strained.

The perineurium protects the nerve bundles by acting as a diffusion barrier to irritants and provides tensile strength and elasticity to a nerve.

In the past, many names have been given to the condition now known universally as CRPS or reflex sympathetic dystrophy (RSD). Because this condition may follow trauma, it is called *posttraumatic pain syndrome.*

RSD consists of an extremity with (1) burning or causalgic pain, (2) limitation of motion, (3) edema with or without pitting, (4) dystrophic skin changes, (5) vasomotor phenomena, and (6) patchy osteoporosis on x-ray examination. This disease is rare in adolescents, but of patients with RSD,

---

TABLE 8-20

SITES OF LUMBOPELVIC SOFT-TISSUE SYNDROMES/ MYOFASCIAL TRIGGER POINTS

Diagnosis	Site of Complaint
Quadratus lumborum syndrome	Gluteal region, anterior iliac spine, greater trochanter of femur
Gluteus maximus or medius syndrome	Sacral and gluteal region, lateral hip
Gluteus minimus syndrome	Lateral hip, thigh, and calf
Chronic lumbar strain (spinal erector muscles)	Laterally to ribs, caudally toward lumbosacral junction
Piriformis syndrome	Sacroiliac region; posterior hip, thigh, calf; possibly sole of foot

Adapted from Brier SR: *Primary care orthopedics,* St Louis, 1999, Mosby.

ORTHOPEDIC GAMUT 8-31

MUSCLE SYNDROMES OF THE LUMBOPELVIC SPINE

Common findings in muscle syndromes of the lumbopelvic spine are as follows:

1. Hip inflexibility, especially hamstring and psoas insufficiency
2. Weakness of the hip and spine extensor mechanism
3. Intersegmental lumbosacral fixation
4. Myofascial trigger points in the spinal erector, quadratus lumborum, gluteal musculature, and psoas muscles
5. Referred zones of pain to the hip, buttocks, thigh, and lateral lower leg
6. Severe tightness of the outward rotators of the hip
7. Muscle hypertonicity
8. Palpable tenderness with pressure or stretch
9. Taut, tender, or ropelike muscle fibers

ORTHOPEDIC GAMUT 8-32

MIXED MOTOR PERIPHERAL NERVE LESION

Effects of a mixed motor (motor, sensory, and sympathetic) peripheral nerve lesion:

1. Flaccid paralysis (motor)
2. Loss of reflexes (motor)
3. Muscle wasting and atrophy (motor)
4. Loss of sensation (sensory)
5. Trophic changes in the skin (sensory), loss of secretions from sweat glands (sympathetic)
6. Loss of pilomotor response (sympathetic)

up to 8% are between 11 and 19 years of age (Buchta, 1983).

The most important clinical finding in RSD is pain. However, the distinguishing feature of the pain in RSD is its severity. The degree of pain is completely out of proportion to the inciting trauma. The nature of the pain varies widely, but early in the condition, the pain is usually described as burning or stinging. Later, the pain is often described as a pressure or cutting pain that becomes constant and unrelenting. Motion severely aggravates the pain, and nearly a complete cessation of voluntary movement of the involved part occurs. Although the pain may start in one area, it rapidly spreads to adjacent sites and eventually involves the entire extremity. In untreated severe cases, the pain progresses to the point that the patient may request amputation of the affected part or even consider suicide. The pain is made markedly worse by attempting active or passive movement of the joints. Severe and excruciating paresthesia may be produced by lightly stroking the skin, even in uninjured areas (Fig. 8-127). Tenderness is always present and is much more severe than one would normally expect.

CRPS-I (previously known as RSD) typically develops after minor trauma with no obvious or a small nerve lesion (e.g., bone fracture, sprains, bruises, skin lesions, surgery). CRPS-I can also develop after remote trauma in the visceral domain or even after a CNS lesion (e.g., stroke). Important features of CRPS-I are that the severity of symptoms is disproportionate to the severity of trauma and that the pain has a tendency to spread distally in the affected limb. The symptoms are not confined to the innervation zone of an individual nerve. Thus all symptoms of CRPS-I may be present irrespective of the type of the preceding lesion. Furthermore, the site of the lesion at the limb does not determine the location of symptoms. CRPS-II (previously known as causalgia) develops after a large nerve lesion (Janig, Baron, 2003).

Although pain is the most prominent symptom, swelling is the most common physical finding. The swelling usually starts in the area of greatest involvement, but it soon spreads proximally and distally to the immediate adjacent areas of the extremity. The swelling is soft initially but turns to brawny edema if the condition persists. The brawny edema often gets so severe that it acts as a mechanical block to motion. This fixed edema eventually gives way to periarticular thickening and to fibrous tendon adhesions. Elevation of the extremity is most effective in reducing swelling when used early in the disease, but this elevation is beneficial any time.

Metabolic changes form an important part of any neurologic disorder and may occur in the skin, nails, subcutaneous tissues, muscles, bones, and joints. In addition to a neuro-

8

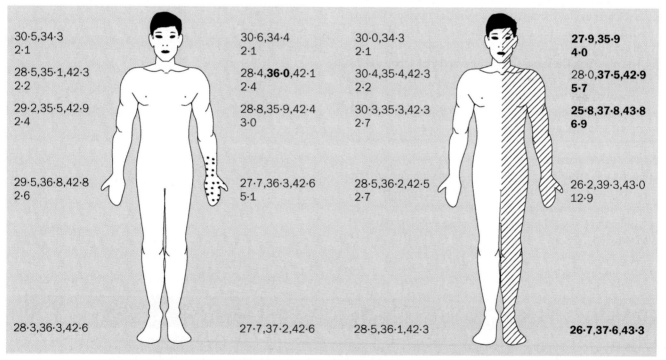

FIG. 8-127 Detection thresholds to cold, warm, and heat stimuli (upper numbers [°C]) and to von Frey filament stimulation (lower rows [g/mm²]) in patients with CRPS I and sensory impairment spatially restricted to the affected limb (left) and in CRPS I patients with generalized sensory impairment (right). Numbers reflect mean values. (Modified from Rommel O, Malin JP, Zenz M, et al: Quantitative sensory testing, neurophysiological and psychological examination in patients with complex regional pain syndrome and hemisensory deficits, *Pain* 93:279-293, 2001. In Janig W, Baron R: Complex regional pain syndrome: mystery explained? *Lancet Neurol* 2[11]:687-697, 2003.)

logic basis, factors such as activity, blood supply, and lymph drainage are involved in the causation of trophic changes. When a peripheral nerve is completely interrupted, the skin loses its delicate indentations and becomes inelastic, smooth, and shiny. When interruption is partial, trophedema occurs. Gradual fibrosis of the subcutaneous tissue occurs, and the overlying skin becomes fissured and prone to heavy folds. This alteration in the quality of the skin produces a *peau d'orange* effect similar to that described for malignant lumps in the female breast. This circumstance is accentuated when the skin is gently squeezed together or when the back is fully extended.

> The idea that patients with CRPS-I have inflammatory processes in the affected region, in particular in the deep somatic tissues including bones, goes back to Sudeck, who believed that this syndrome is an inflammatory bone atrophy (*entzündliche knochenatrophie*). Accordingly, bone scintigraphy revealed periarticular tracer uptake in acute CRPS and synovia biopsies and scintigraphic investigations with radiolabelled immunoglobulins showed protein extravasation, hypervascularity and neutrophil infiltration (Janig, Baron, 2003).

PROCEDURE

- Trophedema is nonpitting to digital pressure. However, when a blunt instrument, such as the end of a matchstick or cotton-tip applicator is used, the indentation produced is clear cut and persists for several minutes, which is distinctly longer than such an indentation would persist in normal skin (Fig. 8-128).
- The matchstick test may be positive and yield deep indentations over an extensive area (commonly over the lower back and hamstrings), or, in mild cases, the test may yield only slight indentations of skin overlying a tender motor point or the neurovascular hilus.

Next Steps/Procedures
Bilateral leg-lowering test, Demianoff sign, double-leg-raise test, hyperextension test, Lewin supine test, Mennell sign, Minor sign, Nachlas test, Quick test, Schober test, sign of the buttock, skin pinch test, spinal percussion test, and Vanzetti sign

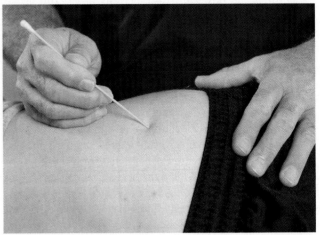

FIG. 8-128 The patient may be in either the prone or the side-lying position. The examiner applies the blunt end of a cotton-tipped applicator to the affected area of skin. The indentations produced are clear-cut and persist for several minutes, which is distinctly longer than when the test is performed on normal skin. The matchstick test is positive if it yields deep indentations over an extensive area (commonly over the lower back and hamstrings) or, in mild cases, if it yields slight indentations of skin overlying a tender motor point or the neurovascular hilus. A positive test is associated with denervation supersensitivity, as seen with a lumbar sprain.

CLINICAL PEARL

Complex regional pain syndrome (CRPS) can occur in any disease that produces pain. This type of dystrophy is a likely secondary condition after 4 months of unrelenting pain from the primary disorder. The earliest sign, other than the symptoms of burning or stinging pain, is localized trophedema. The matchstick test can be applied to any cutaneous area of pain because the test is sensitive to the earliest changes in fluid management in the skin by the sympathetically operated cutaneous vascularity. The result of this test becomes the earliest warning sign of the advancing CRPS type I. An intervertebral disc syndrome with protracted nerve root compression is a common onset mechanism.

MENNELL SIGN

Assessment for Pathologic Involvement of the Sacroiliac Joint Structures

Comment

Blunt pelvic trauma accounts for approximately 10% of all traumatic injuries, occurring at an annual rate of 20 pelvic fractures per 100,000 individuals. Most patients are younger than 40 years, and the incidence is increasing. Although most patients with pelvic injuries annually in the United States have no overt urinary tract injury, disruption of neurovascular and ligamentous structures essential to sexual, urinary, and bowel function might result in impairment that only becomes manifest subsequent to initial hospitalization. The World Health Organization predicts that road traffic accidents will be the third most common cause of disability worldwide by the year 2020, and pelvic fracture associated urologic complications will contribute to this disease burden. Dyspareunia and incontinence in women and erectile dysfunction in men have been reported after pelvic fracture. Pubic diastasis, residual fracture displacement, urethral injury, and patient age are factors associated with dysfunction (Wright et al, 2006).

Fat nodules located on the fascia over muscle or bone may be painful when direct pressure is applied or trunk bending occurs. The aching and radicular sensation that occurs when the nodule is palpated is readily identified with the painful mass. All pain is temporarily relieved with topical anesthesia of the mass.

The panniculitides are a group of heterogeneous inflammatory diseases involving the subcutaneous fat. Classically, the study of the panniculitides has been considered diagnostically challenging for both dermatologists and dermatopathologists for several reasons. First, from clinical point of view, the lesions show a disappointing monotony, and very

different processes involving the subcutaneous fat have the same morphologic features characterized by erythematous nodules generally located on the lower limbs. In addition to this clinical unspecificity, the lesions are located deep in subcutaneous tissue, and large excisional biopsies through subcutaneous fat must be performed for diagnosis. From a histopathologic point of view, the panniculitides, as with other inflammatory diseases of the skin, constitute dynamic processes in which both the composition and the distribution of the inflammatory infiltrate cells change within the course of a few days, and biopsies are often taken from late-stage lesions because of inadequate clinicopathologic correlation. These biopsies usually show nonspecific findings. Furthermore, some authorities believe that "the histologic septal-lobular dichotomy is sometimes diagnostically useful, but more often there is a mixed picture that adds to interpretative difficulties" (Requena, 2007)

The findings obtained are different from those associated with nerve root radiculopathy, but they are easy to confuse. All tender areas in the buttock are not fat nodules. Many tender areas may represent pain referral from an irritated nerve root. For example, a nerve root ganglion or cyst may cause pain in the buttock that is similar to that which occurs with a painful fat nodule that is more proximal.

Fourteen local areas have been identified in which tenderness during palpation is very constant in certain conditions.

Five areas on each side of the back should be examined, one in each buttock and one in the back of each thigh.

S1 radiculopathy is common and is difficult to differentiate from S2 radiculopathy because their myotomal representations overlap almost completely. As with the L5 root, the segmental distribution of the S1 root is diffuse, with both proximal and distal muscle representation.

As with other lumbosacral radiculopathies, bilateral S1 or S2 radiculopathies are relatively common, and most are chronic. Because the symptoms are usually bilateral and involve the feet predominantly, these cases imitate a peripheral polyneuropathy or bilateral tarsal syndromes.

Differentiating these three entities requires meticulous electromyographic examination and is difficult, especially in elderly patients. When typical findings are absent, Tarlov cysts should be considered in the differential diagnoses (Fig. 8-129).

Tarlov's initial descriptions of perineurial cysts were localized primarily to the posterior sacral or coccygeal nerve roots, most often the second or third sacral roots. On very rare occasions, these cysts were also observed in the thoracic spine. These cysts generally occur at the junction of the posterior root and the dorsal ganglion and are located between the perineurium and endoneurium. They are filled

---

ORTHOPEDIC GAMUT 8-33

SACROILIAC PAIN

The radicular component of sacroiliac pain is referred pain similar to pain associated with:

1. The painful tendon attachment
2. Periosteal pain
3. The deep aching associated with compression of a small blood vessel
4. The irritation of a sensory nerve penetrating the fascia
5. Straight leg raising that may be uncomfortable but not radicular

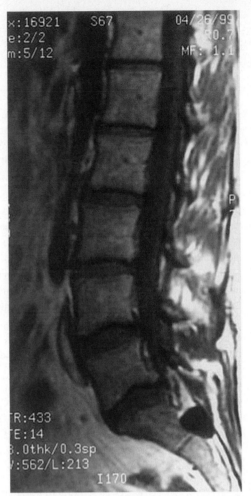

FIG. 8-129 Tarlov cyst within the sacral canal at level S2, with compression of adjacent nerve root. (Adapted from Nadler SF, Bartoli LM, Stitik TP, et al: Tarlov cyst as a rare cause of S1 radiculopathy: A case report, *Arch Phys Med Rehab* 82(5):689-690, 2001.)

with CSF and are static in size. Histologic examination reveals an outer wall composed of vascular connective tissue, and the inner wall is lined with flattened arachnoid. Part of the lining contains nerve fibers and occasionally ganglion cells (Nadler et al, 2001).

PROCEDURE

- The examiner places a thumb over the patient's posterior-superior iliac spine (PSIS), exerts pressure, slides the thumb outward, and then slides it inward (Figs. 8-130 and 8-131).
- The sign is positive if tenderness is increased.
- This result is significant if, when sliding outward, sensitive deposits in structures on the gluteal aspect of the PSIS are noted (Fig. 8-132).
- If, when sliding inward, tenderness is increased, this is a significant result for strain of the superior sacroiliac ligaments.
- Confirmation can be made if tenderness is increased when the examiner posteriorly pulls the anterior-superior iliac spine (ASIS) while standing behind the patient or when the examiner pulls the PSIS forward while standing in front of the patient.
- This test is helpful in determining that tenderness is caused by strained superior sacroiliac ligaments.
- A positive result indicates deposits in the structure or adjacent to the structure of the sacroiliac joint.
- These deposits are the result of ligamentous strain or sprain.

Next Steps/Procedures

Bilateral leg-lowering test, Demianoff sign, double leg-raise test, hyperextension test, Lewin supine test, matchstick test, Minor sign, Nachlas test, Quick test, Schober test, sign of the buttock, skin pinch test, spinal percussion test, and Vanzetti sign

CLINICAL PEARL

This method of tissue examination provides pertinent information, providing the results are accurately interpreted. Palpation of the lumbosacral region, with the patient in either the erect or the prone position, may evoke tender areas in the midline, at the level of the disc lesion, and in the paravertebral area on the side of the nuclear extrusion. The ability to elicit tenderness along the iliac crest or even over the posterior aspect of the sacroiliac joint on the side of an irritated nerve root is not uncommon.

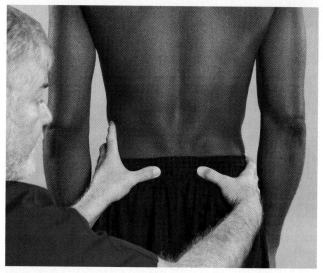

FIG. 8-130 The patient is standing. The examiner places a thumb over the posterior-superior iliac spine on the affected side and exerts pressure.

ORTHOPEDIC GAMUT 8-34

LUMBOPELVIC TENDERNESS

Common areas of palpable lumbopelvic tenderness:

1. Medial to the posterior-superior iliac spine is the most superficial posterior ligament of the sacroiliac joint. Tenderness here suggests a pathologic condition involving the sacroiliac joint.
2. Lateral to the posterior-superior iliac spine is the puny part of the gluteal muscle origin that may be torn by minor trauma. Tenderness here suggests a pathologic condition resulting from a muscle tear.
3. Above the posterior-superior iliac spine is where the sacrospinalis muscle joins its tendon. Muscle fiber tears frequently occur at this junction during minor lifting trauma.
4. Above and medial to the posterior-superior iliac spine is the area over the interlaminar facet joint, where tenderness may be felt if dysfunction is present.
5. Medial and inferior to the posterior-superior iliac spine is the area where local tenderness may be felt from a pathologic condition involving a disc.
6. Tenderness lateral to the ischial tuberosity, where the sciatic trunk emerges from beneath the piriformis muscle, suggests either tightness of the muscle or a pathologic condition of a radicular origin.
7. Tenderness elicited by deeply rolling with the fingers over the sciatic trunk in the back of the thigh indicates neuritis.

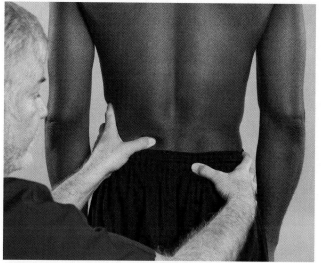

FIG. 8-131 The examiner then slides the thumb upward and inward.

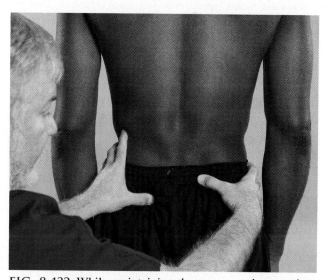

FIG. 8-132 While maintaining the pressure, the examiner moves the thumb downward and outward. The sign is positive if tenderness is increased in either direction. This sign is significant if, when sliding outward, sensitive deposits in structures on the gluteal aspect of the posterior-superior iliac spine are noted. An increase in tenderness when sliding inward indicates inflammation or strain in the superior sacroiliac ligaments. A positive sign indicates involvement of the structure or something adjacent to it, involvement of the sacroiliac joint, or a ligamentous sprain.

MILGRAM TEST

Assessment for Intervertebral Disc Syndrome or Space-Occupying Mass

Comment

The differential diagnosis of back and leg pain is extremely lengthy and complex. It includes diseases intrinsic to the spine and diseases involving adjacent organs that cause pain referred to the back or leg. Lesions can be categorized as extrinsic or intrinsic to the spine.

Extrinsic lesions include diseases of the urogenital system, gastrointestinal system, vascular system, endocrine system, nervous system not localized to the spine, and the extrinsic musculoskeletal system. These factors include infections, tumors, metabolic disturbances, congenital abnormalities, and the associated diseases of aging. LBP can also be associated with pregnancy.

> The lifetime incidence of LBP has been estimated to be between 50% and 80%, and the point prevalence is between 4.4% and 31%. Recent research has demonstrated that LBP is often associated with a prolonged course of recurring episodes and intermittent remissions, making it a major socioeconomic problem. Generalized deep-tissue hyperalgesia has been found in patients with fibromyalgia, whiplash-associated disorders, and OA. In patients with LBP, both hypoalgesia and hyperalgesia to electrical cutaneous stimulation is reported. Recently, hyperalgesia to pressure on the thumbnail was found in idiopathic chronic patients with LBP compared with controls, indicating generalized hyperalgesia (O'Neill et al, 2007).

Intrinsic lesions involve specific diseases that arise primarily in the spine. They include diseases of the spinal musculoskeletal system, the local hematopoietic system, and the local neurologic system. These conditions include trauma, tumors, infections, diseases of aging, and immune diseases affecting the spine or spinal nerves.

The weakest portion of the posterior annulus in the lumbar spine is either side of the midline, where the annulus lacks the reinforcement of the strong central fibers of the posterior longitudinal ligament. Either side of the midline is also the most common site of nuclear protrusions in the lumbar spine. Having penetrated the annulus, the protrusion lodges under the posterior longitudinal ligament. The ligament is stretched commensurate with the size of the fragment and the degree of internal pressure within the disc. In this position, the protrusion is a firm, smooth mound. To accommodate the sequestered fragment, the posterior ligament is lifted off the vertebral bodies. As the nuclear mass increases in size, further stripping of the ligament occurs. The mass may migrate in any direction—cephalad, caudad, medially, or laterally. The mass commonly moves in a lateral

direction close to and parallel to a nerve root, and it may even extend into the IVF. Under the ligament, the mass lies tightly compressed and folded on itself. The mass can be completely free, or it may still be attached to material in the nucleus by strands of irregular, stringy, fibrous tissue. This type of protrusion is by far the most common lesion encountered.

Occasionally, a dissecting protrusion may erode through the posterior ligament at a distance from its site of exit from the annulus. More commonly, the fragment is extruded through the annulus and the ligament. These free sequestra, regardless of their mode of origin, may move in any direction in the spinal canal. The usual course for these sequestra is along one of the extrathecal nerve roots, and they may lodge in the IVF.

The fact that both the dissecting and the extruded nuclear materials can make contact with one of the nerve roots anywhere from the point of exit at the dura to the IVF becomes apparent. In most instances, the nuclear material lodges directly under or slightly to either side of the root, putting it in tension. Because of the lack of elasticity of the roots outside the dura, even a small protrusion is capable of putting tension on the root. In this position, local secondary inflammatory changes bind the root tightly to the underlying nuclear mound; thus, being displaced to one side or the other of the mass is difficult for the root. In cases of long standing, the root may actually become embedded in the heap of local fibrotic tissue that is formed. The root also responds to the abnormal situation by becoming injected, edematous, and cordlike. Within the nerve sheath, granulation tissue appears that, with maturation, is converted to dense fibrous tissue that binds the nerve fasciculi together and in some instances actually destroys the fibers. The neurologic deficits resulting from this process may be permanent.

Chronic pain in general and lumbar intervertebral disk herniations in particular may initiate some common, underlying mechanism such as central sensitization in addition to a possible continuous nociceptive input.

> Pain in the lumbar spine and pelvic region is a frequent complication of pregnancy and delivery. The prevalence of pregnancy-related low back and pelvic pain (PLBP) varies widely from 14.2% to 56%. The pain is mainly located in the sacral area and the area of the symphysis pubis with or without radiation to the groins, thighs, buttocks, and coccygeus region. Several daily activities, such as standing, sitting, forward bending, lifting, climbing stairs, and walking, tend to increase the pain. Although the pain is often quite mild, in 6% to 15% of cases, the pain is considered to be severe, interfering with daily life activities. Pathologic mechanisms underlying PLBP are a matter of debate. According to several authors, dysfunction of the sacroiliac

ORTHOPEDIC GAMUT 8-35

DISORDERS MIMICKING DISC DISEASE

Common disorders that mimic intervertebral disc disease:
1. Ankylosing spondylitis
2. Multiple myeloma
3. Vascular insufficiency
4. Arthritis of the hip
5. Osteoporosis with stress fractures
6. Extradural tumors
7. Peripheral neuropathy
8. Myofascial trigger points and herpes zoster

ORTHOPEDIC GAMUT 8-36

OTHER CAUSES OF SCIATICA

Causes of sciatica not related to disc herniated nucleus pulposus:
1. Synovial cysts
2. Rupture of the medial head of the gastrocnemius
3. Sacroiliac joint dysfunction
4. Lesions in the sacrum and pelvis
5. Fracture of the ischial tuberosity

ORTHOPEDIC GAMUT 8-37

ACTIVE STRAIGHT-LEG-RAISING TEST

- The active straight-leg-raising (ASLR) test is a check for overloading of ligaments of the pelvic ring or lumbopelvic junction or both.
- In this test, performed in supine position, a subject raises one leg (Fig. 8-133), with the knee extended, 20 cm above the examination surface.
- The test is scored, only by the patient, rating the impairment on a 6-point Likert scale.
- The ASLR test is a valid and reliable test to discriminate between patients with pregnancy related low back pain and healthy subjects and to test the severity of pregnancy-related low back pain.
- However, objective measurements are lacking.

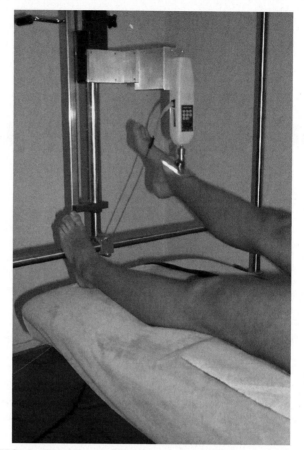

FIG. 8-133 Effort during the active straight-leg-raising test is on a six-point Likert scale: 0 = not difficult at all, 1 = minimally difficult, 2 = somewhat difficult, 3 = fairly difficult, 4 = very difficult, 5 = unable to perform. The scores of both legs are added together, the summed score ranges from 0 to 10. (Adapted from de Groot M, Pool-Goudzwaard AL, Spoor CW, et al: The active straight leg raising test (ASLR) in pregnant women: Differences in muscle activity and force between patients and healthy subjects, *Man Ther* 2008.)

8

joints (SI-joints) plays an important role in PLBP. The primary function of these joints is to transfer the loads from the upper part of the body to the legs and vice versa. SI-joint dysfunction is ascribed to instability, hyper- or hypolaxity, hyper- or hypomobility, or altered stiffness of the joint (de Groot et al, 2008).

PROCEDURE

- The patient is lying supine with both lower limbs straight out and is directed to raise the limbs until the heels are 6 inches off the table (Fig. 8-134).
- The patient holds the position for as long as possible.
- The test is positive if the patient experiences lower back pain (Fig. 8-135).
- Because this maneuver increases the subarachnoid pressure, if the patient can hold the position for 30 seconds without pain, a pathologic condition of intrathecal origin can be ruled out.
- If the test is positive, the patient may have a pathologic condition, such as a herniated disc, in or outside the spinal cord sheath.

Next Steps/Procedures
Antalgia sign, bowstring sign, Cox sign, heel/toe walk test, Kemp test, Lewin punch test, Lewin snuff test, and Neri sign

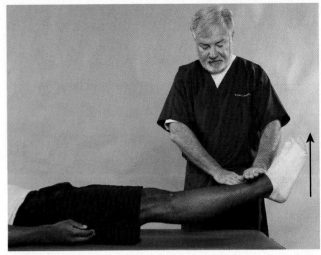

FIG. 8-134 The patient is supine with both legs fully extended. The patient is instructed to raise both legs to a position where the heels are approximately 6 inches from the examination table.

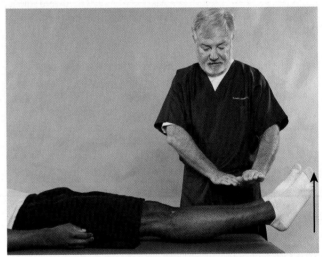

FIG. 8-135 The test is positive if the patient experiences lower back pain that prevents raising of the legs more than 2 to 3 inches, if at all. Because this maneuver increases the subarachnoid pressure, if the patient can hold the position for any length of time without pain, pathologic intrathecal process can be ruled out. A positive test indicates a space-occupying pathologic condition, such as a herniated disc.

CLINICAL PEARL

This test increases thecal pressure. The ability to hold this position for any time rules out a pathologic condition of thecal origin.

Assessment for Sacroiliac Lesions, Lumbosacral Strains and Sprains, Lumbopelvic Fractures, Intervertebral Disc Syndrome, Muscular Dystrophy, and Dystonia

Comment

Muscular or ligamentous injury is a common cause of LBP. It may follow single or multiple traumatic episodes. Incomplete muscular tears or ligament sprains occur and lead to pain and tenderness over the affected area.

Various factors predispose someone to chronic LBP. Obesity, poor muscular tone, cigarette smoking, faulty work habits, the wearing of high-heeled shoes, and the lack of a daily exercise program are among the contributing factors.

A great deal of attention has been directed toward the hypothesis that LBP is caused by vascular insult to the intervertebral discs or joints of the lumbar spine. More specifically, numerous authors have suggested that atherosclerotic occlusion of the lumbar vessels is a primary cause of LBP and lumbar spondylosis. A previous study examined the relationship between lumbar spine disease and single atherosclerotic risk factors. Results showed that cigarette smoking, hypertension, and hypercholesterolemia were associated with the development of lumbar spondylosis. Smoking and hypertension were associated with the development of cLBP. The fact that the presence of multiple risk factors dramatically increases the risk of atherosclerotic occlusion of the coronary arteries and small arteries of the extremities is well known. This circumstance leads to a nearly exponential increase in risk of heart disease and peripheral vascular disease as the number of risk factors increases. It would thus follow, if atherosclerosis of the lumbar vessels is a cause of lumbar spine disease, then increasing the number of atherosclerotic risk factors in an individual would increase his or her odds of developing LBP or lumbar spondylosis (Ahn et al, 2002).

Obesity contributes to cLBP. First, research has shown that intraabdominal pressure aids the erector spinae muscles in keeping the lumbar spine erect and decreases intradiscal pressure. Obese patients have poor abdominal muscular tone. Obese patients also typically have an increase in their lumbar lordosis, which further adds stress to the lower part of the back.

Obesity in the workforce is a considerable problem that shows no indication of slowing. The World Health Organization (1998) has shown that the prevalence of obesity is increasing at a high rate in both developed and developing countries. Obesity is defined using an index called the body mass index (BMI). BMI is calculated as whole body mass in kilograms divided by the square of stature in meters. A BMI between 18.5 and 25 kg/m² is considered normal weight, between 25 and 30 kg/m² is considered overweight, between 30 and 40 kg/m² is obese, and greater than 40 kg/m² is extremely obese. In the United States, obesity has been called an epidemic for both adults and children, with data from 2001 to 2002 showing that 66% of U.S. adults were either overweight or obese, and 5% were extremely obese. These authors also showed that, in the U.S. workforce, the obesity rate for men is 26.1%, and the obesity rate for women is 33.3%. Relevant to the effects of these statistics on occupational safety and health concerns are the results of the study by Hertz and colleagues (2004) that showed that, among both men and women, obese workers are more likely to report work limitations as a result of physical, mental, or emotional problems than their normal-weight counterparts. An area of particular concern may be LBP or lower back disorders because of the additional muscular force required to move the additional body mass while performing various occupational tasks (Xu, Mirka, Hsiang, 2008).

The most commonly overlooked source of lumbar muscle pain may be the quadratus lumborum. This muscle, which not only contributes to the support of the lumbar spine and abdominal cavity, but also is a lateral flexor of the lumbopelvic spine, may be the most active muscle of the lumbar region during activities of daily living. It may possess trigger points that cause localized and referred pain.

The symptom complex of sciatic pain varies widely, and it occurs when a nuclear sequestrum touches one of the nerve roots. In a small percentage of patients, the attack comes on suddenly, and the pain radiates the full length of the limb along the dermatome of the involved nerve root. In a large percentage of patients, the pain comes on slowly and is often felt as an ache that is in one side of the buttocks and that spreads gradually and distally. In some patients, the pain is localized to the posterior or posterolateral aspects of the thigh, depending on whether S1 or L5 nerve roots are implicated. In some patients, the pain may extend as far as the calf (the lateral aspect of the lower leg), the sole of the foot, or the dorsum of the outer three toes, depending on the nerve root affected. From time to time, the presenting complaint is pain that is limited to a small but specific area, such as the buttocks, the back of the thigh, the calf, or the sole of the foot. In rare instances, the pattern of pain spread may be reversed. For example, the pain may begin in the calf or sole of the foot and gradually spread cephalad.

In a small percentage of patients, back pain and sciatica appear simultaneously. Two clinical types of this syndrome are discernible. In one type, the symptoms of back pain and sciatica appear suddenly and simultaneously. In the other type, the onset is gradual. The former is associated with some sudden flexion stress that is applied to the lumbar spine and causes rupture of the annulus and retropulsion of the nuclear material. The latter is consistent with gradual extrusion of the nuclear fragments through the annulus fibrosus. The pain in the back and the sciatica may be of almost equal severity, but in most instances, the intensity of one overshadows the other. When pain in both the back and the leg is severe and the onset is sudden, the patient may be incapacitated and may present a dramatic clinical picture. The pain may be so severe that the affected leg is held in the flexed position, and the patient avoids any maneuver that might extend the limb. The patient complains of severe spasm of the lumbar paravertebral muscles and often exhibits a severe list of the trunk.

Spinal muscular atrophy (SMA) is a neuromuscular disorder caused by degeneration of the anterior horn cells of the spinal cord. This hereditary disease is characterized by muscular weakness, abnormal spinal development, and a disease-related deterioration of respiratory function. The underlying genetic defect on chromosome 5q13 has been identified and characterized. At least three forms of SMA have been identified, often termed type I through type III. These common forms are classified according to the patient's age at the onset of the disease and the maximal motor function achieved. In type I, the most severe form, the onset appears in the patient's first 6 months, and affected individuals never manage to sit unsupported. Type II, the intermediate form, appears before 18 months, and in most cases, the patients never stand or walk independently. In type III, the mildest form, the disease can appear anytime after 18 months and even during adulthood. Type III individuals can learn to walk without support. The prevalence

rate for types II and III is around 12 per million (Armand et al, 2005).

Duchenne muscular dystrophy (DMD) is an X-linked muscle disease caused by an absence of the protein, dystrophin. DMD is also hereditary and is characterized by progressive muscular weakness that can compromise ambulatory status, as well as cardiopulmonary function. The prevalence rate for DMD is approximately 63 per million. Patients with SMA-II and DMD exhibit progressive muscular weakness. In both cases, this weakness is more proximal than distal, affects lower limbs more often than upper limbs, and is characterized more by extensor weakness than flexor weakness (Armand et al, 2005).

PROCEDURE

- Sciatic radiculitis is suggested by how a patient with this condition rises from a seated position (Fig. 8-136).
- The patient supports the body with the uninvolved side by balancing on the healthy leg, placing one hand on the back, and flexing the knee and hip of the affected limb (Fig. 8-137).
- The sign is often present with sacroiliac lesions, lumbosacral strains and sprains, fractures, disc syndromes, dystrophies, and myotonia.

Next Steps/Procedures
Bilateral leg-lowering test, Demianoff sign, double leg-raise test, hyperextension test, Lewin supine test, match stick test, Mennell sign, Nachlas test, Quick test, Schober test, sign of the buttock, skin pinch test, spinal percussion test, and Vanzetti sign

CLINICAL PEARL

With lumbar disc lesions, all movements of the spine—extension, flexion, lateral flexion, and rotation—are affected. With an acute lesion, extension and flexion are seriously restricted, but lateral flexion and rotation are free. The degree of restriction is governed by the phase and severity of the local pathologic process. During an acute attack, the striking feature of the spine is the complete loss of its inherent flexibility. The patient avoids motion in any direction.

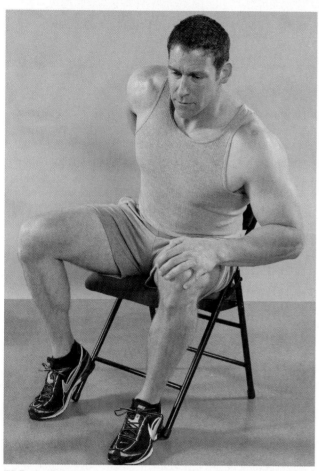

FIG. 8-136 The patient is seated and is asked to stand. The examiner observes how the patient rises from a seated position.

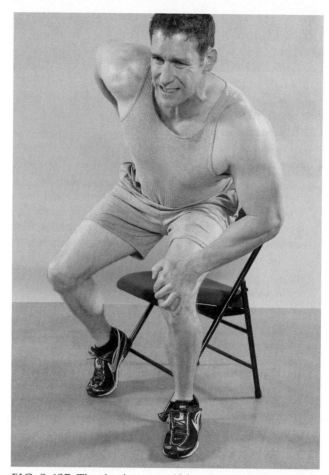

FIG. 8-137 The sign is present if the patient supports weight on the uninvolved side by balancing on the healthy leg, placing one hand on the back, and flexing the knee and hip on the affected side. The sign is often present with sacroiliac lesions, lumbosacral strains and sprains, fractures, disc syndromes, dystrophies, and myotonia.

Assessment for Sacroiliac or Lumbosacral Disorder

Comment

LBP is an extremely common symptom affecting millions of people each year and accounts for a significant number of physician visits in both primary care and specialty pain centers across the world. In the United States, an estimated 90% of adults experience back pain at some time in their life. A growing body of literature suggests that in such cases, psychosocial factors, as well as specific behavioral factors related to fear and avoidance, may be of importance. The structural complexities of the back and the possibility of referred pain from other areas often make precise localization of pain generators difficult. Pain generators may include the vertebral column, surrounding muscles, tendons, ligaments and fascia, or the neural structures (Huntoon, Huntoon, 2004).

A most comprehensive low back differential diagnosis system based on symptoms is that developed by the Quebec Task Force (Table 8-21).

Acute lumbosacral strain is the most common cause of acute LBP. Because of its position in the skeleton, the lumbosacral joint supports the body weight and acts as a fulcrum for this weight in activities that involve bending and lifting. Mechanical damage to this joint is frequent because of the

functional demands placed on the lower back area by everyday activities. In this joint, the traumatic force usually involves lifting or pushing a load when the spine is flexed forward. In this position, the lumbosacral joint is functioning as a fulcrum (Fig. 8-138).

Acute lumbosacral strain occurs when a load is applied while the spine is twisted or rotated or when a sudden force is applied unexpectedly before the back muscles brace to

---

ORTHOPEDIC GAMUT 8-38

DIFFERENTIAL RED FLAGS IN LOW BACK PAIN

- Advanced age
- Bowel or bladder incontinence retention
- Constant progressive pain at night
- Intravenous drug use
- Prior cancer
- Trauma
- Fever
- Prolonged systemic steroid use
- Saddle anesthesia
- Systemic illness or infection
- Unexplained weight loss

TABLE 8-21

DURATION OF SYMPTOMS AND WORKING STATUS CLASSIFICATION OF LOW BACK PAIN DISORDERS

Classification	Symptoms	Duration of Symptoms from Onset	Working Status at Time of Evaluation
1	Pain without radiation	a (<7 days)	W (working)
2	Pain + radiation to extremity, proximally	b (7 days–7 wks)	I (idle)
3	Pain + radiation to extremity, distally	c (>7 wks)	
4	Pain + radiation to upper/lower limb neurologic signs		
5	Presumptive compression of a spinal nerve root on a simple roentgenogram (i.e., spinal instability or fracture)		
6	Compression of a spinal nerve root confirmed by Specific imaging techniques (i.e., computerized		
	Other diagnostic techniques (i.e., electromyography, venography)		
7	Spinal stenosis		
8	Postsurgical status, 1-6 mos after intervention		
9	Postsurgical status, >6 mos after intervention		
	9.1 Asymptomatic		
	9.2 Symptomatic		
10	Chronic pain syndrome		W (working)
11	Other diagnoses		I (idle)

Adapted from Pope MH et al: *Occupational low back pain assessment, treatment and prevention,* St Louis, 1991, Mosby.

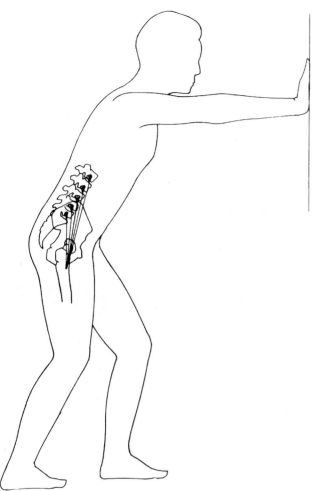

FIG. 8-138 The hip joint must be 'locked' during maximal push by hip flexor muscles, causing compressive and shear forces on lumbar spine. If spinal structures are injured this can be pain producing and may lead to decreased trunk flexion strength. (Adapted from Rantanen P, Nykvist F: Optimal sagittal motion axis for trunk extension and flexion tests in chronic low back trouble, *Clin Biomech* 15(9):665-71, 2000.)

meet it. The latter instance occurs less often than the former.

The importance of shear forces on the human spine is still a matter of debate. Large ranges of estimated joint shear forces and shear strength can be found in the literature. Failure of the pars interarticularis has been shown to occur at joint shear forces ranging from approximately 600 to 4000 N. With respect to the joint shear loading in daily life, estimates of the joint shear forces at the L4-L5 joint during lifting have been reported to be relatively low (i.e., below

300 N) for a range of load weights, load positions, and lifting techniques. At the L5-S1 joint, joint shear forces of much higher magnitude (i.e., between 600 and 1500 N) have been reported during lifting. Joint shear forces of such magnitudes might exceed spinal (intervertebral) shear tolerance (Kingma, Staudenmann, van Dieen, 2007).

The resulting pathologic change is a partial tearing or stretching of the overlying paravertebral muscles, lumbar fascia, and interspinous ligaments. If the injury results in more serious damage to the spine, then by definition it cannot be a lumbosacral strain. Injury to the soft parts initiates paravertebral muscle spasm, which accounts for the clinical picture seen with this condition.

The stimulus for normal tone of the paravertebral muscles is the upright position. These muscles are in normal postural tone only in the standing or seated positions and are completely flaccid in the prone or supine positions. Spasm of the paravertebral muscles involves markedly exaggerated tone that is initiated by the stimulus of overload and is maintained by the stimulus of the upright position. The unspecificity of trunk muscle weakness for low back trouble has not been reported earlier. Immobilization as a result of pain may cause muscular atrophy and weakness. Similarly, a chronic disease may cause depression or fear of pain that may produce a lower degree of effort. Instead, the increase in torque as the sagittal motion axis moves caudally has been reported earlier. This phenomenon has been explained by the increased recruitment of hip flexor and extensor muscles as the rotation axis moves caudally (Rantanen, Nykvist, 2000).

In patients with acute lumbosacral strain, a lag period can always occur between the time the lower back damage was sustained and the onset of the clinical symptoms. This lag period may vary from hours to days and depends on whether the patient remains upright. During this lag period, the paravertebral muscle spasm builds to a point of clinical significance.

The severity of the clinical features of acute lumbosacral strain depends directly on the degree of paravertebral muscle spasm present. The patient gives a history of a twisting or lifting injury to the lower back and states that the onset of symptoms occurred either immediately or, more commonly, after a lag period of several hours or days. The patient walks guardedly and slowly because movement of the spine is painful. The back may be held in flexion or may exhibit a list to one side with a tilted pelvis. The paravertebral muscles feel extremely taut and hard, and the normal lumbar lordotic curve is obliterated. Spinal movements are limited in direct proportion to the amount of muscle spasm present and are associated with a sharp, diffuse, catching type of pain in the lower back, with possible radiation to the buttocks and thighs or upward to the neck.

8

PROCEDURE

- To eliminate lumbosacral muscular influence in this test, the patient is placed prone and relaxed on a rigid table (Fig. 8-139).
- Pain in the lower back and lower extremity is noted during passive flexion of the knee.
- The test is positive if pain is noted in the sacroiliac area or lumbosacral area or if the pain radiates down the thigh or leg (Fig. 8-140).
- A positive test indicates a sacroiliac or lumbosacral disorder.

Next Steps/Procedures
Bilateral leg-lowering test, Demianoff sign, double-leg-raise test, hyperextension test, Lewin supine test, matchstick test, Mennell sign, Minor sign, Quick test, Schober test, sign of the buttock, skin pinch test, spinal percussion test, and Vanzetti sign

CLINICAL PEARL

Intermittent prolapse of nuclear material is called a concealed disc or occult disc. Degenerated nuclear material still within the confines of the annulus, which may be weakened by degenerative process but remains intact, may bulge beyond its normal limits when the spine is subjected to certain stresses. Depending on the stresses, the prolapse appears and then disappears. Extension and hyperextension of the spine favor the prolapse, which can produce a defect in the anterior aspect of a myelographic column of dye. When the spine is relieved of stress, such as when the patient is relaxed and lying in the prone position, the defect disappears.

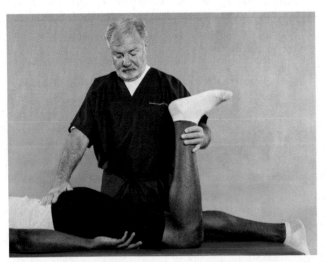

FIG. 8-139 The patient is prone with both legs fully extended. The examiner flexes the knee of the affected leg to 90 degrees.

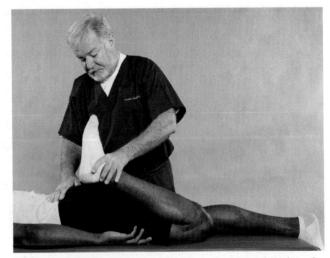

FIG. 8-140 The knee is fully flexed, approximating the heel to the ipsilateral buttock. The test is positive if pain is noted in the sacroiliac area or lumbosacral area or if pain radiates down the thigh or leg. A positive test indicates a sacroiliac or lumbosacral disorder.

Assessment for Lower Intervertebral Disc Syndrome, Lumbosacral and Sacroiliac Strain, or Lumbopelvic Subluxation

Comment

In terms of etiopathologic mechanisms, isthmic spondylolysis involves genetic factors, given that the observation that Caucasians are more frequently affected than African Americans and less affected than some ethnic groups such as the Eskimos. Obviously, a mechanical factor contributes to the development of pars lesion because only bipeds with lumbar lordosis are affected after acquisition of ambulation and because repeated sports-related microtrauma in positions of hyperextension considerably increases the frequency of spondylolysis. Clinically, asymptomatic forms are frequent. Acute low-back pain may involve initial episode of fracture. At a later stage, chronic lower lumbar pain develops; in some patients, sciatica occurs, in most cases by compression of the L5 nerve root. In severe dysplastic spondylolisthesis, this circumstance may even lead to lumbosacral kyphosis with pelvic retroversion. Radiologically, the diagnosis of isthmic spondylolysis is based on oblique lumbar images, CT scans perpendicular to the isthmus, and radionuclide bone scans performed early after initial pains. Spondylolisthesis is assessed using lateral films that allow, for prognosis determination, both the quantification of the degree of slippage and the determination of the lumbosacral kyphosis angle. MRI may reveal recent spondylolysis; it also permits evaluation of the state of discs adjacent to the spondylolis-thesis and can show radicular compromise. The natural history of spondylolisthesis by isthmic spondylolysis depends on the possible collapse of the intervertebral disc. The course of dysplastic spondylolisthesis is more severe, because it affects young subjects before maturity, and the deformity depends on osteocartilaginous growth (Vital, Pedram, 2005).

Surgical treatment of a disc rupture is for the symptomatic relief of leg pain. Patients with predominant back pain may not be relieved of their major complaint—back pain. The best results of 99.5% complete or partial pain relief are obtained when the disc is free in the canal or sequestered. Incomplete herniation or extrusion of disc material into the canal results in complete relief for 82% of patients. Excision of the bulging or protruding disc that is not ruptured through the annulus results in complete relief in 63%, and removal of the normal or minimally bulging disc results in complete relief in 38% (Fig. 8-141).

Although the posterior lumbar interbody fusion (PLIF) procedure has the ability to deal with the degenerate disc, neural impingement, and facet degeneration in one operation, it is technically difficult to perform. PLIF surgery can result in complications such as pseudarthrosis, implant subsidence, epidural bleeding, dural tears, bone graft donor site morbidity, and neurologic complications. The nature of the complications will depend on whether instrumentation is used, the type of instrumentation, and whether cages are used. Neurologic symptoms after PLIF surgery are a potential problem that concerns surgeons. These symptoms are a well-recognized complication after this operation. Reported rates of neurologic complications for PLIF surgery vary between 0% and 15% (Krishna, Pollock, Bhatia, in press).

Traction on anomalous nerve roots has been suggested as a cause of sciatic symptoms without herniation. Sectioning of these roots results in irreversible neurologic damage.

Abnormal physical stresses placed on a degenerated disc may exceed the mechanical strength of the degenerated disc and annulus, resulting in rupture of the annulus. Herniation of nuclear material (either wholly or in fragments) into the spinal canal causes either compression of or tension on a lumbar or sacral spinal nerve root as the root prepares to exit from the spinal canal and is the essential pathologic lesion of the condition known as *herniated intervertebral disc*. The nuclear material may push the posterior longitudinal ligament ahead of it like a sac, or the material may rupture through the posterior longitudinal ligament to extrude directly into the spinal canal.

The general process of intervertebral disc degeneration may extend over a period of years. The clinical picture characteristic of a herniated intervertebral disc does not arise

---

ORTHOPEDIC GAMUT 8-39

ALTERATIONS IN SPINAL BALANCE AND CURVATURE

Alterations of spinal balance and curvature are implicated in the development of a variety of spinal disorders:

- Acute and chronic low back pain
- Disc degeneration
- Spondylosis
- Ossification of spinal ligaments
- Adolescent idiopathic scoliosis
- Scheuermann kyphosis
- Impaired ribcage expansion
- Early osteoarthritis and disc degeneration
- Osteoporosis and vertebral compression fractures
- Spondylolisthesis

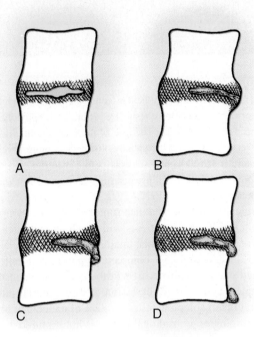

FIG. 8-141 Types of disc herniation. **A,** Normal bulge. **B,** Protrusion. **C,** Extrusion. **D,** Sequestration. (From Canale ST, Beaty JH: *Campbell's operative orthopaedics*, ed 11, Philadelphia, 2008, Mosby.)

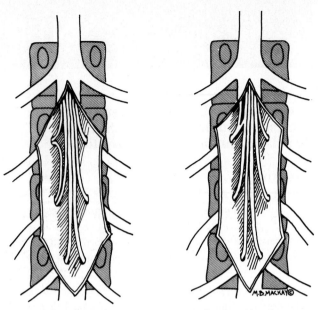

FIG. 8-142 Type-I nerve root anomaly: intradural anastomosis. (From Canale ST: *Campbell's operative orthopaedics*, vol 1-4, ed 9, St Louis, 1998, Mosby.)

ORTHOPEDIC GAMUT 8-40

LUMBAR NERVE ROOT ANOMALIES

- Type I: Intradural anastomosis between rootlets at different levels (Fig. 8-142)
- Type II: Anomalous origin of the nerve roots separated into four subtypes (Fig. 8-143):
  - Cranial origin
  - Caudal origin
  - Combination of cranial and caudal origin
  - Conjoined nerve roots
- Type III: Extradural anastomosis between roots (Fig. 8-144)
- Type IV: Extradural division of the nerve root (Fig. 8-145)

---

until some of the nuclear material herniates or ruptures the posterior longitudinal spinal ligament. This rupture causes pressure on the adjacent spinal nerve root as it passes by and exits from the spine. The actual contact between disc material and the nerve root may be sudden and commonly follows an acute rise in intrathecal pressure that is triggered by sneezing, lifting, twisting, or straining.

Back pain is associated with disc degeneration, but the predominant symptom is sciatic pain that begins when the nuclear material protrudes posterolaterally into the spinal canal and compresses the nerve root. In most instances, a diagnosis of herniated disc is untenable without sciatic leg pain. Many back conditions may be associated with leg pain, but only nerve root irritation at this level produces pain along the distribution of the sciatic nerve. Pain that follows the distribution of the sciatic nerve is associated with signs of a lumbosacral nerve root compression syndrome.

The patient with a herniated intervertebral disc experiences lower back pain that is accompanied by pain radiating into the posterior buttock and leg or just into the leg. When viewed while standing, the patient may exhibit a list of the pelvis or a sciatic scoliosis.

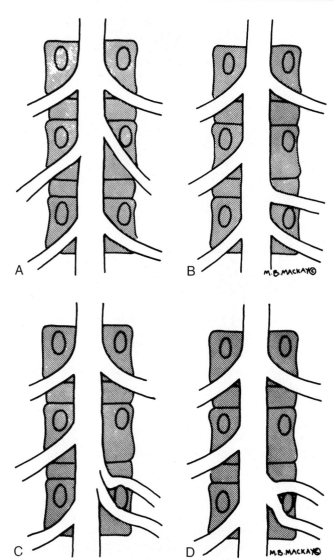

FIG. 8-143 Type II: anomalous origin of nerve roots. **A,** Cranial origin. **B,** Caudal origin. **C,** Closely adjacent nerve roots. **D,** Conjoined nerve roots. (From Canale ST: *Campbell's operative orthopaedics,* vol 1-4, ed 9, St Louis, 1998, Mosby.)

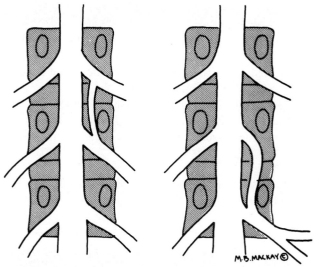

FIG. 8-144 Type-III nerve root anomaly: extradural anastomosis. (From Canale ST: *Campbell's operative orthopaedics,* vol 1-4, ed 9, St Louis, 1998, Mosby.)

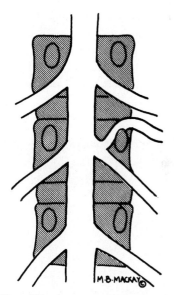

FIG. 8-145 Type-IV nerve root anomaly: extradural division. (From Canale ST: *Campbell's operative orthopaedics,* vol 1-4, ed 9, St Louis, 1998, Mosby.)

PROCEDURE

- While in a standing posture, the patient is directed to bow forward (Figs. 8-146 and 8-147).
- The sign is present when the patient flexes the knee on the affected side (Fig. 8-148).
- The trunk flexion action causes pain in the leg.
- This pain is a common sign with lower disc problems, as well as lumbosacral and sacroiliac strain subluxations.

Procedures

Antalgia sign, bowstring sign, Cox sign, heel/toe walk test, Kemp test, Lewin punch test, Lewin snuff test, and Milgram test

CLINICAL PEARL

Muscle tenderness may be associated with nerve root irritation. With an acute attack, tenderness of the buttock, thigh, and calf on the affected side is often demonstrable. When pain is localized to a specific area along the course of the sciatic nerve, thorough regional examination is essential for ruling out local lesions, such as an abscess, neurofibroma, glomus tumor, lipoma, or sterile abscess, that irritate the sciatic nerve.

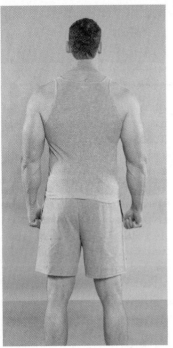

FIG. 8-146 The patient is standing with the arms comfortably at the sides.

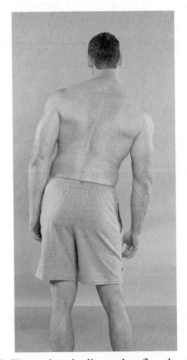

FIG. 8-147 The patient is directed to flex the trunk or bow forward. A lateral antalgic positioning may be noted but does not constitute a positive finding for this test.

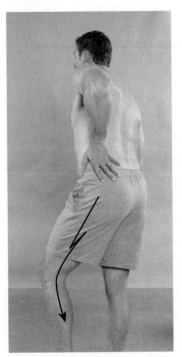

FIG. 8-148 The sign is present if the patient flexes the knee on the affected side and if trunk flexion causes pain in the leg. The sign is present for lower lumbar disc involvement, as well as lumbosacral and sacroiliac strains or subluxations.

PRONE KNEE-BENDING TEST

Assessment for L2 or L3 Nerve Root Lesion, Femoral Nerve Inflammation, or Quadriceps Muscular Strain

Comment

The femoral nerve arises from the L1, L2, L3, and L4 spinal roots and innervates the iliopsoas, sartorius, and quadriceps femoris muscles. Proximal lesions result in weakness of thigh flexion or, more prominently, loss of extension at the knee. The nerve can be injured by pelvic fractures, by surgery, and by direct, penetrating wounds. The nerve can be paralyzed by pressure during childbirth or by arterial aneurysms, retroperitoneal hemorrhage, pelvic neoplasms, or abscesses.

Meralgia paresthetica is a painful mononeuropathy of the LFCN that is characterized clinically by numbness, burning, itching, or pain over the anterior and lateral aspects of the thigh. It is commonly caused by focal entrapment of this nerve as it passes through the inguinal ligament. Meralgia paresthetica typically occurs in isolation and can result from iatrogenic injury to the LFCN during orthopedic procedures that include bone graft harvesting, the insertion of pins in the ASIS during external fixation of the pelvis, and during anterior surgical approaches to the hip and pelvis. In rare instances, meralgia paresthetica has other causes, such as direct trauma to the ilium during accidents, stretch injury, or ischemia. Additional causes include pressure from belts,

---

ORTHOPEDIC GAMUT 8-41

FRANK DEGENERATION OF THE FACETS

Frank degeneration of the facets may be associated with the following three clinically important conditions:

1. Degeneration of the facets is part of the overall process of spinal degeneration and significantly contributes to pain in patients with multilevel spinal osteoarthritis.
2. Degeneration of the facets, with associated development of osteophytes projecting into the lateral recess and central spinal canal, is a significant part of degenerative spinal stenosis.
3. Degeneration of the facets is sometimes associated with a ventrally projecting synovial cyst, which impinges on the nerve root and thus is part of the differential diagnosis of sciatica.

---

braces, trusses and tight trousers (Moucharafieh, Wehbe, Maalouf, in press).

Probably the most common syndrome involving the femoral nerve is the painful mononeuritis that occurs with diabetes. The quadriceps muscle atrophies quickly, and the knee jerk is lost early. Weakness while stepping up and the inability to rise from a one-legged squat are reliable motor signs of quadriceps paralysis. Quadriceps strength can be tested directly. Sensory distribution includes the anteromedial thigh and the anteromedial leg to the foot. Assessing for signs of more widespread deficits would be appropriate before concluding that this nerve alone is paralyzed because similar findings may result from a lesion higher in the lumbar plexus.

Femoral nerve injuries fall into two categories, those distal to the inguinal ligament in the femoral triangle and those proximal and, by definition, intrapelvic. Theoretically, injury to the pelvic portion of the femoral nerve should produce, in addition to quadriceps paralysis and hypesthesia over the anteromedial thigh, a loss of sartorius muscle function. The branch to the sartorius is somewhat variable in origin and course. One of the clearly intrapelvic femoral nerve lesions appears to spare this muscle, whereas several thigh-level lesions may have sartorius loss.

Preservation or loss of this muscle's function does not indicate the level of the femoral nerve involvement.

Only sensory function is mediated by the lateral femoral cutaneous nerve (LFCN). This nerve is not a branch of the femoral nerve, and it follows a different peripheral course. Classic entrapment of the LFCN occurs where it passes under the inguinal ligament medial to the ASIS. This entrapment results in a syndrome of dysesthesia and pain, called *meralgia paresthetica,* along the lateral thigh. Some loss of sensitivity to pain and touch is often typical in a small area. The skin may become sensitive to touch and pinching. No atrophy and no motor or reflex change are seen. Entrapment of the LFCN is distinguished by its common occurrence, curability, and tendency to be easily mistaken for symptoms of L2 and L3 nerve root compression syndromes. This type of entrapment is initiated by obesity or local trauma caused by a belt or truss. Similar to other entrapment neuropathies, LFCN entrapment is apt to occur with metabolic disorders, which may make the peripheral nerves vulnerable to pressure.

Peripheral neuropathy is a common feature of many vasculitic syndromes. In some patients, the neuropathy may be the sole manifestation of vasculitis. Histologic lesions of vasculitis confined to the peripheral nervous system are those of classic polyarteritis nodosa. Neither systemic involvement nor biologic abnormality is observed, which strengthens the role of nerve and muscle biopsy.

ORTHOPEDIC GAMUT 8-42

CAUSES OF MERALGIA PARESTHETICA (LATERAL FEMORAL NERVE COMPRESSION)

A variety of causes for meralgia paresthetica exists (most common in bold type):

- Abdominal distention
- Cholecystectomy
- Direct trauma
- **Iatrogenic complications after thoracoabdominal surgery**
- Idiopathic causes
- **Iliac bone graft harvesting**
- Laparoscopic inguinal hernia repair
- Limb length discrepancy
- Metastatic carcinoma in the iliac crest
- Myomectomy
- Neuropathy involving the lateral cutaneous nerve
- Neuropathy of diabetes mellitus and thyroid diseases
- Obesity and pregnancy
- Rare complication of heart operations
- Retroperitoneal tumors
- Seat belt injury
- **Tight clothing**

PROCEDURE

- The patient is prone as the knees are passively flexed so that the heels touch the buttocks (Fig. 8-149).
- An L2 or L3 nerve root lesion is indicated by unilateral lumbar pain (Fig. 8-150).
- The test stretches the femoral nerve.

Next Steps/Procedures

Ely sign and femoral nerve traction test

CLINICAL PEARL

Prone knee flexion can provide provocative testing for lumbar disc protrusion. The pathophysiologic aspect of this test depends on compression of spinal nerves during hyperextension of the lumbar spine. The compression intensifies intervertebral disc protrusion into the spinal canal. The lumbar intervertebral foramina are narrowed, and the spinal canal cross-sectional area is decreased by lumbar extension. The presence of a protruded disc that has not produced other physical findings may be detected by this test.

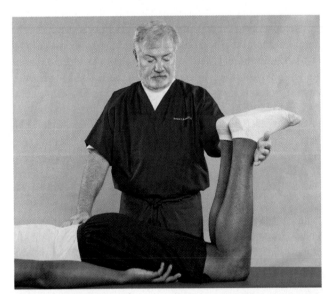

FIG. 8-149 The patient is in the prone position with both knees fully extended. The examiner passively flexes both knees to 90 degrees.

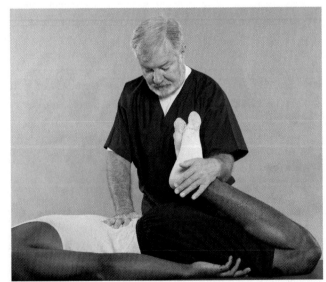

FIG. 8-150 The examiner flexes both knees maximally, approximating the heels to the buttocks. If the examiner is unable to flex the patient's knees past 90 degrees, the test is positive. Unilateral pain in the lumbar area indicates an L2 or L3 nerve root lesion. The test also stretches the femoral nerve. Pain in the anterior thigh indicates tight quadriceps muscles.

Assessment for Lower Back or Lower Extremity Screening

Comment

Back pain is the most common and troublesome complaint because its causes are legion, and exact diagnosis is often difficult. The impairment, with which back pain is usually associated, is often severe and prolonged.

Musculoskeletal pain is a common problem among adults and elderly people. The longitudinal effects of musculoskeletal pain are well known. Moreover, restrictions of physical functioning among elderly people are very important. Some researches into aging and health-related changes have shown that increasing age is associated with a decline in several important musculoskeletal properties that may result in pain or discomfort and decreased physical function. In addition, muscle strength has been shown to be inversely related to age. Loss of bone density and osteoporosis are also a common occurrence during aging and usually lead to skeletal pain. Many health problems result from old age and are related to pain. Previous studies have shown that middle-age and older adults with body pain and physical symptoms are at the risk of prior depression. Several epidemiologic studies have demonstrated that the prevalence of both musculoskeletal pain and balance problems are common in the older population. The overall prevalence of any type of pain or discomfort in the population of older people has been estimated to range from 25% to 75%. More specifically, musculoskeletal pain has been estimated to range from 10% to 71% in the older population. Balance dysfunction in aging population is based on the knowledge of normal aging processes, loss of sensory elements, and lose musculoskeletal function (Yagci et al, 2007).

The mechanical disturbances are clear (osteoporotic spinal fractures, senile kyphosis, spondylolisthesis, Scheuermann disease, spinal osteochondrosis, and, sometimes, OA). In other cases, although the symptoms may be identical in character, the cause cannot be determined with any accuracy. These cases of mechanical LBP formerly attracted many emotive but valueless names, such as lumbago and lower back strain.

Lumbar spinal stenosis is a syndrome in which narrowing of the lumbar spinal canal occurs, which may lead to vague and unusual symptoms. The disorder occurs secondary to a combination of disc degeneration, facet joint arthritis, and subluxation and occasionally to a congenitally small spinal canal.

Roentgenographic examination of the lumbar spine usually reveals degenerative changes throughout the lower part of the back. Electromyographic and myelographic examination may help localize the disorder, and computed axial tomography is often diagnostic (Fig. 8-151). MRI is also helpful.

While taking a history and examining a patient suffering from back pain, the examiner must exhaust the possibility of extraspinal causes; then an attempt should be made to place the patient in one of the three groups described earlier.

ORTHOPEDIC GAMUT 8-43

LOW BACK PAIN

Considering low back pain under three headings is helpful:

1. Back pain may be associated with a spinal pathologic process, such as vertebral infections, tumors, ankylosing spondylitis, polyarthritis, Paget disease, and primary neurologic disease.
2. Back pain may be associated with nerve root pain. The most common causes are intervertebral disc prolapse and compression of nerve roots within the neural canals.
3. Back pain may be caused by disturbance of the mechanics of the spine (mechanical back pain). This group is the largest group of conditions that cause back pain.

PROCEDURE

- The Quick test is accomplished with the patient standing.
- The patient squats down and stands again (Fig. 8-152).
- This action will help the examiner quickly assess the integrity of the ankles, knees, and hips.
- If the patient can fully squat without any symptoms, these joints are free of disease related to the pain complaint.

Next Steps/Procedures

Bilateral leg-lowering test, Demianoff sign, double-leg-raise test, hyperextension test, Lewin supine test, matchstick test, Mennell sign, Minor sign, Nachlas test, Schober test, sign of the buttock, skin pinch test, spinal percussion test, and Vanzetti sign

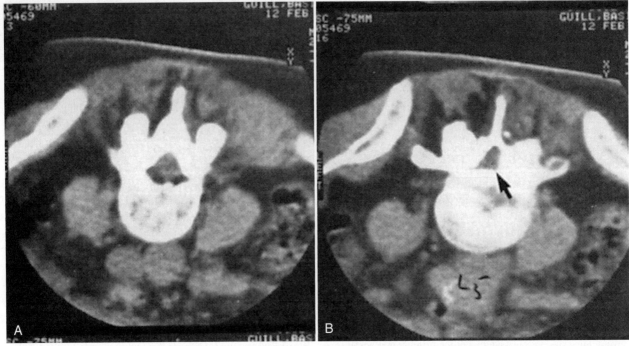

FIG. 8-151 Normal (**A**) and abnormal (**B**) computed tomographic scans of the lumbar spine. (From Mercier LR, Pettid FJ: *Practical orthopedics,* ed 4, St Louis, 1995, Mosby.)

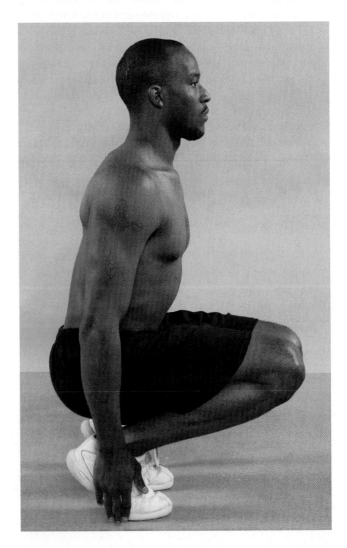

FIG. 8-152 The patient is standing. The patient squats down and stands up again. If the patient can fully squat without any symptoms, the ankles, knees, and hips are free of a pathologic condition. Patients suspected of having arthritis in the lower limb joints should not perform this test, especially pregnant patients and older individuals who exhibit weakness and hypomobility.

CLINICAL PEARL

The Quick test is probably the least demanding screening test for lumbar and lower extremity complaints. In a few, short, and active movements, three major contributors to lower extremity complaints (ankles, knees, and hips) can be ruled in or out of the differential diagnostic process.

Assessment for Lumbar Spine Motion

Comment

LBP and injury are significant public health problems. In the United States, up to 85% of the population suffer LBP at least once in their lifetime, and the total annual cost of back pain in the United States is estimated to range from $20 to $50 billion. Jobs involving flexion tasks and lifting heavy loads have been shown to be associated with a higher incidence of low back injuries. Understanding how subjects perform these flexion and lifting tasks is therefore important to understanding and preventing low back injuries. When examining flexion tasks and the low back, the motion of the spine is a critical component, described as the motion of spinal segments within two regions, the neutral zone where rotation of the spinal segments meets little resistance and the elastic zone where soft-tissue restraints such as ligaments, facet joints (in extension), and the intervertebral disk (in flexion) provide resistance to rotation. At the extremes of the neutral zone, tension in the posterior ligaments (in flexion), moment loading of the intervertebral disc (in flexion), and compression in the facet joints (in extension) are engaged, limiting further motion (Maduri, Pearson, Wilson, in press).

Ankylosing spondylitis is often seen in young adults, usually young men. This condition is characterized by an inflammatory process that involves primarily the soft-tissue elements of the spine. The synovial membranes, capsules, and ligaments of the joints of the spine become swollen, edematous, and thickened. These changes are followed by calcification and eventually ossification. The result is bony ankylosis of all the affected joints. With ankylosing spondylitis, the pathologic process is confined to the intervertebral joints, the posterior articular joints, the sacroiliac joints, and the surrounding ligaments. The peripheral joints of the extremities are spared.

The proliferative process in the soft tissue in and about the IVF (the capsules of the posterior joints, the ligamentum flavum, and the posterior longitudinal ligament) narrows the outlet and may press and irritate the nerve roots that are traversing the bony canals. In addition, the sheaths of the nerves are involved; thus the roots are enmeshed and fixed in a mass of fibrous tissue. The fact that body movements that stretch the roots, such as flexing the leg when extended at the knee, will accentuate the pain in the back and leg becomes apparent.

LBP and sciatica are common complaints in all stages of this disorder, and the incidence of sciatica is greater than formerly realized. In the early stages, diagnostic imaging is not informative; therefore making the diagnosis is difficult.

At this early stage, the clinical picture may mimic that of a disc lesion in the lumbar spine, although the early clinical picture does not unequivocally simulate that of a lumbar disc lesion. LBP is the first manifestation.

The area involved is not only the lumbosacral region, but also the regions of the SI-joints. Pain may be referred to the buttocks and the posterior aspects of the thighs. The syndrome is punctuated by remissions. The pain, which is not of a mechanical nature, is influenced by weather changes. The patient experiences considerable stiffness in the dorsal region and in the thoracic cage. Later, sciatica in one or both legs appears, and all movements of the spine are restricted, especially flexion. As time passes, the lumbar spine is flattened, the patient begins to stoop forward, the cervical curve becomes exaggerated, and flexion contractures of the hips develop. At this point, the clinical picture of ankylosing spondylitis is evident and can be confirmed by diagnostic imaging. Imaging reveals characteristic changes in the posterior articulations and the SI-joints.

Some muscle spasm of the dorsolumbar spine can be demonstrated. Some tenderness can be elicited over the spinous processes and a little to each side of the midline. As the process progresses, the excursions of the thorax become smaller and smaller until the thoracic cage becomes completely rigid and fixed. Throughout the active stages of the disease, the sedimentation rate is always elevated and is a good index to the activity of the process, but serologic tests for rheumatoid factor are usually negative.

Spinal instability (caused by degenerative disc disease) is a clinically symptomatic condition without new injury in which a physiologic load induces abnormally large deformations at the intervertebral joint. Abnormal motion at vertebral segments with degenerative discs and the transmission of the load to the facet joints are usually present in spinal instability.

Instability is demonstrated in the lumbar spine as an anterior slip of 5 mm or more in the thoracic or lumbar spine (Fig. 8-153) or a difference in the angular motion of two adjacent motion segments more than 11 degrees from T1 to L5 and motion greater than 15 degrees at L5–S1 compared with L4–L5.

The diagnosis of LBP remains controversial and uncertain. The terms *nonspecific* or *mechanical* LBP have been commonly used for over a decade, describing a heterogeneous population of patients without specific disease. Clinicians involved in the management of LBP use the physical examination to ascertain management and treatment. The physical examination of patients with LBP consists of many components. Range of movement is a key component of most physical examination processes facilitating the assessment of spinal function, response to therapeutic input, determining work restrictions, functional capacity, or even permanent impairment. Various methods of quantification of range of movement have been advocated. These measures vary in complexity and include observation, tape measurement, goniometry (electrical, electromagnetic, and mechanical), inclinometry (electrical and mechanical), flexible curve lineals, and roentgenographic analysis (Littlewood, May, in press).

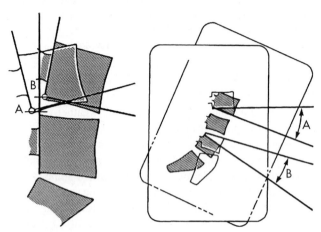

FIG. 8-153 Loss of motion segment integrity. **A,** Translation. **B,** Angular motion. (From Canale ST: *Campbell's operative orthopaedics,* vol 1-4, ed 9, St Louis, 1998, Mosby.)

PROCEDURE

* Schober test is used to assess lumbar spine flexion.
* A point is marked at the spinous process level of S2. Points 0.5 cm below S2 and 10 cm above the S2 level are marked (Fig. 8-154).
* The distance between the two S2 reference points is measured.
* The patient flexes forward. The distance between the S2 reference points is remeasured.
* The difference between the two measurements indicates the amount of lumbar flexion.
* Normally, the S2 reference points should separate at least 5 to 8 cm (Fig. 8-155).

Next Steps/Procedures
Bilateral leg-lowering test, Demianoff sign, double-leg-raise test, hyperextension test, Lewin supine test, matchstick test, Mennell sign, Minor sign, Nachlas test, Quick test, sign of the buttock, skin pinch test, spinal percussion test, and Vanzetti sign

CLINICAL PEARL

For a modification of this test, the patient is placed in a maximal flexion position (seated or standing), and starting from the upper sacral spinous prominence, three 10-cm segments are marked up the spine. The distances between the marks are then remeasured while the patient is erect. The lowest segment should shorten by at least 50%, the middle should shorten by 40%, and the upper should shorten by 30%. The shortening effect will be greater in tall subjects.

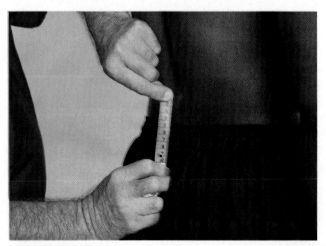

FIG. 8-154 The patient is standing with the arms folded across the chest. Points 0.5 cm below and 10 cm above the S2 level are marked. The span between the two S2 reference points is noted.

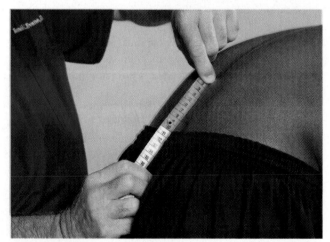

FIG. 8-155 The patient flexes forward. The distances between the two S2 reference points is remeasured. The difference indicates the amount of lumbar flexion. The separation between the S2 reference points should increase at least 5 to 8 cm.

SICARD SIGN

Assessment for Sciatic Radiculopathy

Comment

Spondylolisthesis is a disorder, usually in the lumbar spine, in which one vertebra gradually slips on another. Several types have been described (congenital, degenerative, pathologic, traumatic, and spondylolytic). However, most spondylolisthesis is secondary to spondylolysis, which represents a defect in the pars interarticularis or isthmus of the vertebra (Fig. 8-156). Spondylolisthesis is classified according to the amount of forward slippage of the affected vertebra (Fig. 8-157). LBP, sometimes radiating into the buttocks, occurs with activity and is relieved by rest. Symptoms of nerve root irritation may also be present, along with radiation of the pain into the extremities. These symptoms often progress in severity, especially in the adolescent. Roentgenograms reveal the typical findings of a defect in the pars interarticularis, which may be accompanied by forward slippage (Fig. 8-158).

Characteristic of sciatic pain—increased intraabdominal pressure produced by coughing and sneezing—markedly increases the severity of the pain. Patients with a severe attack will walk with the hip and knee slightly flexed and place the foot slowly on the floor. This carefulness is to prevent any undue traction of the nerve root, which normally

occurs when the extended leg is flexed at the hip. On the other hand, some of the patients exhibit no external malfunction. They do not experience back pain or muscle spasm. Back motion is free and unrestricted, and, in most instances, the patients are able to carry on their daily activities.

A sudden onset of pain usually occurs when a nuclear extrusion touches a nerve root. This phenomenon may occur either during the stage of nuclear sequestration (the interme-

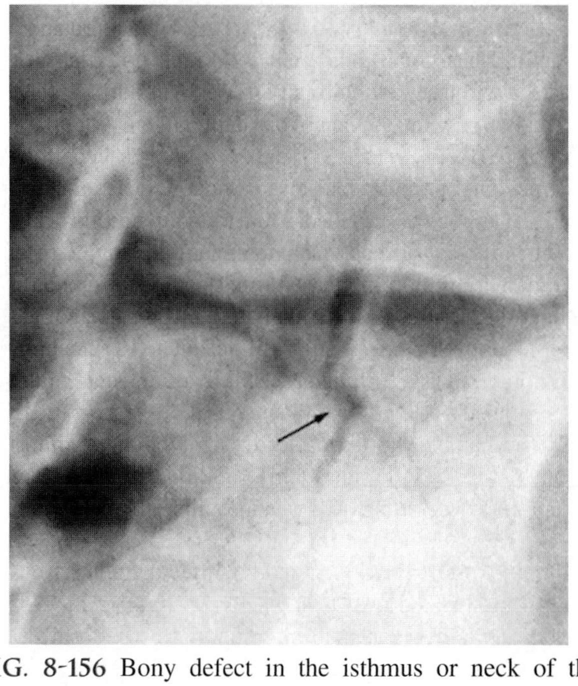

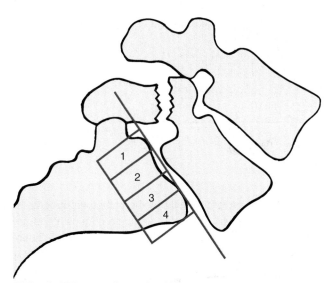

FIG. 8-157 Myerding classification of spondylolisthesis. (From Mercier LR, Pettid FJ: *Practical orthopedics,* ed 4, St Louis, 1995, Mosby.)

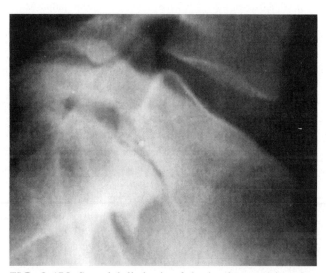

FIG. 8-158 Spondylolisthesis of the lumbosacral junction (note early indication of Knutsson vacuum sign at L5-S1). (From Mercier LR, Pettid FJ: *Practical orthopedics,* ed 4, St Louis, 1995, Mosby.)

FIG. 8-156 Bony defect in the isthmus or neck of the Scottie dog present in spondylolysis. (From Mercier LR, Pettid FJ: *Practical orthopedics,* ed 4, St Louis, 1995, Mosby.)

diate stage) or toward the end of the pathologic process in the nucleus. Fibrosis of the disc is the predominant feature, but fragments of nuclear material that may be extruded may still be present. The distance that the pain spreads along a dermatome is directly proportional to the amount of tension and compression to which the root is subjected.

> Although the mechanical and positional stresses of pregnancy are the primary inciting factors contributing to lumbosacral pain accompanying gestation, in approximately 1 in 10,000 cases, a herniated disk (herniated nucleus pulposus [HNP]) can be identified as the proximal cause of pain. During pregnancy, an MRI evaluation permits a detailed spinal examination without the ionizing effects of x-ray and its acknowledged biologic risk to the developing fetus (LaBan et al, 1995).

An interesting phenomenon is observed in patients with severe sciatica. The pain may suddenly disappear, but the motor and sensory deficits remain, which indicates that the physiologic function of the root is completely interrupted. This lack of pain must not be misconstrued as evidence that the patient is getting better.

Any of the patterns of sciatica may be initiated simply by contact with a sensitive nerve root and without actual herniation of nuclear material. Slight bulging, without rupture, of the annulus may be sufficient to precipitate a sciatic syndrome merely because the bulge touches the hypersensitive nerve root.

> Lumbar disc disease is common, and symptomatic lumbar disc herniation has been recognized for over 70 years. Dandy (1929) was the first to recognize the clinical syndrome of

radicular pain caused by an extradural mass, and Mixter and Barr (1934) were the first to document that extruded disc material caused sciatic pain and detailed a surgical approach to the problem. The most commonly recognized clinical syndrome is that of radiculopathy resulting from posterior or posterolateral disc rupture. Sequestered disc fragments account for 28.6% of all symptomatic disc herniations. Herniated disc fragments are known to migrate within the spinal canal in many directions, including rostral, caudal and lateral, and posterior epidural disc fragment migration has been reported rarely (Mobbs, Steel, 2007).

Once a fragment transgresses the peridural membrane, epidural fat, and the epidural venous plexus, the nerve root itself presumably acts as an impediment to further posterior migration.

PROCEDURE

- While the patient is supine, the extended leg is raised to a point just short of that which produces pain (Fig. 8-159).
- When the sign is present, dorsiflexion of the great toe reproduces sciatic pain (Fig. 8-160).
- The test is significant for sciatic radiculopathy.

Next Steps/Procedures

Bechterew sitting test, Bragard sign, Deyerle sign, Fajersztajn test, Lasègue differential sign, Lasègue rebound test, Lasègue sitting test, Lasègue test, Lewin standing test, Lindner sign, straight-leg-raising test, and Turyn sign

CLINICAL PEARL

The second, third, and fourth nerve roots do not have an increase in tension during straight leg raising, but they do undergo an increase in tension during the femoral stretch tests.

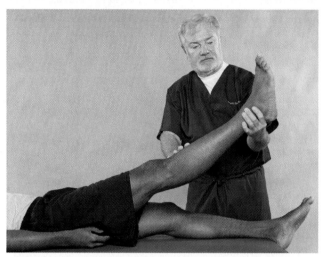

FIG. 8-159 The patient is supine with both legs fully extended. The examiner straight leg raises the affected leg to the point at which symptoms are reproduced.

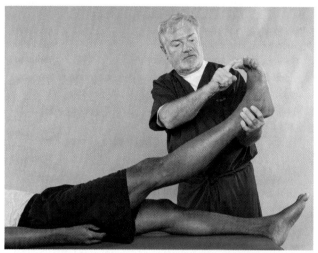

FIG. 8-160 The leg is lowered to a point just below the point at which symptoms are produced, and the examiner sharply dorsiflexes the great toe of the affected foot. The sign is present if toe dorsiflexion reproduces the symptoms. The sign is present with sciatic radiculopathy.

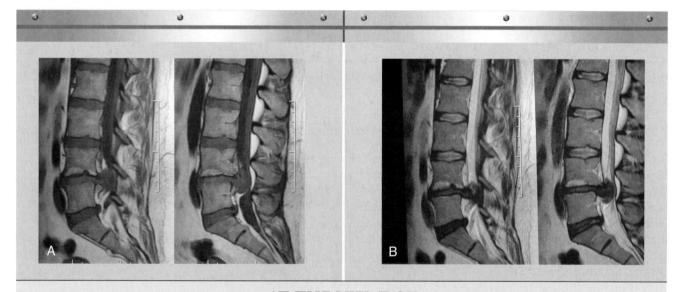

AT THE VIEWBOX

A second patient with a massive disc herniation at L4-5, associated with marked disc space narrowing and retrolisthesis of L4. Not the Modic type 2 fibrofatty subchondral marrow changes. The patient had already consulted a neurosurgeon who recommended surgery. She sought a second opinion, hoping to avoid surgery, but this degree of cauda equina compression is typically considered a surgical emergency. (From the teaching file of Timothy Mick, DC, DACBR)

SIGN OF THE BUTTOCK

Assessment for Gluteal Bursitis, Tumor, or Abscess

Comment

Benign soft-tissue tumors are estimated to be 100 times more common than malignant soft-tissue tumors, with a reported annual clinical incidence of 300 per 100,000. MRI has long been established as the imaging technique of choice for such lesions, but it is limited by the tendency of both benign and malignant soft-tissue masses to demonstrate prolonged T1 and T2 relaxation times. Prediction of the histology of soft-tissue masses from the imaging appearances has been shown to be accurate in only approximately 30% of cases, although lesions in the hand and wrist have been reported as more easily characterized. Lesions with more typical imaging findings include lipomas and their variants, the fibromatoses, hemangiomas, and peripheral nerve sheath tumors (Goodwin, O'Donnell, Saifuddin, in press).

A Morel-Lavallée effusion results as the skin and subcutaneous fatty tissue abruptly separate from the underlying fascia. It is a traumatic lesion pattern that has been termed *closed degloving injury*. This separation creates a cavity that is filled with hematoma, resulting from the disruption of arteries perforating through the fascia, and a mixture of viable and necrotic fat. Morel-Lavallée effusions are particularly common in the trochanteric region and proximal thigh, for which they have been specifically termed *Morel-Lavallée lesions*. Morel-Lavallée described a closed degloving injury in the mid-nineteenth century. Letournel and Judet eventually referred to degloving injuries occurring over the region of the greater trochanter as Morel-Lavallée lesions. These lesions are well known but are rarely mentioned in the medical literature. In addition, these lesions have been listed under different names, including posttraumatic cyst of soft tissue, pseudocyst, Morel-Lavallée extravasation, and Morel-Lavallée effusion. Related posttraumatic entities described as ancient hematoma and chronic expanding hematoma in the literature may have been representing the end stage of some long-standing Morel-Lavallée lesions (Kalaci, Karazincir, Yanat, 2007).

In 1948, Stout first described myxoma as a true mesenchymal neoplasm composed of undifferentiated satellite cells embedded in loose myxoid stroma. Soft-tissue myxoma is a benign neoplasm that may arise from fibroblasts producing an excessive amount of mucopolysaccharide. Most patients with myxoma have a diagnosis of intramuscular compartment origin (82%), the average age of the patients is 55 years, women are slightly predominant, and the tumor has predilection for the thigh (51%), followed by the upper arm (9%), calf (7%), and buttock (7%). The typical appearance

of intramuscular myxoma is a well-defined ovoid tumor with fluid content, with an average size of 7 cm (range, 1.5-17 cm). Most tumors (95%) are characterized by a homogeneous hypointense signal on T1-weighted images and a hyperintense signal on fluid-sensitive MR sequences because of the high water content of mucin, which has been proved histologically (Yao et al, 2007).

The most common injury to the buttocks is from a direct blow, which does not usually cause injury to the skin because of the ample underlying padding. Contusion of the muscle is a common occurrence, but it is usually of little conse-

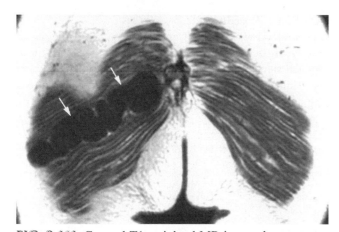

FIG. 8-161 Coronal T1-weighted MR image demonstrates a lobulated tumor *(arrows)* with a homogeneous hypointense signal at the right gluteus muscle. A tumor located along the axis of the gluteus muscle can mimic ganglion cyst of the abductor tendons. (Adapted from Yao MS, Chen CY, Chin-Wei Chien J, et al: Magnetic resonance imaging of gluteal intramuscular myxoma, *Clin Imag* 31(3):214-216, 2007.)

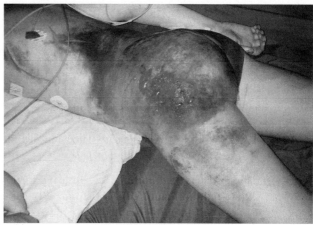

FIG. 8-162 Hemodynamically unstable left buttock contusion and rupture of superior gluteal artery, expanding and spreading to the loins, scrotum and thigh. Within the first 12 hours, the patient received a total of 27 units of blood, 10 units of FFP and 5 units of cryoprecipitate in addition to crystalloid solutions. (Adapted from Haikel S, Willett K. Traumatic rupture of the superior gluteal artery with a stable pelvic fracture, *Injury* 31(5):383-386, 2000.)

quence. In most of the areas of the buttocks, a thick muscle mass is in little danger of being caught between two unyielding objects. As a result, the condition resulting from a blow is diffuse, without gross hematoma formation in the muscle. A tender, painful muscle mass results, and although it may be uncomfortable, the condition is not disabling. During athletic competition, the buttocks are usually not protected by any padding other than that inherent in the athlete's anatomy. Superficial contusion is common, and the examiner should be wary of the condition that is unduly severe or that causes something other than local symptoms.

A contusion of the sciatic nerve may result in pain that begins in the buttock and extends down the back of the thigh into the calf and foot in a way that is similar to sciatic pain from other causes. This pain is nonradicular in character and follows the whole distribution of the sciatic nerve rather than any single nerve root. Straight leg raising causes pain in the area of the contusion. During the acute period, hypesthesia (hypoesthesia) of the skin may be evident in the lower portion of the extremity. This contusion of the sciatic nerve will require no particular treatment other than protection against stretch.

The superior gluteal artery is vulnerable to injury associated with displacement of the fractured pelvic or acetabular fragment or traction injury without any apparent fracture in high-energy trauma; a major disadvantage of late decom-

pression of the buttock is exposure of the hematoma and devitalized muscle to the risk of infection (Fig. 8-162).

Bleeding from the superior gluteal artery may be extensive resulting in compartment syndrome of the buttock. If active bleeding is suspected, urgent arteriography with embolization of the pelvic vessel must be considered prior to fasciotomy. At surgery the hemorrhage may be difficult to arrest because of poor visibility from profuse bleeding and retraction of the proximal vessel into the pelvis. A risk to the sciatic nerve exists if blind clamping of vessels is attempted in the region of the sciatic notch (Haikel, Willett, 2000).

Whether as a result of pelvic fracture, or blunt buttock injury without a fracture, superior gluteal artery rupture is an immediate, potentially life-threatening event (Kligman et al, 2002).

Another area of the buttocks in which a complication of contusion may arise is over the ischial tuberosity. Here the bone is subcutaneous, although it is protected by a layer of muscle of greater or lesser thickness. A contusion here may cause a fracture of the tuberosity, in which case the patient experiences severe pain. The pain is increased by straight leg raising or by any local pressure. More commonly, the result of the blow will be periostitis or fibrositis over the roughened surface of the bone. Other cases will involve the ischial bursa. In the early stages, distinguishing between these conditions is impossible.

8

PROCEDURE

- A passive unilateral straight-leg-raising test is performed on a supine patient (Fig. 8-163).
- When unilateral restriction is encountered, the knee is flexed to determine if hip flexion increases (Fig. 8-164).
- If the lumbar spine is the source of complaint, hip flexion will increase.
- A positive sign of the buttock occurs when hip flexion does not increase with knee flexion.
- The sign is present in bursitis, tumor, or abscess.

Next Steps/Procedures

Bilateral leg-lowering test, Demianoff sign, double-leg-raise test, hyperextension test, Lewin supine test, matchstick test, Mennell sign, Minor sign, Nachlas test, Quick test, Schober test, skin pinch test, spinal percussion test, and Vanzetti sign

CLINICAL PEARL

Trochanteric bursitis causes localized pain and tenderness over the trochanter and occasionally causes pain that radiates down the lateral thigh. The pain is particularly strong when lying on the affected side. Pain from ischio-gluteal bursitis is felt posteriorly and is particularly exacerbated by sitting.

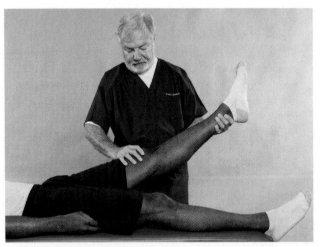

FIG. 8-163 The patient is supine, and the examiner performs a straight-leg-raising test on the affected leg.

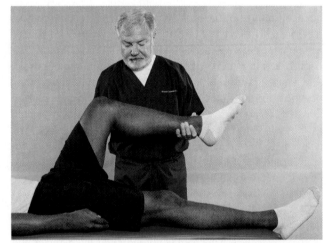

FIG. 8-164 With restriction of the leg movement because of pain or myospasm, the knee is passively flexed. If the disorder is in the lumbar spine, hip flexion increases. If hip flexion does not increase with knee flexion, it is a positive sign of the buttock. A positive sign indicates hip or buttock bursitis, tumor, or abscess.

Assessment for Fibrositic Infiltration

Comment

The most precise definition of true sciatica is pain radiating into the lower limb below the level of the knee in the distribution of a single nerve root and is associated with other neurosensory changes such as numbness, tingling, or weakness (Fig. 8-165). Sciatica usually radiates down one leg in the distribution of the L5 or S1 nerve root. In the case of the S1 nerve root, this pain involves the lateral border of the lower leg and foot, and in the case of the L5 root, the pain involves anterolateral aspect of the leg and dorsum of the foot.

Neurologic claudication is another variant of the peripheral manifestations of lumbar disease. In this condition, pain is felt in the distribution of one or more lumbosacral nerve roots, although the pain is often less well localized than the sciatica or femoral neuritis associated with a disc prolapse. It is often accompanied by neurologic symptoms such as numbness or weakness.

Other clinical findings further help distinguish these two entities (neurogenic claudication versus vascular claudication). Because of the poor circulation in the lower extremities associated with vascular claudication, the feet are cool to the touch and pedal pulses are weak or absent. Other findings include smooth skin and a paucity of hair on the lower legs. Venous stasis and atrophic skin may also be associated with vascular claudication. Noninvasive testing includes measurement of the ankle-brachial index, a ratio of blood pressure in the upper extremity compared with the lower extremity. In most cases, patients will undergo a radiographic imaging study of the lumbar spine. Other tests for nerve root compression (neurogenic claudication) include electromyographic and nerve conduction velocity studies (Gerber et al, 2003).

LBP is a common presenting complaint in emergency departments and primary care clinics. Approximately 90% of adults will experience back pain at some point in their life. Most patients' pain will ultimately resolve spontaneously within 1 to 2 months without a definitive cause of pain and with minimal intervention and a favorable outcome. Multiple causes of back pain must be considered; the patient's age, current and past medical history, and physical examination will guide the clinician toward the appropriate cause in many instances. One entity that may be associated with the complaint of LBP is cauda equina syndrome (CES), which is a relatively rare neurosurgical emergency (Small, Perron, Brady, 2005).

CES is a rare but catastrophic type of low back disease. This condition may arise from a massive lumbar disc herniation, spinal stenosis, tumors, infections, injuries, or other neurologic disease. It is often preceded or accompanied by symptoms of sciatica or neurologic claudication that may be bilateral.

CES is often a neurologic emergency. It has several causes, including lumbar canal stenosis secondary to spondylosis. CES should be considered early in the differential diagnosis of conus medullaris syndrome commonly caused by extrinsic compression of the caudal spinal cord. CES is typically associated with saddle hypoanesthesia, perianal numbness, sphincter disturbance, decreased motor strength, and hypo-

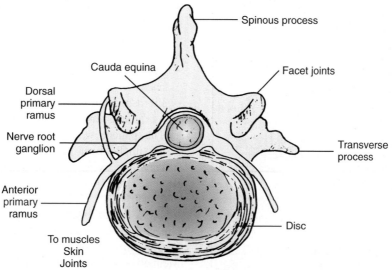

FIG. 8-165 Normal relationships of lumbar nerve roots. (From Pope MH et al: *Occupational low back pain assessment, treatment and prevention*, St Louis, 1991, Mosby.)

reflexia or areflexia. Based on a retrospective review by Kennedy and colleagues, the most important predictor of a favorable outcome in CES is early diagnosis and decompression. Therefore diagnosing CES and instituting appropriate intervention early is imperative to improve outcomes (Lai, Ubogu, in press).

Fibromyalgia syndrome or fibromyositis syndrome really does not present a formidable differential diagnosis, even though it causes symmetric arthralgia and myalgia, which are usually worse after awakening in the morning. Although patients complain of stiffness, unlike persons with RA, they are not stiff. Joint swelling is absent, and tenderness is mild,

except over tense muscles. Muscle atrophy is never seen. No constitutional symptoms, such as fever and weight loss, are observed. The erythrocyte sedimentation rate is normal, and the test for rheumatoid factor is negative. Patients are rarely anemic, and diagnostic imaging of the joints shows normal results. Most patients with the fibromyalgia syndrome are emotionally tense.

> cLBP with radicular symptoms distal to the knee and verified lumbar intervertebral disc herniation is associated with generalized deep-tissue hyperalgesia. This scenario suggests that such chronic pain condition, in addition to the afferent nociceptive barrage, may also be associated with neuroplastic changes (hyperexcitability) (O'Neill et al, 2007).

Nonarticular (soft-tissue) *rheumatism* is a term that encompasses a large group of miscellaneous conditions with a common denominator of musculoskeletal pain and stiffness. This designation is for convenience only and not because of any common etiologic or clinical characteristics. Although some forms of nonarticular rheumatism, such as bursitis and tendinopathy, present well-defined features, the causes of others, including fibrositis and myalgia, are not as clear.

Fibrositis is inflammatory hyperplasia of white connective tissue. It is now a term used rarely in the presence of such real tissue inflammation as arthritis, tendinopathy, or myositis. Among rheumatologists, fibrositis indicates aching, stiffness, tenderness, and pain around joints, muscle fibers, and subcutaneous tissues without the presence of an inflammatory pathologic process. Fibrositis is a local and diffuse idiopathic condition. The symptom complex of fibrositis, with or without connective tissue inflammation, may be a prominent manifestation of many rheumatic diseases, including systemic lupus erythematosus, RA, and subdeltoid bursitis.

ORTHOPEDIC GAMUT 8-47

CAUDA EQUINA SYNDROME

The clinical characteristics of cauda equina syndrome (CES triad of signs) include the following:

1. Anesthesia in the distribution of the S2–S4 nerve roots, which supply the perineum in the distribution of a person sitting on a saddle, leading to the term saddle anesthesia
2. Disturbance of bladder and bowel control with urinary incontinence or retention and fecal incontinence (Any urinary disturbance in a patient with back pain constitutes an emergency and requires urgent investigation.)
3. Lower extremity weakness

ORTHOPEDIC GAMUT 8-48

CAUDA EQUINA SYNDROME DIAGNOSTIC ESSENTIALS

- Presentation
  - Low back pain
  - Radicular symptoms
  - Lower-extremity paresthesias
  - Lower-extremity weakness
  - Urinary or fecal retention, incontinence
  - Gait abnormalities
  - Frequent falls
- Examination
  - Leg weakness
  - Decreased or absent deep-tendon reflexes
  - Saddle anesthesia
  - Decreased or absent sphincter tone
- Tests
  - Positive straight-leg-raising
  - Abnormal sphincter tone
  - Postvoid residual above 100–200 mL
  - Obtain urgent whole spine magnetic resonance imaging

PROCEDURE

- The skin pinch test involves smoothly rolling the skin over the spinous process of the vertebrae by using the forefingers over the advancing thumbs (Fig. 8-166).
- The skin is picked up before rolling it.
- Skin rolling is then performed over each side of the back.
- Fibrositic infiltration and trigger points are demonstrated by tightness and acute tenderness.
- The patient will experience tightness and tenderness maximally over the level at which a pathologic bone condition exists or over the vertebra above the level at which a pathologic oint or disc condition exists.

Next Steps/Procedures

Bilateral leg-lowering test, Demianoff sign, double-leg-raise test, hyperextension test, Lewin supine test, matchstick test, Mennell sign, Minor sign, Nachlas test, Quick test, Schober test, sign of the buttock, spinal percussion test, and Vanzetti sign

CLINICAL PEARL

Trophedematous subcutaneous tissue has a boggy, inelastic texture when rolled between the thumb and finger. This type of tissue is distinguishable from subcutaneous fat. When a patch of skin and subcutaneous tissue a centimeter in diameter is gently squeezed together, instead of immediately forming a fold of flesh, trophedematous tissue does not budge, or it finally yields altogether, with a sudden expanding movement similar to that of inflating a rubber dinghy or air mattress.

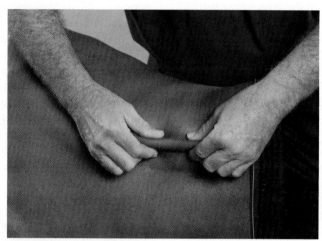

FIG. 8-166 The patient is in either the prone or side-lying position. The examiner picks up an area of skin overlying the affected level of the spine. The examiner performs smooth rolling of the skin over the spinous process of the vertebrae, moving the forefingers over the advancing thumbs. Skin rolling is then performed over each side of the back. The test is positive if tightness and acute tenderness are elicited. A positive test indicates fibrositic infiltration and trigger points.

Assessment for Osseous or Soft-Tissue Injury in the Lumbar Spine

Comment

Fracture risk increases with age, prior fracture at any site, and decreasing BMD. The risk of recurrent fracture is highest in the first 2 years after a fracture (12%), especially in the first year. Early diagnosis and treatment of osteoporosis immediately after fracture is therefore vital (Blonk et al, 2007).

Vehicular accidents are a common source of trauma to the lumbosacral spine and may cause a wide variety of fractures and dislocations. Compression fractures at the anterior edge of the vertebral bodies may be caused by a hyperflexion motion alone or in combination with a vertical compression. The stability of these fractures depends on the degree of vertebral compression and the presence or absence of posterior ligamentous damage.

The question of cord damage is dominant; spine fractures are classified as stable or unstable. In stable fractures, the cord is rarely damaged, and movement of the spine is safe. In unstable fractures, the cord may have been damaged, but if it has escaped damage, it may still be injured by movement.

Stability depends largely on the integrity of the ligaments and in particular the posterior ligament complex. This complex consists of the supraspinous ligament, the interspinous ligaments, the capsules of the facet joints, and possibly the ligamentum flavum. Fortunately, only 10% of the spinal injuries are unstable, and less than 5% are associated with cord damage.

Injuries usually occur when the spinal column is compressed and collapsed in its vertical axis. This injury typically occurs during a fall from a height or when the patient gets trapped under a cave-in; the direction of the force at any level of the spine is determined by the position of the vertebral column during impact. The flexible lumbar segments may also be injured by violent, free movements of the trunk.

Hyperextension is rare in the thoracolumbar spine. When hyperextension occurs, the anterior ligaments and the disc may be damaged, or the neural arch may be fractured. The injury is usually stable, but fracture of the pedicle is often unstable.

If the posterior ligaments remain intact, forced flexion will crush the vertebral body into a wedge. This injury is a stable injury and is by far the most common type of vertebral fracture. If the posterior ligaments are torn, the upper vertebral body may tilt forward on the one below. This type of subluxation is often missed because, by the time the diagnostic image is made, the vertebrae have fallen back into place.

Most serious injuries of the spine are caused by a combination of flexion and rotation. The ligaments and joint capsules, which are strained to the limit, may tear. The facets may fracture, or the top of one vertebra may be sheared off. The result is a forward shift, or dislocation, of the vertebra above, with or without concomitant bone damage. All fracture-dislocations are unstable.

A vertical force acting on a straight segment of the lumbar spine will compress the vertebral body and may cause a comminuted, or burst, fracture. If the vertebra is split, a large fragment may be driven backwards into the spinal canal. This fragment makes these fractures dangerous. Such fractures are associated with a high incidence of neurologic damage.

ORTHOPEDIC GAMUT 8-49

SPINAL TRAUMA MECHANISMS

Spinal trauma mechanisms:
1. Hyperextension
2. Flexion
3. Flexion combined with rotation
4. Axial displacement (compression)

ORTHOPEDIC GAMUT 8-50

OSTEOPOROTIC COMPRESSION FRACTURE CLASSIFICATION

- Type I compression fracture involving the anterior column only
  - Type Ia is a compression fracture with union.
  - Type Ib is a compression fracture with non-union.
- Type II fracture involving both the anterior and middle column
  - Type IIa is a compression fracture with union.
  - Type IIb is a compression fracture with nonunion.
- Type II compression fractures have a higher incidence of non-union than type I.
- In both type I and II non-union groups, fractures achieve greater increase in vertebral body height after vertebroplasty than both type I and type II union group fractures.
- In both non-union groups, fractures achieve a greater reduction of kyphotic angle postvertebroplasty than type I and II union group fractures.

ORTHOPEDIC GAMUT 8-51

ANTERIOR VERTEBRAL COMPRESSION FRACTURES

Roentgenographic findings in anterior vertebral compression fractures:

1. Buckling of the anterior vertebral body cortex
2. Wedge deformity of the fractured vertebral body, with loss of the vertebral body height anteriorly compared with its posterior height (Fig. 8-167)
3. Possibility of some focal increase in kyphosis (Fig. 8-168)
4. A zone of condensation caused by compaction of the trabecular elements of the spongiosa, appearing as a band of increased osseous density through the medullary bone beneath the affected end-plate
5. Vertebral end-plate fractures occur more frequently in the lower thoracic and upper lumbar spines (Fig. 8-169).
6. Vertebral body compression fractures may be suspected when a *frog-face* sign is exhibited on the anteroposterior study (Fig. 8-170).
7. Paraspinal soft-tissue injury is often observed with spinal compression fractures.

In the Chance fracture, a horizontal line may extend through the spinous process, splitting the neural arch (through the laminae, articular pillars, and pedicles) and extending into the posterior body surface. The fracture line divides the vertebra into upper and lower halves.

ORTHOPEDIC GAMUT 8-52

SPINAL FRACTURES

Other forms of spinal fractures may include the following:

1. Lateral body compression-type fractures
2. Pillar fractures
3. Lamina-pedicle fractures
4. Transverse process fractures (Fig. 8-171)

ORTHOPEDIC GAMUT 8-53

INTRA DISCAL PRESSURE

Compressive forces that influencing intra discal pressure:

1. *Standing:* Disc pressure is equal to 100% of body weight.
2. *Supine:* Disc pressure is less than 25% of body weight.
3. *Side lying:* Disc pressure is less than 75% of body weight.
4. *Standing and bending forward:* Disc pressure is approximately 150% of body weight.
5. *Supine with both knees flexed:* Disc pressure is less than 35% of body weight.
6. *Seated in a flexed position:* Disc pressure is approximately 85% of body weight.
7. *Bending forward in a flexed posture and lifting:* Disc pressure is approaching 275% of body weight.

Compression defect of the body of a lumbar vertebra may occur with minimal force in osteoporotic or pathologic bone.

Osteoporotic compression fractures is typically characterized by acute, excruciating back pain, the onset of which does not usually occur as a result of obvious trauma but is precipitated by minor stress such as bending forward. Loss of vertebral body height and kyphotic deformity after osteoporotic compression fractures may cause muscle spasm, stress on ligaments, nerve-root irritation, or any combination, which, in turn, produces chronic back pain. Severe neurologic deficits after osteoporotic fractures are unusual but may develop in the late stages. Fractures, which are frequently multiple, occur most commonly at the thoracolumbar junctions, followed in order of frequency by the middle thoracic and lower lumbar vertebrae (Wu et al, 2006).

8

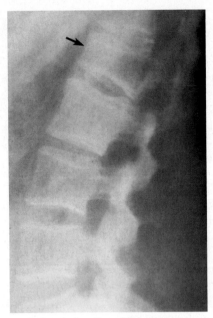

FIG. 8-167 Wedge deformity of the anterior vertebral body height may be indicative of a compression fracture. (From Deltoff MN, Kogon PL: *The portable skeletal x-ray library,* St Louis, 1998, Mosby.)

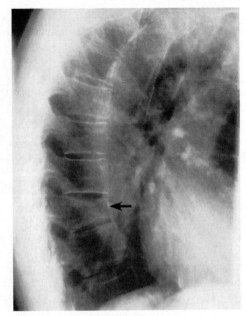

FIG. 8-168 Anterior vertebral body fractures may result in focal or generalized hyperkyphotic angulation of the spine. (From Deltoff MN, Kogon PL: *The portable skeletal x-ray library,* St Louis, 1998, Mosby.)

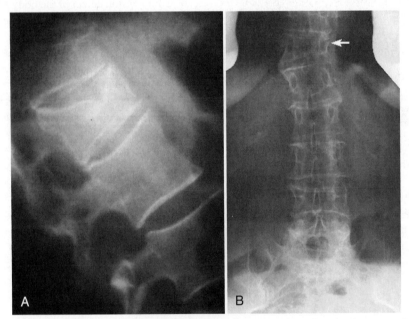

FIG. 8-169 Vertebral body compression fractures occur more often in the upper lumbar or lower thoracic spine.

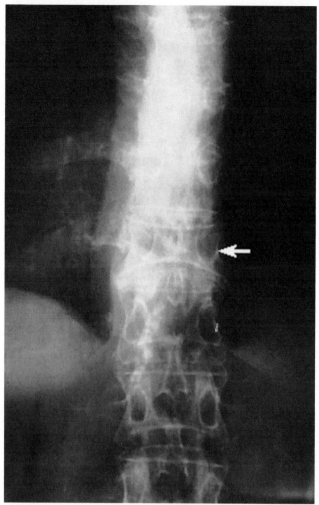

FIG. 8-170 A frog-face sign observed on an anteroposterior radiograph suggests the presence of a vertebral body compression fracture. (From Deltoff MN, Kogon PL: *The portable skeletal x-ray library,* St Louis, 1998, Mosby.)

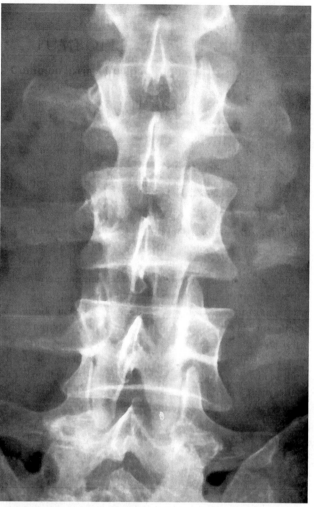

FIG. 8-171 Transverse process fractures at L2, L3, and L4. (From Deltoff MN, Kogon PL: *The portable skeletal x-ray library,* St Louis, 1998, Mosby.)

PROCEDURE

- While the patient is standing and the trunk is slightly flexed, the examiner uses a neurologic hammer to percuss the spinous processes and the associated musculature of each of the lumbar vertebrae (Fig. 8-172).
- Evidence of localized pain indicates a possible vertebra fracture.
- Evidence of radicular pain indicates a possible disc lesion.
- Because of the nonspecific nature of this test, other conditions will also elicit a positive pain response.
- For example, a ligamentous sprain will cause pain when the spinous processes are percussed.
- Percussing the paraspinal musculature will elicit a positive sign for muscular strain (Figs. 8-173 and 8-174).

Next Steps/Procedures

Bilateral leg-lowering test, Demianoff sign, double-leg-raise test, hyperextension test, Lewin supine test, matchstick test, Mennell sign, Minor sign, Nachlas test, Quick test, Schober test, sign of the buttock, skin pinch test, and Vanzetti sign

CLINICAL PEARL

When soft-tissue percussion reproduces the complaint, the examiner may expect the same phenomenon from the use of ultrasound on the tissue. The uses of such therapies may be delayed until the soft tissue is no longer reactive to percussion.

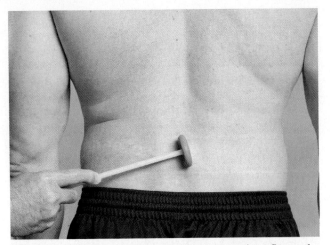

FIG. 8-172 In the standing position, the patient flexes the lumbosacral spine, exposing the spinous processes as much as possible. The examiner percusses the spinous processes of each vertebra. Localized pain is evidence of a fracture or severe sprain. Radiating pain suggests an intervertebral disc syndrome.

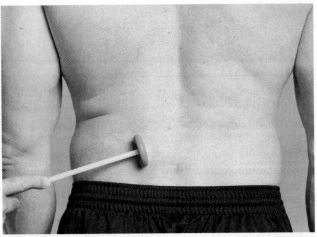

FIG. 8-173 The paravertebral tissues are percussed similarly. Pain elicited in the soft tissues suggests muscular strain and highly sensitive myofascial trigger points.

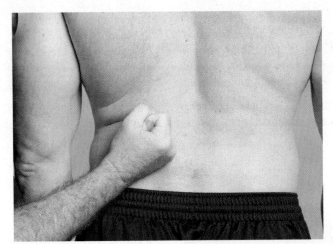

FIG. 8-174 The examiner may perform gross percussion of the lumbar paraspinal tissue. This maneuver is similar to the Lewin punch test. Pain elicited suggests soft-tissue injury.

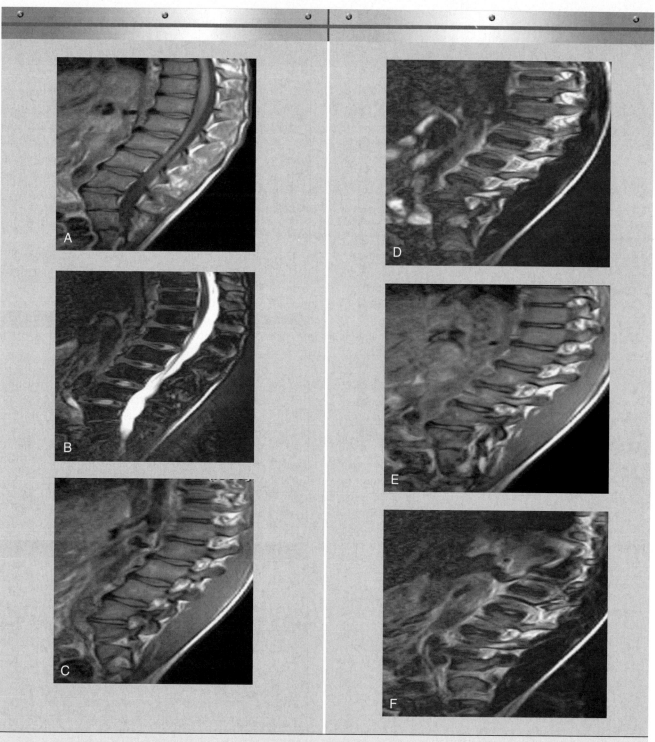

AT THE VIEWBOX

15-year-old male with focal low back pain related to sports activity. Tenderness with spinous process percussion at L5. Midline sagittal MR images are negative (**A, B**), but sagittal images through the pars regions demonstrate diminished T1 and increased T2 signal (bone marrow edema pattern) through the L5 pars regions (**C, D, E, F**), consistent with developing pars stress fractures (spondylolysis). (From the teaching file of Timothy Mick, DC, DACBR)

Assessment for Space-Occupying Mass in the Path of a Nerve Root, Sacroiliac Inflammation, and Lumbosacral Involvement

Comment

The disability caused by LBP leads to a high socioeconomic impact. Despite the growing research addressing assessment and treatment strategies, a considerable percentage of patients continue to be affected by lower back problems. Today, LBP is perceived as a multidimensional problem. Pathoanatomic, physical, neurophysiologic, psychologic, and social factors might influence the disorder (Roussel et al, 2007).

The straight-leg-raising (SLR) test assesses for irritation of the sciatic nerve (L4, L5, S1). Passively raising the leg with the knee extended stretches the sciatic nerve (Fig. 8-175). When the dura is inflamed and stretched, the patient experiences pain along its anatomic course. Dural movement starts at 30 degrees of elevation. Pain of dural origin should not be felt below this degree of elevation. Pain is maximal between 30 and 70 degrees of elevation. Symptoms at greater degrees of elevation may be of nerve root origin but may also be related to mechanical LBP secondary to muscle strain or joint disease.

Normal straight leg raising does not preclude the diagnosis of herniated nucleus pulposus. The response to straight leg raising is generally believed to be caused, in part, by the location of the herniation. Research has shown that straight leg raising causes nerve roots to move distally 0.5 to 5 mm, but the nerve roots also move laterally toward the bone and therefore move into a posterolateral herniation and potentially away from a central herniation. Therefore a midline herniation may not cause sciatica during straight leg raising, and the test will be negative.

The L4 nerve root moves less than L5 and S1 during supine straight leg raising.

Obviously, differentiating sciatica from hamstring tightness during straight leg raising is important. In a classically positive test, sciatica is produced at 30 degrees or less on one side, whereas the other side has full range. In hamstring tightness, leg pain occurs at approximately the same angle on each leg, and pain is confined to the posterior thigh and does not go below the knee.

The SLR test will cause traction on the sciatic nerve, lumbosacral nerve roots, and dura mater. Adhesions within these areas may be caused by herniation of the intervertebral disc or to extradural or meningeal irritation. Pain that the patient feels comes from the dura mater, nerve root, adventitial sheath of the epidural veins, or the synovial facet joints. The test is positive if pain extends from the back down the leg along the sciatic nerve distribution.

In humans, clinical tests such as the SLR test have been developed for patients with low back or leg pain to test for lumbosacral nerve root irritation. The SLR test consists of passive flexion of the hip, with the knee in extension and

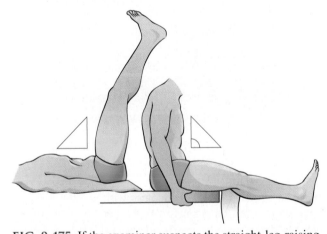

FIG. 8-175 If the examiner suspects the straight-leg-raising test to be unreliable in the supine position, the examiner can surreptitiously raise the leg while the patient is in the sitting position. If the lesion is organic, radiating pain should be experienced in both positions. (From Olson WH et al: *Handbook of symptom-related neurology,* ed 2, St Louis, 1994, Mosby.)

ORTHOPEDIC GAMUT 8-54

UNILATERAL STRAIGHT LEG RAISING

The following are dynamics of unilateral straight leg raising:

1. The slack in sciatic arborization is taken up from 0 to 35 degrees. No dural movement is observed.
2. When approaching 35 degrees, tension is applied to the sciatic nerve roots.
3. In the range of 35 to 70 degrees, the sciatic nerve roots tense over the intervertebral disc. The rate of nerve root deformation diminishes as the angle increases.
4. Above 60 to 70 degrees, practically no further deformation of the root occurs during further straight leg raising, and the pain probably originates in the joint.

the ankle in neutral. The SLR test elongates the nerve bed (the tract formed by the structures that surround the nerve), which increases tension in the nerve roots, the lumbosacral plexus, and the sciatic and tibial nerve. However, the SLR test also loads nonneural structures, such as the hamstring muscles. Sensitizing movements are therefore added to help differentiate neurogenic symptoms from pain from alternative sources, such as musculoskeletal pain. Sensitizing maneuvers aim to increase selectively the mechanical provocation of the peripheral nerve by increasing nerve strain, with minimal effects on other musculoskeletal tissues around the painful area. A change in symptoms after the addition of a sensitizing movement suggests that the symptoms have a neurogenic origin. The most commonly used sensitizing movement in humans is the addition of ankle dorsiflexion to the angle of hip flexion when pain is elicited (Babbage, Coppieters, McGowan, 2007).

The SLR test is commonly used in the assessment of lumbar radiculopathy and is considered a sensitive screening tool for this entity. It should be performed bilaterally and is considered positive with pain referral below the knee. Deville and colleagues determined that the pooled sensitivity for the SLR test was 91% (95% confidence interval [CI], .82-.94), and the pooled specificity was 26% (95% CI, .16-.38). The mean positive predictive value was 89%; the negative predictive value was 33% (Nadler, Malanga, Ciccone, 2004).

PROCEDURE

- The patient lies supine with the legs extended.
- The examiner places one hand under the heel of the patient's affected leg and the other hand on the knee (Fig. 8-176).
- With the limb extended, the examiner flexes the patient's thigh on the pelvis.
- If this maneuver is markedly limited because of pain, the test is positive and may suggest sciatica from lumbosacral or sacroiliac lesions, subluxation syndrome, disc lesions, spondylolisthesis, adhesions, or IVF occlusion.
- The exacerbation of pain by raising the extended leg is further evidence of the effects of traction on a sensitized nerve root (Fig. 8-177).
- Normally, the leg can be raised 15 to 30 degrees before the nerve root is tractioned through the IVF.
- Pain, duplicating sciatica, that is elicited by this maneuver indicates a space-occupying lesion—such as lumbar disc protrusion, tumor, adhesions, edema, and tissue inflammation—at the nerve root level.

Next Steps/Procedures
Bechterew sitting test, Bragard sign, Deyerle sign, Fajersztajn test, Lasègue differential sign, Lasègue rebound test, Lasègue sitting test, Lasègue test, Lewin standing test, Lindner sign, Sicard sign, and Turyn sign

8

CLINICAL PEARL

As many authors have pointed out, the nerve roots have a narrow range of movement for stretching. Most authors also conclude that the nerve roots in normal conditions are not stretched by the straight-leg-raising test until 35 to 70 degrees of angulation have been reached. However, if the nerve exists with a space-occupying mass (protrusion of disc material) that deflects the nerve's normal pathway, the amount of allowable stretch is already used up by the mass. In this case, the positive sign, pain radiating down the sciatic distribution, occurs at a much lower angulation. This pain has been misconstrued by many researchers to indicate the involvement of the sacroiliac joint instead of the sensitive finding that a nerve root compression syndrome exists. Sciatica that is in the leg and produced from 0 to 30 degrees is caused by nerve root compression. *Sciatica that is in the leg and produced from 30 to 60 degrees is probably caused by sacroiliac joint disease. Sciatica that is in the leg and produced above 60 degrees is probably caused by lumbosacral disease.*

A cardinal point is that most, if not all, ranges of movement given for the sciatic nerve roots are based on the absence of a space-occupying mass. The angles change dramatically in the presence of disease. This change is the basis of the Cox sign, which reveals the diseased or compressed nerve root, and Demianoff sign, which reveals the normal nerve root but diseased sacroiliac or lumbosacral musculature.

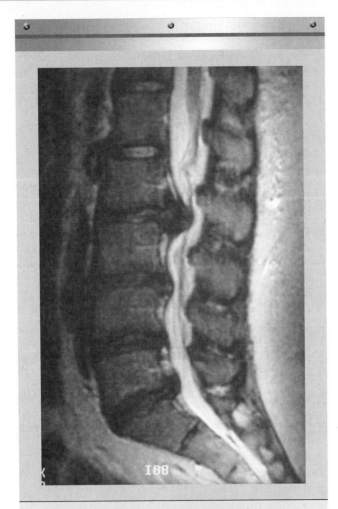

AT THE VIEWBOX

This 19-year-old female has profound discopathy, for age, with evidence of a genomic component. In addition to representing a source of back pain and radiculopathy, disc herniations of this magnitude, at L2–3, must always raise concern for cauda equina syndrome due to marked compression of the cauda equina. This may include bowel and bladder incontinence. Thorough clinical assessment and, if indicated, prompt referral for neurosurgical consultation may prevent catastrophic results, including permanent bowel and bladder dysfunction. (From the teaching file of Timothy Mick, DC, DACBR)

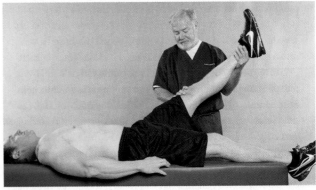

FIG. 8-176 The patient is supine with the legs fully extended. The examiner places one hand under the ankle of the affected leg and the other hand on the knee. The examiner flexes the thigh on the pelvis.

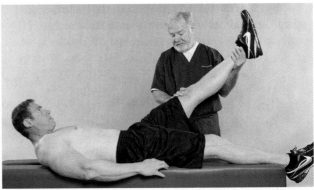

FIG. 8-177 Once the leg reaches the point at which symptoms are reproduced, the patient is instructed to flex the cervical spine and approximate the chin to the chest (Hyndman sign or Brudzinski sign). If this maneuver is markedly limited because of pain, the test is positive. A positive test suggests sciatica from lumbosacral or sacroiliac lesions, subluxation syndrome, disc lesions, spondylolisthesis, adhesions, or intervertebral foramen occlusion. The angle at which symptoms were reproduced is recorded for future testing.

TURYN SIGN

Assessment for Sciatic Radiculopathy

Comment

Various terms are used to describe injuries to the disc. The generally accepted term, *herniated nucleus pulposus,* is rather broad and should be clarified by specific nomenclature to more precisely describe the injury. The three accepted definition categories of HNP are protrusion, extruded, and sequestered. In a disc protrusion, the nucleus bulges against an intact annulus (Fig. 8-178). An extruded disc is characterized by the nucleus extending through the annulus, but the nuclear material remains confined by the posterior longitudinal ligament (Fig. 8-179). Finally, in a sequestered disc, the nucleus is free within the canal (Fig. 8-180).

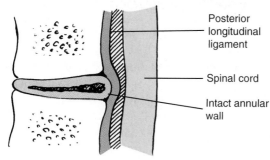

FIG. 8-178 Disc protrusion. (From Shankman GA: *Fundamental orthopedic management for the examiner,* St Louis, 1997, Mosby.)

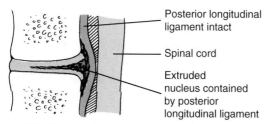

FIG. 8-179 Extruded disc. (From Shankman GA: *Fundamental orthopedic management for the examiner,* St Louis, 1997, Mosby.)

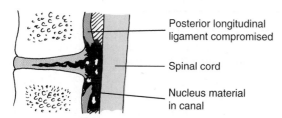

FIG. 8-180 Sequestered disc. (From Shankman GA: *Fundamental orthopedic management for the examiner,* St Louis, 1997, Mosby.)

In buttock claudication with *vascular* pattern (pain worsening quickly with walking but quickly vanishing when stopping) one needs to consider the diagnosis of stenosis of aorta or hypogastric or iliac arteries. Such is also the case for *hip* pain occurring only after some distance. In this respect, as voluminous aneurysms of iliac arteries can induce both an ischemia of the superior gluteal nerve after efforts, and a chronic compression of the nerve, the ongoing weakness of gluteal muscles at rest, should not preclude an arterial cause for pain, as it might be ascribed to the chronic compression of the superior gluteal nerve by the aneurysm (Berthelot et al, 2007).

The clinical picture of posttraumatic (spinal epidural) hematoma is a severe painful episode and then progressive

---

ORTHOPEDIC GAMUT 8-55

LUMBAR DISC DISEASE CLASSIFICATION

Variation of the lumbar disc disease classification model is as follows:
- Disc protrusion
  - Type I: peripheral annular bulge
  - Type II: localized annular bulge
- Disc herniation
  - Type I: prolapsed intervertebral disc
  - Type II: extruded intervertebral disc
  - Type III: sequestered intervertebral disc

ORTHOPEDIC GAMUT 8-56

CATEGORIES OF LOW BACK PAIN

1. *Viscerogenic pain:* Pain that originates from the kidneys, sacroiliac, pelvic lesions, and retroperitoneal tumors. This type of pain is neither aggravated by activity nor relieved by rest.
2. *Neurogenic pain:* Pain commonly caused by neurofibromas, cysts, and tumors of the nerve roots in the lumbar spine.
3. *Vascular pain:* Pain characterized by intermittent claudication from aneurysms and peripheral vascular disease.
4. *Spondylogenic pain:* Pain directly related to the pain originating from soft tissues of the spine and sacroiliac joint.
5. *Psychogenic pain:* Pain that is quite uncommon and ascribed to nonorganic causes.

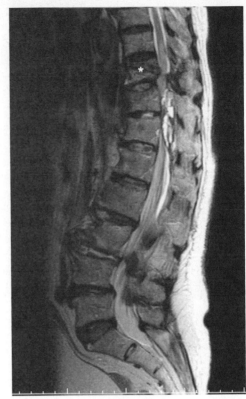

FIG. 8-181 MRI of the thoracic spine demonstrating decreased body height at T10 with deformity, conforming to the diagnosis of a compression fracture, with an epidural mass extending from the T11 to T12 level. (Adapted from Hsieh CT, Chiang YH, Tang CT, et al: Delayed traumatic thoracic spinal epidural hematoma: a case report and literature review, *Am J Emerg Med* 25(1):69-71, 2007.)

symptoms of acute cord compression with neurologic deficits including sensory, motor, or sphincter dysfunction. The duration between onset of symptoms and inciting event varies from minutes to months. Progressive spinal cord compromise can lead to paraplegia, quadriplegia, or even death (Hsieh et al, 2007).

Patients with spinal epidural hematomas can present a baffling history. They may have a negative medical history but experience severe back pain after a recent falling accident. Symptoms may improve without treatment only to be followed by progressive weakness in the bilateral lower limbs. Bilateral lower extremity paraplegia and sensory loss is not uncommon. Physical examination is usually significant for weakness in the bilateral lower extremities (muscle power scores as low as 1/5), hyperreflexia in knee jerks and ankle clonus (4+), and positive Babinski signs, along with urine and fecal incontinence. Differential diagnosis must consider herniated disc, acute vertebral compression, cord edema, cord contusion, and subdural, as well as subarachnoid hemorrhage.

> Human nerves accommodate to limb movement by stretching and gliding to allow for a change in length of the nerve bed. Whereas healthy nerves tolerate compression and strain relatively well, injured or inflamed nerves are extremely sensitive to mechanical stimuli and may become acutely painful with movement. This circumstance explains why a SLR test in a healthy person is not painful, whereas it may

be extremely painful when a nerve root is affected (Babbage et al, 2007).

Pain that radiates down the back of the leg is termed *sciatica,* regardless of whether it is associated with LBP. The pain can be referred from the back along the thigh to the foot and toe. Conversely, sciatica also can be caused by referred pain that radiates in the opposite direction, from the foot upward. In some cases of sciatica, the presence of trigger areas in the lower part of the back can be demonstrated. These trigger areas, when compressed, will set off the pain along the sciatic distribution.

Although herniated intervertebral discs are credited for most cases of sciatica, they do not account for all such symptoms. Diagnosis should be based on careful neurologic evaluation and, when necessary, diagnostic imaging and other tests.

The SLR test is not pathognomonic. Instances occur when, although a disc is central and no symptoms of pressure on the nerve root are present, sciatic radiation of the pain develops, and the prolapsed disc is credited as the cause of sciatica.

Sciatica has a variety of causes, some of which produce this type of posterior leg pain without seeming to involve the sciatic nerve or its contributory roots.

ORTHOPEDIC GAMUT 8-59
SCIATICA

Origins of sciatica:
1. Prolapsed intervertebral disc pressure, infection, and traumatic sciatic neuritis, perineural fibrositis, infections, and tumors of the spinal cord
2. Lumbosacral and sacroiliac sprain and strain, degenerating intervertebral discs, fibrositis, osteomyelitis, hip joint disease, and secondary carcinomatous deposits in bone
3. Nephrolithiasis, prostatic, renal, and anal disease
4. Toxic and metabolic disorders, conversion hysteria, and arterial insufficiency

PROCEDURE

- When the patient is in the supine position with both lower limbs resting straight out on the table, dorsiflexion of the great toe elicits pain in the gluteal region (Figs. 8-182 and 8-183).
- The sign is significant for sciatic radiculopathy.

Next Steps/Procedures
Bechterew sitting test, Bragard sign, Deyerle sign, Fajersztajn sign, Lasègue differential sign, Lasègue rebound test, Lasègue sitting test, Lasègue test, Lewin standing test, Lindner sign, Sicard sign, and straight-leg-raising test

CLINICAL PEARL

A straight-leg-raising test that is positive less than 30 degrees reveals a large disc protrusion. The nerve root is stretched long before it would normally be. The straight-leg-raising test is most useful for identifying L5–S1 disc lesions because the pressures on the nerve root are highest at this level. During straight leg raising, L4–L5 is not as apt to give as much pain as the L5–S1 because the pressure between the disc and the nerve root at L4–L5 is one half that at L5–S1. Therefore the L5–S1 disc lesion gives more pain in the lower back and leg than does the L4–L5 disc lesion. No movement on the nerve root occurs until straight leg raising reaches 30 degrees. No movement on L4 occurs during a straight-leg-raising test. From this circumstance, the presence of a Turyn sign indicates a large disc protrusion at the level of the L5–S1 nerve root.

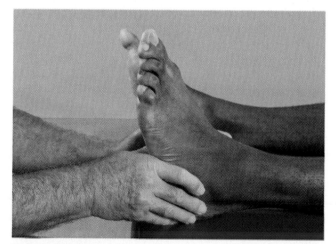

FIG. 8-182 The patient is in the supine position, with both lower limbs fully extended on the examination table.

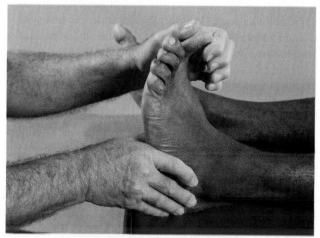

FIG. 8-183 The examiner sharply dorsiflexes the great toe of the affected leg. Pain elicited in the gluteal region is a positive sign. The sign is present in sciatic radiculopathy.

Assessment for Sciatic Scoliosis

Comment

An unlevel sacral base is not synonymous with pelvic tilt. Although sacral unleveling may accompany pelvic obliquity to varying degrees, they are different postural and structural imbalances. Patients with sacral unleveling commonly have a concomitant or resultant lumbar scoliosis, although a certain percentage of individuals with spinal curvatures have compensated through their lumbopelvic articulation (Fig. 8-184).

Scoliosis is a lateral curvature of the spine. For the management of any case, the first and most important determination to make is the presence of any deformity of the vertebrae (structural scoliosis).

Adult scoliosis is defined any curvature of the spine more than 10 degrees in a skeletally mature individual. The term *degenerative de novo scoliosis* refers to scoliotic curves developing after skeletal maturity without previous history of scoliosis. Scoliosis occurs de novo in later life and is associated not only with severe back or leg pain but also with complicated surgical outcomes. Degenerative spondylolisthesis is very common in cases of degenerative scoliosis. In a study of patients with degenerative scoliosis, 55% of them had additional degenerative spondylolisthesis. Rotatory olisthesis coexists in 13% to 34% of adult scoliosis cases. It is a triaxial deformity consisting of axial rotation on the vertical axis, lateral translation toward the convexity of the curve, and anterior translation in the sagittal axis. Trammell and colleagues originally described rotatory olisthesis as the apparent lateral subluxation of one vertebral body on another seen in the anteroposterior films (Ploumis, Transfledt, Denis, in press).

With sciatic scoliosis, the underlying cause is a prolapsed intervertebral disc that impinges on a lumbar or sacral nerve.

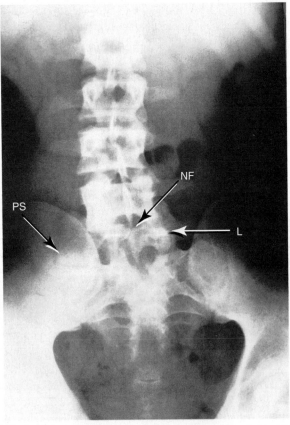

FIG. 8-184 Levorotatory scoliosis with mild pelvic obliquity. *L*, Lumbarization; *NF*, nonfusion defect; *PS*, pseudoarthrosis. (From Brier SR: *Primary care orthopedics*, St Louis, 1999, Mosby.)

ORTHOPEDIC GAMUT 8-60

DEGENERATIVE LUMBAR SCOLIOSIS CLASSIFICATION

- Type I: minimal or no lumbar vertebral rotation
  - Type IA: back pain without radicular symptoms is present.
  - Type IB: sciatic pain (from the lumbosacral hemi curve) back pain may or may not be present.
  - Type IC: femoral pain (from the major curve) back pain may or may not be present.
- Type II: rotatory olisthesis (intersegmental rotation and translation)
  - Type IIA: back pain without radicular symptoms is present.
  - Type IIB: sciatic pain (from the lumbosacral hemi curve) back pain may or may not be present.
  - Type IIC: femoral pain (from the major curve) back pain may or may not be present.
- Type III: rotatory olisthesis and structural coronal
  - More than 4 cm distance from C7 plumb line *or*
  - Positive sagittal imbalance (>2 cm from anterior sacral corner)
  - Type IIIA: back pain without radicular symptoms is present.
  - Type IIIB: sciatic pain (from the lumbosacral hemi curve) back pain may or may not be present.
  - Type IIIC: femoral pain (from the major curve) back pain may or may not be present.

ORTHOPEDIC GAMUT 8-61

SCOLIOSIS

In scoliosis, the deformity is usually one of the following:

1. Compensatory, resulting from tilting of the pelvis from real or apparent shortening of one leg
2. Sciatic, resulting from a unilateral protective muscle spasm, especially accompanying a prolapsed intervertebral disc

The deformity also may be observed in some cases of acute LBP, the pathogenesis of which is not clear. For this type of scoliosis, the curve is in the lumbar region. The abnormal posture is assumed involuntarily in an attempt to reduce the painful pressure on the affected nerve or joint. The predominant feature is severe back pain, or sciatica, that is aggravated by movements of the spine. The onset of this pain is usually sudden. The scoliosis is poorly compensated, and the trunk may be tilted markedly to one side. The curvature is not associated with rotation of the vertebrae.

Structural scoliosis is characterized by an alteration in vertebral shape and mobility, and the deformity cannot be corrected by alteration of posture. A complete history and thorough examination are required to find a cause and give a prognosis. Structural scoliosis may be congenital and may be caused by a hemivertebra, fused vertebrae, or absent or fused ribs.

Traditionally, idiopathic scoliosis has been categorized based on age when the scoliosis was first identified; this is not necessarily the same as the time the curve first appears. Infantile idiopathic scoliosis is defined by the age at onset of younger than 3 years. Juvenile idiopathic scoliosis is defined as idiopathic scoliosis detected between ages 3 to 10 years. Adolescent idiopathic scoliosis is detected between age 10 years and skeletal maturity. These three age groups were theoretically supposed to coincide with periods of increased growth of the spine. Although growth velocity does increase during infancy and adolescence, it is steady during the juvenile period. Because scoliosis curve progression is maximal during the peak periods of growth, Dickson and colleagues believed juvenile-onset scoliosis was rare enough not to warrant a separate category. The authors therefore proposed that idiopathic scoliosis should be divided into two subgroups: early onset (0 to 5 years of age) and late onset (>5 years of age) (Dobbs, Weinstein, 1999).

With paralytic scoliosis, the deformity is secondary to loss of the supportive action of the trunk and spinal muscles, which is almost always a sequel to anterior poliomyelitis.

Neuropathic scoliosis is seen as a complication of neurofibromatosis, cerebral palsy, spina bifida, syringomyelia,

Friedreich ataxia, and neuropathic conditions. Primary disorders of the supportive musculature (muscular dystrophy, arthrogryposis) are responsible for myopathic scoliosis.

Metabolic scoliosis is uncommon but occurs in cystine storage disease, Marfan syndrome, and rickets.

Idiopathic scoliosis is the most common and by far the most important of the structural scolioses. The cause of idiopathic scoliosis remains obscure. Several vertebrae at one or, less commonly, two distinct levels are affected and cause a primary curve. In the area of the primary curve, mobility (the fixed curve) is lost, rotational deformity of the vertebrae is observed (the spinous processes rotate into the concavity, and the bodies that carry the ribs in the thoracic region rotate into the convexity). Above and below the fixed primary curves, secondary curves that are mobile develop to maintain the normal position of the head and pelvis.

The spinal deformity is accompanied by shortening of the trunk, and the patient often experiences impairment of respiratory and cardiac function. In severe cases, this scenario may lead to invalidism and a shortened life expectancy.

Understanding the causes of pelvic obliquity is the key to understanding the most fundamental difference between neuromuscular scoliosis and other deformities. Pelvic obliquity, rotation, and inclination can be caused by contractures of the muscles above or below the pelvis. Because so many muscles attach to the pelvis, understanding the role they play in the production of deformity is fundamental to their correction. To differentiate whether the pelvic obliquity is caused by a contracture of the spinal-femoral, pelvic-femoral, or spinal-pelvic muscles, the patient should be examined in the prone position on the examination table with the hips flexed over the end of the table. By supporting the legs and moving them in an adducted or abducted position, the examiner can note if the pelvic obliquity corrects with hip motion. If the pelvic obliquity is eliminated by abduction or adduction of the hips, pelvofemoral muscle contracture is the cause of the pelvic obliquity, and release of the contracted muscles should alleviate the problem. If the pelvic obliquity persists despite adduction or abduction of the hips, a fixed spinal pelvic obliquity exists (McCarthy, 1999).

PROCEDURE

- With sciatica, the pelvis is always horizontal even though scoliosis exists (Fig. 8-185).
- When scoliosis is present with other spinal lesions, the pelvis will be tilted.

Next Steps/Procedures

Bilateral leg-lowering test, Demianoff sign, double leg-raise test, hyperextension test, Lewin supine test, matchstick test, Mennell sign, Minor sign, Nachlas test, Quick test, Schober test, sign of the buttock, skin pinch test, and spinal percussion test

CLINICAL PEARL

Vanzetti sign allows quick observation of the patient to determine the source of the patient's antalgia before performing the more aggressive assessments of the lumbosacral spine.

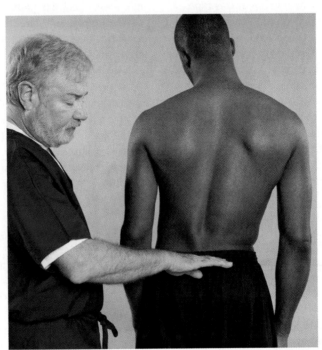

FIG. 8-185 The patient is standing with the arms comfortably at the sides. The examiner assesses the level of the pelvis and sacrum. Despite the antalgia, the pelvis is always horizontal in sciatic conditions. For other spinal lesions, when scoliosis is present, the pelvis is tilted.

CRITICAL THINKING

1. What is a cauda equina syndrome?
2. What are the physical findings of disc herniation at the L3–L4 disc?
3. What are the physical findings of disc herniation at the L4–L5 disc?
4. What are the physical findings of disc herniation at the L5–S1 disc?
5. List *tension* signs associated with lumbar disc herniation.
6. What is antalgia in the lumbar spine?
7. What imaging techniques are used in evaluating lumbar disc disease?
8. What is lumbar spinal stenosis?
9. What is the most common cause for neurologic pain in the aging lumbar spine?
10. What is the hallmark symptom of spinal stenosis?
11. What is spondylolisthesis?
12. What is spondylolysis?
13. List the five classes of spondylolisthesis.
14. Intraspinal cysts in the immediate vicinity of the lumbar zygapophyseal joints are generally accepted as representing either true synovial cysts or ganglion cysts. The cysts are most common at which level?
15. What is the typical presentation of a patient with a low back pain problem?
16. What three imaging procedures are best used to visualize a lumbar spinal-related lesion?
17. The *bowstring* sign is a nerve root tension test. How is it performed?
18. Clinically, what signs and symptoms are consistent with only a single nerve root compression?
19. Why is the degree of lytic spondylolisthesis greater at L4–L5 above the L5 transitional segment than L5 above a S1 transition?
20. What constitutes a positive Cox sign, and what is the significance?
21. The early diagnosis of a disc space infection requires a high level of clinical suspicion on the part of the clinician. What radiographic evidence would be present to establish a disc space infection?
22. Heel-and-toe walking tests are useful in evaluating what disc level and what nerves?
23. What constitutes a positive Kemp sign?
24. What is the significance of localized pain in the Kemp sign maneuver?
25. Kemp sign can be performed seated and standing. Why should it be performed both ways?
26. What signs and symptoms would help differentiate between neurogenic claudication and vascular claudication?
27. Mennell sign is helpful in the evaluation of what condition?
28. What is meralgia paresthetica?
29. What are the symptoms of meralgia paresthetica?
30. What metabolic disorder is associated with meralgia paresthetica?
31. How is Quick test performed?
32. When should the clinician ask the patient to perform the Quick test?
33. What would a negative Quick test indicate?
34. When performing Schober test, where are the marks placed on the patient's back before active forward flexion?
35. What spinal abnormality is considered when performing Schober test?
36. What distance between marks is considered a normal finding in the Schober test?
37. Percussion of the vertebral is segments a necessary part of an evaluation for the senior patient with back pain. Why?
38. Passive straight-leg-raising is done with the knee extended, which will stretch the sciatic nerve. Dural movement starts at what degrees of elevation?
39. In straight-leg-raising, above how may degrees indicates that the back pain is mechanical secondary to spinal muscle strain or joint disease?
40. What type of disc herniation may not cause sciatica during the straight-leg-raise?
41. How is hamstring tightness differentiated from true sciatica?
42. Name the five categories of low back pain and describe the origin.

8

BIBLIOGRAPHY

Abrams WB, Berkow R: *The Merck manual of geriatrics,* Rahway, NJ, 1990, Merck Sharp & Dohme Research Laboratories.

Adams JC, Hamblen DL: *Outline of orthopaedics,* ed 11, Edinburgh, 1990, Churchill Livingstone.

Agency for Health Care Policy and Research, Public Health Service, U.S. Department of Health and Human Services: Diagnostic imaging for low back pain gets mixed review, *Res Activities* 12:3, 1990.

Agency for Health Care Policy and Research, Public Health Services, U.S. Department of Health and Human Services: *Acute low back pain in adults, Clinical Practice Guideline, Number 14,* AHCPR Publication No. 95-0642, Rockville, Md, 1994, The Agency.

Alaranta H et al: A prospective study of patients with sciatica: a comparison between conservatively treated patients and patients who have undergone operation, III, results after one year follow-up, *Spine* 15:1245, 1990.

Alario AJ: *Practical guide to the care of the pediatric patient,* St Louis, 1997, Mosby.

Albeck MJU et al: A controlled comparison of myelography, computed tomography, and magnetic resonance imaging in clinically suspected lumbar disc herniation, *Spine* 20:443, 1995.

Allison D, Strickland N: *Acronyms & synonyms in medical imaging,* Oxford, UK, 1996, ISIS Medical Media.

Allman LF: *Back school program: introduction to back injuries,* Atlanta, 1990, Atlanta Sports Medicine Clinic.

Alricsson M, Werner S: Young elite cross-country skiers and low back pain—a 5-year study. *Phys Ther Sport* 7(4):181-184, 2006.

Altman RD: Musculoskeletal questions and answers, *J Musculoskeletal Med* 7:10, 1990.

American Medical Association: *Guides to the evaluation of permanent impairment,* ed 4, Chicago, 1993, American Medical Association.

American Medical Association: *How to use guides to the evaluation of permanent impairment,* ed 4, Falmouth, Conn, 1993, SEAK.

Ammann W, Matheson GO: Radionuclide bone imaging in the detection of stress fractures, *Clin J Sport Med* 1:115, 1991.

Amundsen T: Lumbar spinal stenosis: clinical and radiologic features, *Spine* 10:1178, 1995.

Anderson KN, Anderson LE: *Mosby's pocket dictionary of medicine, nursing, & allied health,* ed 2, St Louis, 1994, Mosby.

Andersson G: The epidemiology of spinal disorders. In Frymoyer J, editor: *The adult spine,* New York, 1991, Raven.

Apley AG, Solomon L: *Concise system of orthopaedics and fractures,* London, 1988, Butterworth-Heinemann.

Aprill C: Diagnostic disc injection. In Frymoyer JW, editor: *The adult spine: principles and practice,* New York, 1991, Raven.

Avioli LV: Significance of osteoporosis: a growing national health care problem, *Orthop Rev* 21:1126, 1992.

Avramov AI et al: The effects of controlled mechanical loading on group II, III, and IV afferent units from the lumbar facet joint and surrounding tissue: an in vitro study, *J Bone Joint Surg* 74A:1465, 1992.

Barkauskas VH et al: *Health & physical assessment,* ed 2, St Louis, 1998, Mosby.

Batson OV: The function of the vertebral veins and their role in the spread of metastasis, *Ann Surg* 112:138, 1940.

Battie MC, Bigos SJ: Industrial back pain complaints, *Orthop Clin North Am* 22:273, 1991.

Bauer DC et al: Factors associated with appendicular bone mass in older women, *Ann Intern Med* 118:657, 1993.

Beaman D et al: *Substance P innervation of lumbar facet joints.* Proceedings of the seventh annual meeting of North American Spine Society, Boston, July 9-11, 1991.

Bechtel R: Physical characteristics of the axial interosseous ligament of the human sacroiliac joint, *Spine J* 1(4):255-259, 2001.

Bednar DA, Orr FW, Simon GT: Observations on the pathomorphology of the thoracolumbar fascia in chronic mechanical back pain: a microscopic study, *Spine* 20:1161, 1995.

Bell GR, Modic MT: Radiology of the lumbar spine. In Rothman RA, Sinecone FA, editors: *The spine,* ed 3, Philadelphia, 1992, WB Saunders.

Bellah RD et al: Low-back pain in adolescent patients: detection of stress injury to the pars interarticularis with SPECT, *Radiology* 180:509, 1991.

Benzon HT et al: Piriformis syndrome: anatomic considerations, a new injection technique, and a review of the literature, *Anesthesiology* 98(6):1442-1448, 2003.

Berquist T: *MRI of the musculoskeletal system,* ed 3, Philadelphia, 1996, JB Lippincott.

Berthelot J-M et al: Contribution of centralization phenomenon to the diagnosis, prognosis, and treatment of diskogenic low back pain *Joint Bone Spine* (in press, uncorrected proof).

Bischoff RJ et al: A comparison of computed tomography-myelography, magnetic resonance imaging and myelography in the diagnosis of herniated nucleus pulposus and spinal stenosis, *J Spinal Disord* 6:289, 1993.

Boden S et al: Abnormal magnetic resonance scans of the spine in asymptomatic patients, *J Bone Joint Surg* 72A:403, 1990.

Boden SD et al: *The aging spine,* Philadelphia, 1991, WB Saunders.

Bogduk N, Macintosh JE, Pearcy MJ: A universal model of the lumbar back muscles in the upright position, *Spine* 17:897, 1992.

Bogduk N, Twomey LT: *Clinical anatomy of the lumbar spine,* London, 1991, Churchill Livingstone.

Bogduk N: *Pathogenesis of degenerative disc disease,* Toronto, 1991, American Back Society.

Bogduk N: Pathology of lumbar disc pain, *Man Med* 5:72, 1990.

Bond MR: *Pain: its nature, analysis and treatment,* Edinburgh, 1979, Churchill Livingstone.

Borenstein D: Prevalence and treatment outcome of primary and secondary fibromyalgia in patients with spinal pain, *Spine* 20:1055, 1995.

Borenstein DG, Burton JR: Lumbar spine disease in the elderly, *J Am Geriatr Soc* 41:167, 1993.

Borenstein DG et al: *Low back pain: medical diagnosis and comprehensive management,* ed 2, Philadelphia, 1995, WB Saunders.

Bough B et al: Degeneration of lumbar facet joints, *J Bone Joint Surg* 72B:275, 1990.

Bowlus B: *Mosby's regional atlas of human anatomy,* St Louis, 1997, Mosby.

Bozzae A et al: Lumbar disc herniation: MR imaging assessment of natural history in patients treated without surgery, *Radiology* 185:135, 1992.

Bradford FK: Low back sprain and ruptured intervertebral disc, *Med Times* 88:797, 1960.

Brav EA: The diagnosis of low back pain of orthopedic origin: an analysis of sixty-two cases, *Am J Surg* 55(1):57-66, 1942.

Breen A: The reliability of palpation and other diagnostic methods, *J Manipulative Physiol Ther* 15:54, 1992.

Breig A, Troup JDG: Biomechanical considerations in straight-leg-raising test: cadaveric and clinical studies of the effects of medial hip rotation, *Spine* 4:242, 1979.

Brier SR: *Primary care orthopedics,* St Louis, 1999, Mosby.

Brody IA, Williams RH: The signs of Kernig and Brudzinski, *Arch Neurol* 21:215, 1969.

Brooks M, Evans R, Fairclough J: *Sports injuries,* ed 2, London, 1992, Gower Medical.

Brotzman SB: *Clinical orthopaedic rehabilitation,* St Louis, 1996, Mosby.

Brown DE, Neumann RD: *Orthopedic secrets,* Philadelphia, 1995, Hanley & Belfus.

Brudzinski J: A new sign of the lower extremities in meningitis of children (neck sign), *Arch Neurol* 21:216, 1969.

Bucholz RW: *Orthopaedic decision making,* ed 2, St Louis, 1996, Mosby.

Buckwalter J: Spine update: aging and degeneration of the human intervertebral disc, *Spine* 20:1307, 1995.

Budgell B, Noda K, Sata A: Innervation of posterior structures in the lumbar spine of the rat, *J Manipulative Physiol Ther* 20:359, 1997.

Buirski G: Magnetic resonance signal pattern of lumbar discs in patients with low back pain: a prospective study with discographic correlation, *Spine* 17:1205, 1992.

Burkus JK: Spine. In Loth T, editor: *Orthopaedic boards review,* St Louis, 1993, Mosby.

Butler D: *Mobilisation of the nervous system,* Melbourne, 1991, Churchill Livingstone.

Butt S, Saifuddin A: The imaging of lumbar spondylolisthesis, *Clin Radiol* 60(5):533-546, 2005.

Byung-June J et al: Solitary lumbar osteochondroma causing sciatic pain, *Joint Bone Spine* (in press, uncorrected proof).

Cailliet R: *Low back pain syndrome,* ed 3, Philadelphia, 1981, FA Davis.

Cailliet R: *Soft tissue pain and disability,* Philadelphia, 1977, FA Davis.

Campbell JB, Campbell JM: *Mosby's survival guide to medical abbreviations & acronyms prefixes & suffixes symbols Greek alphabet,* St Louis, 1995, Mosby.

Canale ST: *Campbell's operative orthopaedics,* vol 1-4, ed 9, St Louis, 1998, Mosby.

Carcone SM, Keir PJ: Effects of backrest design on biomechanics and comfort during seated work, *Appl Ergon* (in press, corrected proof).

Carragee E et al: Surgical treatment for unstable low-grade isthmic spondylolisthesis in adults: a prospective controlled study of posterior instrumented fusion compared with combined anterior-posterior fusion, *Spine J* 6(5, suppl 1):47S, 2006.

Cats A, Linder SM: Spondyloarthropathies: an overview, *Spine* 4:497, 1990.

Chapman S, Nakielny R: *Aids to radiological differential diagnosis,* ed 3, London, 1995, Bailliere Tindall.

Chappuis JL, Johnson GD, Gines AM: *A source guide for spine care,* Atlanta, 1994, Grater Atlanta Spine Center.

Chavanet P et al: Performance of a predictive rule to distinguish bacterial and viral meningitis, *J Infect* 54(4):328-336, 2007.

Chemmanam T et al: Anhidrosis: a clue to an underlying autonomic disorder, *J Clin Neurosci* 14(1):94-96, 2007.

Chin CH, Chew KC: Lumbosacral nerve root avulsion, *Injury* 28(9-10):674-678, 1997.

Chin KR, Eiszner J, Persaud K: Impact of obesity on the incidence of surgery, outcomes, and complications in low back pain patients, *Spine J* 6(5, suppl 1):158S, 2006.

Chin KR et al: Changes in the iliac crest-lumbar relationship from standing to prone, *Spine J* 6(2):185-189, 2006.

Cipriano JJ: *Photographic manual of regional orthopaedic and neurological test,* ed 3, Baltimore, 1997, Williams & Wilkins.

Cloward RB: Lesions of the intervertebral disc and their treatment by interbody fusion methods: the painful disc, *Clin Orthop* 27:51, 1963.

Cohn RE: *Impairment rating examination and disability evaluation,* ed 3, Wilkesboro, NC, 1994, R Ernest Cohn.

Cole AJ, Herring SA: *The low back pain handbook: a practical guide for the primary care examiner,* Philadelphia, 1997, Hanley & Belfus.

Concannon MJ: *Common hand problems in primary care,* Philadelphia, 1999, Hanley & Belfus.

Connelly C: Easing low back pain, *Postgrad Med* 100:143-156, 1996.

Conwell TD: *Documenting patient progress "daily office charting seminar" thorough accurate quick procedures,* ed 11, Lakewood, Colo, 1990, Timothy D Conwell.

Coppes MH et al: Innervation of annulus fibrosis in low back pain, *Lancet* 336:189, 1988.

Cox JM: *Low back pain mechanism, diagnosis and treatment,* ed 5, Baltimore, 1990, Williams & Wilkins.

Craig Humphreys S et al: Assessing lumbar sagittal motion using videography in an in vivo pilot study, *Int J Ind Ergon* (in press, corrected proof).

Cramer G et al: Comparison of computed tomography to magnetic resonance imaging in the evaluation of the lumbar intervertebral foramina, *Clin Anat* 7:173, 1994.

Cramer GD, Darby SA: *Basic and clinical anatomy of the spine, spinal cord, and ANS,* St Louis, 1995, Mosby.

Crisco JJ, Fujita L, Spenciner DB: The dynamic flexion/extension properties of the lumbar spine in vitro using a novel pendulum system, *J Biomech* (in press, corrected proof).

Crisco JJ, Panjabi MM: The intersegmental and multisegmental muscles of the lumbar spine: a biomechanical model comparing lateral stabilizing potential, *Spine* 16:793, 1991.

Cullinan AM: *Optimizing radiographic positioning,* Philadelphia, 1992, Lippincott.

Cynn H-S et al: Effects of lumbar stabilization using a pressure biofeedback unit on muscle activity and lateral pelvic tilt during hip abduction in sidelying, *Arch Phys Med Rehabil* 7(11):1454-1458, 2006.

Cyrias JH: Lesions discals lombaires, *Acta Orthop Belg* 27:442, 1961.

Cyriax J: *Textbook for orthopaedic medicine, vol 1: diagnosis of soft tissue lesions,* London, 1975, Bailliere Tindall.

Daffner RH et al: The radiology assessment of post-traumatic vertebral stability, *Skeletal Radiol* 19:103, 1990.

Daffner RH: *Clinical radiology: the essentials,* Baltimore, 1993, Williams & Wilkins.

Daffner RH: Thoracic and lumbar vertebral trauma, *Orthop Clin North Am* 21:463, 1990.

Dambro MR, Griffith JA: *Griffith's 5 minute clinical consult,* Baltimore, 1997, Williams & Wilkins.

D'Ambrogio KJ, Roth GB: *Positional release therapy assessment & treatment of musculoskeletal dysfunction,* St Louis, 1997, Mosby.

D'Ambrosia RD: *Musculoskeletal disorders: regional examination and differential diagnosis,* Philadelphia, 1977, JB Lippincott.

Dandy DJ: *Essential orthopaedics and trauma,* Edinburgh, 1989, Churchill Livingstone.

Daniels L, Worthingham C: *Muscle testing: techniques of manual examination,* Philadelphia, 1980, WB Saunders.

Day MO: Spondylolytic spondylolisthesis in an elite athlete, *Chiro Sports Med* 5:91, 1991.

Deen HG et al: Assessment of bladder function after lumbar decompressive surgery for spinal stenosis: a prospective study, *J Neurosurg* 80:971, 1994.

Delamarter RB et al: Experimental lumbar spinal stenosis, *J Bone Joint Surg* 72A:110, 1990.

Delauche-Cavallier MC et al: Lumbar disc herniation: computed tomography scan changes after conservative treatment of nerve root compression, *Spine* 17:927, 1992.

Deltoff MN, Kogon PL: *The portable skeletal x-ray library,* St Louis, 1998, Mosby.

Demeter SL, Andersson GBJ, Smith GM: *Disability evaluation,* St Louis, 1996, Mosby.

DePalma AF, Rothman RH: *The intervertebral disc,* Philadelphia, 1970, WB Saunders.

DeRosa C, Porterfield JA: A physical therapy model for the treatment of low back pain, *Phys Ther* 72:261, 1992.

Deshpande JK, Tobias JD: *The pediatric pain handbook,* St Louis, 1996, Mosby.

Dettenmeier PA: *Radiographic assessment for nurses,* St Louis, 1995, Mosby.

Deyerle WM, May VR: Sciatic tension test, *South Med J* 49:999, 1956.

Deyo R: Nonoperative treatment of low back disorders: differentiating useful therapy. In Frymoryer JW, editor: *The adult spine: principles and practice,* New York, 1991, Raven.

Deyo RA, Loeser JD, Bigos SJ: Herniated lumbar intervertebral disk, *Ann Intern Med* 112(8):598-603, 1990.

Deyo RA, Rainville J, Kent DL: What can the history and physical examination tell us about low back pain? *JAMA* 268:760, 1992.

Doherty M, Doherty J: *Clinical examination in rheumatology,* London, 1992, Wolfe.

Doherty M, George E: *Self-assessment picture tests in rheumatology,* London, 1995, Mosby-Wolfe.

Doherty M: *Color atlas and text of osteoarthritis,* London, 1994, Wolfe.

Dommisse GF, Grobler L: Arteries and veins of the lumbar nerve roots and cauda equina, *Clin Orthop* 115:22, 1976.

Dommisse GF, Louw JA: Anatomy of the lumbar spine. In Floman Y, editor: *Disorders of the lumbar spine,* Rockville, Md, and Tel Aviv, Israel, 1990, Aspen and Freund Publishing House.

Donelson R, McKenzie R: Mechanical assessment and treatment of spinal pain. In Frymoyer JW, editor: *The adult spine: principles and practice,* New York, 1991, Raven.

Dunk NM et al: The reliability of quantifying upright standing postures as a baseline diagnostic clinical tool, *J Manipulative Physiol Ther* 27(2):91-96, 2004.

Dussault R, Lander P: Imaging of the facet joints, *Radiol Clin North Am* 28:1033, 1990.

Dvorak J, Dvorak V: *Manual medicine: diagnostics,* New York, 1990, Thieme.

Dyck P: The femoral nerve traction test with lumbar disc protrusion, *Surg Neurol* 6:163, 1976.

Dyck P: The stoop-test in lumbar entrapment radiculopathy, *Spine* 4:89, 1979.

Edgar MA, Ghadially JA: Innervation of the lumbar spine, *Clin Orthop* 115:35, 1976.

Edgar MS, Park WM: Induced pain patterns on passive straight-leg-raising in lower lumbar disc protrusion, *J Bone Joint Surg* 56B:658, 1974.

Edwards RR et al: Symptoms of distress as prospective predictors of pain-related sciatica treatment outcomes, *Pain* 130(1-2):47-55, 2007.

Ellenberg ME et al: Prospective evaluation of the course of disc herniation in patients with radiculopathy, *Arch Phys Med Rehabil* 74:3, 1993.

Elster AD: *Questions and answers in magnetic resonance imaging,* St Louis, 1994, Mosby.

Epstein BS: *The spine, a radiological text and atlas,* ed 3, Philadelphia, 1969, Lea & Febiger.

Epstein O et al: *Clinical examination,* ed 2, London, 1997, Mosby.

Ericksen MF: Aging in the lumbar spine, *Am J Phys Anthropol* 48:241, 1974.

Fahrni WH: Observations on straight-leg raising with special reference to nerve root adhesions, *Can J Surg* 9:44, 1966.

Faik A et al: Spinal cord compression due to vertebral osteochondroma: report of two cases, *Joint Bone Spine* 72(2):177-179, 2005.

Farfan HF: *Mechanical disorders of the low back,* Philadelphia, 1973, Lea & Febiger.

Farnum CE et al: Volume increase in growth plate chondrocytes during hypertrophy: the contribution of organic osmolytes, *Bone* 30(4):574-581, 2002.

Farrar WE: *Atlas of infections of the nervous system,* London, 1993, Wolfe.

Feldmann E: *Current diagnosis in neurology,* St Louis, 1994, Mosby.

Ferezy JS: *The chiropractic neurological examination,* Gaithersburg, Md, 1992, Aspen.

Fernstrom U, Goldie I: Does granulation tissue in the intervertebral disc provoke back pain? *Acta Orthop Scand* 30:202, 1960.

Fomby EW, Mellion MB: Identifying and treating myofascial pain syndrome, *Phys Sports Med* 25, 1997.

Forbes CD, Jackson WF: *A colour atlas and text of clinical medicine,* Aylesbury, UK, 1993, Wolfe.

Fornage B: *Musculoskeletal ultrasound,* New York, 1995, Churchill Livingstone.

Frank ED et al: *Merrill's atlas of radiographic positioning and procedures,* ed 11, St Louis, 2007, Mosby.

Frymoyer JW: *The adult spine,* New York, 1991, Raven.

Frymoyer JW, Cats-Baril WI: An overview of the incidences and costs of low back pain, *Orthop Clin North Am* 22:263, 1991.

Fulton M: *Lower-back pain: a new solution for an old problem,* Rolling Meadows, NJ, 1992, MedX.

Garcia JH: *Neuropathology: the diagnostic approach,* St Louis, 1997, Mosby.

Garcia-Borreguero D et al: Diagnostic standards for dopaminergic augmentation of restless legs syndrome: report from a world association of sleep medicine—International Restless Legs Syndrome Study Group consensus conference at the Max Planck Institute, *Sleep Med* (in press, corrected proof).

Gartland JJ: *Fundamentals of orthopaedics,* Philadelphia, 1974, WB Saunders.

Gianakopoulos G et al: Inversion devices: their role in producing lumbar distraction, *Arch Phys Med Rehabil* 66:100, 1985.

Giles LGF, Kaveri MJP: Some osseous and soft tissue causes of lumbar stenosis, *J Rheumatol* 17:1374, 1990.

Gilkey DP: Injury prevention in the workplace: a closer look at OSHA's proposed ergonomic standard, *J Am Chiropractic Assoc* 33:25, 1996.

Gillis L: *Diagnosis in orthopaedics,* London, 1969, Butterworths.

Goddard BS, Reid JD: Movements induced by straight-leg-raising in the lumbo-sacral roots, nerves, and plexus and in the intra pelvic section of the sciatic nerve, *J Neurol Neurosurg Psychiatry* 28:12, 1965.

Goldstein JD et al: Spine injuries in gymnasts and swimmers, *Am J Sports Med* 19:463, 1991.

Gracovetsky S: The spine as a motor in sports: application to running and lifting, *Spine* 4:267, 1990.

Granata KP, Rogers E: Torso flexion modulates stiffness and reflex response, *J Electromyogr Kinesiol* 17(4):384-92, 2007.

Greenspan A, Montesano P: *Imaging of the spine in clinical practice,* London, 1993, Wolfe.

Greenspan A: *Orthopedic radiology,* ed 2, Philadelphia, 1992, JB Lippincott.

Greenstein GM: *Clinical assessment of neuromusculoskeletal disorders,* St Louis, 1997, Mosby.

Grobler LS, Wiltse LC: Classification, non-operative, and operative treatment of spondylolisthesis. In Frymoyer JW, editor: *The adult spine: principles and practice,* New York, 1991, Raven.

Groen GJ, Baljet B, Drukker J: Nerves and nerve plexuses of the human vertebral collum, *Am J Anat* 188:282, 1990.

Grossman ZD et al: *Cost-effective diagnostic imaging: the examiner's guide,* ed 3, St Louis, 1995, Mosby.

Guermazi M et al: Traduction en arabe et validation de l'indice d'Oswestry dans une population de lombalgiques Nord-Africains, *Ann Readapt Med Phys* 48(1):1-10, 2005.

Guiheneuc P, Ginet J: Etude du reflexe de Hoffmann obtenu au niveau du muscle quadriceps de sujets humains normaux, *Electroencephalogr Clin Neurophysiol* 3:225-31, 1974.

Gunn CC, Milbrandt WE: Early and subtle signs in low-back sprain, *Spine* 3:267, 1978.

Haher TR, Felmly WT, O'Brien M: Thoracic and lumbar fractures: diagnosis and management. In Bridwell KH, DeWald RL, editors: *The textbook of spinal surgery,* Philadelphia, 1991, JB Lippincott.

Hammer WI: *Functional soft tissue examination and treatment by manual methods: the extremities,* Gaithersburg, Md, 1991, Aspen.

Hammerberg KW: Kyphosis. In Bridwell DH, DeWald RL, editors: *The textbook of spinal surgery,* Philadelphia, 1991, JB Lippincott.

Hanley EN, Phillips ED: Profiles of patients who get spine infections and the type of infections that have a predilection for the spine. In Wiesel SW, editor: *Seminars in spine surgery,* vol 2, Philadelphia, 1990, WB Saunders.

Hansson T et al: The lumbar lordosis in acute and chronic low-back pain, *Spine* 10:154, 1985.

Hardy RW, editor: *Lumbar disc disease,* ed 2, New York, 1992, Raven.

Hass CJ et al: Gait initiation and dynamic balance control in Parkinson's disease, *Arch Phys Med Rehabil* 86(11):2172-2176, 2005.

Hawkins RJ: *An organized approach to musculoskeletal examination and history taking,* St Louis, 1995, Mosby.

Helfet AJ, Gruebel Lee DM: *Disorders of the lumbar spine,* Philadelphia, 1978, JB Lippincott.

Hellstrom M et al: Radiologic abnormalities of the thoracolumbar spine in patients, *Acta Radiol* 31:127, 1990.

Herkowitz HN, Kurz LT: Degenerative lumbar spondylolisthesis with spinal stenosis: a prospective study comparing decompression with decompression and intertransverse process arthrodesis, *J Bone Joint Surg* 73A:802, 1991.

Herlin L: *Sciatic and pelvic pain due to lumbosacral nerve root compression,* Springfield, Ill, 1966, Charles C Thomas.

Herno A et al: The predictive value of preoperative myelography in lumbar spinal stenosis, *Spine* 19:1335-1338, 1994.

Herron LD, Pheasant HC: Prone knee-flexion provocative testing for lumbar disc protrusion, *Spine* 5:65, 1980.

Heuer F et al: Creep associated changes in intervertebral disc bulging obtained with a laser scanning device, *Clin Biomech* (in press, corrected proof).

Hinkle CZ: *Fundamentals of anatomy & movement: a workbook and guide,* St Louis, 1997, Mosby.

Hochschuler SH, editor: *Spine: state of the art review: spinal injuries in sports,* Philadelphia, 1990, Hanley & Belfus.

Hoffman RM, Kent DL, Deyo RA: Diagnostic accuracy and clinical utility of thermography for lumbar radiculopathy: a meta-analysis, *Spine* 16:623, 1991.

Hollinshead WH: *Anatomy for surgeons, vol 3, the back and limbs,* ed 3, Philadelphia, 1982, Harper & Row.

Hopwood MB, Abram SE: Factors associated with failure of lumbar epidural steroids, *Reg Anesth Pain Med* 18:238, 1993.

Hornberger JP: *Exercise physiology therapeutic exercise,* Sarasota, Fla, 1991, Joseph P Hornberger.

Hubbard DR, Berkoff GM: Myofascial trigger points show spontaneous needle EMG activity, *Spine* 18:1803, 1993.

Hudgins WR: The crossed-straight-leg-raising test, *N Engl J Med* 297:1127, 1977.

Hutton WC: The forces acting on a lumbar intervertebral joint, *J Manual Med* 5, 66, 1990.

Jablonski S: *Dictionary of medical acronyms & abbreviations,* ed 3, Philadelphia, 1998, Hanley & Belfus.

Jackson HC, Winkelman KK, Bichel WH: Nerve endings in the human lumbar spine column and related structures, *J Bone Joint Surg* 48A:1272, 1966.

Jarvik JG et al: Interreader reliability for a new classification of lumbar disk disease, *Acad Radiol* 3(7):537-544, 1996.

Jensen MC et al: Magnetic resonance imaging of the lumbar spine in people without back pain, *N Engl J Med* 331:69, 1994.

Johnson RJ: Low-back pain in sports: managing spondylolysis in young patients, *Phys Sports Med* 21:53, 1993.

Johnson RM, Murphy MJ, Southwick WO: Surgical approaches to the spine. In Rothman RH, Simeone FA, editors: *The spine,* ed 3, Philadelphia, 1992, WB Saunders.

Johnsson KE, Rosen I, Uden A: The natural course of lumbar spinal stenosis, *Clin Orthop* 279:82, 1992.

Jonsson B, Stromquist B: Symptoms and signs in degeneration of the lumbar spine, a prospective consecutive study of 300 operated patients, *J Bone Joint Surg* 75B:272, 1993.

Jonsson B, Stromquist B: Symptoms and signs in degeneration of the lumbar spine, *J Bone Joint Surg* 75B:381, 1993.

Kanner R: *Pain management secrets,* Philadelphia, 1997, Hanley & Belfus.

Kapandji IA: *The physiology of the joints, vol 3, the trunk and the vertebral column,* Edinburgh, 1974, Churchill Livingstone.

Katirji B, Weissman JD: The ankle jerk and the tibial H-reflex: a clinical and electrophysiological correlation, *Electromyogr Clin Neurophysiol* 34:331, 1994.

Katirji B: *Electromyography in clinical practice: a case study approach,* St Louis, 1998, Mosby.

Katz WA: *Rheumatic diseases diagnosis and management,* Philadelphia, 1977, JB Lippincott.

Katznelson A, Nerubay J, Level A: Gluteal skyline (G.S.L.): a search for an objective sign in the diagnosis of disc lesions of the lower lumbar spine, *Spine* 7:74, 1982.

Keats TE, Lusted LB: *Atlas of roentgenographic measurements,* ed 6, St Louis, 1990, Mosby.

Keats TE: *An atlas of normal roentgen variants that may simulate disease,* ed 2, Chicago, 1973, Year Book Medical Publishers.

Keim HA: *The adolescent spine,* ed 2, New York, 1976, Springer-Verlag.

Keller TS et al: Influence of spine morphology on intervertebral disc loads and stresses in asymptomatic adults: implications for the ideal spine, *Spine J* 5(3):297-309, 2005.

Kelsey JL: An epidemiological study of acute herniated lumbar intervertebral disc, *Rheum Rehab* 14:144, 1975.

Kendall HO, Kendall FP, Wadsworth GE: *Muscles testing and function,* ed 2, Baltimore, 1971, Williams & Wilkins.

Kent DL et al: Diagnosis of lumbar spinal stenosis in adults: a meta-analysis of the accuracy of CT, MR, and myelography, *AJR Am J Roentgenol* 158:1135, 1992.

Kernig W: Concerning a little noted sign of meningitis, *Arch Neurol* 21:216, 1969.

Kettenbach G: *Writing S.O.A.P. notes,* Philadelphia, 1990, FA Davis.

Khan MA, Linder SM: Ankylosing spondylitis: clinical aspects, *Spine* 4:529, 1990.

Kingston RS: Radiology of the spine. In Watkins RG, editor: *The spine in sports,* St Louis, 1996, Mosby.

Klippel JH, Dieppe PA: *Rheumatology,* vol 1-2, ed 2, London, 1998, Mosby.

Knikou M et al: Pre- and post-alpha motoneuronal control of the soleus H-reflex during sinusoidal hip movements in human spinal cord injury, *Brain Res* 1103(1):123-139, 2006.

Knott R: A 14-year-old boy with metaphyseal dysplasia (Pyle's disease) and low back pain, *Clin Chiropractic* 7(2):73-78, 2004.

Kono H et al: Lumbar juxta-facet cyst after trauma, *J Clin Neurosci* 13(6):694-696, 2006.

Kosteljanetz M, Bang F, Schmidt-Olsen S: The clinical significance of straight-leg raising (Lasègue's sign) in the diagnosis of prolapsed lumbar disc: interobserver variation and correlation with surgical findings, *Spine* 13:393, 1988.

Kostova V, Koleva M: Back disorders (low back pain, cervicobrachial and lumbosacral radicular syndromes) and some related risk factors, *J Neurol Sci* 192(1-2):17-25, 2001.

Kottlors M, Muller K, Glocker FX: Muscle hypertrophy due to compression of the L5 nerve root, *Clin Neurophysiol* 118(4):e61-e62, 2007.

Krodel A, Sturtz H, Siebert CH: Indications for and results of operative treatment of spondylitis and spondylodiscitis, *Arch Orthop Trauma Surg* 110:78, 1991.

Krumova EK et al: Diagnosing complex regional pain syndrome (CRPS) by a comprehensive analysis of long-term skin temperature changes, *Eur J Pain* 11(1, suppl 1):103-104, 2007.

Kurutz M: Age-sensitivity of time-related in vivo deformability of human lumbar motion segments and discs in pure centric tension, *J Biomech* 39(1):147-157, 2006.

Kurutz M: In vivo age- and sex-related creep of human lumbar motion segments and discs in pure centric tension, *J Biomech* 39(7):1180-1190, 2006.

LaFreniere JG: *The low-back patient, procedures for treatment by physical therapy,* New York, 1985, Masson.

Lancourt J, Kettelhut M: Predicting return to work for lower back pain patients receiving worker's compensation, *Spine* 17:629, 1992.

Lauder TD et al: Sports and physical training injury hospitalizations in the Army, *Am J Prevent Med* 18(3, suppl 1):118-128, 2000.

Lavy CBD, Barrett DS: *Questions and answers on Apley's concise system of orthopaedics and fractures,* Oxford, UK, 1991, Butterworth-Heinemann.

Lecuire J et al: 641 operations for sciatic neuralgia due to discal hernia, a computerized statistical study of the results, *Neurochirugie (Stuttg)* 19:501, 1973.

Leffs M: *Back pain in the adolescent athlete,* Toronto, 1991, American Back Society.

Lerner AJ: *The little black book of neurology,* ed 3, St Louis, 1995, Mosby.

Lestini WF, Bell GR: Spinal infections: patient evaluation. In *Seminars in spine surgery,* vol 2, Philadelphia, 1990, WB Saunders.

8

Lewis CB, Knortz KA: *Orthopedic assessment and treatment of the geriatric patient,* St Louis, 1993, Mosby.

Loth TS: *Orthopedic boards review II a case study approach,* St Louis, 1996, Mosby.

Loth TS: *Orthopedic boards review,* St Louis, 1993, Mosby.

Lovett AW: A contribution to the study of the mechanics of the spine, *Am J Anat* 2:457, 1983.

MacLean JJ, Owen JP, Iatridis JC: Role of endplates in contributing to compression behaviors of motion segments and intervertebral discs, *J Biomech* 40(1):55-63, 2007.

MacNab I: *Backache,* Baltimore, 1977, Williams & Wilkins.

Magee DJ: *Orthopedic physical assessment,* ed 3, Philadelphia, 1997, WB Saunders.

Magora A: Investigation of the relation between low back pain and occupation: 4, physical requirements: bending, rotation, reaching and sudden maximal effort, *Scand J Rehabil Med* 5:186, 1973.

Maigne JY, Maigne R, Guerin-Surville H: The lumbar mamillo-accessory foramen: a study of 203 lumbosacral spines, *Surg Radiol Ant* 13:29, 1991.

Malone TR, McPoil TG, Nitz AJ: *Orthopedic and sports physical therapy,* ed 3, St Louis, 1997, Mosby.

Manaster BJ: *Handbooks in radiology skeletal radiology,* Chicago, 1989, Year Book Medical Publishers.

Mandelbaum BR, Gross MC: Spondylolysis and spondylolisthesis. In Reider B, editor: *Sports medicine: the school-age athlete,* Philadelphia, 1991, WB Saunders.

Marcaud V et al: Vascularite restreinte au systeme nerveux peripherique: presentation clinique atypique, *La Revue Med Intern* 23(6):558-562, 2002.

Marchand F, Ahmed A: Investigation of the laminate structure of lumbar disc anulus fibrosus, *Spine* 15:402, 1990.

Martin JH: *Neuroanatomy text and atlas,* ed 2, Stamford, Conn, 1996, Appleton & Lange.

Massie J, Giurea A, Waters S: Antifibrotic gels versus a barrier sheet in the prevention of epidural fibrosis postlaminectomy, *Spine J* 2(2, suppl 1):35, 2002.

Mason M, Currey HLF: *Clinical rheumatology,* Philadelphia, 1970, JB Lippincott.

Mathers LH et al: *Clinical anatomy principles,* St Louis, 1996, Mosby.

Mayo Clinic and Mayo Foundation: *Clinical examinations in neurology,* ed 5, Philadelphia, 1981, WB Saunders.

Mazion JM: *Illustrated manual of neurological reflexes/signs/tests, part I, orthopedic signs/tests/maneuvers for office procedure, part II,* Orlando, Fla, 1980, Daniels Publishing.

McGill S: Quantitative intramuscular myoelectric activity of the quadratus lumborum during a wide variety of tasks, *Clin Biomech* 11:170, 1996.

McGill SM: The influence of lordosis on axial trunk torque and trunk muscle myoelectric activity, *Spine* 17:1187, 1992.

McKenzie RA: *The lumbar spine mechanical diagnosis and therapy,* Wikanae, New Zealand, 1981, Spinal Publications.

McNeil et al: Trunk strengths in attempted flexion, extension, and lateral bending in healthy subjects and patients with low back disorders, *Spine* 5:529, 1980.

McRae R: *Clinical orthopaedic examination,* ed 3, Edinburgh, 1990, Churchill Livingstone.

McRae R: *Practical fracture treatment,* ed 3, New York, 1994, Churchill-Livingstone.

Medical Economics Books: *Patient care flow chart manual,* ed 3, Oradell, NJ, 1982, Medical Economics Books.

Mellion MB: *Office sports medicine,* ed 2, St Louis, 1996, Mosby.

Mellion MB: *Sports medicine secrets,* Philadelphia, 1994, Hanley & Belfus.

Mengel MB, Schwiebert LP: *Ambulatory medicine: the primary care of families,* ed 2, Stamford, Conn, 1996, Appleton & Lange.

Mennell JM: *Back pain,* Boston, 1960, Little, Brown.

Mennell JM: *The musculoskeletal system differential diagnosis from symptoms and physical signs,* Gaithersburg, Md, 1992, Aspen.

Mercier LR, Pettid FJ: *Practical orthopedics,* ed 4, St Louis, 1995, Mosby.

Merkow RL, Lane JM: Paget's disease of bone, *Orthop Clin North Am* 21:171, 1990.

Micheli LJ, Trapman E: Spinal deformities. In Torg S, Welsh RP, Shephard RJ, editors: *Current therapy in sports medicine,* ed 2, St Louis, 1990, Mosby.

Mooney V: Differential diagnosis of low back disorders. In Frymoyer JW, editor: *The adult spine: principles and practice,* New York, 1991, Raven.

Moore KL: *Clinically oriented anatomy,* ed 3, Baltimore, 1992, Williams & Wilkins.

Morris JM, Lucas DB, Bresler B: Role of the trunk in stability of the spine, *J Bone Joint Surg* 43A:327, 1961.

Mosby-Year Book, Inc: *Expert 10-minute physical examination,* St Louis, 1997, Mosby.

Mulleman D et al: Pathophysiology of disk-related sciatica. I. Evidence supporting a chemical component. *Joint Bone Spine* 73(2):151-158, 2006.

Nachemson A: The lumbar spine-an orthopaedic challenge, *Spine* 1:59, 1976.

Nachemson AL: Newest knowledge on low back pain, *Clin Orthop* 279:8, 1992.

Nakagawa H et al: Microendoscopic discectomy (MED) for lumbar disc prolapse, *J Clin Neurosci* 10(2):231-235, 2003.

Nakamura SI: Afferent pathways of discogenic low back pain: evaluation of L2 spinal nerve infiltration, *J Bone Joint Surg* 78B:606, 1996.

Nettina SM: *The Lippincott manual of nursing practice,* ed 6, Philadelphia, 1996, Lippincott.

Neumann WP et al: Trunk posture: reliability, accuracy, and risk estimates for low back pain from a video based assessment method, *Int J Indust Ergon* 28(6):355-365, 2001.

Newton RW: *Color atlas of pediatric neurology,* St Louis, 1995, Mosby-Wolfe.

Nicholas JA, Hershman EB: *The lower extremity & spine in sports medicine,* vol 1-2, ed 2, St Louis, 1995, Mosby.

Nishada T et al: H reflex in S-1 radiculopathy: latency versus amplitude controversy revisited, *Muscle Nerve* 19:915, 1996.

Nitta H et al: Study on dermatomes by means of selective lumbar spinal nerve block, *Spine* 18:1782, 1993.

Nogradi A, Vrbova G: The use of a neurotoxic lectin, volkensin, to induce loss of identified motoneuron pools, *Neuroscience* 50(4):975-986, 1992.

Nordin M, Andersson GBJ, Pope MH: *Musculoskeletal disorders in the workplace: principles and practice,* St Louis, 1997, Mosby.

Nyland J et al: Wrist circumference is related to patellar tendon thickness in healthy men and women, *Clin Imaging* 30(5):335-338, 2006.

O'Connor MI, Carrier BI: Metastatic disease of the spine, *Orthopedics* 15:611, 1992.

O'Donoghue DH: *Treatment of injuries to patients,* ed 4, Philadelphia, 1984, WB Saunders.

Olmarker K, Rydevik B: Pathophysiology of sciatica, *Orthop Clin North Am* 22:223, 1991.

Olson WH et al: *Handbook of symptom-oriented neurology,* ed 2, St Louis, 1994, Mosby.

Omer GE, Spinner M: *Management of peripheral nerve problems,* Philadelphia, 1980, WB Saunders.

O'Young B, Young MA, Stiens SA: *PM&R secrets,* Philadelphia, 1997, Hanley & Belfus.

Padley S et al: Assessment of a single spine radiograph in low back pain, *Br J Radiol* 63:535, 1990.

Pagana KD, Pagana TJ: *Mosby's manual of diagnostic and laboratory tests,* St Louis, 1998, Mosby.

Partheni M et al: Radiculopathy after lumbar discectomy due to intraspinal retained Surgicel: clinical and magnetic resonance imaging evaluation, *Spine J* 6(4):455-458, 2006.

Patten J: *Neurological differential diagnosis,* ed 2, London, 1996, Springer.

Patton KT: *Student survival guide for anatomy and physiology,* St Louis, 1999, Mosby.

Perkin GD: *Mosby's color atlas and text of neurology,* London, 1998, Mosby-Wolfe.

Perrone C et al: Pyogenic and tuberculous spondylodiscitis (vertebral osteomyelitis) in 80 adult patients, *Clin Infect Dis* 19:746, 1994.

Pheasant S: *Ergonomics, work and health,* Gaithersburg, Md, 1991, Aspen.

Phillips LH, Parks TS: Electrophysiologic mapping of the segmental anatomy of the muscles of the lower extremity, *Muscle Nerve* 14:1213, 1991.

Pomeranz SJ, Pretorius HT, Ramsingh PS: Bone scintigraphy and multimodality imaging in bone neoplasia: strategies for imaging in the new health care climate, *Semin Nucl Med* 24:188, 1994.

Pool-Goudzwaard AL et al: Insufficient lumbopelvic stability: a clinical, anatomical and biomechanical approach to 'a-specific' low back pain, *Man Ther* 3(1):12-20, 1998.

Pope MH et al: *Occupational low back pain assessment, treatment and prevention,* St Louis, 1991, Mosby.

Porta M: A comparative trial of botulinum toxin type A and methylprednisolone for the treatment of myofascial pain syndrome and pain from chronic muscle spasm, *Pain* 85(1-2):101-105, 2000.

Porterfield JA, DeRosa C: *Mechanical low back pain: perspectives in functional anatomy,* Philadelphia, 1991, WB Saunders.

Post M: *Physical examination of the musculoskeletal system,* Chicago, 1987, Mosby.

Postacchini F, Cinotti G: Bone regrowth after surgical decompression for lumbar spinal stenosis, *J Bone Joint Surg* 74B:862, 1992.

Rachlin ES: *Myofascial pain and fibromyalgia trigger point management,* St Louis, 1994, Mosby.

Raja SN. 75 Workshop summary: CRPS—a disease with many faces, *Eur J Pain* 11(1, suppl 1):30-31, 2007.

Ramsey M: Results from grade II, III, and IV spondylolisthesis with open reduction and posterior lumbar interbody fusion, *Spine J* 6(5, suppl 1):140S, 2006.

Ranawat VS, Dowell JK, Heywood-Waddington MB: Stress fractures of the lumbar pars interarticularis in athletes: a review based on long-term results of 18 professional cricketers, *Injury* 34(12):915-919, 2003.

Rantanen J, Hurme M, Falck B: The lumbar multifidus muscle five years after surgery for a lumbar intervertebral disc herniation, *Spine* 18:568, 1993.

Ravel R: *Clinical laboratory medicine clinical application of laboratory data,* ed 6, St Louis, 1995, Mosby.

Resnick D, Niwayama G: *Diagnosis of bone and joint disorders,* Philadelphia, 1995, WB Saunders.

Ro CS: Sacroiliac joint. In Cox JM, editor: *Low back pain: mechanism, diagnosis and treatment,* ed 5, Baltimore, 1990, Williams & Wilkins.

Rodnitzky RL: *Van Allen's pictorial manual of neurologic tests: a guide to the performance and interpretation of the neurologic examination,* ed 3, Chicago, 1969, Mosby.

Rossi P et al: Magnetic resonance imaging findings in piriformis syndrome: a case report, *Arch Phys Med Rehabil* 82(4):519-521, 2001.

Rossignol M, Suissa S, Abenhaim L: The evolution of compensated occupational spinal injuries: a three-year follow-up study, *Spine* 17:1043, 1992.

Rothman RH, Simeone FA: *The spine,* ed 3, Philadelphia, 1992, WB Saunders.

Rumack CM, Wilson SR, Charboneau JW: *Diagnostic ultrasound,* vol 1-2, ed 2, St Louis, 1998, Mosby.

Saal JA, Saal JS, Herzog RJ: The natural history of lumbar intervertebral disc extrusions treated nonoperatively, *Spine* 15:683, 1990.

Saidoff DC, McDonough AL: *Critical pathways in therapeutic intervention,* St Louis, 1997, Mosby.

Salovy P et al: Reporting chronic pain episodes on health surveys. In *Vital health statistics,* vol 6, Hyattsville, Md, 1992, National Center for Health Statistics.

Scham SM, Taylor TKF: Tension signs in lumbar disc prolapse, *Clin Orthop* 75:195, 1971.

Schmorl G: *The human spine in health and disease,* ed 2, New York, 1971, Grune & Stratton.

Schofferman J et al: Childhood psychological trauma and chronic refractory low back pain, *Clin J Pain* 9:260, 1993.

Schofferman J, Wassermann S: Successful treatment of low back pain and/or neck pain due to a motor vehicle accident, *Spine* 19:1007, 1994.

Schumacher HR, Klippel JH, Koopman WJ: *Primer on the rheumatic diseases,* ed 10, Atlanta, 1993, Arthritis Foundation.

Schwarzer AC et al: Prevalence and clinical features of lumbar zygapophyseal joint pain: a study in an Australian population with chronic low back pain, *Ann Rheum Dis* 54:100, 1995.

Secher Jensen T et al: Magnetic resonance imaging findings as predictors of clinical outcome in patients with sciatica receiving active conservative treatment, *J Manipulative Physiol Ther* 30(2):98-108, 2007.

Seidel HM et al: *Mosby's guide to physical examination,* ed 4, St Louis, 1999, Mosby.

Shankman GA: *Fundamental orthopedic management for the examiner,* St Louis, 1997, Mosby.

Shin DS, Lee K, Kim D: Biomechanical study of lumbar spine with dynamic stabilization device using finite element method, *Comput Aided Des* 39(7):559-567, 2007.

Simons DG: Muscle pain syndromes, *J Manual Med* 6:3, 1991.

Sledge CB, Poss R: *The year book of orthopedics 1997,* St Louis, 1997, Mosby.

Smith MD, Bohlman HH: Spondylolisthesis treated by a single-stage operation combining decompression with in situ posterolateral and anterior fusion, *J Bone Joint Surg* 72:415, 1990.

Smith SA et al: Straight leg raising: anatomical effects on the spinal nerve root without and with fusion, *Spine* 18:992, 1993.

Snijders CJ et al: Effects of slouching and muscle contraction on the strain of the iliolumbar ligament, *Man Ther* (in press, corrected proof).

Spangfort E: Lasègue's sign in patients with lumbar disc herniation, *Acta Orthop* 42:459, 1971.

Specht NT, Russo RD: *Practical guide to diagnostic imaging,* St Louis, 1998, Mosby.

Spengler DM, Szpalski M: Newer assessment approaches for the patient with low back pain, *Contemp Orthop* 21, 1990.

Starlanyl D, Copeland ME: *Fibromyalgia & chronic myofascial pain syndrome a survival manual,* Oakland, Calif, 1996, New Harbinger Publications.

Stauffer ES et al: Fractures and dislocations of the spine, part II, the thoracolumbar spine. In Rockwood CA, Green DP, Bucholz RW, editors: *Fractures in adults,* ed 3, Philadelphia, 1991, JB Lippincott.

Stedman TL: *Stedman's medical dictionary,* ed 25, Baltimore, 1990, Williams & Wilkins.

Stewart DL, Abeln SH: *Documenting functional outcomes in physical therapy,* St Louis, 1993, Mosby.

Stinson JT: Spondylolysis and spondylolisthesis in the athlete, *Clin Sports Med* 12:517, 1993.

Stith WJ: Exercise and the intervertebral disc, *Spine* 4:259, 1990.

Stoller DW: *Magnetic resonance imaging in orthopaedics & sports medicine,* Philadelphia, 1993, JB Lippincott.

Sward L et al: Anthropometric characteristics, passive hip flexion, and spinal mobility in relation to back pain in patients, *Spine* 15:376, 1990.

Sward L et al: Disc degeneration and associated abnormalities of the spine in elite patients: a magnetic resonance imaging study, *Spine* 16:437, 1991.

Sward L: The thoracolumbar spine in young elite patients, *Sports Med* 13:357, 1992.

Tan JC, Horn SE: *Practical manual of physical medicine and rehabilitation,* St Louis, 1998, Mosby.

Tatarek NE: Variation in the human cervical neural canal, *Spine J* 5(6):623-631, 2005.

8

Taylor JR: The development and adult structure of lumbar intervertebral discs, *J Manual Med* 5:43, 1990.

Thelander U et al: Straight leg raising test versus radiologic size, shape, and position of lumbar disc hernias, *Spine* 17:395, 1992.

Thibodeau GA, Patton KT: *Anatomy & physiology,* ed 4, St Louis, 1999, Mosby.

Thomas NWM: Low back pain, sciatica, cervical and lumbar spondylosis, *Surgery (Oxford)* 25(4):155-159, 2007.

Thompson GH: Back pain in children, *J Bone Joint Surg* 75A:928, 1993.

Thompson JM: *Clinical outlines for health assessment,* St Louis, 1997, Mosby.

Toghill PJ: *Examining patients: an introduction to clinical medicine,* London, 1990, Edward Arnold.

Tollison CD, Satterthwaite JR, Tollison JW: *Handbook of pain management,* ed 2, Baltimore, 1994, Williams & Wilkins.

Torg JS, Shepard RJ: *Current therapy in sports medicine,* ed 3, St Louis, 1995, Mosby.

Traill Z, Richards MA, Moore NR: Magnetic resonance imaging of metastatic bone disease, *Clin Orthop* 312:76, 1995.

Tsuritani I et al: Impact of obesity on musculoskeletal pain and difficulty of daily movements in Japanese middle-aged women, *Maturitas* 42(1):23-30, 2002.

Tumeh SS, Tohmeh AG: Nuclear medicine techniques in septic arthritis and osteomyelitis, *Rheum Dis Clin North Am* 17:559, 1991.

Turek SL: *Orthopaedics principles and their application,* ed 3, Philadelphia, 1977, JB Lippincott.

Twomey L, Taylor JR: Structural and mechanical disc changes with age, *J Manual Med* 5:58, 1990.

Uhthoff J: Prenatal development of the iliolumbar ligament, *J Bone Joint Surg* 75:93, 1993.

Urban LM: The straight-leg-raising test: a review, *J Orthop Sports Phys Ther* 2:117, 1981.

Van Holsbeeck M, Introcaso JH: *Musculoskeletal ultrasound,* St Louis, 1991, Mosby.

Vernon-Roberts B, Perie CJ: Degenerative changes in the intervertebral disc of the lumbar spine and their sequela, *Rheum Rehab* 16:13, 1977.

Vleeming A et al: The posterior layer of the thoracolumbar fascia. Its function in load transfer from spine to legs, *Spine* 20:753, 1995.

Voorhies RM, Jiang X, Thomas N: Predicting outcome in the surgical treatment of lumbar radiculopathy using the Pain Drawing Score, McGill Short Form Pain Questionnaire, and risk factors including psychosocial issues and axial joint pain, *Spine J* (in press, corrected proof).

Waddell G et al: Nonorganic physical signs in low back pain, *Spine* 5:177, 1980.

Waddell G et al: Objective clinical evaluation of physical impairment in chronic low back pain, *Spine* 17:617, 1992.

Wakefield TS, Frank RG: *The examiner's guide to neuro musculoskeletal practice,* Abbotsford, Wis, 1995, Allied Health of Wisconsin, S.C.

Walsh MJ: Evaluation of orthopedic testing of the low back for non-specific low back pain, *J Manipulative Physiol Ther* 21:232, 1998.

Walsh TR et al: Lumbar discography in normal subjects, a controlled, prospective study, *J Bone Joint Surg* 72A:1081, 1990.

Watkins RG: *The spine in sports,* St Louis, 1996, Mosby.

Weineck J: *Functional anatomy in sports,* ed 2, St Louis, 1990, Mosby.

Weinerman SA, Bockman RS: Medical therapy of osteoporosis, *Orthop Clin North Am* 21:109, 1990.

Weinstein SL, Buckwalter JA: *Turek's orthopaedics principles and their application,* ed 5, Philadelphia, 1994, JB Lippincott.

Westmark KD, Weissman BN: Complications of axial arthropathies, *Orthop Clin North Am* 21:427, 1990.

White AA III, Panjabi MM: *Clinical biomechanics of the spine,* Philadelphia, 1978, JB Lippincott.

White AA III, Panjabi MM: The basic kinematics of the human spine, a review of past and current knowledge, *Spine* 3:12, 1978.

White AH, Schofferman JA: *Spine care,* vol 1-2, St Louis, 1995, Mosby.

White G: *Levene's color atlas of dermatology,* ed 2, London, 1997, Mosby-Wolfe.

White G: *Regional dermatology,* London, 1994, Mosby-Wolfe.

Whitmore I, Willan PLT: *Multiple choice questions in human anatomy,* London, 1995, Mosby.

Wicke L: *Atlas of radiologic anatomy,* ed 5, Philadelphia, 1994, Lea & Febiger.

Wiesel SW, Bernini P, Rothman RH: *The aging lumbar spine,* Philadelphia, 1982, WB Saunders.

Wilder DG: The biomechanics of vibration and low back pain, *Am J Ind Med* 23:577, 1993.

Wilkins RH, Brody IA: Lasègue's sign, *Arch Neurol* 21:219, 1969.

Willeford G: *Medical word finder,* West Nyack, NY, 1967, Parker Publishing.

Willis Jr WD, Coggeshall RE: *Sensory mechanisms of the spinal cord,* ed 2, New York, 1991, Plenum.

Windsor RE, Lox DM: *Soft tissue injuries: diagnosis and treatment,* Philadelphia, 1998, Hanley & Belfus.

Woodhall R, Hayes GJ: The well-leg-raising test, *N Engl J Med* 297:1127, 1977.

Xu GL et al: Normal variation of the lumbar facet joint capsules, *Clin Anat* 4:11122, 1991.

Xu GL, Haughton VM, Carrera GF: Lumbar facet joint capsule: appearance at MR imaging and CT, *Radiology* 177:415, 1990.

Yamada K et al: Scoliosis associated with Prader-Willi syndrome, *Spine J* 7(3):345-348, 2007.

Yochum TR, Rowe L: *Essentials of skeletal radiology,* ed 2, Baltimore, 1996, Williams & Wilkins.

Yochum TR: *A closer look at spondylolisthesis,* East Rutherford, NJ, 1990, NYCC Second Multidisciplinary Symposium.

Yoshizawa H, Kobayashi S, Hachiya Y: Blood supply of nerve roots and dorsal root ganglia, *Orthop Clin North Am* 22:195, 1991.

Zacher J, Gursche A: 'Hip' pain, *Best Pract Res Clin Rheum* 17(1):71-85, 2003.

Zatouroff M: *Diagnosis in color physical signs in general medicine,* ed 2, London, 1996, Mosby-Wolfe.

Zitelli BJ, Davis HW: *Atlas of pediatric physical diagnosis,* ed 2, London, 1992, Wolfe.

CITATIONS

Ahn NU et al: Lumbar spine pathology and multiple atherosclerotic risk factors: a 53-year prospective study of 1,337 patients, *Spine J* 2(2, suppl 1):34, 2002.

Allen RP, Earley CJ: Restless legs syndrome: a review of clinical and pathophysiologic features, *J Clin Neurophysiol* 18(2):128-147, 2001.

Armand S et al: A comparison of gait in spinal muscular atrophy, type II and Duchenne muscular dystrophy, *Gait Posture* 21(4):369-378, 2005.

Babbage CS, Coppieters MW, McGowan CM: Strain and excursion of the sciatic nerve in the dog: biomechanical considerations in the development of a clinical test for increased neural mechanosensitivity, *Vet J* 174[2]:330-336, 2007.

Berthelot J-M et al: Buttock claudication disclosing a thrombosis of the superior left gluteal artery: report of a case diagnosed by a selective arteriography of the iliac artery, and cured by per-cutaneous stenting, *Joint Bone Spine* 74(3):289-291, 2007.

Blonk MC et al: The fracture and osteoporosis clinic: 1-year results and 3-month compliance, *Bone* 40(6):1643-1649, 2007.

Brumagne S, Cordo P, Verschueren S: Proprioceptive weighting changes in persons with low back pain and elderly persons during upright standing, *Neurosci Lett* 366(1):63-66, 2004.

Buchta RM: Reflex sympathetic dystrophy in a 14-year-old female, *J Adolesc Health Care* 4(2):121-122, 1983.

Cavanaugh JM et al: Lumbar facet pain: biomechanics, neuroanatomy and neurophysiology, *J Biomech* 29(9):1117-29, 1996.

Chang C-W et al: Measurement of motor nerve conduction velocity of the sciatic nerve in patients with piriformis syndrome: a magnetic stimulation study, *Arch Phys Med Rehabil* 87(10):1371-1375, 2006.

Coudreuse JM, Dupont P, Nicol C: Douleurs musculaires posteffort, *Ann Readapt Med Phys* 47(6):290-298, 2004.

de Groot M et al: The active straight leg raising test (ASLR) in pregnant women: differences in muscle activity and force between patients and healthy subjects, *Man Ther* 13(1):68-74, 2008.

Dilley A, Lynn B, Pang SJ: Pressure and stretch mechanosensitivity of peripheral nerve fibres following local inflammation of the nerve trunk, *Pain* 117(3):462-472, 2005.

Dobbs MB, Weinstein SL: Infantile and juvenile scoliosis, *Orthop Clin North Am* 30(3):331-341, 1999.

Freynhagen R et al: Pseudoradicular and radicular low-back pain—a disease continuum rather than different entities? Answers from quantitative sensory testing, *Pain* (in press, corrected proof).

Gerber MS et al: Cauda equina syndrome and neurogenic claudication. In *Encyclopedia of the neurological sciences,* New York, 2003, Academic Press.

Gillard J et al: Suspected disk space infection with negative microbiological tests—report of eight cases and comparison with documented pyogenic discitis, *Joint Bone Spine* 72(2):156-162, 2005.

Goodwin RW, O'Donnell P, Saifuddin A: MRI appearances of common benign soft-tissue tumours, *Clin Radiol* (in press, corrected proof).

Gradl G et al: Exaggeration of tissue trauma induces signs and symptoms of acute CRPS I, however displays distinct differences to experimental CRPS II, *Neurosci Lett* 402(3):267-72, 2006.

Greenlee JE, Michael JA, Robert BDL Meningitis, viral. In *Encyclopedia of the neurological sciences*, New York, 2003, Academic Press.

Guzey FK et al: Lumbar extradural infiltrating angiolipoma: a case report and review of 17 previously reported cases with infiltrating spinal angiolipomas, *Spine J* (in press, corrected proof).

Haikel S, Willett K: Traumatic rupture of the superior gluteal artery with a stable pelvic fracture, *Injury* 31(5):383-386, 2000.

Hamalainen H et al: Changes in bone mineral density in premenopausal women with rheumatoid arthritis during a two-year follow-up, *Joint Bone Spine* (in press, uncorrected proof).

Hsieh C-T et al: Delayed traumatic thoracic spinal epidural hematoma: a case report and literature review, *Am J Emerg Med* 25(1):69-71, 2007.

Hughes RJ, Saifuddin A: Imaging of lumbosacral transitional vertebrae, *Clin Radiol* 59(11):984-991, 2004.

Huntoon E, Huntoon M: Differential diagnosis of low back pain, *Semin Pain Med* 2(3):138-144, 2004.

Janig W, Baron R: Complex regional pain syndrome: mystery explained? *Lancet Neurol* 2(11):687-697, 2003.

Kalaci A, Karazincir S, Yanat AN: Long-standing Morel-Lavallee lesion of the thigh simulating a neoplasm, *Clin Imaging* 31(4):287-291, 2007.

Kapstad H et al: Changes in pain, stiffness and physical function in patients with osteoarthritis waiting for hip or knee joint replacement surgery, *Osteoarthr Cartil* 15(7):837-843, 2007.

Karachalios T, Karantanas AH, Malizos K: Hip osteoarthritis: what the radiologist wants to know, *Eur J Radiol* 63(1):36-48, 2007.

Kawaguchi Y et al: Adjacent segment disease following expansive lumbar laminoplasty, *Spine J* 7(3):273-279, 2007.

Kingma I, Staudenmann D, van Dieen JH: Trunk muscle activation and associated lumbar spine joint shear forces under different levels of external forward force applied to the trunk, *J Electromyogr Kinesiol* 17(1):14-24, 2007.

Kligman M et al: Hypotension as a delayed complication of rupture of a branch of the superior gluteal artery, following buttock contusion, *Injury* 33(3):285-287, 2002.

Kobayashi S, Yoshizawa H, Yamada S: Pathology of lumbar nerve root compression. Part 1: intraradicular inflammatory changes induced by mechanical compression, *J Orthop Res* 22(1):170-179, 2004a.

Kobayashi S, Yoshizawa H, Yamada S: Pathology of lumbar nerve root compression. Part 2: morphological and immunohistochemical changes of dorsal root ganglion, *J Orthop Res* 22(1):180-188, 2004b.

Krishna M, Pollock RD, Bhatia C: Incidence, etiology, classification, and management of neuralgia after posterior lumbar interbody fusion surgery in 226 patients, *Spine J* (in press, corrected proof).

LaBan MM et al: The lumbar herniated disk of pregnancy: a report of six cases identified by magnetic resonance imaging, *Arch Phys Med Rehabil* 76(5):476-479, 1995.

Lai WWL, Ubogu EE: Chronic inflammatory demyelinating polyradiculoneuropathy presenting as cauda equina syndrome in a diabetic, *J Neurol Sci* (in press, corrected proof).

Langevin HM, Sherman KJ: Pathophysiological model for chronic low back pain integrating connective tissue and nervous system mechanisms, *Med Hypotheses* 68(1):74-80, 2007.

Lariviere C et al: Evaluation of measurement strategies to increase the reliability of EMG indices to assess back muscle fatigue and recovery, *J Electromyogr Kinesiol* 12(2):91-102, 2002.

Li J, Shi R: A device for the electrophysiological recording of peripheral nerves in response to stretch, *J Neurosci Methods* 154(1-2):102-108, 2006.

Littlewood C, May S: Measurement of range of movement in the lumbar spine—what methods are valid? A systematic review, *Physiotherapy* (in press, corrected proof).

Loh J-K et al: Primary spinal tumors in children, *J Clin Neurosci* 12(3):246-248, 2005.

Maduri A, Pearson BL, Wilson SE: Lumbar-pelvic range and coordination during lifting tasks, *J Electromyogr Kinesiol* (in press, corrected proof).

McCarthy RE: Management of neuromuscular scoliosis, *Orthop Clin North Am* 30(3):435-449, 1999.

Millesi H, Zoch G, Rath T: The gliding apparatus of peripheral nerve and its clinical significance, *Ann Chirurgie Main* 9(2):87-97, 1990.

Mobbs RJ, Steel TR: Migration of lumbar disc herniation: an unusual case, *J Clin Neurosci* 14(6):581-584, 2007.

Moucharafieh R, Wehbe J, Maalouf G: Meralgia paresthetica: a result of tight new trendy low cut trousers (`taille basse'), *Int J Surg* (in press, corrected proof).

Nadler SF et al: Tarlov cyst as a rare cause of S1 radiculopathy: a case report, *Arch Phys Med Rehabil* 82(5):689-690, 2001.

Nadler SF, Malanga GA, Ciccone DS: Positive straight-leg raising in lumbar radiculopathy: is documentation affected by insurance coverage? *Arch Phys Med Rehabil* 85(8):1336-1338, 2004.

Nakagawa H et al: Optimal duration of conservative treatment for lumbar disc herniation depending on the type of herniation, *J Clin Neurosci* 14(2):104-109, 2007.

O'Neill S et al: Generalized deep-tissue hyperalgesia in patients with chronic low-back pain, *Eur J Pain* 11(4):415-420, 2007.

Oertel MF et al: Lumbar foraminal and far lateral juxtafacet cyst of intraspinal origin, *Surg Neurol* 66(2):197-199, 2006.

Pau A et al: Redundant nerve roots of the cauda equina, *Surg Neurol* 16(4):245-250, 1981.

Perez RSGM et al: Diagnostic criteria for CRPS I: differences between patient profiles using three different diagnostic sets, *Eur J Pain* (in press, corrected proof).

Ploumis A, Transfledt EE, Denis F: Degenerative lumbar scoliosis associated with spinal stenosis, *Spine J* (in press, corrected proof).

Rabie M, Drory VE: A test for the evaluation of the lateral cutaneous branch of the iliohypogastric nerve using somatosensory evoked potentials, *J Neurol Sci* 238(1-2):59-63, 2005.

Rafii A, Querleu D: Laparoscopic obturator nerve neurolysis after pelvic lymphadenectomy, *J Minim Invasive Gynecol* 13(1):17-19, 2006.

8

Rantanen P, Nykvist F: Optimal sagittal motion axis for trunk extension and flexion tests in chronic low back trouble, *Clin Biomech* 15(9):665-671, 2000.

Rasekhi A et al: Clinical manifestations and MRI findings of patients with hydrated and dehydrated lumbar disc herniation, *Acad Radiol* 13(12):1485-1489, 2006.

Requena L: Normal subcutaneous fat, necrosis of adipocytes and classification of the panniculitides, *Semin Cutan Med Surg* 26(2):66-70, 2007.

Roche P-H et al: Anterior lumbosacral dislocation: case report and review of the literature, *Surg Neurol* 50(1):11-16, 1998.

Roussel NA et al: Low back pain: clinimetric properties of the Trendelenburg test, active straight leg raise test, and breathing pattern during active straight leg raising, *J Manipulative Physiol Ther* 30(4):270-278, 2007.

Sabers SR et al: Procedure-based nonsurgical management of lumbar zygapophyseal joint cyst-induced radicular pain, *Arch Phys Med Rehabil* 86(9):1767-1771, 2005.

Saifuddin A, Blease S, MacSweeney E: Axial loaded MRI of the lumbar spine, *Clin Radiol* 58(9):661-671, 2003.

Sakai T et al: Radiological features of lumbar spinal lesions in patients with rheumatoid arthritis with special reference to the changes around intervertebral discs, *Spine J* (in press, uncorrected proof).

Singh A et al: Mechanical properties of spinal nerve roots subjected to tension at different strain rates, *J Biomech* 39(9):1669-1676, 2006.

Small SA, Perron AD, Brady WJ: Orthopedic pitfalls: cauda equina syndrome, *Am J Emerg Med* 23(2):159-163, 2005.

Smith JA, Hu SS: Management of spondylolysis and spondylolisthesis in the pediatric and adolescent population, *Orthop Clin North Am* 30(3):487-499, 1999.

Solomonow M et al: Flexion-relaxation response to static lumbar flexion in males and females, *Clin Biomech* 18(4):273-279, 2003.

Steffen T et al: Lumbar intradiscal pressure measured in the anterior and posterolateral annular regions during asymmetrical loading, *Clin Biomech* 13(7):495-505, 1998.

Tortolani PJ, Carbone JJ, Quartararo LG: Greater trochanteric pain syndrome in patients referred to orthopedic spine specialists, *Spine J* 2(4):251-254, 2002.

Trummer M et al: Lumbar disc herniation mimicking meralgia paresthetica: case report, *Surg Neurol* 54(1):80-81, 2000.

Vallejo MC et al: Piriformis syndrome in a patient after cesarean section under spinal anesthesia, *Reg Anesth Pain Med* 29(4):364-367, 2004.

van Dun PLS, Girardin MRG: Embryological study of the spinal dura and its attachment into the vertebral canal, *Int J Osteopath Med* 9(3):85-93, 2006.

Vignolo M et al: Fetal spine ossification: the gender and individual differences illustrated by ultrasonography, *Ultrasound Med Biol* 31(6):733-738, 2005.

Vital JM, Pedram M: Spondylolisthesis par lyse isthmique, *EMC—Rhumatologie-Orthopedie* 2(2):125-150, 2005.

Wright JL et al: Specific fracture configurations predict sexual and excretory dysfunction in men and women 1 year after pelvic fracture, *J Urol* 176(4):1540-1545, 2006.

Wu C-T et al: Classification of symptomatic osteoporotic compression fractures of the thoracic and lumbar spine, *J Clin Neurosci* 13(1):31-38, 2006.

Xu X, Mirka GA, Hsiang SM: The effects of obesity on lifting performance, *Appl Ergon* 39[1]:93-98, 2008.

Yagci N et al: Relationship between balance performance and musculoskeletal pain in lower body comparison healthy middle aged and older adults, *Arch Gerontol Geriatr* 45(1):109-119, 2007.

Yao M-S et al: Magnetic resonance imaging of gluteal intramuscular myxoma, *Clin Imaging* 31(3):214-216, 2007.

CHAPTER NINE

PELVIS AND SACROILIAC JOINT

AXIOMS IN ASSESSING THE PELVIS AND THE SACROILIAC JOINTS

- The primary function of the pelvis, including the bones, joints, ligaments, and muscles, is mechanical transfer of weight.
- A secondary function of the bony pelvis is protection of viscera.

INTRODUCTION

The pelvis is a uniquely devised mechanism designed to transfer the body weight from the single weight-bearing axis of the trunk to the bipolar weight bearing of the lower extremities. The spine attaches to the pelvis by a single connection to the sacrum. Weight transfers through the bony ring of the pelvis, from the spinal column to the two lower extremities. Enclosed within the pelvis are the bladder, the female genitalia, the rectum, and the great vessels and nerves that extend to the lower extremities.

Narrow, closely fitted, irregularly shaped, and cartilage-covered surfaces of the posterior and internal ilium and the lateral border of the sacrum form the sacroiliac articulation. The lumbosacral trunk lies anteriorly in direct relationship to the sacroiliac articulation. An inflammatory neuritis is a common accompaniment of sacroiliac arthritis. The anterior ligaments are thin and easily distended by intraarticular swelling.

The upper two thirds of the joint are covered posteriorly by the posterior end of the ilium. The lower third of the joint is covered by the sacroiliac ligaments but can often be palpated in thin individuals.

The conditions that affect the sacroiliac joints (SI-joints) are those that involve any joint. The sacroiliac articulation is a favored site for tuberculous infection and is often the starting point for ankylosing spondylitis. Degenerative arthritic changes are often significant at this joint.

Female genital tuberculosis is a very common disease in developing countries. It tends to lead to menstrual irregularities, infertility, or chronic pelvic or lower abdominal pain and is almost always acquired by hematogenous spread from an extragenital source such as pulmonary or abdominal tuberculosis. The fallopian tubes are the first and most commonly affected genital organs, followed by endometrium, ovary, and cervix. Adhesions among tubes, ovaries, omentum, intestines, liver, and diaphragm (the Fitz-Hugh–Curtis syndrome) are common findings in tuberculosis (Gupta et al, 2007).

The stability of the SI-joint lies in the nature of its articular surfaces and ligaments (Fig. 9-2). Cardinal in this role are the dense, interosseous ligaments lying dorsal to the joint and the ventral sacroiliac ligament covering its anterior aspect.

In ankylosing spondylitis, the patient complains of spinal pain and stiffness. The SI-joints are affected initially; increasing loss of spinal mobility can lead to loss of the lumbar lordosis (Fig. 9-3).

A common tender fatty nodule in the sacroiliac area is sometimes called the **episacroiliac lipoma,** or *back mouse.* In this instance, fatty tissue herniates through the normal deep fascia and become edematous and a source of pain. Clinically, the patient complains of pain in the tender nodules that are palpable and often bilateral. The mass is usually palpable as a mobile soft tumor that slips beneath the examining finger. Such a lipoma mass must be differentiated from the peripelvic serosanguineous cyst.

Peripelvic serosanguineous cysts can develop following pelvic fracture. A serosanguineous cyst develops when shearing forces cause separation of the skin and subcutane-

TABLE 9-1

PELVIS AND SACROILIAC CROSS-REFERENCE TABLE BY ASSESSMENT PROCEDURE

Pelvis Test/Sign	DISEASE ASSESSED					
	Sacroiliac Abnormality	Lumbosacral Syndrome	Sprain	Subluxation	Fracture	Pyogenic Sacroiliitis
Anterior innominate test	•					
Belt test	•	•				
Erichsen sign	•					
Gaenslen test	•	•				
Gapping test	•		•			
Goldthwait sign	•	•				
Hibbs test	•		•	•		
Iliac compression test	•		•	•	•	
Knee-to-shoulder test	•		•	•		
Laguerre test	•		•	•		
Lewin-Gaenslen test	•		•	•		
Piedallu sign	•		•	•		
Sacral apex test	•		•	•		
Sacroiliac resisted-abduction test			•	•		
Smith-Petersen test	•	•				
Squish test			•			
Yeoman test	•		•	•		

TABLE 9-2

PELVIS AND SACROILIAC JOINT CROSS-REFERENCE TABLE BY SYNDROME OR TISSUE

Fracture	Iliac compression test	Sprain	Gapping test
Lumbosacral syndrome	Belt test		Hibbs test
	Gaenslen test		Iliac compression test
	Smith-Petersen test		Knee-to-shoulder test
Pyogenic sacroiliitis	Knee-to-shoulder test		Laguerre test
Sacroiliac abnormality	Anterior innominate test		Lewin-Gaenslen test
	Belt test		Piedallu sign
	Erichsen sign		Sacral apex test
	Gaenslen test		Sacroiliac resisted-abduction test
	Gapping test		Squish test
	Goldthwait sign		Yeoman test
	Hibbs test	Subluxation	Hibbs test
	Iliac compression test		Iliac compression test
	Knee-to-shoulder test		Knee-to-shoulder test
	Laguerre test		Laguerre test
	Lewin-Gaenslen test		Lewin-Gaenslen test
	Piedallu sign		Piedallu sign
	Sacral apex test		Sacral apex test
	Smith-Petersen test		Sacroiliac resisted-abduction test
	Yeoman test		Yeoman test

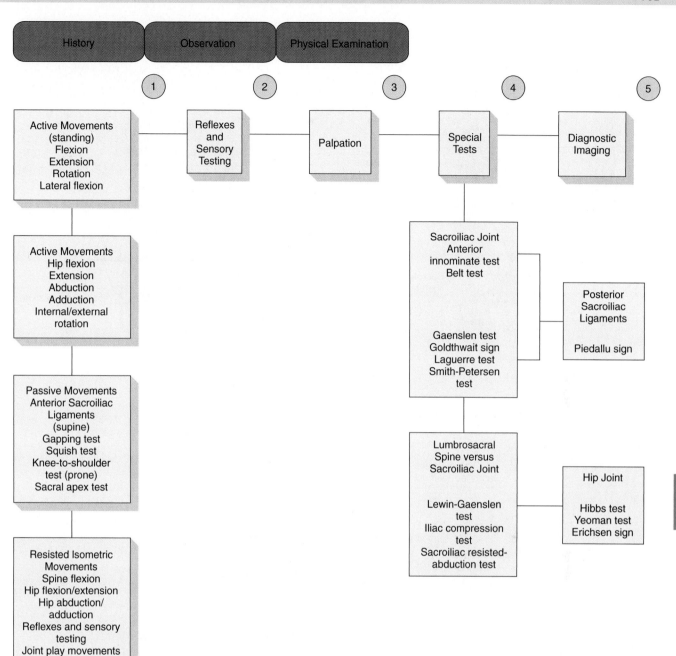

FIG. 9-1 Sacroiliac joint assessment.

ous fat from the **deep fascia** and muscle. The space thus created is filled with serious fluid and blood and is clinically exhibited as soft cystic masses, appearing usually within a day or so or, rarely, after several weeks or months. Most of these lesions resolve spontaneously or after aspiration; however, some may persist, necessitating surgical resection. Computed tomography is the modality of choice for detection and, in specific cysts that require surgery, it is helpful in revealing the exact size and location of these lesions (Rafii et al, 1983).

ESSENTIAL ANATOMY

The two innominate bones (or *hip* bones), the sacrum, and the coccyx (Fig. 9-4) make up the pelvis. The innominate bone consists of the ilium, ischium, and pubis (Fig. 9-5).

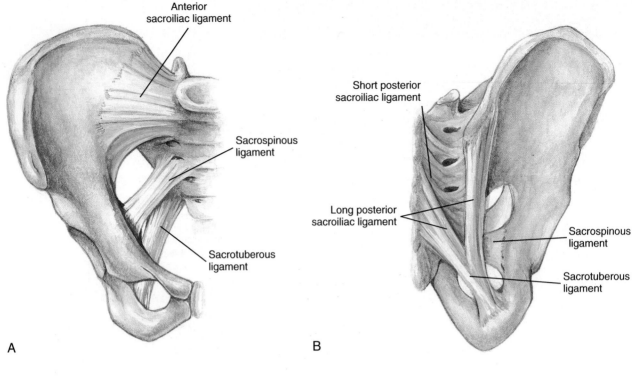

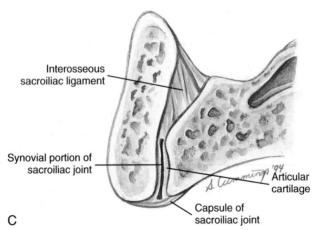

FIG. 9-2 Ligaments of the sacroiliac joint (SIJ) **A,** Anterior view. **B,** Posterior view. **C,** SIJ in horizontal section. (From Cramer GD, Darby SA: *Basic and clinical anatomy of the spine, spinal cord, and ANS*, St Louis, 1995, Mosby.)

ORTHOPEDIC GAMUT 9-1

INNOMINATE BONE

Exterior surfaces of the innominate bones:
1. An upper area, the lateral surface of the ilium
2. A central depressed socket, the acetabulum
3. A lower region, in which curved rami of the pubis and ischium form the obturator foramen

---

ORTHOPEDIC GAMUT 9-2

SUPERIOR HALF OF THE PELVIS

Interior surfaces of the superior half of the pelvis include:
1. Superiorly, the iliac fossa, a shallow depression in the ilium
2. A posterior roughened articular surface
3. Inferiorly, the medial surface of obturator foramen

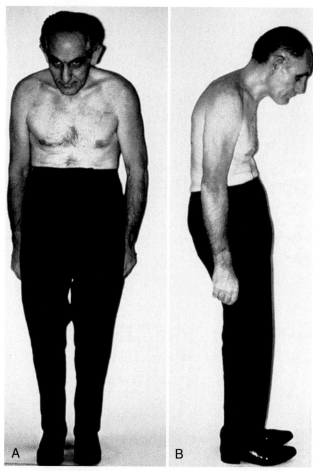

FIG. 9-3 Gross postural changes in man affected by ankylosing spondylitis. (From Seidel HM et al: *Mosby's guide to physical examination*, ed 4, St Louis, 1999, Mosby.)

9

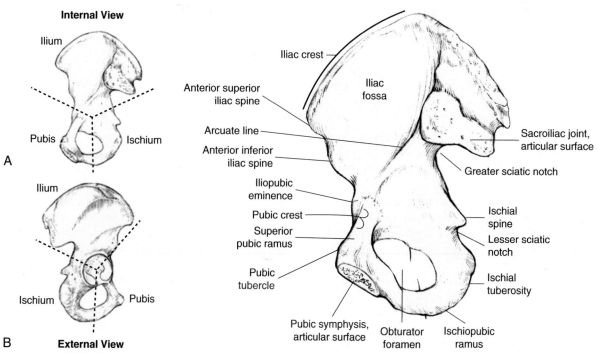

FIG. 9-4 Interior of the pelvis. (From Mathers LH et al: *Clinical anatomy principles*, St Louis, 1996, Mosby.)

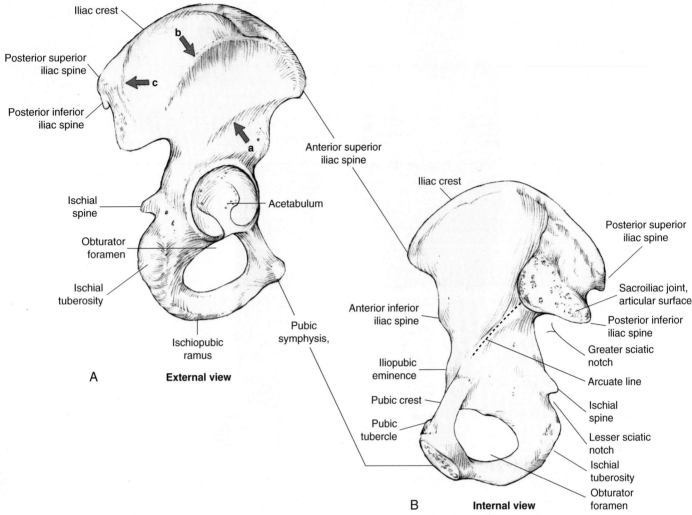

FIG. 9-5 Innominate bone. (From Mathers LH et al: *Clinical anatomy principles*, St Louis, 1996, Mosby.)

The sacrum is the fusion of five sacral vertebrae, separate in embryonic life. The fusion of these vertebrae yields a bony shield, with a shape resembling a curved inverted triangle (Fig. 9-6).

The body of vertebra L5 articulates directly with an upward-facing articular surface on the sacrum (forming the lumbosacral joint). The iliolumbar ligaments connect the transverse processes of L5 to the iliac rests on each side (Fig. 9-7).

The lumbosacral plexus (Fig. 9-8) takes shape on the medial surface of the levator ani muscle (Table 9-3).

The sciatic nerve (L4 to S3), the largest peripheral nerve in the body (Fig. 9-9), divides into the common peroneal and tibial nerves. It exits the pelvis through the greater sciatic foramen inferior to piriformis and lies deep to the gluteus maximus.

ESSENTIAL MOTION ASSESSMENT

Although firmly constrained by its ligaments, the SI-joint exhibits movements that are small in magnitude and complex in nature. The amplitude of nutation of the sacrum is normally not more than 2 mm or 2 degrees.

The SI-joint consequently serves as a stress-relieving joint, the tension that would have otherwise been imposed on bone being absorbed by the sacroiliac ligaments at the expense of slight distracting and sliding movements between the sacrum and ilium.

The pelvis plays an active role in gait, or walking. The femoral heads articulate with the acetabulum on each side, and as one and then the other femur strides forward, the pelvis must *rock* from side to side. Viewed from above, the pelvis appears to rotate its right side anteriorly when the

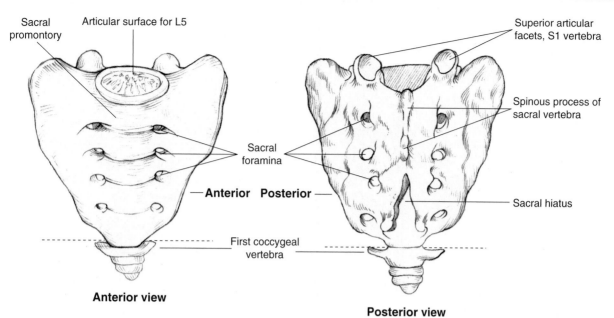

Sacral promontory

Articular surface for L5

Superior articular facets, S1 vertebra

Spinous process of sacral vertebra

Sacral foramina

Anterior   Posterior

Sacral hiatus

First coccygeal vertebra

Anterior view

Posterior view

FIG. 9-6 Sacrum and coccyx. (From Mathers LH, et al: *Clinical anatomy principles*, St Louis, 1996, Mosby.)

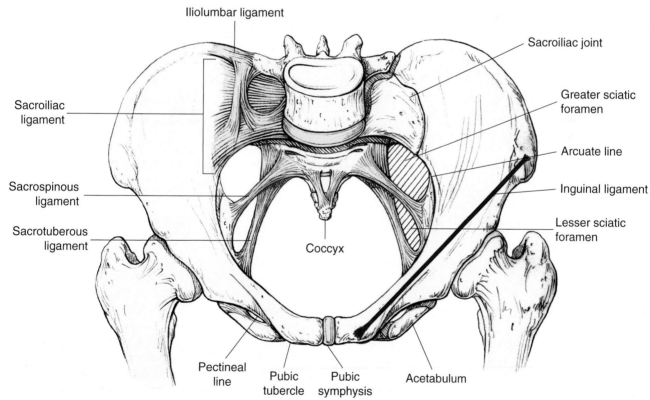

Iliolumbar ligament

Sacroiliac joint

Sacroiliac ligament

Greater sciatic foramen

Arcuate line

Sacrospinous ligament

Inguinal ligament

Sacrotuberous ligament

Lesser sciatic foramen

Coccyx

Pectineal line

Pubic tubercle

Pubic symphysis

Acetabulum

FIG. 9-7 Pelvic ligaments, superoanterior view. (From Mathers LH et al: *Clinical anatomy principles*, St Louis, 1996, Mosby.)

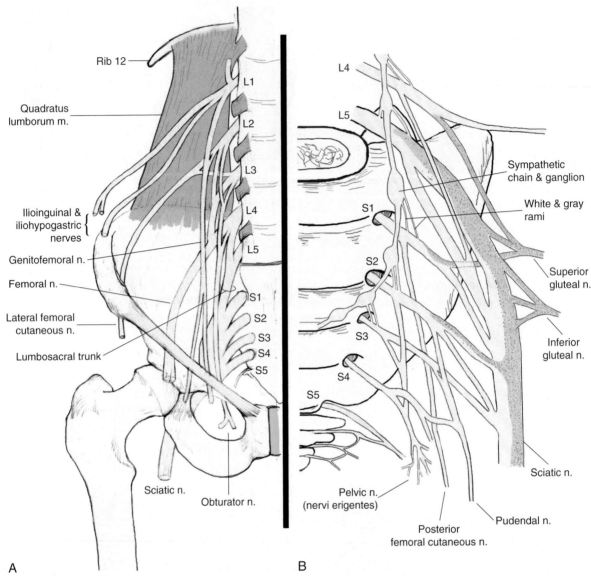

FIG. 9-8 Lumbosacral plexus. (From Mathers LH et al: *Clinical anatomy principles*, St Louis, 1996, Mosby.)

right side lower limb strides forward and the left side of the pelvis moves forward when the left lower limb swings forward.

The pelvis is a major structure within the human body, which in conjunction with the sacrum facilitates the transfer of the weight of the upper body to the hip joints. In addition muscles originating on the cortex of the pelvis allow balance to be maintained about a single hip joint for activities such as walking and running. Experimental studies have found that the resultant force acting through the hip joint during normal walking is around 300% of body weight. The force

required in the abductor muscles to maintain coronal balance during single leg stance can be demonstrated to be around 200% of body weight, with the abductor muscles acting about the hip joint to counteract the weight of the upper body and the weight of the leg not in contact with the ground (Phillips et al, 2007).

If the hip joints should become less mobile, as a result of arthritis for example, the head of the femur will not rotate easily within the acetabulum. This condition results in a limitation on the length of the stride or in pain accompanying gait or both.

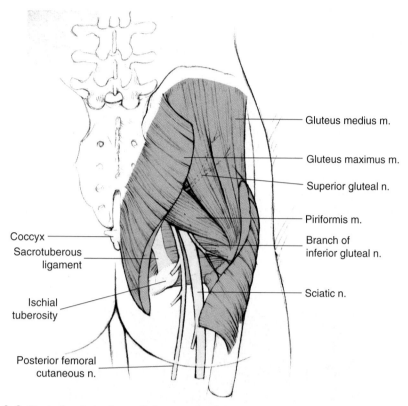

Gluteus medius m.

Gluteus maximus m.

Superior gluteal n.

Piriformis m.

Branch of inferior gluteal n.

Sciatic n.

Coccyx
Sacrotuberous ligament

Ischial tuberosity

Posterior femoral cutaneous n.

FIG. 9-9 Posterior branches of the sacral plexus. (From Mathers LH et al: *Clinical anatomy principles*, St Louis, 1996, Mosby.)

TABLE 9-3

SACRAL PLEXUS

Anterior Divisions	Posterior Divisions
Nerve to quadratus femoris/ inferior gemellus	Nerve to piriformis
Nerve to obturator internus/ superior gemellus	Superior gluteal nerve
Posterior femoral cutaneous nerve*	Inferior gluteal nerve
Tibial nerve	Posterior femoral cutaneous nerve*
Pudendal nerve	Common peroneal nerve
Pelvic splanchnic nerves	Perforating cutaneous nerve
Nerve to levator ani/coccygeus	

*Both divisions contribute to this nerve.
Adapted from Mathers LH et al: *Clinical anatomy principles,* St Louis, 1996, Mosby.

ORTHOPEDIC GAMUT 9-3

LUMBOPELVIC FLEXIBILITY TESTING

Lumbopelvic flexibility testing procedures:

1. *Spinal erector muscles:* With the patient in the supine position, the examiner gently bends the patient's knee to the chest.
2. *Hip flexor muscles:* With the patient prone, the examiner places the patient's affected hip into extension, and then abducts the thigh.
3. *Hamstring muscles:* Placing the patient supine and keeping the patient's hips and buttocks down to the table, the examiner performs a straight leg raise with the knee held in extension.
4. *Gluteal muscles:* The patient should be supine and placed in hip flexion with a bent knee. The lower leg can be internally rotated with thigh adduction to facilitate a stretch of the rotator muscles of the hip, such as the gluteus medius and piriformis.
5. *Quadriceps muscles:* With the patient prone and the examiner's inferior hand on the patient's affected knee, the examiner uses the shoulder to move the patient's lower leg gently toward the ipsilateral buttock to induce knee flexion.

9

ESSENTIAL MUSCLE FUNCTION ASSESSMENT

The gluteal and erector muscles aid in stabilizing the spine and provide extension. To evaluate functional strength in spinal extension, the examiner places the patient in a prone position. The patient raises one arm out straight in front and simultaneously lifts the leg on the opposite side out straight. The patient holds this position for 5 to 10 seconds, and the examiner notes any fatigue or inability to gain a healthy contraction, especially on the side of the leg lift. This side activates the hip and spinal extensor mass. The patient repeats the exercise on the opposite side, and the examiner compares the observations.

ESSENTIAL IMAGING

The pelvis can be well visualized by a routine anteroposterior (AP) roentgenogram (Figs. 9-10 and 9-11). In addition, the sacrum and coccyx may be studied by lateral views (Fig. 9-12) and AP views angled 15 degrees cephalad and caudad (Figs. 9-13 and 9-14).

Radiographic evaluation might play an important role in ruling out an inflammatory arthritis. Conditions such as ankylosing spondylitis can have a clinical presentation similar to other spondyloarthropathies, with referral of pain into the hip and gluteal regions. After pregnancy, conditions such as osteitis condensans ilii can also be identified with plain films. In this case, the soft-tissue findings cannot be evaluated with plain films.

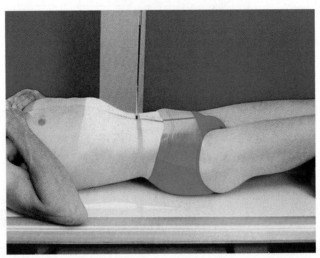

FIG. 9-10 Male anteroposterior abdomen positioning with gonad shield. (From Frank ED et al: *Merrill's atlas of radiographic positioning and procedures,* vol 1-3, ed 11, St Louis, 2007, Mosby.)

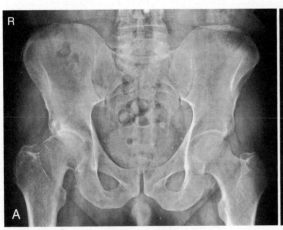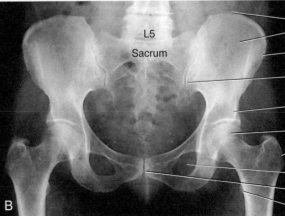

FIG. 9-11 Male anteroposterior pelvis images. (From Frank ED et al: *Merrill's atlas of radiographic positioning and procedures,* vol 1-3, ed 11, St Louis, 2007, Mosby.)

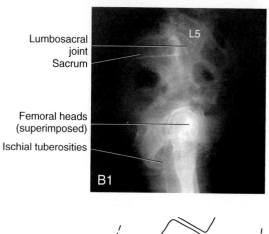

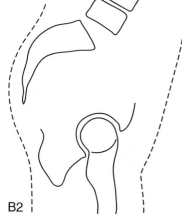

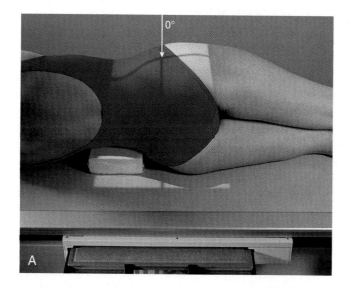

FIG. 9-12 Lateral pelvis positioning and images. (From Frank ED et al: *Merrill's atlas of radiographic positioning and procedures,* vol 1-3, ed 11, St Louis, 2007, Mosby.)

9

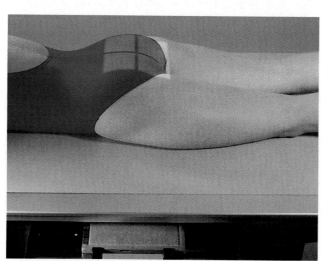

FIG. 9-13 Axial pelvis positioning. (From Frank ED et al: *Merrill's atlas of radiographic positioning and procedures,* vol 1-3, ed 11, St Louis, 2007, Mosby.)

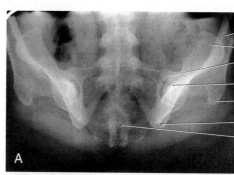

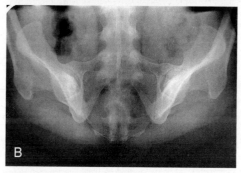

FIG. 9-14 Axial pelvis imaging. (From Frank ED et al: *Merrill's atlas of radiographic positioning and procedures,* vol 1-3, ed 11, St Louis, 2007, Mosby.)

MAZION PELVIC MANEUVER

Assessment for Unilateral Forward Displacement of the Ilia on the Sacrum

Comment

Many cases of acute low back pain that are not correctly identified evolve into a chronic spinal problem with significant disability at the muscular level (Table 9-4). Muscular fixation alone can be the cause of spinal joint dysfunction.

A vast majority of patients with low back pain (LBP) are known to suffer from *mechanical back pain* in which no clear diagnosis is established. Nonetheless, LBP affects up to 70% of the population in developed countries, accounting for an important cause of time off work. The term *sacroiliac-joint dysfunction* is reserved for cases in which no demonstrable abnormality is found in the joint, but the joint is presumed to be biomechanically incompetent in effectively transmitting load to the lower limbs. Experts have argued that this biomechanical abnormality would give rise to pain originating from the SI-joint (Hossain, Nokes, 2005).

The SI-joint is a shock-absorbing link in weight transmission to the lower limb, with all the weight of the upper body transmitted through the two SI joints to the lower limbs. The joint absorbs concussive force at heel strike, transmitting force from the lower limbs to the trunk. Given that the joint surfaces are parallel to the line of weight transmission, the joint ends up bearing shear stress. In spite of the significant joint load, little movement in the joint occurs.

A sprain of the iliosacral ligaments is possible. The injury affects the ligament that extends from the posterior projection of the wing of the ilium to the posterior sacrum. The sprain of this ligament also can have an effect within the pelvis. Many of the conditions identified as sacroiliac sprains are actually other diseases. The sacroiliac ligaments are so strong that ordinary stresses will cause damage to the lumbosacral ligament before they cause damage to the sacroiliac ligaments.

The limitations of provocative maneuvers and SI-joint blocks may stem in part from a contribution of extraarticular ligaments to the genesis of pain believed to originate within the SI-joints. These ligaments include the expansion of the iliolumbar ligaments, the dorsal and ventral sacroiliac ligaments, the sacrospinous ligaments, and the sacrotuberous

---

ORTHOPEDIC GAMUT 9-4

LUMBOPELVIC MUSCLES

Results of lumbopelvic muscle contractures:
1. Contracture of lumbodorsal fascia
2. Anterior pelvic tilt
3. Inappropriate transfer of loads to the lumbar spine
4. Difficulty in attaining the proper biomechanical posture for lifting

---

ORTHOPEDIC GAMUT 9-5

LUMBOPELVIC SPINE MUSCULAR SYNDROMES

Clinical findings of lumbopelvic spine muscular syndromes:
1. Hip inflexibility
2. Weakness of the hip and spine extensor mechanism
3. Intersegmental lumbosacral fixation
4. Myofascial trigger points in the spinal erector, quadratus lumborum, gluteal musculature, and psoas muscles
5. Referred zones of pain to the hip, buttocks, thigh, and lateral lower leg
6. Severe tightness of the outward rotators of the hip
7. Muscle hypertonicity
8. Palpable tenderness with pressure or stretch
9. Taut, tender, or ropelike muscle fibers

TABLE 9-4	
LUMBOPELVIC SYNDROMES	
Diagnosis	**Site of Complaint**
Quadratus lumborum syndrome	Gluteal region, anterior iliac spine, greater trochanter of femur
Gluteus maximus or medius syndrome	Sacral and gluteal region, lateral hip
Gluteus minimus syndrome	Lateral hip, thigh, and calf
Chronic lumbar strain (spinal erector muscles)	Laterally to ribs, caudally toward lumbosacral junction
Piriformis syndrome	Sacroiliac region; posterior hip, thigh, calf; possibly sole of foot

Adapted from Brier SR: *Primary care orthopedics,* St Louis, 1999, Mosby.

ligaments (SI-joint *lato-sensu*). They play a role in locking or in allowing motion of the SI-joints (Berthelot et al, 2006).

After injury of the SI-joint, pain localizes to the articular structures. The patient may also have referred pain to the groin, hamstrings, or back of the thigh. Ordinarily, this pain will not be along the sciatic distribution. Many of the tests that will elicit pain in the SI-joint will also be positive in conditions such as ruptured intervertebral disc, sciatic neuritis, and lumbosacral sprain. The fact that the tests cause pain is of little significance. The significance is in the location of the pain. The common tests—straight leg raising, which puts torsion force on the SI-joint, or the similar test of forward flexion of the trunk while the knees are straight—will cause pain when SI-joint involvement exists. Some tests stress the sacroiliac area specifically. Gaenslen test involves flexing the opposite thigh on the abdomen to immobilize the pelvis in forward flexion. Next, the involved leg is pushed into hyperextension, which causes rotary stress on the SI-joint.

PROCEDURE

- The patient with lower trunk pain is in the standing position and is instructed to place the lower extremity that is opposite the painful side approximately 2 or 3 feet in front of the foot of the other extremity (Fig. 9-15).
- This position is such that the patient appears to be taking a big step forward.
- The patient then bends the upper trunk acutely over the forward extremity so as to put all the weight on the front leg (Fig. 9-16).
- The patient flexes to the point at which the heel of the back foot rises from the floor (Fig. 9-17).
- The production or aggravation of lower trunk pain on the side of the posterior leg indicates a positive test.
- A positive test indicates unilateral forward displacement of the ilia (anterior innominate) in relation to the sacrum.

Next Steps/Procedures
Knee-to-shoulder test, Lewin-Gaenslen test, Piedallu sign, sacral apex test, and sacroiliac resisted-abduction test

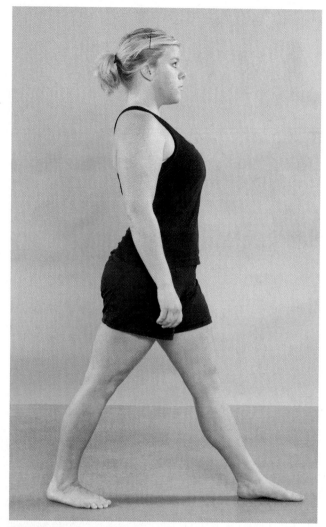

FIG. 9-15 The patient is standing and is instructed to take a big step forward, placing the unaffected leg 2 or 3 feet ahead of the affected leg.

9

CLINICAL PEARL

The sacroiliac joint, most inaccessible to palpation, is difficult to assess clinically. Only florid inflammation or damage to the fibrous portion is likely to result in local posterior tenderness. This tenderness is probably ligamentous.

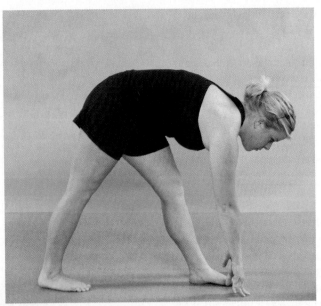

FIG. 9-16 The patient flexes at the waist and tries to touch the floor. This movement places weight onto the forward leg and stretches the affected sacroiliac joint.

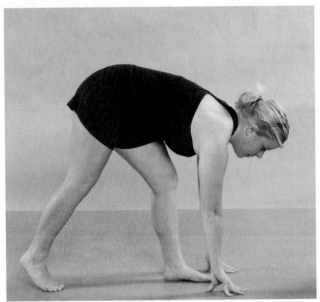

FIG. 9-17 The production of pain in the lower trunk, especially on the affected side, as the heel on the affected side lifts, indicates a positive test. A positive test indicates unilateral forward displacement of the ilium in relation to the sacrum.

BELT TEST

SUPPORTED ADAMS TEST

Assessment for Sprain of the Sacroiliac Ligaments or Lumbosacral Capsular Sprain

Comment

Sacroiliac sprain denotes painful stretching of the ligaments around the joint. The occurrence of this condition is uncommon because the sacroiliac ligaments are very strong. The movements of bending, lifting, and hyperextension that produce torsion strain of the joint are more likely to cause a sprain of the thinner capsular ligaments surrounding the small lumbosacral joints. However, sacroiliac sprain does undoubtedly occur. It is identifiable by its acute onset during a torsion movement and by tenderness over the joint accentuated by a maneuver that reproduces the sprain.

Certain circumstances favor sprain of the sacroiliac ligaments. The ligaments are softened and elongated by pregnancy, prolonged periods of bending and lifting, or degenerative arthritis. The mechanism of injury usually involves the act of straightening up from a stooped position. It is tempting to suppose that muscular incoordination is at fault. The hip flexors hold the ilium forward while the sacrum is rotated backward, or the hamstrings and the gluteus maximus extend the hip, rotating the ilium backward while the sacrum is held forward by the weight of the trunk. This theory has support because a postural defect of pelvic inclination and excessive lumbar lordosis are associated findings.

Biomechanical studies have addressed the loading of separate (spinal) structures and are used to explain risk factors for LBP such as spinal form (hyperlordotic and hyperkyphotic), trunk posture (stooped and asymmetric), or conditions such as vibration and high, repetitive, or unexpected level of load. In addition to loading factors, many biologic influences on LBP have been investigated, including muscle fatigue, disc degeneration caused by age, and malnutrition, as well as psychosocial factors such as work satisfaction and insurance benefits. Although much is known about risk-enhancing conditions, the precise mechanism causing disc herniation and back sprain is still debated. Researchers have suggested that back sprain and disc herniation can be caused by a prolonged or sudden lumbar flexion, even without an elevated axial load on the spine (Snijders et al, 2004).

Sacroiliac subluxation implies that ligamentous stretching has been sufficient to permit the ilium to slip on the sacrum. An irregular prominence of one of the articular surfaces becomes wedged on another prominence of the apposed articular surface. The ligaments are taut, reflex muscle spasms are intense, and pain is severe and continuous until reduction is accomplished.

For most of its extent, the SI-joint is inaccessible to invasive diagnostic procedures. The joint cavity lies deep to the rough and corrugated interosseous surfaces of the sacrum and ilium, which are connected by the dense, interosseous sacroiliac ligament (Fig. 9-18).

PROCEDURE

- The patient with lower back symptoms is in the standing position (Fig. 9-19).
- The patient flexes the dorsolumbar spine while the examiner notes the amount of movement necessary to aggravate the pain (Fig. 9-20).
- While positioned behind the patient, the examiner grasps the patient's iliac crests and braces a hip against the patient's sacrum (Fig. 9-21).
- The patient flexes the spine again as the examiner immobilizes the patient's pelvis (Fig. 9-22).
- If the lesion is of a pelvic nature, flexing the spine with the pelvis immobilized will not reproduce the discomfort.
- If the lesion is of a spinal nature, the pain will be aggravated in both instances.

Next Steps/Procedures
Gaenslen test, Goldthwait sign, and Smith-Petersen test

CLINICAL PEARL

Because of the stabilizing effect of the very strong ligamentous structures, sprain of the sacroiliac ligaments accompanies sacroiliac subluxation and is a subluxation sprain. Posterior subluxation results from a flexion-type injury, which occurs with activities such as lifting or pushing. Anterior subluxation results from extension-type injuries, which occur when falling forward or extending the leg.

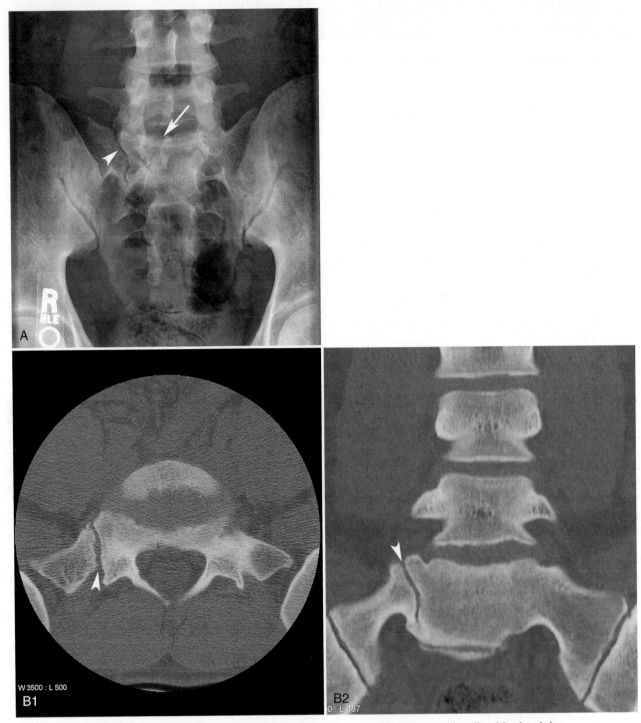

FIG. 9-18 **A,** Plain X-ray film demonstrates a vertical lucency was visualized in the right sacral ala that extended from the superior margin of the sacrum through the second sacral segment. Spina bifida occulta is present at S1 as is a rudimentary disc at the S1–2 level. **B,** CT scan confirmed the presence of a vertical lucency extending through the right sacral ala from anterior to posterior. The lucency had smooth-bordered, sclerotic margins throughout and marginal osteophytes at its inferior aspect. These findings clearly represented a longstanding defect with pseudoarticulation. Spina bifida occulta was also present in the sacrum. (From Green BN, Schultz G, Stanley M: Persistent synchondrosis of a primary sacral ossification center in an adult with low back pain, *Spine J* [in press, corrected proof].)

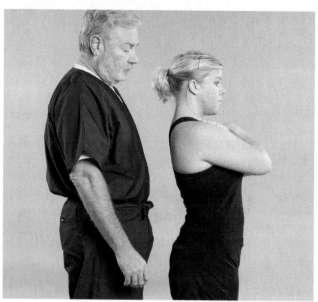

FIG. 9-19 The patient is in the standing position. The examiner, who is positioned behind the patient, notes spinal contours.

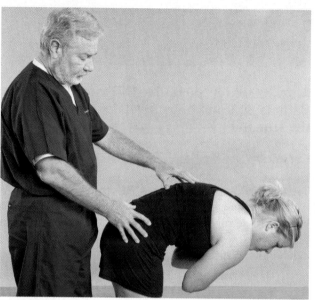

FIG. 9-20 The patient flexes at the waist, as far forward as possible. The examiner notes the amount of flexion necessary to aggravate the lower back or create sacroiliac discomfort.

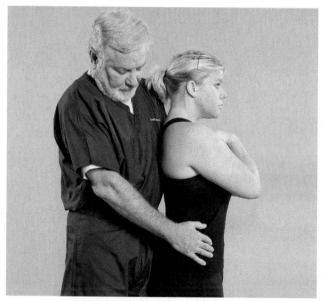

FIG. 9-21 Once the patient stands erect, the examiner grasps the patient's iliac crests and braces a hip against the patient's sacrum.

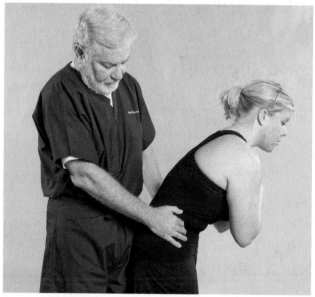

FIG. 9-22 While in this braced position, the patient flexes at the waist. If the source of pain is pelvic, then the move will not reproduce the discomfort because the pelvis is immobilized. Pain of spinal origin will be aggravated in both positions.

9

Assessment for Sacroiliac Disease Versus Pathologic Conditions Involving the Hip Joint

Comment

The stability of the SI-joint lies in the nature of its articular surfaces and ligaments (Fig. 9-23). The sacral articular surface is corrugated; a depression occurs opposite the second sacral segment, whereas the first and third segments exhibit prominences.

Movements that do occur in the SI-joint are those of the pelvis as a whole. During extension, each hemipelvis turns downward about this axis, and during flexion, each one turns upward. Extension of the lower limb involves an upward gliding of the ilium on the sacrum coupled with an element of distraction between the two bones superiorly and anteriorly (Figs. 9-24 and 9-25).

The pelvic curve begins at the lumbosacral joint and ends at the termination of the coccyx. The curve is anteriorly concave and is somewhat tilted downward. The thoracic and pelvic curves are primary curves because they are present in the fetus.

The sacrum is a large triangular bone inserted in a wedge-like manner between the two iliac bones. The base of the sacrum articulates with L5, producing the rather acute lumbosacral angle, formed by increased anterior width of both the body of L5 and the L5–S1 intervertebral disc.

The coccyx is usually a solid bone formed by the fusion of four rudimentary vertebrae. Occasionally, the first coccygeal vertebra exists as a separate segment, and no vertebral canal exists within the coccyx itself.

Articulation of the pelvis with the vertebral column occurs at the interspace between L5 and the sacrum. This articulation is similar in nearly all respects to the articulations that connect the vertebrae with each other. In addition, the iliolumbar ligament connects the pelvis with the vertebral column on either side.

The sacroiliac articulation is an amphiarthrodial, or slightly movable, joint. Cartilaginous plates cover the artic-

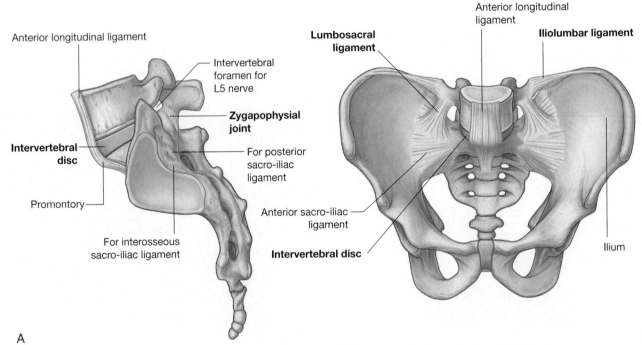

FIG. 9-23 Lumbosacral joints and associated ligaments. **A,** Lateral view. B. Anterior view. **B,** Sacro-iliac joints and associated ligaments: lateral view, anterior view, and posterior view. **C,** Pubic symphysis and associated ligaments. (A-C from Drake RL: *Gray's anatomy for students: with student consult online access,* New York, 2004, Churchill Livingstone.) **D,** A horizontal cross-section of a computed tomography (CT) scan at the level of the sacroiliac joints. Note the irregular articular surfaces. *1,* Rectus abdominis. *2,* psoas major; *3,* iliacus; *4,* gluteus minimus; *5,* gluteus medius; *6,* gluteus maximus; *7,* sacrum; *8,* ilium; *9,* sacroiliac joint. (From Neumann DA: *Kinesiology of the musculoskeletal system: Foundations for physical rehabilitation,* St Louis, 2002, Mosby.)

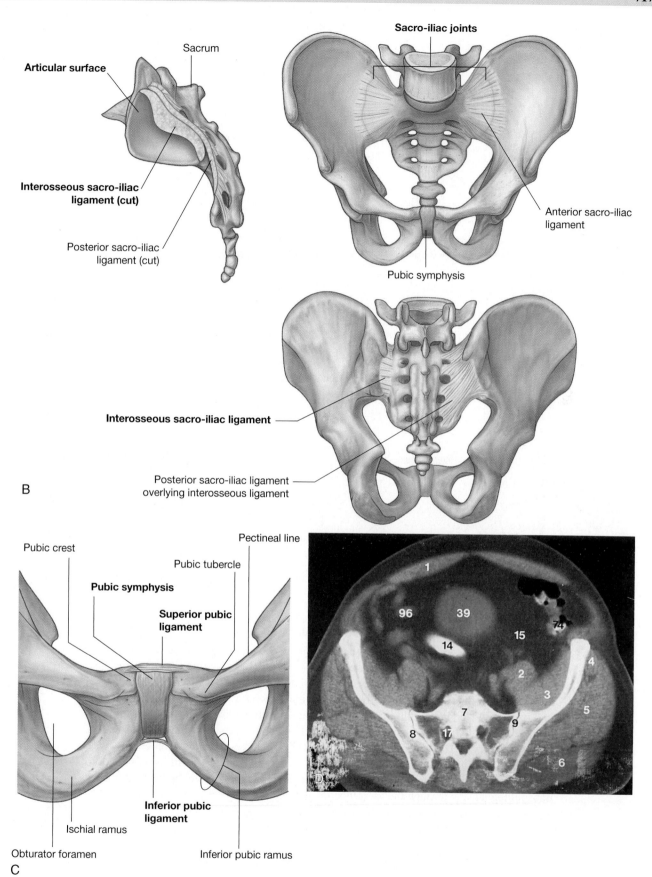

Articular surface

Sacrum

Interosseous sacro-iliac ligament (cut)

Posterior sacro-iliac ligament (cut)

Sacro-iliac joints

Anterior sacro-iliac ligament

Pubic symphysis

Interosseous sacro-iliac ligament

Posterior sacro-iliac ligament overlying interosseous ligament

B

9

Pubic crest

Pectineal line

Pubic tubercle

Pubic symphysis

Superior pubic ligament

Inferior pubic ligament

Ischial ramus

Obturator foramen

Inferior pubic ramus

C

FIG. 9-23, cont'd

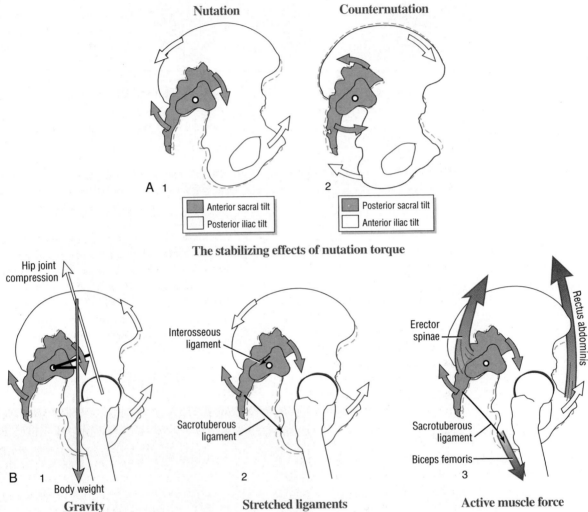

FIG. 9-24 A, The kinematics at the sacroiliac joint. *1,* Nutation; *2,* counternutation (see text for definitions). Sacral rotations are indicated in gray, and iliac rotations in white. The axis of rotation for sagittal plane movement is indicated by the small circle. **B,** Nutation torque increases the stability at the sacroiliac joint. *1,* Two forces originating primarily by gravity—body weight and hip joint compression—generate a nutation torque at the sacroiliac joint. Each force has a moment arm (black lines) that acts from the axis of rotation (circle at joint). *2,* The nutation torque stretches the interosseous and sacrotuberous ligaments that ultimately compresses and stabilizes the sacroiliac joint. *3,* Muscle contraction (red) creates an active nutation torque across the sacroiliac joint. Note the biceps femoris transmitting tension through the sacrotuberous ligament. (A and B from Neumann DA: Kinesiology fothe musculoskeletal system: foundations for physical rehabilitation, St Louis, Mosby, 2002.)

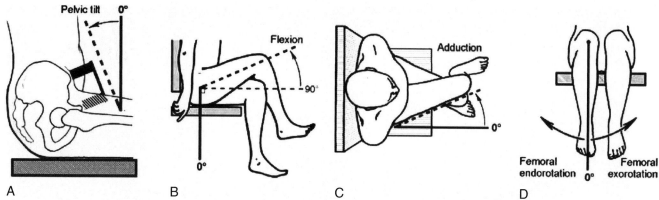

FIG. 9-25 **A,** Pelvic tilt: angle between a plane resting on pubic crest and both anterior superior iliac spines, and the vertical frontal plane. **B,** Flexion of femur: angle between a line from the greater trochanter to the lateral epicondyle and the vertical frontal plane. **C,** Adduction of femur: angle between a line from the greater trochanter to the lateral epicondyle and the vertical sagittal plane. **D,** Axial rotation of femur: angle of the tibia in relation to a vertical plane coinciding with the femoral axis. (From Snijders CJ, Hermans PFG, Kleinrensink GJ: Functional aspects of cross-legged sitting with special attention to piriformis muscles and sacroiliac joints, *Clin Biomech* 21[2]:116-121, 2006.)

ular surfaces of the sacrum and ilium. The cartilaginous plates are in close contact with each other and bound together by fibrous strands.

The sacrococcygeal articulation is a joint similar to the articulation between vertebral bodies. The pubic symphysis is an amphiarthrodial joint formed between the two oval symphyseal surfaces of the pubic bones.

Clinically, the piriformis muscle is related to compression of the sciatic nerve at the greater sciatic foramen with symptoms such as buttock and posterior thigh pain. Sciatica in a large number of patients can be ascribed to spasm of the piriformis muscle. Pain is aggravated by sitting or activity of the lower extremities (Snijders, Hermans, Kleinrensink, 2006).

Fractures of the posterior rim are usually caused by posterior dislocation of the femur (Figs. 9-26 and 9-27). Fractures of the posterior column may also be seen with posterior dislocations of the femur (Fig. 9-28). Fractures involving the quadrilateral plate are more commonly associated with lateral compression forces. Pelvic fractures, healed, are usually marked by significant pelvic deformity and therefore dysfunction at both the lumbosacral articulation and the acetabular-femoral articulation (Fig. 9-29).

In the last few years, great progress has been achieved in the treatment of unstable pelvic fractures. Unstable sacral fractures and sacroiliac dislocations can be complicated by symptomatic malunion and nonunion, especially if treated by conservative means or by external fixation (Oransky, Tortora, 2007).

With successful reduction of a pelvic injury, patients can be expected to lead a normal life in most cases, unless permanent nerve, urologic, or other associated injuries coexist (Tornetta, Matta, 1996).

In an unstable pelvis, more than 10 mm of residual vertical displacement of the posterior pelvic ring represents a poor outcome (Lindahl et al, 1999).

A maximum of 4 to 5 mm of residual displacement is a satisfactory result (Dean Cole, Blum, Ansel, 1996).

ORTHOPEDIC GAMUT 9-6

ACETABULAR FRACTURES

In general, acetabular fractures involve one or more of the following:
1. The posterior rim
2. The posterior column
3. The anterior column
4. The quadrilateral plate

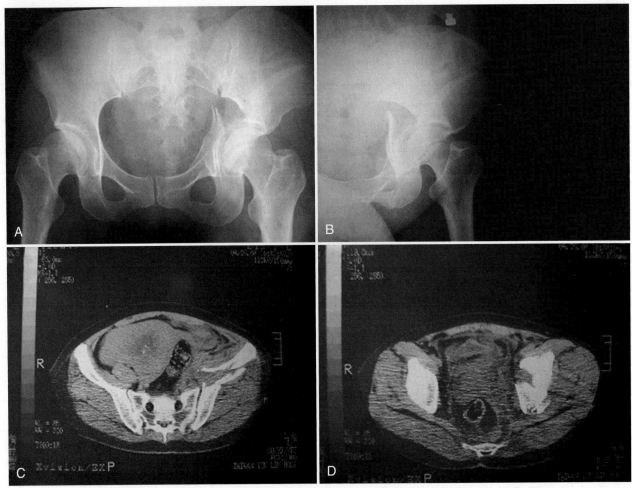

FIG. 9-26 Fracture of the left pelvis and acetabulum. **A,** Anterior–posterior view. **B,** Iliac oblique view, and (**C** and **D**) CT scans of the pelvis and hip joint revealed a widely displaced fracture with comminution of the left acetabulum, left ilium, left pubic bone, and left ischium, as well as a right side shift of the uterus and fetus. *CT,* Computer tomography. (From Chen C-M, Chen W-H, Wong C-S et al: Surgical treatment of a pregnant woman with unstable, displaced pelvic and acetabular fractures, *Injury Extra* 38(11):405-408, 2007.)

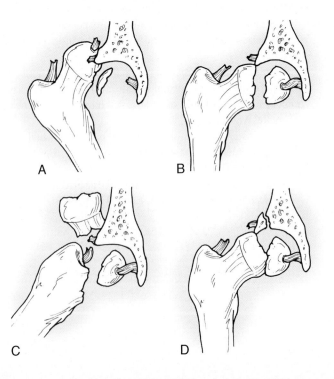

FIG. 9-27 Pipkin classification of posterior dislocation of hip with femoral head fracture. **A,** Type I, femoral head fracture caudad to fovea capitis. **B,** Type II, femoral head fracture cephalad to fovea capitis. **C,** Type III, type I or II fracture with associated femoral neck fracture. **D,** Type IV, type I, II, or III fracture with associated acetabular fracture. (Redrawn from Rockwood CA Jr, Green DP, Bucholz RW, et al (eds): *Rockwood and Green's fractures in adults,* ed 4, Philadelphia, 1996, Lippincott, Williams & Wilkins.) (In Canale ST: *Campbell's operative orthopaedics,* ed 11, St Louis, 2007, Mosby.)

Classification of injury mechanism to the pelvic ring by Young and Burgess

Lateral compression

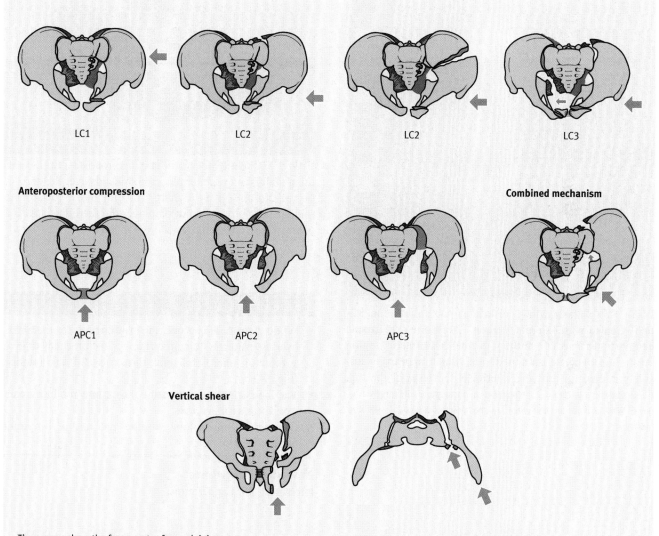

LC1   LC2   LC2   LC3

Anteroposterior compression   **Combined mechanism**

APC1   APC2   APC3

Vertical shear

The arrows show the force vector for each injury.

FIG. 9-28 Young and Burgess classification of injury to the pelvic ring: A classification system that relates the mechanism of injury or the vector of applied force to the pattern of pelvic ring disruption. The four groups of injuries are lateral compression, anteroposterior compression, vertical shear and combined mechanism injuries. (From Nunn T, Pallister I: Fractures of the pelvic ring, *Surgery (Oxford)* 25(10):420-423, 2007.)

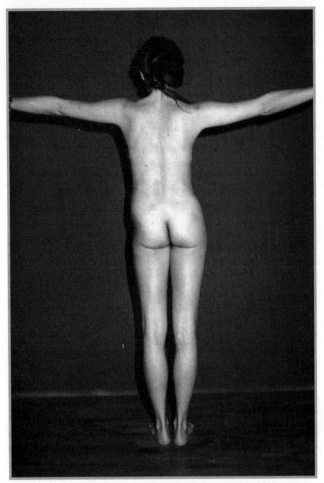

FIG. 9-29 Patient with a dislocated sacroiliac joint, initially treated with external fixation. The shortened left side demonstrates medial shifting of the trochanteric region versus the opposite uninjured side, which appears excessively curved towards the exterior at the level of the hip. (From Oransky M, Tortora M: Nonunions and malunions after pelvic fractures: Why they occur and what can be done? *Injury* 38[4]:489-496, 2007.)

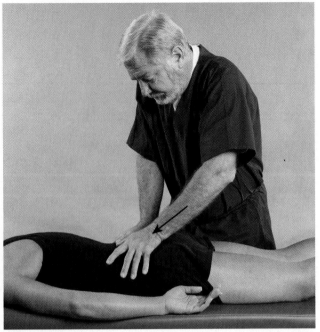

FIG. 9-30 While the patient is lying prone on a firm examining table, the examiner places both hands over the dorsum of the ilia and gives a sharp, forceful thrust toward the midline. The production of pain over the sacroiliac area is a positive sign and indicates sacroiliac joint disease.

PROCEDURE

- While the patient is prone, the examiner places the hands over the patient's dorsum of the ilia and proceeds to give a forceful, sharp, bilateral thrust toward the midline (Fig. 9-30).
- The sign is present when this procedure produces pain over the sacroiliac area.
- Pain is felt in SI-joint disease but not in hip joint disease.

Next Steps/Procedures
Hibbs test and Laguerre test

CLINICAL PEARL

Patients who possess an anomalous relation of the piriformis muscle to the sciatic nerve are particularly susceptible to developing symptoms of sciatic neuritis when the muscle is hypertonic or spastic. Approximately 10% of the population possesses such an anomaly. A reflex spasm of this muscle may occur because of intraarticular sacroiliac subluxation and sacroiliac irritation. Such a spasm is probably the cause of a positive Lasègue test, which is positive in the range of 20 to 45 degrees.

Cross-legged sitting resulted in a relative elongation of the piriformis muscle of 11.7% compared with normal sitting and even 21.4% compared with standing. Application of piriformis muscle force resulted in inward deformation of the pelvic ring and compression of the sacroiliac joints and the dorsal side of the pubic symphysis.

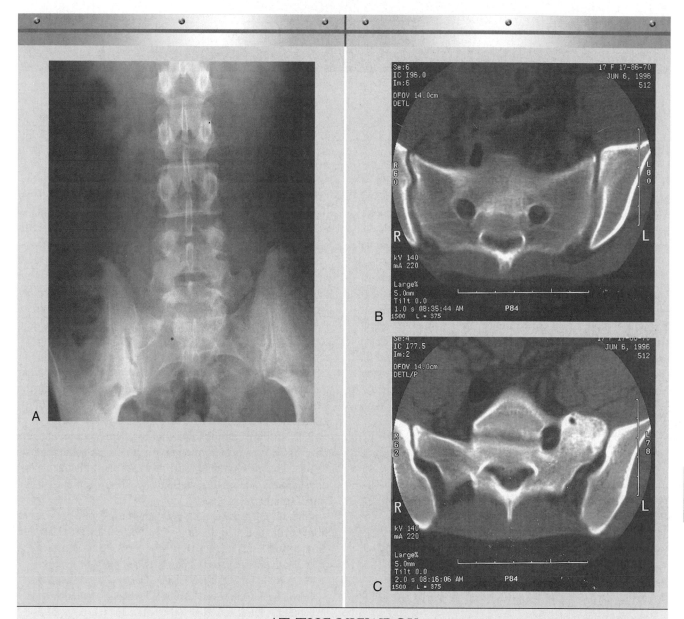

AT THE VIEWBOX

17-year-old female with moderate focal central low back pain. Normal range of motion and no report of stiffness. Patient has been diagnosed with ankylosing spondylitis, but clinical and laboratory findings do not support the diagnosis. CT scan of the sacroiliac joints has been interpreted by the first radiologist as negative, but a second opinion from another radiologist was that findings were compatible with sacroiliitis. Patient is now consulting with a chiropractic physician, resigned to living with ankylosing spondylitis. Plain radiograph (**A**) demonstrates a transitional lumbosacral segment, with unilateral accessory joint on the left (reading left). There is associated developmental sacroiliac joint asymmetry and some reactive sclerosis of the left sacroiliac joint. The CT scan (**B** and **C**) shows no evidence of sacroiliitis but demonstrates mild degenerative joint disease of the left L5–S1 accessory articulation, with reactive sclerosis and subchondral cyst formation. The sacroiliac joints are normal, with incidental note of persistent apophyses of the sacral alae. The patient responded well to chiropractic care and has not demonstrated signs or symptoms of ankylosing spondylitis over a three-year follow-up. (From the teaching file of Timothy Mick, DC, DACBR)

GAENSLEN TEST

Assessment for Sacroiliac Disease

Comment

Because the pelvic ring is complex and involves a total of eight joints (left and right zygapophyseal joints, coxals, and SI-joints, plus the single lumbosacral joint and the pubic symphysis), any change in the trunk or lower extremity is compensated in some way by the complicated dynamic mechanism of the pelvic ring.

The SI-joint is thought to move only 2 mm and 2 degrees, but this small amount of movement is complex. The SI-joints are the keys of the arch between the two pelvic bones. With the symphysis pubis, the joints help transfer the weight from the spine to the lower limbs. This triad of joints also acts as a buffer to decrease the force of jarring and bumping that occurs within the spine and upper body as the lower limbs make contact with the ground. Because of this shock-absorbing function, the structure of the SI-joints and symphysis pubis joints is different from most joints.

ORTHOPEDIC GAMUT 9-7

PELVIC RING

Five distinct different types of joints of the pelvic ring:
1. The lumbosacral zygapophyseal joints
2. The anterior lumbosacral
3. Coxal (hip)
4. Sacroiliac joint
5. Symphysis pubis

ORTHOPEDIC GAMUT 9-8

SACROILIAC JOINTS

Sacroiliac joint movement contributions:
1. Locomotion
2. Spinal and thigh movement
3. Changes of position (e.g., from lying to standing, standing to sitting)

The SI-joints are part synovial and part syndesmosis. A syndesmosis is a type of fibrous joint in which the intervening fibrous connective tissue forms an interosseous membrane or ligament. The synovial portion of the joint is C shaped with the convex iliac surface of the C facing anteriorly and inferiorly. The greater or more acute the angle of the C is, the more stable the joint will be, and the less likely it is for a lesion of the joint to occur. The sacral surface is slightly concave.

The size, shape, and roughness of the articular surfaces vary among individuals. In the child, these surfaces are smooth. In the adult, the surfaces become irregular depressions and elevations that fit into one another. By doing so, the articular surfaces restrict movement at the joint and add to the strength of the joint for transferring weight from the lower limb to the spine. Fibrocartilage covers the articular surface of the ilium. Hyaline cartilage covers the articular surface of the sacrum and is three times thicker than the cartilage of the ilium. In older persons, adhesions may obliterate part of the joint surfaces.

The SI-joints, although mobile in young people, become progressively stiffer with age. In some cases, ankylosis results. The movements occurring in the sacroiliac and symphysis pubis are small in relation to the movements in the spinal joints.

The symphysis pubis is a cartilaginous joint. A disc of fibrocartilage, called the *interpubic disc,* is located between the two joint surfaces.

Near-side motor-vehicle impacts (when the vehicle strikes the driver's side) are the leading cause of pelvic injuries. Pelvic bone fractures are associated with high mortality and morbidity rates, as well as substantial economic costs. Side-impact collisions tend to produce lateral compression fractures of the pelvic ring that involve the pubic rami, sacrum, and acetabulum and, with increased severity, separation at the pubic symphysis and SI-joints. Chronic symphyseal pain is one of the major complications related to symphysis injury (Li et al, in press).

The SI-joints and symphysis pubis have no muscles that directly control their movements. However, the joints are influenced by the action of the muscles that move the lumbar spine and hip because many of these muscles attach to the sacrum and pelvis.

The sacrococcygeal joint is usually a fused line (symphysis) united by a fibrocartilaginous disc. It is located between the apex of the sacrum and the base of the coccyx. Occasionally, the joint is freely movable and synovial. The joints fuse and obliterate with advancing age.

PROCEDURE

- The patient is lying supine.
- The examiner acutely flexes the knee and thigh of the patient's **unaffected** leg to the abdomen.
- This move brings the lumbar spine firmly into contact with the table and fixes both the pelvis and the lumbar spine.
- With the examiner standing at a right angle to the patient, the examiner slowly hyperextends the patient's **affected** thigh (Fig. 9-31).
- This hyperextension is accomplished by gradually increasing the pressure of one hand on top of the knee while the examiner's other hand is on the flexed knee.
- The hyperextension of the affected hip exerts a rotating force on the corresponding half of the pelvis.
- The pull is made on the ilium, through the Y-ligament, and the muscles attached to the anterior iliac spine.
- The test is positive if pain is felt in the sacroiliac area or referred down the thigh.
- The test is performed bilaterally.
- If the test is negative, a lumbosacral lesion is suspected.
- The test is usually contraindicated in older patients.

Next Steps/Procedures
Belt test, Goldthwait sign, and Smith-Petersen test

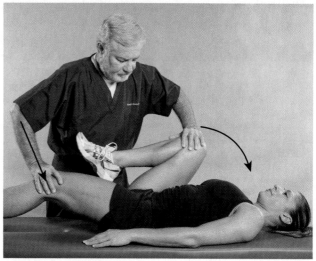

FIG. 9-31 The patient is supine with the affected side of the pelvis well to the side of the table. The unaffected thigh is flexed toward the abdomen. The examiner simultaneously exaggerates the thigh flexion on the unaffected side and the sacroiliac extension on the affected side. The test is positive if pain is felt in the affected sacroiliac joint as it is hyperextended.

9

CLINICAL PEARL

Sacroiliac joint involvement produces local pain over the joint, or pain that is referred to (1) the groin on the same side, (2) the posterior thigh on the same side, and (3) down the leg, which is less often. Pain is often increased by lying on the affected side.

GAPPING TEST

SACROILIAC STRETCH TEST

Assessment for Sprain of the Anterior Sacroiliac Ligaments

Comment

The normal movements that occur at the SI-joints are determined by the direction of the articular surfaces, the muscles acting on the joint, and the symphysis pubis.

The movement is a rotation of the sacrum (or ilia) around the axis of the shortest and strongest part of the posterior interosseous sacroiliac ligament, which is situated in the angle between the posterosuperior and posteroinferior limbs of the auricular surfaces. When anterior rotation of the upper end of the sacrum occurs, the promontory of the sacrum will move in an anteroinferior direction, which narrows the AP diameter of the pelvic inlet. This rotation also increases the coronal width of the pelvic outlet and tightens the sacrotuberous and sacrospinous ligaments. During posterior rotation of the upper end of the sacrum, the reverse movements will occur. These movements produce a widening of the AP diameter of the pelvic inlet, a narrowing of the coronal width of the pelvic outlet, and a relaxation of the sacrotuberous and sacrospinous ligaments. The posterior sacroiliac ligaments will tighten and restrict this posterior rotation of the sacrum on the ilia.

In addition, because the auricular surfaces of the sacrum are inferiorly rather than superiorly closer to the median plane, anterior rotation of the sacrum will result in a slight widening of the symphysis pubis, whereas posterior rotation of the sacrum will result in compression of the symphysis pubis.

When a rotational force is applied to the hip bones in opposite directions—which occurs when extending one thigh while flexing the other, such as in stepping up to a stool—the extended thigh anchors the head of the femur on that side through the iliofemoral and ischiofemoral ligaments and the rectus femoris muscle. The flexed thigh, through the pull of the hamstring muscles, rotates the ilium in a posterior direction. In addition, the sacrum will move with the ilium on the flexed side because the pull of the hamstring muscle is transmitted to it via the sacrotuberous and sacrospinous ligaments. The result is that posterior rotation of the sacrum will occur at the SI-joint on the extended side only.

Although these movements at the SI-joints are small, especially in men, they are definite. The movements are increased when jumping from a height. They are also increased in women, especially toward the end of a preg-

nancy and up to 3 months after pregnancy because of the action of the hormone relaxin.

The finding that directs immediate attention to the SI-joint as a possible cause of pain in the buttock and thigh is that lumbar movements do not affect the gluteal symptom. With acute arthritis, the lumbar movements sometimes mildly increase the pain because, at the extreme of any lumbar motion, an added stress falls on the sacroiliac ligaments. If such an indirect strain on the joint hurts, much more severe pain is produced as soon as the SI-joints are directly tested.

Osteitis pubis is a painful inflammation of the pubic symphysis that is usually self-limited. The cause is unknown, but the condition often develops after urologic procedures or infections after childbirth or after repetitive stresses associated with certain athletic activities (Fig. 9-32). Pain and tenderness over the symphysis pubis are usually present. Coughing may aggravate the pain, which radiates along the adductor and rectus abdominis muscle. Stretching these muscles is painful.

Osteitis pubis (OP) is a serious injury that requires a prolonged rehabilitation period and time away from sports. Full recovery has been reported to take from several months up to years. OP affects predominantly athletes involved in running and kicking sports, and elite youth players appear to be more at risk. OP is generally classified to be an overuse injury believed to be a bony stress reaction involving the pubic symphysis and adjacent bone. It is associated with significant tenderness on palpation, similar to the palpable tenderness along the medial border of the tibia in medial tibia stress syndrome. Although OP is considered an overload injury, the exact cause is still unclear. Little consensus exists regarding the definition of *groin strain* in the literature, and, as such, this lack of consensus can result in difficulties differentiating OP from other groin injuries, such as

---

ORTHOPEDIC GAMUT 9-9

OSTEITIS PUBIS

Primary clinical types of osteitis pubis:
1. Noninfectious osteitis pubis, associated with urologic procedures, gynecologic procedures, and pregnancy
2. Infectious osteitis pubis, associated with local or distant infection loci
3. Athletic or mechanical trauma osteitis pubis
4. Degenerative or rheumatologic osteitis pubis

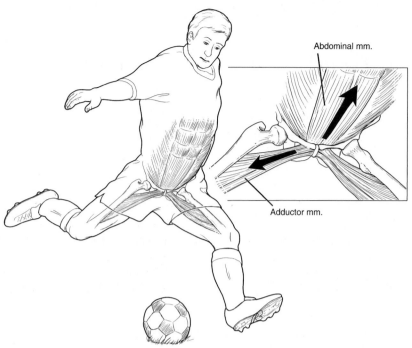

FIG. 9-32 Core imbalance: antagonistic muscle forces centered on the pubic symphysis indicated by the arrows. Muscle imbalance across the pubic symphysis occurs because of eccentric loading and overloading from abdominal muscle pull superiorly and hip flexors, adductors, and abductor muscles pulling inferiorly. (From Mandelbaum B, Mora SA: Osteitis pubis, *Oper Tech Sports Med* 13[1]:62-67, 2005.)

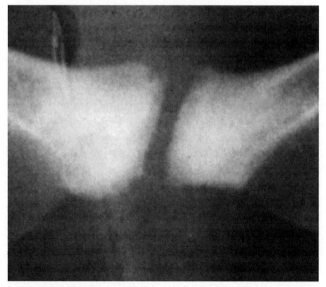

FIG. 9-33 Osteitis pubis. (From Mercier LR, Pettid FJ: *Practical orthopedics*, ed 4, St Louis, 1995, Mosby.)

musculotendinous lesions of the adductor complex. Both OP and muscle strains are load failure–related injuries (Wollin, Lovell, 2006).

Coughing may aggravate the pain, which radiates along the adductor and rectus abdominis muscles. Stretching these muscles is painful.

All factors, such as infections, urologic, gynecologic, and rheumatologic issues, must be taken into consideration when osteitis pubis is being worked up and managed.

Roentgenograms of the pelvis taken early in the disease may be normal. Later, variable amounts of spotty demineralization, widening of the symphysis pubis, and sclerosis are noted (Fig. 9-33).

PROCEDURE

- The patient lies supine, and the examiner places both hands on the patient's anterosuperior spine of each ilium and presses laterally downward.
- Crossing the arms increases the lateral component of the strain on the ligaments (Fig. 9-34).
- The pelvis must not be allowed to rock because the lumbar spine then moves.
- The examiner's hands can cause anterior iliac spine discomfort as a result of compression of the skin against the osseus structures.
- The expected finding is not local pain but rather aggravation of the gluteal symptoms.
- The response to the test is positive only if unilateral gluteal or posterior crural pain is elicited.
- The test is significant for anterior sacroiliac ligament sprain.

Next Steps/Procedure
Yeoman test

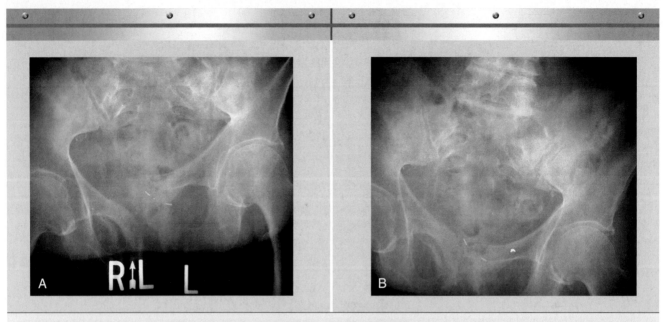

AT THE VIEWBOX

76-year-old female with right hip complaints for 5 years, increasing over the past 5 weeks. Radiographs of the pelvis (**A** and **B**), including stress views demonstrated gross instability of the symphysis pubis, with dislocation, along with asymmetric widening of the left sacroiliac joint, indicating associated sacroiliac instability. Smudgelike opacities in the sacral alae, especially in the context of pelvic instability and osteoporosis, are consistent with sacral insufficiency fractures. These are an under-diagnosed source of sacroiliac region pain in an older population. (From the teaching file of Timothy Mick, DC, DACBR)

CLINICAL PEARL

Stretching the anterior ligaments in the manner described is the most delicate test for the sacroiliac joint. Patients recovering from a sacroiliac injury may say that all pain ceased some days before. Patients walk and bend painlessly; yet for 7 to 10 days after subjective recovery, the straining of the joint that occurs in the gapping test still evokes discomfort. This test clearly applies more stress to sacroiliac ligaments than ordinary daily activities. If a patient has symptoms referable to the sacroiliac joint, this maneuver will elicit them.

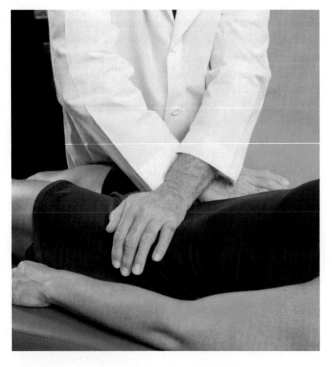

FIG. 9-34 The patient is supine on the examination table. The hips and knees are extended. With crossed arms, the examiner places both hands on the opposite anterosuperior iliac spines of each ilium. A downward and lateral pressure is applied to both ilia. Unilateral gluteal or posterior crural pain is a positive finding and indicates sprain of the anterior sacroiliac ligament.

GOLDTHWAIT SIGN

Assessment for Sacroiliac Joint Sprain Versus a Lumbosacral Spine Abnormality

Comment

Because of their position at the juncture of the skeleton of the trunk and the pelvic girdle, sacroiliac articulations are of importance. In recent years, sacroiliac articulations have been the subject of extensive clinical study. Radiologists are largely the ones who have contributed to the knowledge of these articulations and who have described normal form and pathologic variations.

The radiographic depiction of the sacroiliac synchondrosis is difficult because of its oblique and sinuous form. Severe fractures of the pelvis are sometimes associated with sacroiliac luxations and with marked displacement of the wings of the ilia. The SI-joint may be the site of the infection, especially tuberculosis, with destruction of the articular surfaces and wandering abscess formation. Obliteration or loss of definition of the surface or margins of these joints is an early finding in ankylosing spondylitis.

SI-joint movement is three dimensional and contains several elements. The primary movements are anteroinferior-to-posterosuperior nodding called *nutation* of the sacral base in relation to the ilium (Fig. 9-35, *A*). Movement along an axis that passes longitudinally through the iliac ridge of the SI-joint in rotatory (Fig. 9-35, *B*) and gapping of the superior and inferior aspects of the SI-joint is a third type of SI-joint motion (Fig. 9-35, *C*).

> Load application along the direction of hamstring and gluteus maximus muscles significantly diminishes ventral rotation of the sacrum, implying that loading the sacrotuberous ligament restricts **nutation** of the sacrum. Consequently, muscles that attach to the sacrotuberous ligaments, such as the gluteus maximus and, in certain individuals, the long head of the biceps, can dynamically influence movement and stability of the SI-joints (Vleeming et al, 1989).

The most common morphologic change that is often associated with clinical symptoms is arthrosis deformans, which is demonstrated by marginal osteophyte formation, particularly in the inferior portions of the synchondrosis and by subchondral osteosclerosis. These changes are responsible for a considerable degree of pain, especially with certain movements. These changes occur with advancing age in 90% of men and 77% of women. The healing of pelvic fractures that occurs with poor alignment of the sacroiliac articulations has a significant influence on the spine and the changes that are in these joints and are related to back pain.

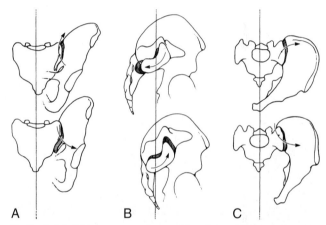

FIG. 9-35 Three types of sacroiliac joint (SIJ) motion. **A,** Superior and inferior aspects of the SIJ are shown gapping. **B,** Anterior and posterior rocking of the sacral base. **C,** Movement of the ilium on the sacrum that takes place in the horizontal plane. The arrows in **A** and **C** show motion of the ilium. The arrows in **B** show sacral motion. These movements are accentuated for demonstrative purposes in this illustration. (From Cramer GD, Darby SA: *Basic and clinical anatomy of the spine, spinal cord, and ANS*, St Louis, 1995, Mosby.)

PROCEDURE

- The patient is supine.
- The patient's affected leg is raised slowly, while one of the examiner's hands is under the lumbar portion of the patient's spine (Fig. 9-36).
- If pain is brought on before the lumbar spine begins to move, a sacroiliac lesion is probably present.
- The lesion may be caused by arthritis or by a sprain of the ligaments that involve the SI-joint (Fig. 9-37).
- If pain does not come on until after the lumbar spine begins to move, the disorder is more likely to have its origin in the lumbosacral area or, less commonly, in the sacroiliac area.
- The test is repeated with the unaffected limb.
- A positive sign of a lumbosacral lesion is elicited if pain occurs at approximately the same height as it did with the affected limb.
- If the unaffected leg can be raised higher than the affected leg, it signifies sacroiliac involvement of the affected side.

Next Steps/Procedures
Belt test, Gaenslen test, and Smith-Petersen test

CLINICAL PEARL

This test is similar to the Lasègue test, the straight-leg-raising test, and Smith-Petersen test. All of these tests have in common the use of the affected leg as a lever to stretch the suspect tissue, whether neural or ligamentous. The key to differentiation is the determination of the moment of L5–S1 separation, reflecting lumbosacral movement.

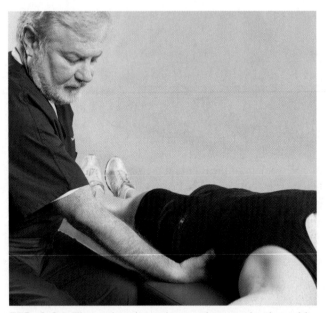

FIG. 9-36 The patient is supine on the examination table. The examiner places one hand under the lumbosacral portion of the patient's spine and palpates the L5 and S1 spinous processes. The examiner maintains contact with these two points.

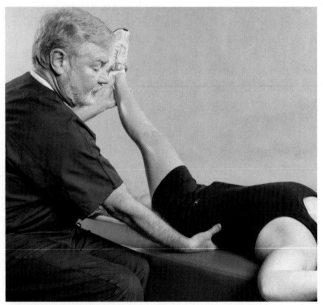

FIG. 9-37 The examiner elevates the affected leg as if performing a straight-leg-raising maneuver. If pain is produced before the L5–S1 spinous processes separate, the lesion involves the sacroiliac joint. If the pain is produced as the L5–S1 spinous processes separate, a spinal lesion likely exists.

Assessment for Sacroiliac Disease

Comment

Evaluation of the SI-joint is challenging for many reasons. First, the SI-joint is subject to a wide range of normal anatomic variation. Second, its unusual location and its oblique position make direct palpation almost impossible.

The seronegative spondyloarthropathies, a class of rheumatic disorders, have several factors in common: radiographic presentation, genetic predisposition, and certain clinical features. Included in this group are the so-called reactive arthritides (e.g., ankylosing spondylitis), along with the associated spondylitic disease, psoriatic arthritis, and inflammatory bowel disease. The benchmark of ankylosing spondylitis, a common cause of LBP and thoracolumbar stiffness, is the presence of sacroiliitis (Fig. 9-38).

Typical magnet resonance (MR) imaging lesions in ankylosing spondylitis and related conditions comprise spondylitis (Romanus lesion), spondylodiscitis (Andersson lesion), arthritis of the apophyseal joints and the costovertebral and costotransverse joints, and insufficiency fractures of the ankylosed vertebral spine (noninflammatory type of Andersson lesion). Sacroiliitis is associated with chronic changes such as sclerosis, erosions, transarticular bone bridges, periarticular accumulation of fatty tissue, and ankylosis. In addition, acute findings include capsulitis, juxtaarticular osteitis, and the enhancement of the joint space after contrast medium administration. Another important sign of spondyloarthritis is enthesitis, which affects the interspinal and supraspinal ligaments of the vertebral spine and the interosseous **ligaments** in the retroarticular space of the SI-joints (Hermann, Bollow, 2004).

Tuberculosis (TB) accounts for 2 million deaths every year globally, and the World Health Organization in 1993 declared TB as *a global emergency*. India accounts for 28% of the global TB burden, and the disease claims more than 1000 lives every day (Navaneeth, Thinagaran, Sulaiman, 2007).

SI-joint involvement has been reported in up to 9.7% of patients with skeletal TB. Lack of awareness of this now uncommon form of infection often leads to diagnostic delay and increased morbidity. Buttock pain is the presenting complaint in all patients. However, radicular pain in the lower back or lower limb is common. SI-joint TB is frequently an isolated phenomenon. Therefore direct sampling of the SI-joint is necessary to establish the diagnosis (Pouchot et al, 1988).

TB infection of the SI-joint often is associated with tuberculosis of the spine at the lumbosacral area and the hip. This association suggests the ease with which TB spreads from the lumbosacral area to the SI-joint by way of the psoas muscle. Destructive caseous lesions are the rule, and they often destroy the joint and form abscesses. The abscess may exhibit dorsally over the joint or intrapelvically, erupting at the inguinal area. Rupture of the abscess results in a resistant sinus and secondary infection. Severe visceral lesions result in a serious condition. If the patient survives, spontaneous bony ankylosis of the SI-joint occurs after 3 or 4 years. The disease may be bilateral.

The disease affects young adults and is rare in infancy and childhood. The onset of the disease is gradual and may follow trauma or pregnancy.

With this type of ankylosis, pain is felt over the SI-joint. Most of the time, this pain is referred to the groin. Less commonly, the pain is referred to the sciatic distribution. The pain is accentuated by direct pressure, such as during recumbency and particularly when turning over in bed. Sitting on the buttock on the affected side is also painful. Sitting on the opposite buttock relieves the pain. Bending forward

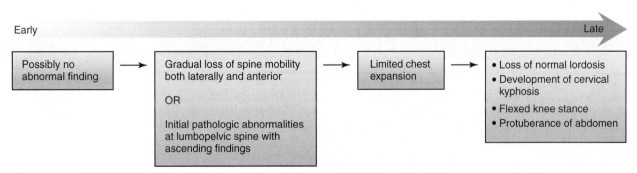

FIG. 9-38 Physical course of ankylosing spondylitis. (From Brier SR: *Primary care orthopedics*, St Louis, Mosby, 1999.)

with the knee extended is painful, but bending forward while the knees are flexed is painless. Jarring that occurs during walking, coughing, or sneezing accentuates the discomfort.

The patient with this disease lists to the opposite side. With the lower extremities extended, forward bending is limited. When the knees and hips are flexed, the hamstrings are relaxed, tension is removed from the pelvis, and farther forward bending is accomplished. Only the lower end of the joint is posteriorly superficial and displays tenderness and a boggy swelling. The swelling and tenderness may be more easily localized during rectal examination. Compressing the iliac crests together causes direct, painful pressure on the joint. Gaenslen test for sacroiliac disease depends on twisting the ilium on the sacrum. The strain this move puts on the inflamed ligamentous structures around the SI-joint produces the pain. The low-grade, inflammatory swelling of a cold abscess or sinus may be present.

PROCEDURE

- While the patient is in the prone position, the examiner stabilizes the patient's pelvis on the nearest side by placing one hand firmly on the dorsum of the iliac bone.
- With the other hand around the patient's ankle, the opposite knee is flexed to a right angle (Fig. 9-39).
- The knee is flexed to its maximum without elevating the thigh from the examination table (Fig. 9-40).
- From this position, the examiner slowly pushes the patient's leg laterally, causing strong internal rotation of the femoral head (Fig. 9-41).
- The test is performed bilaterally.
- The production of pelvic pain is a positive finding.
- The test is significant for a sacroiliac lesion.
- In the absence of hip involvement, stress is transmitted through the hip joints into the sacroiliac mechanism, producing pain.

Next Steps/Procedures
Erichsen sign and Laguerre test

CLINICAL PEARL

Tuberculosis is now rare in developed countries but remains a scourge elsewhere. Complications may be serious because of the formation of sinuses. These sinuses may become secondarily infected and may cause paraplegia (Pott paraplegia) because of (1) pus and intracellular pressure, (2) mechanical injury to the nervous system (cord) caused by bony pressure, or (3) vascular embarrassment of the nervous system where it crosses the bony infection. Hibbs test is not specific for tuberculosis of the sacroiliac joint but is correlated with other systemic findings that may suggest the existence of this type of tuberculosis. At the least, Hibbs test reveals mechanical dysfunction of the sacroiliac joint.

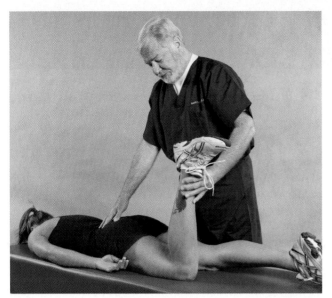

FIG. 9-39 The patient is prone on the examining table. The examiner stabilizes the unaffected side of the pelvis with one hand. With the other hand, the examiner grasps the ankle of the affected leg and flexes the knee to 90 degrees.

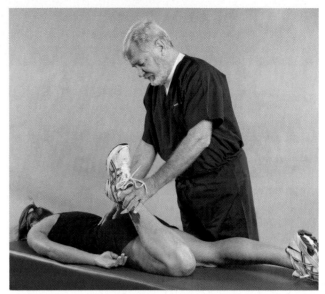

FIG. 9-40 The examiner flexes the patient's knee to its maximum without elevating the thigh from the examination table.

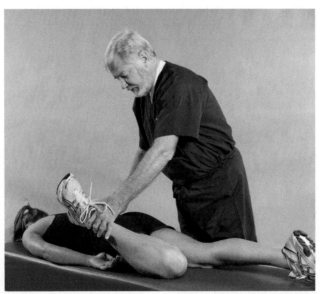

FIG. 9-41 The examiner slowly pushes the leg laterally, causing internal rotation of the femoral head. The production of pelvic pain is a positive finding. Even without a pathologic condition of the hip, the test is significant for a sacroiliac lesion.

COMPRESSION OF THE ILIAC CRESTS

Assessment for Sacroiliac Lesions, Sprain, Inflammation, Subluxation, and Fracture

Comment

The pelvic ring is essentially a rigid circle with very little motion at the interpubic or sacroiliac areas. Fractures involving the ring are generally classified as stable or unstable. Stable fractures are those in which the ring is completely broken only at one point (e.g., superior and inferior pubic ramus fractures on the same side). With unstable fractures, the ring is broken in two or more areas (e.g., both pubic rami on the same side plus a SI-joint dislocation) (Figs. 9-42 and 9-43).

> Traumatic disruption of the pelvic ring is a major cause of life-threatening hemorrhage. The vascular anatomy of the pelvis, coupled with the bulk of cancellous bone, can account for exsanguinating hemorrhage after severe pelvic fractures. Early stabilization, as with other fractures, is a tenet of management, but adequate fracture stabilization of the pelvis is difficult (Croce et al, 2007).

Fractures of the acetabulum occasionally involve the main weight-bearing surface of the hip joint (Fig. 9-44).

Osteoporosis is the usual predisposing cause, but inactivity, long-term steroid use, and other types of metabolic bone disease may also play a role.

Fracture of the wing of the ilium occasionally occurs. When such a fracture occurs, it is usually caused by a direct blow against the wing of the ilium. In most sports in which such an injury is likely, the iliac crest is padded to prevent the occurrence of this injury.

Fracture of the wing of the ilium is a painful injury not only at the time of the blow but also in the period immediately after the injury. This type of fracture is ordinarily recognized as a serious injury. Examination reveals extreme tenderness along the iliac crest and downward onto the wing of the ilium. The area of pain depends on the extent of the fracture. The patient will not usually permit deep enough palpation so that the examiner can actually feel a defect along the rim. Any attempt to use the involved muscles is extremely painful, and involuntary spasms of the abdominal or hip muscles may cause acute distress. The patient should be completely relaxed before a definitive examination can be performed. If a lesion of this severity is suspected, an x-ray examination should be made. The fracture can be completely overlooked in the ordinary AP view of the pelvis. The fracture will be well delineated by an AP view of the ilium rather than of the pelvis.

Lateral compression fractures are caused by forces delivered from the side. They are subdivided into several types

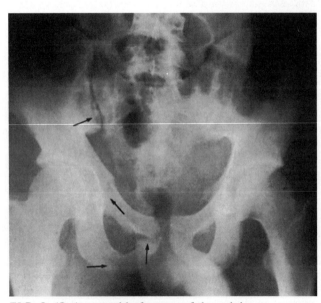

FIG. 9-42 An unstable fracture of the pelvis. (From Mercier LR, Pettid FJ: *Practical orthopedics*, ed 4, St Louis, 1995, Mosby.)

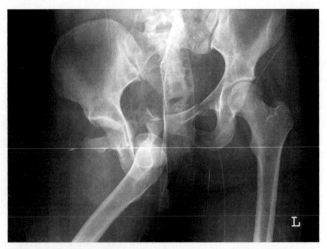

FIG. 9-43 Plain-film view of the pelvis of a hemodynamically unstable young lady after a rollover, demonstrating a vertical shear injury with a transforaminal sacral fracture on the left side and bilateral rami fractures combined with an open anterior hip dislocation on the right side. (From Keel M, Trentz O: Acute management of pelvic ring fractures, *Curr Orthop* 19[5]:334-344, 2005.)

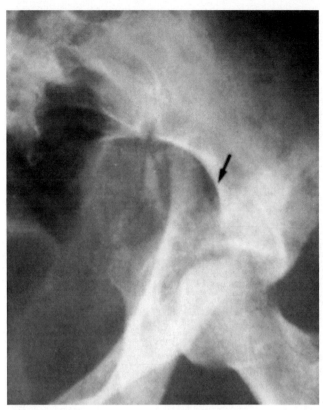

FIG. 9-44 Fracture of the acetabulum. (From Mercier LR, Pettid FJ: *Practical orthopedics*, ed 4, St Louis, 1995, Mosby.)

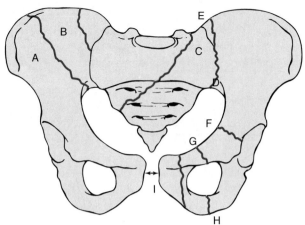

FIG. 9-45 The Letournel and Judet classification of pelvic fractures is anatomic. A, Iliac wing fractures; B, ilium fractures with extension to the sacroiliac joint; C, transsacral fractures; D, unilateral sacral fractures; E, sacroiliac joint fracture-dislocation; F, acetabular fractures; G, pubis ramus fractures; H, ischial fractures; I, pubic symphysis separation. It should be remembered that combinations of all of these injuries could occur. (From Browner: Skeletal trauma: basic science, management, and reconstruction, ed 3, St Louis, 2003, Saunders.)

depending on the severity of the injury and the progressive involvement of the posterior pelvis (Fig. 9-45). Common associations are crush fractures of the sacrum and the medial wall of the acetabulum. The more severe types of AP compression fracture refer to increasing posterior ligamentous injury and subsequent increasing instability (Fig. 9-46). Vertical shear fractures commonly arise from falls from a height. Fractures occur through the pubic rami and posterior pelvis, and they are vertical in orientation (Fig. 9-47). The anterosuperior iliac spine (sartorius), anteroinferior iliac spine (rectus femoris), and ischial tuberosity (hamstrings) are the common sites of avulsion fracture (Fig. 9-48). Sacral insufficiency fracture needs to be ruled out, especially in osteoporotic patients. (Fig. 9-49)

Lourie in 1982 was the first to describe what is now known as sacral insufficiency fracture. Most patients complain of intractable LBP, some might also complain of lower extremity weakness, but signs of neurologic involvement are rare. Routine radiographs of the spine and pelvis are usually inconclusive, and blood biochemistry may show only a raised alkaline phosphatase. Because the patients are often elderly, spinal stenosis, degenerative disc disease, spondylolisthesis, spondylosis, compression fracture or neoplasm are usually the initial diagnosis. Indeed, lumbar spinal degeneration is often considered to be the cause of the patient's symptoms (Schindler, Watura, Cobby, 2003).

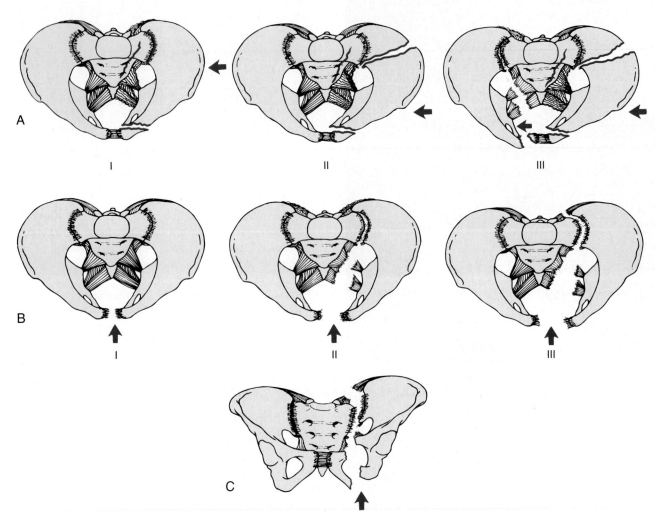

FIG. 9-46 Young and Burgess classification. **A,** Lateral compression force. Type I: a posteriorly-directed force causing a sacral crushing injury and horizontal pubic ramus fractures ipsilaterally. This injury is stable. Type II: a more anteriorly-directed force causing horizontal pubic ramus fractures with an anterior sacral crushing injury and either disruption of the posterior sacroiliac joints or fractures through the iliac wing. This injury is ipsilateral. Type III: an anteriorly-directed force that is continued and leads to a type I or type II ipsilateral fracture with an external rotation component to the contralateral side; the sacroiliac joint is opened posteriorly, and the sacrotuberous and spinous ligaments are disrupted. **B,** Anteroposterior (AP) compression fractures. Type I: an AP-directed force opening the pelvis but with the posterior ligamentous structures intact. This injury is stable. Type II: continuation of a type I fracture with disruption of the sacrospinous and potentially the sacrotuberous ligaments and an anterior sacroiliac joint opening. This fracture is rotationally unstable. Type III: a completely unstable or a vertical instability pattern with complete disruption of all ligamentous supporting structures. **C,** A vertically-directed force or forces at right angles to the supporting structures of the pelvis, leading to the vertical fractures in the rami and disruption of all the ligamentous structures. This injury is equivalent to an AP type III or a completely unstable and rotationally unstable fracture. (A-C redrawn from Young JWR, Burgess AR: *Radiologic management of pelvic ring fractures*, Baltimore, 1987, Urban & Schwarzenberg.) (In Browner: *Skeletal trauma: basic science, management, and reconstruction*, ed 3, St Louis, 2003, Saunders.)

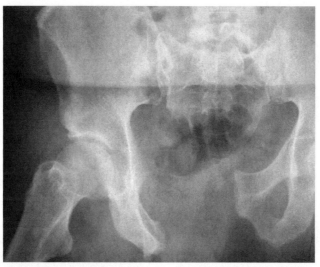

FIG. 9-47 Vertical shear injury with sacroiliac disruption and pubic symphysis disruption. There is an additional fracture of the superior and inferior pubic ramus on the right side with displacement of the right symphyseal segment into the perineum—a tilt fracture. (From Keating J: (v) Delayed reconstruction of pelvic fractures, *Curr Orthop* 19(5):362-372, 2005.)

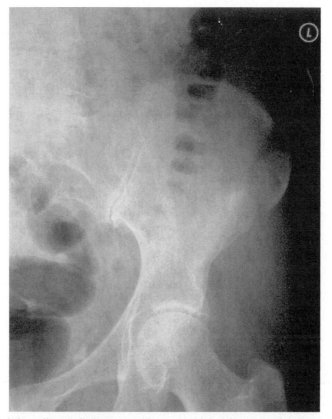

FIG. 9-48 Pelvic radiograph demonstrating an avulsion fracture of the anterior outer iliac crest on the left side. (From Zijderveld SA, ten Bruggenkate CM, van Den Bergh JPA et al. Fractures of the iliac crest after split-thickness bone grafting for preprosthetic surgery: report of 3 cases and review of the literature, *J Oral Maxillofac Surg* 62(7):781-786, 2004).

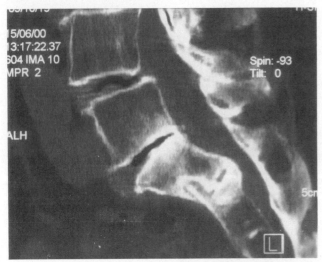

FIG. 9-49 Sagittal reconstruction computed tomographic image of the lumbo-sacral junction, showing sclerosis and resorption around an angulated fracture at the junction of S1 and S2. The appearance is typical for horizontal sacral insufficiency fractures. (From Schindler OS, Watura R, Cobby M: Sacral insufficiency fracture: an under-recognised condition, *Curr Orthop* 17[3]:234-239, 2003.)

PROCEDURE

- The patient is in a side-lying position.
- The examiner compresses the patient's superior ilium toward the floor (Fig. 9-50).
- Forward rolling motion of the sacrum occurs.
- Increased pressure in the SI-joint suggests a sacroiliac lesion.
- This pressure may also indicate a sprain of the posterior sacroiliac ligaments.
- A positive finding is significant for sacroiliac lesions.

Next Steps/Procedure
Diagnostic imaging

CLINICAL PEARL

Fractures of the pelvis are serious in and of themselves and may result in long-term disability. However, even more important is that these fractures are often complicated by damage to the soft tissues, urethra, bladder, bowel, blood vessels, and nerves. These complications can be fatal. Genitourinary complications occur in approximately 20% of pelvic fractures, and the overall mortality is 5%.

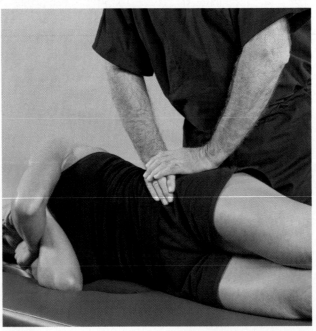

FIG. 9-50 The patient is in the side-lying position on an examination table with a firm surface. The examiner places both hands over the upper part of the superior iliac crest and exerts cautious downward pressure. If the patient experiences an increased feeling of pressure in the sacroiliac joint, the test indicates sacroiliac sprain, inflammation, subluxation, or fracture.

KNEE-TO-SHOULDER TEST

Assessment for Sacroiliac Mechanical Dysfunction and Pyogenic Sacroiliitis
(correlated with systemic findings)

Comment

Septic arthritis is a disease process caused by the direct invasion of a joint space by infectious agents, usually bacteria. Joints become infected by direct penetration spread from contiguous structures or, more often, by hematogenous invasion through the bloodstream. Septic arthritis occurs more often in large peripheral joints than in the lumbosacral spine. When a joint of the axial skeleton is involved, the SI-joint is the one commonly affected.

Pyogenic sacroiliitis is an uncommon illness. Reported incidence rates vary between 1.5% and 10% of all conditions affecting the SI-joint. The disease occurs most commonly in young adult men. The range of age is 20 to 66 years, and the male-to-female ratio is 3:2.

Entry of the organisms into the SI-joint is the initial factor that may result in joint infection. Most commonly, infectious agents reach the SI-joint by traveling through the bloodstream. They lodge in the vascular synovial membrane that lines the lower portion of the SI-joint. The infectious agents grow in the synovium and invade the joint space. The organisms might also lodge in the ilium, the most commonly infected flat bone in the body, and grow into the SI-joint. The symmetric involvement of the ilium and sacrum in pyogenic sacroiliitis suggests that the joint is the initial area affected. Once an infection is established in the joint, rapid destruction may occur because of both the direct, toxic effects that products or organisms have on joint structures and because of the host's inflammatory response to these products or organisms.

Any factor—intravenous drug abuse, skin infections, bone and urinary tract infections, endocarditis, pregnancy, or bowel disease—that promotes blood-borne infection or inhibits the normal defense mechanisms of the synovial joint predisposes the host to infection.

Although the role of trauma in the pathogenesis of pyogenic sacroiliitis is unclear, buttock or hip injuries have been reported in patients before development of pyogenic sacroiliitis. Most patients, however, deny a history of trauma, and its importance as a direct cause of the infection is in question. The histocompatibility typing associated with seronegative spondyloarthropathies, human leukocyte antigen (HLA)-B27, is not associated with pyogenic sacroiliitis.

Another mechanism of joint infection is contamination by local spread from a contiguous suppurative focus. Extension of a pelvic infectious process may cause disruption of the joint capsule or of the periosteum of the ilium or sacrum. Infections spreading beneath the spinal ligaments may gain entry into the SI-joints. Another mechanism of joint infection that is even more uncommon is direct seeding of organisms into the joint during diagnostic or surgical procedures.

ORTHOPEDIC GAMUT 9-10

PATIENT GROUPS SUSCEPTIBLE TO PYOGENIC INFECTION OF THE SACROILIAC JOINT

1. Children
2. Parenteral drug users
3. Immunosuppressed patients
4. Patients with endocarditis
5. Patients with pelvic inflammatory disease
6. Patients with gynecologic infections
7. After uncomplicated pregnancy and labor
8. Patients with sickle cell disease (secondary salmonella) infection
9. Trauma*

---

*Estimated 10% of cases have a history of pelvic trauma.

PROCEDURE

- The patient is supine. The patient's knee and hip are flexed, and the hip is adducted (Fig. 9-51).
- This position rocks the SI-joint (Fig. 9-52).
- The knee is approximated to patient's opposite shoulder (Fig. 9-53).
- A positive test is indicated by pain in the ipsilateral SI-joint.
- A positive test indicates sacroiliac mechanical dysfunction. This may include pyogenic sacroiliitis, when correlated with other system findings.

Next Steps/Procedures
Anterior innominate test, Lewin-Gaenslen test, Piedallu sign, sacral apex test, and sacroiliac resisted-abduction test

CLINICAL PEARL

With acute sacroiliac pyogenic infections, the onset is usually rapid and very painful. Swelling is intense, and tenderness is widespread. The patient resists movement and experiences pyrexia and general malaise. Pyogenic infections occurring in patients with rheumatoid arthritis often have a much slower onset. Although the sacroiliac joint is swollen, other inflammatory changes are often suppressed, especially if the patient is receiving steroids. In the early stages, both modes of onset will mimic simple mechanical injury of the sacroiliac joint.

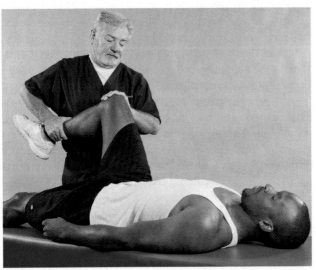

FIG. 9-51 The patient is supine on the examination table. The examiner flexes both the knee and hip of the affected leg to 90 degrees.

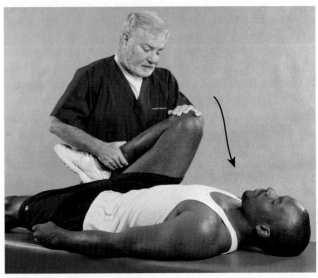

FIG. 9-52 The examiner flexes the patient's hip even farther and toward the patient's abdomen.

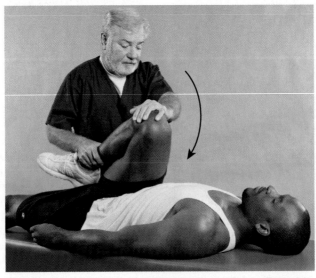

FIG. 9-53 The hip is adducted, approximating the knee of the affected leg to the contra-lateral shoulder. Pain in the sacroiliac joint indicates a positive test.

Assessment for a Sacroiliac Intraarticular Abnormality

Comment

Osteitis condensans ilii is a lesion in which sclerosis of a fairly large area of an ilium adjacent to the SI-joint occurs (Fig. 9-54). It is most common in multiparous women. The importance osteitis condensans ilii lies in distinguishing it from ankylosing spondylitis (Marie-Strumpell disease).

Osteitis condensans ilii is a disease characterized by mild back pain and unilateral or bilateral bony sclerosis of the lower ilium, with sparing of the sacral portion of the SI-joints. The illness is not progressive and is not associated with functional disability. The major difficulty with osteitis condensans ilii is that it is often confused with ankylosing spondylitis.

The prevalence of osteitis condensans ilii has been estimated to be 1.6% in Japanese and 3% in Scandinavians. The typical patient is a woman 30 to 40 years of age. The female-to-male ratio is 9:1 or greater.

The pathogenesis of osteitis condensans ilii is unknown. Urinary tract infections, inflammatory diseases of the SI-joint, and abnormal mechanical stresses have been suggested

as possible causes in this illness. Urinary tract infection may reach the ilium via nutrient arteries, resulting in reactive sclerosis. The absence of a history of urinary tract infection in many individuals makes this mechanism unlikely. Osteitis condensans ilii may be a subset of ankylosing spondylitis. However, histocompatibility testing for HLA-B27 has not documented increased incidence of this antigen in patients with osteitis condensans ilii. In addition, part of the confusion over differentiating osteitis condensans ilii and ankylosing spondylitis is the milder form of the latter illness in women.

A more likely cause of osteitis condensans ilii is mechanical stress across the SI-joint in association with pregnancy and diastasis of the symphysis pubis. A normal physiologic zone of hyperostosis on the anterior iliac margin of the SI-joint may become exaggerated in response to abnormal stresses. Abnormal stresses are placed on the SI-joints during pregnancy. However, these stresses alone would not explain the occasional male patient with osteitis or the female patient who develops osteitis without having been pregnant. Therefore it must be said that the mechanical stresses that cause osteitis condensans ilii are commonly, but not exclusively, associated with pregnancy. Diastasis of the symphysis pubis may explain this clinical occurrence. Diastasis of the pubis commonly occurs during pregnancy and is secondary to the release of relaxin, a product of the corpus pregnancy, which allows greater laxity of the supporting structures (ligaments) of the pelvis. Patients may actually notice movement or a popping sensation in the SI-joints and pubis. Diastasis is not exclusively related to pregnancy because it may occur secondary to trauma. Individuals, both male and female, with diastasis related to trauma may be at risk of developing osteitis condensans ilii. Differentially, radiation osteitis of the pelvis must be considered, especially in patients with a history of gynecologic malignancies.

MR images have been widely used in evaluating residual or recurrent tumor, and postirradiation tissue changes in gynecologic malignancies. In terms of radiation-induced bone change, the early MR signal alteration of irradiated pelvic bone marrow has been previously reported. After radiation therapy, fatty replacement of bone marrow occurs, which produces high signal intensity on T1-weighted images in the region of the radiation port. Radiation osteitis is a delayed skeletal complication of radiation therapy and develops in the pelvis, as well as long bones, chest, and mandible. However, radiation osteitis of SI-joints is rare, and its findings were previously reported using plain-film radiography and computed tomography (Yoshioka et al, 2000).

In radiation osteitis of the pelvis, abnormalities are characterized by mixed areas of dense sclerotic bone together with zones of focal demineralization. The irradiated bones

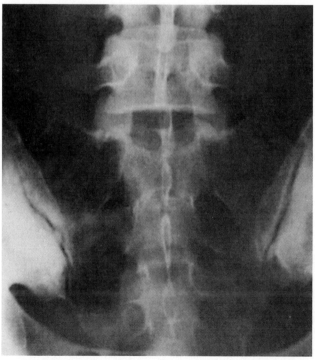

FIG. 9-54 Osteitis condensans ilii. (From Mercier LR, Pettid FJ: *Practical orthopedics*, ed 4, St Louis, 1995, Mosby.)

usually appear osteopenic approximately 1 year after radiation therapy in the pelvis. Attempted bone repair is evident with an area of mottling, sclerosis, osteopenia, and coarsened trabeculae by 2 to 3 years. Radiation-induced changes in the pelvis characteristically begin on the iliac side of the SI-joint and progress to involve the entire joint.

PROCEDURE

- The patient is in a supine position (Fig. 9-55).
- The patient's involved hip is flexed, abducted, and laterally rotated (Fig. 9-56).
- An overpressure at the end of the range of motion is applied.
- The opposite anterior-superior iliac spine is stabilized.
- A positive test is SI-joint pain.
- Because this test approximates a Patrick Fabere procedure, the examiner needs to be alert for coxa signs of disease.

Next Steps/Procedures

Erichsen sign, Hibbs test, and diagnostic imaging

CLINICAL PEARL

Osteitis condensans ilii causes a disturbance of the normal architecture of the ilium in which increased condensations of bone occur in the auricular portion of the ilium without a corresponding change in the sacroiliac joint or the sacrum. Osteitis condensans ilii must be differentiated from ankylosing spondylitis, which also causes condensations around the sacroiliac joint. Laguerre test reveals a mechanical problem of the sacroiliac joint. Involvement of the joint in osteitis condensans ilii can be confirmed only by diagnostic imaging.

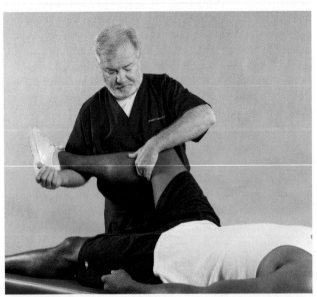

FIG. 9-55 The patient is supine. The examiner flexes and abducts the patient's hip on the affected side. The patient's foot rests on the examiner's forearm.

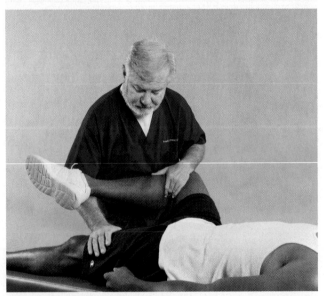

FIG. 9-56 The examiner laterally rotates the hip, applying an overpressure at the end of the range of motion. The contralateral pelvis is stabilized by holding the anterosuperior iliac spine down. Pain in the sacroiliac joint on the affected side constitutes a positive test.

LEWIN-GAENSLEN TEST

Assessment for Sacroiliac Joint Abnormality

Comment

The signs of SI-joint syndrome include tenderness when pressure is applied over the posterior-superior iliac spine (PSIS), in the region of the SI-joint, or in the buttock. Movement of the joint is usually reduced. Normally, the joint moves by rotating in the sagittal plane. Restricted movement can be detected in two ways.

The first way to detect restricted movement is to have the patient stand with one hand resting on the examining table for support. To examine the left SI-joint, the examiner places the thumb of the right hand over the spinous process of L5 and the thumb of the left hand over the left PSIS. The patient then flexes both the left hip and the left knee and lifts the knee toward the chest. As this move is performed, the examiner can detect a small but definite amount of movement. Rotation in the joint causes the iliac spine to move downward in relation to the spinous process of L5. When the SI-joint is fixed in position, this movement of the iliac spine relative to the spinous process is reduced or absent.

Confirmation can be obtained by the second test. To examine the left SI-joint, the examiner places the right thumb over the apex of the patient's sacrum and the left thumb over the ischial tuberosity. In a normal joint, flexing the left knee and hip and bringing the knee toward the chest causes the ischial tuberosity to move laterally, away from the apex of the sacrum. When the joint is fixed in position, the lateral movement does not take place. The SI-joint on the right is examined using the same method.

During forward flexion, the strain falls first on the iliolumbar ligament. Next, the strain is transmitted to the interspinous ligaments from L5 upward and then to the lumbodorsal fascia, particularly to the sacral triangle. During extension, the impingement signs prevail over the tension effects; the articulation comes first and then the interspinous ligaments. The ligamentum flava escapes impingement. During axial rotation, the iliolumbar ligament becomes strained first and then the intertransverse. During lateral flexion, the sequence is quadratus, ligamentum flava, and the interspinous ligament on the convex side.

For screening ambulation, the patient performs the normal movements of walking. The patient should be observed both coming toward the examiner and walking away.

Common causes of postural asymmetry include leg-length difference, pelvic obliquity, and scoliosis. According to current clinical practice, radiologic or ultrasound examination has been used to assess leg-length difference. If differ-

ences in the level of the proximal ends of the femur or the ceiling of the acetabulum are observed, then differences in the bone length of the extremities are presupposed. Pelvic asymmetry is often caused by a dysfunctional SI-joint. Unilateral rotatory malposition of the SI-joint has also been called subluxation, up-slip, or compressed SI-joint rotated anteriorly or posteriorly. Scoliosis (i.e., abnormal lateral curvature of the vertebral column) is considered to be most often of structural and of spinal origin (Timgren, Soinila, 2006).

The SI-joint is subject to several different processes that may damage it. Sprain is common, and SI-joint subluxation can occur. Sprain may occur when heavy loads are placed on the joints, during a fall, or with blows to the SI-joint. The pain that occurs will be felt unilaterally over the SI-joint and can radiate into the ipsilateral hip or buttock. The pain will worsen with movement or axial loading of the joint. During palpation, the joint is extremely tender, particularly near an area just inferomedial to the PSIS. When the patient is being examined for global motions, extending the joint may produce some pain, but flexion is not typically painful. Lateral flexion of the pelvis may be painful but is not universally so, particularly if the motion is very smoothly performed.

Straight-leg-raising tests produce pain at approximately 70 degrees of flexion. No muscular changes are noted, and reflex testing will be normal.

Pain from SI-joint lesions, other than sprain, will typically be dull in nature and perceived in the region of the buttock. The pain may radiate into the area of the anterior groin, the posterior thigh, the knee, or even the lower abdomen, causing possible misdiagnosis as an intraabdominal lesion. A neurologic symptom is rare; thus paresthesia is not often experienced. Patients suffering from mechanical lesions of the SI-joint experience the pain unilaterally. The pain is exacerbated by motions that produce stress on the joint.

ORTHOPEDIC GAMUT 9-11
OBSERVATIONS OF GAIT

1. Equality of stride length
2. Excessive pelvic tilt or lean during ambulation
3. Antalgic lean of the lumbopelvic spine
4. Excessive swayback or hyperlordosis
5. Changes in pelvic inclination (tilt)

ORTHOPEDIC GAMUT 9-12

SACROILIAC JOINT DISORDERS

Classification of disorders of the sacroiliac joint include:
1. Inflammatory lesions
2. Infectious lesions
3. Mechanical lesions
4. Degenerative lesions
5. Osteitis condensans ilii

PROCEDURE

- Lewin-Gaenslen test is a modification of Gaenslen test.
- The patient lies on the unaffected side and pulls the knee of that side to the chest (Figs. 9-57 to 9-59).
- The patient holds the affected thigh in extension for the examiner.
- The examiner, positioned behind the patient, then provides pressure by hyperextending the affected thigh (Fig. 9-60).
- Pain produced in the SI-joint is a positive finding.
- The test is significant for sacroiliac lesions.

Next Steps/Procedures

Anterior innominate test, knee-to-shoulder test, Piedallu sign, sacral apex test, and sacroiliac resisted-abduction test

CLINICAL PEARL

Because of the strength of the sacroiliac ligaments, sprain of these structures is uncommon. Bending movements—such as lifting and hyperextension, which produce a torsion sprain on the joint—are more likely to cause sprain of the thinner capsular ligaments in the small lumbosacral joints.

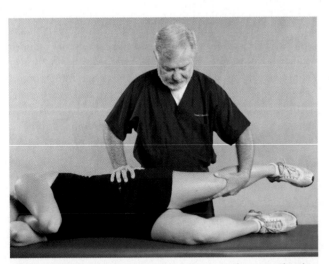

FIG. 9-57 The patient is side-lying on the examination table on the unaffected side. The knee and hip of the unaffected leg are flexed. The examiner abducts the affected leg slightly, supporting its weight with one hand. The examiner's other hand fixes the pelvis to the table with firm downward pressure.

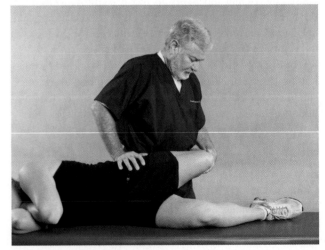

FIG. 9-58 The affected leg is extended by the examiner. Pain elicited during this maneuver constitutes a positive sign and indicates a sacroiliac lesion.

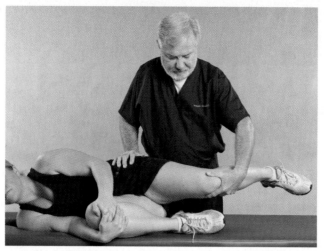

FIG. 9-59 In a slight variation of this test, the patient maximally flexes the thigh of the unaffected leg onto the abdomen and holds it in place.

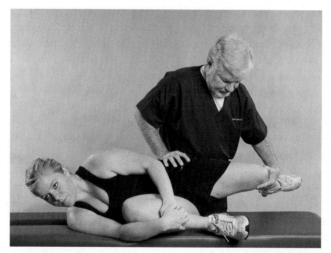

FIG. 9-60 The examiner extends the affected leg, allowing flexion of the knee. With the unaffected thigh in fixed flexion, very little extension motion is required to elicit a pain response in the affected leg.

PIEDALLU SIGN

Assessment for Abnormal Torsion Movement of the Sacroiliac Joint

Comment

Many inflammatory disorders affect the SI-joint. Most of these disorders fall under the general heading of the sero-negative arthropathies, such as ankylosing spondylitis, Reiter syndrome, and psoriatic arthritis. When an inflammatory disorder exists, a combination of radiographic and laboratory tests can be used to confirm the presence of a particular disease. Each disease has it own characteristics, such as a predisposition for ankylosing spondylitis in the SI-joint that migrates superiorly in the spine.

Infections within the SI-joint are most commonly caused by *Staphylococcus* bacteria and by tuberculous or brucellar infection. X-ray examination can once again be used to show typical changes, and bone scans will be useful in demonstrating the hot-spot appearance of such an infection. Aspiration biopsy is needed to culture the organism.

Mechanical lesions of the SI-joint are common and consist of both hypomobility and hypermobility lesions. Causes of hypomobility lesions include rotational stress on the joint, pregnancy, trauma, and unequal leg length. Hypermobility lesions are caused only by an unstable symphysis pubis or by pregnancy, which also affects the symphysis pubis via the release of the hormone relaxin.

Degenerative changes may occur within the SI-joint and in any other joint in the body as well. The changes that occur in the joint are similar to those in other joints. Pitting of the bone occurs accompanied by subchondral sclerosis and osteophytic changes. This condition has a tendency to occur with aging and to occur in concert with greater amounts of stress placed on the joint, such as increasing weight or damage from fracture or biomechanical abnormality.

Osteitis condensans ilii is a condition in which bone condenses along the ilium near the SI-joint. The cause of this condition is not known, but it may be associated with increased stress, ankylosing spondylitis, urinary tract infection, and circulatory problems. Osteitis condensans ilii can lead to LBP. Diagnostic imaging reveals a characteristic triangular area of sclerosis located near the medial ilium.

Sacroiliac subluxation may produce irritative micro-trauma to the articular structures, induction of spinal curvatures, induction of spinal or pelvic subluxation and fixation, and biomechanical abnormalities in stance and locomotion. Evaluation of the SI-joint for the presence of such subluxation or fixation will need to combine both static and dynamic palpation, as well as a plumb-line analysis. Tenderness may be noted during palpation of the PSIS when innominate rotation occurs. A full range-of-motion palpation procedure is needed to evaluate the joint for motion abnormalities or fixation. Both the static and organic procedures need to be performed to evaluate the joint for subluxation or fixation.

In the normal, erect, sitting position, with weight on the thighs, the coccyx does not have pressure against it. With flattening of the lumbar lordosis and sitting in the slumping position, however, the coccyx can reach the seat, and pain may develop over its tip. In coccydynia, pain on sitting is the most common complaint. This pain is aggravated by slumping, sitting on a hard seat, or activity. Many symptoms begin with an injury and may be aggravated by constipation or rectal disease. The symptoms are more common in women than in men. Fractures, when they occur, usually involve the lower part of the sacrum or first sacrococcygeal segments (Fig. 9-61).

Anatomic landmarks on the body surface can be measured with high accuracy by using rasterstereography and surface curvature analysis. The general assumption is that the lumbar dimples are in close relation to the pelvis (in particular to PSISs) and may thus be taken as indicators for pelvis movements. However, a systematic lag of the dimple movements occurred, resulting in a displacement of the dimples of up to ±1.5 mm relative to the pelvis (for ±10-degree pelvis tilt). Either a soft-tissue effect or torsion of the pelvis may be responsible for this behavior. The theory of pelvis torsion is confirmed by the fact that the orientation of the back surface at the locus of the dimples reveals a corresponding torsion of similar magnitude and sign. A torsion angle of approximately ±1.5 degrees in either SI-joint is sufficient to explain the observed dimple lag and the surface torsion (Drerup, Hierholzer, 1987).

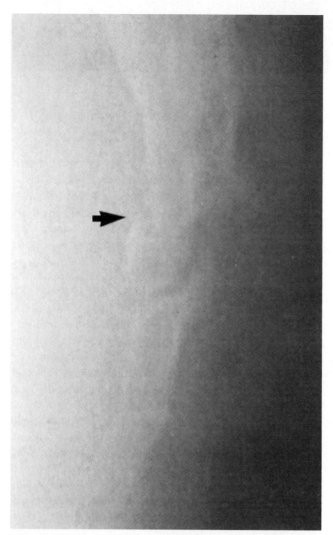

FIG. 9-61 Fracture of the lower portion of the sacrum. (From Mercier LR, Pettid FJ: *Practical orthopedics*, ed 4, St Louis, 1995, Mosby.)

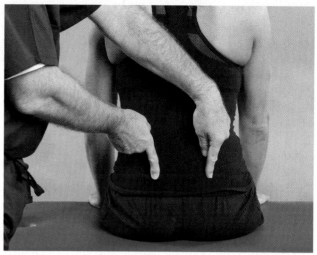

FIG. 9-62 The patient is seated on a hard, flat surface. The examiner notes pelvic symmetry and compares the height of the iliac crests.

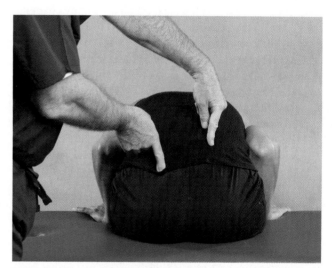

FIG. 9-63 If the posterior-superior iliac spine on the affected side is lower than that of the other, unaffected side, the patient flexes forward while remaining seated. If the lower posterior-superior iliac spine now becomes higher, the test is positive for an abnormality of torsion motion of the sacroiliac joint.

PROCEDURE

- The patient is seated to keep the hamstrings from affecting pelvic-flexion symmetry.
- The PSISs are located and compared for height (Fig. 9-62).
- If one PSIS is lower than the other, the patient flexes forward.
- If the lower PSIS becomes higher during forward flexion, the test is positive.
- The PSIS migration to a higher prominence is the positive sign (Fig. 9-63).
- An abnormality in the torsion motion of the SI-joint is suggested by the positive finding.

Next Steps/Procedures

Anterior innominate test, knee-to-shoulder test, Lewin-Gaenslen test, sacral apex test, and sacroiliac resisted-abduction test

CLINICAL PEARL

In the sacroiliac joint fixation complex, an irregular prominence of one articular surface becomes wedged on another prominence of the opposing articular surface. When reduction is successful, the pain is relieved immediately.

9

SACRAL APEX TEST

Assessment for Abnormal Rotational Shifting of the Sacroiliac Joint

Comment

The SI-joint is made up of thin anterior ligaments that blend in with the true anterior joint capsule and a thick posterior ligament complex with interosseous and accessory components (Fig. 9-64).

The forces for SI-joint motion are gravity, ground-reaction force, and muscle power. SI-joint motion is initiated by the muscles of the vertebral column, thighs, and respiratory system. The vertebral column muscles initiate SI-joint motion of the sacrum, relative to the ilium, by changing posture (lying down, sitting, and standing) and by changing the shape of the spinal column (flexion, extension, lateral flexion, and rotation).

Epidemiologic studies report the lifetime incidence of LBP in industrial workers to be approximately 60%. Yearly incidence has been reported as high as 31%. A significant number of studies have investigated potential predictors of LBP, including physical risk and psychosocial and physiologic factors. A study investigating various physical and psychosocial risk factors over a 1-year period could account for only 12% of serious LBP. Risk has been identified with prolonged sitting, prolonged standing, and lifting, although the exact basis for the risk for sitting is still contentious (O'Sullivan et al, 2006).

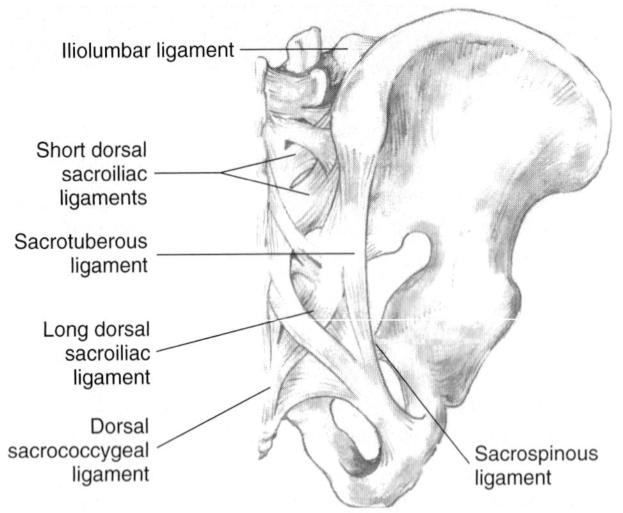

The movement is caused by change in the center of gravity, with the apex of the lordotic curve moving up or down, which causes the sacrum to nutate and the ilium to flare. As a result, the articular surfaces move anterosuperiorly to posteroinferiorly and superomedially to inferolaterally.

The two PSISs will approximate and separate. During lateral flexion, both iliac and sacral auricular surfaces move together but gap at different times in the anterior or posterior part of the joint and the upper or lower margins.

The thigh muscles initiate SI-joint motion of the ilium, relative to the sacrum, again by altering posture and causing motion of the thigh rather than the spine. Here, motions will include thigh flexion, extension, supination, pronation, abduction, and adduction. The two thighs can act together or independently. Abduction and adduction create SI-joint gapping but no shearing of cartilage.

Respiration aids SI-joint motion during inspiration and expiration. During inspiration, the erector spinae muscles contract, and the rectus abdominis relaxes by decreasing abdominal pressure. The pelvic diaphragm also relaxes and decreases abdominal pressure. When the erector group pulls the posterior part of the pelvic ring up and the rectus abdominis is relaxed, the pelvic ring will be tilted anteriorly. This tilt causes the sacral promontory to move backward and superiorly. During expiration, the erector group relaxes and the rectus abdominis contracts, and the pelvic diaphragm contracts. Action of the rectus abdominis pulls the symphysis pubis up and tilts the pelvic ring posteriorly. Abdominal pressure is increased, which causes the sacral promontory to move anteriorly and inferiorly.

FIG. 9-64 L5 sacrum-iliac articulation, posteroanterior view. (From Brier SR: *Primary care orthopedics*, St Louis, 1999, Mosby.)

PROCEDURE

- The patient is prone.
- The examiner places pressure at the apex of the patient's sacrum.
- Pressure is increased, causing a shear of the sacrum on the ilium (Fig. 9-65).
- If pain is produced over the joint, the test is positive.

Next Steps/Procedures

Anterior innominate test, knee-to-shoulder test, Lewin-Gaenslen test, Piedallu sign, and sacroiliac resisted-abduction test

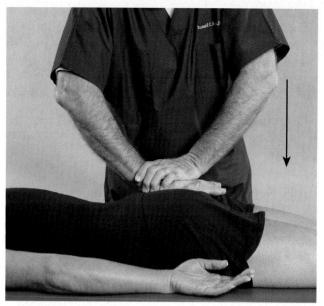

FIG. 9-65 The patient is prone. The examiner places pressure on the apex of the sacrum. Pressure is increased, causing a shear stress of the sacrum on the ilium. Pain produced in a sacroiliac joint is a positive test.

9

CLINICAL PEARL

Sciatic neuritis is a term used to describe pain or other discomfort that is experienced anywhere along the distribution of the sciatic nerve and is caused by a primary disease of the nerve or, more commonly, a mechanical disorder affecting the nerve. A sacroiliac subluxation-sprain may be the true cause of sciatic neuritis. The piriformis muscle is most often affected, and it may involve the L5–S1 and S2 distribution.

SACROILIAC RESISTED-ABDUCTION TEST

HIP-ABDUCTION STRESS TEST

Assessment for Generalized Abductor Muscular Weakness or Sprain or Subluxation of the Sacroiliac Joint

Comment

The SI-joint has well-developed cartilage surfaces, a synovial membrane, strong anterior and posterior ligaments, and a large internal sacroiliac ligament. After the fifth decade of life, fibrosis takes place between the cartilage surfaces. By the sixth or seventh decade, the joint has usually undergone fibrous ankylosis. Bony ankylosis is a rare phenomenon late in life. The joint surfaces can rotate 3 to 5 degrees in the younger, symptom-free patient. The joint has two functions: to provide elasticity to the pelvic ring and to serve as a buffer between the lumbosacral and hip joints.

Sacroiliac syndrome causes pain over one SI-joint in the region of the PSIS. This pain may be accompanied by referred pain in the leg.

The mechanism of injury is not well understood. Until late in middle age, a small amount of movement (3 to 5 degrees) is usually present in the SI-joint. After this age, movement is reduced by articular cartilage degeneration, fibrosis, and, rarely, ankylosis. Minor dysfunction in the SI-joint might leads to pain, but a more reasonable supposition is that pain results from sustained contraction of the muscle overlying the joint. This hypertonicity may accompany dysfunction in the SI-joint or in the L4–L5 or L5–S1 posterior lumbar joints.

A typical symptom is pain that varies in its degree of severity and is over the back of the SI-joint. Another typical symptom is referred pain in the groin, over the greater trochanter, down the back of the thigh to the knee, and, occasionally, down the lateral or posterior calf to the ankle, foot, and toes.

One of the more common results of the peripheral entrapment of the sciatic nerve at the pelvis is piriformis syndrome. A fairly perplexing diagnostic problem, patients with this syndrome have buttock pain in the region of the sciatic notch and down the back of the thigh and leg. The lack of orthopedic and motion findings locally at the spine distinguishes this peripheral entrapment from a lumbar disc lesion. In a small segment of the population, the sciatic nerve splits the piriformis muscle.

Hip flexion with rotation causes pain in an individual with piriformis syndrome because it stretches the piriformis muscle, thereby compromising or irritating the sciatic nerve.

Activities that externally rotate the thigh can strain the piriformis muscle, eventually leading to local swelling and irritation of the sciatic nerve sheath and, eventually, to sciatic neuritis.

This condition is a possible cause of extraspinal sciatica and is often caused by inadequate posture or overuse of the muscle. It leads to reflex hypertonicity of the piriformis and creates pressure on the sciatic nerve. It irritates the nerve and generates neurologic symptoms (Mayrand et al, 2006).

Piriformis syndrome usually generates symptoms such as pain in the buttock, which may radiate to the lower leg and be exacerbated when getting up from a sitting position, by hip adduction and internal rotation, and by prolonged sitting position. Furthermore, local muscle spasm is usually palpable.

ORTHOPEDIC GAMUT 9-13

THREE ELEMENT COMPRISING PIRIFORMIS SYNDROME SYMPTOMS

1. Myofascial referred pain
2. Nerve compression
3. Sacroiliac joint dysfunction

ORTHOPEDIC GAMUT 9-14

FIVE CHARACTERISTICS OF PIRIFORMIS SYNDROME CAUSING SCIATIC PAIN

1. History of local trauma
2. Pain localized to the sacroiliac joint, greater sciatic notch, and piriformis muscle, which extend along the course of the sciatic nerve
3. Acute pain brought on by stooping or lifting and relieved somewhat by traction
4. Palpable spindle mass at the anatomical location of the piriformis muscle
5. Positive Lasègue sign

ORTHOPEDIC GAMUT 9-15

PIRIFORMIS MUSCLE

Trigger points in the piriformis muscle refer pain to the following:
1. Buttocks
2. Toward the hip
3. Posterior thigh
4. Calf
5. The sole of the foot

PROCEDURE

- The patient lies on the unaffected side with the affected leg extended and slightly abducted (Fig. 9-66).
- The unaffected limb can be flexed at the hip and knee to provide stability.
- The examiner then exerts downward pressure on the abducted leg against the patient's resistance (Fig. 9-67).
- The test is repeated on the opposite side.
- If the test elicits pelvic pain near the PSIS, the test is positive (Fig. 9-68).
- The test is specific for a sacroiliac sprain or subluxation.

Next Steps/Procedures

Anterior innominate test, knee-to-shoulder test, Lewin-Gaenslen test, Piedallu sign, and sacral apex test

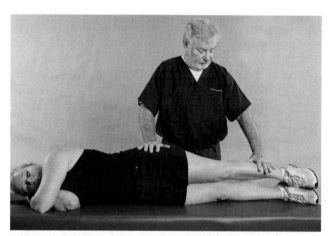

FIG. 9-66 The patient is in a side-lying position on the unaffected side.

CLINICAL PEARL

Slight, unilateral hip-abductor weakness is found in association with lateral pelvic tilt. The abductors are weak on the slightly elevated side of the pelvis. The beginning weakness in the abductors, as seen in nonparalytic individuals, is usually associated with handedness and is a strain weakness from postural or occupational causes.

9

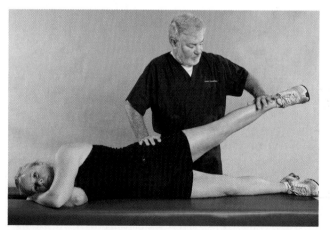

FIG. 9-67 The patient actively abducts the affected leg. At the end of the range of movement, the examiner applies downward pressure on the affected limb. The patient tries to resist this pressure. When it is positive, the test elicits pain at the posterior superior iliac spine. The test is specific for sacroiliac sprain or subluxation.

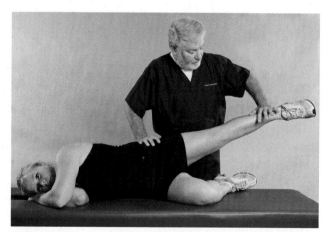

FIG. 9-68 In a slight modification that is only for more stability of the pelvis, the patient may flex the knee of the unaffected leg.

The Smith-Petersen test is often confused with and thought to be synonymous with the Goldthwait sign or Lasègue test.

Assessment for Sacroiliac Joint Involvement versus Lumbosacral Spine Involvement

Comment

Patients with chronic postural or mechanical problems in the lumbar spine or individuals who are vulnerable to repetitive injury may develop a chronic lumbar strain. Similar to the acute traumatic sprain, sacroiliac syndrome commonly causes disability and associated mechanical problems. The patient has sacroiliac tenderness, various fixation patterns, and discomfort or limitation in lumbar flexion and rotation.

SI-joint syndrome refers to the phenomenon of pain emanating from the SI-joint without a readily demonstrable disease such as spondyloarthropathy or crystal or pyogenic arthropathy. The cause of the pain is believed to be mechanical in origin. This diarthrodial joint has been implicated as a primary source of pain (i.e., independent of other conditions) as early as 1905 by Goldthwaite and Osgood (Cheng, Ferrante, 2006).

The incidence of SI-joint syndrome is estimated to be as high as 22% to 30% in centers that specialize in the treatment of LBP. Etiologic factors implicated in the genesis of SI-joint syndrome include trauma, cumulative injury, previous back surgery, or idiopathic causes (Cheng, Ferrante, 2006).

For complete separation of the articular surfaces in a normal SI-joint to be possible, the capsule of the joint must be completely torn through. Therefore, this injury is one that results from considerable violence having been applied to the joint. The soft-tissue damage may cause some residual stiffness because of scarring. At certain sites, where the cavity is shallow, residual capsular laxity may leave an unstable joint. Additionally, an unhealed rent may also lead to recurrent dislocation. Pathologic dislocations may occur in the presence of some inherent ligamentous laxity or abnormal muscle pull, such as in certain neurologic disorders leading to paralytic dislocations. Pathologic dislocations also may occur where the joint lining has been destroyed by an infective process.

Partial displacement of the articular surfaces of the SI-joint, when the bones remain in contact with each other, is a subluxation. In these cases, residual laxity usually persists.

Tears of the capsular lining of the SI-joint may be of a trivial nature, or they may be severe, involving a complete disruption of one of the posterior ligaments. In the latter case, momentary subluxation will have taken place, and unless the ligamentous rent heals, recurrent sprains from minor violence occur.

The fracture of the bony margin of the SI-joint, as it is dislocated, is most commonly seen in the more severe rotational injuries.

ORTHOPEDIC GAMUT 9-16

DIAGNOSTIC CHARACTERISTICS FOR PATIENTS WITH SACROILIAC SYNDROME

1. Pain in the region of the sacroiliac joint, with possible radiation to the groin, medial buttocks, and posterior thigh
2. Reproduction of pain by physical examination techniques that stress the joint
3. Complete elimination of pain with intraarticular injection of local anesthetic
4. An ostensibly morphologically normal joint without demonstrable pathognomonic radiographic abnormalities

---

ORTHOPEDIC GAMUT 9-17

SACROILIAC JOINT INJURIES

Four forms of sacroiliac joint injuries include:
1. Dislocation, in which the articular surfaces are completely displaced from each other
2. Subluxation, in which the articular surfaces remain in contact although they are displaced
3. Sprain, in which a tear of the capsular ligament occurs without a disturbance in its relationship to the opposing surfaces
4. Fracture-dislocation, in which a fracture of part of one of the bones has taken place for the articular surfaces to be completely displaced from each other

PROCEDURE

- The Smith-Petersen test is performed with the patient in the supine posture (Fig. 9-69).
- Straight leg raising is performed slowly while one hand is placed under the lower part of the patient's spine.
- As the hamstrings tighten, leverage is progressively applied to the SI-joint and then to the lumbosacral articulation.
- If pain is brought on before the lumbar spine begins to move, Smith-Petersen considers that a sacroiliac condition is present (Fig. 9-70).
- If, however, pain does not come on until after the lumbar spine begins to move, either sacroiliac or lumbosacral involvement may be present.
- Straight leg raising of both sides should be accomplished.
- If, on the unaffected side, the leg can be raised much higher, sacroiliac involvement is likely.
- If discomfort is elicited when both legs are brought to the same level, lumbosacral involvement is likely.

Next Steps/Procedures
Belt test, Gaenslen test, and Goldthwait test

CLINICAL PEARL

An acute sacroiliac flexion sprain is caused by lifting heavy objects. In many instances, however, the patient with chronic sacral pain has also sustained an ancient fall or flexion sprain. In cases of partial tearing of the sacroiliac ligaments, in which poor healing has taken place, a painful fibrous area persists, resulting in a chronic, weak area of the joint. This area becomes symptomatic when placed under tension and stress.

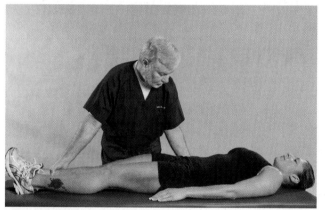

FIG. 9-69 The patient is supine on the examination table. The examiner stands at the side of the table next to the affected leg. The examiner places one hand under the patient's lumbar spine and palpates the L5–S1 spinous processes.

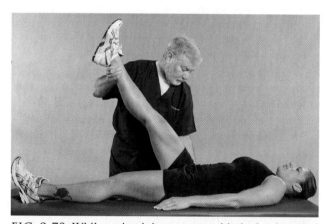

FIG. 9-70 While maintaining contact with the lumbosacral bony landmarks, the examiner performs a straight-leg-raising maneuver on the affected leg. If pain occurs before the L5–S1 spinous processes separate, a sacroiliac lesion is present. If pain occurs as the L5–S1 spinous processes separate, either a sacroiliac lesion or a lumbosacral lesion may be present. The test is performed bilaterally.

9

SQUISH TEST

Assessment for Posterior Sacroiliac Ligament Damage

Comment

Pelvic fractures comprise a spectrum of injuries ranging from stress or insufficiency fractures in osteoporotic bone to life-threatening disruptions of the pelvis ring.

Most acetabular fractures are traumatic, with an overall incidence of 3 in 100,000 patients per year. Unlike acute traumatic fractures, insufficiency fractures are produced by normal stresses applied to bone with diminished mechanical strength. They commonly occur in the spine, pelvis, and lower extremities; osteoporotic vertebral compression fractures are the most common. When in the pelvis, insufficiency fractures usually occur in the pubis, ilium, and sacrum. Atraumatic pelvic insufficiency fractures in the fossa acetabuli are extremely rare (Robinson, Hammoud, Sculco, in press).

In the few reports that exist in the literature, the prototypical patient is a postmenopausal woman with a history of rheumatoid arthritis or pelvic irradiation.

Acetabular insufficiency fractures are extremely difficult to detect on imaging. Routine radiographs are often unsuccessful in identifying these fractures. Computed tomography can provide accurate anatomic images of fractures in the pelvis but is not ideal for detecting impending fractures. Scintigraphy is sensitive for subtle changes in bone, but the findings are nonspecific and require correlation with other studies. MR imaging has been shown to provide the most sensitivity for detecting occult bone injury.

Satisfaction of search (SOS) occurs when an abnormality is missed because another abnormality has been detected. Physicians have long been aware that an injury may draw and hold their attention, diverting it from other injuries. An SOS effect has been demonstrated in which the discovery of a fracture on one image interfered with the detection of a subtle fracture on another image of the same patient (Berbaum et al, 2007).

As with all osseous injuries of the trunk, the possibility of visceral damage must be constantly borne in the examiner's mind. With pelvic injuries, this possibility is particularly applicable because the rectum, bladder, and urethra are contained within the pelvic cavity. Given that the membranous urethra passes through the pelvic diaphragm, this structure is especially vulnerable. A blow hard enough to disrupt the pubic bones is also very capable of rupturing a distended bladder.

Isolated pelvic fractures follow direct blows and therefore occur rather more readily in the more osteoporotic bones of elderly adults. Fractures of the ilium alone, although less common than fractures of the pubic rami, usually result from greater trauma and therefore cause more constitutional upset to the patient. Fractures of the pubic rami on one side are of little significance unless they extend into the hip joint. When both the superior and inferior pubic rami are fractured, and dislocated, the term Malgaigne fracture is appropriate.

The first cases of post-fracture pubic (Malgaigne fracture, named so particularly when bilateral) osteolysis were

---

ORTHOPEDIC GAMUT 9-19

BONY PELVIS

Injuries to the bony pelvis are two types:
1. Isolated fractures of the pubic rami or ilium
2. Double fractures of the pelvic ring

ORTHOPEDIC GAMUT 9-18

FACTORS PREDISPOSING TO PELVIC INSUFFICIENCY FRACTURE

- Female sex
- Osteoporosis
- Degenerative arthritis
- Inflammatory arthritis
- Radiation therapy
- Reconstructive surgery in the lower extremity
- Paget disease
- Regional disuse osteopenia

ORTHOPEDIC GAMUT 9-20

PELVIC RING

The double fractures of the pelvic ring occur in three forms:
1. Type I: The anterior portion of the ring may be broken if all four pubic rami are broken, and the loose portion of the ring will get driven posteriorly.
2. Type II: One side of the pubis may be fractured anteriorly and posteriorly and may roll laterally.
3. Type III: One side of the pelvic ring may be fractured and it may roll laterally and be superiorly displaced as well.

described in 1978 and since then about 50 cases have been reported. Nearly all these patients were women with post-menopausal osteoporosis. Other comorbid conditions included rheumatoid arthritis, hyperparathyroidism, alcohol abuse, and hip replacement. In some patients, the fractures occurred after a fall, a trivial trauma, or unusually strenuous physical activity, whereas in others no precipitating factors were identified. Mechanical groin pain with a limp simulating a hip abnormality was the presenting symptom in most patients. Mean time to healing was 6 months. The fracture lines may be difficult to see on the initial radiographs. However, as part of the search for an explanation to the osteolysis, the fractures are often detected upon careful reexamination of the initial radiographs, if needed under a magnifying glass. The osteolysis may persist for up to 40 months, lasting far longer than the symptoms (Botton et al, 2004).

Detachment of the whole anterior segment of the pubis follows a severe blow on the front of the pelvis. This injury usually results from road accidents or sometimes from falls from a height when the patient lands prone and strikes this region on some hard object.

With lateral disruption of the pelvic ring, the pelvic ring is broken both posterior and anterior to the hip. The natural tendency for the lower limb to roll laterally will open the pelvis anteriorly. The plane of cleavage in the anterior will be either through both pubic rami on the affected side or through the pubic symphysis (diastasis of the symphysis pubis). Posteriorly, the break may be through the ilium, at the SI-joint, or through the ala of the sacrum itself.

The most severe fracture is a combined lateral and superior displacement. With this form of pelvic fracture, the displaced fragment, which is attached to the lower limbs, not only has rolled laterally but is also displaced superiorly.

ORTHOPEDIC GAMUT 9-21

YOUNG AND BURGESS PELVIC FRACTURE CLASSIFICATION

1. Anteroposterior compression injury
2. Injury that results from an anteroposteriorly directed force producing sacroiliac joint opening, which causes external rotation of the hemi pelvis
3. Lateral compression injuries
4. Injury that results from a force parallel to the trabeculae of the sacrum and applied to the lateral aspect of the pelvis (Different lateral compression injuries are found depending on the anteroposterior location of this lateral impacting force.)
5. Vertical shear injury
6. Injury that results from a vertically directed force causing fracture of the pubic rami and disruption of all the ligamentous structures

---

PROCEDURE

- The patient is supine.
- Pressure is placed on the patient's anterosuperior iliac spines. The examiner pushes down at a 45-degree angle (Fig. 9-71).
- Pain indicates a positive test and suggests injury of the posterior sacroiliac ligaments.

Next Steps/Procedures
Gapping test and Yeoman test

9

CLINICAL PEARL

In elderly adults, fractures of the pubic rami and ischial rami are often caused by a trivial fall. The fractures usually occur in pairs. Fracture of one ramus alone is unusual. A positive squish test in an elderly patient indicates a possible fracture of a ramus and a posterior sacroiliac sprain. The fracture can be confirmed with diagnostic imaging.

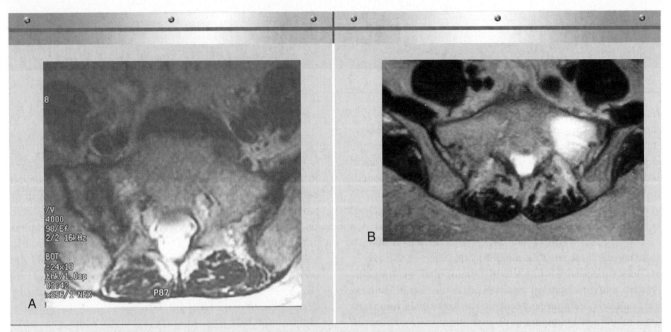

AT THE VIEWBOX

MRI of patient shows linear low signal in the right sacral ala parallel to and subjacent to the right sacroiliac joint (**A**). This is typical of a subacute or chronic sacral stress fracture. In more acute fractures, the fracture line may be obscured on MRI by bone marrow edema, which may mimic neoplasm or an inflammatory process (**B**). This 64-year-old female, the wife of a chiropractic physician had left sacroiliac pain after an extended shopping trip involving an estimated five miles of walking. This did not respond to conservative management, prompting referral for MRI. Plain films were negative. (From the teaching file of Timothy Mick, DC, DACBR)

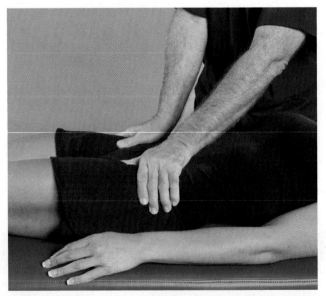

FIG. 9-71 The patient is supine. Pressure is placed on the patient's anterior-superior iliac spines. The examiner pushes inferior and caudal at a 45-degree angle. A positive test indicates sprain of the posterior sacroiliac ligaments.

Assessment for Anterior Sacroiliac Ligament Injury

Comment

Experts have argued that the piriformis muscle may irritate the sciatic nerve as a result of an anatomic abnormality such as a hypertrophic muscle. The term piriformis syndrome first appeared in 1947, and entrapment and irritation of the sciatic nerve in the hip region has largely been ascribed to influence from the piriformis muscle. Anatomic variations such as a bipartite piriformis muscle and the piriformis muscle lying anterior to the nerve have been described as irritating the sciatic nerve. Adhesions between the piriformis muscle and the sciatic nerve have been observed.

A syndrome was described in 1928 by Yeoman in which he proposed that arthritic changes in the SI-joint may cause sciatic pain as a result of secondary inflammatory reaction in the piriformis muscle. Both the piriformis and the internal obturator muscles are external rotators. Passive internal rotation, which stretches the piriformis muscle, will in most cases also stretch the internal obturator muscle. If such stretching triggers pain because of tendinitis, both the piriformis and the internal obturator muscles may therefore be sources of pain during passive internal rotation of the hips (Meknas, Christensen, Johansen, 2003).

A formerly undescribed abnormality affecting the internal obturator muscle and its relationships to the sciatic nerve seems to be responsible for much of the pain and diffuse neurologic symptoms that were first ascribed to a piriformis syndrome. Interestingly, perioperatively, the internal obturator tendon has been found to make contact with the sciatic nerve. Sectioning the internal obturator tendon reduced pain postoperatively.

When certain lumbosacral spinal mesodermal structures —ligaments, periosteum, joint capsule, and the annulus— are subjected to abnormal stimuli, such as excessive stretching, a deep, ill-defined, and dull aching is noted. This aching may be referred into areas of the lumbosacral spine, SI-joint, buttocks, and legs. The referral pattern is to the area designated as the sclerotome, which has the same embryonic origin as the mesodermal tissues stimulated. Although this peripheral pathway can explain the referred pain pattern, the significant individual variations that are encountered necessitate the consideration of central neural pathways. Referred pain distribution depends not only on segmental innervation, but also on the severity of pain and the extent to which an individual is cognizant of the stimulated components of the axial skeleton.

Pain of this type can often present concurrently with radicular pain that results from nerve root tension. The deeper, penetrating pain is usually attributed to distribution along the myotome and sclerotome. The sharper and more localized superficial pain is conveyed via the dermatomes.

The two types of pain may easily be confused. Moreover, sympathetic dystrophic signs and symptoms caused by nerve root encroachment can further confuse the presentation because the causalgia may exist with or without the more classic complaints associated with radiculopathy. Thus, all lower extremity pain is not a result of nerve root compression.

PROCEDURE

- The patient is lying prone.
- With one hand, the examiner applies firm pressure over the patient's suspect SI-joint, fixing the pelvis to the table (Fig. 9-72).
- With the other hand, the examiner flexes the patient's leg on the affected side and hyperextends the thigh by lifting the knee off the examining table (Fig. 9-73).
- If pain is increased in the sacroiliac area, this increase in pain indicates a sacroiliac lesion.
- This pain is caused by the strain placed on the anterior sacroiliac ligaments.
- In a patient without a sacroiliac lesion, pain will not be felt during this maneuver.

Next Steps/Procedures
Gapping test and squish test

CLINICAL PEARL

Ruptured sacroiliac ligaments do not heal soundly, even if they are accurately repaired, because the scar tissue, which forms at the site of the repair, stretches and is never as tough as the original. Surgical repair is often attempted after severe rupture of these ligaments, but conservative management may be equally effective.

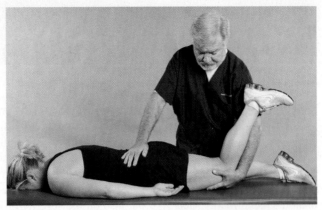

FIG. 9-72 The patient is prone on the examination table. With one hand, the examiner stabilizes the affected sacroiliac joint. The examiner flexes the knee of the affected leg to 90 degrees.

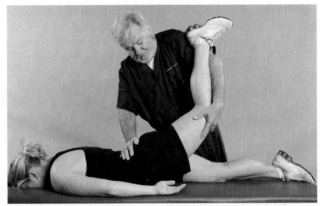

FIG. 9-73 The examiner hyperextends the thigh of the affected leg by lifting it off the examination table. Pressure is maintained over the affected sacroiliac joint. Increased sacroiliac pain constitutes a positive test and indicates a sacroiliac joint lesion.

CRITICAL THINKING

1. What are the seronegative spondyloarthropathies?
2. How is sacroiliitis best demonstrated radiographically?
3. What is osteitis condensans ilii?
4. What are Malgaigne fractures?
5. What are the primary and secondary function of the pelvis bones, joints, ligaments, and muscles?
6. What is the significance of an episacroiliac lipoma?
7. Not uncommonly, injury to the SI-joint results in referred pain. In what areas can this referred pain occur?
8. Why is the piriformis muscle so important in patients with leg pain?
9. What is the significance of side impact collisions to the pelvis?
10. Pain over the symphysis pubis on palpation might indicate what condition?
11. What differentiates sacroiliac involvement from lumbar spine involvement on Goldthwait sign?
12. Osteitis condensans ilii is often confused with what seronegative arthropathy?
13. Why should the clinician perform a squish test in an elderly patient who has undergone a trivial fall?

9

BIBLIOGRAPHY

Abrams WB, Berkow R: *The Merck manual of geriatrics,* Rahway, NJ, 1990, Merck Sharp & Dohme Research Laboratories.

Adams JC, Hamblen DL: *Outline of orthopaedics,* ed 11, Edinburgh, 1990, Churchill Livingstone.

Alario AJ: *Practical guide to the care of the pediatric patient,* St Louis, 1997, Mosby.

Allison D, Strickland N: *Acronyms & synonyms in medical imaging,* Oxford, UK, 1996, ISIS Medical Media.

Altman RD: Musculoskeletal questions and answers, *J Musculoskeletal Med* 7:10, 1990.

American Medical Association: *Guides to the evaluation of permanent impairment,* ed 4, Chicago, 1993, The Association.

American Medical Association: *How to use guides to the evaluation of permanent impairment,* ed 4, Falmouth, Conn, 1993, SEAK.

Anderson KN, Anderson LE: *Mosby's pocket dictionary of medicine, nursing, & allied health,* ed 2, St Louis, 1994, Mosby.

Andersson GBJ: Occupational biomechanics. In Weinstein J, Wiesel SW, editors: *The lumbar spine,* Philadelphia, 1990, WB Saunders.

Andersson GBJ: The epidemiology of spinal disorders. In Frymoyer JW, editor: *The adult spine: principles and practice,* New York, 1990, Raven.

Apley AG, Solomon L: *Concise system of orthopaedics and fractures,* London, 1988, Butterworth-Heinemann.

Apps BK, Cohen BB, Steel CM: *Biochemistry, a concise test for medical students,* ed 5, Iowa City, 1992, Bailliere Tindall.

Aston JN: *A short textbook of orthopaedics and traumatology,* Philadelphia, 1967, JB Lippincott.

Bakkum B, Cramer G: Muscles that influence the spine. In Cramer G, Darby S, editors: *Basic and clinical anatomy of the spine, spinal cord, and ANS,* St Louis, 1995, Mosby.

Barkauskas VH et al: *Health & physical assessment,* ed 2, St Louis, 1998, Mosby.

Battie MC, Bigos SJ: Industrial back pain complaints, *Orthop Clin North Am* 22:273, 1991.

Beal MC: The sacroiliac problem, review of anatomy, mechanics and diagnosis, *J Am Osteopath Assoc* 82:667, 1982.

Berens DL: Roentgen features of ankylosing spondylitis, *Clin Orthop* 74:20, 1971.

Berghs H et al: Diagnostic value of sacroiliac joint scintigraphy with 99 m technetium pyrophosphate in sacroiliitis, *Ann Rheum Dis* 37:190, 1978.

Berthelot J-M et al: Provocative sacroiliac joint maneuvers and sacroiliac joint block are unreliable for diagnosing sacroiliac joint pain, *Joint Bone Spine* 73(1):17-23, 2006.

Bhagavan NV: *Medical biochemistry,* Boston, 1992, Jones and Bartlett.

Boden SD et al: *The aging spine,* Philadelphia, 1991, WB Saunders.

Bogduk N, Amevo B, Pearcy M: A biological basis for instantaneous centers of rotation of the vertebral column, *Proc Inst Mech Eng* 209:177, 1995.

Bogduk N, Macintosh JE, Pearcy MJ: A universal model of the lumbar back muscles in the upright position, *Spine* 17:897, 1992.

Bogduk N, Twomey LT: *Clinical anatomy of the lumbar spine,* ed 2, Melbourne, 1991, Churchill Livingstone.

Bone biopsy of the parasymphyseal region of athletes with osteitis pubis diagnosed by MRI demonstrates new woven bone formation, *J Sci Med Sport* 6(4, suppl 1):95-84, 2003.

Borenstein DG, Wiesel SW: *Low back pain: medical diagnosis and comprehensive management,* Philadelphia, 1989, WB Saunders.

Bowen V, Cassidy JD: Macroscopic and microscopic anatomy of the sacroiliac joint from embryonic life until the eighth decade, *Spine* 6:620, 1981.

Brand C et al: Cryptococcal sacroiliitis: case report, *Ann Rheum Dis* 44:126, 1985.

Braun J, Bollow M, Sieper J: Radiologic diagnosis and pathology of the spondyloarthropathies, *Rheum Dis Clin North Am* 24(4):697-735, 1998.

Breen A: The reliability of palpation and other diagnostic methods, *J Manipulative Physiol Ther* 15:54, 1992.

Brier SR: *Primary care orthopedics,* St Louis, 1999, Mosby.

Brier SR, Nyfield B: A comparison of hip and lumbopelvic inflexibility and low back pain in runners and cyclists, *J Manipulative Physiol Ther* 18:25, 1995.

Brooks M, Evans R, Fairclough J: *Sports injuries,* ed 2, London, 1992, Gower Medical Publishing.

Brotzman SB: *Clinical orthopaedic rehabilitation,* St Louis, 1996, Mosby.

Brown DE, Neumann RD: *Orthopedic secrets,* Philadelphia, 1995, Hanley & Belfus.

Brunner C, Kissling R, Jacob HAC: The efforts of morphology and histopathologic findings on the mobility of the sacroiliac joint, *Spine* 16:1111, 1991.

Bucholz RW: *Orthopaedic decision making,* ed 2, St Louis, 1996, Mosby.

Budgell B, Noda K, Sata A: Innervation of posterior structures in the lumbar spine of the rat, *J Manipulative Physiol Ther* 20:359, 1997.

Burgess A et al: Pelvic ring disruptions: effective classification system and treatment protocols, *J Trauma* 30:848, 1990.

Cammisa M, De Serio A, Guglielmi G: Diffuse idiopathic skeletal hyperostosis, *Eur J Radiol* 27(suppl 1):S7-S11, 1998.

Campbell JB, Campbell JM: *Mosby's survival guide to medical abbreviations & acronyms prefixes & suffixes symbols Greek alphabet,* St Louis, 1995, Mosby.

Canale ST: *Campbell's operative orthopaedics,* vol 1-4, ed 9, St Louis, 1998, Mosby.

Carrera GF et al: CT of sacroiliitis, *AJR Am J Roentgenol* 136:41, 1981.

Cassidy JD: *The pathoanatomy and clinical significance of the sacroiliac joints,* Toronto, 1991, World Chiropractic Congress.

Cats A, Linder SM: Spondyloarthropathies: an overview, *Spine* 4:497, 1990.

Cipriano JJ: *Photographic manual of regional orthopaedic and neurological test,* ed 3, Baltimore, 1997, Williams & Wilkins.

Cohn RE: *Impairment rating examination and disability evaluation,* ed 3, Wilkesboro, NC, 1994, R Ernest Cohn.

Colachis SC: Movement of sacroiliac joint in adult male, *Arch Phys Med Rehabil* 44:490, 1963.

Cole AJ, Herring SA: *The low back pain handbook: a practical guide for the primary care examiner,* Philadelphia, 1997, Hanley & Belfus.

Cox JM: *Low back pain, mechanism, diagnosis and treatment,* ed 5, Baltimore, 1990, Williams & Wilkins.

Coy JT et al: Pyogenic arthritis of the sacroiliac joint: long-term follow-up, *J Bone Joint Surg* 58A:845, 1976.

Craik RL, Oatis CA: *Gait analysis theory and application,* St Louis, 1995, Mosby.

Cramer GD, Darby SA: *Basic and clinical anatomy of the spine, spinal cord, and ANS,* St Louis, 1995, Mosby.

Cullinan AM: *Optimizing radiographic positioning,* Philadelphia, 1992, Lippincott.

Curtis P: In search of the "back mouse," *J Fam Pract* 36:657, 1993.

Cyriax J: *Textbook of orthopaedic medicine, vol. 1, diagnosis of soft tissue lesions,* London, 1982, Bailliere Tindall.

Daffner RH et al: The radiology assessment of post-traumatic vertebral stability, *Skeletal Radiol* 19:103, 1990.

Dambro MR, Griffith JA: *Griffith's 5 minute clinical consult,* Baltimore, 1997, Williams & Wilkins.

D'Ambrogio KJ, Roth GB: *Positional release therapy assessment & treatment of musculoskeletal dysfunction,* St Louis, 1997, Mosby.

D'Ambrosia RD: *Musculoskeletal disorders: regional examination and differential diagnosis,* Philadelphia, 1977, JB Lippincott.

Dandy DJ: *Essential orthopaedics and trauma,* Edinburgh, 1989, Churchill Livingstone.

deBlecourt JJ et al: Hereditary factors in rheumatoid arthritis and ankylosing spondylitis, *Ann Rheum Dis* 20:215, 1961.

DeBosset P et al: Comparison of osteitis condensans ilii and ankylosing spondylitis in female patients: clinical, radiological and HLA typing characteristics, *J Chron Dis* 31:171, 1978.

Delbarre F et al: Pyogenic infection of the sacroiliac joint, *J Bone Joint Surg* 57A:819, 1975.

Deltoff MN, Kogon PL: *The portable skeletal x-ray library,* St Louis, 1998, Mosby.

Demeter SL, Andersson GBJ, Smith GM: *Disability evaluation,* St Louis, 1996, Mosby.

Deshpande JK, Tobias JD: *The pediatric pain handbook,* St Louis, 1996, Mosby.

Dettenmeier PA: *Radiographic assessment for nurses,* St Louis, 1995, Mosby.

Dihlmann W: *Diagnostic radiology of the sacroiliac joints,* New York, 1980, George Thieme Verlag.

Dilsen N et al: A comparative roentgenologic study of rheumatoid arthritis and rheumatoid (ankylosing) spondylitis, *Arthritis Rheum* 5:341, 1962.

Doherty M: *Color atlas and text of osteoarthritis,* London, 1994, Wolfe.

Doherty M, Doherty J: *Clinical examination in rheumatology,* London, 1992, Wolfe.

Doherty M, George E: *Self-assessment picture tests in rheumatology,* London, 1995, Mosby-Wolfe.

DonTigny RL: Anterior dysfunction of sacroiliac joint as a major factor in the etiology of idiopathic low back pain syndrome, *Phys Ther* 70:250, 1990.

Dulhunty JA: Sacroiliac subluxation, facts, fallacies and illusions, *J Aust Chiro Assoc* 15:91, 1985.

Dunn DJ et al: Pyogenic infections of the sacroiliac joint, *Clin Orthop* 118:113, 1976.

Ebraheim N et al: Percutaneous computed tomography guided stabilization of posterior pelvis fractures, *Clin Orthop* 307:222, 1994.

Elliott FA, Schutta HS: The differential diagnosis of sciatica, *Orthop Clin North Am* 2:477, 1971.

Elster AD: *Questions and answers in magnetic resonance imaging,* St Louis, 1994, Mosby.

Epstein MC: Cause of low back problem, *Dig Chiro Econ* 26:52, 1983.

Epstein O et al: *Clinical examination,* ed 2, London, 1997, Mosby.

Failinger MS, McGanety PL: Current concepts review, unstable fractures of the pelvic ring, *J Bone Joint Surg* 74A:781, 1992.

Farfan HF: *Mechanical disorders of the low back,* Philadelphia, 1973, Lea & Febiger.

Farrar WE: *Atlas of infections of the nervous system,* London, 1993, Wolfe.

Feldmann E: *Current diagnosis in neurology,* St Louis, 1994, Mosby.

Ferezy JS: *The chiropractic neurological examination,* Gaithersburg, Md, 1992, Aspen.

Finneson BE: *Low back pain,* ed 2, Philadelphia, 1980, JB Lippincott.

Frank ED et al: *Merrill's atlas of radiographic positioning and procedures,* vol 1-3, ed 11, St Louis, 2007, Mosby.

Freeman MD, Fox D, Richards T: The superior intracapsular ligament of the sacroiliac joint: confirmation of Ill's ligament, *J Manipulative Physiol Ther* 13:374, 1990.

Garcia JH: *Neuropathology the diagnostic approach,* St Louis, 1997, Mosby.

Gatterman MI: Disorders of the pelvic ring. In Gatterman MI, editor: *Chiropractic management of spine-related disorders,* Baltimore, 1990, Williams & Wilkins.

Gibbons K, Soloniuk D, Razack N: Neurological injury and patterns of sacral fractures, *J Neurosurg* 72:889, 1990.

Gifford DB et al: Septic arthritis due to pseudomonas in heroin addicts, *J Bone Joint Surg* 57A:631, 1975.

Gilani SA, Fazal N: Role of TVS in diagnosis of female genital tuberculosis, *Ultrasound Med Biol* 32(5, suppl 1):P92-P93, 2006.

Giles LGF, Kaveri MJP: Some osseous and soft tissue causes of lumbar stenosis, *J Rheumatol* 17:1374, 1990.

Goldberg, J, Kovarsky J: Tuberculous sacroiliitis, *South Med J* 76:1175, 1983.

Goldie BS: *Orthopaedic diagnosis and management: a guide to the care of orthopaedic patients,* ed 2, Oxford, UK, 1998, ISIS Medical Media.

Goldstein MJ et al: Osteomyelitis complicating regional enteritis, *Gut* 10:264, 1969.

Goldstein TS: Treatment of common problems of the hip joint. In Goldstein TS, Lewis CB, series editors: *Geriatric orthopaedics rehabilitative management for common problems,* Gaithersburg, Md, 1991, Aspen.

Gordon G, Kabins SA: Pyogenic sacroiliitis, *Am J Med* 69:50, 1980.

Gorse GJ et al: Tuberculous spondylitis: a report of six cases and a review of the literature, *Medicine (Baltimore)* 62:178, 1978.

Goulet J et al: Comminuted fractures of the posterior wall of the acetabulum: a biomechanical evaluation of fixation methods, *J Bone Joint Surg* 76A:1457, 1994.

Gracovetsky S: Biomechanics of the spine. In White AH, Schofferman JA, editors: *Spine care: diagnosis and conservative treatment,* St Louis, 1995, Mosby.

Greenman PE: Innominate shear dysfunction in sacroiliac syndrome, *J Manual Med* 2:114, 1986.

Greenspan A, Montesano P: *Imaging of the spine in clinical practice,* London, 1993, Wolfe.

Greenstein GM: *Clinical assessment of neuromuscular disorders,* St Louis, 1997, Mosby.

Groen GJ, Baljet B, Drukker J: Nerves and nerve plexuses of the human vertebral column, *Am J Anat* 188:282, 1990.

Gross ML, Nasser S, Finnerman GAM: Hip and pelvis. In DeLee JC, Drez D, editors: *Orthopaedic sports medicine: principles and practice,* vol 2, Philadelphia, 1994, WB Saunders.

Grossman ZD et al: *Cost-effective diagnostic imaging: the examiner's guide,* ed 3, St Louis, 1995, Mosby.

Hassoun A et al: Female genital tuberculosis: uncommon presentation of tuberculosis in the United States, *Am J Med* 118(11):1295-1296, 2005.

Hawkins RJ: *An organized approach to musculoskeletal examination and history taking,* St Louis, 1995, Mosby.

Helfet D, Schmeling G: Management of complex acetabular fractures through single nonextensile exposures, *Clin Orthop* 305:58, 1994.

Hendrix RW, Lin PJP, Kane WJ: Simplified aspiration or injection techniques for the sacroiliac joint, *J Bone Joint Surg* 64A:1249, 1982.

Hinkle CZ: *Fundamentals of anatomy & movement: a workbook and guide,* St Louis, 1997, Mosby.

Hittner VJ: Episacroiliac lipomas, *Am J Surg* 78(3):382-383, 1949.

Hornberger JP: *Exercise physiology therapeutic exercise,* Sarasota, Fla, 1991, Joseph P Hornberger.

Iczkovitz JM, Leek JC, Robbins DL: Pyogenic sacroiliitis, *J Rheumatol* 8:157, 1981.

Isler B: Lumbosacral lesions associated with pelvic ring injuries, *J Orthop Trauma* 4:1, 1990.

Jablonski S: *Dictionary of medical acronyms & abbreviations,* ed 3, Philadelphia, 1998, Hanley & Belfus.

Jenkins DH, Young MH: The operative treatment of sacroiliac subluxation and disruption of the symphysis pubis, *Injury* 10:139, 1978.

Kakarla N, Boswell HB, Zurawin RK: A large pelvic mass in an adolescent patient with granulomatous nephritis: case report and discussion of treatment challenges, *J Pediatr Adolesc Gynecol* 19(3):223-229, 2006.

Kanner R: *Pain management secrets,* Philadelphia, 1997, Hanley & Belfus.

Kapandji LA: *The physiology of the joints, vol 3: The trunk and vertebral column,* New York, 1974, Churchill Livingstone.

Kapoor VK: Abdominal tuberculosis, *Medicine* 35(5):257-260, 2007.

Katirji B: *Electromyography in clinical practice: a case study approach,* St Louis, 1998, Mosby.

9

Katz WA: *Rheumatic diseases diagnosis and management,* Philadelphia, 1977, JB Lippincott.

Keats TE, Lusted LB: *Atlas of roentgenographic measurements,* ed 6, St Louis, 1990, Mosby.

Kelley WN et al: *Textbook of rheumatology,* vol 1, ed 4, Philadelphia, 1993, WB Saunders.

Kellgren JH: The anatomical source of back pain, *Rheumatol Rehab* 16:3, 1977.

Kendall HO, Kendall FP, Wadsworth GE: *Muscles testing and function,* ed 2, Baltimore, 1971, Williams & Wilkins.

Khan MA, Linder SM: Ankylosing spondylitis: clinical aspects, *Spine* 4:529, 1990.

King L: Incidence of sacroiliac joint dysfunction and low back pain in fit college students, *J Manipulative Physiol Ther* 14:333, 1991.

Kingston RS: Radiology of the spine. In Watkins RG, editor: *The spine in sports,* St Louis, 1996, Mosby.

Kirkaldy-Willis WH: *Managing low back pain,* New York, 1983, Churchill Livingstone.

Klippel JH, Dieppe PA: *Rheumatology,* vol 1-2, ed 2, London, 1998, Mosby.

Koenigsberg R: *Churchill's illustrated medical dictionary,* New York, 1989, Churchill Livingstone.

Lavy CBD, Barrett DS: *Questions and answers on Apley's concise system of orthopaedics and fractures,* Oxford, UK, 1991, Butterworth-Heinemann.

Lawrence DJ: Sacroiliac joint, part two, clinical considerations. In Cox JM, editor: *Low back pain: mechanism, diagnosis and treatment,* ed 5, Baltimore, 1990, Williams & Wilkins.

Leffs M: *Back pain in the adolescent athlete,* Toronto, 1991, American Back Society.

Lerner AJ: *The little black book of neurology,* ed 3, St Louis, 1995, Mosby.

LeVeau B: Hip. In Richardson JK, Iglarsh JK, editors: *Clinical orthopaedic physical therapy,* Philadelphia, 1994, WB Saunders.

Lewis CB, Bottomley JM: Orthopaedic treatment considerations. In: *Geriatric physical therapy: a clinical approach,* New York, 1994, Appleton & Lange.

Lewis CB, Knortz KA: *Orthopedic assessment and treatment of the geriatric patient,* St Louis, 1993, Mosby.

Lewkonia RM, Kinsella TD: Pyogenic sacroiliitis: diagnosis and significance, *J Rheumatol* 8:153, 1981.

Lisbona R, Rosenthall L: Observation on the sequential use of 99mTc-phosphate complex and 67Gd imaging in osteomyelitis and septic arthritis, *Radiology* 123:123, 1977.

Longoria RK, Carpenter JL: Anaerobic phygenic sacroiliitis, *South Med J* 76:649, 1983.

Loth TS: *Orthopedic boards review,* St Louis, 1993, Mosby.

Loth TS: *Orthopedic boards review II: a case study approach,* St Louis, 1996, Mosby.

Macintosh JE, Pearcy MJ, Bogduk N: The axial torque of the lumbar back muscles; torsion strength of the back muscles, *Aust N Z J Surg* 63:205, 1993.

Magee DJ: *Orthopedic physical assessment,* ed 3, Philadelphia, 1997, WB Saunders.

Maigne R: *Orthopaedic medicine: a new approach to vertebral manipulation,* Springfield, Ill, 1972, Charles C Thomas.

Maitland GD: *Vertebral manipulation,* ed 5, London, 1986, Butterworth.

Malone TR, McPoil TG, Nitz AJ: *Orthopedic and sports physical therapy,* ed 3, St Louis, 1997, Mosby.

Marchiori DM: *Clinical imaging with skeletal, chest, and abdomen pattern differentials,* St Louis, 1999, Mosby.

Martin JH: *Neuroanatomy text and atlas,* ed 2, Stamford, Conn, 1996, Appleton & Lange.

Martinez Maestre MA, Daza Manzano C, Martinez Lopez R: Postmenopausal endometrial tuberculosis, *Int J Gynecol Obstet* 86(3):405-406, 2004.

Mathers LH et al: *Clinical anatomy principles,* St Louis, 1996, Mosby.

Mazion JM: *Illustrated manual of neurological reflexes/signs/tests, part I, orthopedic signs/tests/maneuvers for office procedure, part II,* Orlando, Fla, 1980, Daniels Publishing.

McCarthy A, Vicenzino B: Treatment of osteitis pubis via the pelvic muscles, *Man Ther* 8(4):257-260, 2003.

McRae R: *Clinical orthopaedic examination,* ed 3, Edinburgh, 1990, Churchill Livingstone.

McRae R: *Practical fracture treatment,* ed 3, New York, 1994, Churchill-Livingstone.

Measured hip joint range of motion loss and its role in the pathogenesis of the athletic groin injury osteitis pubis, *J Sci Med Sport* 6(4, suppl 1):93-84, 2003.

Medical Economics Books: *Patient care flow chart manual,* ed 3, Oradell, NJ, 1982, Medical Economics Books.

Mellion MB: *Sports medicine secrets,* Philadelphia, 1994, Hanley & Belfus.

Mellion MB: *Office sports medicine,* ed 2, St Louis, 1996, Mosby.

Mengel MB, Schwiebert LP: *Ambulatory medicine the primary care of families,* ed 2, Stamford, Conn, 1996, Appleton & Lange.

Mennell JM: *The musculoskeletal system: differential diagnosis from symptoms and physical signs,* Gaithersburg, Md, 1992, Aspen.

Mercier LR, Pettid FJ: *Practical orthopedics,* ed 4, St Louis, 1995, Mosby.

Mester AR et al: Enteropathic arthritis in the sacroiliac joint. Imaging and differential diagnosis, *Eur J Radiol* 35(3):199-208, 2000.

Mirvis SE, Young JWR: *Imaging in trauma and critical care,* Baltimore, 1991, Williams & Wilkins.

Modic MT, Masaryk TJ, Ross JS: *Magnetic resonance imaging of the spine,* ed 2, St Louis, 1994, Mosby.

Mooney V, Robertson J: The facet syndrome, *Clin Orthop* 115:149, 1976.

Mosby-Year Book, Inc: *Expert 10-minute physical examination,* St Louis, 1997, Mosby.

Murphy ME: Primary pyogenic infection of sacroiliac joint, *N Y State J Med* 77:1309, 1977.

Nachemson AL: Newest knowledge on low back pain, *Clin Orthop* 2279:8, 1992.

Nettina SM: *The Lippincott manual of nursing practice,* ed 6, Philadelphia, 1996, JB Lippincott.

Newton RW: *Color atlas of pediatric neurology,* St Louis, 1995, Mosby-Wolfe.

Nicholas JA, Hershman EB: *The lower extremity & spine in sports medicine,* vol 1-2, ed 2, St Louis, 1995, Mosby.

Nordin M, Andersson GBJ, Pope MH: *Musculoskeletal disorders in the workplace: principles and practice,* St Louis, 1997, Mosby.

Norman GF: Sacroiliac disease and its relationship to lower abdominal pain, *Am J Surg* 116:54, 1968.

Numaguci Y: Osteitis condensans ilii, including its resolution, *Radiology* 98:1, 1971.

O'Donoghue DH: *Treatment of injuries to athletes,* ed 3, Philadelphia, 1976, WB Saunders.

Olivieri L et al: Differential diagnosis between osteitis condensans ilii and sacroiliitis, *J Rheumatol* 17:1504, 1990.

Olmarker K, Rydevik B: Pathophysiology of sciatica, *Orthop Clin North Am* 22:223, 1991.

Olson WH et al: *Handbook of symptom-oriented neurology,* ed 2, St Louis, 1994, Mosby.

Omer GE, Spinner M: *Management of peripheral nerve problems,* Philadelphia, 1980, WB Saunders.

Otcenasek M et al: New approach to the urogynecological ultrasound examination, *Eur J Obstet Gynecol Reprod Biol* 103(1):72-74, 2002.

O'Young B, Young MA, Stiens SA: *PM&R secrets,* Philadelphia, 1997, Hanley & Belfus.

Pagana KD, Pagana TJ: *Mosby's manual of diagnostic and laboratory tests,* St Louis, 1998, Mosby.

Panjabi MM: The stabilizing system of the spine, part II, neutral zone and instability hypothesis, *J Spinal Disord* 5:390, 1992.

Panzer DM, Gatterman MI: Sacroiliac subluxation syndrome. In Gatterman MI, editor: *Foundations of chiropractic: subluxation,* St Louis, 1995, Mosby.

Patten J: *Neurological differential diagnosis,* ed 2, London, 1996, Springer.

Pecina MM, Krmpotic-Nemanic J, Markiewitz AD: *Tunnel syndromes,* Boca Raton, Fla, 1991, CRC Press.

Pheasant S: *Ergonomics, work and health,* Gaithersburg, Md, 1991, Aspen.

Polley HF, Hunder GG: *Rheumatologic interviewing and physical examination of the joints,* ed 2, Philadelphia, 1978, WB Saunders.

Poole G, Ward E: Causes of mortality in patients with pelvic fractures, *Orthopedics* 17:691, 1994.

Pope MH, Frymoyer JW, Krag MH: Diagnosing instability, *Clin Orthop* 279:60, 1992.

Pope MH et al: *Occupational low back pain assessment, treatment and prevention,* St Louis, 1991, Mosby.

Rachlin ES: *Myofascial pain and fibromyalgia trigger point management,* St Louis, 1994, Mosby.

Ravel R: *Clinical laboratory medicine clinical application of laboratory data,* ed 6, St Louis, 1995, Mosby.

Ro CS: Sacroiliac joint. In Cox JM editor: *Low back pain: mechanism, diagnosis and treatment,* ed 5, Baltimore, 1990, Williams & Wilkins.

Rogers LR: *Radiology of skeletal trauma,* ed 2, London, 1992, Churchill Livingstone.

Rolak LA: *Neurology secrets,* ed 2, Philadelphia, 1998, Hanley & Belfus.

Rothman RH, Simeone FA, editors: *The spine,* vol 1-2, Philadelphia, 1975, WB Saunders.

Rumack CM, Wilson SR, Charboneau JW: *Diagnostic ultrasound,* vol 1-2, ed 2, St Louis, 1998, Mosby.

Ruwe PA et al: Can MR imaging effectively replace diagnostic arthroscopy? *Radiology* 183:335, 1992.

Saidoff DC, McDonough AL: *Critical pathways in therapeutic intervention,* St Louis, 1997, Mosby.

Saudek CE: The hip. In Gould JA, editor: *Orthopaedic and sports physical therapy,* ed 2, St Louis, 1990, Mosby.

Schafer RC: *Clinical biomechanics,* ed 2, Baltimore, 1987, Williams & Wilkins.

Schlosstein L et al: High association of an HL-A antigen W 27 with ankylosing spondylitis and rheumatoid arthritis, *Ann Rheum Dis* 20:47, 1961.

Schmorl G, Junghanns H: *The human spine in health and disease,* Am ed 2, New York, 1971, Grune & Stratton (Translated by EF Bessmann).

Schumacher HR, Klippel JH, Koopman WJ: *Primer on the rheumatic diseases,* ed 10, Atlanta, 1993, Arthritis Foundation.

Shankman GA: *Fundamental orthopedic management for the physical therapist assistant,* St Louis, 1997, Mosby.

Sharma JB et al: High prevalence of Fitz-Hugh-Curtis syndrome in genital tuberculosis, *Int J Gynecol Obst* (in press, corrected proof).

Simons DG: Muscle pain syndromes, *J Manual Med* 6:3, 1991.

Singal DP et al: HLA antigens in osteitis condensans ilii and ankylosing spondylitis, *J Rheumatol* 4(suppl 3):105, 1977.

Sledge CB, Poss R: *The year book of orthopedics 1997,* St Louis, 1997, Mosby.

Smith-Petersen MN: Painful affections of lower back. In Christopher F, editor: *Textbook of surgery,* ed 5, Philadelphia, 1949, WB Saunders.

Snijders CJ, Vleeming A, Stoeckart R: Transfer of lumbosacral load to iliac bones and legs. Part 1: biomechanics of self-bracing of the sacroiliac joints and its significance for treatment and exercise, *Clin Biomech* 8(6):285-294, 1993.

Specht NT, Russo RD: *Practical guide to diagnostic imaging,* St Louis, 1998, Mosby.

Starlanyl D, Copeland ME: *Fibromyalgia & chronic myofascial pain syndrome: a survival manual,* Oakland, Calif, 1996, New Harbinger Publications.

Stedman TL: *Stedman's medical dictionary,* ed 25, Baltimore, 1990, Williams & Wilkins.

Stewart DL, Abeln SH: *Documenting functional outcomes in physical therapy,* St Louis, 1993, Mosby.

Stoller DW: *Magnetic resonance imaging in orthopaedics & sports medicine,* Philadelphia, 1993, JB Lippincott.

Strange FGS: The prognosis in sacro-iliac tuberculosis, *Br J Surg* 50:561, 1963.

Sutton D: *A textbook of radiology and imaging,* ed 5, London, 1993, Churchill Livingstone.

Sutton D, Young JWR: *A concise textbook of clinical imaging,* ed 2, St Louis, 1995, Mosby.

Swezey RI: Non-fibrositic lumbar subcutaneous nodules: prevalence and clinical significance, *Br J Rheumatol* 30:376, 1991.

Szlachter BN et al: Relaxin in normal and pathologenic pregnancies, *Obstet Gynecol* 59:167, 1982.

Tan JC, Horn SE: *Practical manual of physical medicine and rehabilitation,* St Louis, 1998, Mosby.

Taybi H, Lachman RS: *Radiology of syndromes, metabolic disorders, and skeletal dysplasias,* ed 4, St Louis, 1996, Mosby.

Taylor RW, Sonson RD: Separation of the pubic symphysis, an underrecognized peripartum complication, *J Reprod Med* 31:203, 1986.

Thibodeau GA, Patton KT: *Anatomy & physiology,* ed 3, St Louis, 1996, Mosby.

Thibodeau GA, Patton KT: *Pocket reference to accompany anatomy & physiology,* ed 3, St Louis, 1996, Mosby.

Thompson JM: *Clinical outlines for health assessment,* St Louis, 1997, Mosby.

Toghill PJ: *Examining patients: an introduction to clinical medicine,* London, 1990, Edward Arnold.

Tollison CD, Satterthwaite JR, Tollison JW: *Handbook of pain management,* ed 2, Baltimore, 1994, Williams & Wilkins.

Torg JS, Shepard RJ: *Current therapy in sports medicine,* ed 3, St Louis, 1995, Mosby.

Turek SL: *Orthopaedics principles and their application,* ed 3, Philadelphia, 1977, JB Lippincott.

Van Holsbeeck M, Introcaso JH: *Musculoskeletal ultrasound,* St Louis, 1991, Mosby.

Verrall GM et al: Hip joint range of motion reduction in sports-related chronic groin injury diagnosed as pubic bone stress injury, *J Sci Med Sport* 8(1):77-84, 2005.

Veys EM et al: HLA and infective sacroiliitis, *Lancet* 2:349, 1974.

Vleeming A et al: Mobility in the sacroiliac joints in the elderly: a kinematic and radiological study, *Clin Biomech* 7(3):170-176, 1992.

Vleeming A et al: The posterior layer of the thoracolumbar fascia, its function in load transfer from spine to legs, *Spine* 20:753, 1995.

Wakefield TS, Frank RG: The *examiner's guide to neuro musculoskeletal practice,* Abbotsford, Wis, 1995, Allied Health of Wisconsin, SC.

Wallace R, Cohen AS: Tuberculous arthritis: a report of two cases with review of biopsy and synovial fluid findings, *Am J Med* 61:277, 1976.

Walsh MJ: Evaluation of orthopedic testing of the low back for non-specific low back pain, J Manipulative Physiol Ther 21:232, 1998.

Wang M, Dumas GA: Mechanical behavior of the female sacroiliac joint and influence of the anterior and posterior sacroiliac ligaments under sagittal loads, *Clin Biomech* 13(4-5):293-299, 1998.

Watkins RG: *The spine in sports,* St Louis, 1996, Mosby.

Weiler PJ, King GJ, Geertzbein SD: Analysis of sagittal plane instability of the lumbar spine in vivo, *Spine* 12:1300, 1990.

Weineck J: *Functional anatomy in sports,* ed 2, St Louis, 1990, Mosby.

Weinstein SL, Buckwalter JA: *Turek's orthopaedics principles and their application,* ed 5, Philadelphia, 1994, JB Lippincott.

White AA, Panjabi MM: *Clinical biomechanics of the spine,* ed 2, Philadelphia, 1990, JB Lippincott.

White AH, Schofferman JA: *Spine care,* vol 1-2, St Louis, 1995, Mosby.

Wicke L: *Atlas of radiographic anatomy,* ed 5, Philadelphia, 1994, Lea & Febiger.

Wiesel SW, editor: *The lumbar spine,* Philadelphia, 1990, WB Saunders.

Wiesel SW, Bernini P, Rothman RH: *The aging lumbar spine,* Philadelphia, 1982, WB Saunders.

9

Windsor RE, Lox DM: *Soft tissue injuries: diagnosis and treatment,* Philadelphia, 1998, Hanley & Belfus.

Withrington RH, Sturge RA, Mitchell N: Osteitis condensans ilii or sacro-iliitis? *Scand J Rheumatol* 14:163, 1985.

Wollin M, Lovell G: Osteitis pubis in four young football players: a case series demonstrating successful rehabilitation, *Phys Ther Sport* 7(4):173-174, 2006.

Wray CC, Eason S, Huskinson J: Coccygodynia, aetiology and treatment, *J Bone Joint Surg* 73B:335, 1991.

Young D, Zimmerman G, Toomey M: Osteitis pubis, *J Sci Med Sport* 2(1, suppl 1):94-260, 1999.

Young JWR, Mirvis SE, editors: *Imaging in trauma and critical care,* Baltimore, 1991, Williams & Wilkins.

Zatouroff M: *Diagnosis in color physical signs in general medicine,* ed 2, London, 1996, Mosby-Wolfe.

Zitelli BJ, Davis HW: *Atlas of pediatric physical diagnosis,* ed 2, London, 1992, Wolfe.

CITATIONS

Berbaum KS et al: Satisfaction of search in multitrauma patients: severity of detected fractures, *Acad Radiol* 14(6):711-722, 2007.

Berthelot J-M et al: Provocative sacroiliac joint maneuvers and sacroiliac joint block are unreliable for diagnosing sacroiliac joint pain, *Joint Bone Spine* 73(1):17-23, 2006.

Botton E, Saraux A et al: Post fracture osteolysis of the pubic bone simulating a malignancy. Report of a case, *Joint Bone Spine* 71(3):230-233, 2004.

Botton E et al: Post fracture osteolysis of the pubic bone simulating a malignancy. Report of a case, *J Bone Spine* 71(3):230-233, 2004.

Cheng MB, Ferrante FM: Health-related quality of life in sacroiliac syndrome: a comparison to lumbosacral radiculopathy, *Reg Anesth Pain Med* 31(5):422-427, 2006.

Croce MA et al: Emergent pelvic fixation in patients with exsanguinating pelvic fractures, *J Am College of Surg* 204(5):935-939, 2007.

Dean Cole J, Blum DA, Ansel LJ: Outcome after fixation of unstable posterior pelvic ring injuries, *Clin Orthop Relat Res* 329:160-179, 1996.

Drerup B, Hierholzer E: Movement of the human pelvis and displacement of related anatomical landmarks on the body surface, *J Biomech* 20(10):971-977, 1987.

Gupta N et al: Genital tuberculosis in Indian infertility patients, *Int J Gynecol Obst* 97(2):135-138, 2007.

Hermann K-GA, Bollow M: Magnetic resonance imaging of the axial skeleton in rheumatoid disease, *Best Pract Res Clin Rheumatol* 18(6):881-907, 2004.

Hossain M, Nokes LDM: A model of dynamic sacro-iliac joint instability from malrecruitment of gluteus maximus and biceps femoris muscles resulting in low back pain, *Med Hypotheses* 65(2):278-281, 2005.

Li Z et al: Biomechanical response of the pubic symphysis in lateral pelvic impacts: a finite element study, *J Biomech* (in press, corrected proof).

Lindahl J et al: Failure of reduction with an external fixator in the management of injuries of the pelvic ring. Long-term evaluation of 110 patients, *J Bone Joint Surg* 81(6):955-962, 1999.

Mayrand N al: Diagnosis and management of posttraumatic piriformis syndrome: a case study, *J Manipulative Physiol Ther* 29(6):486-491, 2006.

Meknas K, Christensen A, Johansen O: The internal obturator muscle may cause sciatic pain, *Pain* 104(1-2):375-380, 2003.

Navaneeth BV, Thinagaran K, Sulaiman S: A preliminary report on pulmonary tuberculosis in patient travelers to a rural hospital of South India, *Travel Med Infect Dis* 5(2):142-143, 2007.

O'Sullivan PB et al: The relationship between posture and back muscle endurance in industrial workers with flexion-related low back pain, *Man Ther* 11(4):264-271, 2006.

Oransky M, Tortora M: Nonunions and malunions after pelvic fractures: why they occur and what can be done? *Injury* 38(4):489-496, 2007.

Phillips ATM et al: Finite element modeling of the pelvis: inclusion of muscular and ligamentous boundary conditions, *Med Eng Phys* 29(7):739-748, 2007.

Pouchot J et al: Tuberculosis, of the sacroiliac joint: clinical features, outcome, and evaluation of closed needle biopsy in 11 consecutive cases, *Am J Med* 84(3, part 2):622-628, 1988.

Rafii M et al: Computed tomography of traumatic serosanguineous cysts, *J Comput Tomogr* 7(4):385-388, 1983.

Robinson SP, Hammoud S, Sculco TP: Insufficiency fracture of the acetabular medial wall, *J Arthroplasty* (in press, corrected proof).

Schindler OS, Watura R, Cobby M: Sacral insufficiency fracture: an under-recognised condition, *Curr Orthop* 17(3):234-239, 2003.

Snijders CJ, Hermans PFG, Kleinrensink GJ: Functional aspects of cross-legged sitting with special attention to piriformis muscles and sacroiliac joints, *Clin Biomech* 21(2):116-121, 2006.

Snijders CJ et al: The influence of slouching and lumbar support on iliolumbar ligaments, intervertebral discs and sacroiliac joints, *Clin Biomech* 19(4):323-239, 2004.

Timgren J, Soinila S: Reversible pelvic asymmetry: an overlooked syndrome manifesting as scoliosis, apparent leg-length difference, and neurologic symptoms, *J Manipulative Physiol Ther* 29(7):561-565, 2006.

Tornetta Iii P, Matta JM: Outcome of operatively treated unstable posterior pelvic ring disruptions, *Clin Orthop Relat Res* 329:186-193, 1996.

Vleeming A et al: Load application to the sacrotuberous ligament; influences on sacroiliac joint mechanics, *Clin Biomech* 4(4):204-209, 1989.

Wollin M, Lovell G: Osteitis pubis in four young football players: a case series demonstrating successful rehabilitation, *Phys Ther Sport* 7(3):153-160, 2006.

Yoshioka H et al: MR imaging of radiation osteitis in the sacroiliac joints, *Magn Reson Imaging* 18(2):125-128, 2000.

CHAPTER TEN

HIP

AXIOMS IN ASSESSING THE HIP
- The hip joint is a ball-and-socket synovial joint.
- The hip is an exceptionally strong and stable joint, with a wide range of multiaxial movements.

INTRODUCTION

Hip pain is a common symptom with diverse causes. Typically, hip disease is associated with pain in the groin. The pain may radiate to the anterior, lateral, or medial thigh and occasionally to the knee. Causes of pain in the groin and anterior thigh area include iliopsoas bursitis, adduction tendinopathy, hernias, and pain from retroperitoneal structures and femoroacetabular impingement (Figs. 10-2 and 10-3).

> Femoroacetabular impingement is a relatively recently appreciated *idiopathic* cause of hip pain and degenerative change. Two types of impingement have been described. The first, cam impingement, is the result of an abnormal morphology of the proximal femur, typically at the femoral head–neck junction. Cam impingement is most common in young athletic men. The second, pincer impingement, is the result of an abnormal morphology or orientation of the acetabulum. Pincer impingement is most common in middle-age women (Kassarjian, Brisson, Palmer, in press).

Pain in the trochanteric area aggravated by the lateral decubitus position is highly suggestive of trochanteric bursitis. Pain in the ischiogluteal area aggravated by the sitting position should suggest an ischiogluteal bursitis. Groin pain aggravated by walking and relieved by rest is suggestive of a degenerative hip arthropathy. Pain in the same location, when associated with morning stiffness lasting more than 30 minutes and relieved by activity, is typical of an inflammatory arthropathy. Vascular insufficiency tends to produce buttock pain aggravated by walking and relieved within minutes by rest (Table 10-3).

Hip disease may result in adduction or abduction deformities. An adduction deformity is an upward tilt of the pelvis on the side of the adducted thigh (Fig. 10-4). An abduction deformity is an elevation of the uninvolved side.

Pain in the posterior aspect of the hip is most often referred from the lumbar spine.

Sacroiliac disorders can also cause buttock pain. Mechanical disorders of the thoracolumbar junction (T12 and L1) may refer pain to the greater trochanter area and thus may mimic trochanteric bursitis (Fig. 10-5). Thrombosis or aneurysm formation of branches of the aorta or iliac vessels may give rise to buttock, thigh, or leg pain that may be confused with hip pain. The presence of pain at the extremes of abduction and internal rotation suggests early hip disease caused by arthritis or osteonecrosis. Limitation of hip movements in all directions in a diabetic patient suggests an adhesive capsulitis of the hip joint. The presence of systemic symptoms, such as fatigue, fever, weight loss, or worsening of pain at night, requires baseline laboratory tests and a radio-

---

ORTHOPEDIC GAMUT 10-1
HIP

Loading forces acting on the hip:
1. Standing transfers one third of the body weight to the hip-joint mechanism.
2. Standing on one limb transfers 2.4 to 2.6 times the body weight to the hip-joint mechanism.
3. Walking transfers 1.3 to 5.8 times the body weight on the hip-joint mechanism.

TABLE 10-1

Hip Joint Cross-Reference Table by Assessment Procedure

DISEASE ASSESSED

Test/Sign	Leg Length	Hip Dislocation	Tibial Dysplasia	Fracture	Coxa Abnormality	Tibial/Fibular Fracture	Calcaneal Fracture	Pelvic Obliquity	Meningeal Irritation	Osteoarthritis	Iliotibial Band	Gracilis Contracture	Hip Flexion Contracture	Legg-Calvé-Perthes Disease	Poliomyelitis	Coxa Vara	Subluxation
Actual leg-length test	•							•									
Allis sign		•	•														
Anvil test				•	•	•	•										
Apparent leg-length test	•							•									
Chiene test				•													
Gauvain sign					•												
Guilland sign									•								
Hip telescoping test		•															
Jansen test					•					•							
Ludloff sign				•													
Ober test											•						
Patrick test					•												
Phelps test					•							•					
Thomas test					•								•				
Trendelenburg test		•		•						•				•	•	•	•

TABLE 10-2

Hip Joint Cross-Reference Table for Syndrome or Tissue

Calcaneal fracture	Anvil test	Hip flexion contracture	Thomas test
Coxa abnormality	Anvil test	Iliotibial band	Ober test
	Gauvain sign	Leg length	Actual leg-length test
	Jansen test		Apparent leg-length test
	Patrick test	Legg-Calvé-Perthes disease	Trendelenburg test
	Phelps test	Meningeal irritation	Guilland sign
	Thomas test	Osteoarthritis	Jansen sign
Coxa vara	Trendelenburg test		Trendelenburg test
Fracture	Anvil test	Pelvic obliquity	Actual leg-length test
	Chiene test		Apparent leg-length test
	Ludloff sign	Poliomyelitis	Trendelenburg test
	Trendelenburg test	Subluxation	Trendelenburg test
Gracilis contracture	Phelps test	Tibial dysplasia	Allis sign
Hip dislocation	Allis sign	Tibial/fibular fracture	Anvil test
	Hip telescoping test		
	Trendelenburg test		

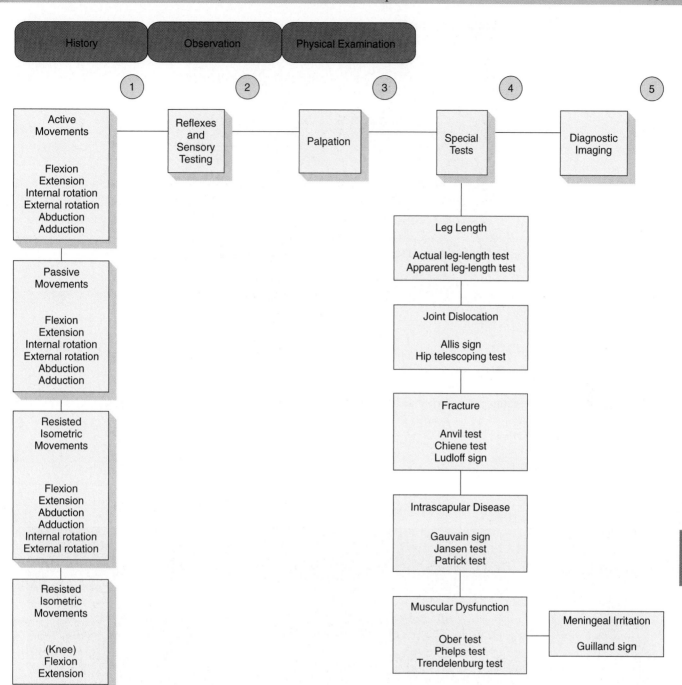

FIG. 10-1 Hip joint assessment.

nuclide bone scan in search of a tumor or an indolent infectious process.

ESSENTIAL ANATOMY

The femur is the longest and strongest bone in the body.

The femoral neck forms an *angle of inclination* with the femoral shaft on the frontal plane. In children, this angle may be up to 150 degrees; in adults, however, it is approximately 125 degrees. Variations in this angle commonly

---

ORTHOPEDIC GAMUT 10-2

PROXIMAL FEMUR

The four major components of the proximal femur are:
1. Greater trochanter
2. Lesser trochanter
3. Femoral neck
4. Femoral head

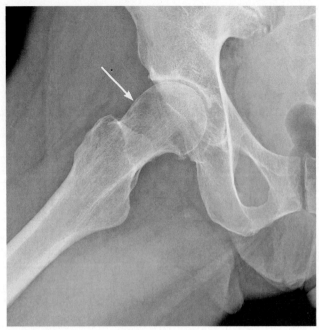

FIG. 10-2 In pure cam type impingement of the hip, the predominant abnormality is in the contour of the anterior/superior femoral head–neck junction with a normal morphology of the acetabulum. Normally, the anterior/superior femoral head–neck junction has a concave configuration. However, this junction is either flattened or convex in cam type impingement. (From Kassarjian A, Brisson M, Palmer WE: Femoroacetabular impingement, *Eur J Radiol* 63[1]:29-35, 2007.)

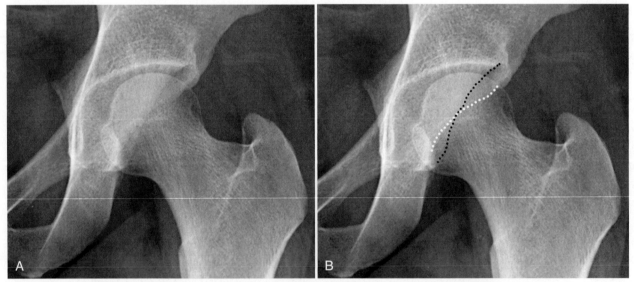

FIG. 10-3 In pure pincer type impingement, the predominant abnormality is with the morphology of the acetabulum with a relatively normal contour of the proximal femur. Abnormalities in acetabular morphology include acetabular retroversion, anterior and/or lateral over-coverage, and protrusio acetabulae. Radiograph (**A**) shows acetabular retroversion as the anterior acetabular rim passes lateral to the posterior acetabular rim. This is called the "crossover sign" as the two rims appear to intersect as indicated by the lines (**B**). (From Kassarjian A, Brisson M, Palmer WE: Femoroacetabular impingement, *Eur J Radiol* 63[1]:29-35, 2007.)

TABLE 10-3

HIP DIAGNOSTIC CONSIDERATIONS

Articular
Inflammatory joint diseases
  Rheumatoid arthritis
  Spondyloarthropathies
  Polymyalgia rheumatica
Degenerative joint diseases
  Primary osteoarthritis
  Secondary osteoarthritis
Metabolic joint diseases
  Gout
  Pseudogout
  Ochronosis
  Hemochromatosis
  Wilson disease
  Acromegaly
Infections
Tumors
  Benign
    Pigmented villonodular synovitis
    Osteochondromatosis
  Malignant
    Synovial sarcoma
    Synovial metastasis
Hemarthrosis
Juvenile
  Transient *toxic* synovitis
  Juvenile chronic arthritis

Periarticular
Bursitis
  Trochanteric
  Iliopsoas
  Ischiogluteal
Tendinitis
  Trochanteric
  Adductor
Acute calcific periarthritis
Heterotropic calcifications
Osseous
Bone lesions
  Fractures, neoplasms, infection, osteonecrosis of the femoral
  head, metabolic bone disease (Paget disease of bone, stress
  fractures, osteomalacia, hyperparathyroidism, renal
  osteodystrophy), reflex sympathetic dystrophy (transient
  migratory osteoporosis)
Juvenile
Congenital dislocation of the hip (usually not painful)
  Acetabular dysplasia
  Coxa vara
  Slipped capital femoral epiphysis
  Legg-Calvé-Perthes disease
  Rickets
Neurologic
Entrapment neuropathies
  Lateral femoral cutaneous nerve (meralgia paresthetica)
Lumbar nerve root compression L2, L3, and L4
Vascular
Atherosclerosis of aorta iliac vessels

Modified from Klippel JH, Dieppe PA: *Rheumatology,* vol 1-2, ed 2, London, 1998, Mosby.

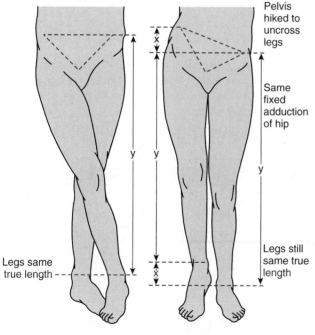

FIG. 10-4 Adduction deformity of the right hip. (From Klippel JH, Dieppe PA: *Rheumatology,* vol 1-2, ed 2, London, 1998, Mosby.)

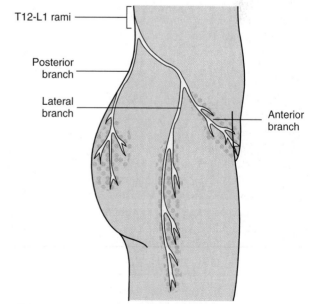

FIG. 10-5 Cutaneous branches originating from the T12–L1 rami. (From Klippel JH, Dieppe PA: *Rheumatology,* vol 1-2, ed 2, London, 1998, Mosby.)

10

occur. An increase in the angle of inclination is known as *coxa valga,* and a reduction in this angle is coxa vara (Fig. 10-6,*A*). The femoral neck is typically aligned anterior to the femoral shaft on the transverse plane. This *angle of anteversion* is approximately 15 degrees in adults. An increase in this angle is known as *excessive femoral anteversion;* a decrease is often called *femoral retroversion* (Fig. 10-6,*B*).

The ligamentum teres (ligamentum capitis femoris) arises from the transverse acetabular ligament and inserts into the fovea capitis in the head of the femur. Important small blood vessels supplying blood to the epiphyseal region of the head of the femur usually travel with this ligament (Fig. 10-7).

The load-bearing capacity of the femoral neck is enhanced by cancellous bone; the complex trabecular arrangement of this bone reinforces this structure to withstand compressive, tensile, and bending forces (Fig. 10-8). By virtue of a complex latticework, these bony columns act to reinforce each other to withstand these forces. Ward's triangle (a small area in the femoral neck with a high content of trabecular bone) often loses its trabecular bone in aged individuals and may be related to hip fractures.

Osteoporosis has long been recognized as a major health problem in women and has more recently gained attention as a condition that affects men significantly as well. Osteoporosis has become an increasingly important problem in men's health, accounting for significant morbidity in the aging male population. Patients with prostatic cancer treated with androgen deprivation therapy are at a high risk of osteoporosis. These patients may have additional morbidity from decreased bone mineralization, such as skeletal fractures.

> The rates of annual bone mass loss in aging men range from 0.5% to 1% compared with 1% to 2% in women. However, during androgen deprivation therapy (ADT), the annual rate of bone loss is much greater, reaching up to 9.6% (Morote et al, 2007).

Bone mineral density decrease is greater during the first year of ADT, with a range of 3.0% to 5.6%, depending on the measured site. After the first year of therapy, the density decreases annually by 1.1% to 2.3%.

The sciatic nerve (Fig. 10-9) leaves the pelvis via the sciatic notch and then passes, usually, under the piriformis muscle, which is covered by the gluteus maximus. In some individuals, the nerve or its peroneal divisions passes through the piriformis muscle and, more commonly, above it. The superior gluteal nerve, which innervates the gluteus medius and minimus and tensor fascia lata, branches off the sciatic trunk before the piriformis. However, the inferior gluteal nerve, which innervates the gluteus maximus, passes under the muscle (Fig. 10-10). Of the lower-extremity mononeuropathies, sciatic mononeuropathy is second in frequency only to peroneal mononeuropathy. The sciatic nerve is predisposed to injury by its proximity to the hip joint and its relatively long course from the sciatic notch to the popliteal fossa.

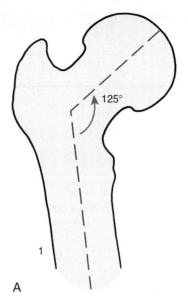

A

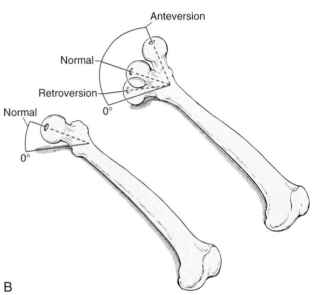

B

FIG. 10-6 **A,** Angle of inclination. **B,** Representation of retroversion and anteversion of the femoral neck. (From Malone TR, McPoil TG, Nitz AJ: *Orthopedic and sports physical therapy,* ed 3, St Louis, 1997, Mosby.)

ORTHOPEDIC GAMUT 10-3
GENDER PREVALENCE FACTORS IN OSTEOPOROSIS

The prevalence of osteoporosis is lower in men than in women for several physiologic reasons:
- A greater accumulation of skeletal mass during growth
- Greater bone size
- Absence of midlife menopause
- A slower rate of bone loss
- A shorter male life expectancy

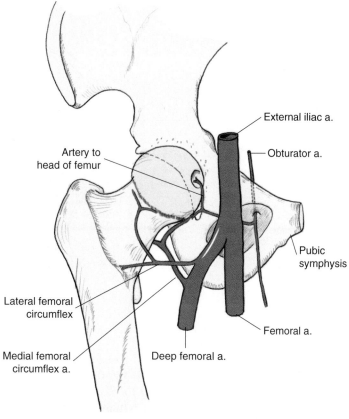

FIG. 10-7 Blood supply to the head of the femur. (From Mathers LH et al: *Clinical anatomy principles*, St Louis, 1996, Mosby.)

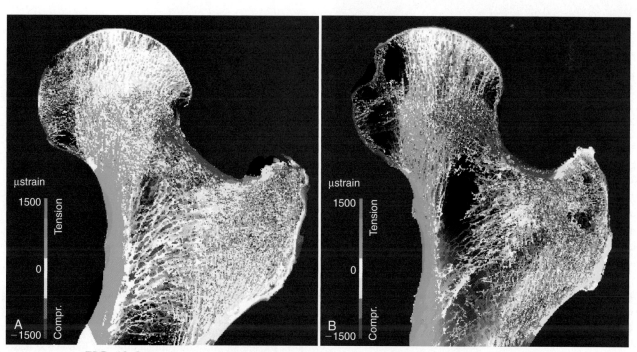

FIG. 10-8 Due to remodeling of bone architecture, an optimal structure is created that minimizes bone mass and maximizes strength. Maximal principal strain in the healthy (**A**) and osteoporotic (**B**) proximal femurs. The posterior halves are shown. (From Verhulp E, van Rietbergen B, Huiskes R: Load distribution in the healthy and osteoporotic human proximal femur during a fall to the side, *Bone* In Press.)

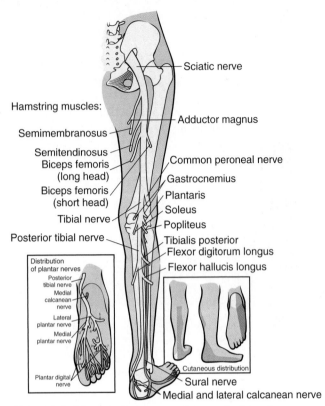

FIG. 10-9 The sciatic nerve and its main branches. (From Katirji B: *Electromyography in clinical practice: a case study approach,* St Louis, 1998, Mosby.)

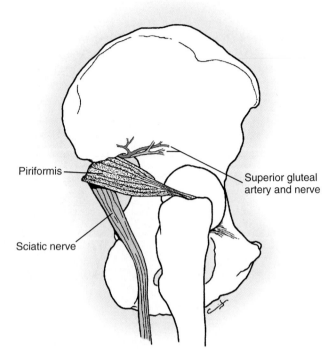

FIG. 10-10 Piriformis divides greater sciatic notch and is key to this region. Sciatic nerve is shown leaving pelvis below this muscle; superior gluteal artery, vein, and nerve are above it. (From Tile M: *Anatomy.* In Tile M: *Fractures of the pelvis and acetabulum,* Baltimore, 1995, Williams & Wilkins.) (Canale ST, Beaty JH: *Campbell's operative orthopaedics,* ed 11, Philadelphia, 2008, Mosby.)

ORTHOPEDIC GAMUT 10-4

HIP BURSAE

The three most clinically important hip bursae are as follows:
1. Trochanteric bursa
2. Iliopsoas bursa
3. Ischiogluteal bursa

ESSENTIAL MOTION ASSESSMENT

When measuring the range of hip movement, the examiner must ensure that the patient's pelvis remains stationary. To accomplish this task, the examiner keeps a hand on the patient's anterosuperior iliac spine to detect any movement.

To test flexion, the examiner should bend the patient's leg, with the knee flexed, into the abdomen. Standing behind the patient and drawing the leg backward until the point at which the pelvis starts to rotate best assesses extension. Abduction is measured by taking the leg outward, again to the point at which, by using the opposite hand, the pelvis is felt to move. Internal and external rotations are tested with the hip and knee flexed to 90 degrees.

Inspection of the hip joint includes an assessment of gait. A smooth and even gait indicates equal leg length and functional hip motion. Antalgic limp is characteristic of disease

---

ORTHOPEDIC GAMUT 10-5

HIP RANGE OF MOTION

In testing range of motion of the hips, the patient performs the following:

While supine
1. Raises the leg above the body with the knee extended
2. Brings the knee to the chest while keeping the other leg straight
3. Swings the leg laterally and medially while keeping the knee straight
4. Places the side of the foot on the opposite knee and moves the flexed knee down toward the examination table (external rotation)
5. Flexes the knee and rotates the leg so that the flexed knee moves inward toward the opposite leg (internal rotation)

While either prone or standing
1. Swings the straightened leg behind the body

that produces pain in a hip joint; the body tilts toward the involved diseased hip in such a way that the weight of the body is directly over the hip. This limp decreases the need for abductor muscle movement and thus may alleviate muscle spasm. If the abductor muscles are weak (i.e., unable to support the pelvis), the unaffected hip may move down-ward in such a way that the weight is borne on that side. This condition is called *Trendelenburg limp.*

Among all of the movements of the hip, abduction and internal rotation are usually the first ones to be painful or limited in the presence of hip abnormality (Figs. 10-11 to 10-16).

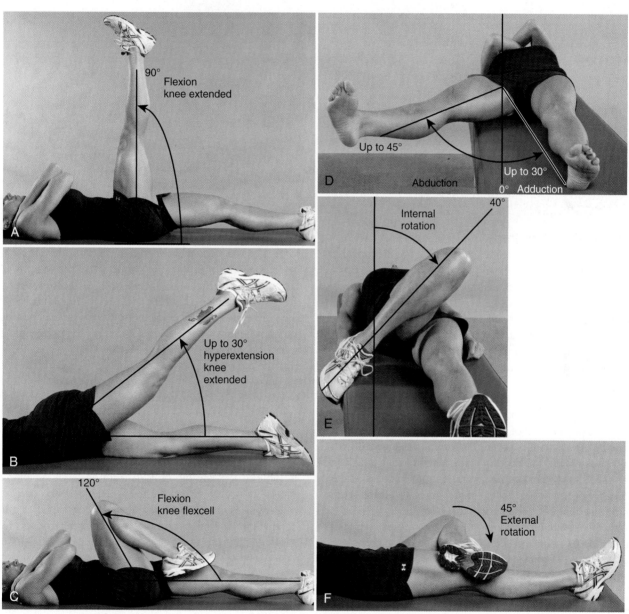

FIG. 10-11 Range of motion of the hip. **A,** Hip flexion with the leg extended. **B,** Hip hyperextension, knee extended. **C,** Hip flexion, knee flexed. **D,** Abduction. **E,** Internal rotation. **F,** External rotation.

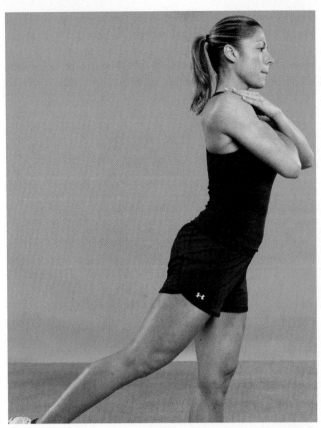

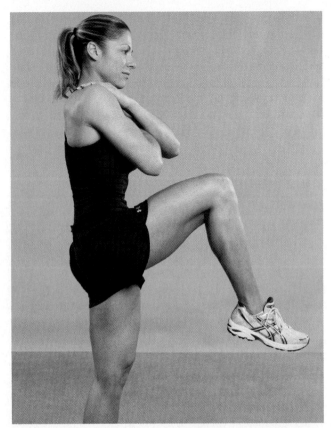

FIG. 10-12 Extension of the hip is defined as the upward (or backward) motion of the hip from the zero starting position. Motion beyond the neutral position (0 degrees) is sometimes alternatively called hyperextension. Extension of the hip is likely to reflect some motion of the back, but this motion is uncommon. Extension normally may measure 10 to 20 degrees less when the patient is prone or supine than when the patient is standing. The difference is attributed to a greater extensor torque, which is created by the weight of the torso, centered slightly posterior to the hip joint in a normal standing position.

In the usual method of clinical examination for extension of the hip, the patient is prone. The examiner applies downward pressure to the sacrum with a flattened hand. The examiner's other hand, which is placed midway against the anterior aspect of the patient's thigh, is used to lift the thigh on the side that is being examined.

With the available methods of eliminating exaggerated lumbar lordosis and accomplishing fixation of the pelvis, 15 degrees of extension or hyperextension of the hip may be obtained. With less adequate fixation or with abnormal laxity of the ligaments of the hip (a rarity), the thigh may be hyperextended approximately 30 to 40 degrees. Retained extension range of motion (standing or prone) of 20 degrees or less is an impairment of the hip in the activities of daily living.

FIG. 10-13 The greatest degree of flexion of the hip while in the standing position is possible when the knee is also flexed. The thigh can be flexed to 120 degrees from the neutral or extended position (0 degrees), if the knee has first been flexed to 90 degrees. Sometimes, the hip can be flexed until the anterior surface of the thigh presses against the anterior abdominal wall.

If the knee cannot be flexed, raising the extended leg off the surface of the examination table can test flexion of the hip. If the knee remains extended, tension of the hamstring muscles will limit flexion of the hip. The angle between the thigh and the long axis of the body, when the hip is normal, may not be more than a right angle (90 degrees).

However, some individuals with apparently normal hips are able to flex the hip only to form an angle of approximately 75 degrees when the leg is extended. In other individuals, the range of motion is much greater than 90 degrees. Retained flexion range of motion of 90 degrees or less is an impairment of hip function in the activities of daily living.

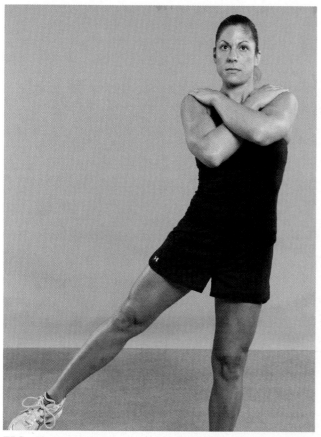

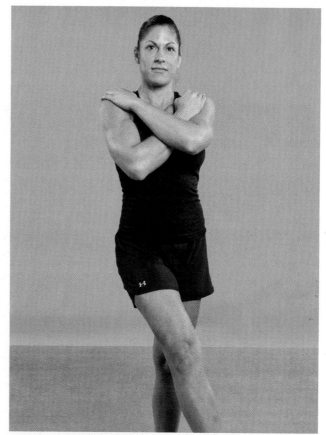

FIG. 10-14 Abduction and adduction are measured while both thighs and legs are in the extended position and are parallel to each other. The patient can be standing or supine. Measurement is made from the angle formed between an imaginary midline that is extended from the long axis of the body and the long axis of the leg. The amount of abduction permitted increases with flexion and decreases with extension of the hip. Normally, when the leg and thigh are extended, the hip abducts to approximately 40 to 45 degrees from the neutral position before the pubofemoral and medial portions of the iliofemoral ligaments restrict this abduction. Retained abduction range of motion of 30 degrees or less is an impairment of the hip in the activities of daily living.

FIG. 10-15 Adduction with the leg straight out is limited by the legs and thighs, which come into contact with each other. When it is possible to adduct the hip with enough flexion to permit crossing one leg over the other and then reversing the procedure, the degree of adduction of the hip of the extremity that is on top can be measured. Adduction is usually possible to approximate 20 to 30 degrees from the neutral (starting) position.

10

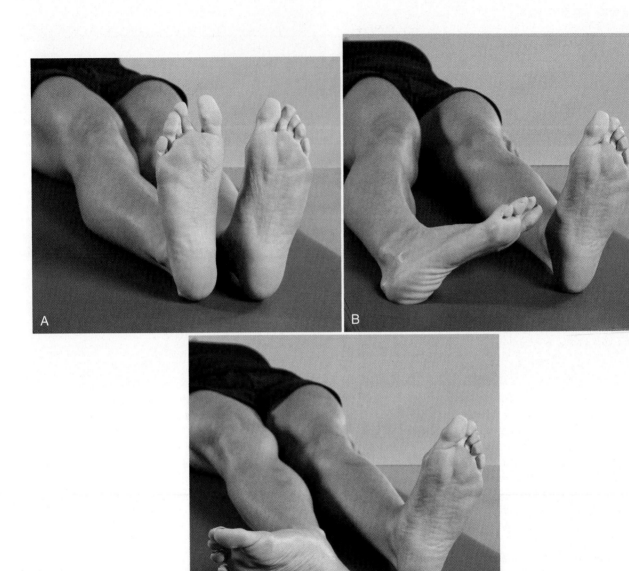

FIG. 10-16 External and internal rotation of the hip can be tested with the patient's hip and knee fully extended while the patient is supine. **A,** Rolling the thigh, leg, and foot inward. **B,** Rolling the thigh, leg, and foot outward. **C,** The hip normally rotates inward approximately 40 degrees and outward approximately 45 degrees. However, the range of motion varies among normal individuals, and both sides should be compared. The lateral band of the iliofemoral ligament limits external rotation. The ischiocapsular ligament limits internal rotation. Rotation of the hip increases with flexion and decreases with extension of the hip. Limitation of internal rotation of the hip is the earliest and most reliable sign of disease of the hip.

Retained internal rotation of 30 degrees or less or retained external rotation range of motion of 40 degrees or less is an impairment of the hip in the activities of daily living.

ESSENTIAL MUSCLE FUNCTION ASSESSMENT

Sciatic palsies are associated with pelvic trauma, injuries to the buttock or thigh, and infiltration by tumor. The muscles supplied by the lateral popliteal component of the nerve tend to be more affected than those supplied by the medial popliteal branch (Fig. 10-17).

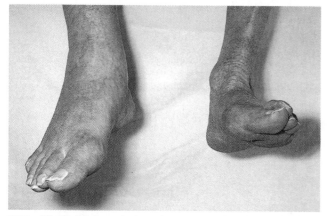

FIG. 10-17 Right sciatic palsy. (From Epstein O et al: *Clinical examination,* ed 2, London, 1997, Mosby.)

Muscles acting at the hip joint may have additional actions on the spine or knee. The psoas major passes from the lumbar spine to the lesser trochanter of the femur. In addition to flexing the hip, it flexes the lumbar spine.

The gluteus maximus, the thickest muscle in the body, forms a soft-tissue barrier to protect the posterior hip and large neurovascular structures of the buttock region (Fig. 10-18). Deep to the gluteus maximus, several smaller muscles that act externally to rotate this joint (Fig. 10-19) span the posterior hip. The iliopsoas muscle passes anterior to the hip joint and acts with the rectus femoris, sartorius, tensor fasciae latae, and anterior hip adductors to create a potential for flexion of the hip against strong resistance.

The innervation of the hip joint follows Hilton's law, which states that a joint is innervated by the same nerves that innervate the muscles acting on it. Thus, branches from the femoral, sciatic, obturator, and superior and inferior gluteal nerves innervate the hip joint. The sclerotome reference for the hip joint is generally considered to be L3. The cutaneous innervation of the hip, buttock, and thigh can be referenced to peripheral nerves or dermatomes (Figs. 10-20 to 10-25).

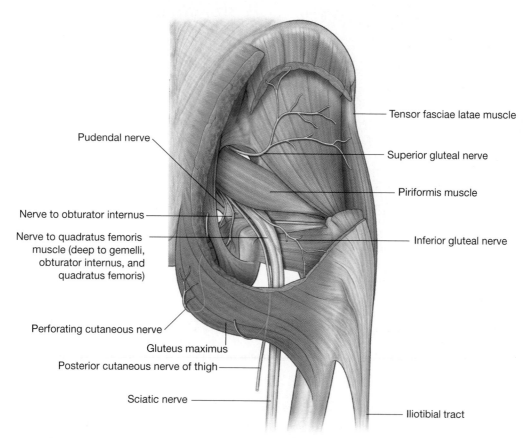

FIG. 10-18 The sciatic nerve enters the gluteal region through the greater sciatic foramen inferior to the piriformis muscle. (From Drake RL: *Gray's anatomy for students: with student consult online access,* New York, 2005, Churchill Livingstone.)

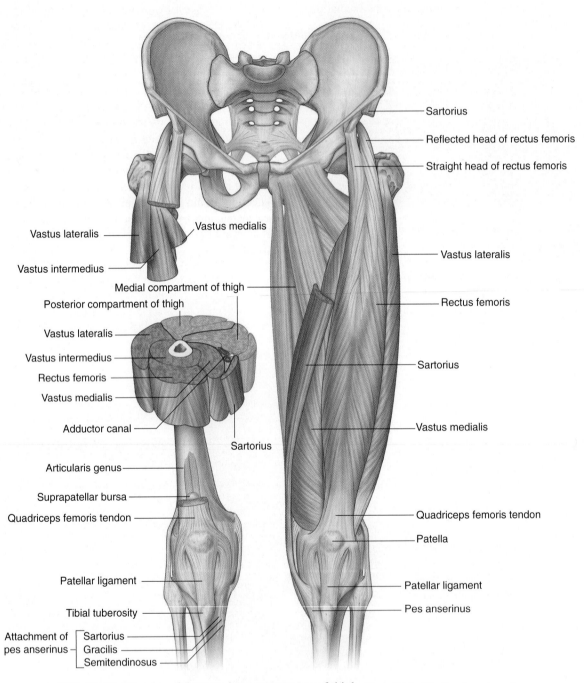

FIG. 10-19 Muscles of the anterior compartment of thigh. (From Drake RL: *Gray's anatomy for students: with student consult online access,* New York, 2005, Churchill Livingstone.)

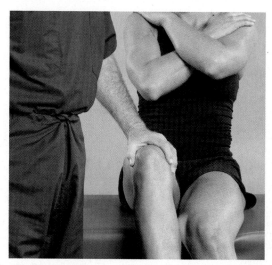

FIG. 10-20 The iliopsoas is the primary flexor of the hip, and it is innervated by the femoral nerve, which contains the L1, L2, and L3 nerve roots. To test the strength of the iliopsoas, the patient is examined while seated on the examination table. The examiner asks the patient to flex the hip against manual resistance, which the examiner provides. Accessory muscles involved are the rectus femoris, sartorius, tensor fasciae latae, pectineus, adductor brevis, adductor longus, and the oblique fibers of the adductor magnus muscle. Flexion of the hip also may be tested while the patient is lying supine with the knee extended. Tension of the hamstring muscles, when they are stretched, may limit flexion and interfere with interpretation of the test.

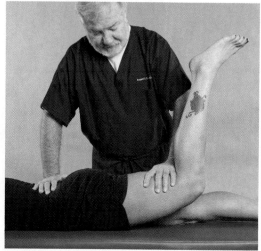

FIG. 10-21 Prime movers in extension of the hip are the gluteus maximus (inferior gluteal nerve, L5, S1, and S2), semitendinosus (tibial branch of sciatic nerve, L4, L5, S1, and S2), and semimembranosus (tibial branch of sciatic nerve, L5, S1, and S2) muscles, as well as the long head of the biceps femoris (tibial branch of the sciatic nerve, S1, S2, and S3) muscle. To measure the strength of the gluteus maximus, the patient is placed prone on the examination table and is directed to extend the hip against the examiner's hand, which is placed on the thigh and pelvis.

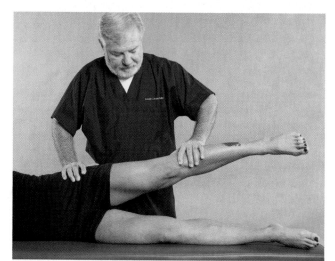

FIG. 10-22 The gluteus medius muscle (superior gluteal nerve, L4, L5, and S1) is the prime mover in abduction of the hip. The gluteus minimus, tensor fasciae latae, and upper fibers of the gluteus maximus muscles are accessory to this motion. The strength of these can be estimated by observing the patient's gait and using Trendelenburg's test. An additional test can be performed by placing the patient in a side-lying position on the examination table and having the patient abduct the hip against resistance provided by the examiner.

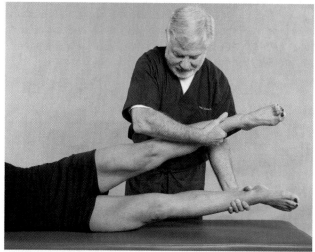

FIG. 10-23 Prime movers in adduction of the hip are the adductor magnus (obturator and sciatic nerves, L3, L4, L5, and S1), adductor brevis (obturator nerve, L3, and L4), adductor longus (obturator nerve, L3, and L4), pectineus (femoral nerve, L2, L3, L4, and occasionally obturator nerve, L3, and L4), and gracilis (obturator nerve, L3, and L4) muscles. Adduction is tested while the patient is lying on one side with the legs extended. The upper leg, which is supported by one of the examiner's hands, is held in approximately 25 degrees of abduction. The patient then adducts the lower leg off the table, toward the elevated leg, without rotating the leg or tipping the pelvis. The examiner's free hand provides graded resistance proximal to the knee joint.

10

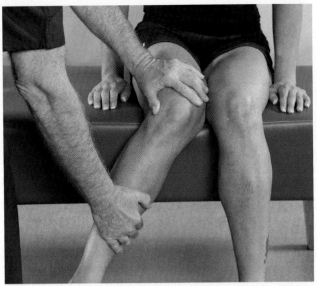

FIG. 10-24 Prime movers in external rotation of the hip are
the obturator externus (obturator nerve, L3, and L4), obturator internus (sacral plexus, L4, L5, and S1), piriformis
(sacral plexus, S1, and S2), gemellus superior (sacral plexus,
L5, S1, and S2), gemellus inferior (sacral plexus, L4, L5,
and S1), and the gluteus maximus (inferior gluteal nerve,
L5, S1, and S2) muscles. The sartorius muscle is accessory
to this motion. Lateral rotation of the hip is tested while the
patient sits with the legs hanging over the edge of the table.
The examiner places one hand over the lateral aspect of the
thigh, just above the knee, and applies counterpressure to
the thigh to prevent abduction and flexion of the hip. The
patient can grasp the edge of the table to help stabilize the
pelvis. The patient then rotates the hip and thigh laterally,
and the lower leg rotates medially while the examiner's
other hand applies graded resistance above the ankle against
the motion being tested.

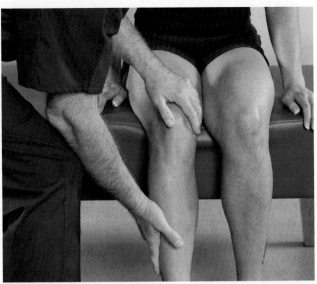

FIG. 10-25 Prime movers in internal rotation of the hip are
the gluteus minimus (superior gluteal nerve, L4, L5, and S1)
and the tensor fasciae latae (superior gluteal nerve, L4, L5,
and S1) muscles. Anterior fibers of the gluteus medius, semimembranosus, and semitendinosus muscles are accessory to
this motion. Medial rotation of the hip is tested while the
patient sits with the legs over the edge of a table as if testing
lateral rotation of the hip. The examiner uses one hand to
apply counterpressure above the knee and over the medial
aspect of the thigh to prevent adduction of the hip. The
patient holds the edge of the table to stabilize the pelvis. The
patient then rotates the thigh medially and rotates the lower
leg laterally while the examiner's other hand provides graded
resistance above the ankle joint.

ORTHOPEDIC GAMUT 10-6
BASIC HIP IMAGING STUDY

The basic hip plain-film imaging study:
1. AP pelvic (Figs. 10-26 and 10-27) view
2. AP spot hip (Fig. 10-28) view
3. Lateral (frog-leg) spot view of the side of complaint
   (Figs. 10-29 and 10-30)

ORTHOPEDIC GAMUT 10-7
OSSEOUS DEFORMITIES OF THE PROXIMAL FEMUR

Four common osseous deformities of the proximal
femur are:
1. Coxa vara
2. Coxa valga
3. Femoral anteversion
4. Femoral retroversion

ESSENTIAL IMAGING

The major part of the pelvis is typically visualized with a
single anteroposterior (AP) view. Both lower extremities are
internally rotated approximately 20 degrees to elongate the
femoral necks and take the trochanteric processes out of
superimposition with the femoral necks.

The AP pelvic view allows comparative assessment of
the various paired structures of the pelvic girdle and hip
regions, and the spot AP view brings the central ray to the
area of interest, allowing better projection advantage.

The lateral frog-leg spot view offers a 90-degree or true
lateral analysis of the proximal femur. Occasionally, a bilat-

eral frog projection can be performed as an expedient survey, particularly to rule out slipped capital femoral epiphysis.

Whether occurring unilaterally or bilaterally, each of these conditions can result in alterations in load bearing throughout the lower limb and spine and thus are of great importance.

Excessive femoral anteversion is a condition in which the angle between the femoral neck and the femoral shaft on the transverse plane is greater than approximately 12 degrees in adults. When this deformity is present, the ipsilateral lower limb appears to be excessively internally rotated when the femoral head is in the neutral position within the acetabulum (Fig. 10-31). The range of motion of hip internal rotation is usually greater than external rotation (Fig. 10-32). Craig test is typically positive.

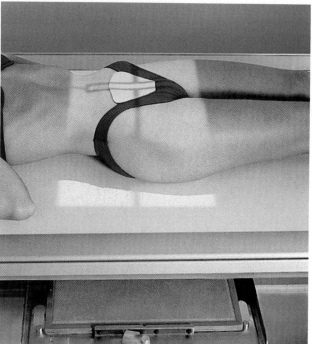

FIG. 10-26 Female anteroposterior pelvis positioning with gonad *(shadow)* shield. (From Frank ED et al: *Merrill's atlas of radiographic positioning and procedures*, vol 1-3, ed 11, St Louis, 2007, Mosby.)

ORTHOPEDIC GAMUT 10-8
COXA VARA

The developmental and acquired conditions that can resulting in coxa vara are:
1. Intertrochanteric fracture
2. Slipped capital femoral epiphysis
3. Legg-Calvé-Perthes disease
4. Congenital hip dislocation
5. Rickets
6. Paget disease

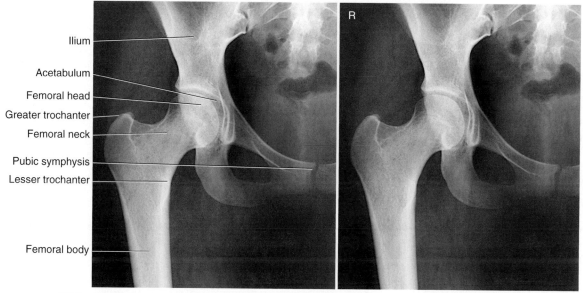

Ilium
Acetabulum
Femoral head
Greater trochanter
Femoral neck
Pubic symphysis
Lesser trochanter
Femoral body

FIG. 10-27 Anteroposterior hip images. (From Frank ED et al: *Merrill's atlas of radiographic positioning and procedures*, vol 1-3, ed 11, St Louis, 2007, Mosby.)

10

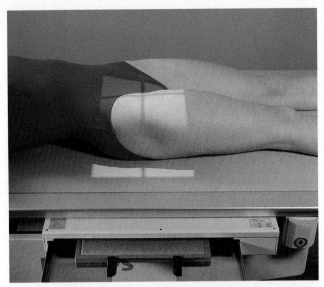

FIG. 10-28 Anteroposterior hip positioning. (From Frank ED et al: *Merrill's atlas of radiographic positioning and procedures*, vol 1-3, ed 11, St Louis, 2007, Mosby.)

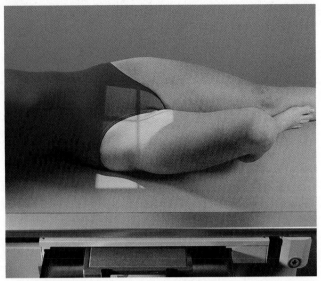

FIG. 10-29 Unilateral anteroposterior oblique femoral neck positioning: modified Cleaves method. (From Frank ED et al: *Merrill's atlas of radiographic positioning and procedures*, vol 1-3, ed 11, St Louis, 2007, Mosby.)

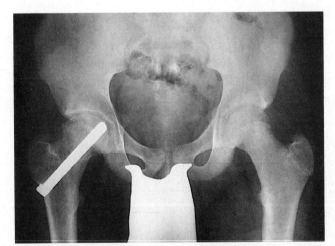

FIG. 10-30 Anteroposterior oblique femoral neck images. Note fixation device in right hip and gonad shield. (From Frank ED et al: *Merrill's atlas of radiographic positioning and procedures*, vol 1-3, ed 11, St Louis, 2007, Mosby.)

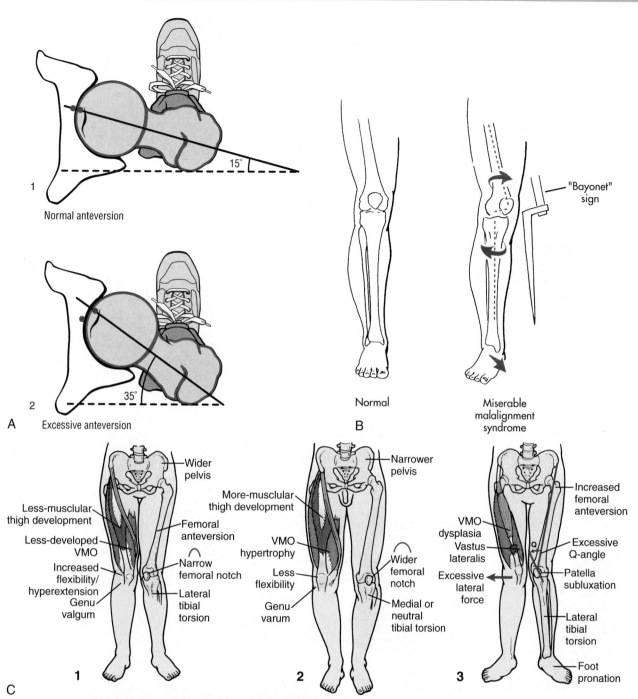

FIG. 10-31 **A,** A superior view showing the angle of torsion of the right hip. *1,* The 15-degree anterior projection of the femoral head is considered normal anteversion of the hip. *2,* Excessive anteversion of the right hip. (From Neumann DA: *Kinesiology of the musculoskeletal system: foundations for physical rehabilitation,* St Louis, 2002, Mosby.) **B,** Miserable malalignment syndrome. Anatomic alignment is assessed in the standing position. The miserable malalignment syndrome is characterized by combined femoral anteversion, "squinting patellae," external tibial torsion, and foot pronation. (From Shankman GA: *Fundamental orthopedic management for the physical therapist assistant,* ed 2, St Louis, 2004, Mosby.) **C,** *1,* Normal female alignment with wider pelvis, femoral anteversion, genu valgum, hyperflexibility, lateral tibial torsion, and narrow notch. *2,* Normal male alignment demonstrates a narrower pelvis, more developed musculature, genu varum, medial or neutral tibial torsion, and wider notch. *3,* Miserable malalignment syndrome is a term coined to describe patients who have increased femoral anteversion, genu valgum, vastus medialis obliquus (VMO) dysplasia, lateral tibial torsion, and forefoot pronation. These factors create excessive lateral forces and contribute to patellofemoral dysfunction. (From Griffin LY, editor: *Rehabilitation of the injured knee,* St Louis, 1995, Mosby–Year Book.)

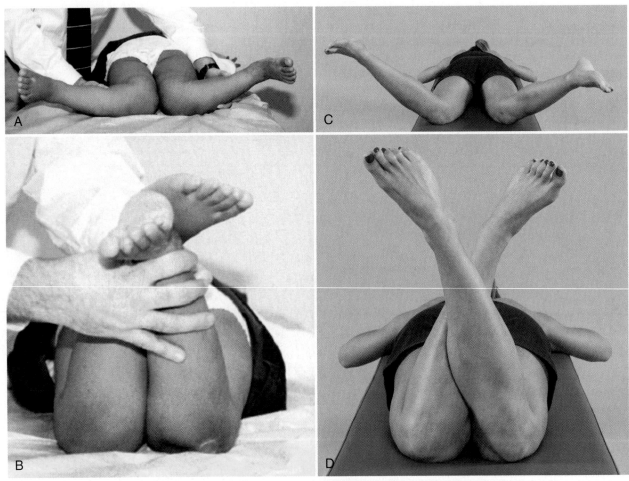

FIG. 10-32 Anteversion measured by medial rotation of hip (**A**) and lateral rotation of
hip (**B**). (From Kliegman: Nelson textbook of pediatrics, ed 18, Philadelphia, 2007 Saunders.) **C** and **D**,
The typical range of motion pattern of the hips without bilateral femoral anteversion.
C, Internal rotation; **D,** external rotation.

Assessment for True Leg-Length Discrepancy

Comment

In terms of millimeters, large amounts of anatomic leg-length inequality are infrequent. In a population of 2.68 million, the ratio is 1 person in 1000 with leg-length inequality of more than 20 mm (approximately 0.75 inch) (Guichet et al, 1991).

The initial assessment of leg-length inequality begins with the physical examination. In the standing position on a flat floor, symmetry of the gluteal folds and transverse popliteal skin creases of both legs are inspected, as well as other findings such as pelvic tilting, scoliosis, and leg or foot deformities. Younger children are examined in the supine position on a firm, flat surface, with the feet held in a flat plane on the examining surface and the knees flexed to 90 degrees. In this position, determination of whether the femur or tibia of the affected limb is longer or shorter than the opposite one is accomplished (*Galeazzi test*).

Methods of measuring the lower limbs are often confusing. Accuracy in measurement is of more than academic significance. Accurate measurement is of practical importance when corrective operations or adjustments to the shoes are contemplated. Limb length can be measured clinically within an error of 1 cm. If greater accuracy is needed, radiographic measurement (scanography) is recommended (Fig. 10-33).

The first required step is to measure the real, or true, length of each limb. Second, the examiner must determine the existence of any apparent, or false, discrepancy in the length of the limbs as a result of fixed pelvic tilt. Measuring the true leg length is always necessary. Also necessary is to measure apparent discrepancy only when a correctable pelvic tilt is observed.

The anterosuperior iliac spine is far lateral to the axis of hip movement. This positioning does not matter if the angle between the limb and the pelvis is the same on each side.

The measurements will be fallacious if the angle between limb and pelvis is not the same for each side. Abduction of a hip brings the medial malleolus nearer to the corresponding anterosuperior iliac spine. Adduction of the hip carries the medial malleolus away from the anterosuperior iliac spine. Thus, if measurements are made while the patient lies with one hip adducted and the other abducted (a common posture in cases of hip disease), inaccurate readings will be obtained. The length will be exaggerated on the adducted side and diminished on the abducted side.

Obtaining an accurate comparison of true length by surface measurement requires that the two limbs be placed in comparable positions relative to the pelvis. If one limb is adducted and cannot be brought out to the neutral position, the other limb must be adducted through a corresponding angle by crossing it over the first limb before the measurements are taken. Similarly, if one hip is in fixed abduction, the other hip must be abducted to the same angle before the measurements of true length are made.

In fixing the tape measure to the anterosuperior iliac spine, a flat metal end is essential. The metal end is placed immediately distal to the anterosuperior iliac spine, and this end is pushed up against the spine. The thumb is then pressed firmly backward against the bone and the tape end. This procedure provides rigid fixation of the tape measure against the bone.

When taking the reading at the medial malleolus, the tip of the index finger should be placed immediately distal to the medial malleolus and should be pushed up against it. The thumbnail is brought down against the tip of the index finger, pinching the tape measure between them. The thumbnail indicates the point of measurement.

If measurements reveal real shortening of a limb, the examiner must determine whether the shortening is above the trochanteric level (suggesting an affection in or near the hip) or below the trochanteric level (suggesting an affection of the limb bones).

In principle, Bryant triangle is nothing more than a method of comparing the distance between the greater tro-

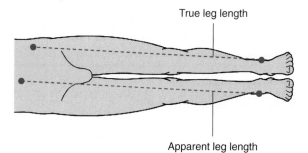

True leg length

Apparent leg length

FIG. 10-33 Leg length measurement. (From Klippel JH, Dieppe PA: *Rheumatology*, vol 1-2, ed 2, London, 1998, Mosby.)

ORTHOPEDIC GAMUT 10-9

LEG-LENGTH DEFICIENCY

Tests to determine leg-length deficiency occurring above the trochanteric level include:
1. Measurement of Bryant triangle
2. Construction of Nélaton line
3. Construction of Shoemaker line

chanter and the wing of the ilium on the two sides. While the patient is lying supine, a perpendicular is dropped from the anterosuperior spine of the ilium toward the examination table. A second line is projected upward from the tip of the greater trochanter to meet the first line at a right angle. The second line is the important line of the triangle because it is measured and compared bilaterally. The third side of the triangle is unimportant. This third line joins the anterosuperior iliac spine to the tip of the greater trochanter. Measurement of Bryant triangle allows for comparison of the distance between the pelvis and the trochanter on each side. Relative shortening on one side indicates that the femur is displaced upward as a result of a lesion in or near the hip. If a possibility exists that both sides are abnormal, measurement of Bryant triangle is not helpful.

Nélaton line is measured while the patient is lying on the unaffected side. A tape measure or string is stretched on the affected side from the tuberosity of the ischium to the anterosuperior spine of the ilium. Normally, the greater trochanter lies on or below this tape measure line. If the trochanter lies above the line, the femur has been displaced upward.

Shoemaker line is a similar test involving projection of two lines, one on each side of the body, from the greater trochanter through and beyond the anterosuperior iliac spine. Normally, the two lines meet in the midline above the umbilicus. If one femur is displaced upward because of shortening above the greater trochanter, the lines will meet away from the midline on the opposite side. If both femora are displaced, the lines will meet at or near the midline but below the umbilicus.

True shortening is sometimes caused by an abnormality such as a congenital defect of development, impaired epiphyseal growth, congenital vascular malformations, or previous fracture with overlapping of the fragments that occurs below the trochanteric level (Fig 10-34). To investigate this possibility, the examiner should obtain measurements of the femur (tip of the greater trochanter to the line of the knee joint) and of the tibia (line of the knee joint to the medial malleolus) on each side.

Leg-length discrepancy (LLD) has been reported as a sequela of congenital vascular malformations affecting the lower extremity and may result in disfigurement, gait disturbance, pelvic tilting, scoliosis, or back pain. In the general population, the prevalence of LLD of less than 2 cm has been reported to be 40% to 70%. In contrast, an LLD of greater than 2 cm has been reported to be very rare. In addition, the reported prevalence of LLD varies according to the definition and methods of assessment, and various cutoff points have been used as criteria for surgical or nonsurgical intervention of LLD by orthopedic surgeons (Kim et al, 2006).

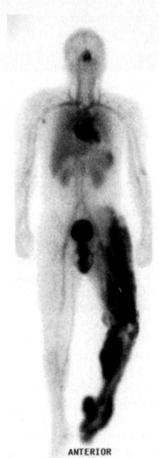

ANTERIOR

FIG. 10-34 Extent of the congenital vascular malformation lesion. Whole-body blood pools scan in a patient with venous malformation that involves the left whole leg. (From Kim YW, Lee SH, Kim DI, et al: Risk factors for leg length discrepancy in patients with congenital vascular malformation, *J Vasc Surg* 44[3]:545-53, 2006.)

PROCEDURE

- The patient is lying supine with the feet together, the knees and hips straight, and the anterosuperior iliac spines and the iliac crests exposed.
- The examiner, by way of palpation, marks the apex of the anterior iliac spines and the crests of the ilia.
- The examiner then measures the distance between these features and the medial malleolus (Fig. 10-35).
- The distance is recorded and compared with the opposite side.
- These distances represent the actual leg length.
- Actual LLDs are caused by an abnormality above or below the trochanter level.

Next Steps/Procedure
Apparent leg-length measurements

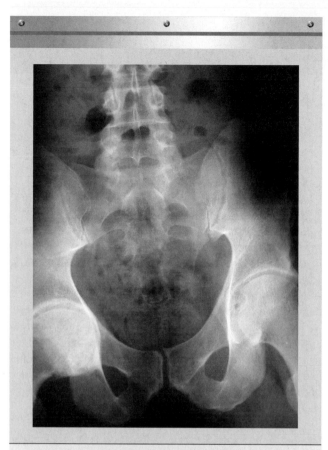

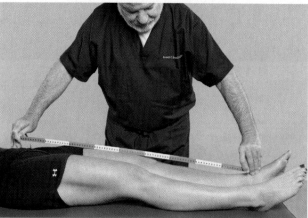

FIG. 10-35 The patient is lying supine with the feet together. The knees and hips are straight. With a tape measure, the examiner measures the length of the affected leg from the apex of the anterosuperior iliac spine to the medial malleolus. The distance is recorded and compared with the opposite leg. Actual leg-length shortening is caused by an abnormality above or below the trochanter level.

AT THE VIEWBOX

35-year-old male with right hip pain and diminished range of motion. There is marked pelvic obliquity due to marked leg length discrepancy, low on the right (reading left). The lower lumbar spine lists to the right, demonstrating lack of proper compensation for the pelvic obliquity. Lower extremity deficiency may be a source of low back and lower extremity pain. (From the teaching file of Timothy Mick, DC, DACBR)

10

CLINICAL PEARL

Causes of true shortening above the trochanter include (1) coxa vara, resulting from neck fractures, slipped epiphysis, Perthes disease, and congenital coxa vara; (2) loss of articular cartilage from infection or arthritis; and (3) dislocation of the hip. Rarely does lengthening of the other limb give relative, true shortening. This relative, true shortening may be caused by (1) stimulation of bone growth from increased vascularity, which may occur after long bone fracture in children or bone tumor, and (2) coxa valga, which follows polio.

ALLIS SIGN

ALSO KNOWN AS GALEAZZI SIGN

Assessment for Femoral Portion Structural Deficiency or Tibial Portion Structural Deficiency

Comment

Even though the cause of osteonecrosis at the femoral head is unclear, the widely accepted belief is that the process is initiated by vascular occlusion, which may be the result of trauma or occur spontaneously and is intermittent (Fig. 10-36). Trauma may include inflammation, as well as endocrine and nutritional disturbances.

At the beginning of the last century, Legg, Calvé, and Perthes independently identified a special type of osteonecrosis of the femoral head seen in children. This disease was subsequently named Legg-Calvé-Perthes disease (LCPD). It is now known to occur in children mainly between the age of 2 and 14 years, with an incidence of 0.05% to 0.11%, a boy-to-girl ratio of 5:1, and with 15% of the patients suffering bilateral disease. The cause if LCPD remains a factor of discussion, although it has now become generally accepted to be initiated by an intermittent vascular occlusion, the precise origin of which and its underlying mechanism still remaining unclear. Theories have suggested trauma, inflammation, and endocrine and nutritional disturbances to be causative, and more recently an elevated platelet count or abnormality in their function has been advanced but as yet remains unproven (Eijer, 2007).

The classic diagnostic findings include an obvious limp and often a complaint of ipsilateral, medial thigh, and knee pain. The affected hip is usually limited in internal rotation and abduction. The radiographic findings vary with the stage of the disorder. The classic crescent is a sign of osteonecrosis (Fig. 10-37).

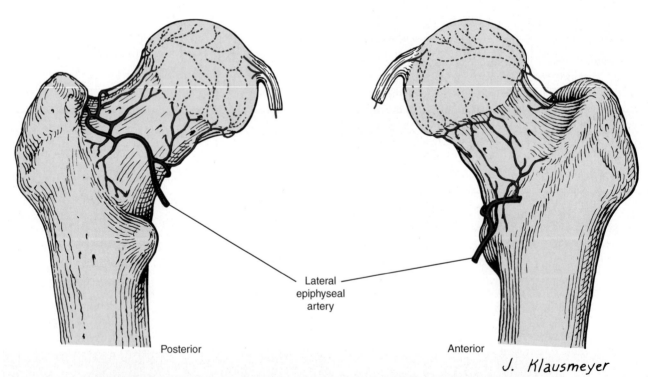

Lateral epiphyseal artery

Posterior

Anterior

J. Klausmeyer

FIG. 10-36 Arterial blood supply to the proximal end of the femur in an adult. The lateral epiphyseal artery supplies most of the weight-bearing surface of the femoral head in more than 90% of adults. Note the lack of significant arterial supply from the region of insertion of the anterior capsule. In the etiology of Legg-Calvé-Perthes disease, acetabular retroversion may cause abnormal loading of dorsal femoral head-neck junction with restricted blood supply to the femoral epiphysis. (From Browner BD: *Skeletal trauma: basic science, management, and reconstruction,* ed 3, Philadelphia, 2003, WB Saunders.)

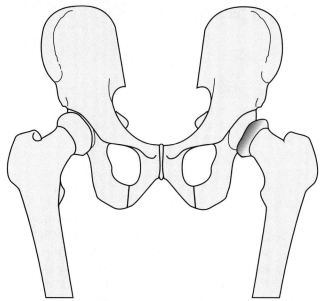

FIG. 10-37 A schematic anteroposterior view of the hips demonstrating changes occurring with Legg-Calvé-Perthes disease. The darkened area in the left hip represents necrosis and flattening of the femoral head. (From Malone TR, McPoil TG, Nitz AJ: *Orthopedic and sports physical therapy*, ed 3, St Louis, 1997, Mosby.)

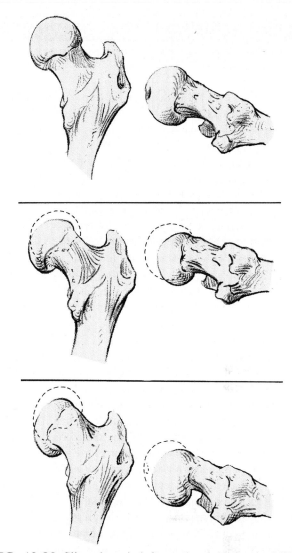

FIG. 10-38 Slipped capital femoral epiphysis. **A,** Mild. **B,** Moderate. **C,** Severe. (From Malone TR, McPoil TG, Nitz AJ: *Orthopedic and sports physical therapy*, ed 3, St Louis, 1997, Mosby.)

ORTHOPEDIC GAMUT 10-10

FORMS OF CONGENITAL HIP DISLOCATION

1. Congenital hip dysplasia
2. Acetabular dysplasia
3. Congenital subluxation

A slipped capital femoral epiphysis occurs when shear forces lead to a displacement of the epiphysis of the femoral head and cause it to *slip* inferiorly and posteriorly relative to the neck of the femur (Fig. 10-38). This condition is most common in children ages 10 to 16 years and is seen more often in boys than in girls. Congenital dislocation of the hip can be caused by a variety of conditions that result in dysplasia of the femur or acetabulum.

> The physical examination should include observing the child walk after removing all clothing other than the diaper or underwear. The child should walk a sufficient distance so that several complete gait cycles can be observed. This observation will determine if the child actually has a gait disturbance such as toe walking, in-toeing, or out-toeing, or a true limp (Myers, Thompson, 1997).

Congenital dislocation of the hip is a spontaneous dislocation of the hip that occurs before, during, or shortly after birth. Clearly, several factors are implicated as causative agents. Some of the factors are genetic and some environ-

---

ORTHOPEDIC GAMUT 10-11

DIAGNOSING CONGENITAL HIP DYSPLASIA

1. Neonatal (birth to 1 month): Barlow test, Ortolani test
2. Infancy (1 month to 2 years): limited hip abduction with the hips flexed to 45 degrees, shortening on the affected side with hips and knees flexed (Galeazzi sign), Trendelenburg sign
3. Age 2 to 6 years: obvious limp, Trendelenburg sign, limb shortening if unilateral
4. Older than 6 years: limp, limited hip abduction

10

CATEGORIES OF PEDIATRIC LIMPING

I. An antalgic limp is one that is painful, and a child with an antalgic limp spends a greater portion of the gait cycle on the asymptomatic leg than the symptomatic leg.

II. A Trendelenburg limp is not painful but is caused by muscle weakness or instability of the hip joint such as in unilateral developmental dysplasia of the hip. A child with a Trendelenburg gait tilts the pelvis away from the involved side. In a single-limb stance on the affected side, the patient shifts the trunk over the involved side to stabilize the hip.

III. A child with bilateral developmental dysplasia of the hip has a waddling gait.

Lateral pillar classification

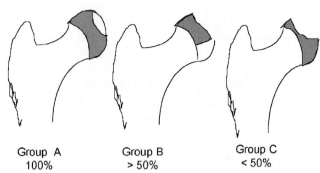

FIG. 10-39 The lateral pillar classification of Herring was published in 1992. Femoral heads are classified into three groups, depending on the maintenance of height of the lateral pillar of the femoral head, compared to the height of the lateral pillar on the opposite normal side. Maintenance of lateral femoral head height is associated with a reduction in deformity and prevention of extrusion. The advantages of the lateral pillar classification is that it requires only an AP radiograph and the measurements are easy to perform and to understand. The disadvantages are that the definitive measurement must be made at the fullest extent of fragmentation (i.e. well into the course of the disease and therefore after the most suitable time for intervention), that it is not suitable for bilateral disease, and that femoral heads may progress from one category to the other. Children in Group A and younger children in Group C have better result. (From Hunter JB: (iv) Legg Calve Perthes' disease, *Curr Orthop* 18[4]:273-283, 2004.)

mental. One such factor, acting alone, may not always be sufficient by itself to bring about dislocation, and a combination of factors may often be at work.

Generalized ligamentous laxity is found in some patients, and it may also be present in a parent or relative. This laxity leads to a lack of stability at the hip; therefore, dislocation may occur easily in certain positions of the joint.

In girls, a ligament-relaxing hormone (relaxin) may possibly be secreted by the fetal uterus in response to estrogen and progesterone that reaches the fetal circulation. The release of relaxin may cause instability, as does genetically determined joint laxity. Also possible is that laxity of the hip ligaments from this cause might help explain the greater incidence of dislocation in girls.

Defective development of the acetabulum and the femoral head can be inherited. The defect appears always to be bilateral and is probably as common in boys as in girls. Defective development of the acetabulum predisposes a fetus to hip dislocation, which may indeed occur before birth. If dislocation does not occur, the defect may show itself in adult life in the form of an unduly shallow acetabulum that has a tendency to subluxate. Later, osteoarthritis (acetabular dysplasia) may occur.

The incidence of congenital hip dislocation is slightly higher when an infant is delivered by a breech rather than normal delivery. The act of extending the hips during delivery may possibly precipitate dislocation when a predisposition already exists to it from ligamentous laxity or acetabular dysplasia.

Two distinct types of congenital dislocation of the hip may exist. The first type of dislocation is caused by ligamentous laxity, whether genetically determined or hormonal. With this type of dislocation, the dislocation occurs almost accidentally when some precipitating movement, such as extension of the hips during delivery, occurs. This dislocation is the type that is often unilateral and readily correctable. The second type of dislocation is caused by genetically determined dysplasia of the acetabulum, which is always bilateral and often much more difficult to treat.

Treatment usually involves surgical intrusion. The outcome of surgery is readily assessed by changes in gait and stance and with the *Lateral Pillar Classification,* the *Mose Sphericity Measurement,* and the *Stulberg Outcome Grades* (Figs. 10-39, 10-40, 10-41).

MOSE SPHERICITY MEASUREMENT

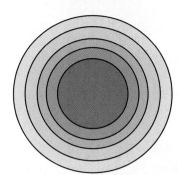

- Concentric ring template
- 2 mm spacing
- Exact fit 1 circle = Good
- < 2 mm = Fair
- > 2 mm = Poor

FIG. 10-40 Mose method of grading results with concentric circles. The long-term complication for patients with Perthes disease is osteoarthritis. The long-term follow-up demonstrates that at 40 years of follow-up (i.e., patients in their late 40s and 50s), 40% had had a joint replacement, 10% had disabling arthritis that warranted a joint replacement. The factors affecting the prognosis have historically been given as the age at onset and the shape of the femoral head at maturity. Female gender was thought to be a poor prognostic fracture, but the evidence for this is limited and if the ages of girls with Perthes are corrected for skeletal maturity, their prognosis appears to be much the same as boys. An onset of Perthes before the age of 5 appears to have a good prognosis with an onset after the age of 8 carrying a poor prognosis. This leaves a considerable indeterminate area and Snyder and others have reported poor results even in very young patients with Perthes. Much effort has focused on judging the shape of the femoral head at maturity. Two methods are commonly used, the classification of Stulberg and the concentric ring method of Mose. (From Hunter JB: (iv) Legg Calve Perthes' disease, *Curr Orthop* 18[4]:273-283, 2004.)

- The patient is lying supine with the knees flexed and the soles of the feet flat on the table, the great toes and malleoli being approximated bilaterally.
- The examiner observes the heights of the knees from a viewpoint at the foot of table (Fig. 10-42).
- If one knee is lower than the other, ipsilateral hip dislocation or severe coxa disorder is indicated (Fig. 10-43).
- Tibial-length discrepancies are also discerned in this position.
- From viewing the position from the side, the examiner can assess femoral-length discrepancies (Figs. 10-44 and 10-45).

Next Steps/Procedures
Hip telescoping test and diagnostic imaging

10

CLINICAL PEARL

Congenital dislocation of the hip is a condition in which one or both hips are dislocated at birth or are dislocated in the first few weeks of life. The disorder has a familial tendency and a well-established geographic distribution. It may occur with other congenital defects.

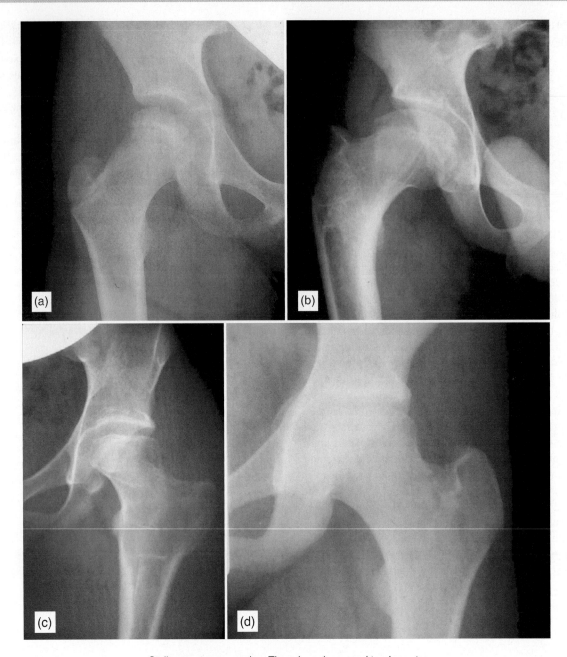

Stulberg outcome grades. There is an increased tendency to premature osteoarthritis with increasing grade.

Stulberg outcome grades.
I Completely normal
II Spherical with coxa magna/short neck/steep acetabulum
III Not spherical but not flat ie umbrella or mushroom shaped
IV Flat head with abnormal head/neck/acetabulum
V Flat head with normal head/neck/acetabulum

FIG. 10-41 Example Stulberg outcome grades. (a), Grade 2; (b), grade 3; (c), grade 4; and (d), grade 5. Stulberg outcome grades. There is an increased tendency to premature osteoarthritis with increasing grades. (From Hunter JB: (iv) Legg Calve Perthes' disease, *Curr Orthop* 18[4]:273-83, 2004.)

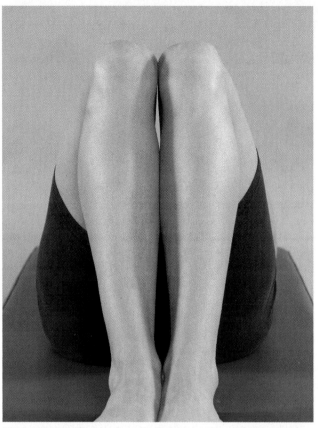

FIG. 10-42 The patient is lying supine. The knees are flexed, and the feet are flat on the examination table. The great toes and malleoli are approximated bilaterally.

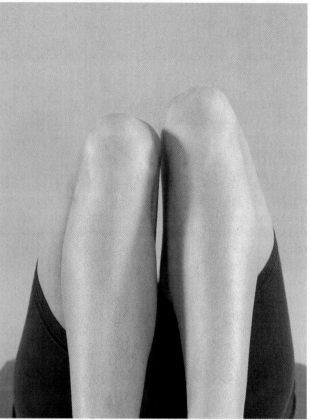

FIG. 10-43 From the foot of the table, the examiner observes the height of the knees. If one is lower than the other, a femoral deficiency that is caused by a pathologic condition of the ipsilateral coxa (dislocation) is indicated. This finding may also indicate a tibial-length discrepancy.

10

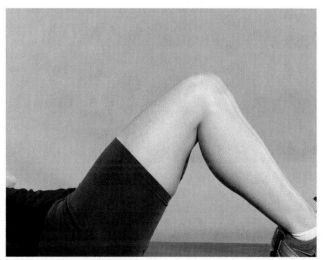

FIG. 10-44 From the side of the table, the examiner observes the position of the patient's knees. Again, the great toes and malleoli are approximated bilaterally.

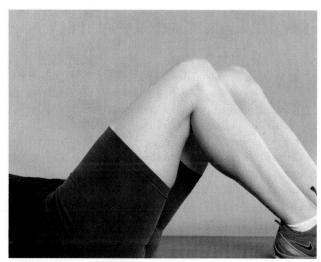

FIG. 10-45 If one knee is ahead of the other, it indicates femoral-length discrepancy (dysplasia) or an ipsilateral coxa abnormality (dislocation).

Assessment for Fracture of the Femoral Neck or Head

Comment

All fracture-dislocations of the hip have a history of severe trauma in common. The type of trauma and the mechanism of injury are extremely important in identifying the fracture-dislocations. Physical examination and simple observation of the attitude of the limp will aid in differentiating the type of fracture-dislocation even before diagnostic imaging. Laboratory data are usually of no help unless the patient has extremely low hemoglobin and hematocrit counts. When these counts are low, the possibility of pelvic fracture must be a paramount consideration because enormous quantities of blood can be lost in the retroperitoneal area from pelvic fractures.

Fractures of the head of the femur usually occur in association with a dislocation of the head of the femur but have been known to occur without a dislocation. Nothing about the presentation of these fractures that aids in their differentiation is unique. The examiner must rely on diagnostic imaging for help in identifying the type of fracture (Fig. 10-46). The examiner should look for fractures of the superior aspect of the head of the femur with anterior dislocation and fractures of the inferior aspect with posterior dislocations.

Fractures of the neck of the femur may be displaced or undisplaced. The undisplaced fractures are caused by stress, which usually occurs in young athletic individuals; by impaction, which usually occurs in instances of minor trauma and associated osteoporosis; or by postirradiation of the pelvis, which occurs after treatments for cervical cancer (Fig. 10-47). The patient experiences mild to moderate pain in the groin and no rotational deformity or length discrepancy of the extremity. The patient often is able to walk but has an antalgic gait. Routine AP diagnostic imaging of the hip will often be normal. Oblique X-ray studies and tomograms are indicated.

On the other hand, displaced fractures of the neck of the femur have a usual mode of presentation. These fractures occur in osteoporotic individuals, usually older women, and are associated with a minor fall or severe trauma, although the latter circumstance is rare. These patients experience severe pain throughout the hip, and the leg is held in external rotation and mild abduction. Some shortening occurs. Radiographs are diagnostic and make fractures readily apparent with the displacement and disruption of Shenton's line.

In older people, the average age being 70 years, intertrochanteric fractures occur more often than femoral neck fractures. These neck fractures are more common in women, in a ratio of 8:1 over men. Neck fractures usually occur in a major fall or an associated motor-vehicle injury, with both direct and indirect forces acting on the hip. The indirect forces are the iliopsoas, with its attachment on the lesser trochanter, and the abductors, with their attachment on the greater trochanter. These indirect forces explain why separate fragments often occur within this type of injury. External rotation of the extremity will be marked, especially in the comminuted fracture, with the foot often resting on its lateral surface. This rotation occurs because of the attachment of the iliopsoas, which can now rotate the shaft of the femur externally because of the fracture. The leg shortening varies with the degree of comminution.

Osteoporosis-related fractures result in disability and death in a significant proportion of men who suffer fractures. One third of all hip fractures in the United States occur in men. Low bone mineral density (BMD) is a risk factor for hip fracture in men and women; each standard deviation decrease in femoral neck BMD was associated with a two- to three-fold increase in the relative risk of hip fracture. Osteoporosis was reported in 6% of U.S. white men age 50 years and older when it was defined as femoral neck T-score at or below −2.5 compared with the National Health and Nutritional Examination Survey (NHANES) III, young male reference peak BMD (SD) 0.93 g/cm^2 (0.136). The lifetime risk for a hip, forearm, or vertebral fracture after age 50 years in men was estimated to be 13%. Thus millions of older U.S. men have osteoporosis or low BMD and are at

---

ORTHOPEDIC GAMUT 10-13

MSCORE (MALE, SIMPLE CALCULATED OSTEOPOROSIS RISK ESTIMATION)

- MSCORE is based on bone mineral density at the femoral neck
- MSCORE is derived from five variables independently associated with osteoporosis
- MSCORE = [2 × (patient age in decades) − (weight in lb ÷ 10) + 4 with gastrectomy, + 4 with emphysema, + 3 with two or more prior fractures + 14]
- Increased osteoporosis risk is reflected in higher MSCORE values
  - Low (<9)
  - Moderate (9-13)
  - High (>13)

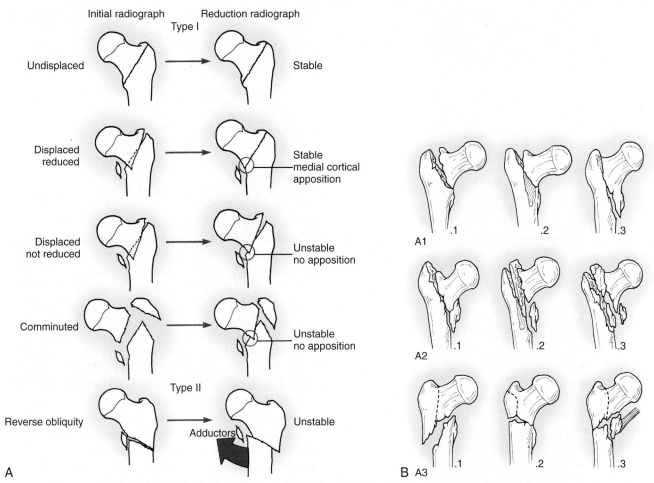

FIG. 10-46 Hip fractures are primarily classified into intra- and extra-capsular according to their relationship to the capsular attachment of the hip. Extra-capsular fractures comprise about half of all the hip fractures and may be subdivided into those in the trochanteric region (also termed per- or inter-trochanteric) and those below the level of the lesser trochanter (subtrochanteric). Various classification systems have been used to classify extra-capsular hip fractures. The most frequently used system is the Jensen and Michaelsen's modification of Evans classification (**A**). (From DeLee JC: *Fractures and dislocations of the hip.* In Rockwood CA Jr, Green DP, eds: *Fractures in adults*, ed 2, Philadelphia, 1984, Lippincott.) **B,** AO classification of trochanteric fractures. Group A1, simple two-part fracture; group A2, fracture extends over two or more levels of medial cortex; group A3, fracture extends through lateral cortex of femur. (Redrawn from Müller ME, Nazarian S, Koch P, et al: *The comprehensive classification of fractures of long bones*, Berlin, 1990, Springer-Verlag.) (Canale ST, Beaty JH: *Campbell's operative orthopaedics*, ed 11, Philadelphia, 2008, Mosby.)

increased risk of suffering a hip fracture (Zimering et al, in press).

Patients with subtrochanteric fractures are usually younger than those with femoral neck or intertrochanteric fractures. More force is needed to produce a subtrochanteric fracture than an intertrochanteric fracture. The physical findings are the same, and only diagnostic imaging can make the differentiation.

PROCEDURE

- While the patient is lying supine, the inferior calcaneus is struck with the examiner's fist (Fig. 10-48).
- Localized pain in the thigh indicates a femoral fracture or a severe pathologic condition of the joint.
- Localized pain in the leg indicates a tibial or fibular fracture.
- Pain localized to the calcaneus indicates calcaneal fracture.

Next Steps/Procedures
Chiene test, Ludloff sign, and diagnostic imaging

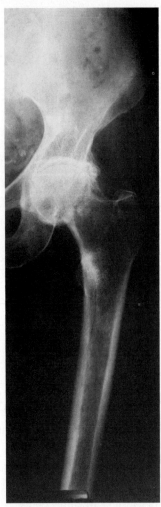

FIG. 10-47 Longitudinal fracture of the femoral shaft, radiograph demonstrating callus and fracture line. (From Soubrier M, Dubost JJ, Boisgard S, et al: Insufficiency fracture. A survey of 60 cases and review of the literature, *Joint Bone Spine* 70(3):209-218, 2003.)

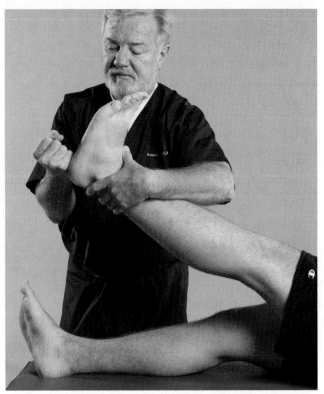

FIG. 10-48 The patient is lying supine. The examiner elevates the affected leg while keeping the knee extended. The inferior calcaneus is struck with the examiner's fist. Localized pain in the thigh indicates a femoral fracture or a severe pathologic condition involving the joint. Localized pain in the leg indicates a tibial or fibular fracture. Pain localized to the calcaneus indicates calcaneal fracture. Markedly reactive patients may be tested with the affected leg resting completely on the examination table.

CLINICAL PEARL

Two questions must be answered in the assessment of a hip fracture. Does a fracture exist? Is the fracture displaced? The break usually becomes obvious when viewed with diagnostic imaging, but an impacted fracture can be missed. The assessment is important because impacted or undisplaced fractures have a good prognosis. Displaced fractures have a high rate of non-union and avascular necrosis.

APPARENT LEG-LENGTH TEST

Assessment for Apparent Leg-Length Discrepancy

Comment

The degree of LLD that is clinically significant remains controversial. Although generally assumed to be of little clinical significance, LLD of as little as 5 mm has been reported to be associated with low back or hip pain. A simulated LLD of as little as 10 mm can lead to a significant shift of the mean center-of-pressure position and an increase in postural sway while standing quietly. In children with a LLD of 5.5% or greater of the longer leg side, more mechanical work is performed by the long extremity, and the vertical displacement of the body's center of mass is greater (Hanada et al, 2001).

Measurements of the patient's leg length can be made while the patient is standing, measuring from the anterior-superior iliac spine to the floor and from the posterior-superior iliac spine to the floor bilaterally. If the anterior-superior and posterior-superior iliac spines are lower on one side, an anatomic LLD exists. If the anterior-superior iliac spine is lower and posterior-superior iliac spine is higher on the same side, a functional LLD exists.

Apparent, or false, discrepancy in limb length is caused entirely by sideways tilting of the pelvis. The usual cause is an adduction deformity in one hip, which gives an appearance of shortening on that side, or an abduction deformity, which gives an appearance of lengthening. An exception is a fixed pelvic obliquity that is caused by severe lumbar scoliosis.

To measure apparent discrepancy, the limbs must be placed parallel to one another and in line with the trunk. Measurement is made from any fixed point in the midline of the trunk (e.g., the xiphisternum) to each medial malleolus. True length must be evaluated when apparent discrepancy is determined.

Measurement is made bilaterally from the umbilicus or xiphisternum to the apex of the medial malleolus. This measurement is an index of the functional length of the lower extremities. An abduction contracture deformity causes apparent lengthening of the limb, and an adduction contracture deformity causes an apparent shortening. Because the pelvis is tilted sideways to make the legs

---

ORTHOPEDIC GAMUT 10-15

ANATOMIC LEG-LENGTH DIFFERENCE

Causes of an anatomic leg-length difference include:
1. Poliomyelitis of the lower limb
2. Fracture of the femur or tibia
3. Bone growth problems of the lower extremity (epiphyseal plate damage)

ORTHOPEDIC GAMUT 10-16

LEG-LENGTH MEASUREMENTS

Leg-length measurement landmarks include:
1. Iliac crest to greater trochanter to determine whether coxa vara is present
2. Greater trochanter to knee for femur length
3. Knee joint line to medial malleolus for tibial length

ORTHOPEDIC GAMUT 10-14

SEQUELAE ASSOCIATED WITH LEG LENGTH DISCREPANCY

A high proportion of the normal population has at least a mild leg-length discrepancy. A leg-length discrepancy of sufficient magnitude may lead to several problems, including:
- Increased energy expenditure in gait
- Cosmetically disturbing gait
- Equinus contracture of the ankle on the short leg side
- Late degenerative arthritis of both the long-leg hip and knee (long-leg arthropathy)
- Low back pain
- Compensatory scoliosis

ORTHOPEDIC GAMUT 10-17

FUNCTIONAL LEG-LENGTH DIFFERENCE

Causes of a functional leg-length difference include:
1. One pronated foot or one supinated foot
2. Muscle spasms in one hip
3. Hip capsule tightness
4. Adductor muscle spasm on one side
5. More genu valgus on one side
6. Femoral anteversion on one side

parallel, the heel of the shorter side cannot be placed on the ground when the knees are straight. The difference between the lower limbs is caused only by pelvic obliquity, and measuring for a structural short leg is highly inaccurate when performed in this manner.

- Measurement is made bilaterally from the umbilicus or xiphisternum to the apex of the medial malleolus (Fig. 10-49).
- This measurement is an index of the functional length of the lower extremities.

Next Steps/Procedure
Actual leg-length measurements

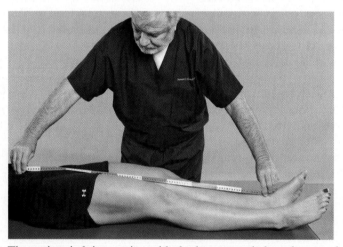

FIG. 10-49 The patient is lying supine with the legs extended on the examination table. With a tape measure, the examiner measures the length of the affected leg from the medial malleolus to the umbilicus. The distance is recorded and compared with the measurement obtained for the opposite leg. The difference in the length of the legs is probably the result of pelvic obliquity.

CLINICAL PEARL

Pelvic tilting accompanied by a heel discrepancy indicates apparent shortening of the limb. This apparent shortening may be accompanied by some true shortening. The discrepancy at the heels provides a measure of its degree.

Assessment for Fracture of the Neck of the Femur; Hip Dislocation

Comment

Although fractures generally occur in all age groups, hip fractures are most common among elderly women.

The vascular supply to the femoral head and neck may be significantly compromised with certain fracture patterns and levels of severity (Fig. 10-50). Generally, hip fractures can be classified by location and described by severity (simple or comminuted).

Fracture about the hip is unusual in the adolescent and young adult because the bone is exceptionally resilient. In young patients, the hip is much more likely to dislocate than it is to break.

If a fracture does occur, it is a major injury and should be treated as a medical emergency. The patient with a broken hip is completely disabled at once. The patient has severe pain in the hip and resists any attempt to manipulate the limb. The extremity is usually held with the thigh internally rotated and adducted while the knee rests above and against its fellow on the opposite side. The trochanter appears prominent. Any attempt to move the thigh from this position of flexion adduction and internal rotation causes pain. Diagnosis is confirmed by diagnostic imaging, and the images should be carefully studied to be sure that an accompanying fracture exists in the femoral shaft or acetabulum. The posterior acetabular margin, vulnerable in the adult, is seldom broken in the adolescent or young adult.

Femoral neck fractures account for less than 1% of all children's fractures. The femoral neck in children is tough, dense bone with a thick, strong periosteum that requires high-energy trauma to fracture compared with the commonly seen hip fractures in the elderly osteoporotic popula-

---

ORTHOPEDIC GAMUT 10-18

HIP FRACTURES

Typical locations of fractures of the hip include:
1. Extracapsular or trochanteric (Fig. 10-51)
2. Femoral neck or subcapital areas (These areas are intracapsular.) (Fig. 10-52)
3. Proximal femoral shaft or subtrochanteric areas (Fig. 10-53; Fig. 10-54)

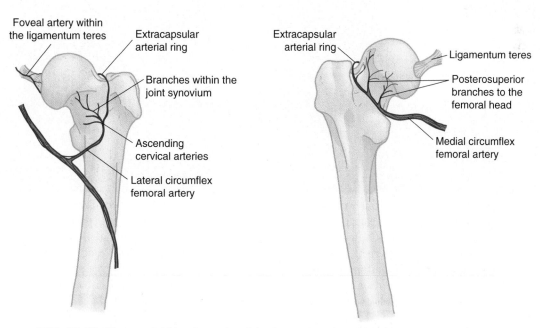

FIG. 10-50 The arterial blood supply of the femoral neck and head is provided to varying degrees by three sources: the ascending cervical arteries, the arterial branches within the marrow (not illustrated), and the dubious foveal artery within the ligamentum teres. (From Marx JA, Hockberger RS, Walls RM, et al: *Rosen's emergency medicine: concepts and clinical practice,* ed 6, St Louis, 2006, Mosby.)

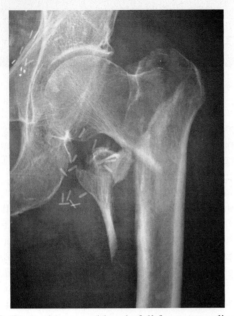

FIG. 10-51 An 81-year-old male fell from a standing height and sustained an unstable left intertrochanteric hip fracture (AO 31A-2.2). (Adapted from Gardner MJ, Briggs SM, Kopjar B, et al: Radiographic outcomes of intertrochanteric hip fractures treated with the trochanteric fixation nail, *Injury* 38[10]:1189-1196, 2007.)

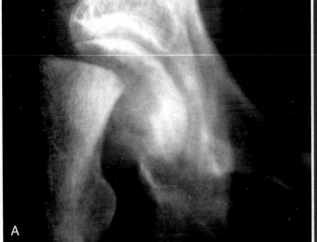
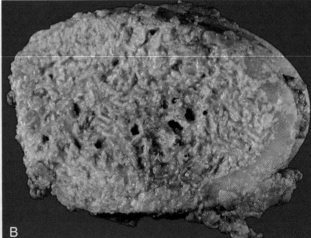

FIG. 10-52 A 61-year-old woman with a pancreatic tumor and two liver masses. She underwent a distal pancreatectomy combined with liver resections. Six weeks postoperatively, she complained of right hip pain with no history of trauma and a radiograph showed a fractured neck of the right femur combined with a dislocation, **(A)**. The bone marrow of the right femur was uniformly grey and necrotic **(B)**. Histologic findings revealed IMFN (intramedullary fat necrosis). (From Hashimoto M, Miki K, Beck Y, et al: Femoral neck fracture as a complication of lipase-secreting pancreatic acinar cell carcinoma, *Surgery* 142[5]:779-780, 2007.)

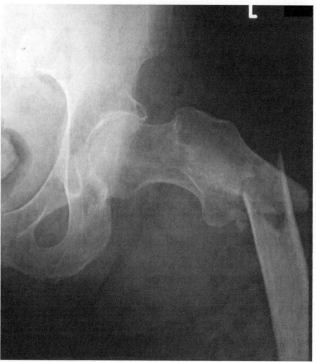

FIG. 10-53 Subtrochanteric hip fracture. Biomechanical analyses demonstrate a high concentration of stress and bending moments in the subtrochanteric region generated by the body weight and hip muscles. Just raising the leg while lying in bed can produce forces two to three times the body weight and walking up to five times the body weight. These fractures occur predominantly in cortical bone, which tends to take longer to heal than cancellous bone. The uneven pull of the hip abductors, adductors, and iliopsoas causes fracture displacement. The proximal fragment abducts, externally rotates and if the lesser trochanter is still attached to the upper femur the pull of the iliopsoas muscle causes flexion. The adductors and hamstrings lead to shortening and a varus deformity. In addition, the fractures are often comminuted with a defective medial buttress. (From Heinert G, Parker MJ: Intramedullary osteosynthesis of complex proximal femoral fractures with the Targon PF nail, *Injury* 38[11]:1294-1299, 2007.)

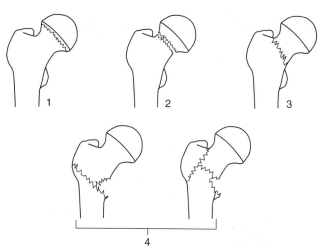

FIG. 10-54 Delbet simple classification is the most widely used and accepted (approximate percentage of incidence). Type 1, Transphyseal, with or without dislocation of the femoral head (3%); type 2, transcervical, displaced, or undisplaced (50%); type 3, cervico-intertrochanteric (37%); type 4, intertrochanteric (10%). (From Holton C, Foster P, Templeton P: Fractures of the femoral neck in children, *Curr Orthop* 20[5]:361-366, 2006.)

tion. Fracture patterns and classification differ in children compared with adults in part because of the different anatomy. A more precarious vascular anastomosis between the femoral neck and head leads to a higher incidence of avascular necrosis after displaced fractures within the paediatric population. Growth disturbance is an important complication of surgical fixation owing to the presence of the physeal plate (Holton, Foster, Templeton, 2006).

Additional complicating factors that may be present include avascular necrosis of the femoral head, which appears on diagnostic images as density changes and collapse of the head, and osteoarthritis that may restrict the mobility of the head of the acetabulum.

PROCEDURE

- The examiner determines whether a fracture of the neck of the femur has occurred by using a tape measure.
- The patient is supine with the legs extended on the examination table.
- Using a tape measure, the examiner measures the circumference of the thigh, passing the tape over the level of the greater trochanter (Fig. 10-55).
- The distance is recorded and compared with that of the opposite leg.
- An increased diameter indicates that the trochanter has rolled laterally.
- This increased measurement correlates with fracture of the neck of the femur.

Next Steps/Procedures
Anvil test, Ludloff sign, and diagnostic imaging

ORTHOPEDIC GAMUT 10-21

FEMORAL NECK FRACTURE NON-UNION

Non-union of femoral neck fractures occurs in approximately 15% of the cases. Reasons for nonunion are:
1. Meager blood supply
2. Inaccurate approximation and rigid fixation of the fragments

10

ORTHOPEDIC GAMUT 10-22

FACTORS INFLUENCING THE OCCURRENCE OF AVASCULAR NECROSIS IN PEDIATRIC PROXIMAL FEMUR FRACTURE

- Ligamentum teres contributes very little blood supply to the head until the age of 8; as an adult, it serves only 20%.
- Medial and lateral circumflex metaphyseal vessels that traverse the femoral neck predominately supply the head at birth. These later become virtually nonexistent by the age of 4, owing to the development of the cartilaginous physis that forms a barrier to these penetrating vessels.
- As the metaphyseal vessels diminish their supply to the femoral head, the lateral epiphyseal vessels become the main blood supply as they bypass the physeal barrier. These vessels can be identified as the posteroinferior and posterosuperior branches of the medial circumflex artery that supply the femoral head throughout the rest of its life.

ORTHOPEDIC GAMUT 10-23

CLINICAL FEATURES OF NON-UNION OF FEMORAL NECK FRACTURES

1. Pain in the hip when bearing weight
2. Shortening and external rotation of the limb
3. Grating or crepitus in the hip during motion

CLINICAL PEARL

A fracture of the neck of the femur occurs mainly among elderly women whose bones are osteoporotic. The patient may fall, but the patient more often catches a foot on something and ends up twisting the hip. The femoral neck is broken by rotational force. In most cases, the fracture is markedly displaced and completely unstable. In some cases, the fragments are impacted, and the patient may even walk about, albeit with some pain.

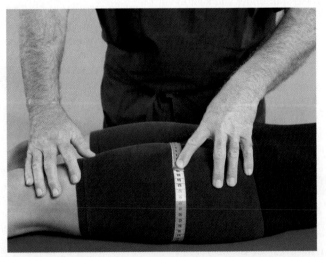

FIG. 10-55 The patient is lying supine with the legs extended on the examination table. Using a tape measure, the examiner measures the circumference of the thigh by passing the tape over the level of the greater trochanter. The distance is recorded and compared with the measurement obtained for the opposite leg. An increased diameter indicates that the trochanter has rolled laterally. This result correlates with fracture of the neck of the femur.

GAUVAIN SIGN

Assessment for Tuberculous Arthritis of the Hip Joint or Adult-Onset Osteonecrosis of the Femoral Head

Comment

Osteonecrosis is a common cause of hip pain in young and middle-age patients and ultimately results in severe degeneration of the hip joint. The exact pathogenesis of osteonecrosis is unknown, but interference of the blood supply to the femoral head is the common pathway.

Various skeletal conditions can occur during pregnancy and may involve the hip joint, leading mainly to transient osteoporosis of the hip (TOH) and osteonecrosis of the femoral head (Steib-Furno et al, in press).

Hip diseases, at least those resulting in significant clinical impairment, appear infrequent during pregnancy and early postpartum. Physical exercise is usually recommended to pregnant women, with the risk of worsening symptoms that can evolve into severe impairment and ultimately into complications such as spontaneous fracture of the femoral neck. TOH is the most frequently encountered pregnancy-related hip disease. Pregnancy-related osteonecrosis is not frequent. Stress fractures of the femoral head appear as an important cause of pregnancy-related hip disease. The clinical features of occult stress fractures of the femoral head share many similarities with TOH, and only thorough examination with magnetic resonance imaging (MRI) can differentiate between them. Diagnosis of pregnancy-related occult fractures of the femoral head is important because it might reveal an underlying bone disease.

Renal transplantation (RT) may improve the bone metabolism disturbances of end-stage renal disease. However, avascular or ischemic osteonecrosis and osteoporosis are the most common osseous complications after RT. Avascular osteonecrosis results from necrosis of marrow cells, trabecular cells, and osteocytes unrelated to bacterial infection. The femoral head is most commonly affected. The incidence of osteonecrosis has been more than 20%; corticosteroids have been considered to contribute to both osteoporosis and osteonecrosis among renal transplant recipients. Since the introduction of anticalcineurin agents and lowered cumulative glucocorticoid doses, the incidence has been reduced to 5%. Bone pain and functional restriction are major clinical problems. X-rays can be normal at the early stage of bone disease, whereas MRI is more sensitive and specific for the diagnosis of avascular necrosis (Hedri et al, 2007).

The rise in the prevalence of tuberculosis, as well as an increase in its extrapulmonary manifestations, has been a significant in the last decade. Drug-resistant strains, human immunodeficiency virus infection, chronic diseases,

---

ORTHOPEDIC GAMUT 10-24

OSTEONECROSIS

Common causes of osteonecrosis include:
1. Steroid use
2. Alcohol use
3. Trauma
4. Gout
5. Metabolic problems
6. Genetic problems

ORTHOPEDIC GAMUT 10-25

HIP PAIN

Other causes of hip pain producing symptoms similar to osteonecrosis include:
1. Gout
2. Femoral or inguinal hernia
3. Pigmented villonodular synovitis
4. Stress fracture of femoral neck
5. Rheumatoid arthritis

ORTHOPEDIC GAMUT 10-26

RADIOGRAPHIC STAGES OF OSTEONECROSIS AIDING PROGNOSIS

Osteonecrosis is classified into several radiographic stages that aid with prognosis:

Stage 0: No change on plain radiographs, but a positive magnetic resonance imaging scan

Stage I: Mottled densities or osteopenia

Stage II: Areas of increased density in the femoral head (Fig. 10-56) crescent sign with subchondral fracture (Fig. 10-57)

Stage III: Depression of femoral head (Fig. 10-58)

Stage IV: Flattening and collapse of femoral head (Fig. 10-59)

Stage V: Degenerative arthrosis

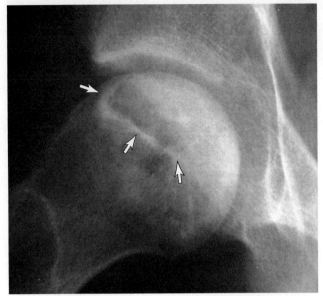

FIG. 10-56 Osteonecrosis stage II: increased density in the area of maximum loading of the femoral head. A young adult male patient with a history of renal transplantation and right hip pain for the last 3 months. The plain radiograph shows a sclerotic rim *(arrows)* surrounding a lysis which corresponds to the necrotic area. (From Malizos KN, Karantanas AH, Varitimidis SE, et al: Osteonecrosis of the femoral head: Etiology, imaging and treatment, *Eur J Radiol* 63[1]:16-28, 2007.)

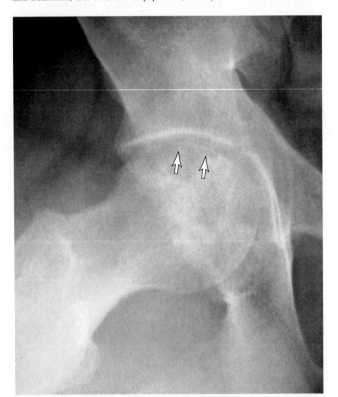

FIG. 10-57 Osteonecrosis stage IIA: the "crescent sign" with subchondral fracture. Patient with idiopathic hip osteonecrosis. The frog leg radiograph shows the lucent "crescent" sign *(arrows)* which represents a subchondral fracture. The femoral head contour is intact. (From Malizos KN, Karantanas AH, Varitimidis SE, et al: Osteonecrosis of the femoral head: Etiology, imaging and treatment. *Eur J Radiol* 63[1]:16-28, 2007.)

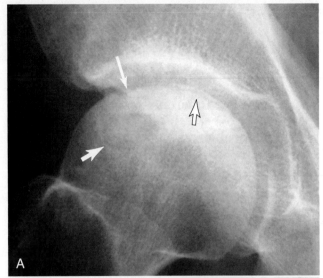

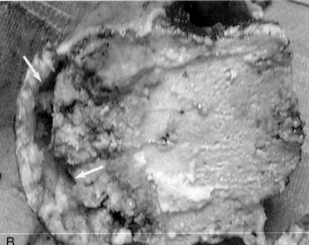

FIG. 10-58 Osteonecrosis stage III; flattening of the femoral head. A middle-aged male patient with right hip osteonecrosis and recent deterioration of pain. **(A)** The plain radiograph shows the reactive sclerotic rim surrounding the lytic necrotic area *(thick arrow)*, the subchondral fracture *(small arrow)*, and a segmental articular collapse *(long arrow)* in keeping with advanced osteonecrosis. The joint space width is normal. **(B)** The patient underwent total hip replacement 4 years later. The sagittally sliced gross section of a femoral head obtained at surgery, shows the subchondral fracture *(crescent sign) (arrows)*. (From Malizos KN, Karantanas AH, Varitimidis SE, et al: Osteonecrosis of the femoral head: Etiology, imaging and treatment, *Eur J Radiol* 63[1]:16-28, 2007.)

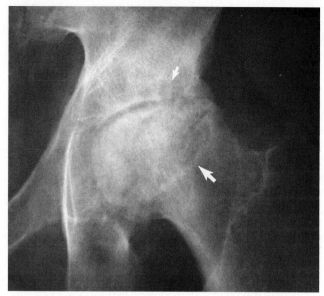

FIG. 10-59 Osteonecrosis stage IV; collapse of the femoral head and loss of normal contour. Advanced osteonecrosis. The plain AP radiograph shows the sclerotic rim of the necrotic lesion *(arrow)*, the articular collapse, the severe joint space narrowing and the subchondral cyst formation in the acetabulum *(thin arrow)* suggesting secondary osteoarthritis. (From Malizos KN, Karantanas AH, Varitimidis SE, et al: Osteonecrosis of the femoral head: Etiology, imaging and treatment, *Eur J Radiol* 63[1]:16-28, 2007.)

malignancy, transplantation, and other immunosuppressive conditions have contributed to this process. However, breast tuberculosis is a rare form of tuberculosis. The incidence in Western countries varies from 0.025% to 0.1% of all surgically treated breast disease. The incidence in developing countries is 3% to 4.5% of all surgically diagnosed breast disease (Ursavas et al, in press).

Tuberculosis of the hip joint may appear at any age, but it occurs most commonly in children. An intermittent limp is the first, constant sign. At first, tuberculosis of the hip may come on after exercise, but later it is present after rest, such as in the early morning. Initially, pain may be only a slight discomfort that occurs in the groin or the knee and thigh (referred pain). Startling pain at night occurs at a later stage and is caused by relaxation of the protective muscle contrac-

tion. At an even later stage, the patient may experience stiffness of the joint.

In the early stages of the disease, when it is limited to the synovium or bone, the position of the joint is that of slight flexion, abduction, and lateral rotation (greatest fluid capacity). At a later stage, when arthritis supervenes, the leg becomes flexed, adducted, and internally rotated. At an early stage, muscle wasting is not a very pronounced sign, but soon afterward, it becomes obvious. In a long-standing case, atrophy of the quadriceps and glutei becomes very pronounced. At a later stage, swelling that is caused by the formation of an abscess may be present. This abscess commonly points anteriorly. Apparent lengthening may be present in the active stage because of fixed abduction. Apparent shortening occurs later and is caused by fixed adduction.

In the early stage, deep tenderness can often be elicited in the groin. At a later stage, if an abscess is present, a soft swelling may be palpable. Atrophy of the muscles occurs later, and the trochanter may be raised on the affected side.

At first, only the extremes of movement are limited and painful. The Thomas test becomes positive at an early stage and reveals concealed flexion contracture. Limitation of extension is also a valuable sign. Later, when arthritis supervenes, movements are restricted by muscular spasm, and attempted movement becomes very painful.

General malaise and pallor accompany tuberculous arthritis, and slight evening pyrexia is not uncommon. In the healing stage, the general condition improves, and the joint is no longer painful.

PROCEDURE

- The patient is lying supine or in a side-lying position with the affected thigh extended (Fig. 10-60).
- The examiner carefully rotates the patient's thigh (Fig. 10-61).
- The sign is positive if contraction of the abdominal muscles is noted on the same side that is being maneuvered (Fig. 10-62).
- The sign is significant for reflex muscle spasm, which is commonly elicited in tuberculosis of the coxa, or adult-onset osteonecrosis.

Next Steps/Procedures
Jansen test, Patrick test, and diagnostic imaging

10

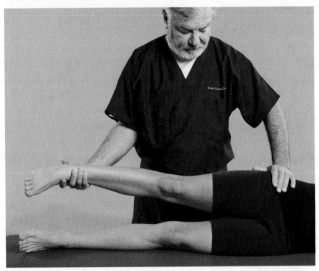

FIG. 10-60 The patient is in a side-lying position on the unaffected hip. The affected leg is extended, and the examiner slightly abducts the affected leg.

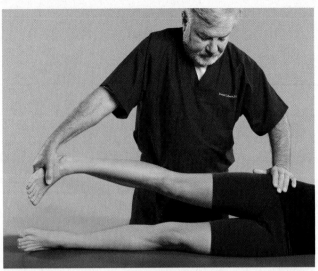

FIG. 10-61 The examiner cautiously externally rotates the leg (externally rotates the femoral head).

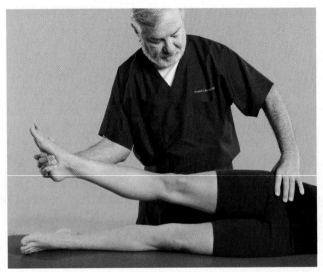

FIG. 10-62 Next, the examiner internally rotates the leg (internally rotating the femoral head). If abdominal muscular contraction occurs on the same side, the sign is positive. The sign indicates reflex muscle spasm caused by tuberculosis of the hip or adult-onset osteonecrosis of the femoral head. Tuberculosis of the hip is usually not common after adolescence.

CLINICAL PEARL

A resurgence in tuberculosis (TB) has occurred worldwide. Approximately 2 billion people have latent infection, 8 million develop active TB annually, and 2 to 3 million die as a result of TB. With this resurgence, cases with extrapulmonary TB have also shown an increase. Approximately 10% to 11% of extrapulmonary TB involves joints and bones, which is approximately 1% to 3% of all TB cases. The global prevalence of latent joint and bone TB is approximately 19 to 38 million. TB arthritis most commonly leads to monoarthritis of weight-bearing joints in the hip or the knee. A child infected with this disease walks with a limp and often complains of pain in the groin or knee. Night pain is another feature. In early cases, complete resolution may be hoped for with antituberculous therapy, bed rest, and traction. In the advanced case, joint debridement is carried out with efforts to obtain a bony fusion of the joint.

Assessment for Meningeal Irritation

Comment

Viruses, bacteria, spirochetes, and fungi may infect the meninges and subarachnoid space (Fig. 10-63). The relative incidence of these causes varies enormously in different areas of the world, and viral and bacterial infections sometimes show a seasonal variation.

Drug-induced aseptic meningitis is relatively rare but should always be considered in the appropriate clinical setting. Several nonsteroidal antiinflammatory drugs, including ibuprofen, are known to produce meningeal inflammation. Several other drugs, including antibiotics and isoniazid, have also been shown to produce chemical meningitis. The exact mechanism of such meningitis is not clear, but the proposed theories are a delayed hypersensitivity–type reaction and direct meningeal irritation (Thomas, Krishnamoorthy, Kapilamoorthy, 2006).

In senescence, the features that make the diagnosis difficult may include an apyrexial course or neurologic symptoms dominated by confusion and delirium or focal signs caused by cerebral venous thrombosis, mimicking a cerebrovascular accident (Fig. 10-64).

A wide range of viruses can cause meningitis; most cases are caused by enteroviruses (70% to 90%), genital herpes simplex virus, or mumps. The typical syndrome of viral meningitis comprises acute onset of fever, headache, and

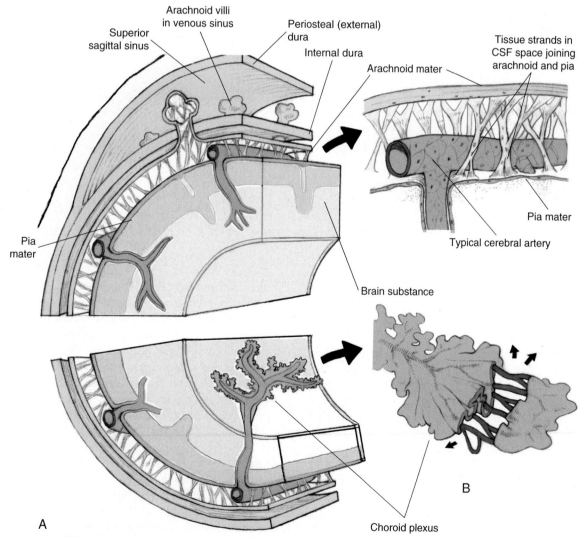

FIG. 10-63 Choroid plexus and arachnoid granulations. *CSF,* Cerebrospinal fluid. *(From Mathers LH et al: Clinical anatomy principles, St Louis, 1996, Mosby.)*

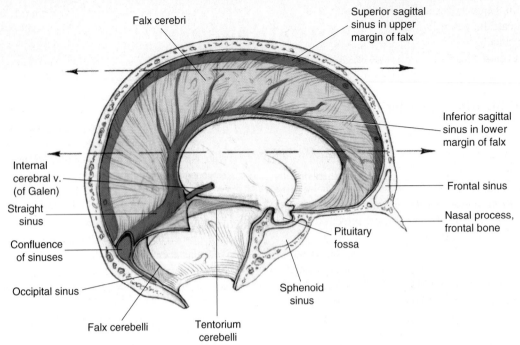

FIG. 10-64 Falx cerebri and sagittal sinuses. (From Mathers LH et al: *Clinical anatomy principles*, St Louis, 1996, Mosby.)

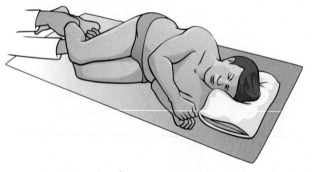

FIG. 10-65 Kernig sign. (From Olson WH et al: *Handbook of symptom-oriented neurology*, ed 2, St Louis, 1994, Mosby.)

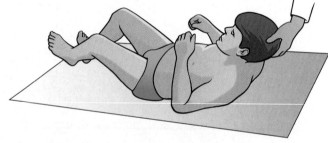

FIG. 10-66 Brudzinski sign. (From Olson WH et al: *Handbook of symptom-oriented neurology*, ed 2, St Louis, 1994, Mosby.)

accompanying signs of meningeal irritation (photophobia, neck stiffness, Kernig sign and jolt accentuation of headache). The outlook for most patients with viral meningitis is excellent (Rice, 2005).

The signs and symptoms of meningitis may develop explosively de novo or may appear in the waning stages of an infection that is localized elsewhere. Headache, backache, nausea, and vomiting are common symptoms, and nuchal rigidity occurs in more than 80% of patients. Kernig/Brudzinski sign is often present (Figs. 10-65 and 10-66). Only in the neonate and very young infant is meningitis often unattended by evidence of increased pressure and meningeal irritation. At this stage, even fever may be absent. Photophobia may be a prominent, early symptom and is related in some way to the meningeal inflammation.

Disturbances in mental status occur in nearly all cases of acute bacterial meningitis. Irritability, confusion, delirium, and stupor are common. Coma occurs in approximately 10%

of the cases and indicates a poor prognosis. Focal or generalized seizures occur in approximately one fourth of all patients with meningitis. Seizures are encountered much more often in infants who have a greater susceptibility to them. Signs of cerebral dysfunction, other than altered consciousness and seizures, are uncommon in cases of acute bacterial meningitis. The signs of cerebral dysfunction appear most often when treatment has been delayed. These signs include a disturbed conjugate gaze, dysphagia, paresis of extremities, and visual field defects. Striking and persistent signs are usually caused by infarction of tissue as a result of cortical venous thrombosis. This complication commonly develops during the second week of the disease, when signs of infection and meningeal irritation are subsiding. Bilateral neurologic signs and convulsions occurring first on one side then on the other always suggest an associated thrombosis of the superior sagittal sinus. Prominent and slowly progressive focal signs appearing early in the meningitis should indicate an associated focus of sepsis such as subdural endocarditis with cerebral embolism.

Between 5% and 20% of the patients with bacterial meningitis will develop cranial nerve palsies during the acute stage of the disease. Impaired ocular movement, deafness, and labyrinthine dysfunction are most frequently seen. Blindness and facial paralysis also occur. Most cranial nerve palsies are probably attributable to the meningeal exudate, but the eighth nerve complex may be damaged by bacteria or their toxins, which act directly on the inner ear. Although the cerebrospinal fluid pressure is usually elevated in patients with bacterial meningitis, papilledema is rare and is more characteristic of a brain abscess, subdural empyema, or venous sinus thrombosis. The uncommon occurrence of

papilledema in uncomplicated meningitis is probably explained by the short duration of the increased pressure.

PROCEDURE

- While the patient is in a supine position, a brisk flexion of the hip and the knee occurs when the quadriceps muscle on the opposite limb is irritated, such as by a firm pinch (Figs. 10-67 to 10-69).
- The sign is present in cases of meningeal irritation.

Next Steps/Procedures
Kernig/Brudzinski sign, clinical laboratory assessment, and neurologic assessment

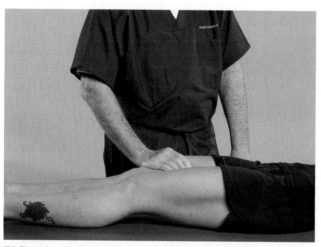

FIG. 10-67 The patient is lying supine with the legs extended on the examination table. The examiner firmly irritates (pinches) one of the quadriceps muscles.

CLINICAL PEARL

Acute meningitis (associated with cortical encephalitis and often with ventriculitis) is an emergency and should be suspected in any patient with the acute onset of nonlocalizing central nervous system signs. Fever, nuchal rigidity, headache, altered mental status, vomiting, and photophobia are typically present. The absence of fever is not uncommon. Meningeal signs are not usually present in infants younger than 6 months. Acute signs may also be less apparent in elderly, alcoholic, immunocompromised, or comatose patients.

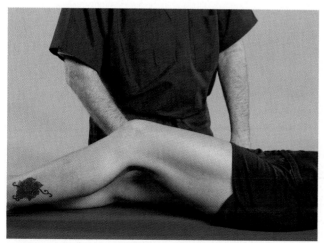

FIG. 10-68 If the sign is present, brisk flexion of the opposite hip and knee occurs. The sign is present only in meningeal irritation.

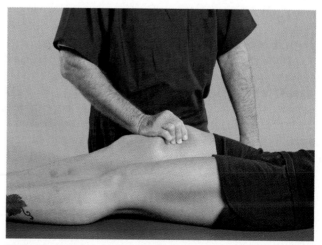

FIG. 10-69 The sign is not exclusive to brisk flexion of the contralateral hip and knee. Ipsilateral flexion, as a function of spasmophilia caused by meningeal irritation, can occasionally be observed.

Assessment for Congenital Dislocation of the Hip Articulation

Comment

Congenital dislocation of the hip (CDH) occurs as the result of underlying dysplasia of the joint. Several theories have been offered as to the origin of this type of dislocation, but the precise cause is still unknown. The disorder exhibits familial and racial tendencies and is often seen in Mediterranean and Scandinavian countries.

CDH is more correctly termed *developmental dysplasia of the hip* (DDH) because few hips are truly dislocated at birth. Hip dislocations in the neonate are thought to be caused by teratologic factors. The incidence of late DDH is approximately 2 per 1000 live births compared with neonatal hip instability of 5 to 20 per 1000. The majority of these cases spontaneously stabilize. For 60% of neonates with hip instability, no known risk factor can be identified. In 20% of cases, both hips are unstable. However, risk factors such as a positive family history, female sex, firstborn children, oligohydramnios, high birth weight, and breech presentation have been well documented. Girls are affected more than boys at a ratio of 5:1. Breech presentation, particularly with extended knees, increases the incidence by a factor of 10. Other congenital anomalies such as torticollis, metatarsus adductus, congenital talipes equinovarus, congenital vertical talus, and calcaneovalgus are associated with DDH (Dare, Clarke, 2007).

The two general degrees of the pathologic condition are complete dislocation and subluxation. Subluxation is the more common type, and, if the condition goes untreated, it may develop into complete dislocation.

As a consequence of a defective acetabulum, the roof of the acetabulum slopes vertically instead of lying in its normal horizontal position. The acetabulum is shallow, and the labrum (limbus) may be folded into the cavity. The femoral head is dislocated upward and laterally out of the acetabulum. Forward torsion of the axis of the femoral neck (anteversion) is usually marked. Adaptive changes take place in the capsule and muscles, and the acetabulum is filled with fatty tissue.

Dislocation is much more common in girls than in boys, and it is often bilateral. In the infant, the obvious clinical findings in unilateral cases are the asymmetric skin folds on the medial aspect of the thigh, the exaggerated vertical angle of the inguinal crease, and the shortening of the affected extremity. The lengths of the patient's femurs are compared while the hips and knees are flexed at 90 degrees. Shortening is readily apparent from the lower level of the knee on the involved side. Abduction of the flexed thigh, which is normally possible up to approximately 90 degrees, is sharply limited. While the thigh is flexed to 90 degrees, a telescopic movement may be apparent by a gentle push-pull technique. During palpation, the absence of the femoral head in Scarpa's triangle and its abnormal posterior position are noted. A click may be felt as the femoral head passes in and out of the acetabulum when the flexed hip is abducted or adducted.

After walking starts, an abnormality of gait is noted. If the condition is unilateral, the child walks with an abduction lurch, and if the condition is bilateral, the child walks with a typical duck-waddling gait.

Congenital subluxation of the hip is associated with clinical findings of asymmetric skin folds and limited abduction of the flexed hip. The diagnosis of congenital subluxation is established by diagnostic imaging. The acetabular roof shows an obliquity and the underdeveloped capital epiphysis, which lies slightly lateral and superior, although in the acetabulum.

Slipped femoral capital epiphysis, which may be chronic, occurs in adolescent children and is probably related to trauma. It represents a variety of Salter-Harris type I fracture of the epiphyseal plate. It is most commonly seen in boys approaching puberty, particularly those who are overweight and sexually immature (Fig. 10-70).

ORTHOPEDIC GAMUT 10-27

SLIPPED FEMORAL CAPITAL EPIPHYSIS

Radiographic signs of slipped femoral capital epiphysis include the following:
1. Blurring of the epiphyseal line
2. Increased width of the epiphyseal plate
3. Prolongation of the superior neck fails to cut epiphysis
4. Loss of height of the epiphysis in comparison with a normal contralateral hip

---

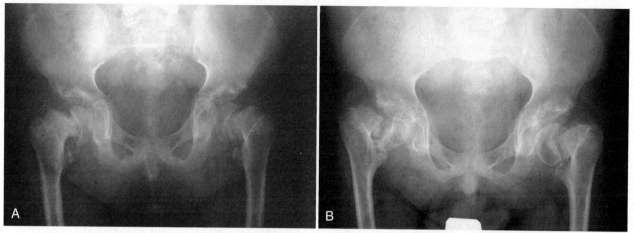

FIG. 10-70 **A,** Plain AP radiograph showing bilateral SUFE, in a Down syndrome patient. **B,** Three years have elapsed. The slips were not pinned. Note there is no evidence of AVN and remodeling has occurred. (From Parsons SJ, Barton C, Banerjee R, et al: Slipped upper femoral epiphysis, *Curr Orthop* 21[3]:215-228, 2007.)

PROCEDURE

- The patient is in a supine position.
- The hip and knee are both flexed to 90 degrees.
- The femur is pushed down toward the examination table (Fig. 10-71a).
- The leg is lifted from the examination table (Fig. 10-71b).
- Movement in hip dislocation will be considerable.
- This is hip telescoping.

Next Steps/Procedures

Allis sign and diagnostic images

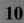

10

CLINICAL PEARL

When treatment in childhood for congenital dislocation of the hip has been unsuccessful, or even when the condition has not been diagnosed, a patient may seek help during the third and fourth decades of life. Symptoms may arise from the hips or the spine. In the hips, secondary arthritic changes occur in the false joint that may form between the dislocated femoral head and the ilium. In the spine, osteoarthritic changes are the result of long-standing scoliosis. The telescoping test may remain positive for as long as the cause of the dislocation goes untreated.

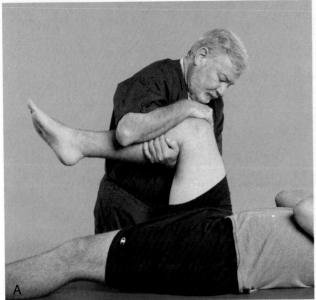

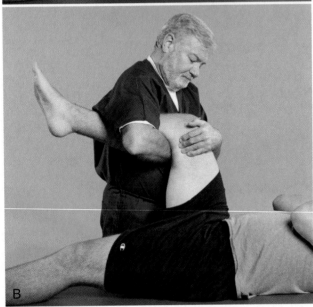

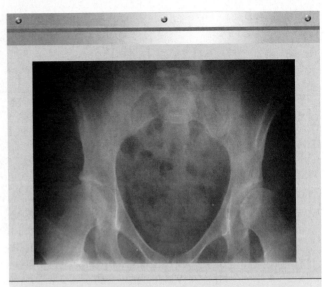

AT THE VIEWBOX

23-year-old female with low back pain and bilateral hip pain with sensation of popping and clicking, associated with pain with hip orthopedic and range of motion tests. There are shallow acetabuli, with altered orientation of the acetabular roofs, which are slightly superiorly angled, laterally. Associated superolateral subluxation with lateral uncovering of the femoral heads, more obvious on the left (reading right). The findings are typical of a mild form of developmental dysplasia of the hips (aka congenital hip dislocation/ hip dysplasia). (From the teaching file of Timothy Mick, DC, DACBR)

FIG. 10-71 The patient is supine. The examiner flexes the affected hip to 90 degrees and the knee to 90 degrees. The femur is pushed toward the examining table and then pulled up from the table. If the test is positive, a distinct pistoning of the hip is noted. The positive finding indicates dislocation of the hip. Although this test is usually used with neonates, the effect of the test may be observed throughout adult life in individuals with untreated or undiagnosed congenital hip dislocations.

Assessment for Osteoarthritis of the Hip Joint

Comment

Osteoarthritis (OA) is the most common joint affection worldwide. According to estimates of the World Health Organization, 190 million people are suffering worldwide from symptomatic OA. It is frequently associated with pain und functional impairment. In recent years, health-related quality of life (HRQL) has increasingly become an important outcome measure in clinical trials and treatment. The Arthritis Impact Measurement Scale, developed by Meenan and colleagues in 1980 for rheumatoid arthritis, was one of the first self-administered questionnaires to assess functional status and HRQL (Rosemann, Szecsenyi, in press).

OA involves a few joints, thus symptoms and signs are localized in nature. Early in the disease, OA is associated with few or no symptoms. Pain is usually the earliest symptom, and it comes on with use, particularly after prolonged inactivity of the joint, and is relieved by rest. The pain is usually a low-grade ache that is often difficult for the patient to localize. As the disease progresses in severity, pain occurs even during rest. Cold, damp weather exacerbates the pain. In some patients, pain may be aggravated by heat. The pain that is experienced by patients with OA is of multiple origins. The pain may result from periosteal elevation associated with cartilage and bone proliferation, from pressure on exposed bone, from microfractures of bone, or from trauma to the synovium. Synovitis occurs in advanced cases of the disease and may cause pain as a result of inflammation. Spasm of muscles or pressure on nerves in the region of the joint may also be a major source of pain.

Stiffness is another common complaint, and it is usually more severe when a patient awakens in the morning or after inactivity during the day. Pain and stiffness are often worse just before changes in the weather. Although stiffness is an important symptom in other forms of connective tissue disease, the stiffness, or fibrositis, associated with osteoarthritis is short lived and usually lasts less than 15 minutes. Limited joint motion eventually develops as a result of abnormalities in the joint surface, muscle spasm, contracture of soft tissues, and the interfering effect of spurs and loose bodies.

During physical examination, the joints may show slight tenderness, and pain occurs as the joint is moved. Palpation of the joint will often reveal crepitus—a sensation of grating as the joint is moved. Joint enlargement is seen, primarily as a result of proliferative reactions in cartilage and bone. Later, both deformity and subluxation become more apparent.

OA of the hip usually occurs in older persons, but it may begin at an earlier age. OA is progressive in nature, and bilateral involvement is not uncommon. Pain is often associated with a limp early on in the disease. Hip pain is felt at the side or the front of the joint or along the inner aspect of the thigh. Errors in diagnosis often arise because pain that originates in the hip may be referred to other regions and may be felt elsewhere. Hip pain may occur in the buttocks or sciatic region. In many individuals, pain is referred along the obturator nerve, down the front of the thigh and knee. In some patients, most or all the pain of the hip disease is felt in the knee. The pain in this area may be so severe that its hip origin is overlooked. Conversely, pain in the region of the hip may originate elsewhere, such as in the lumbosacral spine. Varying degrees of limited hip motion can be noted during examination when OA is present. For example, the leg is held in external rotation with the hip flexed and adducted. Functional shortening may occur. Walking is awkward, and the patient finds difficulty sitting, rising from a seated position, and ascending stairs. Sexual intercourse becomes a stressful activity.

A discussion of hip OA and subsequent sciatic nerve lesions is not complete without referring to the piriformis syndrome. Leg pain (sciatic) may be caused by compression of the sciatic nerve by the piriformis muscle at the pelvic outlet. In healthy individuals, the sciatic nerve passes underneath the piriformis muscle in 85% to 90% of patients; in 9% to 32% of instances, the peroneal division passes only above or through the muscle; and in 1% to 2% of persons, the entire sciatic nerve pierces the piriformis muscle.

The clinical manifestations of the piriformis syndrome include buttock and leg pain that worsens during sitting (without low back pain) and that is exacerbated by internal rotation or abduction and external rotation of the hip (and the straight-leg-raising test) and exquisite local tenderness in the buttock. These symptoms are caused by sciatic nerve compression by the piriformis muscle.

ORTHOPEDIC GAMUT 10-28
PIRIFORMIS SYNDROME AXIOMS

1. Symptoms of piriformis syndrome are not usually substantiated by clinical or electrophysiologic findings.
2. Denervation in the sciatic nerve distribution is usually caused by aberrant fascial bands rather than piriformis muscle.

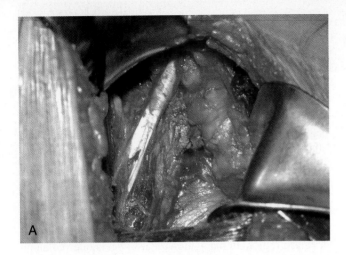

A

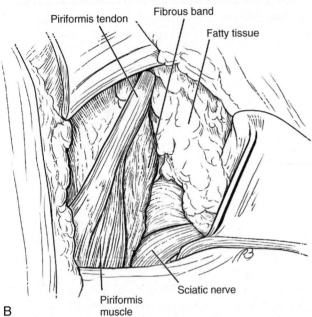

Piriformis tendon   Fibrous band

Fatty tissue

Sciatic nerve

B

Piriformis
muscle

FIG. 10-72 **A** and **B**, The gluteus maximus muscle fibers have been split in line with the incision and are retracted, revealing the underlying structures. The piriformis tendon is isolated, and its muscular fibers are seen overlying the sciatic nerve. In this case, an aberrant fibrous band parallels the piriformis on its deep surface, contributing to compression of the sciatic nerve. Distally, the layer of fat that normally overlies the nerve is seen. This tissue is preserved to reduce the risk of perineural adhesions. (From Byrd JWT: Piriformis syndrome, *Operat Tech Sports Med* 13[1]:71-79, 2006.)

Patients with lumbosacral or buttock pain and those who have referred pain to the thigh in the symptomatic side when ascending inclines and reproduction of the pain on needling provide tacit support for recognizing the piriformis muscle as a contributing factor to the pain (Broadhurst, Simmons, Bond, 2004).

The pattern of denervation is useful; the gluteus medius and tensor fascia lata, both innervated by the superior gluteal nerve, which branches from the sciatic trunk before the piriformis muscle, are normal (Fig. 10-72).

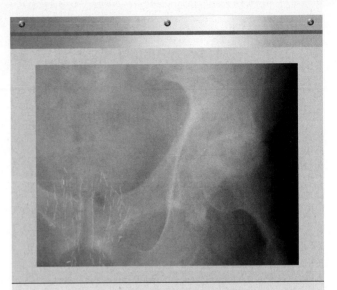

AT THE VIEWBOX

Senior adult male with left hip pain, increased during the year following treatment of prostate cancer with implanted radioactive "seeds." There is end-stage osteoarthritis of the hip joint, with bone on bone appearance at the superior compartment, along with lucency and sclerosis, in a pattern consistent with avascular necrosis of the femoral head. The possible relationship of avascular necrosis to the chronic, low grade radiation therapy might be questioned, but could not be firmly established. (From the teaching file of Timothy Mick, DC, DACBR)

PROCEDURE

- In osteoarthritis deformans of the hip, the patient is asked to cross the legs, with a point just above the ankle resting on the opposite knee (Figs. 10-73 and 10-74).
- If significant disease exists, this test and motion are impossible.

Next Steps/Procedure
Gauvain sign, Patrick test, and diagnostic imaging

CLINICAL PEARL

Primary osteoarthritis of the hip occurs in middle-age and elderly patients and is often associated with obesity and overuse. However, in many instances, no obvious cause can be found. The symptoms of secondary osteoarthritis of the hip are identical to those of primary osteoarthritis. The condition most commonly occurs as a sequel to congenital hip dislocation.

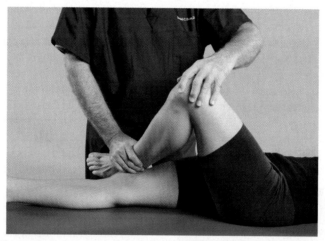

FIG. 10-73 The patient is lying supine. The examiner flexes and externally rotates the affected hip, crossing the patient's ankle over the contralateral knee.

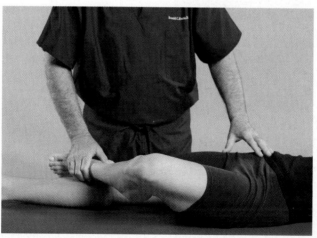

FIG. 10-74 The hip is allowed to abduct and extend passively. The distance between the lateral surface of the thigh and the examination table is noted. The distance is compared with the distance obtained on the opposite side. The test is positive when the motion is impossible to complete. A positive test indicates osteoarthritis of the hip joint.

10

Assessment for Traumatic Separation of the Lesser Trochanter

Comment

Occasionally, the tip of the greater trochanter is cracked as a result of a direct blow. Other than protecting the limb by avoiding weight bearing for a few weeks until the reaction to the trauma has settled down, no specific treatment is required for such a trochanteric crack.

> Isolated lesser trochanter fractures are a rare presentation of hip fractures in elderly adults. Classically, lesser trochanter fractures in adults are associated with tumors and result from little or no trauma (Bonshahi, Knowles, Hodgson, 2004).

The lesser trochanter may be avulsed by the pull of the psoas muscle (Fig. 10-75). By itself, this avulsion is of no importance, but it sometimes occurs because the bone at this level is weakened through pathologic change or a secondary neoplastic deposit. The examiner must bear this possibility in mind and should perform a biopsy if necessary.

Many varieties of malignant tumors have been identified. The picture of any of them may vary depending on the age of the patient, the site, and duration of the lesion. A picture common for one tumor at one stage may be similar to that of a different tumor at a different stage. The examiner does not encounter enough examples of a rare tumor to make generalizations.

Two points are imperative for the examiner to remember. A constant need exists to be aware of the possibility that a malignant lesion may be present. Additionally, a need exists to simplify the problem. These needs can be accomplished, but even so, the examiner should maintain the attitude that the diagnosis, although highly probable, does not become established until the tissue is actually examined.

Although any metastatic tumor may appear in bone, for many tumors, such is the case only when they have existed long enough and are in the terminal stage. Tumors of this type should have been recognized much earlier. Several of the tumors are so rare that the whole group represents less than 2% of the cases involving the structural tissues.

These considerations serve to reduce the list of malignant lesions for practical purposes to approximately 13 varieties, and two of these, metastatic carcinomas of the breast and prostate, are differentiated by the sex of the patient.

These few lesions can be separated into conveniently small groups when the usual age of onset of the particular disease is considered.

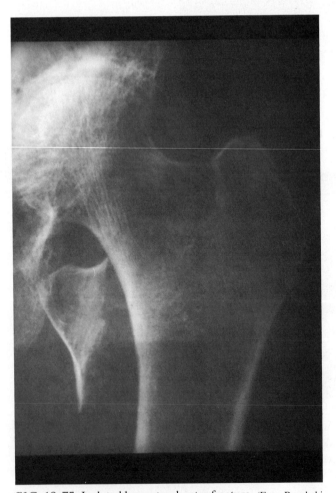

FIG. 10-75 Isolated lesser trochanter fracture. (From Bonshahi AY, Knowles D, Hodgson SP: Isolated lesser trochanter fractures in elderly–a case for prophylactic DHS fixation: A case series, *Injury* 35[2]:196-198, 2004.)

ORTHOPEDIC GAMUT 10-29

MALIGNANT LESIONS

The 13 common malignant tissue lesions are:

1. Neuroblastoma
2. Ewing sarcoma
3. Lymphoma
4. Primary osteogenic sarcoma or chondroma
5. Secondary osteogenic sarcoma or chondroma
6. Metastatic carcinoma of the thyroid
7. Metastatic carcinoma of the breast in women
8. Metastatic carcinoma of the prostate in men
9. Metastatic carcinoma of the bronchus
10. Metastatic carcinoma of the kidneys
11. Hypernephroma
12. Myeloma
13. Neurogenic carcinoma

PROCEDURE

- In traumatic separation of the epiphysis of the lesser trochanter, swelling, and ecchymosis are present at the base of Scarpa triangle, and the patient cannot raise the thigh when in the seated position (Figs. 10-76 and 10-77).

Next Steps/Procedures

Anvil test, Chiene test, and diagnostic imaging

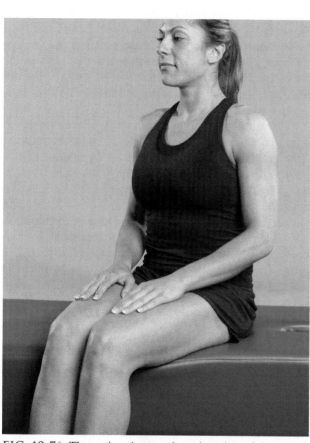

FIG. 10-76 The patient is seated on the edge of the examination table. The feet may touch the floor.

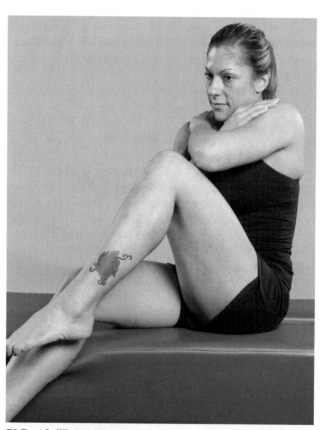

FIG. 10-77 While remaining seated, the patient tries to raise the affected thigh from the table surface. The sign is present when this move cannot be accomplished. When accompanied by swelling and ecchymosis in Scarpa's triangle, this sign indicates fracture of the lesser trochanter.

CLINICAL PEARL

As with femoral neck fractures, this fracture is common in elderly, osteoporotic women. However, in sharp contrast to the intracapsular neck fractures, the extracapsular trochanteric fractures unite very easily and seldom cause avascular necrosis.

Assessment for Iliotibial Band Contracture

Comment

Muscle strains commonly occur in the pelvis and thigh. The two primary causes of muscle injury are acute trauma and overuse trauma. A common mechanism is acute trauma. Single traumatic events, which are usually high-velocity eccentric contractions in which the muscle is rapidly forced into an elongated position, cause the so-called pulled muscle.

The greater trochanteric bursa separates the tendon of the gluteus maximus from the superior portion of the greater trochanter; the trochanteric bursa lies between the tendon of the gluteus medius and the anterosuperior portion of the greater trochanter (Fig. 10-78).

During the clinical examination, the patient typically indicates a localized area of tenderness near the superoposterior tip of the greater trochanter. This area is often quite tender, and the patient may be unable to lie on the affected side for prolonged periods. A positive Ober sign is often present, as is weakness of the hip abductors when tested in an antigravity position.

The iliotibial band is a thickened portion of the tensor fascia latae along its lateral aspect. The tensor fascia latae arises from the coccyx, the sacrum, the iliac crest, Poupart's ligament, and the pubic ramus. Between two layers, the band encloses the gluteus maximus and the tensor fasciae femoris, giving attachment to the latter muscle and most of the former. The fibers of the fasciae converge to form the iliotibial band along the lateral side of the thigh. The iliotibial band is continuous medially with the lateral intermuscular septum, which attaches to the linea aspera. Distally, the band gives origin to the short head of the biceps. At the level of the knee joint, the band spreads out and attaches to the lateral tibial condyle and the head of the fibula. The iliotibial band lies in a plane anterior to the hip joint and posterior to the knee.

Involvement of the attached muscles is responsible for increased tension. The band is placed under the attached muscles during the acute and convalescent stages. The taut band is perceived by deep palpation while adducting and extending the thigh. Resistance to passive flexing of the hip while the knee is fully extended demonstrates spasm in the gluteus maximus. Spasm in the short head of the biceps is demonstrated by flexing the hip, which relaxes the iliopsoas band, and by finding resistance to extension of the knee. The patient assumes the most comfortable position in which the thigh is flexed, abducted, and externally rotated at the hip while the knee is flexed. This position relaxes the tension of

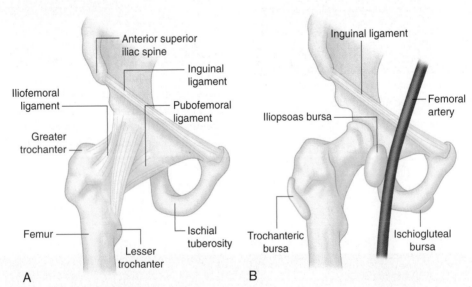

FIG. 10-78 Musculoskeletal anatomy of the hip. **A,** Anterior aspect of the hip joint and bony structures. **B,** Relationship of the distended iliopsoas, trochanteric, and ischiogluteal bursae (shown in blue) to the hip joint and adjacent structures. (Modified from Raney R, Brashear H, Shands A, editors: *Shands' handbook of orthopaedic surgery,* St Louis, 1971, Mosby.) (In Malone TR, McPoil TG, Nitz AJ: *Orthopedic and sports physical therapy,* ed 3, St Louis, 1997, Mosby.)

the band. If tension is not overcome by stretching during the acute stage, band contracture becomes progressive, and permanent deformity ensues.

Iliotibial band contracture is part of the natural history of Duchenne muscular dystrophy (DMD).

DMD consists of the ambulatory and wheelchair phase. Most of the patients become ambulant just after 18 months. Muscle strength initially increases, remains constant, but decreases rapidly from 5 or 6 years of age. Additionally, the time required to perform the Gowers' maneuver (Gowers' time) first decreases, remains constant, and then increases rapidly. The patients lose their ability to stand up from the floor usually at 7 to 8 years of age. The increasing muscle weakness and the development of progressive contractures leads to frequent falls and finally to the loss of ambulation at 9.5 years on average (Forst, Forst, 1999).

The asymmetric retraction of the iliotibial band can be measured reliably only by performing the dangling-leg test. This test shows a spontaneous but asymmetric abduction of both hips. Additionally, the adduction capacity of both hips measured from the neutral position is markedly reduced because the retraction of the iliotibial band the pelvis and the trunk are tilted forward when the patient tries to stand with the feet close together. The alignment of pelvis and trunk is restored if the patient stands with his legs apart.

PROCEDURE

- The patient is in a side-lying position on the unaffected hip and thigh.
- The examiner places one hand on the patient's pelvis to steady it and grasps the patient's ankle lightly with the other hand, holding the knee flexed at a right angle (Fig. 10-79).
- The thigh is abducted and extended in the coronal plane of the body.
- In the presence of iliotibial band contracture, the leg will remain abducted; the degree of abduction depends on the amount of contracture present (Figs. 10-80 and 10-81).
- The sign is present both in the conscious and in the anesthetized patient.
- Ober calls attention to the frequency of a negative roentgenogram in the presence of clinical signs and symptoms of irritation of the sacroiliac or lumbosacral joints.
- He refers to the importance of the iliotibial band as a factor to consider in the occurrence of lumbosacral spinal disorders with or without associated sciatica.

Next Steps/Procedures
Phelps test, Thomas test, and Trendelenburg test

10

CLINICAL PEARL

Transient synovitis of the hip is the most common cause of an irritable hip and can produce a limp and a positive Ober test. The patient sometimes has a history of preceding minor trauma, which in some cases is at least coincidental. Radiographs of the hip sometimes give confirmatory evidence of synovitis, but no other pathologic condition is demonstrable.

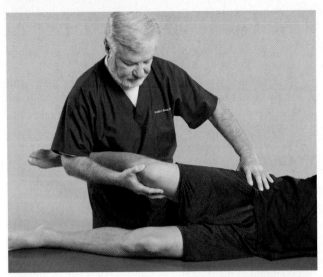

FIG. 10-79 The patient is in a side-lying position on the unaffected hip. The affected leg is extended. The examiner slightly abducts the affected leg.

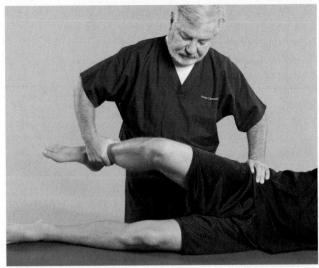

FIG. 10-80 The examiner stabilizes the pelvis with one hand and grasps the ankle of the affected leg with the other hand. The examiner flexes the knee to 90 degrees. The thigh is abducted and extended. The test is positive if the leg remains abducted. A positive test indicates iliotibial band contracture.

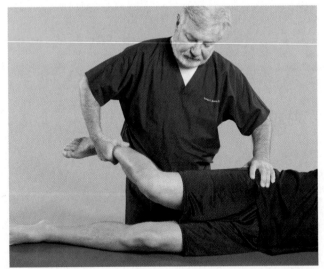

FIG. 10-81 The same procedure used on a normal hip demonstrates the normal adduction movement of the leg.

PATRICK TEST

ALSO KNOWN AS FABERE SIGN (FLEXION, ABDUCTION, EXTERNAL ROTATION, EXTENSION)

Assessment for Intracapsular Coxa Pathologic Conditions

Comment

Death of the subchondral bone of the femoral head as a result of vascular impairment is known as *avascular necrosis* (AVN), *aseptic necrosis*, or *osteonecrosis*. This severely disabling condition can affect individuals of all ages. The clinical picture typically includes persistent inguinal pain and limping. In many cases, the patient is unable to report a recent injury or precipitating event but, when questioned in detail, may report one or more of the risk factors mentioned previously. The diagnosis is confirmed with radiographic evaluation. In many cases, the classic finding of the crescent sign is apparent on AP films (Fig. 10-82).

Articular cartilage is not innervated. As the OA progresses, capsular fibrosis and shortening occur; the typical pattern results in limited extension, abduction, and internal rotation of the hip. The capsule can be painfully stretched during the middle and late stance phases of gait, which require the hip to assume these positions. This action results in muscle guarding by the hip intrinsic muscles, further restricting motion and causing pain.

Rheumatoid arthritis (RA) is a disabling, autoimmune, systemic connective tissue disease that is present to different degrees in more than 3.6 million Americans. This disease is characterized by chronic swelling, pain, and progressive deformity of multiple joints.

Degenerative arthritis that is confined to the hip joint is a common affliction that occurs in the middle and later years of adult life. The cause of degenerative arthritis is not completely understood, but obesity, trauma, CDH, AVN of the femoral head, and slipped capital femoral epiphysis are all factors in its onset.

ORTHOPEDIC GAMUT 10-30
HIP OSTEOARTHRITIS

Classic radiographic findings of hip osteoarthritis include:
1. Loss of joint space
2. Sclerosis of subchondral bone of the femoral head
3. Osteophytes around the joint margins
4. Bone cysts in the subchondral bone (Fig. 10-83)

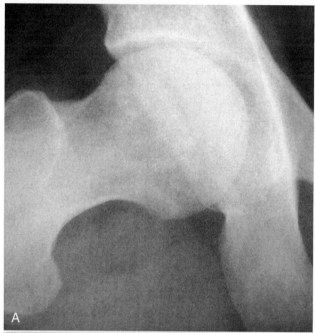

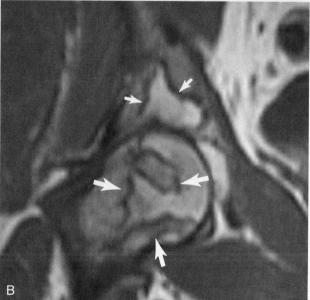

FIG. 10-82 A 27-year-old man with right hip osteonecrosis. The lateral radiograph (**A**) of the right hip is unremarkable. The coronal T1-weighted MR image (**B**) reveals a large osteonecrotic lesion stage ICC according to ARCO classification (arrows). A large osteonecrotic lesion, not visible on plain radiograph, is also shown in the acetabulum (small arrows). (From Zibis AH, Karantanas AH, Roidis NT et al: The role of MR imaging in staging femoral head osteonecrosis, *Eur J Radiol* 63(1):3-9, 2007.)

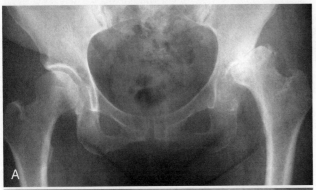

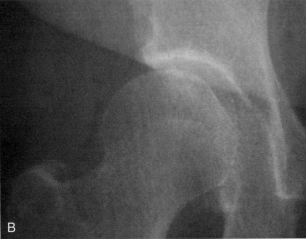

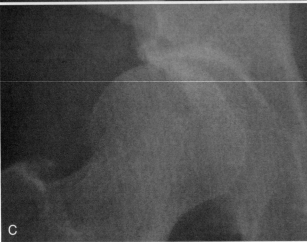

FIG. 10-83 Radiographs of a 58-year-old woman who was diagnosed with rapidly destructive arthrosis of the left hip. (A) Anteroposterior radiograph obtained at the time of the left THA (total hip arthroplasty) shows subluxation and flattening of the left femoral head. The right hip joint appears to be normal except for the presence of developmental dysplasia of the acetabulum (AHI (acetabular head index), 69%; CE (center-edge) angle, 15 degrees). (B) Anteroposterior radiograph of the right hip obtained 2.3 years after THA shows mild joint space narrowing. (C) Anteroposterior radiograph obtained 3.4 years after THA shows a rapid loss of joint space mainly at the superolateral portion of the femoral head. (From Motomura G, Yamamoto T, Nakashima Y, et al: Outcome of the contralateral hip in rapidly destructive arthrosis after total hip arthroplasty: A preliminary report, *J Arthroplasty* 21(7):1026-1031, 2006.)

Pathologically, the articular cartilage becomes progressively thinned and worn away. New bone proliferation around the femoral head and acetabulum occurs. The synovium becomes chronically thickened and congested.

In global radiologic classifications of OA such as the Kellgren-Lawrence score, the notion of a certain sequence of degeneration is implicit: narrowing of joint space precedes the development of osteophytes, which precedes subchondral sclerosis, which precedes the formation of cysts, which precedes deformation of the femoral head and acetabulum. Croft's widely used update of the Kellgren-Lawrence classification does not have this premise of a causal chain of degeneration; one is able to choose two to four out of five different radiographic features in characterizing the level of degeneration. This ability to choose is an advantage; a certain sequence of degenerative bone reaction has not been documented in the literature (Jacobsen et al, 2004).

The clinical course is gradual, and both hips may be affected. The onset of symptoms may be precipitated by a minor injury. Pain after activity and stiffness after rest are characteristic. The stiffness often subsides with activity, and the pain usually subsides with rest. The pain is often referred to the knee joint region. With the passage of time, the pain increases, sometimes even occurring during rest. Crepitus and grating in the hip may develop, and a painful limp is common.

Numerous special tests can be performed in the supine position to clarify the involved tissues. Gentle, manual spinal distraction may reduce low back pain and assist the examiner in the differential diagnosis. The nature of the passive motion of the hip can be further appreciated with inferior glide, lateral glide, and *perimeter* scouring (Fig. 10-84).

Examination reveals tenderness over the anterior and posterior hip joint and restriction of motion, especially internal rotation and abduction. Pain is usually present at the extremes of motion, and a flexion contracture often develops. This contracture can be measured by the Thomas test.

PROCEDURE

- Patrick test is of particular value in geriatric cases because it indicates hip joint disease.
- The patient lies supine, and the examiner grasps the patient's ankle and the flexes knee (Fig. 10-85).
- The thigh is flexed, abducted, externally rotated, and extended (Figs. 10-86 and 10-87).
- The first letters of these words form the acronym FABERE.
- Pain in the hip during the maneuver, particularly on abduction and external rotation, is a positive sign of a coxa pathologic condition.

Next Steps/Procedures
Gauvain sign, Jansen test, and diagnostic imaging

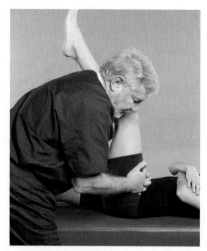

FIG. 10-84 *Perimeter scouring* of the hip.

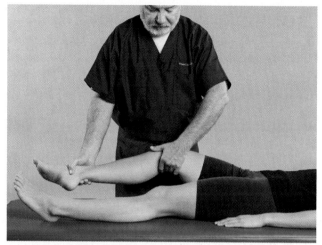

FIG. 10-85 The patient is lying supine on the examination table. The examiner grasps the affected leg.

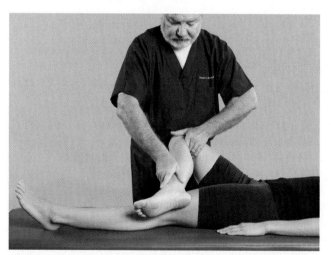

FIG. 10-86 The examiner flexes the hip, abducts the thigh, crosses the ankle over the contralateral knee, and externally rotates the hip.

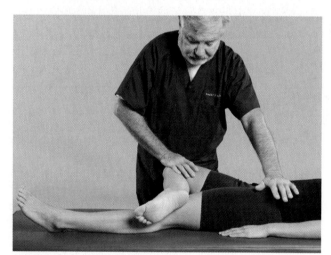

FIG. 10-87 The examiner then extends the hip by applying downward pressure on the knee. The contralateral side of the pelvis is fixed to the table and not allowed to rock upward. Pain during abduction and external rotation is a positive finding and indicates a coxa pathologic condition.

10

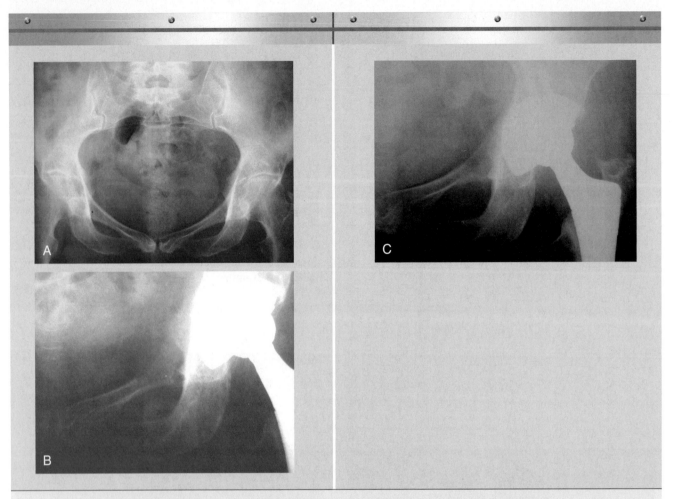

AT THE VIEWBOX

66-year-old female with left anterior groin pain, treated with left hip joint replacement, but with ongoing left hip pain over the following year. History of breast cancer, with lumpectomy 3 years ago. Pre-operative X-ray (**A**) demonstrates an ill-defined, rounded lucency in the left (reading right) supra-acetabular region, along with non-uniform left hip joint space narrowing. There are also mild degenerative changes of the symphysis pubis and sacroiliac joints. Continued left hip pain prompted a follow-up radiograph by the orthopedist, to assess for loosening of a left hip arthroplasty (**B**). This was interpreted as negative for loosening. Subtle cortical destruction and ill-defined lucency in the superior pubic ramus was not recognized. A follow-up radiograph of the left hip joint (**C**) demonstrates more obvious osteolytic destruction of the left superior pubic ramus, due to osteolytic breast metastasis. The patient passed away shortly thereafter from the metastatic disease. It is recognized that "hip" complaints may arise from a wide variety of etiologies and sites of origin. (From the teaching file of Timothy Mick, DC, DACBR)

CLINICAL PEARL

An intracapsular fracture, which can cause a positive Patrick test, can cut off the blood supply to the femoral head completely, which can lead to aseptic necrosis, non-union, or both. Because the fracture line is inside the capsule, blood is contained within it. This trapped blood raises the intracapsular pressure, damaging the femoral head still further, and prevents visible bruising because the blood cannot reach the subcutaneous tissues.

Assessment for Contracture of the Gracilis Muscle Associated with a Pathologic Condition of the Hip Joint

Comment

Piriformis syndrome is a condition in which the piriformis muscle contributes to entrapment or irritation of the adjacent nerves. Numerous pain-sensitive structures course in the small interval created by the inferior margin of the piriformis and the superior gemellus muscle (Fig. 10-88). The clinical picture of piriformis syndrome includes a complaint of buttock pain, which often refers posteriorly to the ipsilateral thigh and occasionally to the calf. If a patient has an observable internal rotation of one or both lower limbs, excessive femoral anteversion may be present. More range of motion

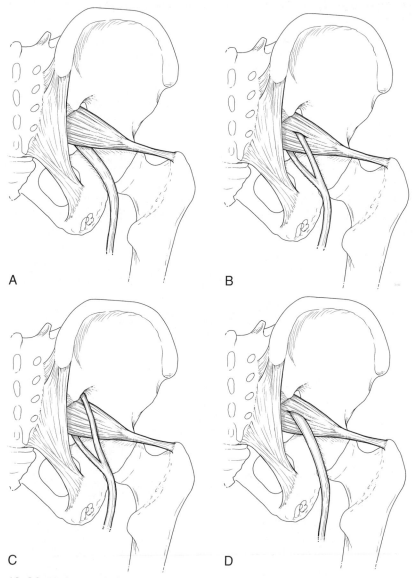

FIG. 10-88 Various relationships of the piriformis muscle and the sciatic nerve as described by Beaton and Anson. **A,** Most commonly, the undivided nerve exits the greater sciatic notch below the piriformis muscle (84.2%). **B,** Second most common, divisions of the sciatic nerve pass between and below the bifid muscle belly of the piriformis (11.7%). **C,** Divisions of the nerve pass above and below an undivided muscle (3.3%). **D,** An undivided nerve passes between the bifid muscle bellies of the piriformis (0.8%). (From Byrd JWT: Piriformis syndrome, *Operat Tech Sports Med* 13[1]:71-79, 2005.)

is usually present in internal than in external rotation of the hip in these patients.

The presence of excessive femoral anteversion can be corroborated by Craig test (Fig. 10-89). To perform this procedure, the examiner flexes the prone patient's knee to 90 degrees. The examiner then rotates the patient's hip while palpating the greater trochanter. When the greater trochanter is felt to be in a mid position, such as parallel to the floor, the examiner then views the angle of the tibia relative to the long axis of the body. In a normal adult hip, it should be roughly perpendicular to the floor. Excessive anteversion is present if the tibia is pointing outward, away from the midline of the patient's body.

Most patients seeking help because of a hip-joint problem may do so because of pain, stiffness, a limp, or a deformity.

Pain of a hip-joint origin may be localized to the groin and from there may radiate down the medial or anterior aspect of the thigh. The pain also may arise in the region of the greater trochanter and radiate laterally along the course of the tensor fasciae latae toward the knee. Hip-joint pain may be evident posteriorly in the region of the ischial tuberosity and must be carefully differentiated from the complaint of sciatica. The pain often is referred to the lower back or knee and can be reproduced or accentuated by movements of the hip joint.

Subjective stiffness of the hip joint may be noted by the patient after periods of immobility, such as after prolonged sitting or on arising from bed in the morning. In more advanced degenerative states affecting the hip joint, objective stiffness may be noted by the examiner. In degenerative arthritis of the hip joint, for example, the patient will lose hip-joint motion sequentially, with the ability to rotate the hip being lost first, followed by abduction and adduction

loss, and finally hip flexion loss. For this reason, many patients with degenerative arthritis of the hip describe difficulty in putting a shoe or stocking on the affected leg because this action usually requires the ability to rotate the hip joint externally.

A restricted hip range of motion has been described in many of the diagnostic entities used to categorize sports-related chronic groin injury (CGI). A lower range of hip-joint motion has been detected in athletes diagnosed with osteitis pubis and in athletes with pubic bone stress injury. A lower range of motion in hip abduction has been associated with athletes diagnosed as having groin strain and adductor-related groin pain (Verrall et al, in press).

Hip-joint range-of-motion restriction precedes the development of CGI and may be a risk factor for this condition.

A limp is a pathologic asymmetric gait, and several mechanisms, singly or in combination, may be operating on the hip joint to produce it. Shortening of the lower extremity and marked stiffness of the hip joint may be sufficient to alter gait pattern. The limp may be protective because of weight-bearing pain. This type of abnormal gait, called an *antalgic gait,* is characterized by a very short stance phase. However, the gait most characteristic of hip-joint disease is called a *gluteal lurch,* and it relates directly to a structural or functional weakness of the gluteus medius on the affected side. Any abnormality of the pelvic-femoral lever arm may weaken the gluteus medius muscle. If this weakening occurs, the muscle can no longer support the pelvis and trunk on the lower extremity, and the patient's trunk lurches to the affected side during weight bearing.

Visible deformity of the lower extremity is often associated with injuries or disease affecting the hip joint. A patient with a fracture of the hip joint usually holds the lower extremity in marked external rotation. A patient who has

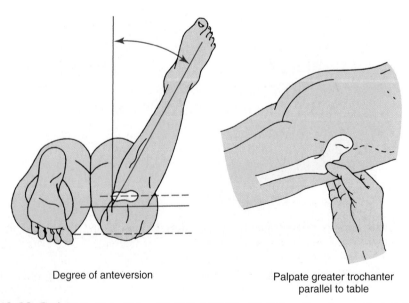

Degree of anteversion

Palpate greater trochanter parallel to table

FIG. 10-89 Craig test. (From Malone TR, McPoil TG, Nitz AJ: *Orthopedic and sports physical therapy,* ed 3, St Louis, 1997, Mosby.)

sustained a traumatic dislocation of the hip joint usually holds the lower extremity in internal rotation. Degenerative arthritis of the hip joint is often associated with flexion-adduction external-rotation contractures. Flexion and adduction contractures about the hip, external-rotation position of the lower extremity, shortening of the leg, and a limp are characteristic deformities that may be produced by hip-joint disorders.

PROCEDURE

- The patient is lying prone, the knees are extended, and the thighs are maximally abducted (Fig. 10-90).
- Pain and resistance should be used as criteria for maximal abduction.
- The patient's knees are flexed bilaterally to a right angle (Fig. 10-91).
- The examiner notes if the maneuver allows more hip abduction.
- The test is positive if knee flexion increases or knee extension decreases hip abduction.
- The test indicates contracture of the gracilis muscle.

Next Steps/Procedures
Ober test, Thomas test, and Trendelenburg test

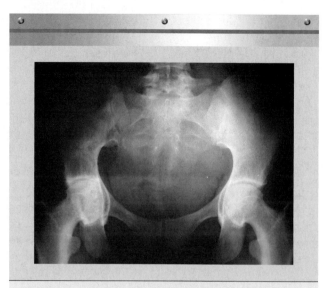

AT THE VIEWBOX

26-year-old female with bilateral hip pain. There is bilateral, symmetric invagination of the medial acetabuli, typical of a primary, developmental form of protrusio acetabulum. There is associated premature osteoarthritis, with non-uniform joint space narrowing and osteophyte formation at the femoral head-neck junctions. Secondary forms of protrusio acetabuli include any cause of bone softening, such as chronic inflammatory arthritis and osteomalacic conditions.
(From the teaching file of Timothy Mick, DC, DACBR)

10

CLINICAL PEARL

Two nonspecific gait abnormalities commonly result from hip disease. The antalgic gait usually indicates a painful hip. The patient shortens the stance phase on the affected hip, leaning over the affected side, to prevent painful contraction of the hip abductors. Trendelenburg gait, or abductor limp, indicates weakness of the abductors on the affected side. During the stance phase, on the affected side, the contralateral pelvis dips down, and the body leans to the unaffected side. If the condition is bilateral, a waddling gait is produced.

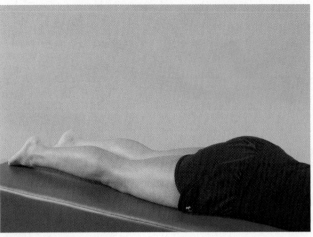

FIG. 10-90 The patient is lying prone with the knees extended. The thighs are maximally abducted as far as the patient can tolerate.

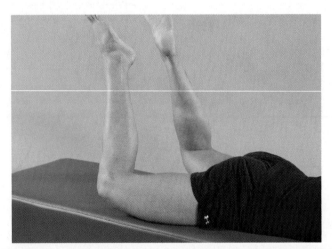

FIG. 10-91 The knees are flexed actively or passively to 90 degrees. If flexion of the knees allows more hip abduction, the test is positive. A positive test indicates gracilis muscle contracture.

THOMAS TEST

Assessment for Flexion Contracture Involving the Iliopsoas

Comment

The Thomas test is designed to evaluate the presence of a flexion contracture of the hip (Fig. 10-92).

Age and sex largely limit osteochondritis deformans juvenilis, or coxa plana. Legg (1910), Perthes (1910), and Calvé (1910) described the disease separately in the United States, Germany, and France. It is seen almost exclusively in children 3 to 12 years of age, but the disease has been reported in children as young as 2 and in others as old as 18. More boys than girls are affected by a ratio of 4:1. The disease is usually unilateral, and a familial history of the disease is present in 20% of the cases.

The most widely accepted cause for the disease is interruption of the blood supply to the head of the femur. This interrupted blood supply is thought to be produced by excessive fluid pressure of a synovial effusion in the hip joint. The head of the femur is at risk between the ages of 3 and 10 because, of the three blood supplies to the femoral head, only the lateral epiphyseal vessels are functional during this period. The blood supply to different segments of the head of the femur varies. For instance, the blood supply to the posterior segment is more generous than the supply to the anterior segment. The posterior portion of the head of the femur is often spared from this disease.

Subchondral fractures occur early in the disease, and these may be the initiating factor in a sequence of events that results in LCPD. Abnormal blood-clotting processes, caused by substances that create a state of hypercoagulability, are thought to result in formation of platelet aggregations and fibrin thrombi that might block the limited vascular supply to the head of the femur. This process has a relationship with previous transient synovitis or other inflammatory processes because of the presence of thickened blood vessels and capsules.

During physical examination, pain can range from mild to severe and will be felt in the groin, thigh, and often the knee. This pain is associated with a limp or slightly abnormal gait. The gait is an antalgic one, in which the patient tries to protect the hip by rapidly shifting body weight off the foot of the involved side.

> Crouch gait is one of the most prevalent walking patterns in children with cerebral palsy characterized by increased and excessive knee flexion, increased ankle dorsiflexion, and hip trajectory ranging from almost normal to excessively flexed throughout the gait cycle. Crouch gait can develop as a consequence of surgical lengthening of Achilles' tendon or as a result of weakness of triceps surae. However, in most cases, crouch gait originates from contractured or tightened hamstrings, which are often combined with hip flexors deformity (Matjacic, Olensek, 2007).

The iliopsoas muscle is a uniarticular hip flexor and exerts hip-flexion moment. Therefore, contracture of the

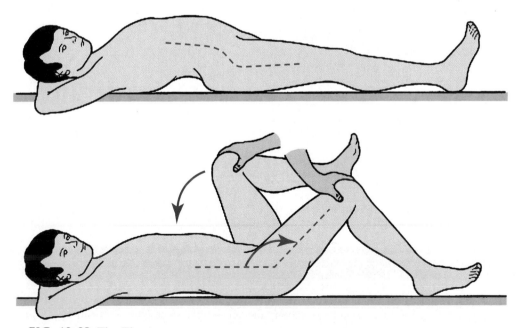

FIG. 10-92 The Thomas test. (From Klippel JH, Dieppe PA: *Rheumatology*, vol 1-2, ed 2, London, 1998, Mosby.)

iliopsoas directly forces the hip into flexion. The iliopsoas can also dynamically act to accelerate the knee into flexion. This excessively flexed hip posture reduces influence of iliopsoas contracture at initial contact and loading response and postpones it into terminal stance. Given that the iliopsoas dynamically acts to accelerate the knee into flexion, this acceleration must be controlled.

With a flexion contracture (positive Thomas test), motion—particularly abduction, internal rotation, extension, and flexion—at the hip is limited. A patient may experience muscle spasm of the adductor and psoas muscle and muscle wasting of the thigh and buttock. The anterior and posterior aspects of the hip joint may also be tender.

The erythrocyte sedimentation rate might be elevated, but the results of other laboratory investigations are normal.

PROCEDURE

- The patient lies supine, and the thigh is flexed with the knee bent toward the abdomen (Fig. 10-93).
- The patient's lumbar spine should normally flatten, or flex.
- If the spine maintains a lordosis, the test is positive and indicates hip flexion contracture, as from a shortened iliopsoas muscle (Fig. 10-94).

Next Steps/Procedures
Ober test, Phelps test, and Trendelenburg test

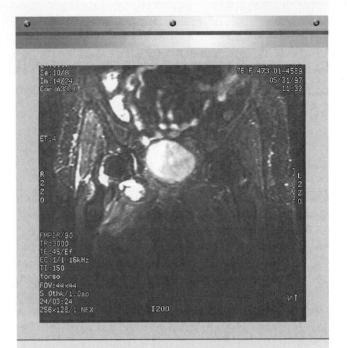

AT THE VIEWBOX

76-year-old female with right hip pain. A fluid collection at the inferomedial aspect of the femoral head-neck junction on this inversion recovery (fluid-weighted) image is typical of iliopsoas bursitis. This may be an isolated finding or may be associated with intrinsic hip joint abnormality. The normal urinary bladder lies superomedial to the bursal fluid collection. (From the teaching file of Timothy Mick, DC, DACBR)

CLINICAL PEARL

Restricted hip flexion may be compensated by an increase in lumbar lordosis. This increase masks the fixed flexion deformity. Fixed flexion, external rotation, and abduction accumulate sequentially as the hip disease progresses.

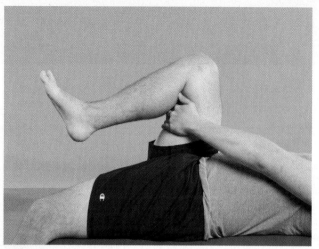

FIG. 10-93 The patient is lying supine on the examination table. The thigh of the unaffected leg is actively flexed toward the abdomen. The patient holds the leg in this position with both hands. The examiner observes the posture of the lower back and the affected leg. The lumbar spine should flatten, and the opposite leg should remain flat on the table.

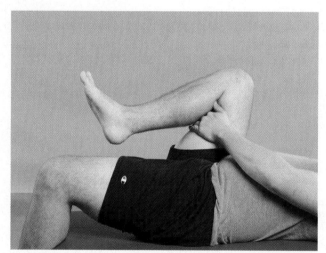

FIG. 10-94 If the lumbar spine maintains a lordosis, if the affected leg flexes, and if the patient is unable to lay the leg flat on the table, the test is positive. A positive test indicates a shortened iliopsoas muscle.

10

Assessment for Insufficiency of the Hip Abductor System

Comment

The unilateral leg stand or Trendelenburg test is a useful procedure for detecting hip-joint dysfunction. A positive Trendelenburg sign is identified when the patient is unable to maintain the pelvis horizontal to the floor while standing first on one foot and then on the other foot (Fig. 10-95).

The Trendelenburg test was developed to assess the function of the hip joint. The test was performed in the standing position, based on the description provided by Hardcastle and Nade. The patient was asked to flex one hip to 30 degrees and to lift the pelvis of the nonstance side above the transiliac line. This position was maintained for 30 seconds. The pelvis should not tilt or rotate as the weight is shifted to the supporting leg. The patient was allowed to touch the table with one finger to correct for potential balance problems. If the patient was not able to hold the test position, or if the pelvis of the nonstance side could not be elevated above the transiliac line, then the test was scored positive by the examiner. In addition, after performing the test, the patient was asked to score the perceived effort to perform the test (Roussel et al, 2007).

Trendelenburg test investigates stability of the hip and particularly the ability of the hip abductors (gluteus medius and gluteus minimus) to stabilize the pelvis on the femur.

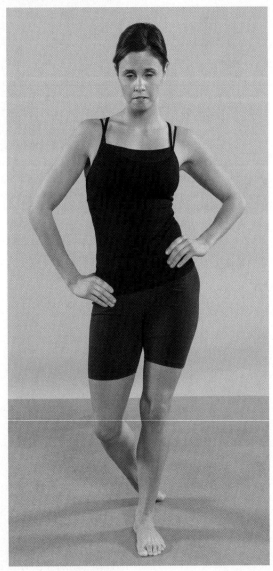

FIG. 10-95 A positive, uncompensated Trendelenburg test indicates weakness of the left hip abductor mechanism.

ORTHOPEDIC GAMUT 10-31

POSITIVE TRENDELENBURG TEST

Fundamental causes for a positive Trendelenburg test include:

1. Paralysis of the abductor muscles, which can occur with poliomyelitis
2. Marked approximation of the insertion of the muscles to their origin by upward displacement of the greater trochanter causing the muscles to be slack (This slackening may occur in severe coxa vara or congenital dislocation of the hip.)
3. Absence of a stable fulcrum causes a positive test (This result occurs in the ununited fracture of the femoral neck.)
4. Sometimes, a combination of two of the aforementioned factors

Normally, when one leg is raised from the ground, the pelvis tilts upward on that side because of the action of the hip abductors of the supporting limb. This automatic mechanism allows the lifted leg to clear the ground while walking. If the abductors are inefficient, they are unable to sustain the pelvis against the body weight. The result is that the pelvis tilts downward instead of rising on the side of the lifted leg.

For instance, upward dislocation of the hip is associated with an unstable fulcrum and approximation of the origin of the abductor muscles to their insertion.

PROCEDURE

- The patient with a suspected hip involvement stands on one foot, on the side of the involvement, and raises the other foot and leg for thigh flexion and knee flexion.
- If the hip and its muscles are normal, the iliac crest will be low on the standing side and high on the side of the elevated leg (Fig. 10-96).
- If hip joint and muscle weakness are involved, the iliac crest will be high on the standing side and low on the side of the elevated leg (Fig. 10-97).
- The test is commonly positive in a developing LCPD, poliomyelitis, muscular dystrophy, coxa vara, Otto pelvis, epiphyseal separation, coxa ankylosis, dislocation, fracture, or subluxation.

Next Steps/Procedures
Ober test, Phelps test, and Thomas test

CLINICAL PEARL

Trendelenburg test is positive as a result of (1) gluteal paralysis or weakness (from polio), (2) gluteal inhibition (from pain arising in the hip joint), (3) gluteal insufficiency from coxa vara, or (4) congenital dislocation of the hip. Nevertheless, false-positive results have been recorded in approximately 10% of the patients with hip pain.

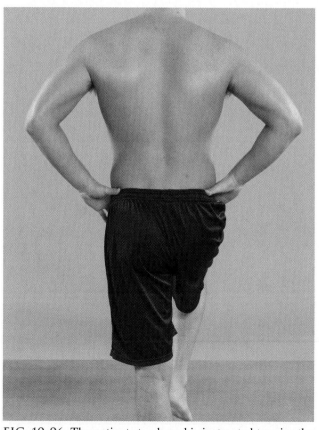

FIG. 10-96 The patient stands and is instructed to raise the foot of the unaffected leg off the floor. If normal, the iliac crest may be low on the standing side and high on the side of the elevated leg.

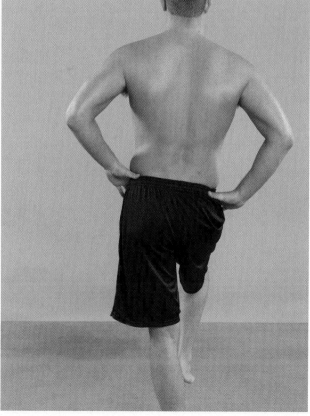

FIG. 10-97 If the test is positive, the iliac crest will be high on the standing side and low on the side of the elevated leg. A positive test indicates a coxa pathologic condition.

CRITICAL THINKING

1. Where is most of the pain in degenerative arthritis of the hip?
2. What is the Thomas test?
3. What is Trendelenburg test?
4. List the three specific tests for hip abnormality in an infant.
5. What is slipped capital femoral epiphysis?
6. What is Legg-Calvé-Perthes disease?
7. What is a hip dislocation?
8. What is the mechanism for an avulsion fracture?
9. What is iliotibial band syndrome?
10. When might slipped capital femoral epiphysis be present?
11. What are the causative factors of stress fractures of the femoral neck?
12. How can increased femoral anteversion cause problems in the lower extremity?
13. How can the presence of femoral anteversion or retroversion be determined?
14. Limitation of hip movements in all directions in a diabetic patient suggests what hip-joint abnormality?
15. Greater trochanteric bursitis creates pain in the hip joint. What spinal level may refer pain to the area of the greater trochanter?
16. What are the three clinically relevant hip bursae?
17. Branches of what nerve or nerves innervate the hip joint?
18. What is the sclerotome referenced for the hip joint?
19. Name six developmental and acquired conditions that can result in coxa vara.
20. A child has a waddling gait. What is the suspected cause?
21. Your patient has a history of hip joint fracture that occurred several months ago. The presenting complaints are pain in the hip when weight bearing, shortening and external rotation of the limb, and a grating or crepitus of the hip during motion. What condition is suspected?
22. Name the most common causes of osteonecrosis of the hip joint.
23. What is the origin of the iliotibial band?
24. Describe Chiene test for assessment of possible fracture of the neck of the femur.

BIBLIOGRAPHY

Abrams WB, Berkow R: *The Merck manual of geriatrics,* Rahway, NJ, 1990, Merck Sharp & Dohme Research Laboratories.

Adams JA: Transient synovitis of the hip joint in children, *J Bone Joint Surg* 45B:471, 1963.

Adams JC: *Standard orthopaedic operations,* Edinburgh, 1985, Churchill Livingstone.

Adams JC, Hamblen DL: *Outline of orthopaedics,* ed 11, Edinburgh, 1990, Churchill Livingstone.

Adams RD: *Diseases of muscle,* ed 3, London, 1975, Henry Kimpton.

Alario AJ: *Practical guide to the care of the pediatric patient,* St Louis, 1997, Mosby.

Alexander CJ: The etiology of femoral epiphyseal slipping, *J Bone Joint Surg* 48B:299, 1966.

Allison D, Strickland N: *Acronyms & synonyms in medical imaging,* Oxford, UK, 1996, ISIS Medical Media.

American Academy of Orthopaedic Surgeons: *Atlas of limb prosthetics,* St Louis, 1981, Mosby.

American Academy of Orthopaedic Surgeons: *Instructional course lectures,* vol 37, Chicago, 1988, The Academy.

American Medical Association: *Guides to the evaluation of permanent impairment,* ed 4, Chicago, 1993, The Association.

American Medical Association: *How to use guides to the evaluation of permanent impairment,* ed 4, Falmouth, Conn, 1993, SEAK.

American Orthopaedic Association: *Manual of orthopaedic surgery,* Chicago, 1972, The Association.

Anderson GH et al: Preoperative skin traction for fractures of the proximal femur, a randomized prospective trial, *J Bone Joint Surg* 75B:794, 1993.

Anderson KN, Anderson LE: *Mosby's pocket dictionary of medicine, nursing, & allied health,* ed 2, St Louis, 1994, Mosby.

Apley AG, Solomon L: *Concise system of orthopaedics and fractures,* London, 1988, Butterworth-Heinemann.

Arokoski JPA et al: Postural control in male patients with hip osteoarthritis *Gait Posture* 23(1):45-50, 2006.

Aston JN: *A Short textbook of orthopaedics and traumatology,* Philadelphia, 1967, JB Lippincott.

Aydogan M et al: Severe erosion of lumbar vertebral body because of a chronic ruptured abdominal aortic aneurysm, *Spine J* (in press, corrected proof).

Baker PA, Watson SB: Functional gracilis flap in thenar reconstruction, *J Plast Reconstr Aesth Surg* (in press, corrected proof).

Barkauskas VH et al: *Health & physical assessment,* ed 2, St Louis, 1998, Mosby.

Barlow TG: Congenital dislocation of the hip, *Hosp Med* 2:571, 1968.

Barnes R: Fracture of the neck of the femur, *J Bone Joint Surg* 49B:607, 1967.

Batt AK, Braham RA, Goodman C: Selected physical capacity norms for Australian football players at the non-elite level, *J Sci Med Sport* 10(2):119-126, 2007.

Beattie P et al: Validity of derived measurements of leg-length differences obtained by the use of a tape measure, *Phys Ther* 70:150, 1990.

Beeson PB, McDermott W: *Textbook of medicine,* ed 13, Philadelphia, 1971, WB Saunders.

Ben-Galim P et al: Hip-spine syndrome: the effect of total hip replacement surgery upon low back pain in patients with severe osteoarthritis of the hip, *Spine J* 6(5, suppl 1):31S-32S, 2006.

Bennett JT, MacEwen GD: Congenital dislocation of the hip: recent advances and current problems, *Clin Orthop* 247:15, 1989.

Benson MKD, Evans DCJ: The pelvis osteotomy of Chiari, *J Bone Joint Surg* 58B:164, 1976.

Berkeley ME et al: Surgical therapy for congenital dislocation of the hip in patients who are twelve to thirty-six months old, *J Bone Joint Surg* 66A:412, 1984.

Bharam S: Labral tears, extra-articular injuries, and hip arthroscopy in the athlete, *Clin Sports Med* 25(2):279-292, 2006.

Bierbaum BE et al: Late complications of total hip replacement. In Steinberg ME, editor: *The hip and its disorders,* Philadelphia, 1991, WB Saunders.

Bijlsma JWJ, Knahr K: Strategies for the prevention and management of osteoarthritis of the hip and knee, *Best Pract Res Clin Rheumatol* 21(1):59-76, 2007.

Birch R: The place of microsurgery in orthopaedics. In: *Recent advances in orthopaedics,* ed 5, Edinburgh, 1987, Churchill Livingstone.

Blockey NJ: Derotation osteotomy in the management of congenital dislocation of the hip, *J Bone Joint Surg* 66B:485, 1984.

Boling MC et al: Outcomes of a weight-bearing rehabilitation program for patients diagnosed with patellofemoral pain syndrome, *Arch Phys Med Rehabil* 87(11):1428-1435, 2006.

Bombelli R: *Osteoarthritis of the hip: pathogenesis and consequent therapy,* New York, 1976, Springer-Verlag.

Bonalaski JS, Schumacher HR: Arthritis and allied conditions. In Steinberg M, editor: *The hip and its disorders,* Philadelphia, 1991, WB Saunders.

Bottin A et al: Non-invasive assessment of the gracilis muscle by means of surface electromyography electrode arrays, *J Surg Res* 134(2):265-269, 2006.

Bowen JR, Foster BK, Hartzell C: Legg-Calve-Perthes disease, *Clin Orthop* 185:97, 1984.

Bradley GW et al: Resurfacing arthroplasty: femoral head viability, *Clin Orthop* 220:137, 1987.

Brashear HR, Raney RB: *Shands' handbook of orthopaedic surgery,* St Louis, 1978, Mosby.

Bringnall CG, Stainsby GD: The snapping hip: treatment by Z-plasty, *J Bone Joint Surg* 73B:253, 1991.

Brooks M, Evans R, Fairclough J: *Sports injuries,* ed 2, London, 1992, Gower Medical.

Brotzman SB: *Clinical orthopaedic rehabilitation,* St Louis, 1996, Mosby.

Brown DE, Neumann RD: *Orthopedic secrets,* Philadelphia, 1995, Hanley & Belfus.

Bruno PA, Bagust J: An investigation into motor pattern differences used during prone hip extension between subjects with and without low back pain, *Clin Chiropr Edu* 10(2):68-80, 2007.

Bucholz RW: *Orthopaedic decision making,* ed 2, St Louis, 1996, Mosby.

Burnett W: *Clinical science for surgeons,* London, 1981, Butterworth.

Burwell RG, Harrison HM, editors: Perthes disease (symposium), *Clin Orthop* 209:2, 1986.

Butler WT et al: Diagnostic and prognostic value of clinical and laboratory findings in cryptococcal meningitis, *N Engl J Med* 270:59, 1964.

Caffey J: The early roentgenographic changes in essential coxa plana, their significance in pathogenesis, *Am J Roentgenol* 103:620, 1968.

Callaghan JJ: The clinical results and basic science of total hip arthroplasty with porous coated prosthesis, *J Bone Joint Surg* 75A:299, 1993.

Cameron HU: *The technique of total hip arthroplasty,* St Louis, 1992, Mosby.

Camp WA: Sarcoidosis of the central nervous system: a case with postmortem studies, *Arch Neurol* 7:432, 1962.

Campbell JB, Campbell JM: *Mosby's survival guide to medical abbreviations & acronyms prefixes & suffixes symbols Greek alphabet,* St Louis, 1995, Mosby.

Campbell WC: *Operative orthopaedics,* ed 7, London, 1981, Henry Kimpton.

Campion GV, Dixon A: *Rheumatology,* Oxford, UK, 1989, Blackwell.

Canale ST: *Campbell's operative orthopaedics,* vol 1-4, ed 9, St Louis, 1998, Mosby.

Carney BT, Weinstein SL, Nuhe J: Long term follow up of slipped capital femoral epiphysis, *J Bone Joint Surg* 73A:667, 1991.

10

Carter CO, Wilkinson JA: Genetic and environmental factors in the etiology of congenital dislocation of the hip, *Clin Orthop* 33:119, 1964.

Catterall A: The natural history of Perthes disease (symposium), *J Bone Joint Surg* 53B:37, 1971.

Catterall A: *Recent advances in orthopaedics,* ed 5, Edinburgh, 1987, Churchill Livingstone.

Catterall M: Perthes disease. In Steinberg ME, editor: *The hip and its disorders,* Philadelphia, 1991, WB Saunders.

Chahidi N et al: Gracilis free muscle flap for coverage of palmar defects, *J Hand Surg Eur Vol* 32(suppl 1):59, 2007.

Chao EY et al: Biomechanics of malalignment, *Orthop Clin North Am* 25:379, 1994.

Chapman S, Nakielmy R: *Aids to radiological differential diagnosis,* ed 3, London, 1995, Bailliere Tindall.

Charnley J: Total hip replacement by low-friction arthroplasty, *Clin Orthop* 72:7, 1970.

Chell J, Dhar S: Perthes disease, *Surgery (Oxford)* 22(1):18-20, 2004.

Chibnall JT, Tait R: The pain disability index: factor structure and normative data, *Arch Phys Med Rehabil* 75:1082, 1994.

Cipriano JJ: *Photographic manual of regional orthopaedic and neurological test,* ed 3, Baltimore, 1997, Williams & Wilkins.

Clarke NMP, Clegg J, Al-Chalabi AN: Ultrasound screening of hips at risk for congenital dislocation, *J Bone Joint Surg* 71B:9, 1989.

Coates CJ, Paterson JM, Woods KR: Femoral osteotomy in Perthes disease: results at maturity, *J Bone Joint Surg* 72B:581, 1990.

Cohn RE: *Impairment rating examination and disability evaluation,* ed 3, Wilkesboro, NC, 1994, R Ernest Cohn.

Cole MH, Grimshaw PN: Electromyography of the trunk and abdominal muscles in golfers with and without low back pain, *J Sci Med Sport* (in press, corrected proof).

Collins DN, Nelson CL: Infections of the hip. In Steinberg M, editor: *The hip and its disorders,* Philadelphia, 1991, WB Saunders.

Collo MC et al: Evaluating arthritic complaints, *Nurse Pract* 16:9, 1991.

Colosimo AJ, Ireland ML: Thigh compartment syndrome in a football athlete: a case report and review of the literature, *Med Sci Sports Exerc* 24:958, 1992.

Cook C et al: Interrater reliability and diagnostic accuracy of pelvic girdle pain classification, *J Manipulative Physiol Ther* 30(4):252-258, 2007.

Cooper DE, Warren RF, Barnes R: Traumatic subluxation of the hip resulting in aseptic necrosis and chondrolysis in a professional football player, *Am J Sports Med* 19:322, 1991.

Copperman DR, Stulberg SD: Ambulatory containment treatment in Perthes disease, *Clin Orthop* 203:289, 1986.

Cormack, DH: *Essential histology,* Philadelphia, 1993, Lippincott.

Craik RL, Oatis CA: *Gait analysis theory and application,* St Louis, 1995, Mosby.

Crenshaw AH editor: *Campbell's operative orthopaedics,* vol 3, ed 8, St Louis, 1992, Mosby.

Cruess RL, Rennie W: *Adult orthopaedics,* New York, 1987, Churchill Livingstone.

Currey HLF: *Essentials of rheumatology,* ed 2, Edinburgh, 1988, Churchill Livingstone.

Cyriax JH: *Textbook of orthopaedic medicine,* ed 8, London, 1983, Bailliere, Tindall.

Daffner RH: *Clinical radiology: the essentials,* Baltimore, 1993, Williams & Wilkins.

Dalinka MK, Neustadter LM: Radiology of the hip. In Steinberg ME, editor: *The hip and its disorders,* Philadelphia, 1991, WB Saunders.

Dambro MR, Griffith JA: *Griffith's 5 minute clinical consult,* Baltimore, 1997, Williams & Wilkins.

D'Ambrogio KJ, Roth GB: *Positional release therapy assessment & treatment of musculoskeletal dysfunction,* St Louis, 1997, Mosby.

D'Ambrosia RD: *Musculoskeletal disorders: regional examination and differential diagnosis,* Philadelphia, 1977, JB Lippincott.

Dandy DJ: *Essential orthopaedics and trauma,* Edinburgh, 1989, Churchill Livingstone.

Dasch B et al: Fracture-related hip pain in elderly patients with proximal femoral fracture after discharge from stationary treatment, *Eur J Pain* (in press, corrected proof).

de Groot IB et al: Validation of the Dutch version of the hip disability and osteoarthritis outcome score, *Osteoarthr Cartil* 15(1):104-109, 2007.

de Groot M et al: The active straight leg raising test (ASLR) in pregnant women: differences in muscle activity and force between patients and healthy subjects, *Man Ther* (in press, corrected proof).

Deltoff MN, Kogon PL: *The portable skeletal x-ray library,* St Louis, 1998, Mosby.

Demeter SL, Andersson GBJ, Smith GM: *Disability evaluation,* St Louis, 1996, Mosby.

Demoulin C et al: Spinal muscle evaluation using the Sorensen test: a critical appraisal of the literature, *Joint Bone Spine* 73(1):43-50, 2006.

DeRosa GP, Feller N: Treatment of congenital dislocation of the hip, management before walking age, *Clin Orthop* 225:77, 1987.

Deshpande JK, Tobias JD: *The pediatric pain handbook,* St Louis, 1996, Mosby.

Dettenmeier PA: *Radiographic assessment for nurses,* St Louis, 1995, Mosby.

Dickinson WH, Duwelius PJ, Colville MR: Muscle strength following surgery for acetabular fractures, *J Orthop Trauma* 7:39, 1993.

Dixon AS et al: A double-blind controlled trial of Rumalon in the treatment of painful osteoarthrosis of the hip, *Ann Rheum Dis* 29:193, 1970.

Dobbs HS: Survivorship of total hip replacements, *J Bone Joint Surg* 62B:168, 1980.

Dodge PR, Swartz MN: Bacterial meningitis: special neurologic problems, postmeningitic complications and clinicopathologic correlations, *N Engl J Med* 272:954, 1965.

Doherty M: *Color atlas and text of osteoarthritis,* London, 1994, Wolfe.

Doherty M, Doherty J: *Clinical examination in rheumatology,* London, 1992, Wolfe.

Doherty M, George E: *Self-assessment picture tests in rheumatology,* London, 1995, Mosby-Wolfe.

Doria AS et al: Contrast-enhanced power Doppler sonography: assessment of revascularization flow in Legg-Calve-Perthes' disease, *Ultrasound Med Biol* 28(2):171-182, 2002.

Doward DA, Troxell ML, Fredericson M: Synovial chondromatosis in an elite cyclist: a case report, *Arch Phys Med Rehabil* 87(6):860-865, 2006.

Dunk NM, Callaghan JP: Gender-based differences in postural responses to seated exposures, *Clin Biomech* 20(10):1101-1110, 2005.

Duthie RB, Bentley G, editors: *Mercer's orthopaedic surgery,* ed 8, London, 1983, Edward Arnold.

Dutkowski JP: Nontraumatic bone and joint disorders. In Crenshaw AH, editor: *Campbell's operative orthopaedics,* ed 8, vol 3, St Louis, 1992, Mosby.

Eastcott HHG: *Arterial surgery,* ed 2, London, 1973, Pitman.

Echternach J, editor: *Clinics in physical therapy of the hip,* New York, 1990, Churchill Livingstone.

Eftekhar NS, editor: Low friction arthroplasty, *Clin Orthop* 211:2, 1986.

Egund N, Wingstrand H: Legg-Calve-Perthes disease: imaging with MR, *Radiology* 179:89, 1991.

Elster AD: *Questions and answers in magnetic resonance imaging,* St Louis, 1994, Mosby.

Engesaeter LB et al: Ultrasound and congenital dislocation of the hip, *J Bone Joint Surg* 72B:202, 1990.

Epstein O et al: *Clinical examination,* ed 2, London, 1997, Mosby.

Eslam Pour A et al: Back pain and total hip arthroplasty: a prospective natural history study, *J Arthroplasty* 22(2):314, 2007.

Esterhai JL et al: Adult septic arthritis, *Orthop Clin North Am* 22:503, 1991.

Eyre-Brook A: Septic arthritis of the hip and osteomyelitis of upper end of the femur in infants, *J Bone Joint Surg* 42B:11, 1960.

Eyre-Brook AL, Jones DA, Harris FC: Pemberton's acetabuloplasty for congenital dislocation of subluxation of the hip, *J Bone Joint Surg* 60B:18, 1978.

Farr D et al: Arthroscopic bursectomy with concomitant iliotibial band release for the treatment of recalcitrant trochanteric bursitis, *Arthroscopy* (in press, corrected proof).

Farrar WE: *Atlas of infections of the nervous system,* London, 1993, Wolfe.

Feldmann E: *Current diagnosis in neurology,* St Louis, 1994, Mosby.

Ferezy JS: *The chiropractic neurological examination,* Gaithersburg, Md, 1992, Aspen.

Ferguson AB Jr: The pathology of degenerative arthritis of the hip and the use of osteotomy in its treatment, *Clin Orthop* 77:118, 1971.

Fisk JW, Balgent ML: Clinical and radiological assessment of leg length, *N Z Med J* 81:477, 1975.

Foldes K et al: Nocturnal pain correlates with effusions in diseased hips, *J Rheumatol* 19:1756, 1992.

Fornage B: *Musculoskeletal ultrasound,* New York, 1995, Churchill Livingstone.

Frank ED et al: *Merrill's atlas of radiographic positioning and procedures,* vol 1-3, ed 11, St Louis, 2007, Mosby.

French HP: Physiotherapy management of osteoarthritis of the hip: a survey of current practice in acute hospitals and private practice in the Republic of Ireland, *Physiotherapy* (in press, corrected proof).

Frick SL: Evaluation of the child who has hip pain, *Orthop Clin North Am* 37(2):133-140, 2006.

Fricker PA, Taunton JE, Ammann W: Osteitis pubis in athletes; infection, inflammation, or injury, *Sports Med* 12:266, 1991.

Frost A, Bauer M: Skier's hip: a new clinical entity? proximal femur fractures sustained in cross-country skiing, *J Orthop Trauma* 5:47, 1991.

Frymoyer J, editor: *Orthopedic knowledge update No. 4,* Rosemont, Ill, 1993, American Academy of Orthopedic Surgery.

Fuss FK, Bacher A: New aspects of the morphology and function of the human hip joint ligaments, *Am J Anat* 192:1, 1991.

Gage JR, Winter RB: Avascular necrosis of the capital femoral epiphysis as a complication of closed reduction of congenital dislocation of the hip, *J Bone Joint Surg* 54A:373, 1972.

Galasko CSB, editor: *Neuromuscular problems in orthopaedics,* Oxford, UK, 1987, Blackwell.

Galasko CSB, Nobel J, editors: *Current trends in orthopaedic surgery,* Manchester, UK, 1988, Manchester University Press.

Galpin RD et al: One-stage treatment of congenital dislocation of the hip in older children, *J Bone Joint Surg* 71A:734, 1989.

Garbuz DS, Xu M, Sayre EC: Patients' outcome after total hip arthroplasty: a comparison between the Western Ontario and McMaster Universities Index and the Oxford 12-Item Hip Score, *J Arthroplasty* 21(7):998-1004, 2006.

Garcia JH: *Neuropathology the diagnostic approach,* St Louis, 1997, Mosby.

Garrick J, Webb DR: Pelvis, hip, thigh injuries. In Garrick J, Webb DR, editors: *Sports injuries: diagnosis and management,* Philadelphia, 1990, WB Saunders.

Gartland JJ: *Fundamentals of orthopaedics,* ed 2, Philadelphia, 1974, WB Saunders.

Gartland JJ: Orthopaedic clinical research, *J Bone Joint Surg* 70A:1357, 1988.

Gerard JA, Kleinfield SL: *Orthopaedic testing,* New York, 1993, Churchill Livingstone.

Gillis L: *Diagnostic in orthopaedics,* London, 1969, Butterworth.

Giuliani G et al: CT scan and surgical treatment of traumatic iliacus hematoma with femoral neuropathy: case report, *J Trauma* 30:229, 1990.

Glick JM: Hip arthroscopy. In Mcginty JB et al, editors: *Operative arthroscopy,* New York, 1991, Raven.

Goldie BS: *Orthopaedic diagnosis and management a guide to the care of orthopaedic patients,* ed 2, Oxford, UK, 1998, ISIS Medical Media.

Goldman GA et al: Idiopathic transient osteoporosis of the hip in pregnancy, *Int J Gynaecol Obstet* 46:317, 1994.

Goldstein TS: Treatment of common problems of the hip joint. In Goldstein TS, Lewis CB, series editors: *Geriatric orthopaedics rehabilitative management of common problems,* Gaithersburg, Md, 1991, Aspen.

Golightly YM et al: Relationship of limb length inequality with radiographic knee and hip osteoarthritis *Osteoarthr Cartil* (in press, corrected proof).

Gombatto SP et al: Gender differences in pattern of hip and lumbopelvic rotation in people with low back pain, *Clin Biomech* 21(3):263-271, 2006.

Goodman CG, Snyder TE: Systemic origins of musculoskeletal pain: associated signs and symptoms. In: *Differential diagnosis in physical therapy,* Philadelphia, 1990, WB Saunders.

Gordon M: *Nursing diagnosis: process and application,* ed 3, St Louis, 1994, Mosby.

Graham S et al: The Chiari osteotomy, *Clin Orthop* 208:249, 1986.

Grauer JD et al: Resection arthroplasty of the hip, *J Bone Joint Surg* 71A:669, 1989.

Greenspan A: *Orthopedic radiology,* ed 2, Philadelphia, 1992, JB Lippincott.

Greenstein GM: *Clinical assessment of neuromusculoskeletal disorders,* St Louis, 1997, Mosby.

Greenwald AS: Biomechanics of the hip. In Steinberg ME, editor: *The hip and its disorders,* Philadelphia, 1991, WB Saunders.

Gregory DE, Brown SHM, Callaghan JP: Trunk muscle responses to suddenly applied loads: do individuals who develop discomfort during prolonged standing respond differently? *J Electromyogr Kinesiol* (in press, corrected proof).

Gross ML, Nasser S, Finnerman GAM: Hip and pelvis. In DeLee JC, Drez D, editors: *Orthopaedic sports medicine: principles and practice,* vol 2, Philadelphia, 1994, WB Saunders.

Grossman ZD et al: *Cost-effective diagnostic imaging the clinician's guide,* ed 3, St Louis, 1995, Mosby.

Gruebel-Lee DM: *Disorders of the hip,* Philadelphia, 1983, JB Lippincott.

Hadlow V: Neonatal screening for congenital dislocation of hip, *J Bone Joint Surg* 70B:740, 1988.

Hall AJ: Perthes disease: progression in aetiological research. In Catterall P, editor: *Recent advances in orthopaedics,* ed 5, Edinburgh, 1987, Churchill Livingstone.

Halland AM et al: Avascular necrosis of the hip in systemic lupus erythematosus: the role of magnetic resonance imaging, *Br J Rheumatol* 32:972, 1993.

Hammer WI: *Functional soft tissue examination and treatment by manual methods the extremities,* Gaithersburg, Md, 1991, Aspen.

Hananouchi T et al: Interventional therapy for hip ganglion using open MRI, *Eur J Radiol Extra* 60(1):43-47, 2006.

Hansson G: Congenital dislocation of the hip joint: problems in diagnosis and treatment, *Curr Orthop* 2:104, 1988.

Hansson G et al: Radiographic assessment of coxarthrosis following slipped capital femoral epiphysis, *Acta Radiol* 34:117, 1993.

Hardinge K: The etiology of transient synovitis of the hip in childhood, *J Bone Joint Surg* 52B:100, 1970.

Harris CM, Baum J: Involvement of the hip in juvenile rheumatoid arthritis, *J Bone Joint Surg* 70A:821, 1988.

Harris WH: Etiology of osteoarthritis of the hip, *Clin Orthop* 213:20, 1986.

Hartley A: *Practical joint assessment lower quadrant,* ed 2, St Louis, 1995, Mosby.

Harty M: Hip anatomy. In Steinberg ME, editor: *The hip and its disorders,* Philadelphia, 1991, WB Saunders.

Hawkins RJ: *An organized approach to musculoskeletal examination and history taking,* St Louis, 1995, Mosby.

Heikkila E, Ryoppy S, Louchimo I: The management of primary acetabular dysplasia, *J Bone Joint Surg* 67B:25, 1985.

Heinmann WG, Freiberger RH: Avascular necrosis of the femoral and humeral heads after high-dosage corticosteroid therapy, *N Engl J Med* 263:627, 1960.

10

Henderson RS: Osteotomy for unreduced congenital dislocation of the hip in adults, *J Bone Joint Surg* 52B:468, 1970.

Hernandez RS, Cornell RG, Hensinger RN: Ultrasound diagnosis of neonatal congenital dislocation of the hip, *J Bone Joint Surg* 76A:539, 1994.

Hernigou P et al: Deformities of the hip in adults who have sickle-cell disease and had avascular necrosis in childhood, *J Bone Joint Surg* 73:91, 1991.

Herrera A et al: Management of types III and IV acetabular deficiencies with the longitudinal oblong revision cup, *J Arthroplasty* 21(6):857-864, 2006.

Hertling D, Kessler R: *Management of common musculoskeletal disorders,* ed 2, Philadelphia, 1990, JB Lippincott.

Hiehle JF, Kneeland JB, Dalinka MK: Magnetic resonance imaging of the hip with emphasis on avascular necrosis, *Rheum Dis Clin North Am* 17:669, 1991.

Hinkle CZ: *Fundamentals of anatomy & movement: a workbook and guide,* St Louis, 1997, Mosby.

Hirsch C, Frankel VH: Analysis of forces producing fractures of the proximal end of the femur, *J Bone Joint Surg* 42B:633, 1960.

Hoeksma HL et al: A comparison of the OARSI response criteria with patient's global assessment in patients with osteoarthritis of the hip treated with a non-pharmacological intervention, *Osteoarthr Cartil* 14(1):77-81, 2006.

Hornberger JP: *Exercise physiology therapeutic exercise,* Sarasota, Fla, 1991, Joseph P Hornberger.

Hudson ZL, Darthuy E: Iliotibial band tightness and patellofemoral pain syndrome a case-control study, *Phys Ther Sport* 7(4):173-271, 2006.

Hughes S, Benson MKD, Colton CL: *The principles and practice of musculoskeletal surgery,* Edinburgh, 1987, Churchill Livingstone.

Hughes SS et al: Extrapelvic compression of the sciatic nerve, *J Bone Joint Surg* 74A:1533, 1992.

Inerot S et al: Proteoglycan alterations during developing experimental osteoarthritis in a novel hip joint model, *J Orthop Res* 9:658, 1991.

Jablonski S: *Dictionary of medical acronyms & abbreviations,* ed 3, Philadelphia, 1998, Hanley & Belfus.

Jacobson T, Allen W: Surgical connection of the snapping iliopsoas tendon, *Am J Sports Med* 18:470, 1990.

Jehl J, Crummy P: *Essentials of radiologic surgery,* ed 6, Philadelphia, 1993, JB Lippincott.

Jette AM: Using health-related quality of life measures in physical therapy outcomes research, *Phys Ther* 73:528, 1993.

Johnson I: Iliacus stretching for symptomatic relief of femoral mononeuropathy, *Clin Chiro* 10(2):97-100, 2007.

Johnson KE: *Histology and cell biology,* ed 2, Baltimore, 1991, Williams & Wilkins.

Jones DA: Irritable hip and campylobacter infection, *J Bone Joint Surg* 71B:227, 1989.

Jones JP Jr, Engelman EP: Osseous avascular necrosis associated with systemic abnormalities, *Arthritis Rheum* 5:728, 1966.

Jones M: Clinical reasoning in manual therapy, *Phys Ther* 72:875, 1992.

Junqueira LC, Carneiro J, Kelly RO: *Basic histology,* ed 7, Norwalk, Conn, 1992, Appleton & Lange.

Kampa K: Mortality of hip fracture patients within one year of fracture, an overview, *Geritopics* 14:10, 1991.

Kanner R: *Pain management secrets,* Philadelphia, 1997, Hanley & Belfus.

Kapstad H et al: Changes in pain, stiffness and physical function in patients with osteoarthritis waiting for hip or knee joint replacement surgery, *Osteoarthr Cartil* (in press, corrected proof).

Kassarjian A, Brisson M, Palmer WE: Femoroacetabular impingement, *Eur J Radiol* (in press, corrected proof).

Katirji B: *Electromyography in clinical practice: a case study approach,* St Louis, 1998, Mosby.

Katirji MB, Wilbourn AJ: High sciatic lesions mimicking peroneal neuropathy at the fibular head, *J Neurosci* 121:172, 1994.

Katz WA: *Rheumatic diseases diagnosis and management,* Philadelphia, 1977, JB Lippincott.

Keats TE: *Atlas of roentgenographic measurement,* ed 6, St Louis, 1990, Mosby.

Keats TE: *Atlas of normal roentgen variants,* ed 6, St Louis, 1996, Mosby.

Kedroff L, Amis A, Newham D: Do patients with patellofemoral pain syndrome exhibit alterations in steadiness on hip and knee flexion? *Gait Posture* 24(suppl 2):S269-S70, 2006.

Kendell RP, McCreary EK, Provance PG: *Muscles: testing and function,* ed 4, Baltimore, 1993, Williams & Wilkins.

Keret D et al: Coxa plana: the fate of the physis, *J Bone Joint Surg* 66A:870, 1984.

Kessler RM, Hertling D: The hip. In Hertling D, Kessler RM, editors: *Management of common musculoskeletal disorders,* ed 2, Philadelphia, 1990, JB Lippincott.

Kim Y-W et al: Risk factors for leg length discrepancy in patients with congenital vascular malformation, *J Vasc Surg* 44(3):545-553, 2006.

Klippel JH, Dieppe PA: *Rheumatology,* vol 1-2, ed 2, London, 1998, Mosby.

Knutson GA: Examination of two subjects with severe, quantified anatomic leg length inequality using unloaded "functional" leg checks, *Clin Chir* 9(2):76-80, 2006.

Koenigsberg R: *Churchill's illustrated medical dictionary,* New York, 1989, Churchill Livingstone.

Koval KJ, Zuckerman JD: Functional recovery after fracture of the hip, current concepts review, *J Bone Joint Surg* 76A:751, 1994.

Koyama Y et al: A study of the reality of daily life among patients with osteoarthritis of the hip undergoing conservative treatment, *J Orthop Nurs* (in press, corrected proof).

Kramer PA, Sarton-Miller I: The energetics of human walking: is Froude number (Fr) useful for metabolic comparisons? *Gait Posture* (in press, corrected proof).

Kuklo TR, Mackenzie WG, Keeler KA: Hip arthroscopy in Legg-Calve-Perthes Disease, *Arthroscopy* 15(1):88-92, 1999.

Lafforguw P et al: Early-stage avascular necrosis of the femoral head: MR imaging for prognosis in 31 cases with at least 2 years of follow-up, *Radiology* 187:199, 1993.

Langlais F et al: Hip pain from impingement and dysplasia in patients aged 20-50 years. Workup and role for reconstruction, *Joint Bone Spine* 73(6):614-623, 2006.

Latke PA: Soft tissue afflictions. In Steinberg ME, editor: *The hip and its disorders,* Philadelphia, 1992, WB Saunders.

Laude F, Boyer T, Nogier A: Anterior femoroacetabular impingement, *Joint Bone Spine* 74(2):127-132, 2007.

Lavy CBD, Barrett DS: *Questions and answers on Apley's concise system of orthopaedics and fractures,* Oxford, UK, 1991, Butterworth-Heinemann

Lawrence JS: Generalized osteoarthrosis in a popular sample, *Am J Epidemiol* 90:381, 1969.

Lehner JT, Miller T, Mills A: Comparison of intermediate-term status in Legg-Calve-Perthes Disease patients treated with varus derotational osteotomy with or without subsequent epiphysiodesis of the greater trochanter, *J Am Coll Surg* 199(3, suppl 1):50, 2004.

Lennox IA, McLauchlan J, Murali R: Failures of screening and management of congenital dislocation of the hip, *J Bone Joint Surg* 75B:72, 1993.

Lerner AJ: *The little black book of neurology,* ed 3, St Louis, 1995, Mosby.

Les RD, Gerhardt JJ: Range-of-motion measurements, *J Bone Joint Surg* 77A:784, 1995.

Lesher J et al: Hip joint pain referral patterns: a descriptive study, *Arch Phys Med Rehabil* 87(11):e23-e35, 2006.

Letourmeau L, Dessureault M, Carette S: Rheumatoid iliopsoas bursitis presenting as unilateral femoral nerve palsy, *J Rheumatol* 18:462, 1991.

LeVeau B: Hip. In Richardson JK, Iglarsh JK, editors: *Clinical orthopaedic physical therapy,* Philadelphia, 1994, WB Saunders.

Lewis CB, Bottomley JM: Orthopaedic treatment considerations. In Lewis CB, Bottomley JM, editors: *Geriatric physical therapy: a clinical approach,* New York, 1994, Appleton & Lange.

Lewis CB, Knortz KA: *Orthopedic assessment and treatment of the geriatric patient,* St Louis, 1993, Mosby.

Liebenson C: Hip dysfunction and back pain, *J Bodywork Mov Ther* 11(2):111-115, 2007.

Lloyd-Roberts GG: Suppurative arthritis in infancy, *J Bone Joint Surg* 42B:706, 1960.

Locher S et al: Radiological anatomy of the obturator nerve and its articular branches: basis to develop a method of radiofrequency denervation for hip joint pain, *Eur J Pain* 10(suppl 1):s136-s137, 2006.

Lorber J: Long-term follow-up of 100 children who recovered from tuberculous meningitis, *Pediatrics* 28:778, 1961.

Loth TS: *Orthopedic boards review II: a case study approach,* St Louis, 1996, Mosby.

Loth TS: *Orthopedic boards review,* St Louis, 1993, Mosby.

Love BRT, Stevens PM, William PF: A long-term review of shelf arthroplasty, *J Bone Joint Surg* 62B:321, 1980.

Lu T-W, Chen H-L, Wang T-M: Obstacle crossing in older adults with medial compartment knee osteoarthritis, *Gait Posture* (in press, corrected proof).

Lynch AF: Tuberculosis of the greater trochanter, *J Bone Joint Surg* 64B:185, 1982.

MacAusland WR Jr, Mayo RA: *Orthopedics: a concise guide to clinical practices,* Boston, 1965, Little, Brown.

MacEwen GD: Treatment of congenital dislocation of the hip in older children, *Clin Orthop* 225:86, 1987.

Magee DJ: *Orthopedic physical assessment,* ed 3, Philadelphia, 1997, WB Saunders.

Malone TR, McPoil TG, Nitz AJ: *Orthopedic and sports physical therapy,* ed 3, St Louis, 1997, Mosby.

Marchiori DM: *Clinical imaging with skeletal, chest, and abdomen pattern differentials,* St Louis, 1999, Mosby.

Martin JH: *Neuroanatomy text and atlas,* ed 2, Stamford, Conn, 1996, Appleton & Lange.

Mathers LH et al: *Clinical anatomy principles,* St Louis, 1996, Mosby.

Maxted MJ, Jackson RK: Innominate osteotomy in Perthes' disease, *J Bone Joint Surg* 67B:399, 1985.

Mayrand N et al: Diagnosis and management of posttraumatic piriformis syndrome: a case study, *J Manipulative Physiol Ther* 29(6):486-491, 2006.

Mazion JM: *Illustrated manual of neurological reflexes/signs/tests, part I, orthopedic signs/tests/maneuvers for office procedure, part II,* Orlando, Fla, 1980, Daniels Publishing.

McAndrew MP, Weinstein SL: A long-term follow-up of Legg-Calve-Perthes disease, *J Bone Joint Surg* 66A:860, 1984.

McCarthy GM, McCarthy DJ: Intrasynovial corticosteroid therapy, *Bull Rheum Dis* 43:2, 1994.

McCarty DJ, Koopman WJ, editors: *Arthritis and allied conditions,* ed 12, Philadelphia, 1993, Lea & Febiger.

McDonald D et al: Total joint reconstruction. In: *Orthopedic boards review,* St Louis, 1993, Mosby.

McGann WA: History and physical examination. In Steinberg ME, editor: *The hip and its disorders,* Philadelphia, 1991, WB Saunders.

McKean KA et al: Gender differences exist in osteoarthritic gait, *Clin Biomech* 22(4):400-409, 2007.

McKee GK: Development of total prosthetic replacement of the hip, *Clin Orthop* 72:85, 1970.

McKibbin B: Anatomical factors in the stability of the hip joint in the newborn, *J Bone Joint Surg* 52B:148, 1970.

McKibbin B, editor: *Recent advances in orthopaedics,* ed 4, Edinburgh, 1983, Churchill Livingstone.

McRae R: *Clinical orthopaedic examination,* ed 3, Edinburgh, 1990, Churchill Livingstone.

McRae R: *Practical fracture treatment,* ed 3, New York, 1994, Churchill-Livingstone.

Medical Economics Books: *Patient care flow chart manual,* ed 3, Oradell, NJ, 1982, Medical Economics Books.

Meenan RF, Gertman PM, Mason JH: Measuring health status in arthritis: the arthritis impact measurement scales, *Arthritis Rheum* 23(2):146-152, 1980.

Mellion MB: *Sports medicine secrets,* Philadelphia, 1994, Hanley & Belfus.

Mellion MB: *Office sports medicine,* ed 2, St Louis, 1996, Mosby.

Mendez AA, Eyster RL: Displaced nonunion stress fracture of the femoral neck treated with internal fixation and bone graft, *Am J Sports Med* 20:230, 1992.

Menelaus MB: Lessons learned in the management of Legg-Calve-Perthes disease, *Clin Orthop* 209:41, 1986.

Mengel MB, Schwiebert LP: *Ambulatory medicine: the primary care of families,* ed 2, Stamford, Conn, 1996, Appleton & Lange.

Mennell JM: *The musculoskeletal system: differential diagnosis from symptoms and physical signs,* Gaithersburg, Md, 1992, Aspen.

Mens J et al: Possible harmful effects of high intra-abdominal pressure on the pelvic girdle, *J Biomech* 39(4):627-635, 2006.

Mercier LR, Pettid FJ: *Practical orthopedics,* ed 4, St Louis, 1995, Mosby.

Meyer HM Jr et al: Central nervous system syndromes of viral etiology: a study of 713 cases, *Am J Med* 29:334, 1960.

Milgram JW et al: Resection arthroplasty for septic arthritis of the hip in ambulatory and nonambulatory adult patients, *Clin Orthop* 272:181, 1991.

Miller M: Adult reconstruction and sports medicine. In Miller M, editor: *Review of orthopaedics,* Philadelphia, 1992, WB Saunders.

Mitchell S et al: The need for a falls prevention programme for patients undergoing hip and knee replacement surgery, *J Orthop Nurs* (in press, corrected proof).

Modic MT, Masaryk TJ, Ross JS: *Magnetic resonance imaging of the spine,* ed 2, St Louis, 1994, Mosby.

Mohagheghi AA et al: Differences in gastrocnemius muscle architecture between the paretic and non-paretic legs in children with hemiplegic cerebral palsy, *Clin Biomech* (in press, corrected proof).

Moll JMH: *Manual of rheumatology,* Edinburgh, 1987, Churchill Livingstone.

Monzon DG, Iserson KV, Vazquez JA: Single fascia iliaca compartment block for post-hip fracture pain relief, *J Emerg Med* 32(3):257-262, 2007.

Moore FH: Examination of infant's hips: can it do harm? *J Bone Joint Surg* 71B:4, 1989.

Moore FJ et al: The relationship between head-neck-shaft angle, calcar width, articular cartilage and bone volume in arthrosis of the hip, *Br J Rheumatol* 35:432, 1994.

Moore KL: *Clinically oriented anatomy,* ed 3, Baltimore, 1992, Williams & Wilkins.

Moosabhoy MA, Gard SA: Methodology for determining the sensitivity of swing leg toe clearance and leg length to swing leg joint angles during gait, *Gait Posture* 24(4):493-501, 2006.

Mosby-Year Book, Inc: *Expert 10-minute physical examination,* St Louis, 1997, Mosby.

Mosler AB, Blanch PD, Hiskins BC: The effect of manual therapy on hip joint range of motion, pain and eggbeater kick performance in water polo players, *Phys The Sport* 7(3):128-136, 2006.

Mourad LA: *Orthopedic disorders,* St Louis, 1991, Mosby.

Muirhead-Allwood W, Catterall A: The treatment of Perthes disease, *J Bone Joint Surg* 64B:282, 1982.

Mulford K: Greater trochanteric bursitis, *J Nurs Pract* 3(5):328-332, 2007.

Murphy DR et al: Interexaminer reliability of the hip extension test for suspected impaired motor control of the lumbar spine, *J Manipulative Physiol Ther* 29(5):374-377, 2006.

Murray AW, Robb JE: Pelvic osteotomy for the management of hip displacement in neuromuscular disorders, *Cur Orthop* (in press, corrected proof).

10

Nettina SM: *The Lippincott manual of nursing practice,* ed 6, Philadelphia, 1996, JB Lippincott.

Neumann DA, Hase AD: The electromyographic analysis of the hip abductors during load carriage: implications for hip joint protection, *J Orthop Sports Phys Ther* 19:296, 1994.

Neumann DA et al: An electromyographic analysis of hip abductor muscle activity when subjects are carrying loads in one or both hands, *Phys Ther* 72:207, 1992.

Neumann G et al: Prevalence of labral tears and cartilage loss in patients with mechanical symptoms of the hip: evaluation using MR arthrography, *Osteoarthr Cartil* (in press, corrected proof).

Newton RW: *Color atlas of pediatric neurology,* St Louis, 1995, Mosby-Wolfe.

Nicholas JA, Hershman EB: *The lower extremity & spine in sports medicine,* vol 1-2, ed 2, St Louis, 1995, Mosby.

Nobel J, Galasko CSB: *Recent developments in orthopaedic surgery,* Manchester, UK, 1987, Manchester University Press.

Noble HB, Hajek MR, Porter M: Diagnosis and treatment of iliotibial band tightness in runners, *Sports Med* 10:67, 1982.

Nordin M, Andersson GBJ, Pope MH: *Musculoskeletal disorders in the workplace: principles and practice,* St Louis, 1997, Mosby.

Noriyasu S et al: On the morphology and frequency of Weitbrecht's retinacula in the hip joint, *Okajimas Folia Anat Jpn* 70:87, 1993.

Nunn D: The ring uncemented plastic-on-metal total hip replacement, *J Bone Joint Surg* 70B:40, 1988.

Ober FB: The role of the iliotibial and fascia lata as a factor in the causation of low-back disabilities and sciatic, *J Bone Joint Surg* 18:105, 1936.

O'Donoghue DH: *Treatment of injuries to athletes,* ed 3, Philadelphia, 1976, WB Saunders.

Olson WH et al: *Handbook of symptom-oriented neurology,* ed 2, St Louis, 1994, Mosby.

Omer GE, Spinner M: *Management of peripheral nerve problems,* Philadelphia, 1980, WB Saunders.

O'Sullivan M et al: Iliopsoas tendonitis: a complication after total hip arthroplasty, *J Arthroplasty* 22(2):166-170, 2007.

O'Sullivan PB et al: The relationship between posture and back muscle endurance in industrial workers with flexion-related low back pain, *Man Ther* 11(4):264-271, 2006.

Owen R, Goodfellow J, Bullough P, editors: *Scientific foundations of orthopaedics and traumatology,* London, 1980, Heinemann.

O'Young B, Young MA, Stiens SA: *PM&R secrets,* Philadelphia, 1997, Hanley & Belfus.

Pagana KD, Pagana TJ: *Mosby's manual of diagnostic and laboratory tests,* St Louis, 1998, Mosby.

Pardiwala DN, Nagda TV: Arthroscopic chondral cyst excision in a Stiff Perthes' hip, *Arthroscopy* (in press, corrected proof).

Parker MJ, Pryor GA: *Hip fracture management,* Boston, 1993, Blackwell.

Paterson D, Salvage JP: The nuclide bone scan in the diagnosis of Perthes disease, *Clin Orthop* 209:23, 1986.

Patten J: *Neurological differential diagnosis,* ed 2, London, 1996, Springer.

Patterson RJ, Bickel WH, Dahlin DC: Idiopathic avascular necrosis of the head of the femur: a study of fifty-two cases, *J Bone Joint Surg* 42A:267, 1964.

Persselin JE: Diagnosis of rheumatoid arthritis, medial and laboratory aspects, *Clin Orthop* 265:73, 1991.

Philippon MJ, Schenker ML: Arthroscopy for the treatment of femoroacetabular impingement in the athlete, *Clin Sports Med* 25(2):299-308, 2006.

Planner AC, Donaghy M, Moore NR: Causes of lumbosacral plexopathy: *Clin Radiol* 61(12):987-995, 2006.

Polley HF, Hunder GG: *Rheumatologic interviewing and physical examination of the joints,* Philadelphia, 1978, WB Saunders.

Post M: *Physical examination of the musculoskeletal system,* Chicago, 1987, Mosby.

Poul J et al: Early diagnosis of congenital dislocation of the hip, *J Bone Joint Surg* 53B:56, 1971.

Pratt NE: *Clinical musculoskeletal anatomy,* Philadelphia, 1991, JB Lippincott.

Radin EL: The physiology and degeneration of joints, *Arthritis Rheum* 2:245, 1972.

Ranawat CS: Surgery for rheumatoid arthritis: the hip, *Curr Orthop* 3:146, 1989.

Ranawat CS, Figgie MP: Early complications of total hip replacement. In Steinberg ME, editor: *The hip and its disorders,* Philadelphia, 1991, WB Saunders.

Rang M, editor: *The growth plate and its disorders,* Edinburgh, 1969, Livingstone.

Rao JP, Bronstein R: Dislocation following arthroplasties of the hip: incidence, prevention and treatment, *Orthop Rev* 20:261, 1991.

Rat A-C et al: Development and testing of a specific quality-of-life questionnaire for knee and hip osteoarthritis: OAKHQOL (osteoarthritis of knee hip quality of life), *Joint Bone Spine* 73(6):697-704, 2006.

Ratliff AHC: Perthes disease: a study of thirty-four hips observed for thirty years, *J Bone Joint Surg* 49B:102, 1967.

Ravel R: *Clinical laboratory medicine: clinical application of laboratory data,* ed 6, St Louis, 1995, Mosby.

Reginster J-Y: Managing the osteoporotic patient today, *Bone* 40(5, suppl 1):S12-S18, 2007.

Reid DC: *Problems of the hip, pelvis, and sacroiliac joint, sports injury assessment and rehabilitation,* New York, 1992, Churchill Livingstone.

Reid DC: *Sports injury assessment and rehabilitation,* New York, 1992, Churchill Livingstone.

Reikeras O: Is there a relationship between femoral anteversion and leg torsion? *Skeletal Radiol* 10:409, 1991.

Renne JW: The iliotibial band friction syndrome, *J Bone Joint Surg* 57A:1110, 1975.

Renshaw TS: *Pediatric orthopaedics,* Philadelphia, 1987, WB Saunders.

Resnick D, Niwayama G: *Diagnosis of bone and joint disorders,* Philadelphia, 1995, WB Saunders.

Rhodes I, Matzinger F, Matzinger MA: Transient osteoporosis of the hip, *Can Assoc Radiol J* 44:399, 1993.

Ring PA: Complete replacement arthroplasty of the hip by the ring prosthesis, *J Bone Joint Surg* 50B:720, 1968.

Rizzo PF et al: Diagnosis of occult fractures about the hip, magnetic resonance imaging compared with bone scanning, *J Bone Joint Surg* 75A:395, 1993.

Roach HI, Shearer JR, Archer C: The choice of an experimental model: a guide for research workers, *J Bone Joint Surg* 71B:549, 1989.

Roach KE, Miles T: Normal hip and knee active range of motion: the relationship to age, *Phys Ther* 71:656, 1991.

Robinson D, On E, Halperin N: Anterior compartment syndrome of the thigh in athletes: indications for conservative treatment, *J Trauma* 32:183, 1992.

Rockwood CA, Green DP, Bucholz RW, editors: *Rockwood and Green's fractures in adults,* vol II, ed 3, Philadelphia, 1991, JB Lippincott.

Rogers AW: *Textbook of anatomy,* New York, 1992, Churchill-Livingstone.

Rolak LA: *Neurology secrets,* ed 2, Philadelphia, 1998, Hanley & Belfus.

Rooser B: Acute compartment syndrome from anterior thigh muscle contusion: report of eight cases, *J Orthop Trauma* 5:55, 1991.

Rumack CM, Wilson SR, Charboneau JW: *Diagnostic ultrasound,* vol 1-2, ed 2, St Louis, 1998, Mosby.

Russotti GM, Conventry MB, Stauffer RN: Cemented total hip arthroplasty with contemporary techniques, *Clin Orthop* 235:141, 1988.

Saidoff DC, McDonough AL: *Critical pathways in therapeutic intervention,* St Louis, 1997, Mosby.

Saji MJ, Upakhyay SS, Leong JCY: Increased femoral neck-shaft angles in adolescent idiopathic scoliosis, *Spine* 20:303, 1995.

Sammarco GJ, Stephens MM: Neuropraxia of the femoral nerve in a modern dancer, *Am J Sports Med* 19:413, 1991.

Saudek CE: The hip. In Gould JA, editor: *Orthopaedic and sports physical therapy,* ed 2, St Louis, 1990, Mosby.

Schapira D: Transient osteoporosis of the hip, *Semin Arthritis Rheum* 22:98, 1992.

Schmalzried TP: The infected hip: telltale signs and treatment options, *J Arthroplasty* 21(4, suppl 1):97-100, 2006.

Schmalziried TP, Amstutz HC, Dorey FJ: Nerve palsy associated with total hip replacement, risk factors and prognosis, *J Bone Joint Surg* 73A:1074, 1991.

Schulte KR et al: The outcome of Charnley total hip arthroplasty with cement after a minimum of twenty year follow-up, *J Bone Joint Surg* 75A:961, 1993.

Schulz BW, Ashton-Miller JA, Alexander NB: Maximum step length: relationships to age and knee and hip extensor capacities, *Clin Biomech* (in press, corrected proof).

Schumacher HR, Klippel JH, Koopman WJ: *Primer on the rheumatic diseases,* ed 10, Atlanta, 1993, Arthritis Foundation.

Scott JT, editor: *Copeman's textbook of the rheumatic diseases,* ed 6, Edinburgh, 1986, Churchill Livingstone.

Segal A, Krauss ES: Infected total hip arthroplasty after intravesical Bacillus Calmette-Guerin therapy, *J Arthroplasty* (in press, corrected proof).

Sells LL, German DC: An update on gout, *Bull Rheum Dis* 43:4, 1994.

Shankman GA: *Fundamental orthopedic management for the physical therapist assistant,* St Louis, 1997, Mosby.

Sherlock DA, Gibson PH, Benson MKD: Congenital subluxation of the hip, *J Bone Joint Surg* 67B:390, 1985.

Sledge CB, Poss R: *The yearbook of orthopedics 1997,* St Louis, 1997, Mosby.

Smith ET, Pevey JK, Shindler TO: The erector spinae transplant: a misnomer, *Clin Orthop* 20:144, 1963.

Smith G et al: Hip pain caused by buttock claudication: relief of symptoms by transluminal angioplasty, *Clin Orthop* 284:176, 1992.

Solomon L: Patterns of osteoarthritis of the hip, *J Bone Joint Surg* 58B:176, 1976.

Somerville EW: A long-term follow-up of congenital dislocation of the hip, *J Bone Joint Surg* 60B:25, 1978.

Specht NT, Russo RD: *Practical guide to diagnostic imaging,* St Louis, 1998, Mosby.

Staheli LT: Medial femoral torsion, *Orthop Clin North Am* 11:39, 1980.

Stedman TL: *Stedman's medical dictionary,* ed 25, Baltimore, 1990, Williams & Wilkins.

Steinberg ME, Steinberg DR: Avascular necrosis of the femoral head. In Steinberg ME, editor: *The hip and its disorders,* Philadelphia, 1991, WB Saunders.

Steinbert ME, Steinberg DR: Evaluation and staging of avascular necrosis, *Semin Arthroplasty* 2:175, 1991.

Stevens A, Lowe J: *Histology,* New York, 1992, Gower Medical.

Stewart DL, Abeln SH: *Documenting functional outcomes in physical therapy,* St Louis, 1993, Mosby.

Stewart JDM, Hallett JP: *Traction and orthopaedic appliances,* Edinburgh, 1983, Churchill Livingstone.

Stock G: *The book of questions,* New York, 1985, Workman Publishing.

Stoller DW: *Magnetic resonance imaging in orthopaedics & sports medicine,* Philadelphia, 1993, JB Lippincott.

Stratford PW et al: Measurement properties of the WOMAC LK 3.1 pain scale, *Osteoarthr Cartil* 15(3):266-272, 2007.

Strickland E et al: In vivo contact pressures during rehabilitation, part 1: acute phase, *Phys Ther* 72:691, 1992.

Susuke S et al: Diagnosis by ultrasound of congenital dislocation of the hip joint, *Clin Orthop* 217:171, 1987.

Sutton D, Young JWR: *A concise textbook of clinical imaging,* ed 2, St Louis, 1995, Mosby.

Swartout R, Compere EL: Ischiogluteal bursitis: the pain in the arse, *JAMA* 227:551, 1974.

Swartz MN, Dodge PR: Bacterial meningitis: general clinical features, special problems and unusual meningeal reactions mimicking bacterial meningitis, *N Engl J Med* 272:725, 1965.

Swointkowski MF: Intracapsular fractures of the hip, *J Bone Joint Surg* 76A:129, 1994.

Tachdjian MO: *Pediatric orthopedics,* Philadelphia, 1972, WB Saunders.

Tan JC, Horn SE: *Practical manual of physical medicine and rehabilitation,* St Louis, 1998, Mosby.

Taybi H, Lachman RS: *Radiology of syndromes, metabolic disorders, and skeletal dysplasias,* ed 4, St Louis, 1996, Mosby.

Terjesen T: Ultrasonography in the primary evaluation of Perthe's disease, *J Pediatr Orthop* 13:437, 1993.

Terjesen T, Berdland T, Berg V: Ultrasound for hip assessment in the newborn, *J Bone Joint Surg* 71B:767, 1989.

Teshima R, Otsuka T, Yamamoto K: Effects of nonweight bearing on the hip, *Clin Orthop* 279:149, 1992.

Tetsworth K, Paley D: Malalignment and degenerative arthropathy, *Orthop Clin North Am* 25:367, 1994.

Thibodeau GA, Patton KT: *Anatomy & physiology,* ed 3, St Louis, 1996, Mosby.

Thibodeau GA, Patton KT: *Pocket reference to accompany anatomy & physiology,* ed 3, St Louis, 1996, Mosby.

Thompson JM: *Clinical outlines for health assessment,* St Louis, 1997, Mosby.

Timgren J, Soinila S: Reversible pelvic asymmetry: an overlooked syndrome manifesting as scoliosis, apparent leg-length difference, and neurologic symptoms, *J Manipulative Physiol Ther* 29(7):561-565, 2006.

Toalt V et al: Evidence for viral aetiology of transient synovitis of the hip, *J Bone Joint Surg* 75B:973, 1993.

Toghill PJ: *Examining patients: an introduction to clinical medicine,* London, 1990, Edward Arnold.

Tollison CD, Satterthwaite JR, Tollison JW: *Handbook of pain management,* ed 2, Baltimore, 1994, Williams & Wilkins.

Toohey AK et al: Iliopsoas bursitis; clinical features, radiographic findings, and disease associations, *Semin Arthritis Rheum* 10:41, 1990.

Torg JS, Shepard RJ: *Current therapy in sports medicine,* ed 3, St Louis, 1995, Mosby.

Tronzo RG, editor: *Surgery of the hip joint,* Philadelphia, 1973, Lea & Febiger.

Turek SL: *Orthopaedics principles and their application,* ed 3, Philadelphia, 1977, JB Lippincott.

Ursavas A et al: Breast and osteoarticular tuberculosis in a male patient, *Diagn Microbiol Infect Dis* (in press, corrected proof).

Van Dillen LR et al: Symmetry of timing of hip and lumbopelvic rotation motion in 2 different subgroups of people with low back pain, *Arch Phys Med Rehabil* 88(3):351-360, 2007.

Van Holsbeeck M, Introcaso JH: *Musculoskeletal ultrasound,* St Louis, 1991, Mosby.

Verrall GM et al: Hip joint range of motion restriction precedes athletic chronic groin injury, *J Sci Med Sport* (in press, corrected proof).

Viere RG et al: Use of the Pavlik harness in congenital dislocation of the hip, an analysis of failures of treatment, *J Bone Joint Surg* 72A:238, 1990.

Vignon E et al: Osteoarthritis of the knee and hip and activity: a systematic international review and synthesis (OASIS), *Joint Bone Spine* 73(4):442-455, 2006.

Vingard E et al: Sports and osteoarthritis of the hip: an epidemiologic study, *Am J Sports Med* 21:195, 1993.

Vrahas MS et al: Contribution of passive tissues to the intersegmental moments at the hip, *J Biomech* 23:357, 1990.

Wainwright D: The shelf operation for hip dysplasia in adolescence, *J Bone Joint Surg* 58B:159, 1976.

Wakefield TS, Frank RG: *The clinician's guide to neuromusculoskeletal practice,* Abbotsford, Wis, 1995, Allied Health of Wisconsin, SC.

Walter F, Haynes MB, Markel DC: A randomized prospective study evaluating the effect of patellar eversion on the early functional outcomes in primary total knee arthroplasty, *J Arthroplasty* (in press, corrected proof).

Wang T-G et al: Assessment of stretching of the iliotibial tract with Ober and modified Ober tests: an ultrasonographic study, *Arch Phys Med Rehabil* 87(10):1407-1411, 2006.

10

Weineck J: *Functional anatomy in sports,* ed 2, St Louis, 1990, Mosby.

Weinstein SL, Buckwalter JA: *Turek's orthopaedics principles and their application,* ed 5, Philadelphia, 1994, JB Lippincott.

Weir J, Abrahams PH: *Imaging atlas of human anatomy,* version 2.0 [CD-ROM], London, 1997, Mosby.

Weisl H: Intertrochanteric osteotomy for osteoarthritis, *J Bone Joint Surg* 62B:37, 1980.

Weiss JM, Ramachandran M: Hip and pelvic injuries in the young athlete, *Oper Tech Sports Med* 14(3):212-217, 2006.

Weiss W, Flippen HJ: The changing incidence and prognosis of tuberculous meningitis, *Am J Med Sci* 250:46, 1965.

Weller IMR, Kunz M: Physical activity and pain following total hip arthroplasty, *Physiotherapy* 93(1):23-29, 2007.

Wenger DR, Ward WT, Herring JA: Legg-Calve-Perthes disease, *J Bone Joint Surg* 73A:778, 1991.

Whitmore I, Willan PLT: *Multiple choice questions in human anatomy,* London, 1995, Mosby.

Whyte Ferguson L: Knee pain: addressing the interrelationships between muscle and joint dysfunction in the hip and pelvis and the lower extremity, *J Bodywork Mov Ther* 10(4):287-296, 2006.

Wijnhoven HAH, de Vet HCW, Picavet HSJ: Explaining sex differences in chronic musculoskeletal pain in a general population, *Pain* 124(1-2):158-166, 2006.

Williams PF, editor: *Orthopaedic management in childhood,* Oxford, UK, 1982, Blackwell.

Windsor RE, Lox DM: *Soft tissue injuries: diagnosis and treatment,* Philadelphia, 1998, Hanley & Belfus.

Wingstrand H, Wingstrand A, Krantz P: Intracapsular and atmospheric pressure in the dynamics and stability of the hip, *Acta Orthop Scand* 61:231, 1990.

Winter D: *Biomechanics and motor control of human movement,* ed 2, New York, 1990, John Wiley & Sons.

Winternitz WA et al: Acute compartment syndrome of the thigh in sports related injuries not associated with femoral fractures, *Am J Sports Med* 20:476, 1992.

Woerman AL, Binder-Macleod SA: Leg-length discrepancy assessment: accuracy and precision in five clinical methods of evaluation, *J Orthop Sports Phys Ther* 5:230, 1984.

Wynne-Davis R: Acetabular dysplasia and familial joint laxity: two etiological factors in congenital dislocation of the hip, *J Bone Joint Surg* 52B:704, 1970.

Yagci N et al: Relationship between balance performance and musculoskeletal pain in lower body comparison healthy middle aged and older adults, *Arch Gerontol Geriatr* 45(1):109-119, 2007.

Yang RS, Tsuang YH, Liu TK: Traumatic dislocation of the hip, *Clin Orthop* 265:218, 1991.

Yochum TR, Rowe LJ: Measurements in skeletal radiology. In Yochum TR, Rowe LJ, editors: *Essentials of skeletal radiology,* vol 1, Baltimore, 1987, Williams & Wilkins.

Yogasakaran S, Menezes F: Acute neuropathic pain after surgery: are we treating them early/late? *Acute Pain* 7(3):145-149, 2005.

Yuen EC, Olney RK, So YT: Sciatic neuropathy: clinical and prognostic features in 73 patients, *Neurology* 44:1669, 1994.

Yuen EC, So YT, Olney RK: The electrophysiologic features of sciatic neuropathy in 100 patients, *Muscle Nerve* 18:414, 1995.

Zitelli BJ, Davis HW: *Atlas of pediatric physical diagnosis,* ed 2, London, 1992, Wolfe.

CITATIONS

Bonshahi AY, Knowles D, Hodgson SP: Isolated lesser trochanter fractures in elderly—a case for prophylactic DHS fixation: a case series, *Injury* 35(2):196-168, 2004.

Broadhurst NA, Simmons DN, Bond MJ: Piriformis syndrome: correlation of muscle morphology with symptoms and signs, *Arch Phys Med Rehabil* 85(12):2036-2039, 2004.

Dare CJ, Clarke NMP: Proximal femoral osteotomy in childhood, *Curr Orthop* 21(2):115-121, 2007.

Eijer H: Towards a better understanding of the aetiology of Legg-Calve-Perthes' disease: acetabular retroversion may cause abnormal loading of dorsal femoral head-neck junction with restricted blood supply to the femoral epiphysis, *Med Hypotheses* 68(5):995-997, 2007.

Forst J, Forst R: Lower limb surgery in Duchenne muscular dystrophy, *Neuromusc Disord* 9(3):176-181, 1999.

Guichet JM et al: Lower limb-length discrepancy: an epidemiologic study, *Clin Orthop Relat Res* 272:235-241, 1991.

Hanada E et al: Measuring leg-length discrepancy by the "iliac crest palpation and book correction" method: reliability and validity, *Arch Phys Med Rehabil* 82(7):938-942, 2001.

Hedri H et al: Avascular osteonecrosis after renal transplantation, *Transplant Proc* 39(4):1036-1038, 2007.

Holton C, Foster P, Templeton P: Fractures of the femoral neck in children, *Curr Orthop* 20(5):361-366, 2006.

Jacobsen S et al: The relationship of hip joint space to self reported hip pain: a survey of 4,151 subjects of the Copenhagen City Heart Study: the Osteoarthritis Substudy, *Osteoarthr Cartil* 12(9):692-697, 2004.

Kassarjian A, Brisson M, Palmer WE: Femoroacetabular impingement, *Eur J Radiol* (in press, corrected proof).

Kim Y-W et al: Risk factors for leg length discrepancy in patients with congenital vascular malformation, *J Vasc Surg* 44(3):545-553, 2006.

Matjacic Z, Olensek A: Biomechanical characterization and clinical implications of artificially induced crouch walking: differences between pure iliopsoas, pure hamstrings and combination of iliopsoas and hamstrings contractures, *J Biomech* 40(3):491-501, 2007.

Morote J et al: Prevalence of osteoporosis during long-term androgen deprivation therapy in patients with prostate cancer, *Urology* 69(3):500-504, 2007.

Myers MT, Thompson GH: Imaging the child with a limp, *Pediatr Clin North Am* 44(3):637-658, 1997.

Rice P: Viral meningitis and encephalitis, *Medicine* 33(4):60-63, 2005.

Rosemann T, Szecsenyi J: Cultural adaptation and validation of a German version of the Arthritis Impact Measurement Scales (AIMS2), *Osteoarthr Cartil* (in press, corrected proof).

Roussel NA et al: Low back pain: clinimetric properties of the Trendelenburg test, active straight leg raise test, and breathing pattern during active straight leg raising, *J Manipulative Physiol Ther* 30(4):270-278, 2007.

Steib-Furno S et al: Pregnancy-related hip diseases: incidence and diagnoses, *Joint Bone Spine* (in press, uncorrected proof).

Thomas B, Krishnamoorthy T, Kapilamoorthy TR: Contrast enhanced FLAIR imaging in ibuprofen induced aseptic meningitis, *Eur J Radiol Extra* 60(3):97-99, 2006.

Ursavas A et al: Breast and osteoarticular tuberculosis in a male patient, *Diagn Microbiol Infect Dis* (in press, corrected proof).

Verrall GM et al: Hip joint range of motion restriction precedes athletic chronic groin injury, *J Sci Med Sport* (in press, corrected proof).

Zimering MB et al: Validation of a novel risk estimation tool for predicting low bone density in Caucasian and African American men veterans, *J Clin Densitometry* (in press, corrected proof).

KNEE

AXIOMS IN ASSESSING THE KNEE

- The knee consists of two joints: the patellofemoral and the tibiofemoral.
- Knee pain can arise from the joint itself, from periarticular tissues, or from the hip or femur.

INTRODUCTION

Pain is the most common presenting symptom of knee abnormalities. The causes of knee pain tend to be age related. A convenient way to classify knee pain complaints is by age group and by whether the pain is intraarticular, periarticular, or referred (Table 11-3).

The rounded contour of the femoral condyles furnishes little stability, and the flat tibial plateaus, deepened by the semilunar cartilages. The quadriceps muscle and its tendinous expansions are great contributors to the stability and function of the knee. The earliest clinical indication of internal knee derangement is atrophy of the quadriceps.

ORTHOPEDIC GAMUT 11-1
KNEE STABILITY

Knee stability depends on four ligaments:
1. Tibial collateral
2. Fibular collateral
3. Anterior cruciate
4. Posterior cruciate

ORTHOPEDIC GAMUT 11-2
KNEE

Parts of a knee vulnerable to injury:
- Ligaments
- Muscle tendon
- Capsule
- Meniscus
- Cartilage
- Bone
- Bursae
- Any combination of these

The knee is not a true hinge joint. The tibia navigates a helical course on the condyles of the femur. Most cases of traumatic arthritis of the knee in middle-age and elderly people result from minor derangements of the soft tissues, especially the menisci.

The knee lacks the stability of the hip, which has its ball and socket, or the ankle, which has its mortise and tendon. Both the hip and ankle have structures that give some degree of bony stability. In the knee joint, the socket of the top of the tibia is so minimal that the lateral tibial plateau may be flat or even convex. The little bit of buffering provided by the menisci gives minimal increase in stability because the menisci are unstable themselves. For stability, the knee must depend largely on the soft tissues, ligaments, capsule, and muscles.

Making an accurate diagnosis about the exact nature of the patient's knee injury is extremely important. Examina-

TABLE 11-1

KNEE JOINT CROSS-REFERENCE TABLE BY ASSESSMENT PROCEDURE

DISEASE ASSESSED

Test/Sign (Knee Joint)	Medial Collateral Ligament	Lateral Collateral Ligament	Medial Meniscus	Lateral Meniscus	Patellar Dislocation	Chondromalacia Patellae	Anterior Cruciate Ligament	Posterior Capsule	Iliotibial Band	Posterior Cruciate Ligament	Arcuate-Popliteus Complex	Posterior Oblique Ligament	Patellar Fracture	Patellar Syndromes (Soft Tissue)	Anterolateral Rotary Syndrome	Effusion	Valgus Deformity	Quadriceps	Osteochondritis
Abduction stress test	•																		
Adduction stress test		•																	
Apley compression/ distraction test			•	•															
Apprehension test for the patella					•														
Bounce home test																			
Childress duck waddle test			•	•															
Clarke test			•	•		•								•					
Drawer test	•						•	•	•	•	•	•							
Dreyer sign													•						
Fouchet sign						•													
Lachman test							•				•	•							
Lateral pivot shift maneuver		•					•	•	•		•								
Losee test															•				
McMurray sign			•	•															
Noble compression test									•										
Patella ballottement test																•			
Payr sign			•																
Q-angle test					•	•								•	•		•		
Slocum test	•	•					•	•	•	•	•	•							
Steinmann sign			•	•															
Thigh circumference test																		•	
Wilson sign																			•

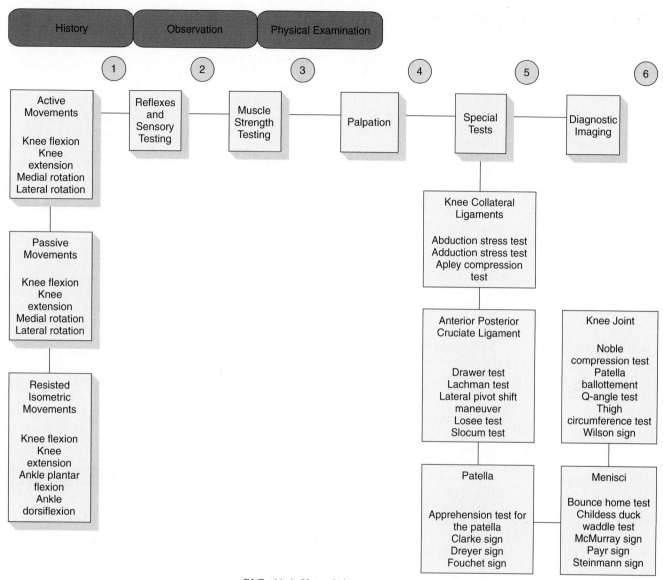

FIG. 11-1 Knee-joint assessment.

11

tion must determine what part of the knee is injured and how bad the injury is.

ESSENTIAL ANATOMY

The knee joint is the articulation of the femur, patella, and tibia (Fig. 11-2). The fibula is not involved in this articulation. The knee allows for flexion and extension and for rotation when the knee is in complete flexion (but not if the knee is fully extended).

In both the lateral and the medial compartments of the joint is a C-shaped, flattened cartilaginous meniscus (Fig. 11-3) loosely attached to the superior surface of the tibial plateau.

The anterior cruciate ligament (ACL) prevents excessive anterior *sliding* of the tibia with respect to the femur; the posterior cruciate ligament (PCL) prevents excessive poste-

rior sliding of the tibia on the femur. The posterior medial corner of the knee aids in medial stability (Fig 11-4).

The superficial medial collateral ligament (MCL), or tibial collateral ligament (TCL), consists of parallel, longitudinal fibers anteriorly and an oblique array of fibers posterior to this. These posterior fibers follow a course at 25 degrees to the longitudinal fibers and have been termed the posterior oblique ligament (POL) of the knee. The POL is the first of the structures that make up the posterior third of the medial aspect of the knee, or posteromedial corner. The other intimately related and closely interacting components are the semimembranosus insertion, the posterior third of the medial meniscus, the oblique popliteal ligament (OPL) and the meniscotibial ligament (House, Connell, Saifuddin, 2007).

The patella enhances quadriceps strength. The articulating surface is divided by a median ridge into lateral and

TABLE 11-2

KNEE CROSS-REFERENCE TABLE BY SUSPECTED SYNDROME OR TISSUE

Anterior cruciate ligament	Drawer test
	Lachman test
	Lateral pivot shift maneuver
	Slocum test
Arcuate-popliteus complex	Drawer test
	Lachman test
	Lateral pivot shift maneuver
	Slocum test
Anterolateral rotary syndromes	Losee test
	Q-angle test
Chondromalacia patella	Clarke test
	Fouchet sign
	Q-angle test
Effusion	Patella ballottement test
Iliotibial band	Drawer test
	Lateral pivot shift maneuver
	Noble compression test
	Slocum test
Lateral collateral ligament	Adduction stress test
	Lateral pivot shift maneuver
	Slocum test
Lateral meniscus	Apley compression/distraction test
	Bounce home test
	Clarke test
	McMurray sign
	Steinmann sign
Medial collateral ligament	Abduction stress test
	Drawer test
	Slocum test
Medial meniscus	Apley compression/distraction test
	Bounce home test
	Clarke test
	McMurray sign
	Payr sign
	Steinmann sign
Osteochondritis	Wilson sign
Patellar dislocation	Apprehension test for the patella
	Q-angle test
Patellar fracture	Dreyer sign
Patellar syndromes	Clarke test
	Fouchet sign
	Q-angle test
Posterior capsule	Drawer test
	Lateral pivot shift maneuver
	Slocum test
Posterior cruciate ligament	Drawer test
	Slocum test
Posterior oblique ligament	Drawer test
	Fouchet sign
	Slocum test
Quadriceps	Thigh circumference test
Valgus deformity	Q-angle test

TABLE 11-3

INTRAARTICULAR KNEE PAIN DIFFERENTIATED BY AGE

Age	Intraarticular
Juvenile (2–10 yrs)	Juvenile chronic arthritis
	Osteochondritis dissecans
	Septic arthritis
	Torn discoid lateral meniscus
Adolescent (10–18 yrs)	Osteochondritis dissecans
	Torn meniscus
	Anterior knee pain syndrome
	Patellar malalignment
Early adult (18–30 yrs)	Torn meniscus
	Instability
	Anterior knee pain syndrome
	Inflammatory conditions
Adult (30–50 yrs)	Degenerate meniscal tears
	Early degeneration after injury or meniscectomy
	Inflammatory arthropathies
Mature (>50 yrs)	Osteoarthritis
	Inflammatory arthropathies

Adapted from Klippel JH, Dieppe PA: *Rheumatology*, vol 1-2, ed 2, London, 1998, Mosby.

ORTHOPEDIC GAMUT 11-3

FABELLA

A fabella can be a source of:
- Fabellar pain syndrome
- Chondromalacia
- Fractures
- Symptomatic dislocation (Fig. 11-6)
- Osteoarthritis
- Hypertrophy causing peroneal nerve paralysis

---

medial facets. Six types of patella are described based on shape (Wiberg types) (Fig. 11-5). Types I and II are considered most stable, whereas the other types, because of unbalanced forces, are prone to lateral subluxations.

The fabella *(little bean)* is a sesamoid bone that is present in approximately 10% to 30% of the general population (Fig. 11-6). This bone can only occasionally act as a source of atypical knee pain, often mistaken for a more common cause of clinical symptoms, such as an intraarticular loose body or an osteophyte.

A painful fabella belongs to a wide range of conditions that can cause pain in or malfunctioning of the knee and therefore may lead to delay in diagnosis and uncritical use of arthroscopy (Franceschi et al, 2007).

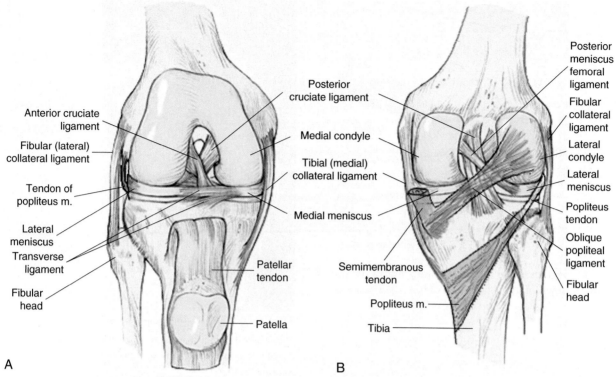

FIG. 11-2 Knee joint opened, anterior **(A)** and posterior **(B)** view. (From Mathers LH et al: *Clinical anatomy principles*, St Louis, 1996, Mosby.)

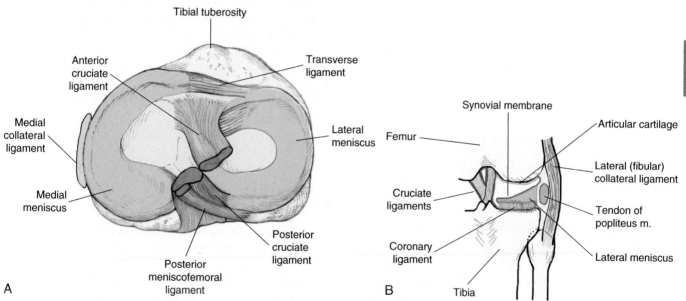

FIG. 11-3 Superior end of the right tibia. (From Mathers LH et al: *Clinical anatomy principles*, St Louis, 1996, Mosby.)

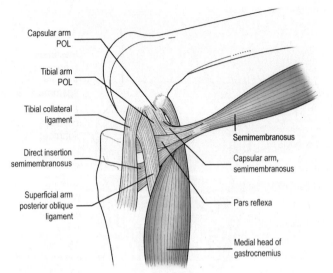

FIG. 11-4 Diagram of the supporting structures of the posteromedial corner of the knee. (From House CV, Connell DA, Saifuddin A: Posteromedial corner injuries of the knee, *Clin Radiol* 62[6]:539-46, 2007.)

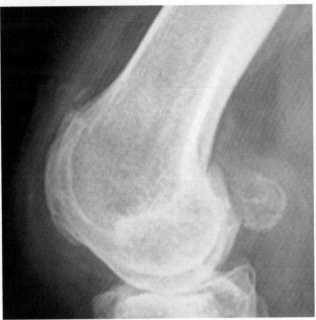

FIG. 11-6 Radiograph demonstrates a hypertrophic, dislocated fabella. (From Franceschi F, Longo UG, Ruzzini L, et al: Dislocation of an enlarged fabella as uncommon cause of knee pain: A case report, *Knee* 14[4]:330-332, 2007.)

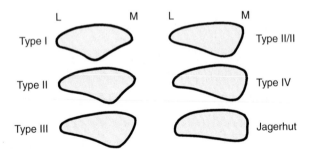

FIG. 11-5 Wiberg and Baumgartl patellar types. (From Scott WN: *The knee*, vol 1-2, St Louis, 1994, Mosby.)

ORTHOPEDIC GAMUT 11-4

THIGH MUSCLES

The three thigh muscles that attach to the medial side of the tibia (supplied by three different nerves) are the following:
1. Gracilis (obturator nerve)
2. Sartorius (femoral nerve)
3. Semitendinosus (tibial nerve)

ESSENTIAL MOTION ASSESSMENT

The flexion-extension movement of the knee is not a simple hinge motion (Figs. 11-7 and 11-8). As the knee passes through its degrees of flexion and extensions, the imaginary mediolateral axis through which the movement occurs shifts up and down on the femur (Fig. 11-9).

With the foot planted on the ground and the knee fully extended, the knee is said to be *locked* in such a way that muscles of the thigh and leg can relax for short periods without making the joint too unstable.

ESSENTIAL MUSCLE FUNCTION ASSESSMENT

The examiner tests the muscles responsible for knee flexion and extension, the hamstrings and quadriceps, respectively (Figs. 11-10 and 11-11).

Quadriceps weakness and wasting can accompany joint disease. In a normal joint, unilateral quadriceps weakness suggests either a femoral neuropathy or an L3 root syndrome (Fig. 11-12). Femoral neuropathy leads to weakness and wasting of the quadriceps, loss of the knee jerk, and sensory change over the anterior thigh and the medial aspect of the lower leg (Fig. 11-13).

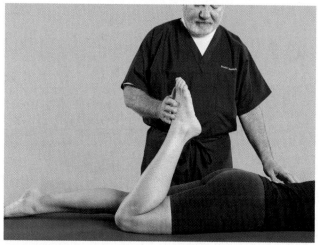

FIG. 11-7 The normal angle of knee flexion ranges from 130 to 150 degrees. A simple and useful but less-precise method for comparing the flexion of both knees can be used. This method involves comparing the distance between the heel and buttock when both knees are maximally flexed. Less than 140 degrees of retained active flexion range of motion is an impairment of the knee joint in the activities of daily living.

Flexion contractures (limitation of extension) of the knee often complicate chronic involvement of the joint. Varying degrees of subluxation or dislocation of the knee are most often the result of posterior displacement of the tibia on the femur or are occasionally from destruction of one condyle and the supporting plate of the tibia. When, as a result of such destruction, the tibia is dislocated laterally or medially, abnormal lateral or medial mobility is present, although the range of flexion and extension of the knee is limited.

A catch or jerky motion can sometimes be felt or seen during passive flexion and extension of the knee when the joint space harbors loose bodies. When the motion is repeated, the catch occurs at the same position in the arc of movement. The knee may lock or become suddenly fixed in partial extension while flexion from the point of limitation may remain unrestricted. A catching or jerky motion also may result from the absence of both menisci, whether from surgical removal or from disintegration that is secondary to articular inflammatory diseases, such as rheumatoid arthritis.

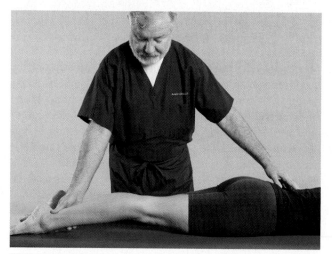

FIG. 11-8 The knee should normally extend to a straight line (0 degrees) and occasionally can be hyperextended up to 15 degrees. The degree of extension is determined by measuring the angle formed between the thigh and the leg. A flexion angle that is 10 degrees or greater in the fully extended knee is an impairment of the knee in the activities of daily living.

ORTHOPEDIC GAMUT 11-5

SCIATIC NERVE

The sciatic nerve innervates the following:
1. Hip joint
2. Biceps femoris
3. Semitendinosus
4. Semimembranosus
5. Ischial head of the adductor magnus

11

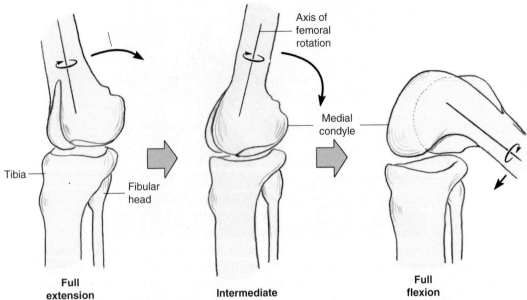

FIG. 11-9 Rotation at the knee. (From Mathers LH et al: *Clinical anatomy principles*, St Louis, 1996, Mosby.)

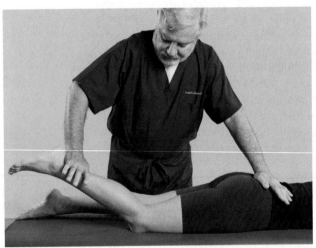

FIG. 11-10 The prime movers involved in flexion of the knee are the biceps femoris (sciatic nerve, tibial branch, S1, S2, and S3 to the long head; peroneal branch, L4, L5, S1, and S2 to the short head), semitendinosus (sciatic nerve, tibial branch, L4, L5, S1, S2, and S3), and the semimembranosus (sciatic nerve, tibial branch, L4, L5, S1, S2, and S3) muscles. Accessory muscles to this motion are the popliteus, sartorius, gracilis, and gastrocnemius. Flexion of the knee is tested while the patient is lying in a prone position with the knees extended. The examiner places one hand over the lateral aspect of the pelvis to immobilize it and applies graded resistance just proximal to the ankle with the other hand. The patient flexes the knee through its range of motion. If knee flexion is tested with the ankle rotated laterally, the biceps femoris is tested more directly because it is placed in better alignment. If knee flexion is tested with the ankle rotated medially, the semimembranosus and semitendinosus muscles are tested more directly during flexion. To prevent substitution by the gastrocnemius muscle, plantar flexion of the foot should not be allowed during knee flexion.

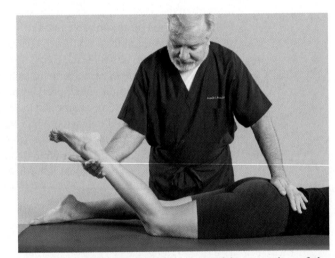

FIG. 11-11 The prime mover involved in extension of the knee is the quadriceps femoris (rectus femoris, vastus intermedius, vastus medialis, and vastus lateralis) muscle (innervated by the femoral nerve, L2, L3, and L4). Extension of the knee is tested while the patient is lying in a prone position with the knees flexed. The examiner places one hand over the lateral aspect of the pelvis to immobilize it and applies graded resistance just proximal to the ankle with the other hand. The patient extends the knee through its range of motion. As an alternative, the examiner can observe quadriceps femoris weakness if the patient is not able to rise from a low chair (height less than 65 cm) or from a squatting to a standing position without using the hands or other supports.

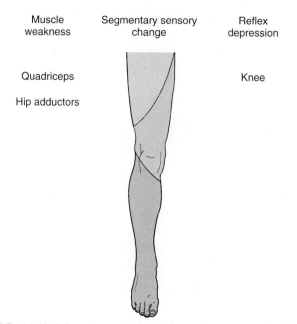

FIG. 11-12 L3 root syndrome. Motor, sensory, and reflex abnormalities. (From Epstein O et al: *Clinical examination*, ed 2, London, 1997, Mosby.)

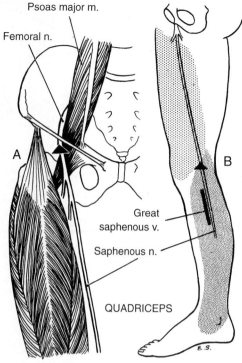

FIG. 11-13 Femoral nerve compression. This nerve has a close anatomic relation with the psoas muscle and inguinal ligament (**A**). Compression at the groin may cause quadriceps weakness and sensory impairment in the nerve's distribution at the thigh (*lightly stippled area*) and in the saphenous branch (*heavily stippled area*). Pressure at the knee (**B**) or surgery to the saphenous veins may affect the saphenous nerve. (From Dyck PJ, Thomas PK, Lambert EH: *Peripheral neuropathy,* Philadelphia, 1975, WB Saunders.)

ESSENTIAL IMAGING

The typical knee study consists of an anteroposterior (AP) (or posteroanterior [PA]) and a lateral view (Figs. 11-14 to 11-17). Many examiners will include tangential, tunnel, or oblique views for further evaluation. The tangential view provides an axial depiction of the patella and its relationship with the femur. The tunnel view allows excellent visualization of the intercondylar region of the femoral-tibial articulation (Figs. 11-18 and 11-19).

Typically, an AP knee radiograph is taken, but if the patella were the primary area of concern, a PA view would be useful (Figs. 11-20 and 11-21).

The lateral film is most sensitive for evaluating effusion of the joint (Fig. 11-22).

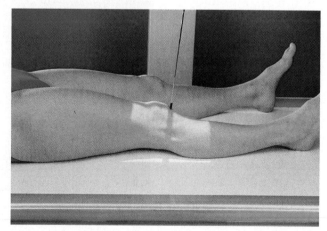

FIG. 11-14 Anteroposterior knee positioning. (From Frank ED et al: *Merrill's atlas of radiographic positioning and procedures*, vol 1-3, ed 11, St Louis, 2007, Mosby.)

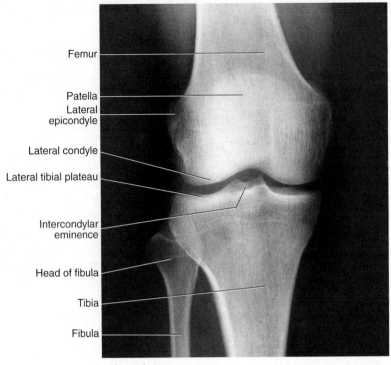

Femur

Patella

Lateral
epicondyle

Lateral condyle

Lateral tibial plateau

Intercondylar
eminence

Head of fibula

Tibia

Fibula

FIG. 11-15 Anteroposterior knee image. (From Frank ED et al: *Merrill's atlas of radiographic positioning and procedures*, vol 1-3, ed 11, St Louis, 2007, Mosby.)

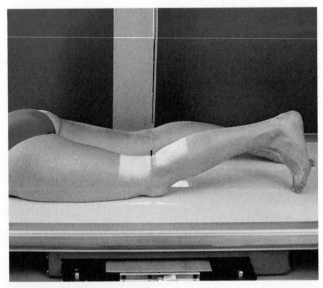

FIG. 11-16 Posteroanterior knee positioning. (From Frank ED et al: *Merrill's atlas of radiographic positioning and procedures*, vol 1-3, ed 11, St Louis, 2007, Mosby.)

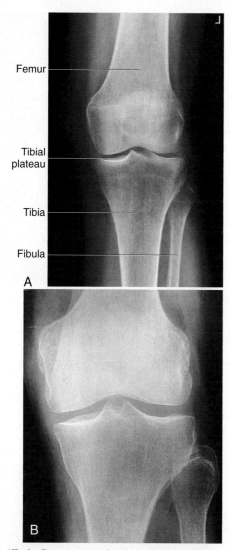

Femur

Tibial plateau

Tibia

Fibula

A

B

FIG. 11-17 **A,** Posteroanterior knee image. **B,** Posteroanterior knee image showing epiphyses of teenager. (From Frank ED et al: *Merrill's atlas of radiographic positioning and procedures*, vol 1-3, ed 11, St Louis, 2007, Mosby.)

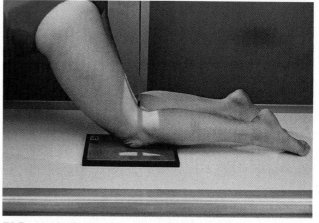

FIG. 11-18 Posteroanterior axial intercondylar fossa positioning: kneeling on radiographic table. (From Frank ED et al: *Merrill's atlas of radiographic positioning and procedures*, vol 1-3, ed 11, St Louis, 2007, Mosby.)

11

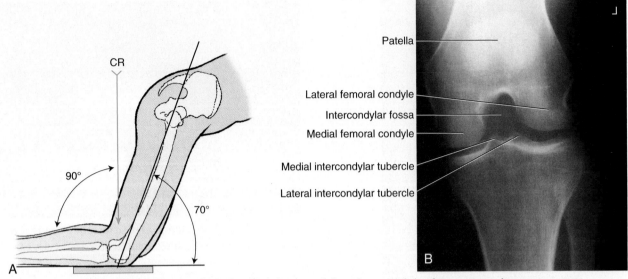

FIG. 11-19 Alignment relationships for any of three intercondylar fossa approaches. (From Frank ED et al: *Merrill's atlas of radiographic positioning and procedures*, vol 1-3, ed 11, St Louis, 2007, Mosby.)

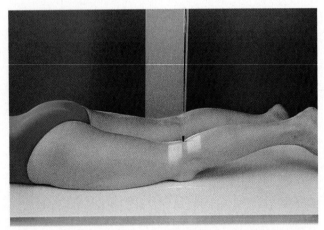

FIG. 11-20 Posteroanterior patella positioning. (From Frank ED et al: *Merrill's atlas of radiographic positioning and procedures*, vol 1-3, ed 11, St Louis, 2007, Mosby.)

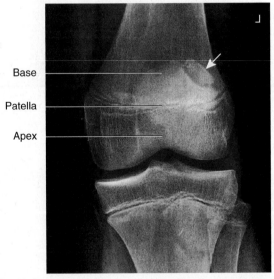

FIG. 11-21 Posteroanterior patella image. (From Frank ED et al: *Merrill's atlas of radiographic positioning and procedures*, vol 1-3, ed 11, St Louis, 2007, Mosby.)

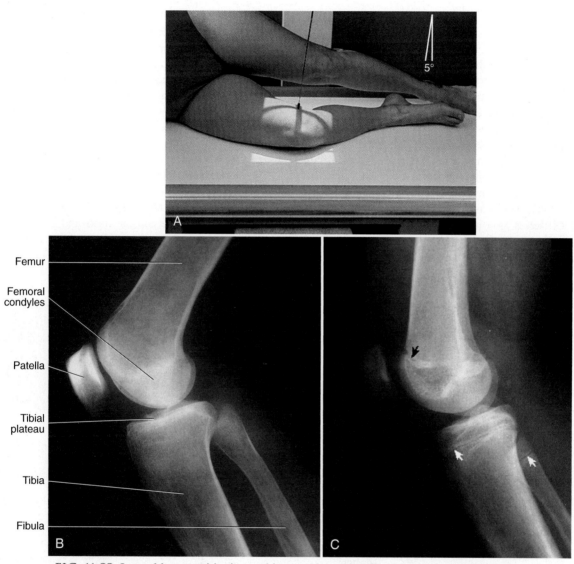

FIG. 11-22 Lateral knee positioning and images demonstrating 5 degrees cephalad angulation of central ray. (From Frank ED et al: *Merrill's atlas of radiographic positioning and procedures*, vol 1-3, ed 11, St Louis, 2007, Mosby.)

ALSO KNOWN AS VALGUS STRESS TEST

Assessment for Medial Collateral Ligament Injury

Comment

Injuries to the medial collateral are the most common ligament injuries seen in the knee. An intimate anatomic relationship exists between the MCL and the medial meniscus of the knee. O'Donoghue is credited with describing the *unhappy triad* as a combined injury to the MCL, ACL, and medial meniscus. Because the MCL and medial meniscus are strongly attached to one another, clearly the meniscus may become injured, along with more severe MCL injuries (Fig. 11-23). However, the more common triad is the MCL, ACL, and lateral meniscus.

The MCL serves as a primary stabilizer against valgus stresses to the knee. The MCL complex consists of three layers. The most superficial layer is an extension of the crural fascia, which covers the quadriceps muscles. The next layer, which is often termed the superficial layer of the MCL, is the TCL. The deepest layer is known as the capsular ligament or the deep MCL. This deep MCL layer acts as part of the joint capsule and consists of the meniscofemoral and meniscotibial (or coronary) ligaments. An MCL bursa has been demonstrated to lie between the TCL and the capsular ligament layers. The MCL complex also includes the POL. The TCL is thought to be the strongest and the most important portion for posterior medial knee stabilization and rotatory stabilization of the knee. The TCL is the portion of the MCL complex that is most easily seen on magnetic resonance imaging (MRI) (Wen et al, 2007).

The medial ligament is the main strut of the capsular tissues of the knee. The deep portion of the ligament is a thickened part of the capsule itself and is adherent to the medial meniscus. The superficial part forms a strong, broad, and triangular strap. Originating from a point just distal to

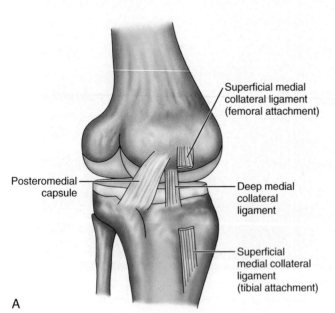

A

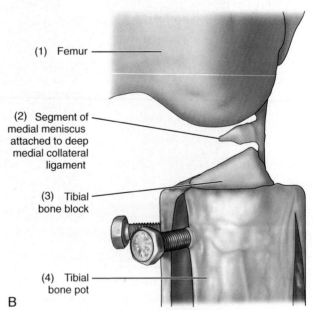

(1) Femur

(2) Segment of medial meniscus attached to deep medial collateral ligament

(3) Tibial bone block

(4) Tibial bone pot

Superficial medial collateral ligament (femoral attachment)

Deep medial collateral ligament

Posteromedial capsule

Superficial medial collateral ligament (tibial attachment)

B

FIG. 11-23 The medial meniscus can also become injured in conjunction with the medial collateral ligament (MCL) because of its intimate anatomic relationship with the MCL. **(A)** The MCL complex. The longitudinal fibres of the superficial medial collateral ligament (sMCL) have been divided to show the deep medial collateral ligament (dMCL) beneath. (1) The longitudinal fibers of the sMCL–femoral attachment. (2) The dMCL. (3) The posteromedial capsule (PMC). (4) sMCL–tibial attachment. **(B)** Deep MCL in the tensile testing rig. The segment of meniscus to which the ligament is attached has been retained. (1) Femur, (2) segment of medial meniscus attached to deep MCL, (3) tibial bone block, and (4) tibial bone pot. (Adapted from Robinson JR, Bull AMJ, Amis AA: Structural properties of the medial collateral ligament complex of the human knee, *J Biomech* 38[5]:1067-1074, 2005.)

ORTHOPEDIC GAMUT 11-6

MEDIAL COLLATERAL LIGAMENT INJURY CLASSIFICATIONS

Grade I: 0 to 5 mm of joint opening with no instability

Grade II: 5 to 10 mm of joint opening with some degree of instability

Grade III: 10 to 15 mm of joint opening with moderate instability

Grade IV: Greater than 15 mm of joint opening with gross ligament instability

---

the adductor tubercle, the ligament keeps free of the meniscus and the joint margins and has an extensive insertion into the medial surface of the tibia—at least 1.5 inches below the joint level. The posterior border of the ligament has continuity with the strong posterior capsule of the knee joint. Anterior to this structure are fibrous connections with the quadriceps expansion and the patellar ligament. The medial capsule, which is accompanied by its ligament, is adequately designed to take strong control of the tibia in all movements of the knee, both by structure and by the intimate connections that the capsule forms with the anterior and posterior muscles of the thigh.

A ligament is a fibrous structure designed to prevent abnormal motion of a joint. Any ligamentous injury that is caused by an abnormal motion may be defined as a sprain. A sprain can vary from a complete dislocation of the joint, accompanied by total loss of ligament integrity, to a slight tearing of a few isolated fibers, with no loss of function. A sprain should include avulsion of the ligament from the bone, with or without a small fragment (sprain-fracture); partial avulsion of the ligament from the bone; or tearing (transversely, obliquely, or longitudinally) of the ligament within its substance. In the last instance, the ligament will be elongated, although it will still be intact. The function of the ligament depends not only on its strength but also on its length. A ligament that is elongated does not carry out its function of preventing abnormal motion of the joint. The

severity of the injury is of more significance than the exact location or type of tear.

Injuries to the MCL are usually thought to occur as a result of sudden traumatic valgus stress to the knee, which produces tensile overload to the fibers of the MCL, which, in turn, leads to their disruption. The deep capsular layer is thought to be the weakest layer and hence the first to be disrupted. The stronger TCL becomes disrupted when additional force is applied. More severe clinical grades of MCL injury are often associated with concurrent injuries of the ACL. The ACL serves as an important secondary stabilizer of the knee against valgus stress (Wen et al, 2007).

Medial ligament syndrome is an ill-defined syndrome in which the patient complains of pain at the site of insertion of the medial ligament. Examination reveals tenderness over the insertion of the ligament, and valgus stress may exacerbate the pain. It is more common in women than in men and is associated with valgus knees and the pain amplification syndrome. Differentiating anserine bursitis and pes anserinus tendinopathy may be difficult. The cause is obscure; however, in some cases, an inflammatory arthropathy, such as ankylosing spondylitis, is present.

PROCEDURE

- While the patient is lying supine and the knee is in complete extension, the examiner, who is on the ipsilateral side, places one palm against the lateral aspect of the patient's knee at the joint line.
- While the other hand is gripping the ankle, the examiner laterally draws the leg to open the medial side of the joint (Fig. 11-24).
- If the patient is indifferent to this action, the examiner repeats it while the knee is in approximately 30 degrees of flexion, a position of lesser stability.
- This maneuver makes the medial joint vulnerable to torsion stress.
- The production or increase of pain, especially below, above, or at the joint line, is evidence of MCL injury.

Next Steps/Procedures

Adduction stress test and Apley compression/distraction test

11

CLINICAL PEARL

The knee is an unusual joint because it contains ligaments deep within the joint. Medial and lateral collateral menisci in the joint can also be damaged. Finally, the normal motions of the knee are very complex, including two planes of rotation. Multiple and complex injuries are common.

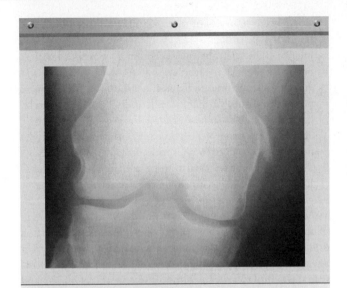

AT THE VIEWBOX

History of severe knee injury while skiing years ago. Clinical findings of internal knee derangement with gross instability. Ossification at the femoral attachment site of the medial collateral ligament is typical of Pellgrini-Steiada disease. This post-traumatic hemorrhagic bone formation indicates a chronic tear of the medial collateral ligament and is typically associated with medial meniscus and anterior cruciate ligament tears. (From the teaching file of Timothy Mick, DC, DACBR)

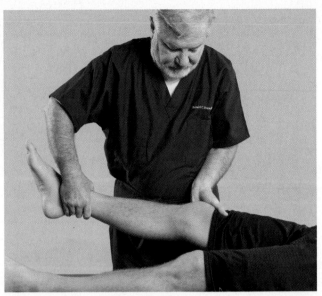

FIG. 11-24 The patient is lying supine, and the knee is in complete extension. The examiner, who is on the ipsilateral side, places one palm against the lateral aspect of the patient's knee at the joint line. With the other hand gripping the ankle, the examiner draws the leg laterally to open the medial side of the knee joint. The production or increase of pain—especially below, above, or at the joint line—is evidence of medial collateral ligament injury.

ADDUCTION STRESS TEST

ALSO KNOWN AS VARUS STRESS TEST

Assessment for Lateral Collateral Ligament Injury

Comment

Pain along the lateral side of the knee must be thoroughly evaluated because the anatomy and biomechanics of this region are very complex. Lateral knee pain syndrome includes lateral meniscal abnormalities, iliotibial band syndrome, lateral collateral ligament (LCL) sprain, and popliteus tendonitis. On the other hand, the proximal tibiofibular joint abnormalities have received little attention in the evaluation of lateral knee pain (Bozkurt et al, 2004).

The proximal tibiofibular joint is vulnerable to dysfunction of both static and dynamic structures and is often seen in patients with lateral knee pain. Knee, thigh, and low back pain are the most common symptoms.

The lateral ligament extends in two layers from the lateral condyle of the femur to the head of the fibula, where the ligament inserts on the biceps tendon. The tendon of the popliteus and often a bursa separates the ligament from the knee joint and the lateral meniscus. The only connection the ligament has with the fibrous capsule is at the posterior border of the lateral ligament, which is continuous with the fascia covering the popliteus and is therefore continuous with that muscle's attachments to the posterior horn of the lateral meniscus. The lateral ligament plays its part in stability of the leg on the thigh through the superior tibiofibular joint. The lateral ligament is independent of rotary movements of the tibia. Where the ligament attaches to the lateral meniscus, rotation is prevented, and flexion of the knee is restricted. The lateral capsule is thinner and weaker than the one on the medial side.

ORTHOPEDIC GAMUT 11-7

PROXIMAL TIBIOFIBULAR JOINT DYSFUNCTION SYMPTOMS

- Dull ache at the lateral aspect of the knee
- Pain radiating distally or proximally or both
- Hamstring tightness
- Knee and ankle movements that exacerbate the pain
- Pain that is relieved by rest
- Painful fibular head
- Full knee extension restricted or absent owing to hamstring tightness or pain

---

Ligament instability may be defined as abnormal rotational or translational motion of the tibial plateaus in relation to the femoral condyles. This rotational or translational motion occurs around one or more axes or in one or more planes of motion and results in a functional deficit. The key to evaluating ligament instability is the term *functional deficit*. Although two patients may have identical degrees of ligamentous instability, the functional deficit in each is not the same because the demands each patient places on the knees are different. A moderate amount of instability in an individual who wants to take part in vigorous physical activity may create a serious handicap, but a more sedentary patient may find that the same degree of instability is not a serious problem.

Stability of the knee is provided by static and dynamic elements that work together as an integrated mechanism. Static support is a function of the ligaments, capsule, menisci, and bony contour of the joint. Dynamic support is the function of the surrounding muscles. Attempting to assign a specific function to each ligament has led to confusion in evaluating ligamentous instability. The examiner must bear in mind that the static stabilizers are an integral part of a mechanism that must provide support to an inherently unstable joint that is subject to a variety of forces. Rarely does an injury affect only one element in this complex system. An injury usually influences more than one other structure either directly or indirectly. The knee joint is not merely a hinge joint that allows flexion and extension. The joint also has the element of rotation and even some valgus and varus motion.

Even with normal ligaments, knee stability is a rather tenuous situation because the knee does not have the dynamic support of the various thigh and calf muscles, which protect the static elements. The static structures define the limits of motion, and the musculotendinous structures control the motion through voluntary and kinesthetic mechanisms. These structures create appropriate motion and simultaneously serve as energy-absorbing mechanisms for extrinsic and intrinsic forces that might otherwise injure the static structures.

The LCL is rarely injured in isolation; it is usually torn in association with damage to the posterolateral ligament complex (lateral capsule, arcuate ligament, and popliteus tendon). The cruciate ligaments may also be damaged. The mechanism of injury is usually a varus force on a flexed knee. The ligament usually ruptures at its fibular insertion, or it may avulse the fibular styloid. Peroneal nerve palsy may be associated with a LCL tear and should be looked for at the time of the injury. Little functional instability arises from an isolated tear of the LCL.

PROCEDURE

- While the patient is lying supine and the knee is in complete extension, the examiner, who is on the ipsilateral side, places one palm against the medial aspect of the patient's knee, at the joint line.
- While the examiner's other hand grasps the ankle, the examiner draws the leg medially to open the lateral side of the joint (Fig. 11-25).
- If the patient is indifferent to this procedure, the examiner repeats it with the knee in approximately 30 degrees of flexion.
- An initiation or increase of pain above, below, or at the joint line is evidence of LCL injury.

Next Steps/Procedures

Abduction stress test and Apley compression/distraction test

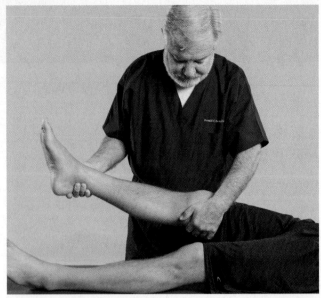

FIG. 11-25 The patient is lying supine, and the knee is in complete extension. The examiner, who is standing on the ipsilateral side, places one palm against the medial aspect of the patient's knee at the joint line. With the other hand gripping the ankle, the examiner draws the leg medially to open the lateral side of the knee joint. The production or increase of pain that is above, below, or at the joint line is evidence of lateral collateral ligament injury.

CLINICAL PEARL

Little congruency exists between the articular surfaces of the tibia and the femur. As a result, the knee has a well-developed system of ligaments for stability and an arrangement of intraarticular menisci that reduce the contact loading between the femur and the tibia.

ALSO KNOWN AS APLEY DISTRACTION TEST AND APLEY GRINDING TEST

Assessment for Collateral Ligament Injury and Meniscus Tears

Comment

Meniscus tears are often associated with a traumatic event, but they can also occur because of the cartilage degeneration process in osteoarthritis (OA).

When bearing weight, the tibia rotates laterally as the knee joint extends, and it rotates medially as the knee flexes. If this synchrony is forcibly prevented, such as by the weight of the patient's falling body, the rotator mechanism of the knee is injured. Certain cartilage tears are caused by this disruption of the rotator mechanism of the knee. In a geriatric patient, the transverse fracture of the fibrotic medial meniscus, which takes place at the junction of the anterior two thirds and the posterior one third, may be the result of pressure and grinding between the femur and the tibia. All other tears can be explained by the violent stretching that must occur if medial rotation of the tibia is prevented when the knee is flexed or if lateral rotation is prevented when the knee is extended. Similar forces are brought into play when weight is taken on while squatting or kneeling. For example, a sudden twisting may occur without extension or further flexion, or the tibia may twist laterally while the body lurches backward and increases flexion of the knee.

At first, the meniscus straightens. To allow it to do so, transverse or oblique splits form in the shorter or free edge. This minor split is the most common finding and is usually deeper in the lateral meniscus than in the medial meniscus because of the longer curve of the latter. If no more damage occurs, the knee might be symptomless after recovery from the acute injury, but the split itself would not heal. However, the split occasionally extends obliquely to form a mobile tag, which causes an irritating, recurring, and painful catch in the knee.

The split usually occurs at the apex of the curve or in the anterior portion of the meniscus. This location is to be expected because the straightening under tension would take place first in the more mobile portion. The posterior segments are more firmly fixed to the capsule.

If the range of unaccommodated movement is greater, it is achieved both by pulling the cartilage away from its attachments to the anterior cruciate and from its capsular moorings at the back or by splitting the cartilage longitudinally to allow the free border to bowstring across the joint.

The medial meniscus is more often injured than the lateral. The two tests commonly used to aid in the diagnosis of a torn meniscus are Apley test and the McMurray test.

The menisci of the knee are crescent-shaped fibrocartilaginous washers that protect articular cartilage by maximizing contact area and minimizing contact stress within the tibiofemoral joint. When a meniscus is torn, the contact mechanics of the tibiofemoral joint are altered, which disrupts the homeostasis of articular cartilage metabolism, placing the knee at risk for early OA. Biomechanical studies have clearly shown that joint contact mechanics are altered after meniscectomy and meniscal transplantation (Bowers et al, in press).

ORTHOPEDIC GAMUT 11-8

INDICATIONS OF PATHOLOGIC CONDITIONS OF THE MENISCUS

1. Pain or tenderness on the lateral surfaces of the knee joint
2. Popping, snapping, or grating sounds with movement
3. Inability to fully extend the knee *(locking)*

PROCEDURE

- The test involves four steps, and if any or all of them elicit knee pain or clicking, the test is positive.
- The patient is lying prone with the lower limbs straight and the ankles hanging over the end of the examination table.
- The examiner grasps the foot of the involved lower extremity, strongly rotates the leg internally, and flexes the knee past 90 degrees (Fig. 11-26).
- This maneuver is repeated with the leg strongly rotated in external rotation (Fig. 11-27).
- The examiner anchors the patient's thigh to the examination table by placing a knee in the patient's popliteal space.
- A small pillow or towel should be used for cushioning.
- The examiner strongly distracts the patient's knee joint by lifting the foot (Fig. 11-28).
- This move is followed by rapidly rotating the leg, both internally and externally.
- This procedure is repeated with strong downward pressure on the patient's foot.
- An intermediate maneuver may be performed.
- The examiner flexes the patient's knee to 90 degrees and rapidly rotates the foot and leg both internally and externally without anchorage to rule out a rotational strain or collateral ligament tear.
- The test is significant for meniscus tear.

Next Steps/Procedures

Abduction stress test, adduction stress test, bounce home test, Childress duck waddle test, McMurray sign, Payr sign, and Steinmann sign

CLINICAL PEARL

The phrase *internal derangement of the knee* is a common provisional diagnosis for any patient with mechanical symptoms of the knee. The initials of this phrase, *IDK*, also stand for "I don't know," and the temptation to use these initials, instead of making a complete diagnosis, must be avoided.

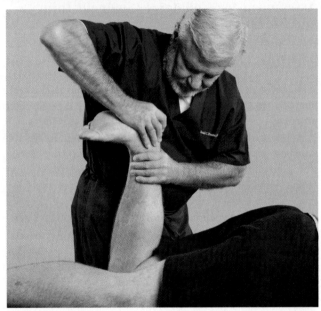

FIG. 11-26 The patient is lying prone with the leg extended and the ankles hanging over the table edge. The examiner grasps the foot and strongly *internally rotates* the leg, bringing the knee into 90 degrees.

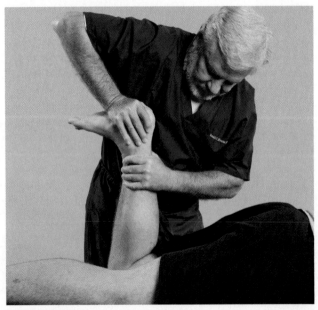

FIG. 11-27 The examiner repeats the maneuver described in Fig. 11-26 while the leg is strongly *rotated externally and strong downward pressure* is applied to the patient's foot. The production of pain is significant for meniscus tear.

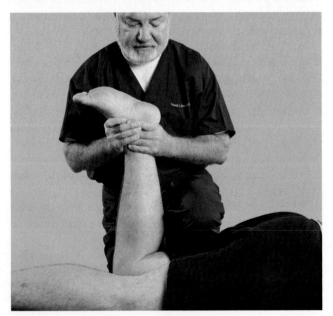

FIG. 11-28 The examiner anchors the patient's thigh to the table by placing a knee in the patient's popliteal space, which can be cushioned by a small pillow or towel. The examiner *strongly distracts* the patient's knee joint by lifting the foot. This maneuver is followed by rapid *rotation, both internally and externally,* of the leg. Pain elicited is significant for collateral ligament tear.

Assessment for Vulnerability to Recurrent Dislocation of the Patella

Comment

Disorders of the patellofemoral joint are common in children and adolescents.

Recurrent subluxation of the patella is a common disorder that is often undiagnosed because the symptoms are similar to other derangements of the knee. The patella usually subluxates or dislocates laterally. The condition may follow an acute patellar dislocation that fails to heal properly. The disorder is often bilateral and is more common in women than in men.

Roentgenographic studies are usually helpful. A merchant (*sunrise*) view taken with the knee relaxed in slight flexion will often reveal lateral displacement (Fig. 11-29).

Congenital dislocation occurs in infancy and involves irreducible lateral displacement of the patella. It is associated with genu valgum, a small patella, hypoplasia of the lateral femoral condyle, and tethering of the lateral capsule.

Isolated patella aplasia-hypoplasia without associated clinical or radiologic anomalies, first described by Kutz in 1949, is an extremely rare autosomal-dominant disorder. This entity is different from small patella syndrome, Meier-Gorlin syndrome, or nail-patella syndrome, in which patella aplasia-hypoplasia as an essential feature is accompanied by other abnormalities. Patients with congenital patella aplasia or hypoplasia often have knee instability, recurrent patella luxations or subluxations, alone or in combination with knee pain resulting from secondary patellofemoral dysfunction, chondromalacia, or gonarthrosis (Nomura, Inoue, Kobayashi, in press).

In habitual dislocation, lateral displacement of the patella occurs every time the knee is flexed. It is caused by contracture of the vastus lateralis and iliotibial band (ITB), with an abnormal insertion of the ITB into the patella.

Recurrent dislocation, or subluxation, of the patella that occurs to the lateral side while the knee is flexed is commonly encountered in adolescents. This type of dislocation is often bilateral, and it occurs in women more often than in men.

The first dislocation is initiated by trauma. A mild hypoplasia of the anterior surface of the lateral femoral condyle and genu valgum are predisposing factors. This type of trauma usually occurs while the patient is engaged in an active sport. The patient falls and strikes the medial aspect of the patella, forcing it laterally over the condyle. Pain is severe, and the patient is unable to straighten the leg. The displacement may be reduced immediately, either by the patient or a companion, or spontaneously.

After this type of fall, some patients have no further difficulty. In other cases, dislocation occurs more and more frequently, and the patient complains that the knee is unstable and gives way. Occasionally, a patient is able to describe the maneuver by which the dislocation can be reduced. This maneuver involves straightening the knee and forcing the lateral border of the patella in a medial direction. After reduction, the knee is usually painful for 2 or 3 days. Mild effusion may also be present. With recurrent episodes, degenerative changes develop on the undersurface of the patella and on the femoral condyle.

When the patient is examined after recurrent episodes of dislocation, tenderness occurs along the medial aspect of the patella and suggests a partial tear of the insertion of the vastus medialis. Effusion of the knee and slight quadriceps atrophy also occurs. The range of knee motion is normal.

ORTHOPEDIC GAMUT 11-9

PREDISPOSING FACTORS FOR PATELLAR DISLOCATION

- High Q-angle
- Patella dysplasia
- Shallow trochlea
- Patella alta
- Lateral structure tightness
- Vastus medialis insufficiency
- Generalized joint laxity
- Femoral or tibial torsion
- Valgus knee

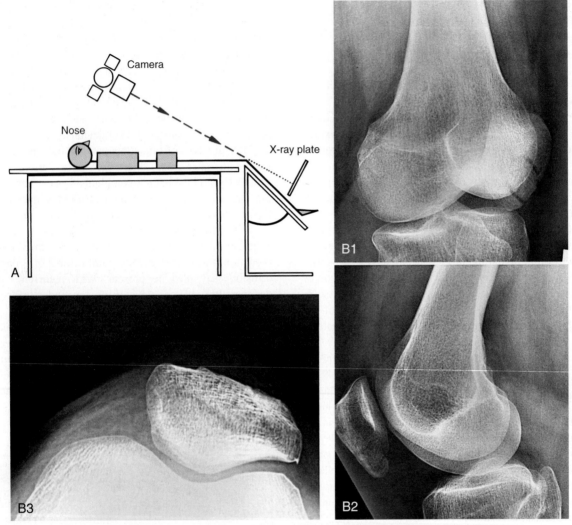

FIG. 11-29 **A,** Merchant tangential view of the patella is made with the knee flexed 45 degrees and the radiograph exposed as shown (see text). **B,** Patellar fracture of the middle and inferior pole is best seen on the oblique view (1). (2) Lateral and (3) Merchant (sunrise) views. (From Johnson: *Atlas of emergency radiology*, St Louis, 2001, W.B. Saunders.) (From Resnick D, Niwayama G: Diagnosis of bone and joint disorders, ed 2, Philadelphia, 1988, WB Saunders.)

PROCEDURE

- The apprehension test for the patella is a test for vulnerability to recurrent dislocation of the patella.
- For the test, the patient is either supine or seated, with the quadriceps muscles relaxed (Fig. 11-30).
- The knee is flexed to at least 30 degrees.
- The examiner carefully and slowly pushes the patella laterally (Fig. 11-31).
- If the patella feels as if it is about to dislocate, the patient will contract the quadriceps muscles and bring the patella back into line.
- This action indicates a positive test.
- The patient will also exhibit a look of apprehension.

Next Steps/Procedures
Clarke sign, Dreyer sign, and Fouchet sign

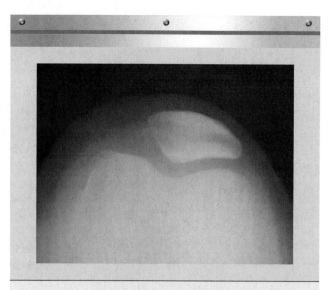

AT THE VIEWBOX

Adult female with history of patellar dislocation. There is a small fracture fragment adjacent to the medial facet of the patella, indicating patellar dislocation with reduction. The fracture occurs when the medial facet impacts on the articular margin of the lateral femoral condyle, during relocation. This may be the only imaging sign of prior dislocation. Patellar dislocations are far more common in patients who have had a prior dislocation. (From the teaching file of Timothy Mick, DC, DACBR)

11

CLINICAL PEARL

The examiner should observe for genu recurvatum and the position of the patella in relation to the femoral condyles. A high patella (*patella alta*) is a predisposing factor to recurrent lateral dislocation of the patella. The recurrent dislocation of the patella is also most common in women with the genu valgum deformity.

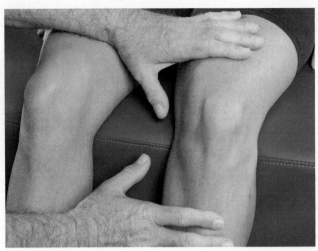

FIG. 11-30 The patient is seated, with the quadriceps muscles relaxed and the knee flexed to approximately 30 degrees.

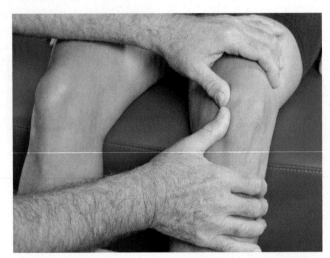

FIG. 11-31 The examiner carefully and slowly pushes the patella laterally. If the patella feels as if it is about to dislocate, the patient will contract the quadriceps muscle to bring the patella back into line. This action indicates a positive test. A positive test indicates a vulnerability or predisposition for recurrent dislocation of the patella.

Assessment for Meniscal Tears

Comment

The congenital discoid meniscus typically involves the lateral meniscus, and it often presents symptoms in childhood. With this defect, the meniscus is not in the usual semilunar form but rather is shaped more as the letter *D*, with its central edge extending toward the tibial spines. The meniscus may produce a very pronounced clicking from the lateral compartment, a block to the extension of the joint and other derangement signs.

The discoid meniscus is a morphologic abnormality of the knee occurring almost exclusively on the lateral side. The discoid lateral meniscus was first described by Young in 1889, and the prevalence of discoid meniscus has been reported to range from 0.4% to 20% among patients undergoing arthroscopy. Classic symptoms of discoid menisci include pain, popping, snapping, and decreased knee extension.

The lateral meniscus plays an important role in the transmission of load across the knee joint. Discoid lateral menisci are thicker and have poorer vascularity than normal lateral menisci. In addition, some discoid lateral menisci have unstable peripheral attachments (Wrisberg type in the classification of Watanabe and colleagues). These factors have been shown to lead to increased susceptibility of discoid menisci to tearing as a result of mechanical and shear forces in the tibiofemoral joint (Good et al, 2007).

The most common cause of meniscal tears in young adults is a sporting injury, such as when a twisting strain is applied to the flexed, weight-bearing leg. In this case, the entrapped meniscus often splits longitudinally, and its free edge may displace inward toward the center of the joint. This type of tear is called a *bucket-handle tear* (Fig. 11-32). This type of tear also prevents full extension (locking), and if an attempt is made to straighten the knee, a painful, elastic resistance (a springy block to full extension) is felt. The

---

ORTHOPEDIC GAMUT 11-10
CLASSIFICATIONS OF DISCOID MENISCUS
1. Complete, disk-shaped meniscus thin center; covers the tibial plateau
2. Incomplete, semilunar-shaped meniscus; partial tibial plateau coverage
3. Wrisberg-type, hypermobile meniscus caused by deficient posterior tibial attachment

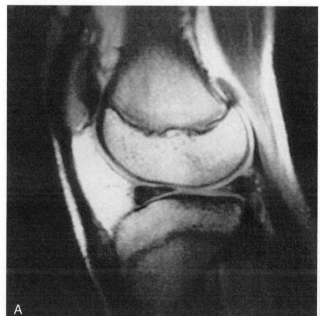
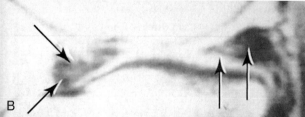

FIG. 11-32 Magnetic resonance image of a 14-year-old male hockey player's knee. **A,** Linear tear of the anterior horn of the lateral meniscus. **B,** Complex tear of the posterior horn. (From Brier SR: *Primary care orthopedics,* St Louis, 1999, Mosby.)

injury of the medial meniscus, which involves prolonged loss of full extension, may lead to stretching and eventual rupture of the ACL. Lateral meniscus tears are often associated with cysts that restrict the mobility of the meniscus. Major meniscus tears are treated by excision of the meniscus. However, with bucket-handle tears, the removal of only the central portion may decrease the risk of late, secondary OA. In some lesions involving the periphery of the meniscus, repair by direct suture is sometimes attempted.

Loss of elasticity in the menisci through degenerative changes associated with the aging process may cause horizontal cleavage tears within the substance of the meniscus. These tears may not be associated with any remembered incident. Sharply localized tenderness in the joint line is a common feature.

Soft-tissue masses within the cavity of the knee joint—also known as intraarticular ganglia, intercondylar cysts, intraarticular synovial cysts, intraarticular cystic masses, or cruciate ganglionic cysts—are uncommon and are mostly incidental findings on MRI and arthroscopy. Even if ganglia and cysts differ in their histologic and etiologic features, the two terms are used interchangeably because their clinical significance is equivalent. Synovial cysts are fibrous or synovial membrane lined, or filled, with synovial fluid, and usually communicate with the joint cavity. Ganglia show a dense connective-tissue capsule with thick viscous content and may communicate with the joint space (Roidis et al, 2007).

The reported incidence in arthroscopic studies ranges from 0.27% for medial meniscal cysts to 1.5% for lateral meniscal cysts. In the development of lateral meniscal cysts, the patient often has a history of a blow on the side of the knee, over the meniscus. The cysts are tender, and because they restrict mobility of the menisci, the cysts render them more susceptible to tears. Medial meniscus cysts must be carefully differentiated from ganglion cysts that arise from the pes anserinus (the insertion of the sartorius, gracilis, and semitendinosus).

PROCEDURE

- The patient is supine.
- The patient's knee is flexed completely (Fig. 11-33).
- The knee is allowed to drop into extension (Fig. 11-34).
- If the extension is not complete, the test is positive.
- The positive finding suggests a torn meniscus.

Next Steps/Procedures
Childress duck-waddle test, McMurray sign, Payr sign, and Steinmann sign

CLINICAL PEARL

Meniscus lesions are the most common internal derangement. Although the menisci are damaged by trauma, the incident is often so trivial that the patient cannot remember any injury at all. Because of this circumstance, patients with meniscal injuries are rarely seen in emergency rooms.

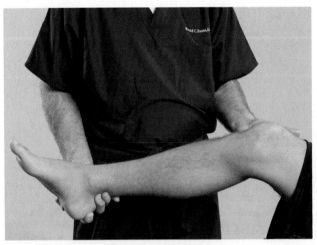

FIG. 11-33 The patient is supine. The examiner grasps the patient's leg at the ankle. The patient's knee is flexed.

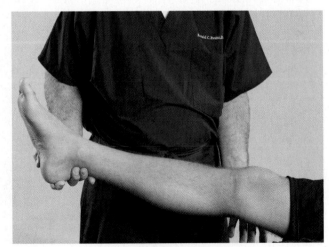

FIG. 11-34 The knee is allowed to drop into extension. If the extension is not complete, the finding is positive. This finding indicates a torn meniscus.

CHILDRESS DUCK WADDLE TEST

Assessment for Medial or Lateral Meniscus Tears

Comment

The term *internal derangement* is used to group a variety of knee joint conditions, usually of traumatic origin, in which the internal structure of the joint is affected to such an extent that its function and mechanics are compromised.

A rotary force applied to the knee joint may trap a meniscus between the femur and the tibia and produce the familiar torn-cartilage lesion. A meniscus cannot be torn while the knee is in extension. To produce a tear, the knee joint must be first rotated in the flexed position to trap the meniscus and then extended to produce the tearing force on the tissue. This combination of motions is commonly encountered on the football field or basketball court.

Tears of the medial meniscus are encountered about nine times more frequently than tears of the lateral meniscus. This difference in frequency is believed to be because the medial meniscus is attached to the deep layer of the MCL and because the mechanisms that cause the tearing are more frequently applied to the medial aspect of the joint.

A tear of the medial meniscus is associated with pain that is referred to the medial side of the joint and is accompanied by synovial effusion. The pain caused by the torn meniscus is often aggravated by forced rotation of the foot and leg. Pain or a clicking may be produced by testing for the McMurray sign. Locking of the joint may or may not be present, depending on the location of the tear.

Spontaneous osteonecrosis (SON) of the knee is a well-defined clinical entity, but the exact cause and natural history is unknown. Although MRI is a useful diagnostic tool, in some circumstances, initial symptoms of SON can correlate with negative findings, and pain can be attributed to a meniscal lesion that frequently presents in older patients (Muscolo et al, 2006).

Tears similar to those seen in the medial meniscus may involve the lateral meniscus, but these tears are less common. On the other hand, cystic degeneration is much more common in the lateral meniscus than in the medial meniscus. In this condition, multiple cysts containing gelatinous material appear within the peripheral border of the meniscus. Repeated trauma causes the appearance of these cysts. Once developed, cartilage cysts may cause pain and often can be seen and palpated along the lateral border of the knee joint.

A discoid meniscus is a congenitally abnormal lateral meniscus, in which the structure assumes a thickened and rounded shape. Because of its thickness, the meniscus does not glide smoothly between the femur and the tibia. Rather, the meniscus must force its way through. As a result, a loud clicking noise is heard when the knee flexes or extends, but locking does not occur.

PROCEDURE

- The patient stands with the feet somewhat apart and the legs in maximal internal rotation (Fig. 11-35).
- A full squat is attempted (Fig. 11-36).
- During this maneuver, the patient's heels may come up from the floor, with weight bearing passing to the balls of the feet.
- The maneuver is repeated, with the lower limbs in maximal external rotation (Figs. 11-37 and 11-38).
- A positive test consists of pain, inability to fully flex the knee, or a clicking sound on either posterior side of the joint.
- The test is significant during internal rotation for a medial meniscus tear or during external rotation for a lateral meniscus tear.

Next Steps/Procedures

Bounce home test, McMurray sign, Payr sign, and Steinmann sign

---

ORTHOPEDIC GAMUT 11-11

COMMON MENISCAL TEARS TYPE

1. Type I: splitting of the meniscus, along its longitudinal axis, producing the so-called bucket-handle tear
2. Type II: a tear along transverse axis of the meniscus

CLINICAL PEARL

The menisci are important parts of the load-bearing mechanism of the knee because they absorb the downward thrust of the convex femoral condyles. The menisci are so effective that, if they are removed, the force that is taken by the articular cartilage during peak loading increases approximately five times. Therefore, a meniscectomy exposes the articular cartilage to much greater forces than normal. Evidence of degenerative osteoarthritis is seen in 75% of patients 10 years after a total meniscectomy.

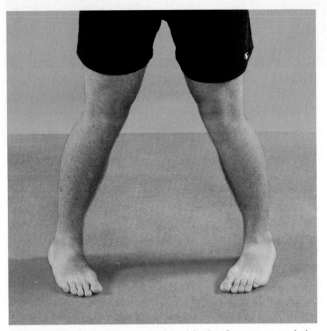

FIG. 11-35 The patient stands with the feet apart and the legs in maximal internal rotation.

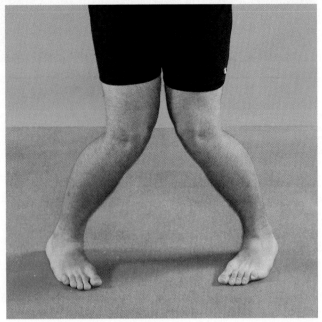

FIG. 11-36 The patient attempts a full squat. During this maneuver, the patient's heels may come up from the floor and weight may be shifted to the balls of the feet.

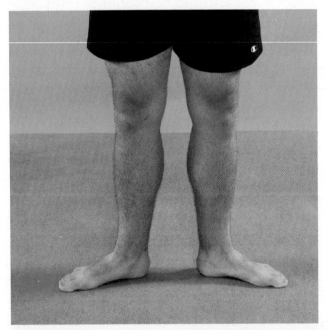

FIG. 11-37 The maneuver is repeated with the lower limbs in maximal external rotation.

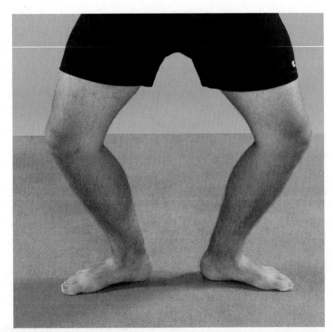

FIG. 11-38 A full squat is attempted again. A positive test consists of pain, inability to fully flex the knee, or a clicking sound on either posterior side of the joint. With internal rotation, the test is significant for a medial meniscus tear. During external rotation, the test is significant for a lateral meniscus tear.

CLARKE SIGN

Assessment for Chondromalacia Patellae

Comment

Anterior knee pain in the adolescent continues to be one of the more difficult problems to treat in musculoskeletal medicine for two main reasons. The first reason is that the patient can experience pain, patellofemoral instability, or both. Patients and clinicians frequently have a difficult time discriminating between pain and instability, especially when instability leads to pain. The second reason is that the sources of pain are poorly understood and that multiple painful sites are frequently present. This kind of confusion leads to imprecise diagnoses and generic, *one size fits all,* treatment interventions (Gerbino, 2006).

The term *patellofemoral syndrome* is imprecise and has been used interchangeably with patellofemoral pain syndrome, anterior knee pain, and chondromalacia patella. Anterior knee pain refers to all pain about the anterior knee, and chondromalacia patella means actual damage to the patella cartilage that may or may not be associated with specific knee pain. The term *patellar malacia* has been used as a catchall term to include the many processes that involve the undersurface of the patella. True malacia is a softening or breaking down of a part of the tissue. When chronic synovitis of the knee causes the patellar cartilage to break down and the bed to eburnate so that denuded bone is exposed, the condition is called *malacia.* This condition is the same one that occurs in a young individual who has fragmentation of the patellar cartilage with no signs of arthritis.

Thorough evaluation of the anatomic development of the knee may give a definite indication of the cause of the idiopathic malacia. Patella alta is prone to alter the mechanism of the gliding surface of the patella on the trochlear groove and to contribute to the malacia. Lateral subluxation of the patella, as the knee comes into complete extension, may cause malacia of the patella without actually giving any evidence of gross displacement.

ORTHOPEDIC GAMUT 11-12

THREE GROUPS OF PATELLAR MALACIA

1. Group I: Trauma related.
   a. A chondral fracture or infraction may exist caused either by acute trauma or by repeated, lesser traumata to the patella.
   b. Infraction of the patellar cartilage causes irritation of the patellar groove on the femur, and gradual changes supervene with fissuring, absorption, and fragmentation of the cartilage.
2. Group II: Disturbance of the rhythm of the patellar function.
   a. These disturbances are commonly called *tracking disorders.*
   b. This type of malacia accompanies intrinsic injury to the knee.
   c. Any condition that causes a disturbance in the rhythm of the knee action often results in involvement of the undersurface of the patella.
   d. The knee is checked abruptly, motion is reversed, and the patella is driven against the femur.
   e. A relationship exists between the locking of the knee and the degree of malacia present.
   f. These two factors are much more important for indicating the amount of malacia present than is the age of the patient.

   g. The exact mechanism of the breakdown of the patella has never been wholly explained.
   h. This condition also probably occurs as the result of various other causes, including direct trauma and synovitis of the joint and general chondrolytic changes.
   i. The particular pathologic changes described usually accompany other intrinsic conditions of the knee.
3. Group III: Primary malacia of the patella, usually a bilateral condition, without any demonstrable etiologic factor.
   a. These cases are puzzling.
   b. The examiner cannot rule out the effect of repeated trauma because young patients are usually very physically active.
   c. These patients should be expected to traumatize the patella repeatedly.
   d. However, the simultaneous involvement of both knees, with relative lack of involvement of other chondral surfaces equally susceptible to trauma, prompts the examiner to seek a cause other than a simple contusion.

ORTHOPEDIC GAMUT 11-13
ETIOLOGY OF CHONDROMALACIA PATELLA

- Any injury or anatomic abnormality that predisposes the area to an irregular pattern of movement of the patella
- Meniscus injuries that alter normal tibiofemoral motion
- Recurrent subluxation of the patella
- Quadriceps imbalance
- Patella alta
- Angular deformities of the knee
- Direct trauma to the patella

PROCEDURE

- The patient's knee is extended fully (Fig. 11-39).
- The examiner compresses the quadriceps muscles at the superior pole of the patella (Fig. 11-40).
- The patient gently contracts the quadriceps muscles as the examiner resists the movement of the patella (Fig. 11-41).
- Retropatellar pain and failure to hold the contraction is considered positive.
- A positive test suggests chondromalacia patella.
- To test different parts of the patella, the knee should be tested in 30, 60, and 90 degrees of flexion and in full extension.

Next Steps/Procedures

Apprehension test for the patella, Dreyer sign, and Fouchet sign

CLINICAL PEARL

In examining the patella, the examiner should note any tenderness over the anterior surface and whether a bipartite ridge is present. Upper and lower pole tenderness occurs in Sinding-Larsen-Johansson disease and jumper's knee (an extensor apparatus traction injury).

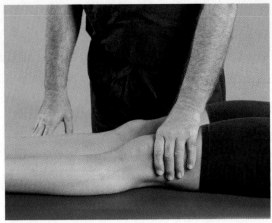

FIG. 11-39 The patient is lying supine with the affected knee extended. The examiner presses down with the web of the hand at a site that is slightly proximal to the upper pole or base of the patella.

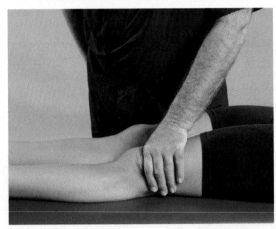

FIG. 11-40 The examiner pushes the patella into an inferior position, which stretches the quadriceps muscle and tendon.

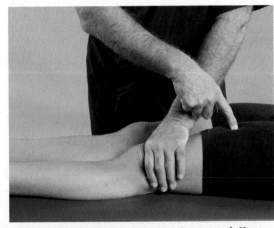

FIG. 11-41 The patient is instructed to *carefully* contract the quadriceps muscle as the examiner restricts the movement of the patella by continuing to push down. If this maneuver causes retropatellar pain and the patient cannot hold the contraction, the test is positive. A positive test is significant for chondromalacia patellae.

Assessment for Injury to Some Degree of (1) the Anterior Cruciate Ligament, Especially the Anteromedial Bundle, (2) the Posterolateral Capsule, (3) the Posteromedial Capsule, (4) the Medial Collateral Ligament, Especially the Deep Fibers, (5) the Iliotibial Band, (6) the Posterior Oblique Ligament, (7) the Arcuate-Popliteus Complex, and (8) the Posterior Cruciate Ligament (in Testing Posterior Drawer Movements)

Comment

Ligament injuries of the knee refer to various degrees of sprains that may lead to frank ruptures of the ligament exhibited by loss of joint function. Knee ligament sprains and joint instability are complex and sophisticated problems involving various degrees of straight plane, either isolated or with combined rotatory instability.

Degrees of anterior cruciate instability are graded similarly to degrees of ligament sprains.

Injuries involving the ACL of the knee joint present major problems to high-demand (level I or II activities) athletes and usually confine them to level III and IV activities only.

ORTHOPEDIC GAMUT 11-14
GRADES OF KNEE LIGAMENT SPRAINS

1. Grade I (mild)—first-degree ligament sprain: an incomplete stretching of collagen ligament fibers resulting in minimal pain, minimal or no swelling, no loss of joint function, and no clinical or functional instability.
2. Grade II (moderate)—second-degree ligament sprain: a partial loss of ligament fiber continuity. A few collagen ligament fibers may be completely torn; however, most of the ligament remains intact. This degree of sprain is characterized by moderate (more intense than a first-degree sprain) pain, moderate swelling, some loss of joint function, and some loss of joint stability.
3. Grade III (severe)—third-degree sprain (rupture): the entire collagen ligament fiber bundles are completely torn. No continuity exists within the body of the ligament. This injury is usually characterized by profound pain, intense swelling, loss of joint function, and instability.

The ACL may be injured by contact (e.g., lacrosse, ice hockey, gymnastics, football, rugby) or noncontact (e.g., basketball, competitive badminton, volleyball, alpine skiing, football, rugby) mechanisms. Injuries of the ACL from martial arts, although possible, occur much less frequently than in other sports (Huang, Hsu, Wang, 2007).

Damage to the ACL most commonly occurs as a sequel to tears of the medial meniscus. Many longitudinal meniscus tears produce a block to extension of the joint. Attempts to obtain full extension lead to attrition rupture of the ligament. ACL tears may also accompany severe collateral ligament injuries.

Isolated ruptures of the ACL are uncommon and are not usually treated surgically unless they are accompanied by avulsion of the bone at the anterior tibial attachment. When the tear accompanies a meniscus lesion, the meniscus is preserved, if possible, to reduce the risks of tibial subluxation and secondary osteoarthritic changes. Nevertheless, the damage may be such that excision cannot be avoided. When an acute tear is associated with damage to the collateral ligaments, a combined repair or reconstruction is usually attempted. Problems from tibial subluxation are common, particularly when anterior cruciate tears are accompanied by damage to the medial or lateral structures, which can be assessed with the **Lysholm Knee Scale** instrument (Fig. 11-42). When anterior tibial subluxation is the main source of symptoms, surgical reconstruction may be indicated if simple measures, such as quadriceps strengthening, are not successful.

The Lysholm Knee Scale was originally developed to evaluate outcome after ACL injury but has been used for a variety of other conditions, including articular cartilage lesions. The Lysholm Knee Scale consists of eight items: pain, instability, locking, stair climbing, limp, support, swelling, and squatting. Kocher and colleagues provided evidence for reliability, validity, and responsiveness of the Lysholm Knee Scale in patients with articular cartilage lesions (Irrgang, 2006).

ORTHOPEDIC GAMUT 11-15
HUGHSTON KNEE INSTABILITIES INDEX

1. Mild instability: graded 1+ (5 mm or less of joint surface separation)
2. Moderate instability: graded 2+ (joint surface separation of 4 to 10 mm)
3. Severe instability: graded 3+ (joint surface separation of 10 mm or more)

Lysholm Scoring Scale

	Points
Limp (5 points)	
None	5
Slight or periodic	3
Severe and constant	0
Support (5 points)	
Full support	5
Stick or crutch	3
Weight bearing impossible	0
Stair Climbing (10 points)	
No problems	10
Slightly impaired	6
One step at a time	2
Unable	0
Squatting (5 points)	
No problems	5
Slightly impaired	4
Not past 90°	2
Unable	0
Walking, Running, and Jumping (70 points)	
Instability	
Never giving way	30
Rarely during athletic or other severe exertion	25
Frequently during athletic or other severe exertion (or unable to participate)	20
Occasionally in daily activities	10
Often in daily activities	5
Every step	0
Pain	
None	30
Inconstant and slight during severe exertion	25
Marked on giving way	20
Marked during severe exertion	15
Marked on or after walking more than 2 km	10
Marked on or after walking less than 2 km	5
Constant and severe	0
Swelling	
None	10
With giving way	7
On severe exertion	5
On ordinary exertion	2
Constant	0
Atrophy of Thigh (5 points)	
None	5
1–2 cm	3
More than 2 cm	0
Total Score	100

Modified from Lysholm J, Gillquist J: Evaluation of knee ligament surgery results with special emphasis on use of a scoring scale, *Am J Sports Med* 10:150–154, 1982.

ORTHOPEDIC GAMUT 11-16

POSITIVE ANTERIOR DRAWER TEST

In a positive anterior drawer test, the following structures may have been injured to some degree:
- Anterior cruciate ligament, especially the anteromedial bundle
- Posterolateral capsule
- Posteromedial capsule
- Medial collateral ligament, especially the deep fibers
- Iliotibial band
- Posterior oblique ligament
- Arcuate-popliteus complex

The PCL is the primary restraint against straight posterior translation of the tibia at all positions of the knee. Early studies on the natural history of PCL injury found that conservative treatment achieved satisfactory function outcomes. However, patients with grade 3 (the tibial plateau displaced posterior to the femoral condyle between 10 and 15 mm) or grade 4 (posterior displacement more than 15 mm) PCL injuries are at high risk of functional disability because of recurrent pain, instability, and knee degeneration (Wu et al, 2007).

PCL tears are produced when the tibia is forcibly pushed backward while the knee is flexed (e.g., in a motor-vehicle accident in which the upper part of the leg strikes the dashboard). Surgical repair is always advised if the injury is seen at the acute stage. The persisting instability and OA are the usual sequelae in the untreated case.

In this group of conditions, which are characterized by rotary instability in the knee, the tibia may subluxate forward or backward on either the medial or lateral side when the knee is stressed. This subluxation may cause pain and a feeling of instability in the joint.

Clinical examination of the PCL can be confusing. In the first test, the anterior and posterior drawer test, the tibia *sags* or subluxates posteriorly relative to the femur if the PCL is torn (Fig. 11-43). The examiner may produce a *false-positive* anterior drawer sign, wherein the posterior tibial sag is actually being reoriented to the neutral position rather than a true anterior translation occurring (Fig. 11-44).

FIG. 11-42 Lysholm Knee Scoring Scale. The Lysholm scale or questionnaire is constituted of eight questions, with closed answers alternatives, of which final score is expressed nominally and ordinally, with a score ranging from 95 to 100 points = "excellent"; 84 to 94 points = "good"; 65 to 83 points = "fair"; and less than or equal to 64 points = "poor." (From Peccin MS CR, Cohen M: Specific questionnaire for knee symptoms—the "Lysholm Knee Scoring Scale": translation and validation into Portuguese, *Acta Orthop* 14[5] 268-272, 2006.)

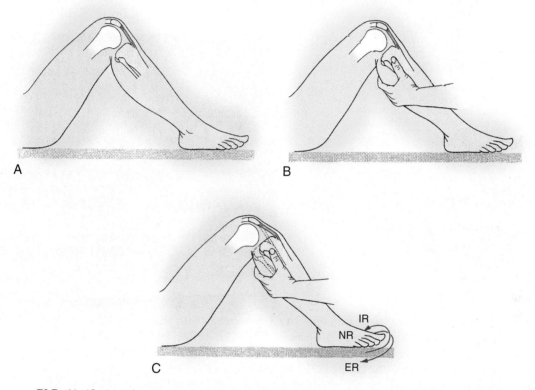

FIG. 11-43 Anterior drawer test. **A,** In resting position, tibial plateau is held in normal position by intact posterior cruciate ligament. **B** and **C,** With anterior cruciate insufficiency, tibia can be pulled forward against force of gravity and tone of flexors. (From Muller W: *The knee: form, function, and ligament reconstruction*, New York, 1983, Springer-Verlag.)

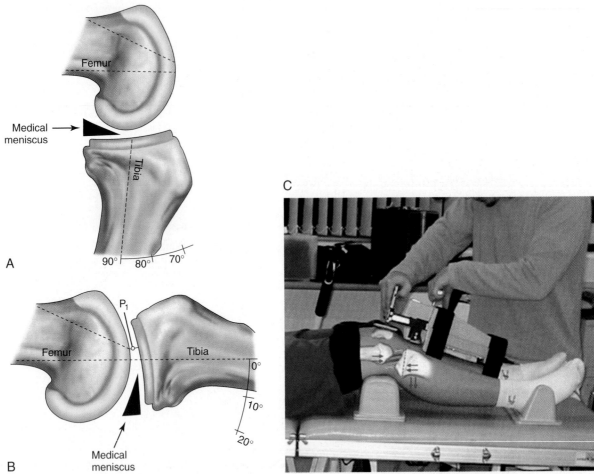

FIG. 11-44 An anterior drawer sign 6 to 8 mm greater than that of the opposite knee indicates a torn anterior cruciate ligament. *However*, before applying anterior drawer stress, the examiner must make sure that the tibia is not sagging posteriorly as a result of laxity of the posterior cruciate ligament. In such knees, an apparent sign of anterior drawer instability simply may be the return of the tibia to the neutral starting point; posterior instability frequently is misdiagnosed because of this fact. Even if a positive anterior drawer sign is not accompanied by a pivot shift phenomenon, a posterior cruciate ligament insufficiency exists until proved otherwise. Any tendency of one tibial plateau to rotate abnormally should be noted as the test is carried out. **A,** With knee flexed to 90 degrees for classic anterior drawer sign, medial meniscus, being attached to tibia, abuts against acutely convex surface of medial femoral condyle and has "door-stopper" effect, preventing or hindering anterior translation of tibia. **B,** With knee extended, relationships are changed. Comparatively flat weight-bearing surface of femur does not obstruct forward motion of meniscus and tibia when anterior stress is applied. (A and B from Torg JS, Conrad W, Kalen V: *Am J Sports Med* 4:84, 1976.) **C,** During a simulated anteroposterior laxity test, ligament forces and contact forces were found to increase with posterior tilt. (From Hohmann E, Bryant A: Closing or Opening Wedge High Tibial Osteotomy: Watch out for the Slope, *Operat Tech Orthop* 17[1]:38-45, 2007.)

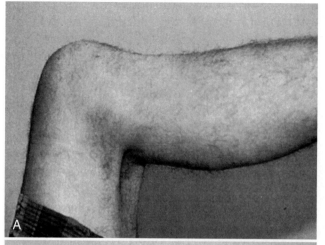

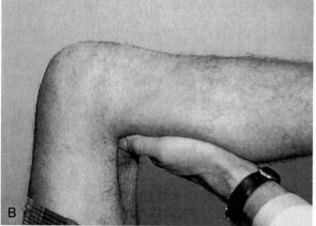

FIG. 11-45 Posterior sag sign (Godfrey tibial sag sign). **A,** Posterior subluxation of the tibia on the femur is noted with the hip and the knee flexed to 90 degrees. **B,** Anteriorly applied force reduces the subluxation, suggesting a significant injury to the posterior cruciate ligament. (From Swenson TM, Harner CD: Knee ligament and meniscal injuries: current concepts, *Orthop Clin North Am* 26:529-546, 1995.)

The second test, the Godfrey posterior tibial sag test, is more sensitive. The patient is supine with the hip and knee of the affected limb held at 90 degrees. The examiner holds the heel of the affected limb and allows the tibia to translate, subluxate, or sag posteriorly by gravity (Fig. 11-45).

ORTHOPEDIC GAMUT 11-17

COMMON TYPES OF POSTERIOR CRUCIATE LIGAMENT TEARS

- The medial tibial condyle subluxates anteriorly (anteromedial instability).
- The lateral tibial condyle subluxates anteriorly (anterolateral rotary instability).
- The lateral tibial condyle subluxates posteriorly (posterolateral rotary instability).
- Combinations of these lesions may be found.

ORTHOPEDIC GAMUT 11-18

POSITIVE POSTERIOR DRAWER TEST

In a positive posterior drawer test, the following structures may have been injured to some degree:
- Posterior cruciate ligament
- Arcuate-popliteus complex
- Posterior oblique ligament
- Anterior cruciate ligament

PROCEDURE

- The patient's knee is flexed to 90 degrees.
- The patient's foot is held on the table by the examiner.
- The tibia is pulled forward on the femur by placing hands around the tibia (Fig. 11-46).
- Normal movement is approximately 6 mm.
- When the tibia moves forward more than 6 mm on the femur, the test is positive.
- To test the PCL, the tibia is pushed back on the femur (Fig. 11-47).
- The test is positive when excessive movement is noted.

Next Steps/Procedures

Lachman test, lateral pivot shift maneuver, Losee test, and Slocum test

11

CLINICAL PEARL

A tibia that is already displaced backward, as a result of a posterior cruciate tear, may give a false-positive result when the examiner is testing the anterior cruciate. This false-positive test may also occur with the Lachman test.

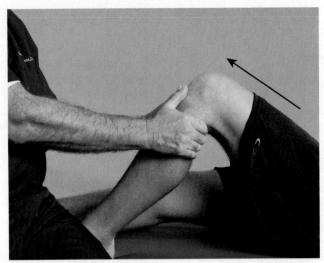

FIG. 11-46 The patient is lying supine; the knee is flexed to 90 degrees. The patient's foot is held on the table by the examiner. The tibia is pulled forward on the femur. Normal movement is approximately 6 mm. If the tibia moves forward more than 6 mm on the femur, the test is positive.

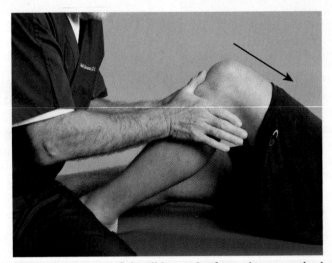

FIG. 11-47 Posterior movement of the tibia on the femur is assessed when the tibia is pushed posterior on the femur. If the test is positive, which is demonstrated by a large amount of posterior movement, (1) the posterior cruciate ligament, (2) the arcuate-popliteus complex, (3) the posterior oblique ligament, or (4) the anterior cruciate ligament may have been damaged.

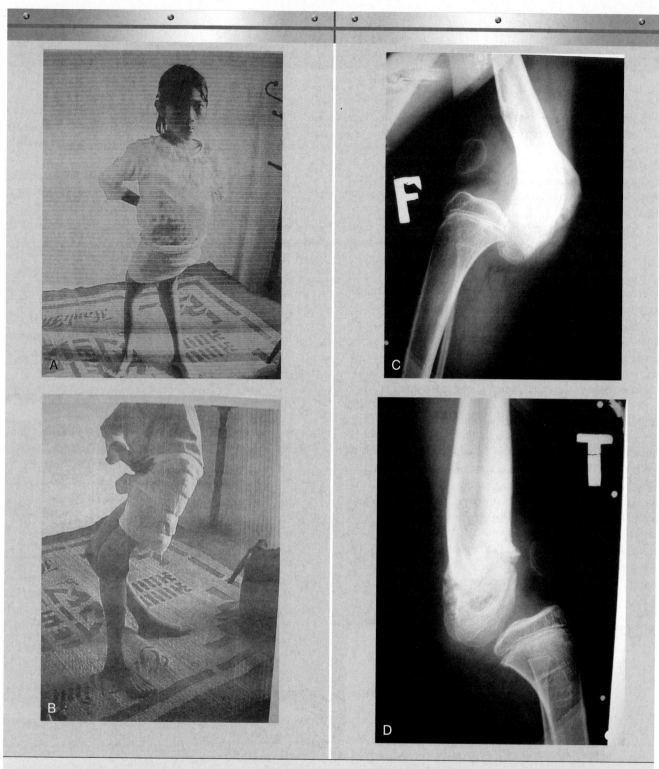

AT THE VIEWBOX

Young Vietnamese girl with marked genu recurvatum **(A, B).** Knee deformity and dysfunction, since infancy, increasing since walking and now markedly limiting her activity. She is being assessed for possible orthopedic intervention. Plain films demonstrate dislocation or near dislocation of both femorotibial joints, with posterior displacement of the femora on the tibiae **(C, D).** Gross insta- bility with the drawer test indicates lack of integrity of the anterior cruciate ligaments (ACLs), in this case due to rare congenital absence of the ACLs. Most often, the positive drawer test would indicate tear of the ACL from one or more traumatic events. (From the teaching file of Timothy Mick, DC, DACBR)

Assessment for Fracture of the Patella

Comment

Fractures of the patella usually result from a direct blow to the knee. They are classified as undisplaced or displaced (Fig. 11-48).

Fracture of the patella is not as common as chondral fractures of the patella. Fractures of either the superior or inferior pole or along the medial or lateral margins are usually either strain fractures or sprain fractures. The examiner should suspect chondral fracture to accompany stellate fracture of the patella without displacement.

Fracture of the patella by direct contusion is not uncommon. The fracture usually involves the lateral portion of the patella because the bone is thinner in this area. A fracture of the patella differs from the avulsion type, in which the fragment is torn away by the tension on the fragment. The avulsion fracture is usually on the medial side and occurs as the patella is forced laterally. A patellar fracture also differs from the explosive type of fracture that is caused by a forceful blow against the patella while the quadriceps is in violent contraction. This situation may occur when the knee hits the dashboard in a motor-vehicle accident. The contusion fracture results from to a sharp blow in a localized area. This same force may cause chondral damage.

The bipartite or tripartite patella should not be confused with acute injury. The partite patella is usually bilateral and symmetric and is asymptomatic. Thorough examination will demonstrate that the symptoms are not in the area of the anomaly. It is possible for the quadriceps lateralis to avulse or partially avulse the separate piece, in which the condition will be symptomatic.

Bipartite patella occurs when the ossification centers of the patella fail to fuse. The defect is seen as a lucent line, usually at the superolateral corner of the patella, where it may be mistaken for a fracture. Occasionally, the synchondrosis may fracture as a result of repetitive stress and cause pain and tenderness.

Patellar fracture is the second most frequent periprosthetic fracture of the knee joint after the femur and may occur in both unresurfaced and resurfaced cases. Multiple etiologic factors such as limb or prosthesis malalignment, lateral release, patellar component design, and excessive resection of bone have been implicated in the pathogenesis of fracture (Chalidis et al, 2007).

PROCEDURE

- While lying supine with the knee extended, the patient is unable to raise the leg (Fig. 11-49).
- When the examiner applies compression to the thigh, by using the hands to give anchorage to the quadriceps, the patient is able to lift the leg (Fig. 11-50).
- When this force is removed, the patient is again unable to raise the leg.
- The test is significant for a fracture of the patella.

Next Steps/Procedures

Apprehension test, Clarke sign, Fouchet sign, and diagnostic imaging

FIG. 11-48 Displaced fracture of the patella. (From Mercier LR, Pettid FJ: *Practical orthopedics*, ed 4, St Louis, 1995, Mosby.)

ORTHOPEDIC GAMUT 11-19

ORTIGUERA AND BERRY CLASSIFICATION OF PERIPROSTHETIC FRACTURES OF THE PATELLA

- Type I: intact extensor mechanism; stable implant
- Type II: disruption of extensor mechanism; with or without implant in place
- Type III: intact extensor mechanism:
  - Loosening of patellar component
  - Reasonable remaining bone stock
  - Poor bone stock

CLINICAL PEARL

The quadriceps muscle gains insertion into the tibia through the medium of the patella, which is enclosed within the quadriceps expansion and the patellar tendon. Complete rupture may occur as a disruption through the patella. This area is the usual site of rupture for a common variety of fractured patella. The injury occurs mainly in adults of middle age.

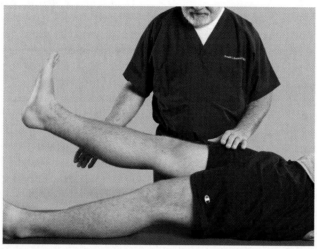

FIG. 11-49 The patient is lying supine with the knee extended. The patient attempts to raise the leg. In the presence of patellar fracture, this raising motion is painful and difficult to accomplish.

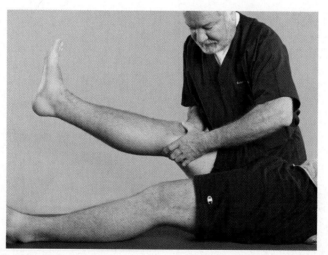

FIG. 11-50 The examiner applies forceful, circumferential grasp to the thigh with the hands, which give anchorage to the quadriceps. The patient attempts to lift the leg. The sign is present when the patient can lift the leg with minimal distress with the force applied, However, when this force is removed, the inability to raise the leg recurs. The presence of the sign is significant for a fracture of the patella.

Assessment for Patellar Tracking Disorder, Peripatellar Syndrome, or Patellofemoral Dysfunction

Comment

Pain arising from the anterior aspect of the knee joint is common in adolescence. Specific conditions, such as patella malalignment, osteochondritis dissecans, Osgood-Schlatter disease, and trauma, may be responsible.

> Anterior knee pain, diagnosed as patellofemoral pain syndrome (PFPS), is claimed to be one of the most common musculoskeletal disorders. PFPS is the main cause of chronic knee pain in active young adults and may affect as many as 15% of young men and women in military service (Jensen et al, in press).

The patella is a pulley, and its excursion is controlled by the direction of action of the quadriceps group of muscles and the position of the tibial tubercle, which carries the patellar ligament.

The movements of the patellofemoral joint are complex. In full extension, only the distal part of the patellar articular surface is in contact with the femoral groove. As flexion proceeds, the contact area on the patella sweeps proximally until, at 90-degree flexion, the proximal part is in contact with the distal groove. From 90-degree flexion, the odd facet (the most medial) articulates with the lateral edge of the medial femoral condyle, and the lateral facet articulates with the medial edge of the lateral femoral condyle. The medial facet lies in contact with the synovium overlying the ACL (Donell, 2006).

The articular surface of the patella is divided into a large lateral and a small medial area. These areas are separated by a vertical, rounded ridge. During full extension, the shape of the patella fits into the trochlear surface of the femur. The ridge then lies in the hollow, or trough, of the trochlear surface. When the knee is flexed, the patella is carried downward and backward on the under aspect of the femur, where the trochlear surface is prolonged onto the inner condyle. During flexion, the patella tilts away from the lateral condyle;

ORTHOPEDIC GAMUT 11-20

PATHOMECHANICS OF PATELLOFEMORAL DISORDERS

- Q-angle (Fig. 11-51)
- Lateral retinacular tightness (Fig. 11-52)
- Vastus medialis obliquus deficiency (Fig. 11-53)
- Lateral deviation of the patella at terminal extension (J sign) (Fig. 11-54)
- Patella alta or infera (Fig. 11-55)
- Trochlear depth (Fig. 11-56,*A*)
- Congruence of the patellofemoral joint (Fig. 11-56,*B*)

ORTHOPEDIC GAMUT 11-21

DEJOUR CLASSIFICATION OF EXTENSOR MECHANISM MALALIGNMENT

- Major patellar instability; more than one documented dislocation
- Objective patellar instability; one dislocation with associated anatomic abnormalities
- Potential patellar instability; patellar pain with associated radiologic abnormalities

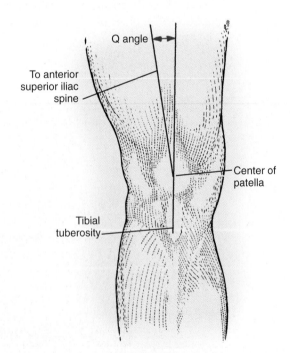

FIG. 11-51 The Q angle. The quadriceps mechanism has a normal valgus alignment. This angle is measured by drawing a line from the anterior superior iliac spine to the center of the patella. The angle that this line makes with a line drawn along the center of the longitudinal axis of the patella and then from the center of the patella to the center of the tibial tubercle is called the Q angle. (From Green RB: *Skeletal trauma in children,* ed 3, Philadelphia, 2003, Saunders.)

Text continued on p. 886

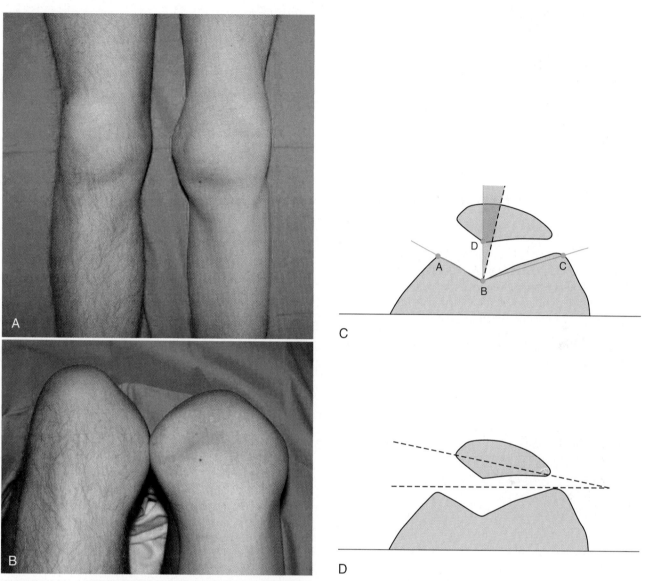

FIG. 11-52 (A) Standing and (B) seated views of the 14-year-old boy 2 years after arthroscopic lateral release resulting from generalized ligamentous laxity with a locked lateral patella dislocation. (From Freitag S, Lill H, Hepp P et al: Locked lateral patella dislocation with generalized ligamentous laxity after arthroscopic lateral release of the knee. Arthroscopy: *J Arthrosc Relat Surg* 21[5]:628.e1-.e4, 2005.) **C,** Method used to measure patellar congruence. The sulcus angle, ABC, is bisected (dotted line). A second line BD is drawn from the sulcus to the apex of the patella. The shaded area represents the congruence angle (congruence angle, is used to measure the medial/lateral displacement of the patella in reference to the trochlear groove. In the original study, Merchant described that a congruence angle of greater than 16 degrees was associated with patellar subluxation). **D,** Method used to measure patellar tilt angle. The angle is measured between the coronal axis of the patella and a line tangent to the medial and lateral trochlear ridges (patellar tilt is a radiographic measurement originally described for native knees and is now commonly used to evaluate patellofemoral alignment in patients after TKA; 5 degrees of lateral patellar tilt is the upper limit of normal). (From Benjamin J, Chilvers M: Correcting lateral patellar tilt at the time of total knee arthroplasty can result in overuse of lateral release, *J Arthroplasty* 21[6, Suppl 1]:121-126, 2006.)

11

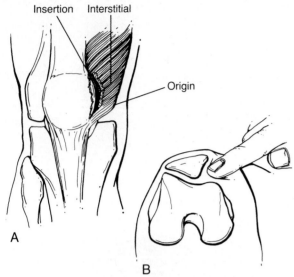

FIG. 11-53 Rupture of the vastus medialis obliquus muscle with acute patellar dislocation. **A,** Possible sites of vastus medialis obliquus rupture. The majority will be interstitial. However, most significant is the insertional rupture, which can be sutured surgically. When insertional rupture occurs, **(B)** shows how skin and soft tissues can be easily invaginated into the joint through the site of rupture. This should aid in making the diagnosis. (From DeLee JC, Drez D, Miller MD: *DeLee and Drez's orthopaedic sports medicine,* ed 2, Philadelphia, 2003, Saunders.)

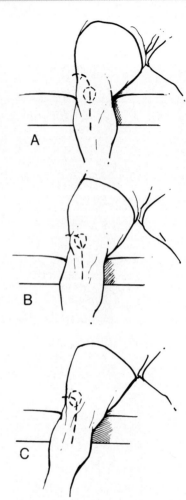

FIG. 11-54 J sign. As the knee is extended from a 90-degree flexed position **(A)** to a fully extended position **(C),** the patella describes an exaggerated inverted J-shaped course, indicating predominance of laterally directed forces. (From DeLee JC, Drez D, Miller MD: *DeLee and Drez's orthopaedic sports medicine*, ed 2, Philadelphia, 2003, Saunders.)

FIG. 11-55 The Insall–Salvati index is computed by dividing the length of the patellar ligament (L_{pl}) by the longest diagonal length of the patella (L_p). Insall–Salvati ratios greater than or equal to 1.2 indicated the presence of patella alta, while indices between 0.80 and 1.19 identified subjects as having normal patellar position. (From Ward SR, Powers CM: Influence of patella alta on patellofemoral joint stress during normal and fast walking, *Clin Biomech* 19[10]:1040-1047, 2004.)

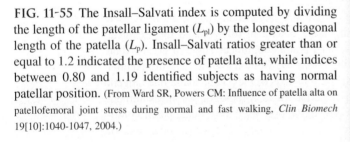

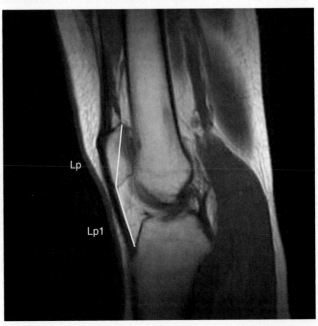

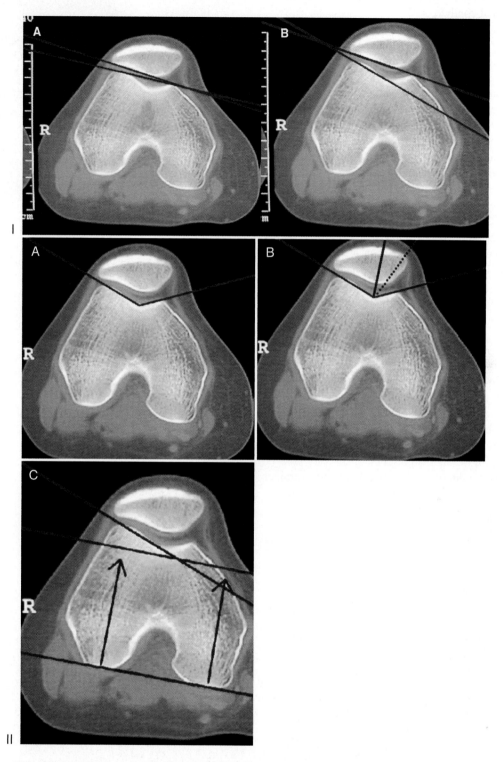

FIG. 11-56 (I) The lateral patellofemoral angle (α) is determined by the junction of a line across the femoral condyles and another line drawn across the lateral patellar facet. **(II)** CT scan angles. *(A)* Sulcus angle between both femoral facets. *(B)* Congruence angle between halving sulcus angle and line between sulcus and inferior dome of patella *(dotted line)*. *(C)* Condyle-lateral angle between lateral femoral facet and line over posterior condyles. (From Alemparte J, Ekdahl M, Burnier L, et al: Patellofemoral evaluation with radiographs and computed tomography scans in 60 knees of asymptomatic subjects, *Arthroscopy* 23[2]:170-177, 2007.)

therefore, only the inner part of its articular surface rests against the medial condyle.

So long as the tibial tubercle rotates smoothly, the patella travels its short course smoothly and under even tension. However, any derangement of the joint that prevents lateral rotation of the tibia during extension of the knee would affect the normal tension because contraction of the quadriceps would force the inner border of the patella against the medial condyle of the femur. This forced meeting explains the patellar symptoms and signs produced by certain cartilage injuries. Some of these symptoms and signs include retropatellar pain experienced during climbing and descending stairs, tenderness of the medial border of the patella, and the pattern of cartilage erosion that develops only on the medial surfaces of the patella and the femur. This pattern differs from that produced by retropatellar arthritis, which complicates recurring dislocation, when the lateral surface of the patellar cartilage undergoes fibrillation. Later, the medial surface is damaged from repeated drag over the lateral condyle of the femur during reduction. This repeated dragging results in erosion of the articular cartilage. By this time, both sides of the patella are tender.

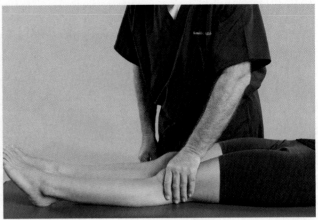

FIG. 11-57 The patient is lying supine, and the affected knee is in full extension. With the flat of a hand, the examiner compresses the patella against the femur. If this produces point tenderness and pain at the patellar margin, the sign is present. If no pain is produced, the patella is then rubbed transversely, against the femur. Audible or palpable grating and pain confirm the presence of the sign. The sign is significant for patellar tracking disorders, peripatellar syndrome, or patellofemoral dysfunction.

PROCEDURE

- While the patient is lying supine and the knee is in full extension, the examiner uses the flat of a hand to compress the patella against the femur (Fig. 11-57).
- If this action produces point tenderness and pain at the patellar margin, the sign is present.
- If pain is not produced by this maneuver, the examiner then rubs the patella transversely against the femur.
- Audible or palpable grating and pain confirm the presence of the sign.
- When the patella has peripheral tenderness on medial or lateral displacement, this is known as Perkins sign.
- Perkins sign is significant for patellar tracking disorder, peripatellar syndrome, or patellofemoral dysfunction.

Next Steps/Procedures
Apprehension test for the patella, Clarke sign, Dreyer sign, and diagnostic imaging

CLINICAL PEARL

Placing a palm of the hand over the patient's patella and the thumb and index finger along the joint line as the joint is flexed and extended will distinguish the source of the crepitus from damaged articular surfaces.

LACHMAN TEST

Assessment for Injury to Some Degree of (1) the Anterior Cruciate Ligament, Especially the Posterolateral Bundle, (2) the Posterior Oblique Ligament, and (3) the Arcuate-Popliteus Complex

Comment

Ligamentous injuries to the knee are among the most serious of all knee disorders. Because of the importance of the ligaments in stabilizing the joint, early diagnosis of the injury is mandatory. Any delay in diagnosis and treatment may lead to a chronically unstable knee, which predisposes the individual's knee to early traumatic arthritis.

The mechanism is usually one of forceful stress against the knee while the extremity is bearing weight. A valgus stress against the knee may sprain or tear the MCL; a varus stress will injure the LCL. Tears of the cruciate ligaments, menisci, and capsule also may occur with the collateral ligament injury.

The history of a ligamentous injury is often difficult to reconstruct, but it will provide clues to the type of force applied to the knee. After the injury, the extremity's ability to bear weight is often lost. Swelling from an acute ligament or capsular tear is usually immediate and results from hemorrhage. A pop or tearing sensation may be heard or felt. Incomplete tears or sprains are often more painful than complete ligamentous ruptures.

Patients with chronically unstable knees from old injuries often complain of the knee going out or giving way or crepitus when walking and of being unable to depend on the extremity. These symptoms are always most noticeable during vigorous activities. A chronic effusion is often present.

With an acute injury, the examination is of utmost importance. Any swelling or discoloration is noted. The lesion can often be localized by palpation alone. The palpation should begin away from the suspected area to promote patient cooperation. A point of maximal tenderness is often present along the course of the collateral ligament or capsule.

The knee should always be tested for stability while the patient is in a relaxed, supine position. If the examination cannot be adequately performed because of pain or hamstring spasm, it may have to be repeated while the patient is under local or general anesthesia. The injured knee is always compared with the opposite, uninvolved knee.

The Lachman test is similar to the anterior drawer test. However, in this test, the knee is held in 20 degrees of flexion, and the tibia is pulled forward on the femur (Fig 11-58). An increase in this anterior translation suggests an

ACL tear (Fig. 11-59). The Lachman test is thought to be a better indicator of injury to the ACL than the anterior drawer test. If a soft or *mushy* feel is noted and the infrapatellar slope disappears when the tibia is moved forward on the femur, the Lachman test is positive. This sign indicates damage to the ACL, especially the posterolateral band.

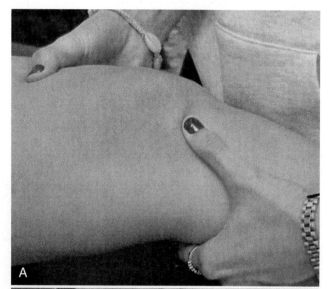

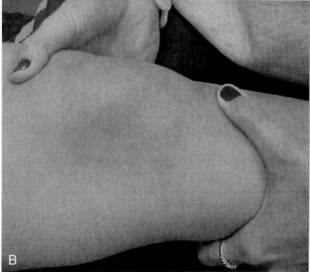

FIG. 11-58 Typical examiner grip configurations adapted 2 cm below knee joint, achieving greater accuracy of assessment than placing a grip 8 cm or more below knee joint. (From Hurley WL, Boros RL, Challis JH: Influences of variation in force application on tibial displacement and strain in the anterior cruciate ligament during the Lachman test, *Clin Biomechanics* 19[1]:95-98, 2004.)

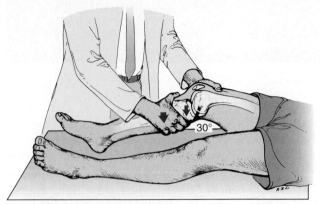

FIG. 11-59 The posterior Lachman test. (From Tria AJ, Klein KS: *Illustrated guide to the knee*, New York, 1991, Churchill Livingstone.)

Tests of ligamentous stability are commonly included as part of the clinical examination of patients with knee injuries. Stress tests, such as the Lachman test, remain the mainstay of knee injury evaluation. Skillful performance of the Lachman test is fundamental to accurate knee evaluation albeit the results of the test are determined subjectively and its efficacy is thought to be highly dependent on the skill and experience of the clinician (Hurley, Boros, Challis, 2004).

PROCEDURE

- The patient is supine.
- The patient's knee is held between full extension and 30 degrees of flexion.
- The patient's femur is stabilized with one hand as the tibia is moved forward (Fig. 11-60).
- A mushy, or soft, end-feel when the tibia is moved forward on the femur and the infrapatellar tendon slope disappears is a positive sign.
- A positive sign suggests damage to (1) the ACL, especially the posterolateral bundle, (2) the POL, and (3) the arcuate-popliteus complex.

Next Steps/Procedures
Drawer test, lateral pivot shift maneuver, Losee test, and Slocum test

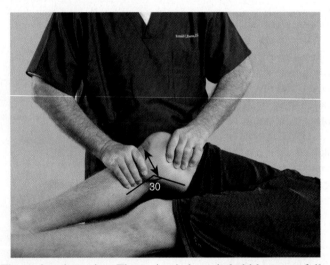

FIG. 11-60 The patient is supine. The patient's knee is held between full extension and 30 degrees of flexion. The patient's femur is stabilized with one hand as the tibia is moved forward. A mushy or soft end-feel when the tibia is moved forward on the femur and the infrapatellar tendon slope disappears is a positive sign.

CLINICAL PEARL

When medial and lateral or anterior and posterior, as well as the medial and lateral, compartments are torn, combined complex instability exists. Transitory dislocation, or at least subluxation of the knee, is a preliminary symptom. In many instances, the peroneal nerve has been injured.

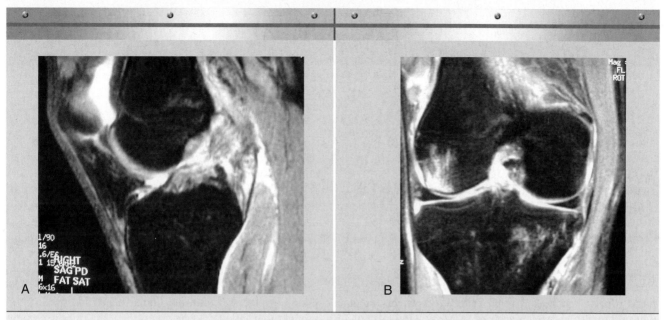

AT THE VIEWBOX

24-year-old male with soccer injury. MRI demonstrates disruption of the anterior cruciate ligament (ACL) characteristic of a full thickness, mid-substance ACL tear (*arrow*). There is an associated joint effusion (**A**). Fluid-weighted coronal MR image (**B**) demonstrates increased signal in the subchondral bone of the femoral condyle and tibial plateau. This bone marrow edema pattern is compatible with subchondral contusions or occult fractures, which often accompany ACL tears. (From the teaching file of Timothy Mick, DC, DACBR)

11

Assessment for Injury to Some Degree of (1) the Anterior Cruciate Ligament, (2) the Posterolateral Capsule, (3) the Arcuate-Popliteus Complex, (4) the Lateral Collateral Ligament, and (5) the Iliotibial Band

Comment

Lateral instabilities of the knee may involve both varus and rotational instabilities. The rotation instabilities are anterolateral rotary instability, which involves a lateral tibial plateau that displaces anteriorly, and posterolateral instability, which involves a lateral tibial plateau that displaces posteriorly. The most commonly encountered lateral instability is the anterolateral rotary instability. A lateral rotary instability is called the *lateral pivot shift,* which should not be confused as something other than anterolateral rotary instability. Clinically, this instability is characterized by a sensation that the knee *gives way* as the patient decelerates suddenly and pivots on the involved extremity.

Anterolateral instability is created by incompetency of the ACL, incompetency of the mid lateral capsule, some degree of laxity of the arcuate ligament, and occasionally laxity of the iliotibial tract. If the iliotibial tract has been stretched or injured, the McIntosh-type testing for anterolateral rotary instability will not be positive in eliciting the classic jumping sensation. With most anterolateral instabilities, the iliotibial tract is intact, and the instability can be more graphically demonstrated with some form of the McIntosh test.

The lateral pivot shift maneuver is the primary test used to assess anterolateral rotary instability of the knee. During this test, the tibia moves away from the femur on the lateral side and moves anteriorly in relation to the femur.

The McIntosh test (lateral pivot shift maneuver) is a duplication of the anterior subluxation-reduction phenomenon that occurs during the normal gait cycle when the ACL is torn. The test illustrates a dynamic subluxation. This shift occurs at between 20 and 40 degrees of flexion. (Zero degrees occur when the knee is in the extended position.) This phenomenon is the one that gives the patient the clinical description of feeling that the knee gives way.

The pivot shift test begins with the knee in full extension. The tibia is held in internal rotation with valgus force. The thumb is placed behind the fibular head, and the knee is brought into flexion. As flexion occurs, the tibia is brought forward on the anterolateral side. With further flexion, the tibia reduces with a clunk (Fig. 11-61).

Losee modified the jerk test (Fig. 11-62) in an attempt to accentuate the subluxation. The knee begins in flexion but with the tibia externally rotated. The valgus force is applied, and then the knee is extended with gradual internal rotation of the tibia (reverse pivot shift) (Fig. 11-63). The clunk of the reduction occurs in the last few degrees from full extension.

> The pivot shift test is specific for injury to the ACL. It can be very uncomfortable and, in general, should be conducted only when examining the knee under anesthesia. The examiner internally rotates the foot and applies a valgus stress to the knee with his other hand. The knee is gently flexed. A positive test results if the ACL is ruptured and the lateral femoral condyle appears to jerk anteriorly on the tibia. The lateral femoral condyle appears to jerk posteriorly (as the tibia sub luxes) as the knee is extended (Smith, Moran, 2006).

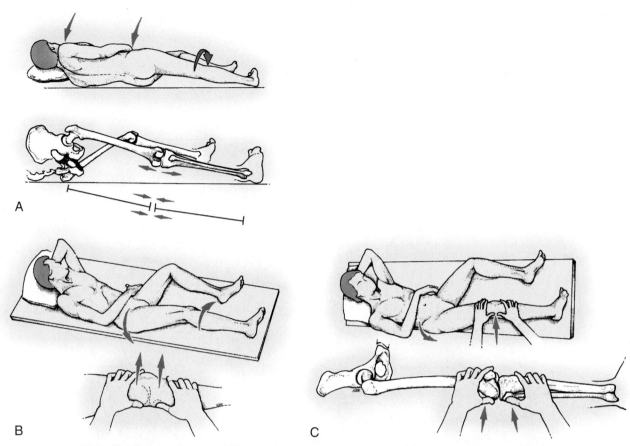

FIG. 11-61 Lateral pivot shift test. **A,** Position of patient for test on right knee. Weight of right lower extremity is borne on right heel. **B,** Same position viewed from above. Right thumb of examiner is placed behind fibular head, and index finger palpates anterior aspect of subluxated lateral tibial plateau. Left thumb is placed behind lateral femoral condyle. **C,** With knee unsupported in valgus and tibia internally rotated on femur, knee is flexed by pushing anteriorly with both thumbs. Tibia is reduced from its anteriorly subluxated position by tension of iliotibial band as knee reaches 25 to 45 degrees of flexion. Reduction should be readily palpable. (Redrawn from Slocum DB et al: *Clin Orthop* 118:63, 1976.)

11

FIG. 11-62 Jerk test. Several methods of this test have been described. In Hughston method, with the patient supine, the lower extremity is supported by the examiner while the knee is flexed to 90 degrees and the tibia is rotated internally. When the right knee is being examined, the foot is grasped with the right hand and the tibia is internally rotated while valgus stress is exerted with the left hand over the proximal end of the tibia and fibula. Then the knee is extended gradually, maintaining the internal rotation and valgus stress. When the test is positive, the lateral tibia spontaneously subluxes forward in the form of a sudden jerk at approximately 30 degrees of flexion. (Courtesy JC Houston, M.D., redrawn. In Canale ST: *Campbell's operative orthopaedics,* ed 10, St Louis, 2003, Mosby.)

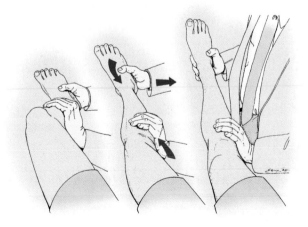

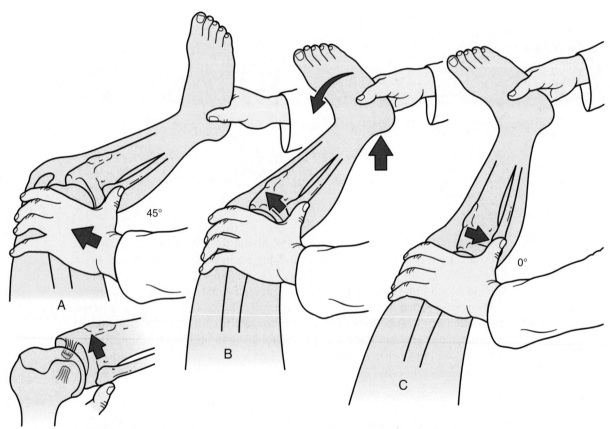

FIG. 11-63 The Losee test begins with the knee in flexion and the tibia in lateral rotation and valgus stress. As the knee is extended, the foot is allowed to medially rotate, and the previously subluxated tibia reduces as the knee approaches full extension. A palpable "clunk" correlates with anterior cruciate ligament tear. (Redrawn from Scott WN, editor: *Ligament and extensor mechanism injuries of the knee: diagnosis and treatment,* St Louis, 1991, Mosby.)

PROCEDURE

- The patient is supine.
- The examiner flexes the knee slightly (5 degrees) (Fig. 11-64).
- A valgus stress is applied to the knee while maintaining a medial rotation torque on the tibia and at the ankle (Fig. 11-65).
- The leg is flexed 30 to 40 degrees. The tibia reduces or jogs backward.
- The patient experiences the sensation of the knee *giving way*.
- This sensation is the positive finding.
- To some degree, (1) the ACL, (2) the posterolateral capsule, (3) the arcuate-popliteus complex, (4) the LCL, or (5) the ITB has been injured.

Next Steps/Procedures
Drawer test, Losee test, and Slocum test

CLINICAL PEARL

Normally, the knee's center of rotation changes constantly through its range of motion as a result of the shape of the femoral condyles, the ligamentous restraint, and the muscle pull. A positive pivot shift test usually suggests damage to the anterior cruciate, the posterior capsule, or the lateral collateral ligament.

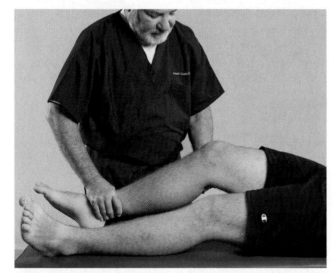

FIG. 11-64 The patient is supine. The examiner flexes the knee slightly (5 degrees). A valgus stress is applied to the knee while maintaining medial rotation torque on the tibia and the ankle.

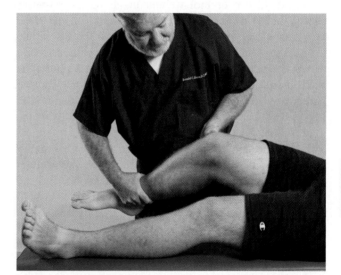

FIG. 11-65 The leg is flexed 30 to 40 degrees. The tibia reduces or jogs backward. The patient experiences the knee *giving way*. If the test is positive, the following structures have been injured: (1) the anterior cruciate ligament, (2) the posterolateral capsule, (3) the arcuate-popliteus complex, (4) the lateral collateral ligament, or (5) the iliotibial band.

11

Assessment for Anterolateral Rotary Instability of the Knee

Comment

Ligaments of the knee have four primary mechanisms of injury. Valgus stress with the knee in slight flexion is by far the most common pattern (Fig. 11-66). The ACL is torn in the mid substance in 75% of cases (Fig. 11-67). The next most common injury is hyperextension. The third most common pattern occurs with the knee flexed and with a posteriorly directed force to the anterior aspect of the knee (Fig. 11-68). The fourth pattern is the varus stress (Fig. 11-69).

The most serious injuries to the knee involve instability. Forceful overrotation of the flexed knee while the leg is fixed may disrupt many parts of the knee.

Simple instability denotes that only one compartment of the knee is involved. The medial complex structures, such as the MCL, can be torn without involving the posterior capsule and can produce a valgus deformity or one-plane laxity. This laxity can result from a blow to the side of the leg or from a fall from a height. Immediate pain, a feeling of weakness, and valgus laxity are the cardinal signs. The MCL usually tears at its upper pole. Motion may not be particularly affected for the first 12 hours, but motion is later impeded by hemarthrosis. Clinically, medial laxity of the joint is what determines the diagnosis.

Lateral instability of the simple type involves primarily varus rather than rotational laxity. However, pure lateral instability is unusual. When present, the lateral ligament and usually the ITB and the popliteal tendon are torn. In both instances, the patient feels a pop, and the knee becomes quite wobbly. Pain during flexion is localized to the upper end of the fibula and over the joint line. The lateral side of the knee is slightly lax in flexion.

Acute anterolateral instability occurs when the leg is hit from the posterior side, while the foot is planted, with the tibia internally rotated and the strain placed on the lateral side. This circumstance can produce irreducible knee dislocation (Fig 11-70). A part of the lateral complex, the anterior cruciate and the lateral meniscus, are torn. Internal-external rotation is increased, but an intact PCL prevents backward tibia displacement. An anterior drawer test will be positive, and lateral laxity is present.

Posterolateral instability (PLI) of the knee is from a complicated injury that involves a complex array of static and dynamic structures of the posterolateral corner. PLI overlooked at the acute state can result in marked disability. Because injuries to the posterolateral corner commonly have combined with cruciate ligament tears (PCL or ACL or both), inappropriate management of PLI can lead to late

failure of cruciate reconstruction. The principal anatomic structures of the posterolateral corner of the knee include the LCL, popliteus complex, including the popliteofibular ligament, the short lateral ligament, the fabellofibular ligament, and the posterolateral capsule (Kim et al, 2004).

Irreducible knee dislocation has been reported in the literature as rare cases. The majority of instances are posterolateral dislocations. The dimple sign has been reported as a characteristic sign and possibly pathognomonic. Irreducibility results from the interposition of the anteromedial capsule and ligaments into the medial compartments (Said, Learmonth, 2007).

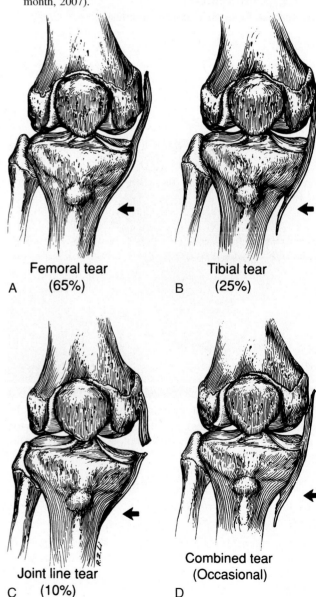

A   **Femoral tear (65%)**

B   **Tibial tear (25%)**

C   **Joint line tear (10%)**

D   **Combined tear (Occasional)**

FIG. 11-66 The distribution of medial collateral ligament disruptions. (From Scott WN: *The knee*, vol 1-2, St Louis, 1994, Mosby.)

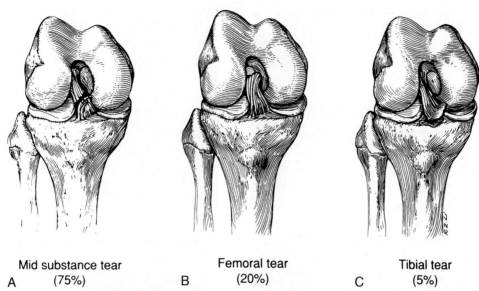

Mid substance tear	Femoral tear	Tibial tear
A (75%)	B (20%)	C (5%)

FIG. 11-67 The distribution of anterior cruciate ligament disruptions. (From Scott WN: *The knee*, vol 1-2, St Louis, 1994, Mosby.)

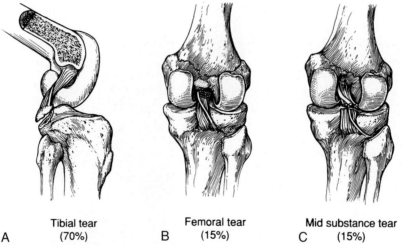

Tibial tear	Femoral tear	Mid substance tear
A (70%)	B (15%)	C (15%)

FIG. 11-68 The distribution of posterior cruciate ligament disruptions. (From Scott WN: *The knee*, vol 1-2, St Louis, 1994, Mosby.)

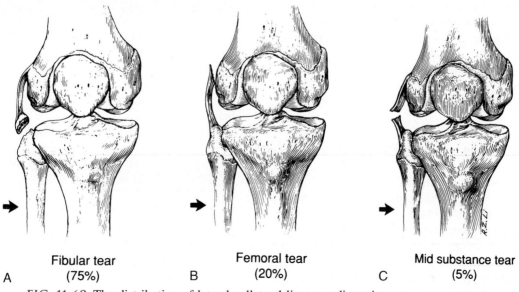

Fibular tear	Femoral tear	Mid substance tear
A (75%)	B (20%)	C (5%)

FIG. 11-69 The distribution of lateral collateral ligament disruptions. (From Scott WN: *The knee*, vol 1-2, St Louis, 1994, Mosby.)

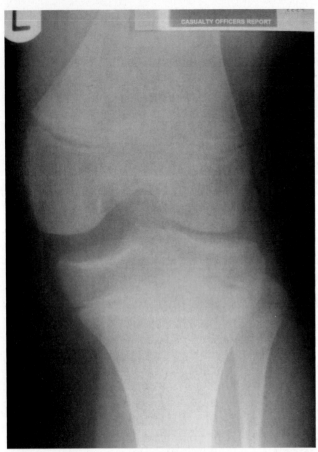

FIG. 11-70 Lateral subluxation of the tibia with widening of the medial joint space. (From Said HG, Learmonth DJA: *Chronic irreducible posterolateral knee dislocation: two-stage surgical approach,* Arthroscopy 23[5]:564.e1-564.e4, 2007.)

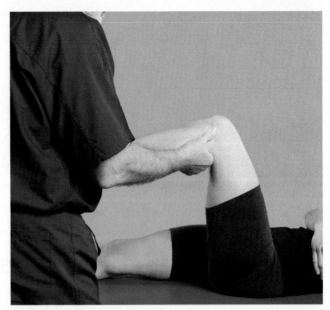

FIG. 11-71 The patient is lying supine, and the knee is extended and relaxed. The examiner holds the patient's leg externally rotated. The knee is then flexed to 30 degrees.

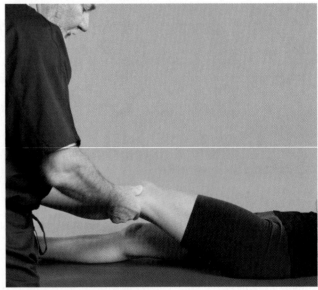

FIG. 11-72 The examiner hooks a thumb behind the fibular head. A valgus force is applied to the knee. The examiner extends the patient's knee and applies forward pressure behind the fibular head with the thumb. The leg is allowed to move into medial rotation. If a *clunk* is heard or felt just before full extension of the knee, the test is positive. This clunk means that the tibia has subluxed anteriorly.

PROCEDURE

- The patient is in a supine position.
- The patient's leg is externally rotated.
- The patient's knee is flexed to 30 degrees (Fig. 11-71).
- The examiner hooks a thumb behind the patient's fibular head.
- A valgus force is applied to the knee.
- The knee is extended, and forward pressure is applied behind the fibular head with the examiner's thumb (Fig. 11-72).
- The leg moves into medial rotation.
- If a *clunk* forward is noted just before full extension of the knee, the test is positive.
- This clunk means that the tibia has subluxed anteriorly and indicates injury to the same structures listed with the lateral pivot shift maneuver.
- The Losee test assesses anterolateral rotary instability.

Next Steps/Procedures
Drawer test, lateral pivot shift maneuver, and Slocum test

CLINICAL PEARL

If rotary instability is present, then as full extension is reached, a dramatic clunk will occur as the lateral tibial condyle subluxates forward. The patient should relate this information to the sensations experienced during activity.

Assessment for Medial or Lateral Meniscus Injury

Comment

The normal function of the knee joint depends on the presence of smooth surface with a low friction index. Such a surface is provided by articular cartilage. However, its vulnerability to various types of lesions may restrict the proper knee function and may lead to OA (Widuchowski, Widuchowski, Trzaska, 2007).

Injuries of the menisci are common in men younger than 45. A tear is usually caused by a twisting force while the knee is semi flexed or flexed. This tear is usually the result of an athletic injury, but it is also common among men who work in a squatting position, such as coal miners and flooring installers. The medial meniscus is torn much more often than the lateral.

Three types of tears have been identified. All of these tears begin as longitudinal splits. If this split extends throughout the length of the meniscus, it becomes a bucket-handle tear, in which the fragments remain attached at both ends. This tear is the most common type. The bucket handle, the central fragment, is displaced toward the middle of the joint; thus, the condyle of the femur rolls on the tibia through the rent in the meniscus. Because of the shape of the femoral condyle, it requires the most space when the knee is straight. The main effect of a displaced bucket-handle fragment is that it limits full extension (locking).

If the initial longitudinal tear emerges at the concave border of the meniscus, a pedunculated tag is formed. With a posterior horn tear, the fragment remains attached at the posterior horn. With an anterior horn tear, the fragment remains attached to the anterior horn. A transverse tear through the meniscus is nearly always an artifact.

The menisci are almost avascular. Consequently, when the menisci are torn, no effusion of blood occurs into the joint. However, an effusion of synovial fluid does occur, which is secreted in response to the injury. Major tears of the menisci do not heal spontaneously, probably because the torn surfaces are separated by fluid (Fig. 11-73).

In addition to the surroundings muscles, the joint has passive stabilizers such as the ligaments, menisci, and the joint capsule that play important roles in stabilizing the joint. When secondary stabilizers in the knee are injured during a sports accident, it can lead to an overuse of other internal knee structures (Majewski, Susanne, Klaus, 2006).

Statistics have demonstrated that 32.6% of all sports injuries involve the knee, and 20% to 25% of all knee injuries occur while performing sports. Interestingly, the level of injury caused by sports is similar to that of injuries caused by motor-vehicle accidents but occurring at twice the rate of traffic accidents. Soccer and skiing show a high number of sports injuries, with the rate of injury caused by skiing rising in the last 20 years, making skiing the most routinely performed sport with the highest risk of injury among adults. Among athletes who perform in competitions, the triathletes have the highest rates of injury (Majewski et al, 2006).

The patient is usually 18 to 45 years of age. This history is characteristic, especially with bucket-handle tears. In consequence of a twisting injury, the patient falls and has pain at the anteromedial aspect of the joint. The patient is either unable to continue the activity or does so with difficulty. The patient is unable to straighten the knee fully. The next day, the patient notices swelling of the whole knee. The knee is rested, and during the next 14 days, the swelling decreases. The knee straightens, and the patient resumes activities. Within weeks or months, the knee suddenly gives way again during a twisting movement. Pain and swelling occur as before. Similar incidents occur repeatedly.

Locking means inability to extend the knee fully and is not a true jamming of the joint because free range of flexion exists. Locking is a common feature of a torn medial meniscus, but the limitation of extension is often so slight that the patient does not notice it. Persistent locking can occur only in bucket-handle tears. Tag tears cause momentary catching but not locking in the true sense.

The meniscal tears described are uncommon in patients older than 50, which is when the menisci begin to show degenerative changes. A degenerative meniscus suffers a different type of lesion. The medial meniscus, in particular, may split horizontally at a point that is often near the middle of its convexity. Such a split is usually of small dimensions. Because fragments do not separate, natural healing can occur.

Clinically, the patient complains of troublesome and persistent pain at the medial aspect of the knee at the joint level. The pain may be noticed after a minor injury, but it often comes on spontaneously, without any preceding incident. In the early stages, effusion of fluid into the joint is usually small.

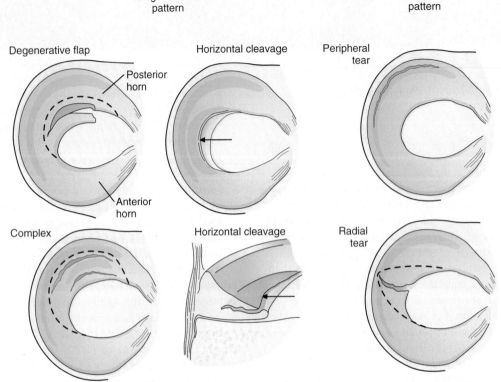

Degenerative pattern

Traumatic pattern

Degenerative flap

Posterior horn

Anterior horn

Horizontal cleavage

Peripheral tear

Complex

Horizontal cleavage

Radial tear

FIG. 11-73 Depending on the pattern, the meniscus can be reparable or nonreparable. Because of the essential role of the meniscus in sharing load and preventing the progression of degenerative arthritis, salvageable meniscus tears should always be repaired. Usually, reparable meniscus tears are vertical and peripheral and occur in a younger population. Degenerative, flap, parrot beak, and small radial tears are not amenable to repair and generally require simple débridement. (From Rakel RE: *Textbook of family medicine,* ed 7, Philadelphia, 2007, Saunders.)

PROCEDURE

- The patient is lying supine, and the thigh and leg are flexed until the heel approaches the buttock (Fig. 11-74).
- One of the examiner's hands is on the knee, and the other is on the heel (Fig. 11-75).
- The examiner internally rotates and slowly extends the leg (Fig. 11-76).
- The examiner then externally rotates and slowly extends the leg.
- McMurray sign is present if, at some point in the arc, a painful click or snap is heard.
- This sign is significant in meniscal injury.
- The point in the arc at which the snap is heard locates the site of injury of the meniscus.
- If noted with internal rotation, the lateral meniscus will be involved.
- The higher the leg is raised when the snap is heard, the more posterior the lesion is in the meniscus.
- If noted with external rotation, the medial meniscus will be involved.

Next Steps/Procedures
Bounce home test, Childress duck waddle test, Payr sign, and Steinmann sign

CLINICAL PEARL

The examiner should observe for tenderness in the joint line and test for a springy block to full extension of the knee. These two signs, in association with evidence of quadriceps atrophy, are the most consistent and reliable signs of a torn meniscus.

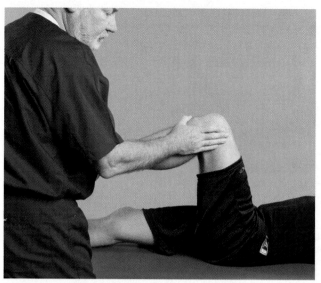

FIG. 11-74 The patient is lying supine. The examiner flexes the thigh and leg to 90 degrees.

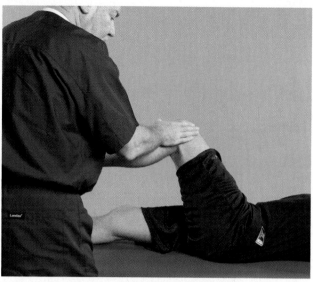

FIG. 11-75 The examiner places one hand on the knee; the other hand grasps the patient's heel.

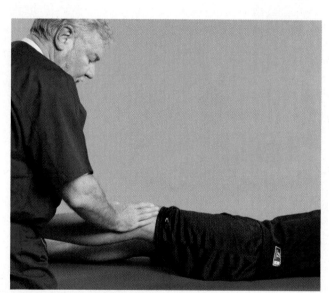

FIG. 11-76 The examiner internally rotates the lower leg and then slowly extends the knee, applying valgus pressure to the joint. The examiner then *externally rotates* the leg and slowly extends it. The test is positive if, at some point in the arc, a click or snap that causes pain is heard. This test is significant for a meniscal injury. If the click is noted with *internal rotation*, the lateral meniscus is involved. If the click is noted with external rotation, the medial meniscus is involved. The higher the leg is raised when the snap is heard, the more posterior the lesion is.

11

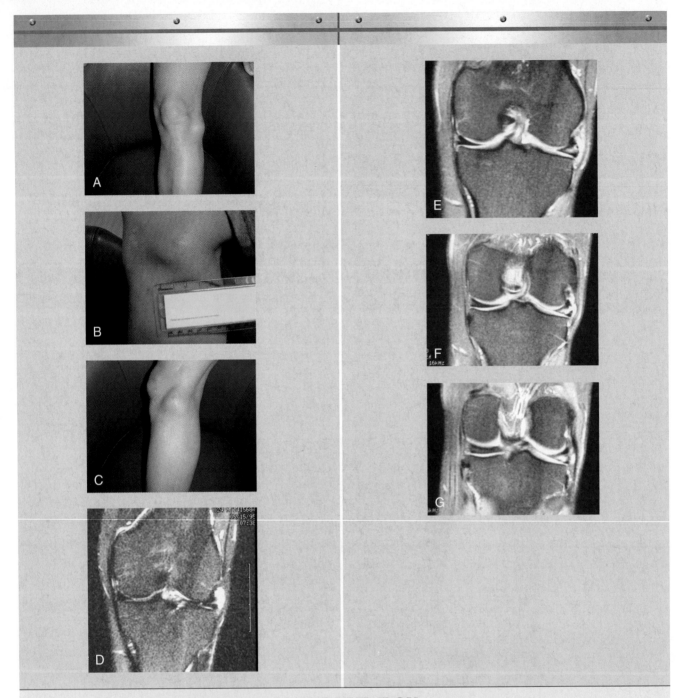

AT THE VIEWBOX

Active adult female with history of multiple knee injuries and surgeries. Recurrence of severe knee pain following recent injury is accompanied by a slowly growing, firm, tender mass at the joint line (**A, B, C**). MRI demonstrated a meniscal cyst, extending from a large meniscal tear. Another patient, a 23-year-old male active in soccer, had a similar palpable mass with relatively mild knee pain. There was clinical concern for a neoplasm, but MRI demonstrated a similar meniscal cyst, arising from a large lateral meniscal tear (**D, E, F, G**). (From the teaching file of Timothy Mick, DC, DACBR)

Assessment for Iliotibial Band Friction Syndrome

Comment

The biceps femoris and the ITB are both active in stabilizing the fully extended knee. Contraction of these muscles is a preliminary to strong action by the extensors of the knee. In the initial stages of contraction, until the quadriceps group of muscles has shortened sufficiently to exert full power, the position and stability of the knee must be controlled by the action of the biceps femoris and the ITB. The biceps femoris tendon is inserted into the head of the fibula with the fibular collateral ligament, but the ITB finds insertion into the tibia through the lateral capsule and into the fibula through the lateral ligament. The biceps femoris muscle is also a flexor of the knee, and both the biceps femoris and ITB play a part in external rotation of the tibia. With paralytic contracture of the knee, the ITB may indeed be the main contributor to the flexion–external rotation deformity.

However, the most important function of the biceps femoris and ITB is probably to stabilize the fibular component of the leg during weight bearing. Through their attachments, the biceps femoris and ITB exert control on the superior tibiofibular joint. When the knee is fully extended, rotation of the tibia on the femur is impossible. In addition, the weight-bearing knee cannot indulge in any change of its exact ratio of flexion-extension to rotation. The flexion and extension movements of the ankle and inversion and eversion of the foot do not take place in isolation in the ankle and the subtalar and midtarsal joints. The foot and ankle movements require a component of rotation in the leg. This necessary movement must take place in the inferior and superior tibiofibular joints, a factor more easily appreciated when it is realized that the increasing width of the articular surface of the talus needs posterior changing accommodation in the ankle mortise. Indeed, one might generalize by saying that most actions of the weight-bearing leg are accomplished by adaptive movements of all the joints of the leg, from the hip downward. The coordination of the joints, whether stationary or in motion, is a fundamental part of bodily posture and movement.

ITB syndrome is widely recognized as an overuse injury that is a common cause of exercise-related lateral knee pain in running and other sports. The diagnosis is based on the symptoms of exercise-related tenderness over the lateral femoral epicondyle and on a clinical examination confirming the location of pain and absence of other pathologies. Patients frequently complain of a sharp, burning pain when the practitioner performs an Ober's test; that is, the practitioner presses on the epicondyle as the patient's knee is

flexed and extended, with the hip in abduction. Experts generally consider that ITB syndrome is associated with inflammation caused by the movement of the tract across the lateral epicondyle during knee flexion and extension. The recurrent movement is suggested as causing frictional force, considered to be most acute when the knee is flexed to 30 degrees, and is responsible for inflaming the ITB, particularly the posterior fibers, and for an associated bursitis (Fairclough et al, 2007).

ITB friction syndrome *(runner's knee)* occurs in runners as a result of overuse. It tends to occur in patients with genu varum and planus feet. The symptoms are of pain over the lateral epicondyle of the femur during running come from friction between the ITB and the femur and may be caused by an inflamed bursa. Tenderness is found over the lateral epicondyle. The symptoms usually settle with rest, but in resistant cases, a corticosteroid injection into the tender site may help.

The cause of ITB friction syndrome is multifactorial, with representation of both intrinsic and extrinsic factor. ITB friction syndrome in a nontraumatic overuse injury caused by friction or rubbing of the distal portion of the ITB over the lateral femoral epicondyle with repeated flexion and extension of the knee. Orchard and associates describe an *impingement zone,* which occurs at approximately 30 degrees of knee flexion during foot-strike and early stance phase. At approximately 30 degrees and greater of knee flexion, the ITB passes over and posterior to the lateral femoral epicon-

---

ORTHOPEDIC GAMUT 11-22

EXTRINSIC AND INTRINSIC CAUSATIVE FACTORS OF ILIOTIBIAL BAND FRICTION SYNDROME

Extrinsic Factors
1. Running or cycling on an oblique surface causing a pelvic tilt
2. Sudden increase in running or cycling distance
3. Improper seating with cleats too far internally rotated or a saddle that is not well positioned

Intrinsic Factors
1. Varus knee deformity that predisposes the area for this friction syndrome between the lateral femoral epicondyle and the overriding iliotibial band
2. Leg-length discrepancy
3. Forefoot pronation

dyle. During the impingement period, eccentric contraction of the tensor fascia lata and gluteus maximus to decelerate the leg whilst running, exert great tension through the ITB. Orchard and colleagues described a similar impingement zone for cycling (Ellis, Hing, Reid, in press).

In sports in which repetitive knee flexion past 30 degrees is required, the ITB is especially susceptible to irritation. Therefore this syndrome is typically observed in runners and has been described as the *jogger's knee,* but football players and cyclists also present this exertional pain syndrome. Most often, the initiation of the pain syndrome is related to running or cycling as part of training.

PROCEDURE

- The patient is in a supine position.
- The patient's hip and knee are flexed 90 degrees (Fig. 11-77).
- The examiner applies thumb pressure to the lateral femoral condyle (Fig. 11-78).
- The patient's knee is extended as the thumb pressure is maintained.
- In the positive test, the patient will complain of severe pain over the lateral femoral condyle, near 30 degrees of flexion (Fig. 11-79).
- This pain indicates ITB syndrome.

Next Steps/Procedures

Patella ballottement test, Q-angle test, thigh circumference test, and Wilson sign

CLINICAL PEARL

This syndrome produces a line of tenderness that extends from the anterolateral tibia, across the joint line, and up the side of the thigh. Tenderness is usually maximal over the lateral femoral condyle, and a painful arc occurs at approximately 30 degrees of flexion.

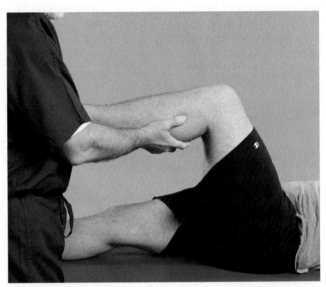

FIG. 11-77 The patient is supine. The patient's knee and hip are flexed to 90 degrees.

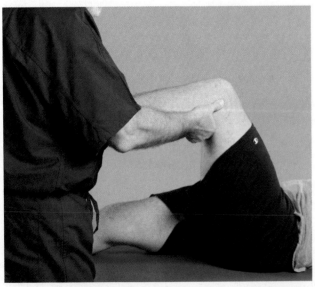

FIG. 11-78 The examiner applies thumb pressure to the lateral femoral condyle.

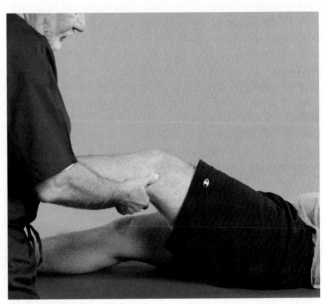

FIG. 11-79 The patient's knee is extended as thumb pressure is maintained. In the positive test, the patient will complain of severe pain over the lateral femoral condyle near 30 degrees of flexion. This indicates iliotibial band syndrome.

PATELLA BALLOTTEMENT TEST

Assessment for Joint Effusion

Comment

The swollen knee is the result of conditions that create an inflammatory response of the synovial membrane. The basic inflammatory process in each condition is similar, and if left to proceed unhindered, the process results in secondary degenerative changes of the joint. The differential diagnosis of these conditions is difficult at the onset. However, with sufficient information, the diagnosis usually becomes apparent.

> Joint effusion commonly follows acute trauma, chronic degenerative joint disease, and surgical intervention. Reflex inhibition of the quadriceps after an acute knee joint effusion is well documented. This neuromuscular response, termed *arthrogenic muscle inhibition,* is accompanied by an increased neuromuscular drive to the soleus (Palmieri et al, 2003).

Undoubtedly, trauma is the most common cause of effusion within the knee joint. Effusion is caused by intrinsic factors, such as internal derangements that damage the synovial membrane, creating bleeding within the joint, or from extrinsic factors, such as a direct blow to the knee or a twisting injury. In most instances of trauma, the history is sufficient to make a diagnosis of a traumatic effusion or hemarthrosis. However, such a history may not be apparent in the infant or young child who is unable to communicate. It also is not apparent in the adult in whom the effusion is secondary to microtrauma. The microtrauma may be secondary to some activity related to the patient's occupation, such as one requiring the repeated use of the knee to perform a certain maneuver or repeated minor blows to the knee, which may not be of any significance to the patient.

Effusion can have its beginnings as a traumatic synovitis, which creates synovial effusion that leads to rest and immobility with resultant quadriceps atrophy. The loss of muscle protection makes the knee more susceptible to the minor trauma of everyday use. Recurring injury creates repeated synovial effusions and sets up a vicious cycle that promotes chronic synovitis. A patient with this condition experiences a painful, swollen knee that is held in a semiflexed position, the position of maximal comfort. The suprapatellar pouch may be distended and quite tense. The patella is ballotable. The knee may be somewhat warm, but it does not give the appearance of a septic joint. Motion is resisted because attempts at flexion or extension create more tension, which causes pain within the joint.

The test for small effusions in the knee joint is called the *bulge sign.* The medial aspect of the knee is *milked* upward two to three times to displace fluid. The lateral margin of the knee is pressed (Fig. 11-80). A positive bulge sign will demonstrate a swelling or bulge of fluid in the area medial to the patella. The bulge sign, useful for assessing small effusions, is often absent in large effusions.

Differentiating traumatic hemarthrosis from traumatic synovitis can be a diagnostic problem. Swelling from a traumatic hemarthrosis begins within a few minutes after the injury, whereas a traumatic synovial effusion begins several hours after the injury and progresses more slowly. The aspiration of blood from the joint confirms a traumatic hemarthrosis, and fat globules that float in the blood indicate an interarticular fracture as well. A traumatic synovial reaction may have synovial fluid that appears normal but, in some instances, is tinged with blood. The joint is somewhat warmer to the touch than usual but does not have the warmth or redness of the skin that is found with acute septic arthritis.

Rheumatoid arthritis of the knee should be evaluated and treated in the context of a systemic disease involving multiple organs and joints (Fig. 11-81). Rarely are the knee symptoms the initial presentation, and patients are most often taking medication for rheumatoid arthritis.

Other causes of acute inflammation should be excluded. These conditions include crystal arthropathy, hemophilia, and infection. Acute infection is not uncommon in the knee joint in patients taking immunosuppressive medication for rheumatoid arthritis, and knee aspiration with culture of the joint fluid may be indicated. Synovial cysts are fluid collection in the bursas of the articular spaces. This category

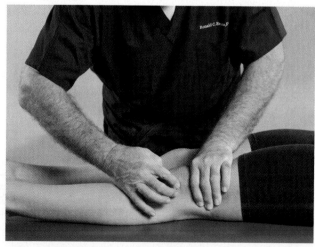

FIG. 11-80 Testing for the bulge sign. After *milking* the medial aspect of the knee, the lateral side of the patella is tapped. The medial side is then observed for the presence of a bulge.

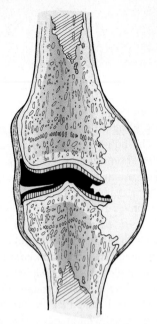

FIG. 11-81 Diagram of the knee showing hypotrophy of the synovium and bony erosion and osteoporosis seen in rheumatoid arthritis. (From Bucholz RW: *Orthopaedic decision making*, ed 2, St Louis, 1996, Mosby.)

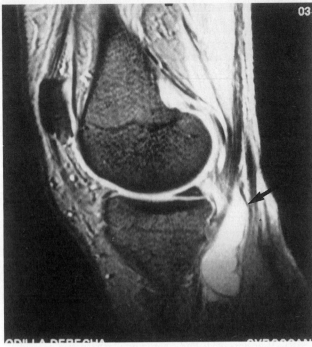

FIG. 11-82 Sagittal magnetic resonance image showing normal joint fluid and a massive Baker cyst *(arrow)*. (From Marti-Bonmati L et al: MR imaging of Baker cysts—prevalence and relation to internal derangements of the knee, *Magn Reson Materials Biol Phys Med* 10[3]:205-210, 2000.)

includes popliteal or Baker cyst, the most frequently encountered versions (Fig. 11-82).

The articular cavity is lined by a fine membrane, the synovium, with the exception of cartilage areas and the central portion of the menisci. The main function of the synovium is to secrete a mucoid substance into the articular fluid. In normal joints, the quantity of fluid is small, close to 4 ml. Synovial cysts are fluid collection in the bursas of the articular spaces. Although several bursas are located in the knee, popliteal or Baker cyst is the most frequently encountered. This cyst is produced as a consequence of a communication of the posterior articular capsule and the bursa located between the medial head of the gastrocnemius and the semimembranous tendons. Fluid enters inside the Baker cyst from the articular cavity (Marti-Bonmati et al, 2000).

- The patient's knee is extended.
- A slight tap or pressure is applied over the patella (Fig. 11-83).
- This test is positive if a large amount of swelling in the knee is detected.

Next Steps/Procedures
Fouchet test, Q-angle test, thigh circumference test, and Wilson sign

CLINICAL PEARL

If popliteal swelling is found, confirming communication with the joint is possible by massaging its contents back into the main synovial cavity while the knee is in flexion. The examiner maintains pressure on the patient's popliteal fossa, extends the patient's knee, and then removes the pressure. The swelling will not reappear until the patient flexes the knee several times, confirming a valve-like communication between the main cavity and the cyst.

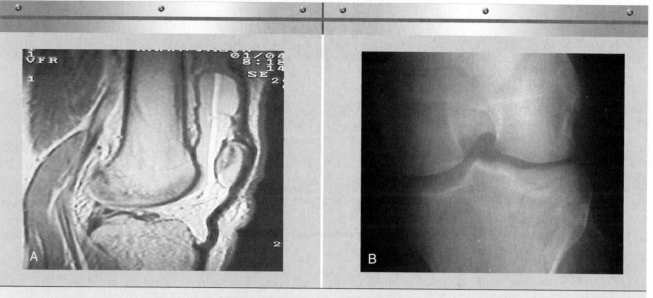

AT THE VIEWBOX

Adult female with skiing injury, involving landing hard on the outside edge of the ski, while coming off of a mogul. Knee pain and swelling with limited motion. MRI demonstrates an effusion, with suprapatellar bursal distension **(A).** Note the layered appearance of the fluid, with distinct fat-blood-serum levels, described as an "FBI" sign (fat-blood interface). This is usually, though not invariably, associated with an intra-articular fracture, which may be subtle or occult on plain films. Classically, this involves the tibial plateau. Plain film demonstrates slight depression of the lateral tibial plateau, with minimal cortical disruption **(B).** This has been described as a "bumper fracture." (From the teaching file of Timothy Mick, DC, DACBR)

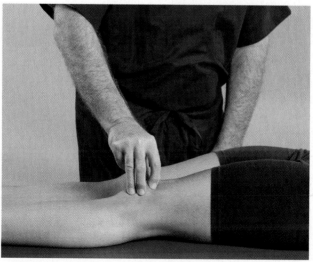

FIG. 11-83 The patient is supine with the knee extended. Pressure is applied over the patella. A floating sensation of the patella is a positive finding and indicates a large amount of swelling in the knee.

Assessment for Injury of the Posterior Horn of the Medial Meniscus

Comment

The medial meniscus is shaped similar to the letter *C*. Its anterior attachment is on top of the tibia near the midline and in front of the tibial spines. The posterior attachment is on top of the tibia, behind the tibial spines. In each case, the attachment is near the periphery of the tibia, thus the two ends are widely separated from each other. The meniscus is attached by the coronary ligament, which has its origins around the top of the tibia, to the MCL, and then to the tibia. This attachment is firm, and although it does allow a little movement, extensive motion is not permitted in the normal medial meniscus. A meniscal flounce is a single fold in the free inner margin of the meniscus (Fig 11-84).

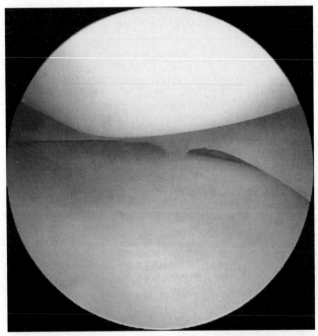

FIG. 11-84 Normal small flounce in zone 3 of the medial meniscus. (From Williams AM et al: The meniscal flounce: a valuable arthroscopic sign, *Knee* 13[4]:337-341, 2006.)

The meniscal flounce is produced when stress maneuvers are applied to the tibiofemoral joint, resulting in distraction and some rotation of the compartment being assessed. During these stress maneuvers, meniscal motion and configuration are influenced by the capsular and ligamentous attachments, relative tibiofemoral movement, and loading of the knee joint. When the meniscus is stressed, the peripheral attachments cause differential stresses within the body of the intact meniscus. These stresses are characterized by *buckling* of the free inner margin of the meniscus, known as the *meniscal flounce*. Disease affecting the integrity of the meniscus or its attachments can alter the appearance of this flounce (Williams et al, 2006).

In sprain of the MCL, the tibia and femur separate on the medial side, and stress is applied in the area of the attachment of the meniscus to the MCL. The cartilage may be forced to accompany either the femur or the tibia, depending on the location of the ligament injury. Because the structure of the meniscus does not allow much flexion stress, it will tear transversely or, more commonly, split around its periphery. If the tear is actually in the attachment to the ligament, it may heal. If the tear is within the substance of the meniscus, it will not. Meniscus injury accompanies repeated sprains of the knee more often than it does the initial, single sprain. With an acute injury, the examiner has no way to determine whether the meniscus is torn unless the knee is locked. If the knee is locked and the ligaments are stable, the episode is the first. If the meniscus has been detached at its periphery, this attachment may heal. This possibility is much more likely if the meniscus has slipped into the knee, locked, and then immediately unlocked.

PROCEDURE

- The patient is in the cross-legged, Yoga-seated position, with the feet and ankles crossed (Fig. 11-85).
- The examiner applies downward pressure on the knee joint (Fig. 11-86).
- Pain is elicited on the medial side of the joint when the sign is present.
- The test is significant when a lesion of the posterior horn of the medial meniscus is present.

Next Steps/Procedures

Bounce home test, Childress duck waddle test, McMurray sign, and Steinmann sign

CLINICAL PEARL

Meniscal cysts lie in the joint line, feel firm during palpation, and are tender to deep pressure. Cysts of the menisci may be associated with tears. Lateral meniscus cysts are by far the most common. Cystic swellings on the medial side are sometimes caused by ganglions that arise from the pes anserinus (insertion of the sartorius, gracilis, and semitendinosus).

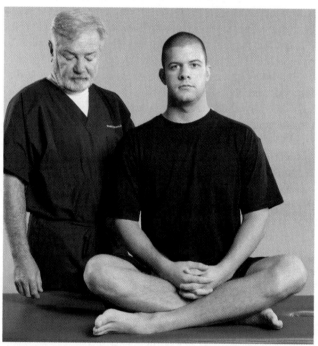

FIG. 11-85 The patient is in a yoga Lotus seated position, with the feet and ankles crossed as comfortably as possible.

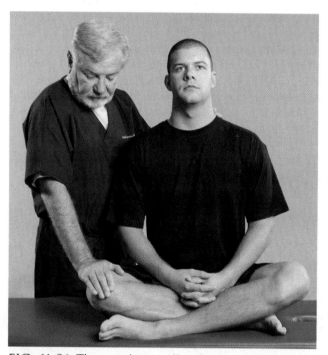

FIG. 11-86 The examiner applies downward pressure on the affected knee joint. Pain is elicited on the medial side of the joint when the sign is present. The sign is present when there is a lesion of the posterior horn of the medial meniscus.

11

Q-ANGLE TEST

Assessment for Patellofemoral Dysfunction, Patella Alta, Subluxating Patella, Increased Femoral Anteversion, Genu Valgum, or Increased Lateral Tibial Torsion

Comment

The true, congenital dislocation of the patella implies actual and constant dislocation of the patella. This dislocation is usually lateral to the femoral condyle. If fully developed, this condition will interdict athletic participation. Of much greater importance is the dislocation that occasionally occurs under certain circumstances. This type of dislocation results from repeated episodes of acute dislocation in a normal knee. Although no true congenital dislocation exists, certain physical characteristics predispose an individual to subluxation or luxation. One predisposing anatomic condition is an abnormally acute angle between the axis of the patellar tendon and the axis of the quadriceps mechanism, the quadriceps angle (Q-angle).

> Noncontact ACL injury rates in female athletes are reported to be three to eight times greater than those of male athletes. Skeletal alignment differences between sexes, such as a greater hip width to femoral length ratio and a larger Q-angle) are thought to contribute to excessive amounts of knee valgus (lateral angulation or abduction of the tibia with respect to the femur). The combination of knee valgus (tibial

abduction) and external rotation positions contribute to ACL impingement and injury (Pantano et al, 2005).

The angle formed by a line drawn from the anterosuperior iliac spine to the center of the patella and a line drawn from the center of the patella to the tibial tubercle is called the Q-angle (Fig. 11-87). In a normal knee, the Q-angle measures approximately 15 degrees, and an angle exceeding 20 degrees is abnormal. A Q-angle greater than 15 to 20 degrees is more prevalent in women than in men.

If the patellar tendon tends to angulate sharply and laterally to reach its tibial attachment, this angulation, combined with a quadriceps mechanism that tends to angulate medially at the knee, results in an increased angle between the patellar tendon and the long axis of the quadriceps tendon. As the quadriceps muscle is contracted, this angle tends to straighten by slipping the patella laterally. This action may be inhibited anteriorly by the prominence of the lateral femoral condyle. The general tendency is for the patella to slide laterally with each forceful extension of the knee. The female athlete, with a widened pelvis and internally angulated femora, is much more prone to patellar subluxation or dislocation than the male athlete. A similar situation arises in patients with tibial torsion or genu valgum. A dislocated patella in a patient with genu varum is uncommon because, in such a patient, the axis of the patellar tendon and the quadriceps muscle is parallel. However, in some patients with genu varum, this bow is part of the internal torsion of

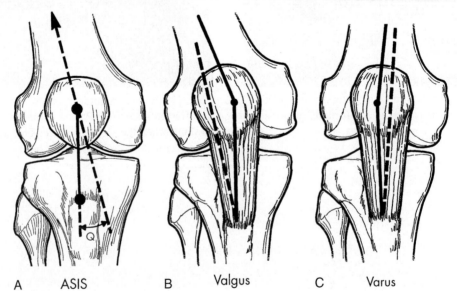

FIG. 11-87 **A,** The Q-angle, which may indicate patellar tracking problems, is formed by two lines, one drawn from the anterior superior iliac spine through the center of the patella, and the second line drawn from the tibial tubercle to the center of the patella. **B,** Valgus and **(C)** varus measurement of the Q-angle. (From Scott WN: *The knee,* vol 1, St Louis, 1994, Mosby.)

the femur; therefore, the femoral condyles are rotated toward the midline. Such a patient often has an associated external rotation of the tibia to compensate and straighten the long axis of the leg. In this instance, the Q-angle may be markedly more acute as the patellar tendon moves from the internally rotated patella down to the externally rotated patellar tubercle.

CLINICAL PEARL

In children, an increased Q-angle is associated with genu valgum. The examiner must note whether the genu valgum is unilateral or, as is usual, bilateral. The severity of the deformity is recorded by measuring the intermalleolar gap. The examiner grasps the child's ankles and rotates the legs until the patellae are vertical. The legs are brought together to touch lightly at the knees. A measurement is made between the malleoli. Serial measurements, often every 6 months, are used to check progress. Note that, with growth, a static measurement is an angular improvement.

PROCEDURE

- To determine the Q-angle, a line is drawn from the antero-superior iliac spine to the midpoint of the patella and from the tibial tubercle to the midpoint of the patella (Fig. 11-88).
- The angle formed by the intersection of these two lines is the Q-angle (Fig. 11-89).
- Normally, the Q-angle is 13 to 18 degrees. The normal angle for men is 13 degrees, and for women it is 18 degrees.
- Less than 13 degrees suggests patellofemoral dysfunction or patella alta.
- Greater than 18 degrees suggests patellofemoral dysfunction, subluxating patella, increased femoral anteversion, genu valgum, or increased lateral tibial torsion.

Next Steps/Procedures
Noble compression test, patella ballottement test, thigh circumference test, and Wilson sign

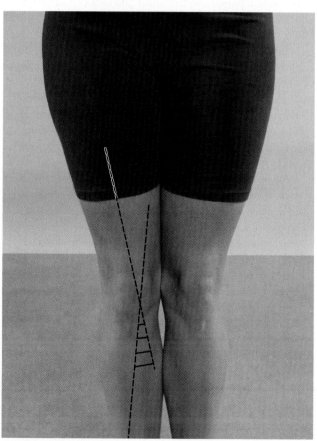

FIG. 11-88 To determine the Q-angle, a line is drawn from the anterosuperior iliac spine to the midpoint of the patella and from the tibial tubercle to the midpoint of the patella. The angle formed by the intersection of these two lines is the Q-angle. Normally, the Q-angle is 13 to 18 degrees (13 degrees for men and 18 degrees for women). Less than 13 degrees suggests patellofemoral dysfunction or patella alta.

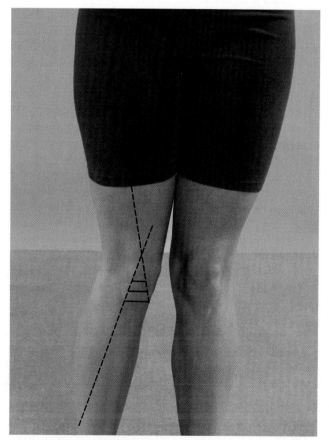

FIG. 11-89 Greater than 18 degrees suggests patellofemoral dysfunction, subluxating patella, increased femoral anteversion, genu valgum, or increased lateral tibial torsion.

11

SLOCUM TEST

Assessment for Anterolateral Rotary Instability, with Injury to Some Degree of (1) the Anterior Cruciate Ligament, (2) the Posterolateral Capsule, (3) the Arcuate-Popliteus Complex, (4) the Lateral Collateral Ligament, (5) the Posterior Cruciate Ligament, and (6) the Iliotibial Band (Tensor Fascia Lata)

Comment

The fact that women are at a greater risk than men to rupture the ACL is well known. Based on a scientific review by leading experts in the area, the suggested opinion is that neuromuscular and biomechanical factors are crucial to help explain the injury rate differential. Current theory suggests that women perform athletic tasks in a manner that exposes the knee joint to greater amounts of ligamentous strain (Schmitz et al, 2007).

Anterolateral rotatory instability is the most common type of instability to occur with ACL rupture. When the ligament is ruptured, the tibia is able to move forward and internally rotate on the femur. This subluxation of the lateral tibial condyle occurs at between 15 and 20 degrees of knee flexion, causing the pivot shift phenomenon. *Pivot shift* is simply the term used to describe the phenomenon of subluxation or reduction of the tibia on the femur in a knee with anterolateral rotary instability. This subluxation is what the patient describes as the knee *giving way.*

The cruciate ligaments are valuable stabilizers of the knee. These ligaments not only assist in knee flexion and extension but also limit rotation, extension, and flexion. The ACL varies in length. The ligament is taut when the knee is in full extension and when the knee is externally rotated at the femorotibial joint. The ligament remains taut until 5 to 20 degrees of flexion, at which point it relaxes. The ligament is most relaxed at 40 to 50 degrees of flexion and becomes taut again when the knee flexes to 70 to 90 degrees.

Internal rotation increases the tension of the ACL even when the knee is flexed to 40 or 50 degrees. External rotation increases the tautness of the ligament, as does abduction of the knee. Anterior shear of the tibia on the femur is permitted to 5 mm of distance but is then checked. Excessive external rotation can tear the ACL, especially if added abduction occurs. Hyperextension and anterior shear may tear this ligament. With the knee flexed to 90 degrees and externally rotated, the first limiting soft tissue that tears is the medial capsular ligament. With further rotation and abduction, the next tissue to tear is the tibial MCL, and then the ACL tears. Isolated tears of the ACL, when they do happen, probably occur from a posterior force, which causes shear stress but also may occur from internal rotation.

The ACL can be torn as an isolated injury resulting from an acute deceleration from a sharp stop-and-cut movement. As the forward motion of the patient is abruptly halted, the quadriceps muscle decelerates the leg and simultaneously pulls the tibia forward on the femur. This shearing disrupts the ACL. With the abrupt stop, the patient often makes a rapid rotation, or cut, to form the direction of movement. This rotation places anterior shear and rotatory stress on the knee. The rotational stress depends on the direction of the cut.

After a jump, the knee absorbs the impact by being slightly flexed. Thus, shear also occurs at this point because of deceleration.

During landing, the lower extremity musculature must function in concert to dissipate the kinetic energy and bring the body's downward momentum to zero. Single-leg landings are performed primarily in the sagittal plane; hence controlled flexion of the joints is likely the primary mechanism through which the impulse is applied. Current literature is lacking to address the role of the combined joint energetics of a single extremity to control the body's momentum in a single-leg landing. Although current focus is on the cause of knee injuries through applied forces, the examiner needs to consider the role of all lower extremity joints in controlling the body as the joints of the lower extremity act in concert to modulate the transfer of mechanical energy absorption during the landing process (Schmitz et al, 2007).

The patient who makes the stop and cuts or jumps feels a pop as the knee gives way. Swelling occurs within 3 or 4 hours.

PROCEDURE

- The patient is sitting or in a supine position.
- The knee is flexed to 80 or 90 degrees; the hip is flexed to 45 degrees.
- The foot is internally rotated.
- The foot is held as the tibia is pulled anteriorly.
- Movement will occur on the lateral side of the knee if the test is positive.
- This movement indicates anterolateral rotatory instability.
- Excessive movement suggests injury to (1) the ACL, (2) the posterolateral capsule, (3) the arcuate-popliteus complex, (4) the LCL, (5) the PCL, or (6) the ITB.
- The test also may be performed while the patient is seated with the knees flexed over the edge of the examination table.
- The examiner pulls or pushes the tibia to the knee while medially or laterally rotating the foot (Fig. 11-90).
- Pulling on the tibia tests for anterior rotary instability. Pushing the tibia tests for posterior rotary instability.

Next Steps/Procedures
Drawer test, lateral pivot shift maneuver, Losee test, and Lachman test

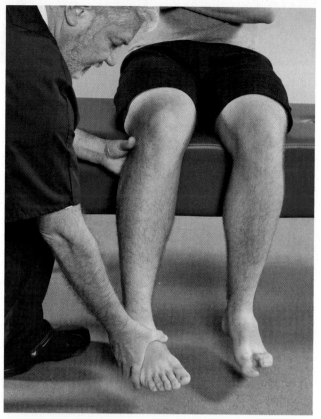

FIG. 11-90 The patient is seated with the knees flexed and hanging over the edge of the examination table. The examiner pulls or pushes the tibia while the foot is medially or laterally rotated. Anterior tibial force tests for anterior rotary instability. Posterior tibial force tests for posterior rotary instability. Excessive movement is a positive test, which indicates cruciate ligament instability.

11

CLINICAL PEARL

This maneuver tightens the lateral capsule, giving enough stability to eliminate the anterior drawer sign. If the anterior drawer sign is still positive while the patient is in this position (most anterior movement occurring on the lateral side), the lateral capsule (or lateral collateral ligament) is likely also damaged.

STEINMANN SIGN

ALSO KNOWN AS STEINMANN TENDERNESS DISPLACEMENT TEST

Assessment for Lateral or Medial Meniscus Tear

Comment

An accurate clinical diagnosis of a meniscal tear can be difficult, especially when another concomitant intraarticular disease is present. Many signs and symptoms associated with meniscal tears have been described in the literature, with variable reported rates of diagnostic accuracy. No single test is pathognomonic for a torn meniscus, and therefore, in addition to a complete history, the physician must rely on a collection of physical findings derived from a variety of reliable tests (Lowery et al, 2006).

Although MRI and arthroscopy have become important in the diagnosis and management of meniscal abnormalities, a complete history and physical examination remain essential. More than 20 meniscal tests have been described for diagnosing tears. Although joint line tenderness is one of the oldest and best known of these tests, little has been reported concerning its accuracy and value (Eren 2003).

During normal movements of the knee, the anterior mobile portion of the medial semilunar cartilage slides slightly backward, into the interior of the joint, as flexion occurs. If the joint is simultaneously abducted, the medial side of the joint is opened, and the mobility of the cartilage is increased further. Turning of the trunk toward the opposite side produces a movement of external rotation on the fixed tibia in relation to the femur. The medial meniscus is forced toward the back of the joint, and the MCL becomes taut.

The ligament initially steadies the posterior part of the cartilage. If the MCL can withstand the strain, the anterior mobile part of the meniscus is injured, and either of the following may occur. The anterior part of the ligament may be detached where it joins with the fixed posterior portion. The ligament may sustain any variety of transverse or oblique tears.

A fragment may slip into the interior of the joint. When the knee is extended and an attempt is made to screw the condyle home, the fragment is impacted between the condyles, and the joint locks. When the medial rotator strain is more severe, the collateral ligament is stretched to such an extent that the attachment between it and the meniscus is destroyed. With even more severe strain, the ligament may become avulsed from its tibial attachment and from the cartilage. In either of the two cases, the whole cartilage slips into the interior of the joint. When the knee is extended, the free border is trapped between the condyles, and a longitudinal split occurs in the substance of the meniscus to form the bucket-handle tear.

Detachment or longitudinal tears of the posterior horn are caused by forceful lateral rotation of the femur on the fixed tibia, when the rotation is combined with flexion.

Although the lateral semilunar cartilage is much less frequently injured than the medial cartilage, tears and displacements do occur. The mechanism is the opposite of that which damages the medial cartilage.

Joint line tenderness as a test for lateral meniscal tears is accurate (96%), sensitive (89%), and specific (97%). However, for medial meniscal tears, rates are lower. Specificity reflects the ability of the test to determine correctly that a lesion is not present. The greater the specificity is, the more likely it is that patients who do not have the lesion will be excluded by the test. Sensitivity is defined as the ability of a test to detect an abnormality.

> **ORTHOPEDIC GAMUT 11-23**
>
> ### FACTORS CONTRIBUTING TO MENISCUS TEAR
>
> - The knee must be bearing weight.
> - The knee must be flexed.
> - A rotation strain is required.

PROCEDURE

- Knee pain moves anteriorly when the knee is extended (Fig. 11-91) and moves posteriorly when the knee is flexed (Fig. 11-92).
- The movement of pain is the positive sign.
- This sign indicates a meniscus tear.
- Medial pain is elicited by lateral rotation.
- Lateral pain is elicited by medial rotation.

Next Steps/Procedures

Bounce home test, Childress duck waddle test, McMurray sign, and Payr sign

CLINICAL PEARL

Patients use the term locking to describe episodes of severe pain in the knee or even collapsing of the knee. Curiously, the word is not applied in this way to any other joints. Locking denotes mechanical jamming of the knee joint and nothing more.

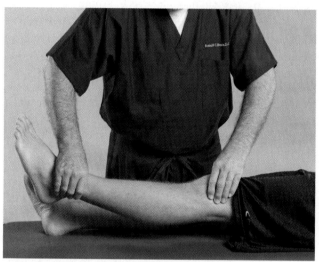

FIG. 11-91 The patient is lying supine with the knee extended. With one hand, the examiner grasps the leg at the ankle and palpates for tenderness at the knee joint with the other hand.

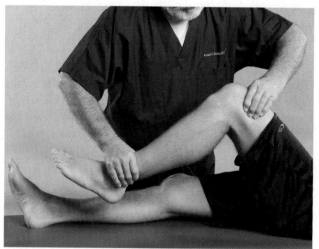

FIG. 11-92 If the pain is found during initial palpation while the knee is extended and if the pain moves posteriorly as the knee is flexed, the sign is present. The sign indicates a meniscal tear.

11

THIGH CIRCUMFERENCE TEST

Assessment for Muscle Hypertonicity or Hypotonicity of the Thigh

Comment

Ruptures of the patellar or quadriceps tendon are rare injuries requiring immediate repair to reestablish knee extensor continuity and to allow early motion. Early operative treatment has been reported to reestablish normal knee function in most patients. Ruptures of the quadriceps tendon are more commonly seen in patients older than 40 years and are often associated with degenerative changes of the tendon (Ramseier, Werner, Heinzelmann, 2006).

Quadriceps rupture occurs 1 to 2 cm away from the upper patellar pole, corresponding to the avascular region of the tendon. Patellar tendon ruptures occur in younger patients, usually as a result of direct trauma, and occur in the proximal part of the tendon close to the inferior patellar pole.

The quadriceps and, to a lesser extent, the hamstrings rapidly atrophy after injury to the cartilage and the ligaments of the knee. This reaction varies in degree and is caused by disturbance of the neurotrophic relationships between the joint and its controlling musculature. Muscle bulk, tone, and control are diminished rapidly and in some instances severely. This diminishment is not caused by muscle inactiv-

ity alone, although this factor does aggravate both atrophy and weakness. Conscientious muscle exercise cannot prevent but does minimize muscle atrophy. Although effusion remains, atrophy is generalized, but the tendency is for the medial vasti to show greater atrophy in sympathy with a medial meniscus injury. Lateral ruptures are associated with atrophy of the lateral vastus.

The vastus medialis obliquus is often the first part of the muscle to waste. The circumference of the thigh 10 cm above the upper pole of the patella should be measured and compared with the other side; this assessment gives an objective measure of thigh wasting. The presence of swellings around the knee should be noted. Swelling within the synovial cavity is seen above the patella and on either side of the patella and patella tendon (Fig. 11-93).

Although muscle weakness is present, effusion persists and is increased with any activity beyond the power and the endurance of the residual muscle bulk. In turn, the effusion affects the trophic reflexes, and further atrophy occurs.

Displacement of a meniscus remains and, despite arduous exercise, muscle bulk and tone cannot recover significantly. If the cartilage is reduced or removed so that the knee recovers full movement, then exercise will increase both power and bulk of the muscle.

The bulk of the quadriceps muscle is a sensitive guide to the presence of knee-joint disease. If necessary, the examiner measures the thigh of each leg at a comparable distance from the joint margin. In effusion, swelling will extend from the suprapatellar region down either side of the patella (Fig. 11-94). In OA, bony swellings around the joint and secondary quadriceps wasting are common (Fig. 11-95). The popliteal fossa is the site for posterior synovial protrusions (Baker cysts) (Fig. 11-96).

A varus deformity means that the distal component of a joint is deviated toward the midline. In contrast, a valgus deformity means that the distal member of a joint is deviated away from the midline (Fig. 11-97).

ORTHOPEDIC GAMUT 11-24

RISK FACTORS FOR PATELLAR OR QUADRICEPS RUPTURE

- Diabetes mellitus
- Gout
- Repetitive microtrauma
- Endocrine disorders

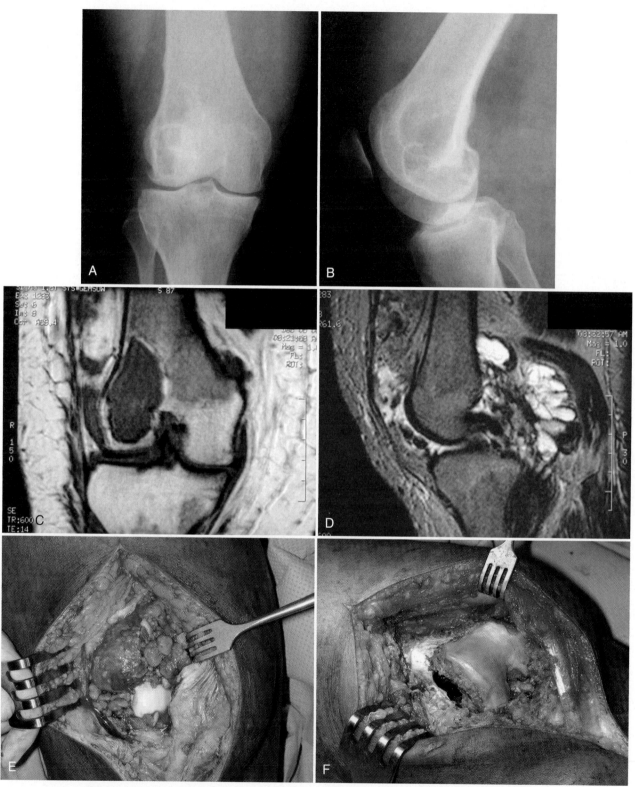

FIG. 11-93 Anteroposterior (**A**) and lateral (**B**) radiographs of right knee of 31-year-old woman with pigmented villonodular synovitis show lytic lesion in distal femur and degenerative changes in knee. MRI shows effusion with intraarticular and intraosseous masses that are dark on T1-weighted (**C**) and T2-weighted (**D**) images. **E,** Intraoperative photograph of pigmented villonodular synovitis. **F,** Intraoperative photograph after synovectomy. (From Canale ST, Beaty JH: *Campbell's operative orthopaedics*, ed 11, Philadelphia, 2007, Mosby.)

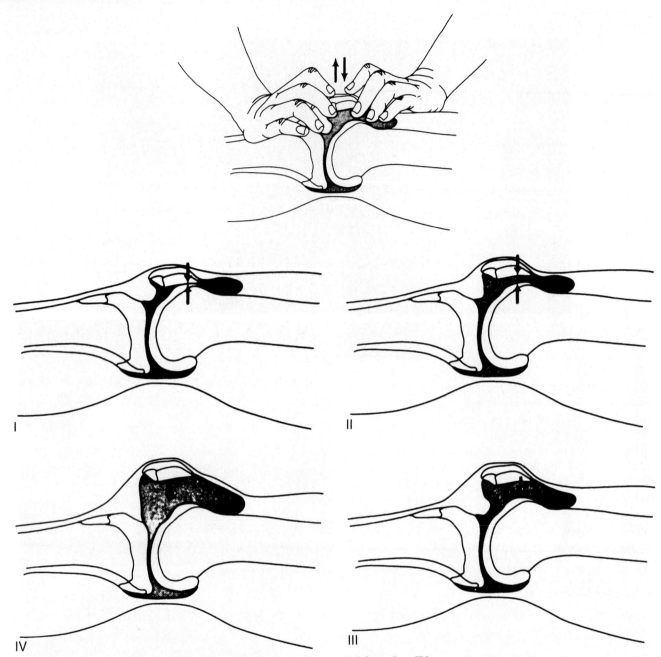

FIG. 11-94 Effusions of the knee can be graded from I to IV. (From Scott WN: *The knee*, vol 1, St Louis, 1994, Mosby.)

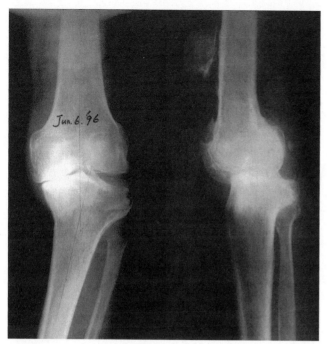

FIG. 11-95 Left knee X-rays of a 64-year-old man who first sustained a fall with trauma of his left knee in 1957 when he was 25 years old. Patellar tendon rupture was diagnosed at that time, and surgical repair was performed at a local hospital. Symptoms of knee pain and limping gait exacerbated; and in May 1996, radiographs of the left knee showed severe degenerative change with narrowing of the medial knee joint space. Surprisingly, a 10-cm proximal migration of the patella was found. The intact patella was palpable over his lower anterior thigh. Crepitus was noted, with passive motion of the left knee and compression of the patella. The range of motion (ROM) of the left knee was from 35 degrees to 100 degrees. (From Chen CF, Chen WM, Lee KS et al: Advanced osteoarthritic knee with neglected patellar tendon rupture treated with total patellectomy and total knee arthroplasty, *J Arthroplasty* 19[6]:793-796, 2004.)

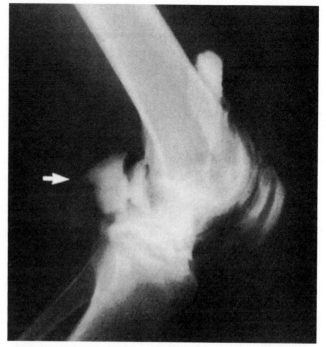

FIG. 11-96 Arthrogram revealing a large popliteal cyst. (From Mercier LR: *Practical orthopedics*, ed 5, St Louis, 2000, Harcourt Health Sciences.)

PROCEDURE

- An area of the thigh 10 cm above the patella is identified (Fig. 11-98).
- The circumference of the leg at that point is measured and compared with the opposite leg (Fig. 11-99).

Next Steps/Procedures
Noble compression test, patella ballottement test, Q-angle test, and Wilson sign

11

CLINICAL PEARL

Although all the quadriceps muscle atrophies uniformly, atrophy of the bulky vastus medialis (particularly in a fit young man) may be the most conspicuous. Quadriceps atrophy is a difficult sign to detect, particularly in the middle-age, elderly, and female patients. Some asymmetry of muscle bulk is common.

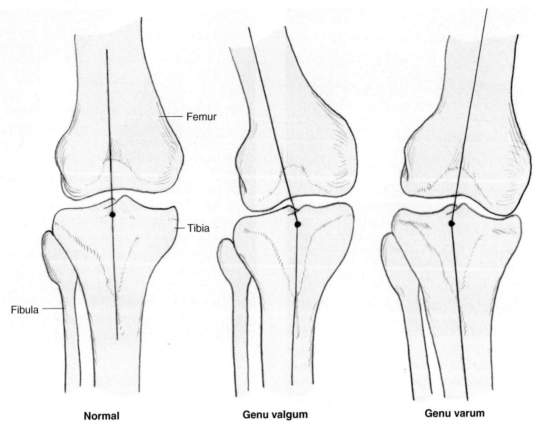

Normal   **Genu valgum**   **Genu varum**

FIG. 11-97 Valgus and varus deformities at the knee joint. A valgus deformity is one in which the distal element of a joint is deviated laterally (away from the midline). A varus deformity is one in which the distal element of a joint is deviated medially (toward the midline). (From Mathers LH et al: *Clinical anatomy principles*, St Louis, 1996, Mosby.)

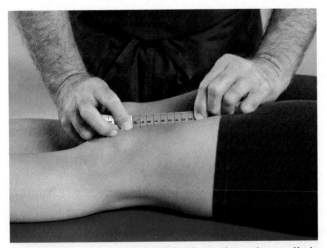

FIG. 11-98 An area of the thigh 10 cm above the patella is identified.

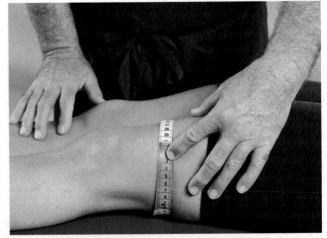

FIG. 11-99 The circumference of the muscle at that point is measured and recorded. This leg is compared with the uninvolved leg.

WILSON SIGN

Assessment for Osteochondritis Dissecans of the Knee

Comment

Osteochondritis dissecans (OCD) is a condition in which a section of articular cartilage and underlying bone separates from the joint surface. It can arise in many joints, although 75% of reported cases occur in the knee. Within the knee, approximately three quarters of lesions occur on the medial femoral condyle (Murray et al, 2007).

Loose bodies, or joint mice, are most commonly osteo-cartilaginous fragments of traumatic origin. They are typically from tangential osteochondral fractures. However, joint mice can also originate from pathologic processes, such as OCD. Other types of loose bodies may consist of chondral fragments (pieces of articular cartilage), remnants of menisci, foreign bodies, fibrous tissues, and interarticular tumors. Some loose bodies may obtain a synovial attachment, but they more commonly remain loose in the joint. A tangential osteochondral fragment, with its normal bone, is more likely to become attached to the synovium than is a fragment from OCD, with its necrotic bone fragment. Fragments of articular cartilage can enlarge as these are nourished by the synovial fluid. Small, loose bodies are more likely to cause symptoms than larger ones because the former may be more easily impinged between the articular surfaces.

On diagnostic imaging, a fragment of avascular bone is seen that is demarcated from the adjacent femur by a radiolucent line. Occasionally, a loose body may be present (Fig. 11-100).

OCD is an ischemic condition that involves the subchondral bone and is probably either the result of or in association with repeated trauma to the area. The involved area of ischemic bone demarcates and may eventually separate with the overlying articular cartilage. This separation leaves behind a defect, a fragment that becomes a loose body within the joint. The knee is the most commonly involved joint, and the incidence is higher in men than in women.

OCD occurs at the classic site and is caused by repeated trauma to the area from contact with a prominent medial tibial spine. The central lesions in the femoral condyles are usually associated with a meniscal lesion that traumatizes the area. The patient often has a family history of OCD, and involvement of knees is not unusual.

Classically, the problem occurs in a teenage boy who complains of pain and a giving way of the knee. The patient may experience effusion and transient episodes of locking as opposed to the more persistent locking that is seen with a torn meniscus. Before the fragment separates, the complaints are nondiagnostic. After the fragment separates, episodes of transient locking are frequent, and the patient may be aware of something loose in the knee.

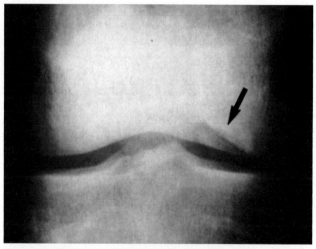

FIG. 11-100 Osteochondritis dissecans of the knee. (From Mercier LR, Pettid FJ: *Practical orthopedics*, ed 4, St Louis, 1995, Mosby.)

ORTHOPEDIC GAMUT 11-25

COMMON ORIGINS OF A LOOSE BODY IN THE KNEE

- Osteochondritis dissecans at the lateral border of the medial femoral condyle (men)
- Marginal fracture that is from the lateral margin of the lateral femoral condyle and is secondary to direct trauma or patellar dislocation (men)
- Medial tangential osteochondral fracture of the patella from dislocation (men)
- This order is reversed in the female patient.

ORTHOPEDIC GAMUT 11-26

COMMON SITES FOR OSTEOCHONDRITIS DISSECANS

1. The lateral border of the medial femoral condyle
2. The inferior, central area of the lateral femoral condyle
3. The inferior, central region of the medial femoral condyle

PROCEDURE

- The patient is in a supine position.
- The patient's knee is flexed to 90 degrees by the examiner.
- The knee is extended with the tibia medially rotated.
- Near 30 degrees of flexion, pain in the knee increases (the patient often stops the rotating movement) (Fig. 11-101).
- If the tibia is rotated laterally, the pain disappears, which is a positive test (Fig. 11-102).
- The positive test indicates osteochondritis dissecans of the femur.

Next Steps/Procedures

Noble compression test, patella ballottement test, Q-angle test, and thigh circumference test

CLINICAL PEARL

Patients often give a classic account of a loose fragment in the knee and are usually able to describe its size and shape. Loose bodies are sometimes called joint mice, which is an appropriate description because these loose bodies can be recognized instantly, but they disappear and may be impossible to find again. Loose bodies should not be called foreign bodies. Foreign bodies, including bullets and bits of gravel, come from outside the body and are rare in joints.

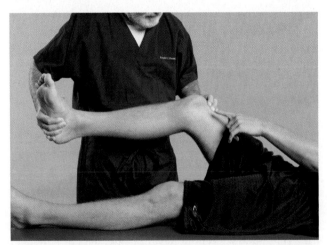

FIG. 11-101 The patient is supine. The knee is flexed to 90 degrees by the examiner. The knee is extended with the tibia medially rotated. Near 30 degrees of flexion, the pain in the knee increases. The patient attempts to stop the movement.

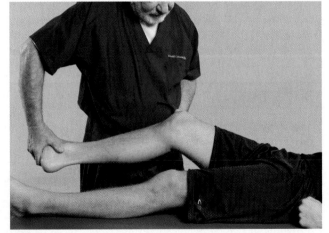

FIG. 11-102 The tibia is rotated laterally, and the pain disappears. This disappearance of pain indicates that the sign is present, which suggests osteochondritis dissecans of the femur.

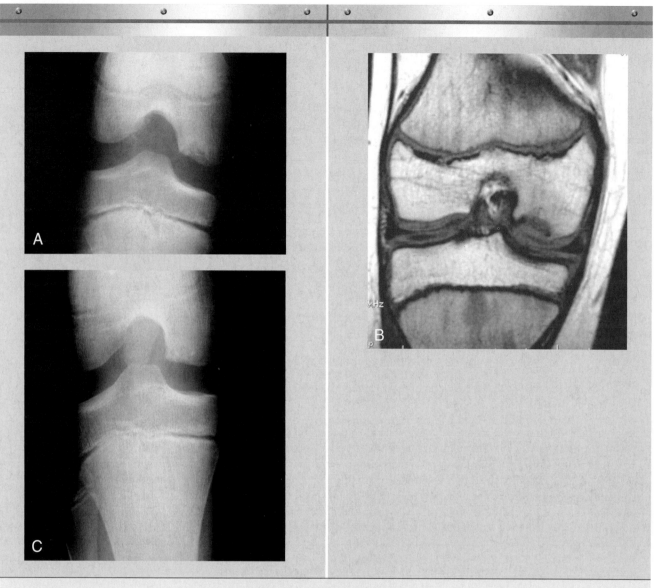

AT THE VIEWBOX

Adolescent male, active in sports, with ongoing knee pain, with transient episodes of a locking sensation. A tunnel view of the knee (**A**) demonstrates a large, irregular defect in the medial femoral condyle, characteristic of osteochondritis dissecans. MRI allows excellent visualization of the lesion, along with assessing the menisci and ligaments, including the medial and lateral collateral ligaments (**B**). The patient was managed conservatively, with restriction of activities and non-weight bearing for six weeks, with gradual resolution of pain and eventual return to activity. Follow-up radiograph (**C**) showed evidence of healing, including decrease in articular surface irregularity. The degree of change in imaging findings varies considerably and does not necessarily correlate with the clinical course of osteochondritis dissecans. (From the teaching file of Timothy Mick, DC, DACBR)

CRITICAL THINKING

1. Classify disruptions of knee ligamentous structures.
2. What is the triad of O'Donoghue?
3. How is the Q-angle measured?
4. How is posterior cruciate ligament injury tested?
5. What is the usual mechanism of injury for a meniscal tear?
6. What is the most common meniscal tear?
7. How is the McMurray test performed?
8. What is the most common congenital meniscal anomaly?
9. How is the Lachman test performed?
10. What is the posterior sag test?
11. What is varus deformity?
12. What is valgus deforming of the knee?
13. What is osteochondritis dissecans?
14. List the common sites of osteochondritis dissecans in the body.
15. Describe the cause of patellar fracture.
16. What is a convenient way to classify knee pain?
17. Knee stability depends on what four major ligaments and what tendon?
18. What is the name of the sesamoid bone that is present in approximately 10% to 30% of the general population? Why is it significant when present?
19. The three thigh muscles that attach to the medial side of the tibia are supplied by three different nerves. What nerve supplies which medial thigh muscle?
20. How many plain-film views of the knee are a common study for the clinician to evaluate the knee joint?
21. What is the most commonly injured ligament in the knee?
22. Describe the *unhappy triad* of the knee.
23. The severity of medial collateral ligament injuries can be classified by the amount of joint opening. List the four grades and the distance of joint opening to indicate the degree of instability.
24. What two tests are commonly used to aid in the diagnosis of a torn meniscus? List three indications of disease of the meniscus.
25. What condition is a predisposing factor to recurrent lateral dislocation of the patella?
26. What is a *bucket-handle tear,* and what is the mechanism?
27. Classify the three groups of patellar malacia.
28. What structures may be injured in a patient with a positive anterior drawer test?
29. A positive posterior drawer test might indicate injury what structures?
30. Iliotibial band (ITB) syndrome is caused primarily by what type of injury? What is the typical symptom presentation of ITB? Name the test that is helpful in arriving at your diagnosis.
31. Noncontact anterior cruciate ligament injury rates in women are reported to be three to eight times greater than that of men. Why?
32. Ruptures of the quadriceps and patellar tendon are more commonly seen in patients older than 40 years and are often associated with degenerative changes of the tendon. Name four conditions that are considered risk factors for this degeneration to occur.

BIBLIOGRAPHY

Abrahams S, Kern JH: Anterior knee pain: plica syndrome, the forgotten pathology? *Physiotherapy* 87(10):523-528, 2001.

Abrams WB, Berkow R: *The Merck manual of geriatrics,* Rahway, NJ, 1990, Merck Sharp & Dohme Research Laboratories.

Adachi N et al: The complete type of suprapatellar plica in a professional baseball pitcher: consideration of a cause of anterior knee pain, *Arthroscopy* 20(9):987-991, 2004.

Adams JC, Hamblen DL: *Outline of orthopaedics,* ed 11, Edinburgh, 1990, Churchill Livingstone.

Aegerter E, Kirkpatrick JA: *Orthopaedic diseases,* ed 3, Philadelphia, 1968, WB Saunders.

Alario AJ: *Practical guide to the care of the pediatric patient,* St Louis, 1997, Mosby.

Allison D, Strickland N: *Acronyms & synonyms in medical imaging,* Oxford, UK, 1996, ISIS Medical Media.

American Medical Association: *Guides to the evaluation of permanent impairment,* ed 4, Chicago, 1993, American Medical Association.

American Medical Association: *How to use guides to the evaluation of permanent impairment,* ed 4, Falmouth, Conn, 1993, SEAK.

Anderson KN, Anderson LE: *Mosby's pocket dictionary of medicine, nursing, & allied health,* ed 2, St Louis, 1994, Mosby.

Andrikoula SI et al: Intra-articular ganglia of the knee joint associated with the anterior cruciate ligament: a report of 4 cases in 3 patients, *Arthroscopy* (in press, corrected proof).

Aniel DM, Fritschy D: Anterior cruciate ligament injuries. In DeLee JC, Drez D, editors: *Orthopaedic sports medicine: principles and practice,* vol 2, Philadelphia, 1994, WB Saunders.

Apley AG, Solomon L: *Concise system of orthopaedics and fractures,* London, 1988, Butterworth-Heinemann.

Arnbjornson A et al: The natural history of recurrent dislocation of the patella, long-term results of conservative and operative treatment, *J Bone Joint Surg* 74B:140, 1992.

Assimakopoulos A et al: The innervation of the human meniscus, *Clin Orthop* 275:232, 1992.

Baker CL, Norwood LA, Hughston JC: Acute combined posterior and posterolateral instability of the knee, *Am J Sports Med* 12:204, 1984.

Barkauskas VH et al: *Health & physical assessment,* ed 2, St Louis, 1998, Mosby.

Barnett CH, Davies DV, MacConaill MA: *Synovial joints: their structure and mechanics,* New York, 1961, Longmans Green.

Barrack RL, Skinner HB: The sensory function of knee ligaments. In Daniel D et al, editors: *Knee ligaments: structure, function, injury and repair,* New York, 1990, Raven.

Bennell K et al: The nature of anterior knee pain following injection of hypertonic saline into the infrapatellar fat pad, *J Orthop Res* 22(1):116-121, 2004.

Bennett JG: Rehabilitation of patellofemoral joint dysfunction. In Greenfield BH, editor: *Rehabilitation of the knee: a problem solving approach,* Philadelphia, 1994, FA Davis.

Berry JD, Rowbotham MC, Petersen KL: Complex regional pain syndrome-like symptoms during herpes zoster, *Pain* 110(1-2):8-9, 2004.

Beynnon BD et al: Anterior cruciate ligament strain behavior during rehabilitation exercises in vivo, *Am J Sports Med* 23:24, 1995.

Brooks M, Evans R, Fairclough J: *Sports injuries,* ed 2, London, 1992, Gower Medical.

Brotzman SB: *Clinical orthopaedic rehabilitation,* St Louis, 1996, Mosby.

Brown DE, Neumann RD: *Orthopedic secrets,* Philadelphia, 1995, Hanley & Belfus.

Bucholz RW: *Orthopaedic decision making,* ed 2, St Louis, 1996, Mosby.

Butler DL, Noyes FR, Grood ES: Ligamentous restraints to anterior-posterior drawer in the human knee, *J Bone Joint Surg* 622A:259, 1980.

Cailliet R: *Knee pain and disability,* ed 2, Philadelphia, 1983, FA Davis.

Campbell JB, Campbell JM: *Mosby's survival guide to medical abbreviations & acronyms prefixes & suffixes symbols Greek alphabet,* St Louis, 1995, Mosby.

Canale ST: *Campbell's operative orthopaedics,* vol 1-4, ed 9, St Louis, 1998, Mosby.

Chhabra A et al: The arthroscopic appearance of a normal anterior cruciate ligament in a posterior cruciate ligament-deficient knee: the posterolateral bundle (PLB) sign, *Arthroscopy* 21(10):1267.e1-1267.e3, 2005.

Childress HM: Popliteal cysts associated with undiagnosed posterior lesions of the medial meniscus, *J Bone Joint Surg* 52A:1487, 1970.

Chow JW et al: Reliability of a technique for determining sagittal knee geometry from lateral knee radiographs, *Knee* 13(4):318-323, 2006.

Cipriano JJ: *Photographic manual of regional orthopaedic and neurological test,* ed 3, Baltimore, 1997, Williams & Wilkins.

Clancy WG: Tendon trauma and overuse injuries. In Leadbetter WB, Buckwalter JA, Gordon SL, editors: *Sports-induced inflammation: clinical and basic science concepts,* Park Ridge, Ill, 1990, AAOS.

Clancy WG: Repair and reconstruction of the posterior cruciate ligament. In Chapman MW, editor: *Operative orthopaedics,* vol 2, Philadelphia, 1993, JB Lippincott.

Cohn RE: *Impairment rating examination and disability evaluation,* ed 3, Wilkesboro, NC, 1994, R Ernest Cohn.

Cormack DH: *Essential histology,* Philadelphia, 1993, Lippincott.

Corso SJ, Thal R, Forman D: Locked patellar dislocation with vertical axis rotation, *Clin Orthop* 279:190, 1992.

Covey DC, Sapega AA: Current concepts review, injuries of the posterior cruciate ligament, *J Bone Joint Surg* 75A:1376, 1993.

Crawford EJ, Emery RJ, Archrogh PM: Stable osteochondritis dissecans-does the lesion unite? *J Bone Joint Surg* 72B:320, 1990.

Crenshaw AH, editor: *Campbell's operative orthopedics,* ed 8, St Louis, 1992, Mosby.

Crosby EB, Insall J: Recurrent dislocation of the patella, *J Bone Joint Surg* 58A:9, 1976.

Dambro MR, Griffith JA: *Griffith's 5 minute clinical consult,* Baltimore, 1997, Williams & Wilkins.

D'Ambrogio KJ, Roth GB: *Positional release therapy: assessment & treatment of musculoskeletal dysfunction,* St Louis, 1997, Mosby.

D'Ambrosia RD: *Musculoskeletal disorders: regional examination and differential diagnosis,* Philadelphia, 1977, JB Lippincott.

Dandy DJ: *Essential orthopaedics and trauma,* Edinburgh, 1989, Churchill Livingstone.

Dandy DJ, Jackson RW: The impact of arthroscopy on the management of disorders of the knee, *J Bone Joint Surg* 57B:346, 1975.

Daniels DM, Stone ML: KT-1000 anterior-posterior displacement measurements. In Daniels DM, Akeson WH, O'Connor JJ, editors: *Knee ligament: structure, function, injury and repair,* New York, 1990, Raven.

DeLee JC, Drez D, editors: *Orthopedic sports medicine: principles and practice,* Philadelphia, 1994, WB Saunders.

Del Notaro C, Hug T: Intra-articular hemangioma of the knee as a cause of knee pain, *Arthroscopy* 19(6):e12-e14, 2003.

Deltoff MN, Kogon PL: *The portable skeletal x-ray library,* St Louis, 1998, Mosby.

Demeter SL, Andersson GBJ, Smith GM: *Disability evaluation,* St Louis, 1996, Mosby.

Deshpande JK, Tobias JD: *The pediatric pain handbook,* St Louis, 1996, Mosby.

Detenbeck LC: Function of the cruciate ligaments in knee stability, *Am J Sports Med* 2:217, 1974.

Dettenmeier PA: *Radiographic assessment for nurses,* St Louis, 1995, Mosby.

11

Diamantopoulos A et al: The posterolateral corner of the knee: evaluation under microsurgical dissection, *Arthroscopy* 21(7):826-833, 2005.

Dijkstra PU et al: Phantom pain and risk factors: a multivariate analysis, *J Pain Symptom Manage* 24(6):578-585, 2002.

Dinham JM: Popliteal cysts in children, *J Bone Joint Surg* 57B:69, 1975.

Doherty M: *Color atlas and text of osteoarthritis,* London, 1994, Wolfe.

Doherty M, George E: *Self-assessment picture tests in rheumatology,* London, 1995, Mosby-Wolfe.

Donell S: Patellofemoral dysfunction—extensor mechanism malalignment, *Curr Orthop* 20(2):103-111, 2006.

Doucette SA, Goble EM: The effect of exercise on patellar tracking in lateral patellar compression syndrome, *Am J Sports Med* 20:434, 1992.

Dunaway DJ et al: The sartorial branch of the saphenous nerve: its anatomy at the joint line of the knee, *Arthroscopy* 21(5):547-551, 2005.

Ehrlich M, Hulstyn M, D'Amoto C: Sports injuries in children and the clumsy child, *Pediatr Clin North Am* 39:433, 1992.

Eifert-Mangine M et al: Patellar tendinitis in the recreational athlete, *Orthopedics* 15:1359, 1992.

Elias DA, White LM: Imaging of patellofemoral disorders, *Clin Radiol* 59(7):543-557, 2004.

Elster AD: *Questions and answers in magnetic resonance imaging,* St Louis, 1994, Mosby.

Engle RP, Meade TD, Canner BC: Rehabilitation of posterior cruciate ligament injuries. In Greenfield BH, editor: *Rehabilitation of the knee: a problem solving approach,* Philadelphia, 1993, FA Davis.

Epstein O et al: *Clinical examination,* ed 2, London, 1997, Mosby.

Fanelli GC, Orcutt DR, Edson CJ: The multiple-ligament injured knee: evaluation, treatment, and results, *Arthroscopy* 21(4):471-486, 2005.

Federico DJ, Lynch JK, Jokl P: Osteochondritis dissecans of the knee: a historical review of etiology and treatment, *Arthroscopy* 6:190, 1990.

Fetto JF, Marshall JL: Injury to the anterior cruciate ligament producing the pivot shift sign: an experimental study on cadaver specimens, *J Bone Joint Surg* 61A:710, 1979.

Ficat RP, Hungerford DS: *Disorders of the patello-femoral joint,* Baltimore, 1977, Williams & Wilkins.

Firer P: Aetiology and results of treatment of iliotibial band friction syndrome, *J Bone Joint Surg* 72B:742, 1990.

Frank ED et al: *Merrill's atlas of radiographic positioning and procedures,* ed 11, St Louis, 2007, Mosby.

Franz WB III: Overuse syndromes in runners. In Mellion MB, Walsh WM, Shelton GL, editors: *Sports injuries and athletic problems,* Philadelphia, 1990, Hanley & Belfus.

Fu FH, Baratz M: Meniscal injuries. In DeLee JC, Drez D, editors: *Orthopaedic sports medicine: principals and practice,* vol 2, Philadelphia, 1994, WB Saunders.

Fulkerson JP, Hungerford DS: *Disorders of the patellofemoral joint,* Baltimore, 1990, Williams & Wilkins.

Fulkerson JP, Shea KP: Current concepts review disorders of patellofemoral alignment, *J Bone Joint Surg* 72A:1424, 1990.

Furman W, Marshall JL, Girgis FG: The anterior cruciate ligaments: a functional analysis based on postmortem studies, *J Bone Joint Surg* 58A:179, 1976.

Gaine WJ, Mohammed A: Osteophyte impingement of the popliteus tendon as a cause of lateral knee joint pain, *Knee* 9(3):249-252, 2002.

Galland O et al: An anatomical and radiological study of the femoropatellar articulation, *Surg Radiol Anat* 12:119, 1990.

Galway HR, MacIntosh DL: The lateral pivot shift: symptoms and sign of anterior cruciate ligament insufficiency, *Clin Orthop* 147:45, 1980.

Garret JC: Osteochondritis dissecans, *Clin Orthop Sports Med* 10:569, 1991.

Garth WB: Current concepts regarding the anterior cruciate ligament, *Orthop Rev* 21:565, 1992.

Gartland JJ: *Fundamentals of orthopedics,* ed 2, Philadelphia, 1974, WB Saunders.

Gatehouse PD et al: Magnetic resonance imaging of the knee with ultra-short TE pulse sequences, *Magn Reson Imaging* 22(8):1061-1067, 2004.

George M, Wall EJ: Locked knee caused by meniscal subluxation: magnetic resonance imaging and arthroscopic verification, *Arthroscopy* 19(8):885-888, 2003.

Gerard JA, Kleinfield SL: *Orthopaedic testing,* New York, 1993, Churchill Livingstone.

Gillis L: *Diagnosis in orthopaedics,* London, 1969, Butterworths.

Girgis FG, Marshall JL, Al Monajem ARS: The cruciate ligaments of the knee joint: anatomical, functional and experimental analysis, *Clin Orthop* 106:216, 1975.

Goldie BS: *Orthopaedic diagnosis and management: a guide to the care of orthopaedic patients,* ed 2, Oxford, UK, 1998, ISIS Medical Media.

Goldstein RS: Geriatric orthopaedics, rehabilitative management of common problems. In Lewis CB, editor: *Aspen series in physical therapy,* Gaithersburg, Md, 1991, Aspen.

Goodfellow J, Hungerford DS, Woods C: Patello-femoral joint mechanics and pathology: chondromalacia patella, *J Bone Joint Surg* 58B:291, 1976.

Goodfellow J, Hungerford DS, Zindel M: Patello-femoral joint mechanics and pathology: functional anatomy of the patello-femoral joint, *J Bone Joint Surg* 58B:287, 1976.

Greenstein GM: *Clinical assessment of neuromusculoskeletal disorders,* St Louis, 1997, Mosby.

Grelsamer RP, Meadows S: The modified Insall-Salvati ratio for assessment of patellar height, *Clin Orthop* 282:170, 1992.

Grelsamer RP, Proctor CS, Bazos AN: Evaluation of patellar shape in the sagittal plane: a clinical analysis, *Am J Sports Med* 22:61, 1994.

Grelsamer RP, Tedder JL: The lateral trochlear sign: femoral trochlear dysplasia as seen on a lateral view roentgenograph, *Clin Orthop* 281:159, 1992.

Grossman ZD et al: *Cost-effective diagnostic imaging: the clinician's guide,* ed 3, St Louis, 1995, Mosby.

Guzzanti V et al: Patellofemoral malalignment in adolescents: computerized tomographic assessment with or without quadriceps contraction, *Am J Sports Med* 22:55, 1994.

Halperin JL: Evaluation of patients with peripheral vascular disease, *Thromb Res* 106(6):V303-V311, 2002.

Hammer WI: *Functional soft tissue examination and treatment by manual methods: the extremities,* Gaithersburg, Md, 1991, Aspen.

Handelberg FM, Shahabpour M, Casteleyn PP: Chondral lesions of the patella evaluated with computed tomography, magnetic resonance imaging, and arthroscopy, *Arthroscopy* 6:24, 1990.

Harner CD et al: Loss of motion after anterior cruciate ligament reconstruction, *Am J Sports Med* 20:499, 1992.

Hartley A: *Practical joint assessment: lower quadrant,* ed 2, St Louis, 1995, Mosby.

Hawkins RJ: *An organized approach to musculoskeletal examination and history taking,* St Louis, 1995, Mosby.

Hede A, Hempel-Poulson S, Jensen JS: Symptoms and level of sports activity in patients awaiting arthroscopy for meniscal lesions of the knee, *J Bone Joint Surg* 72A:550, 1990.

Helfet AJ: *Disorder of the knee,* Philadelphia, 1974, JB Lippincott.

Henigan SP et al: The semimembranosus-tibial collateral ligament bursa, *J Bone Joint Surg* 76A:1322, 1994.

Henry JH: Conservative treatment of patellofemoral subluxation, *Clin Sports Med* 8:261, 1989.

Hinkle CZ: *Fundamentals of anatomy & movement: a workbook and guide,* St Louis, 1997, Mosby.

Hornberger JP: *Exercise physiology therapeutic exercise,* Sarasota, Fla, 1991, Joseph P Hornberger.

Hughston J: *Knee ligaments: injury and repair,* St Louis, 1993, Mosby.

Hughston JC et al: The classification of knee ligament instabilities. Part I. The medial compartment and cruciate ligaments, *J Bone Joint Surg* 58A:159, 1976.

Hughston JC, Norwood LA: The posterolateral drawer and external rotational recurvatum test for posterolateral rotary instability of the knee, *Clin Orthop* 147:82, 1980.

Hughston JC, Walsh WM, Puddu G: *Patellar subluxation and dislocation,* Philadelphia, 1984, WB Saunders.

Hughston JC et al: The classification of knee ligament instabilities. Part II. The lateral compartment, *J Bone Joint Surg* 58A:173, 1976.

Inaba Y et al: Provoked anterior knee pain in medial osteoarthritis of the knee, *Knee* 10(4):351-355, 2003.

Indelicato PA, Hermansdorfer J, Huegel M: The nonoperative management of complete tears of the medial collateral ligament of the knee in intercollegiate football players, *Clin Orthop* 256:174, 1990.

Indelicato PA et al: Clinical comparison of freeze-dried/fresh frozen patella tendon allografts for anterior cruciate ligament reconstruction of the knee, *Am J Sports Med* 18:335, 1990.

Ingebretsen L et al: A prospective, randomized study of three surgical techniques for treatment of acute ruptures of the anterior cruciate ligament, *Am J Sports Med* 18:585, 1990.

Insall J, Falvo KA, Wise DW: Chondromalacia patella, *J Bone Joint Surg* 58A:1, 1976.

Jablonski S: *Dictionary of medical acronyms & abbreviations,* ed 3, Philadelphia, 1998, Hanley & Belfus.

Jackson RW, Kunkel SS, Taylor GJ: Lateral retinacular release for patellofemoral pain in the older patient, *Arthroscopy* 7:283, 1991.

Jakob RP, Hassler H, Staeubli HU: Observations on rotary instability of the lateral compartment of the knee, *Acta Orthop Scand Suppl* 191:1, 1981.

James SL: Running injuries to the knee, *J Am Acad Orthop Surg* 3:309, 1995.

Jensen R et al: Quantitative sensory testing of patients with long lasting patellofemoral pain syndrome, *Eur J Pain* (in press, corrected proof).

Johansson H, Sjolander P, Sojka P: A sensory role for the cruciate ligaments, *Clin Orthop* 268:161, 1991.

Johnson DP, Eastwood DM, Witherow PJ: Symptomatic synovial plicae of the knee, *J Bone Joint Surg* 75A:1485, 1992.

Jonsson T et al: Clinical diagnosis of ruptures of the anterior cruciate ligament: a comparative study of the Lachman test and the anterior drawer sign, *Am J Sports Med* 10:100, 1982.

Junqueira LC, Carneiro J, Kelly RO: *Basic histology,* ed 7, Norwalk, Conn, 1992, Appleton & Lange.

Kalebo P et al: Ultrasonography in the detection of partial patellar ligament ruptures (jumper's knee), *Skeletal Radiol* 20:285, 1991.

Kanner R: *Pain management secrets,* Philadelphia, 1997, Hanley & Belfus.

Karlson J et al: Partial rupture of the patellar ligament, *Am J Sports Med* 19:403, 1992.

Katirji B: *Electromyography in clinical practice: a case study approach,* St Louis, 1998, Mosby.

Kato S et al: Glomus tumor beneath the plica synovialis in the knee: a case report, *Knee* 14(2):164-166, 2007.

Katz WA: *Rheumatic diseases diagnosis and management,* Philadelphia, 1977, JB Lippincott.

Kaufman RL: Popliteal aneurysm as a cause of leg pain in a geriatric patient, *J Manipulative Physiol Ther* 27(6):427-557, 2004.

Keats TE: *Atlas of roentgenographic measurement,* ed 6, St Louis, 1990, Mosby.

Kendall HO, Kendall RP, Wadsworth GE: *Muscles: testing and function,* ed 3, Baltimore, 1992, Williams & Wilkins.

Kennedy JC: *The injured adolescent knee,* Baltimore, 1979, Williams & Wilkins.

Kerimoglu S et al: Bucket-handle tear of medial plica, *Knee* 12(3):239-241, 2005.

King JB et al: Lesions of the patellar ligament, *J Bone Joint Surg* 72B:46, 1990.

Klippel JH, Dieppe PA: *Rheumatology,* vol 1-2, ed 2, London, 1998, Mosby.

Koenigsberg R: *Churchill's illustrated medical dictionary,* New York, 1989, Churchill Livingstone.

Kolowich PA et al: Lateral release of the patella: indications and contraindications, *Am J Sports Med* 18:359, 1990.

Koshino T: Changes in patellofemoral compressive force after anterior or anteromedial displacement of tibial tuberosity for chondromalacia patellae, *Clin Orthop* 266:133, 1991.

Koskinen SK, Hurme M, Kujala UM: Restoration of patellofemoral congruity by combined lateral release and tibial tuberosity transposition as assessed by MRI analysis, *Int Orthop* 15:363, 1991.

Krauspe R, Schmidt M, Schaible H: Sensory and innervation of the anterior cruciate ligament, *J Bone Joint Surg* 74A:390, 1992.

Kujula UM et al: Scoring of patellofemoral disorders, *Arthroscopy* 9:159, 1993.

Kursunoglu-Brahme S, Resnick D: Magnetic resonance imaging of the knee, *Orthop Clin North Am* 21:561, 1990.

Lakdawala A, El-Zebdeh M, Ireland J: Excision of a ganglion cyst from within the posterior septum of the knee—an arthroscopic technique, *Knee* 12(3):245-247, 2005.

Lange AK et al: Degenerative meniscus tears and mobility impairment in women with knee osteoarthritis, *Osteoarthr Cartil* 15(6):701-708, 2007.

Laskin RS: Total condylar knee replacement in patients who have rheumatoid arthritis, *J Bone Joint Surg* 72A:529, 1990.

Laurin CA et al: The abnormal lateral patellofemoral angle: a diagnostic roentgenographic sign of recurrent patellar subluxation, *J Bone Joint Surg* 60A:55, 1978.

Lavy CBD, Barrett DS: *Questions and answers on Apley's concise system of orthopaedics and fractures,* Oxford, UK, 1991, Butterworth-Heinemann.

Lee CC, Vainchenker U, Crupi RS: Ten-year-old boy with a swollen knee: unusual cause of knee pain, *J Emerg Med* 25(4):449-450, 2003.

Leon HO et al: Intercondylar notch stenosis in degenerative arthritis of the knee, *Arthroscopy* 21(3):294-302, 2005.

Lerner AJ: *The little black book of neurology,* ed 3, St Louis, 1995, Mosby.

Lewallen DG et al: Effects of retinacular release and tibial tubercle elevation in patellofemoral degenerative joint disease, *J Orthop Res* 8:856, 1990.

Lewis CB, Knortz KA: *Orthopedic assessment and treatment of the geriatric patient,* St Louis, 1993, Mosby.

Linton RC, Indelicato PA: Medial ligament injuries. In DeLee JC, Drez D, editors: *Orthopedic sports medicine: principles and practice,* vol 1, Philadelphia, 1994, WB Saunders.

Lipscomb PR Jr., Lipscomb PR Sr, Bryan RS: Osteochondritis dissecans of the knee with loose fragments, *J Bone Joint Surg* 60A:235, 1978.

Liu P-C et al: Snapping knee symptoms caused by an intra-articular ganglion cyst, *Knee* 14(2):167-168, 2007.

Losee RE, Ennis TRJ, Southwick WO: Anterior subluxation of the lateral tibial plateau: a diagnostic test and operative review, *J Bone Joint Surg* 60A:1015, 1978.

Loth TS: *Orthopedic boards review II: a case study approach,* St Louis, 1996, Mosby.

Lougher L, Southgate CRW, Holt MD: Coronary ligament rupture as a cause of medial knee pain, *Arthroscopy* 19(10):e157-e158, 2003.

MacAusland WR, Mayo RA: *Orthopedics: a concise guide to clinical practices,* Boston, 1965, Little, Brown.

Magee DJ: *Orthopedic physical assessment,* ed 3, Philadelphia, 1997, WB Saunders.

Main WK, Scott WN: Knee anatomy. In Scott WN, editor: *Ligament and extensor mechanism injuries of the knee, diagnosis and treatment,* St Louis, 1991, Mosby.

Malone TR, McPoil TG, Nitz AJ: *Orthopedic and sports physical therapy,* ed 3, St Louis, 1997, Mosby.

Maquet PGJ: *Biomechanics of the knee: with application of the pathogenesis and the surgical treatment of osteoarthritis,* New York, 1976, Springer-Verlag.

11

Marchiori DM: *Clinical imaging with skeletal, chest, and abdomen pattern differentials,* St Louis, 1999, Mosby.

Mariani PP, Mauro CS, Margheritini F: Arthroscopic diagnosis of the snapping popliteus tendon, *Arthroscopy* 21(7):888-892, 2005.

Martin AF: The pathomechanics of the knee joint, *J Bone Joint Surg* 42A:13, 1960.

Martin JH: *Neuroanatomy text and atlas,* ed 2, Stamford, Conn, 1996, Appleton & Lange.

Mathers LH et al: *Clinical anatomy principles,* St Louis, 1996, Mosby.

Mazion JM: *Illustrated manual of neurological reflexes/signs/tests, part I, orthopedic signs/tests/maneuvers for office procedure, part II,* Orlando, Fla, 1980, Daniels Publishing.

McMurray TP: *The Robert joint birthday volume,* London, 1928, Humphrey Milford.

McMurray TP: The semilunar cartilages, *Br J Surg* 29:407, 1942.

McPherson A et al: Imaging knee position using MRI, RSA/CT and 3D digitisation, *J Biomech* 38(2):263-268, 2005.

McPherson T: Benign tumors of fibrous tissue and adipose tissue of the hand, *J Hand Ther* 18(1):53-54, 2005.

McRae R: *Clinical orthopaedic examination,* ed 3, Edinburgh, 1990, Churchill Livingston.

McRae R: *Practical fracture treatment,* ed 3, Edinburgh, 1994, Churchill-Livingstone.

Medical Economics Books: *Patient care flow chart manual,* ed 3, Oradell, NJ, 1982, Medical Economics Books.

Mellion MB: *Sports medicine secrets,* Philadelphia, 1994, Hanley & Belfus.

Mellion MB: *Office sports medicine,* ed 2, St Louis, 1996, Mosby.

Mengel MB, Schwiebert LP: *Ambulatory medicine: the primary care of families,* ed 2, Stamford, Conn, 1996, Appleton & Lange.

Mennell JM: *The musculoskeletal system: differential diagnosis from symptoms and physical signs,* Gaithersburg, Md, 1992, Aspen.

Merchant AC: Patellofemoral malalignment and instabilities. In Ewing JW, editor: *Articular cartilage and knee joint function: basic science and arthroscopy,* New York, 1990, Raven.

Merchant AC: Patellofemoral disorders, biomechanics, diagnosis, and non-operative treatment. In McGinty JB, editor: *Operative arthroscopy,* New York, 1991, Raven.

Merchant AC: Radiologic evaluation of the patellofemoral joint. In Aichroth PM, Cannon WD, editors: *Knee surgery,* London, 1992, Martin Dunitz.

Mercier LR, Pettid FJ: *Practical orthopedics,* ed 4, St Louis, 1995, Mosby.

Miller M: *Review of orthopaedics,* Philadelphia, 1992, WB Saunders.

Minns RJ: The role of gait analysis in the management of the knee, *Knee* 12(3):157-162, 2005.

Mirkopulos N, Myer TJ: Isolated avulsion of the popliteus tendon, *Am J Sports Med* 19:417, 1991.

Moore KL: *Clinically oriented anatomy,* ed 3, Baltimore, 1992, Williams & Wilkins.

Mori Y et al: Lateral retinaculum release in adolescent patellofemoral disorders: its relationship to peripheral nerve injury in the lateral retinaculum, *Bull Hosp J Dis Orthop* 51:218, 1991.

Mosby-Year Book, Inc: *Expert 10-minute physical examination,* St Louis, 1997, Mosby.

Muller W: *The knee: form, function and ligament reconstruction,* New York, 1983, Springer-Verlag.

Munetea T et al: Computerized tomographic analysis of tibial tubercle position in the painful female patellofemoral joint, *Am J Sports Med* 22:67, 1994.

Munuera L, Reinoso F, Martinez-Moreno E: *The innervation of the anterior cruciate ligament and the patellar ligament of the knee* [thesis], Madrid, 1992, Universidad Autonoma.

Murray KJ: Hypermobility disorders in children and adolescents, *Best Pract Res Clin Rheumatol* 20(2):329-351, 2006.

Myllymaki T et al: Ultrasonography of jumper's knee, *Acta Radiol* 31:47, 1990.

Neumann RD: Traumatic knee injuries. In Mellion MB, editor: *Sports medicine secrets,* Philadelphia, 1994, Hanley & Belfus.

Neuschwander D, Drez D, Finney T: Lateral meniscal variant with absence of the posterior coronary ligament, *J Bone Joint Surg* 74A:1186, 1992.

Nicholas JA: The five-one reconstruction for anteromedial instability of the knee, *J Bone Joint Surg* 55A:899, 1973.

Nicholas JA, Hershman EB: *The lower extremity & spine in sports medicine,* vol 1-2, ed 2, St Louis, 1995, Mosby.

Niitsu M: Moving knee joint: technique for kinematic MR imaging, *Radiology* 174:569, 1990.

Noble HB, Hajek MR, Porter M: Diagnosis and treatment of iliotibial band tightness in runners, *Sports Med* 10:67, 1984.

Nordin M, Andersson GBJ, Pope MH: *Musculoskeletal disorders in the workplace: principles and practice,* St Louis, 1997, Mosby.

Noyes FR et al: Clinical paradoxes of anterior cruciate instability and a new test to detect its instability, *Orthop Trans* 2:36, 1978.

Noyes FR et al: The anterior cruciate ligament-deficient knee with varus alignment, *Am J Sports Med* 20:707, 1992.

Noyes FR et al: Posterior subluxations of the medial and lateral tibiofemoral compartments: an in vitro ligament sectioning study in cadaveric knees, *Am J Sports Med* 21:407, 1993.

O'Connor J et al: Geometry of the knee. In Daniel D, editor: *Knee ligaments: structure, function, injury and repair,* New York, 1990, Raven.

O'Donoghue DH: *Treatment of injuries to athletes,* ed 3, Philadelphia, 1976, WB Saunders.

Ogilvie-Harris DJ, Basinski A: Arthroscopic synovectomy of the knee for rheumatoid arthritis, *Arthroscopy* 7:91, 1991.

Olson WH et al: *Handbook of symptom-oriented neurology,* ed 2, St Louis, 1994, Mosby.

Omer GE, Spinner M: *Management of peripheral nerve problems,* Philadelphia, 1980, WB Saunders.

Pagana KD, Pagana TJ: *Mosby's manual of diagnostic and laboratory tests,* St Louis, 1998, Mosby.

Pagnani M, Cooper D, Warren R: Extrusion of the medial meniscus: case report, *Arthroscopy* 7:297, 1991.

Palumbo RC et al: Ligamentous injuries to the knee: a retrospective analysis, *Orthop Trans* 16:321, 1992.

Patten J: *Neurological differential diagnosis,* ed 2, London, 1996, Springer.

Peace KAL, Lee JC, Healy J: Imaging the infrapatellar tendon in the elite athlete, *Clin Radiol* 61(7):570-578, 2006.

Peat G et al: How reliable is structured clinical history-taking in older adults with knee problems?: Inter- and intraobserver variability of the KNE-SCI, *J Clin Epidemiol* 56(11):1030-1037, 2003.

Pecina MM, Krmpotic-Nemanic J, Markiewitz AD: *Tunnel syndromes,* Boca Raton, Fla, 1991, CRC.

Pfeiffer WH, Gross JL, Seeger LL: Osteochondritis dissecans of the patella, *Clin Orthop* 271:207, 1991.

Pheasant S: *Ergonomics, work and health,* Gaithersburg, Md, 1991, Aspen.

Polley HF, Hunder GG: *Rheumatologic interviewing and physical examination of the joints,* ed 2, Philadelphia, 1978, WB Saunders.

Pope CF: Radiologic evaluation of tendon injuries, *Clin Sports Med* 11:579, 1992.

Rajadhyaksha AD, Mont MA, Becker L: An unusual cause of knee pain 10 years after arthroscopy, *Arthroscopy* 22(11):1253.e1-1253.e3, 2006.

Ravel R: *Clinical laboratory medicine: clinical application of laboratory data,* ed 6, St Louis, 1995, Mosby.

Renne JW: The iliotibial band friction syndrome, *J Bone Joint Surg* 57A:1110, 1975.

Rethnam U, Sinha A: Instability of the proximal tibiofibular joint, an unusual cause for knee pain, *Injury Extra* 37(5):190-192, 2006.

Ricklin P, Ruttiman A, Del Buono MA: *Meniscus lesions: practical problems of clinical diagnosis, arthrography and therapy,* New York, 1971, Grune & Stratton.

Rizzello G et al: Para-articular osteochondroma of the knee, *Arthroscopy* (in press, corrected proof).

Robertson A et al: The fabella: a forgotten source of knee pain? *Knee* 11(3):243-245, 2004.

Rockwood CA, Green DP, Bucholz R, editors: *Rockwood and Green's fractures in adults,* vol 2, ed 3, Philadelphia, 1991, JB Lippincott.

Rolak LA: *Neurology secrets,* ed 2, Philadelphia, 1998, Hanley & Belfus.

Royle SC et al: The significance of chondromalacic changes on the patella, *Arthroscopy* 7:158, 1991.

Rumack CM, Wilson SR, Charboneau JW: *Diagnostic ultrasound,* vol 1-2, ed 2, St Louis, 1998, Mosby.

Saidoff DC, McDonough AL: *Critical pathways in therapeutic intervention,* St Louis, 1997, Mosby.

Satterfield WH, Johnson DL: Arthroscopic patellar "bankart" repair after acute dislocation, *Arthroscopy* 21(5):627.e1-627.e5, 2005.

Schenck RC, Heckman JD: Injuries of the knee, *Clin Symp* 45(1):1-32, 1993.

Schindler OS: Synovial plicae of the knee, *Curr Orthop* 18(3):210-219, 2004.

Schumacher HR, Klippel JH, Koopman WJ: *Primer on the rheumatic diseases,* ed 10, Atlanta, 1993, Arthritis Foundation.

Scott WN: *The knee,* vol 1-2, St Louis, 1994, Mosby.

Scranton PE et al: Mucoid degeneration of the patellar ligament in athletes, *J Bone Joint Surg* 74A:435, 1992.

Sebast C, Denelli WJ: Osteochondrosis. In DeLee JC, Drez D, editors: *Orthopedic sports medicine: principles and practice,* vol 1, Philadelphia, 1994, WB Saunders.

Sebastianelli WJ et al: Isolated avulsion of the biceps femoris insertion, *Clin Orthop* 259:200, 1990.

Seto JL, Brewster CE: Rehabilitation of meniscal injuries. In Greenfield BH, editor: *Rehabilitation of the knee: a problem-solving approach,* Philadelphia, 1993, FA Davis.

Shankman GA: *Fundamental orthopedic management for the physical therapist assistant,* St Louis, 1997, Mosby.

Shea KG, Nilsson K, Belzer J: Patellar dislocation in skeletally immature athletes, *Oper Tech Sports Med* 14(3):188-196, 2006.

Shelbourne KD, Nitz PA: The O'Donoghue triad revisited, *Am J Sports Med* 19:474, 1991.

Shelbourne KD, Porter DA: Anterior cruciate ligament-medial collateral ligament injury: non-operative management of medial collateral ligament tears with anterior cruciate reconstruction, *Am J Sports Med* 20:283, 1992.

Shelbourne KD et al: Arthrofibrosis in acute anterior cruciate ligament reconstructions, *Am J Sports Med* 19:332, 1991.

Shellock FG et al: Evaluation of patients with persistent symptoms after lateral retinacular release by kinematic magnetic resonance imaging of the patellofemoral joint, *Arthroscopy* 6:226, 1990.

Shelton GL, Thigpen LK: Rehabilitation of patellofemoral dysfunction: a review of literature, *J Orthop Sports Phys Ther* 14:243, 1991.

Shino K et al: Reconstruction of the anterior cruciate ligament using allogenic tendon, *Am J Sports Med* 18:457, 1990.

Simmons E, Cameron JC: Patella alta and recurrent dislocation of the patella, *Clin Orthop* 274:265, 1992.

Sisk TD: Knee realignment and replacement in the recreational athlete. In DeLee JC, Drez D, editors: *Orthopaedic sports medicine: principals and practice,* vol 2, Philadelphia, 1994, WB Saunders.

Slocum DB, Larson RL: Rotary instability of the knee, *J Bone Joint Surg* 50A:211, 1968.

Slocum DB et al: A clinical test for anterolateral rotary instability of the knee, *Clin Orthop* 118:63, 1976.

Smillie IS: *Injuries of the knee joint,* Edinburgh, 1970, E & S Livingstone.

Smillie IS: *Diseases of the knee joint,* New York, 1974, Longmans.

Solomonow M, D'Ambrosia R: Neural reflex arcs and muscle control of knee stability and motion. In Scott NW, editor: *Ligament and extensor mechanism injuries of the knee, diagnosis and treatment,* St Louis, 1991, Mosby.

Specht NT, Russo RD: *Practical guide to diagnostic imaging,* St Louis, 1998, Mosby.

Spring H et al: *Stretching and strengthening exercises,* New York, 1991, Thieme.

Stanitski CL: Anterior knee pain syndromes in the adolescent, *J Bone Joint Surg* 75A:1407, 1993.

Staubli HU, Birrer S: The popliteus tendon and its fascicles at the popliteal hiatus: gross anatomy and functional arthroscopic evaluation with and without anterior cruciate ligament deficiency, *Arthroscopy* 6:209, 1990.

Stedman TL: *Stedman's medical dictionary,* ed 25, Baltimore, 1990, Williams & Wilkins.

Steensen RN, Dopirak RM, Maurus PB: Minimally invasive "crescentic" imbrication of the medial patellofemoral ligament for chronic patellar subluxation, *Arthroscopy* 21(3):371-375, 2005.

Steinkamp LA et al: Biomechanical consideration in patellofemoral joint rehabilitation, *Am J Sports Med* 21:438, 1993.

Stewart DL, Abeln SH: *Documenting functional outcomes in physical therapy,* St Louis, 1993, Mosby.

Stoller DW: *Magnetic resonance imaging in orthopaedics & sports medicine,* Philadelphia, 1993, JB Lippincott.

Strum GM et al: Acute anterior cruciate reconstructions, *Clin Orthop* 253;184, 1990.

Suh J-T, Cheon S-J, Choi S-J: Synovial hemangioma of the knee, *Arthroscopy* 19(7):e77-e80, 2003.

Sutton D, Young JWR: *A concise textbook of clinical imaging,* ed 2, St Louis, 1995, Mosby.

Tamea CD, Henning CD: Pathomechanics of the pivot shift maneuver, *Am J Sports Med* 9:31, 1981.

Tan JC, Horn SE: *Practical manual of physical medicine and rehabilitation,* St Louis, 1998, Mosby.

Taybi H, Lachman RS: *Radiology of syndromes, metabolic disorders, and skeletal dysplasias,* ed 4, St Louis, 1996, Mosby.

Taylor JC: Fractures of the lower extremity. In Crenshaw AH, editor: *Campbell's operative orthopedics,* ed 8, St Louis, 1992, Mosby.

Tenuta JJ, Arciero RA: Arthroscopic evaluation of meniscal repairs: factors that affect healing, *Am J Sports Med* 22:797, 1994.

Theruvil B et al: Vascular malformations in muscles around the knee presenting as knee pain, *Knee* 11(2):155-158, 2004.

Thibodeau GA, Patton KT: *Anatomy & physiology,* ed 3, St Louis, 1996, Mosby.

Thibodeau GA, Patton KT: *Pocket reference to accompany anatomy & physiology,* ed 3, St Louis, 1996, Mosby.

Timm K: Knee. In Richardson JK, Iglarsh ZA, editors: *Clinical orthopaedic physical therapy,* Philadelphia, 1994, WB Saunders.

Toghill PJ: *Examining patients: an introduction to clinical medicine,* London, 1990, Edward Arnold.

Tollison CD, Satterthwaite JR, Tollison JW: *Handbook of pain management,* ed 2, Baltimore, 1994, Williams & Wilkins.

Torg JS, Shepard RJ: *Current therapy in sports medicine,* ed 3, St Louis, 1995, Mosby.

Torres L et al: The relationship between specific tissue lesions and pain severity in persons with knee osteoarthritis, *Osteoarthr Cartil* 14(10):1033-1040, 2006.

Turek SL: *Orthopaedics principles and their application,* ed 3, Philadelphia, 1977, JB Lippincott.

Vail TP, Malone TR, Basset FH: Long-term functional results in patients with anterolateral rotatory instability treated by iliotibial band transfer, *Am J Sports Med* 20:274, 1992.

Vallejo MC et al: Piriformis syndrome in a patient after cesarean section under spinal anesthesia, *Reg Anesth Pain Med* 29(4):364-367, 2004.

Van Holsbeeck M, Introcaso JH: *Musculoskeletal ultrasound,* St Louis, 1991, Mosby.

Van Kampen A, Huiskes R: The three-dimensional tracking pattern of the human patella, *J Orthop Res* 8:372, 1990.

Vignon E et al: Osteoarthritis of the knee and hip and activity: a systematic international review and synthesis (OASIS), *Joint Bone Spine* 73(4):442-455, 2006.

Voight ML, Wieder DL: Comparative reflex response times of vastus medialis obliquus and vastus lateralis in normal subjects and subjects with

11

extensor mechanism dysfunction: an electromyographic study, *Am J Sports Med* 19:131, 1991.

Waldron VD: A test for chondromalacia patella, *Orthop Rev* 12:103, 1983.

Walsh WM: Patellofemoral joint. In DeLee JC, Drez D, editors: *Orthopaedic sports medicine: principles and practice,* vol 2, Philadelphia, 1994, WB Saunders.

Walsh WM, Helzer-Julin MJ: Patellar tracking problems in athletes, *Prim Care* 19:303, 1992.

Waseem M, Jari S, Paton RW: Glomus tumour, a rare cause of knee pain: a case report, *Knee* 9(2):161-163, 2002.

Watanabe Y et al: Functional anatomy of the posterolateral structures of the knee, *Arthroscopy* 9:57, 1993.

Waters P, Kasser J: Infection of the infrapatellar bursa, *J Bone Joint Surg* 72A:1095, 1990.

Weineck J: *Functional anatomy in sports,* ed 2, St Louis, 1990, Mosby.

Weinstein SL, Buckwalter JA: *Turek's orthopaedics principles and their application,* ed 5, Philadelphia, 1994, JB Lippincott.

Whitmore I, Willan PLT: *Multiple choice questions in human anatomy,* London, 1995, Mosby.

Wilk KE: Rehabilitation of medial capsular injuries. In Greenfield BH, editor: *Rehabilitation of the knee: a problem solving approach,* Philadelphia, 1993, FA Davis.

Wilson RM, Fowler P: Arthroscopic anatomy. In Scott WN, editor: *Arthroscopy of the knee: diagnosis and treatment,* Philadelphia, 1990, WB Saunders.

Windsor RE, Lox DM: *Soft tissue injuries: diagnosis and treatment,* Philadelphia, 1998, Hanley & Belfus.

Wiss DA: Supracondylar and intercondylar fractures of the femur. In Rockwood CA, Green DP, Bucholz RW, editors: *Rockwood and Green's fractures in adults,* ed 3, Philadelphia, 1991, JB Lippincott.

Woodland LH, Francis RS: Parameters and comparisons of the quadriceps angle of college-aged men and women in the supine and standing positions, *Am J Sports Med* 20:209, 1992.

Yates PJ et al: Early MRI diagnosis and non-surgical management of spontaneous osteonecrosis of the knee, *Knee* 14(2):112-116, 2007.

Zatouroff M: *Diagnosis in color physical signs in general medicine,* ed 2, London, 1996, Mosby-Wolfe.

Zitelli BJ, Davis HW: *Atlas of pediatric physical diagnosis,* ed 2, London, 1992, Wolfe.

CITATIONS

Bowers ME et al: Quantification of meniscal volume by segmentation of 3 T magnetic resonance images, *J Biomech* (in press, corrected proof).

Bozkurt M et al: The evaluation of the proximal tibiofibular joint for patients with lateral knee pain, *Knee* 11(4):307-312, 2004.

Chalidis BE et al: Management of periprosthetic patellar fractures: a systematic review of literature, *Injury* 38(6):714-724, 2007.

Donell S: Patellofemoral dysfunction—extensor mechanism malalignment, *Curr Orthop* 20(2):103-111, 2006.

Ellis R, Hing W, Reid D: Iliotibial band friction syndrome—a systematic review, *Man Ther* (in press, corrected proof).

Eren OT: The accuracy of joint line tenderness by physical examination in the diagnosis of meniscal tears, *Arthroscopy* 19(8):850-854, 2003.

Fairclough J et al: Is iliotibial band syndrome really a friction syndrome? *J Sci Med Sport* 10(2):74-76, 2007.

Franceschi F et al: Dislocation of an enlarged fabella as uncommon cause of knee pain: a case report, *Knee* 14(4):330-332, 2007.

Gerbino PG: Adolescent anterior knee pain, *Oper Tech Sports Med* 14(3):203-211, 2006.

Good CR et al: Arthroscopic treatment of symptomatic discoid meniscus in children: classification, technique, and results, *Arthroscopy* 23(2):157.e1-163.e1, 2007.

House CV, Connell DA, Saifuddin A: Posteromedial corner injuries of the knee, *Clin Radiol* 62(6):539-546, 2007.

Huang K-C, Hsu W-H, Wang T-C: Acute injury of anterior cruciate ligament during karate training, *Knee* 14(3):245-248, 2007.

Hurley WL, Boros RL, Challis JH: Influences of variation in force application on tibial displacement and strain in the anterior cruciate ligament during the Lachman test, *Clin Biomech* 19(1):95-98, 2004.

Irrgang JJ: Clinical outcomes after cartilage injury and repair, *Oper Tech Orthop* 16(4):286-2891, 2006.

Jensen R et al: Quantitative sensory testing of patients with long lasting patellofemoral pain syndrome, *Eur J Pain* (in press, corrected proof).

Kim S-J et al: New technique for chronic posterolateral instability of the knee: posterolateral reconstruction using the tibialis posterior tendon allograft, *Arthroscopy* 20(suppl 2):195-200, 2004.

Lowery DJ et al: A clinical composite score accurately detects meniscal pathology, *Arthroscopy* 22(11):1174-1179, 2006.

Majewski M, Susanne H, Klaus S: Epidemiology of athletic knee injuries: a 10-year study, *Knee* 13(3):184-188, 2006.

Marti-Bonmati L et al: MR imaging of Baker cysts—prevalence and relation to internal derangements of the knee, *MAGMA* 10(3):205-210, 2000.

Murray JRD et al: Osteochondritis dissecans of the knee; long-term clinical outcome following arthroscopic debridement, *Knee* 14(2):94-98, 2007.

Muscolo DL et al: Medial meniscal tears and spontaneous osteonecrosis of the knee, *Arthroscopy* 22(4):457-460, 2006.

Nomura E, Inoue M, Kobayashi S: Bilateral recurrent patellar dislocation in a patient with isolated patella aplasia-hypoplasia, *Arthroscopy* (in press, corrected proof).

Palmieri RM et al: The effect of a simulated knee joint effusion on postural control in healthy subjects, *Arch Phys Med Rehabil* 84(7):1076-1079, 2003.

Pantano KJ et al: Differences in peak knee valgus angles between individuals with high and low Q-angles during a single limb squat, *Clin Biomech* 20(9):966-972, 2005.

Ramseier LE, Werner CML, Heinzelmann M: Quadriceps and patellar tendon rupture, *Injury* 37(6):516-519, 2006.

Roidis N et al: Tumor-like meniscal cyst, *Arthroscopy* 23(1):111.e1-111.e6, 2007.

Said HG, Learmonth DJA: Chronic irreducible posterolateral knee dislocation: two-stage surgical approach, *Arthroscopy* 23(5):564.e1-564.e4, 2007.

Schmitz RJ et al: Sex differences in lower extremity biomechanics during single leg landings, *Clin Biomech* 22(6):681-688, 2007.

Smith A, Moran C: Soft tissue injuries of the knee, *Surgery (Oxford)* 24(11):376-381, 2006.

Wen DY et al: MRI description of knee medial collateral ligament abnormalities in the absence of trauma: edema related to osteoarthritis and medial meniscal tears, *Magn Reson Imaging* 25(2):209-214, 2007.

Widuchowski W, Widuchowski J, Trzaska T: Articular cartilage defects: study of 25,124 knee arthroscopies, *Knee* 14(3):177-182, 2007.

Williams AM et al: The meniscal flounce: a valuable arthroscopic sign, *Knee* 13(4):337-341, 2006.

Wu C-H et al: Arthroscopic reconstruction of the posterior cruciate ligament by using a quadriceps tendon autograft: a minimum 5-year follow-up, *Arthroscopy* 23(4):420.e2-477.e2, 2007.

CHAPTER TWELVE

LOWER LEG, ANKLE, AND FOOT

ORTHOPEDIC GAMUT 12-1

IMPORTANT SHOE DESIGN FEATURES

1. The arch support can reduce muscle fatigue in the calf and disperse arch pressure.
2. Outsoles with 1.5-cm thickness in the metatarsal zone tend to produce lower metatarsal pressure and vertical impact force and reduce low back discomfort.
3. A shoe upper with soft leather and mid sole made with ethylene vinyl acetate or polyurethane materials are helpful in increasing whole-body and foot comfort.
4. An outsole with heel height between 1.8 and 3.6 cm tends to generate lower heel pressure and vertical impact force in the forefoot and to reduce ankle discomfort.

AXIOMS IN ASSESSING THE LOWER LEG, ANKLE, AND FOOT

- Pain in the ankle and foot can arise from the bones and joints, periarticular soft tissues, nerve roots and peripheral nerves, or vascular structures.
- Pain in the foot can also be referred from the lumbar spine or knee joint.
- The greatest majority of painful foot conditions result from inappropriate footwear, weak intrinsic muscles, foot deformities, or static disorders.

INTRODUCTION

The leg, ankle, and foot are subject to static deformities more than any other skeletal unit. The weight-transmitting and propulsive functions of these structures are restricted daily by nonyielding foot coverings. Anatomic variations in the shape and stability of joint surfaces may predispose, resist, or modify the deforming force of common footwear.

Modern civilization disregards the physiologic features of the ankle and foot. Fashion and eye appeal rather than function determine shoe design, especially in the fore part of the shoe where most disabilities and deformities of the foot occur.

The restrictive force of poorly fitting shoes produces little deformity on the tarsus because the tarsus is made up of short, heavy bones. Normal movement in the tarsal joints is limited because the articular surfaces of the tarsal joints are flat (Fig. 12-2). However, the phalanges and metatarsals are long, thin bones with a normally wide range of joint motion. Restrictive force on these bones produces most of the static deformities of the forefoot. These static deformities include first metatarsophalangeal joint deformities, hammertoe, tailor's bunion, overlapping toes, and many other conditions that are deviations from normal (Table 12-3).

The human foot is uniquely specialized. The metatarsals and toes enable the body to stand erect. The versatility of the forefoot permits the human to retain an upright stance and allows for grace during walking, dancing, and athletics.

A well-developed and strong foot withstands surprising abuse. Morbid changes take place only when maltreatment becomes excessive. An underdeveloped and frail foot, ankle, and lower-leg mechanism may fail under ordinary stress and strain.

The ankle and foot are inspected in both the resting and the standing positions for evidence of swelling

TABLE 12-1

LOWER LEG, ANKLE, AND FOOT CROSS-REFERENCE TABLE BY ASSESSMENT PROCEDURE

Lower Leg, Ankle, and Foot Test/Sign	DISEASE ASSESSED											
	Talofibular Ligament	Vascular	Atrophy	Peroneal Nerve Paralysis	Foot Pronation	Calcaneus Fracture	Thrombophlebitis	Fibular Fracture	Neuroma	Metatarsalgia	Achilles' Tendon	Tarsal Tunnel Syndrome
Anterior drawer sign of the ankle	•											
Buerger test		•										
Calf circumference test			•									
Claudication test		•										
Duchenne sign				•								
Foot tourniquet test		•										
Helbings sign					•							
Hoffa test						•						
Homans sign		•					•					
Keen sign								•				
Morton test									•	•		
Moszkowicz test		•										
Moses test		•										
Perthes test		•										
Strunsky sign										•		
Thompson test						•					•	
Tinel foot sign												•

ORTHOPEDIC GAMUT 12-2

ETIOLOGY OF ACHILLES TENDON SWELLING

1. Tendon rupture
2. Calcaneal bursitis
3. Rheumatoid nodules
4. Urate tophi

TABLE 12-2

LOWER LEG, ANKLE, AND FOOT CROSS-REFERENCE TABLE BY SYNDROME OR TISSUE

Achilles tendon	Thompson test
Atrophy	Calf circumference test
Calcaneus fracture	Hoffa test
	Thompson test
Fibular fracture	Keen sign
Foot pronation	Helbings sign
Metatarsalgia	Morton test
	Strunsky sign
Neuroma	Morton test
Peroneal nerve paralysis	Duchenne sign
Talofibular ligament	Anterior drawer sign of the ankle
Tarsal tunnel syndrome	Tinel foot sign
Thrombophlebitis	Homans sign
	Moses test
Vascular	Buerger test
	Claudication test
	Foot tourniquet test
	Homans sign
	Moszkowicz test
	Moses test
	Perthes test

(Fig. 12-3), deformity (Fig. 12-4), or skin abnormalities such as edema, erythema, tophi, subcutaneous nodules (Fig. 12-5), and ulcers. Abnormalities of gait are observed while the patient is walking. The gait or walking cycle can be divided into two phases: the stance, or weight-bearing phase, and the swing, or non–weight-bearing phase.

In the standing position, the calcaneus normally maintains the line of the Achilles tendon. Deformities of the subtalar joint, resulting in eversion (calcaneovalgus) or

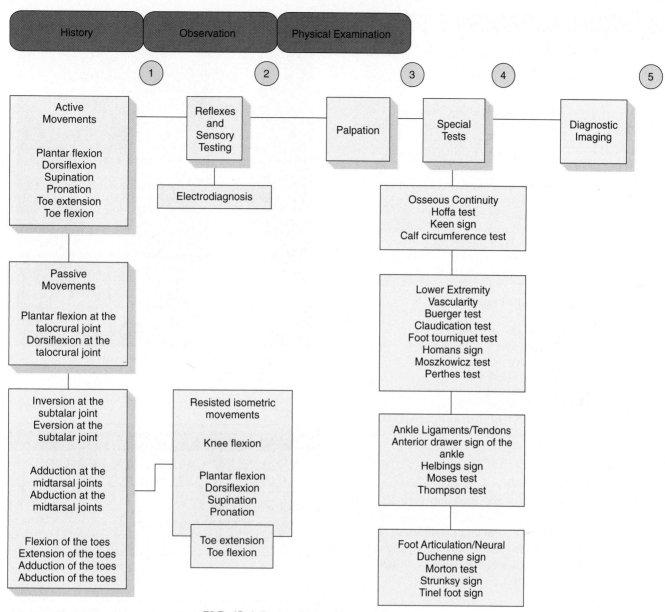

FIG. 12-1 Lower leg, ankle, and foot assessment.

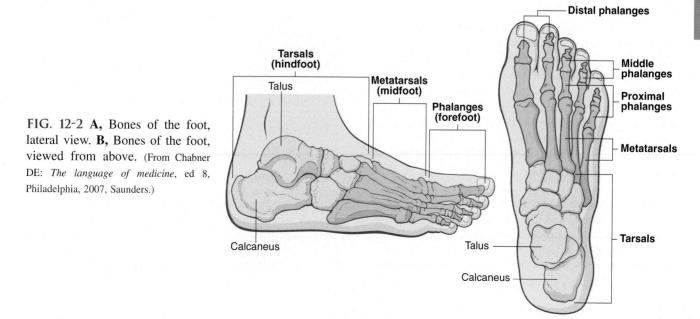

FIG. 12-2 **A,** Bones of the foot, lateral view. **B,** Bones of the foot, viewed from above. (From Chabner DE: *The language of medicine*, ed 8, Philadelphia, 2007, Saunders.)

12

TABLE 12-3

ANKLE AND FOOT DIFFERENTIATION BY ONSET

Articular	Trauma, sprain
	Arthritis
	Metatarsalgia
	Congenital disorders (e.g., clubfoot)
Neurologic	Entrapment of lumbosacral nerve roots form herniated lumbar disc
	Entrapment of the lateral popliteal nerve behind the neck of the fibula
	Tarsal tunnel syndrome (posterior tibial nerve)
	Interdigital (Morton) neuroma
	Peripheral neuropathy and insensitive foot
Periarticular	Cutaneous and subcutaneous
	Plantar fascia
	Tendons and tendon sheaths
	Bursitis
	Acute calcific periarthritis
Osseous	Fracture
	Epiphysitis (osteochondritis)
	Bone neoplasms, infection
	Painful accessory ossicles
Vascular	Ischemic foot pain
	Vasospastic disorders with Raynaud phenomenon
	Cholesterol embolization with *purple toes*

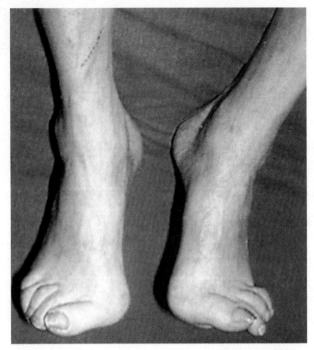

FIG. 12-3 Hallux valgus. (From Moll JMH: *Rheumatology,* ed 2, London, 1997, Churchill Livingstone.)

---

inversion (calcaneovarus) of the heel, are best observed from behind (Fig. 12-6). *Equinus* and *calcaneus* refer to angulation of the ankle in plantar and dorsiflexion, respectively. Inspection while the patient is standing may reveal lowering of the longitudinal arch (pes planus) or increased height of the arch (pes cavus).

ESSENTIAL ANATOMY

The leg is divided by fascial septa into posterior, lateral, and anterior compartments (Fig. 12-7). Because they have a common nerve supply, the anterior and lateral compartments are often considered to be one. The posterior compartment is further divided into a superficial and deep area. Although each compartment of the leg has a specialized vascular and nerve supply, the nerves and vessels are sometimes not physically within the compartment they supply (e.g., the lateral compartment is supplied by the peroneal artery, which lies in the posterior compartment).

The anterior leg muscles (Fig. 12-8) attach to the area between the tibia and fibula.

The anterior tibial compartment is one of the commonest sites affected by muscle herniation, which usually occurs along the lateral border of the tibia at the fascial insertion. Trauma can cause rupture of the fascia, allowing muscle to herniate through the defect. It is also seen as a result of regular vigorous exercise. This defect leads to muscle

---

ORTHOPEDIC GAMUT 12-3

MUSCLE OF THE ANTERIOR COMPARTMENT OF THE LEG

1. Tibialis anterior
2. Extensor hallucis longus
3. Extensor digitorum longus

ORTHOPEDIC GAMUT 12-4

ANKLE JOINT

Structures crossing the ankle joint (Fig. 12-10):

Anteriorly
- Tendons of the tibialis anterior
- Extensor hallucis longus
- Anterior tibial vessels
- Deep peroneal nerve
- Extensor digitorum longus
- Peroneus tertius

Posteromedially
- Tibial vessels
- Tibial nerve
- Flexor hallucis longus

Posterolaterally
- Tendons of the peroneus longus and brevis

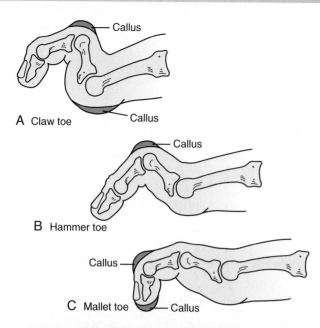

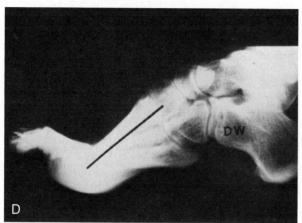

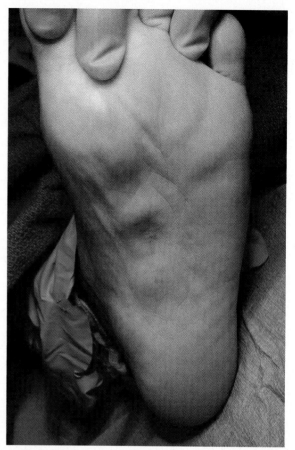

FIG. 12-5 Typical size and appearance of plantar fibromas along medial border of plantar fascia. (From Coughlin MJ, Mann RA: *Surgery of the foot and ankle*, vol 1-2, ed 7, St Louis, 1999, Mosby.)

FIG. 12-4 Digital deformities. **A,** Claw toe, with additional flexion contraction of distal interphalangeal joint (DIPJ). **B,** Hammer toe deformity, with extension contracture of metatarsophalangeal joint (MPJ) and flexion contracture of proximal interphalangeal joint (PIPJ). **C,** Mallet toe, with single flexion contraction at distal interphalangeal joint. (From McGlamry ED, ed: *Comprehensive textbook of foot surgery*, Baltimore, 1987, Williams & Wilkins.) (From Noble: *Textbook of primary care medicine*, ed 3, St Louis, 2001, Mosby.) **D,** Plantar-flexed first metatarsal. (© M. J. Coughlin. Used with permission.) (From DeLee: *DeLee and Drez's orthopaedic sports medicine*, ed 2, St Louis, 2003, Saunders.)

hypertrophy and increased compartmental pressures, which subjects the fascia to chronic stress, with eventual hernia formation (Williams, Hassan, 2007).

The muscles in the anterior and lateral compartments can be injured with a traumatic blow to the lateral leg. This trauma damages the common peroneal nerve. The most noticeable deficits to result from such an injury are weakness in extension (dorsiflexion) of the ankle and a dragging of the toes *(foot drop)* in walking. One of the more difficult

complications to traumatic injury of the leg is compartment syndrome. The fascial enclosures of the three compartments are so strong that hemorrhage, major tissue injury, and edema within one or another of these compartments cause pressure to increase. This compartmental hyperextension decreases the blood flow. Structures distal to the injury become ischemic and are usually permanently injured.

The ankle is the joint between the malleoli of the tibia and fibula, which combine to form a mortise. The talus is a tarsal bone that fits into this mortise (Fig. 12-9).

The flexor retinaculum connects the medial malleolus to the calcaneus and plantar aponeurosis posteroinferiorly. This passage is also called the *tarsal tunnel*, and compression and pressure can produce a tarsal tunnel syndrome comparable to the carpal tunnel syndrome of the wrist (Fig. 12-10).

ESSENTIAL MOTION ASSESSMENT

For the sake of simplicity, motions are tested along three different axes. Dorsiflexion and plantar flexion are movements at the ankle joint that occur around a transverse axis

12

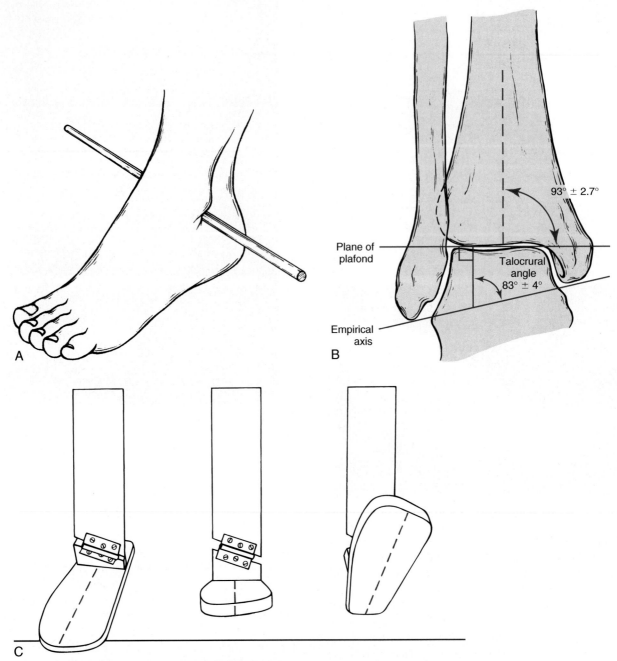

FIG. 12-6 **A,** A line joining the tips of the medial and lateral malleoli is a close approximation of the axis of the ankle joint, called the empirical axis of the ankle. **B,** The tibiotalar articular surface (plafond) usually has a slight lateral tilt, averaging 3 degrees. The empirical axis is in a relatively varus position, as indicated by the talocrural angle, formed by the intersection of a line perpendicular to the plafond with the empirical axis. This averages 83 ± 4 degrees and is a reliable radiographic indicator of the relationship among malleoli and plafond. It should be similar to that of the opposite ankle. **C,** The obliquity of the ankle axis produces relative medial deviation of the foot (internal rotation) with plantar flexion and relative lateral deviation of the foot (external rotation) with dorsiflexion. (Redrawn from Mann R: *Surgery of the foot,* ed 5, St Louis, 1986, Mosby) (In Browner BD: *Skeletal trauma: basic science, management, and reconstruction,* ed 3, Philadelphia, 2003, Saunders.)

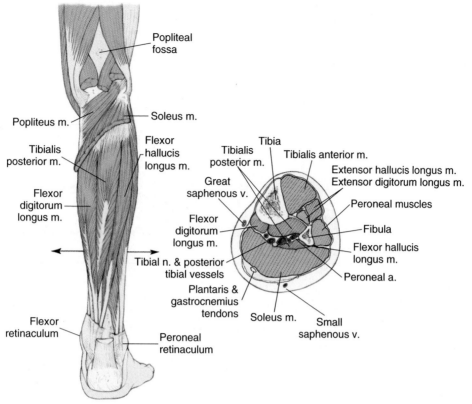

FIG. 12-7 Right leg muscles, posterior view, deep layers. (From Mathers LH et al: *Clinical anatomy principles*, St Louis, 1996, Mosby.)

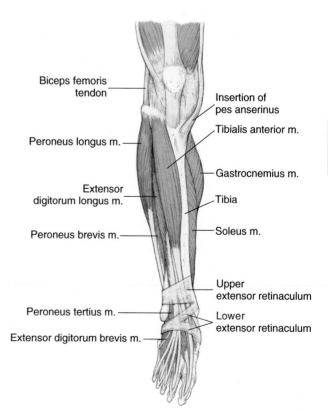

FIG. 12-8 Right leg muscles, anterior view. (From Mathers LH et al: *Clinical anatomy principles*, St Louis, 1996, Mosby.)

12

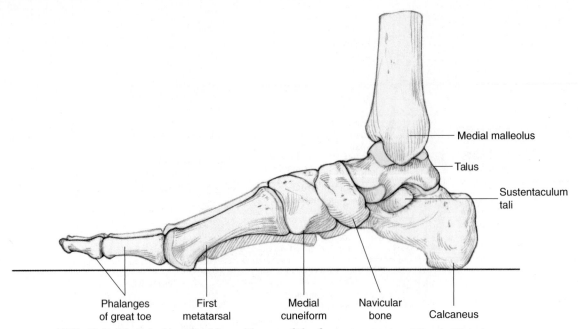

FIG. 12-9 Medial view of ankle and bones of the foot. (From Mathers LH et al: *Clinical anatomy principles*, St Louis, 1996, Mosby.)

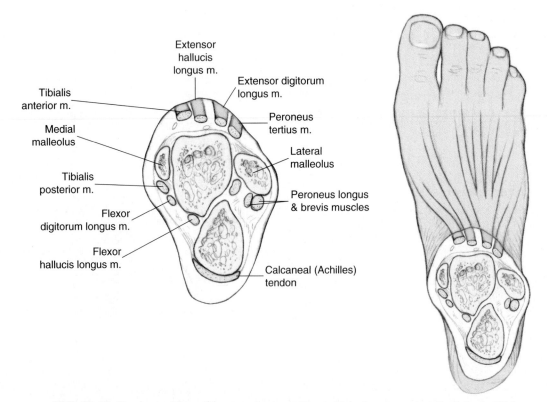

FIG. 12-10 Tendons at the ankle. (From Mathers LH et al: *Clinical anatomy principles*, St Louis, 1996, Mosby.)

ORTHOPEDIC GAMUT 12-5

ANKLE AND FOOT

Activities for testing range of motion of the ankle and foot (Fig. 12-11):
1. Point the foot up toward the ceiling.
2. Point the foot down toward the floor.
3. With the foot bent at the ankle, point the medial side of the foot toward the floor (eversion) and repeat with the lateral side (inversion).
4. Rotate the ankle, turning the foot away from and then toward the other foot.

that passes through the body of the talus. Inversion and eversion are movements of rotation of the foot along its long axis. Abduction and adduction of the forefoot, occurring along a vertical axis, are movements of the midtarsal joints. Pronation and supination refer to a weight-bearing foot. The complex movements of eversion and inversion indicate changes in the form of the whole foot when it is not bearing weight.

Forefoot adduction and abduction occur mainly at the midtarsal joints and are tested passively. The examiner moves the forefoot laterally and medially in relation to the calcaneus and then compares the range of motion with that of the opposite foot.

The other joints that allow significant motion in the forefoot are the metatarsophalangeal and interphalangeal joints. Of particular importance are the joints of the great toe. Normal dorsiflexion of the great toe is approximately 50 degrees. Plantar flexion of the metatarsophalangeal and interphalangeal joints of the great toe is approximately 30 degrees. Retained dorsiflexion of the great toe that is 40 degrees or less is an impairment of the foot in the activities of daily living. Retained plantar flexion of the great toe that is 20 degrees or less is an impairment of the foot in the activities of daily living.

Movements of the lesser toes can be measured in a similar manner. Clinically, it is adequate to note whether fixed contractures are present or if the joints are supple. Restriction of joint motion can be the result of soft-tissue contractures, bony abutment, or intraarticular adhesions. Motion may be restricted because of pain that results from inflammation or injuries (Figs. 12-12 and 12-13).

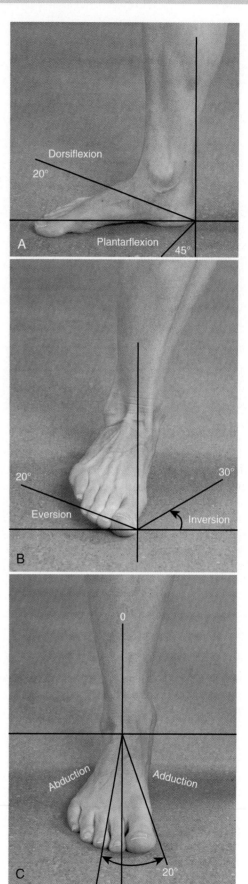

FIG. 12-11 Range of motion of the ankle and foot.

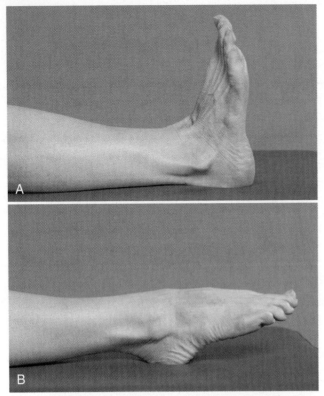

FIG. 12-12 When testing the dorsiflexion and plantar flexion of the ankle joint, neutral position for the ankle is when the lateral border of the foot is at 90 degrees in relation to the leg and the knee is in full extension. A normal ankle allows 20 degrees of dorsiflexion (A) and 40 degrees of plantar flexion from this position (B). Retained dorsiflexion of 10 degrees or less and retained plantar flexion range of motion of 30 degrees or less are impairments of the ankle for the activities of daily living. The measurements of dorsiflexion and plantar flexion can be repeated while the knee is held in 45 degrees of flexion. If the arc of motion is different from the previous finding, the presence of Achilles' tendon tightness is indicated. For all practical purposes, movements of the ankle joint are considered limited to dorsiflexion and plantar flexion. In some individuals with hypermobility of the ankle joint, medial tilt of the talus can occur within the ankle mortise. This tilt is the result of a congenital laxity of the lateral collateral ligaments and predisposes the patient to recurrent ankle sprains.

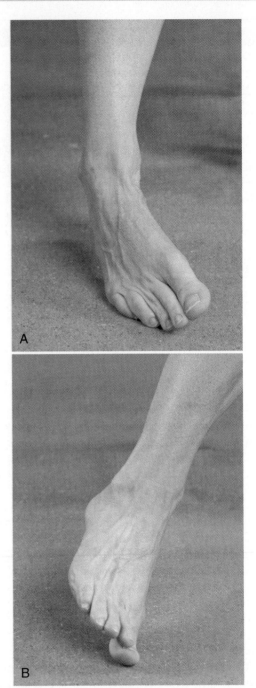

FIG. 12-13 Inversion and eversion of the foot occur mainly at the subtalar joint and are tested while the patient is lying supine. The ankle is first dorsiflexed to a neutral position. The patient rocks the foot into inversion (A) and eversion (B). A normal joint allows 20 degrees of eversion and approximately 30 degrees of inversion. Retained inversion range of motion that is 20 degrees or less and retained eversion range of motion that is 10 degrees or less are impairments of the foot-ankle mechanism in the activities of daily living.

ESSENTIAL MUSCLE FUNCTION ASSESSMENT

The main muscles of the calf are the soleus and gastrocnemius. The soleus acts purely as a flexor of the ankle, and the gastrocnemius flexes both the ankle and the knee. The flexor digitorum longus and flexor hallucis longus flex the toes and great toe, respectively. The anterior compartment muscles include the tibialis anterior, extensor digitorum longus, and extensor hallucis longus (Fig. 12-14). The tibialis anterior inverts the foot and dorsiflexes the ankle.

The examiner should test the individual muscles involved with movement at the ankle and foot, starting with the plantar and dorsiflexors of the ankle and then of the toes (Fig. 12-15). The extensor of the big toe, extensor hallucis longus, should be specially tested. Finally, the examiner should test the evertors and invertors of the foot. Variations of the arch need to be assessed (Fig. 12-16).

The motions in the ankle joint are plantar flexion and dorsiflexion. The muscles in the posterior compartment, which are innervated by the tibial nerve, are responsible primarily for plantar flexion motion. The major muscles for plantar flexion are the gastrocnemius and soleus, and they are supplemented by the tibialis posterior, peroneus longus, flexor digitorum longus, and hallucis longus. The power of the gastrocnemius-soleus group is weakened when the knee is in flexion because the gastrocnemius is a two-joint muscle. However, while the knee is in flexion, the passive range of ankle dorsiflexion increases slightly. The muscles of the anterior compartment, innervated by the deep peroneal nerve, are responsible primarily for dorsiflexion motion. Dorsiflexion is performed by the tibialis anterior and the extensor digitorum longus. When these two muscles

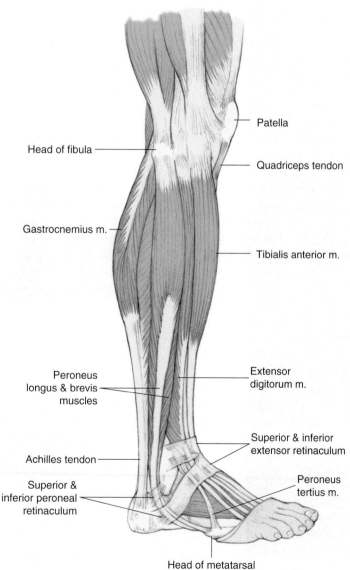

FIG. 12-14 Right leg muscles, lateral view. (From Mathers LH: *Principles of clinical anatomy,* St Louis, 1996, Mosby.)

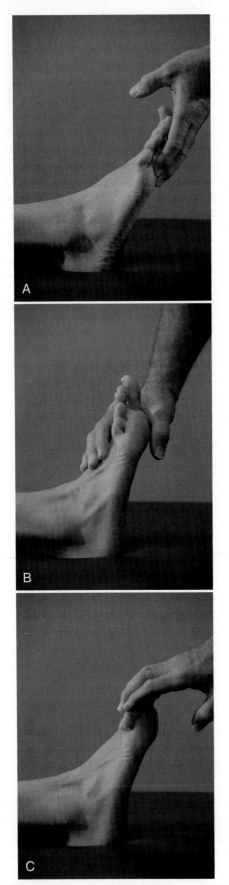

FIG. 12-15 Testing (**A**) plantar flexion and dorsiflexion of the ankle (**B**) and dorsiflexion of the toes (**C**).

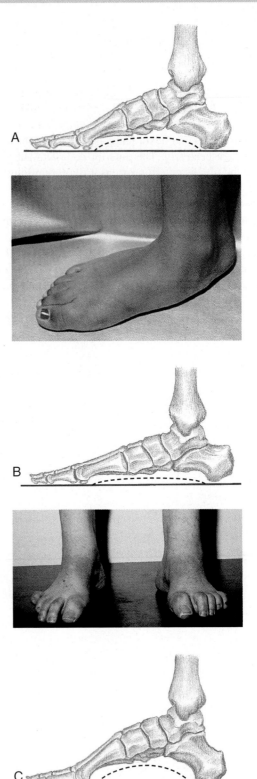

FIG. 12-16 Variations in the longitudinal arch of the foot. **A,** Expected arch. **B,** Pes planus (flatfoot). **C,** Pes cavus (high instep). (From Seidel HM: *Mosby's guide to physical examination,* ed 4, St Louis, 1999, Mosby.)

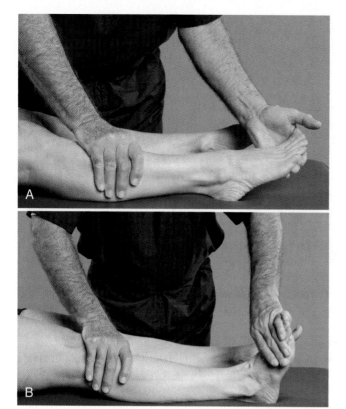

FIG. 12-17 The soleus and gastrocnemius should be evaluated separately. The soleus is evaluated by applying a dorsiflexion force to the foot while the patient plantar flexes the foot (**A**). The maneuver is performed with the knee in extension to evaluate the muscle power of the gastrocnemius. The tibialis anterior is tested by exerting a counter force to the dorsiflexion and inversion movement of the foot and ankle (**B**).

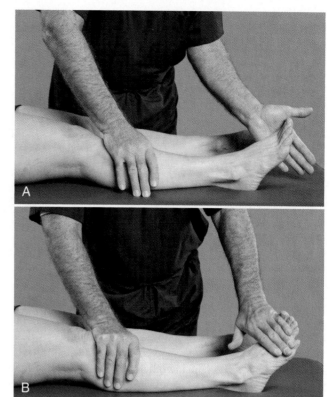

FIG. 12-18 The prime motions at the intertarsal joints are inversion and eversion, and these motions occur primarily at the subtalar joint. Inversion is achieved principally by the tibialis posterior and the tibialis anterior, but it is supplemented by the long toe flexors and gastrocnemius soleus muscle. Eversion is achieved primarily by the peroneus brevis and peroneus longus, which are innervated by the superficial peroneal nerve, and is supplemented by the extensor digitorum longus and peroneus tertius. The tibialis posterior is evaluated by exerting a counter force to the foot while the patient inverts and plantar flexes the foot (**A**). The peroneus longus is tested by exerting a counter force to a foot that is held in plantar flexion while the patient actively everts it (**B**). The peroneus brevis is evaluated the same way, but the foot is held in the neutral position.

12

act together, their individual actions of inversion and eversion are neutralized. The extensor hallucis longus and peroneus tertius also aid in dorsiflexion (Figs. 12-17 to 12-20).

ESSENTIAL IMAGING

The standard views of the ankle are the anteroposterior (AP) (Figs. 12-21 and 12-22), medial oblique (mortise view), and lateral views (Figs. 12-23 and 12-24). The AP ankle view includes the collimate field from the distal tibia and fibula

through the talocalcaneal junction. The primary purpose of the AP ankle view is to illustrate the coronal relationship of the talocrural articulation and its surrounding bony elements of the tibia, fibula, and talus. The AP and oblique projections of the ankle are sensitive for ruling out sites of injury along the lower tibia and fibula. The lateral ankle view includes the lower tibia and fibula. In cases of suspected ligamentous instability, eversion and inversion stress views can be performed. Inversion will test the lateral collateral ligament, whereas eversion will check the medial collateral (deltoid) ligament (Fig. 12-25).

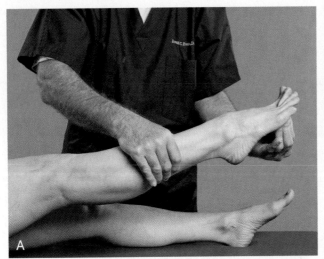
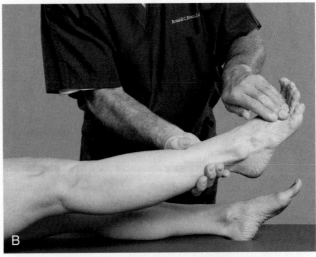

FIG. 12-19 The main motions at the metatarsophalangeal and interphalangeal joints are extension and flexion. Flexion of the metatarsophalangeal joint is achieved primarily by the lumbricales, interossei, and flexor hallucis brevis, which are augmented by the flexor hallucis longus and the flexor digitorum longus and brevis (A). Extension of these joints is achieved primarily by the extensor digitorum longus and the extensor hallucis longus, which are supplemented by the extensor digitorum brevis and the extensor hallucis brevis (B). The interphalangeal joints are hinge joints that allow flexion and extension but more flexion than extension. Flexion is achieved by the flexor digitorum longus at the distal interphalangeal joint and is supplemented by the flexor digitorum brevis at the proximal interphalangeal joints.

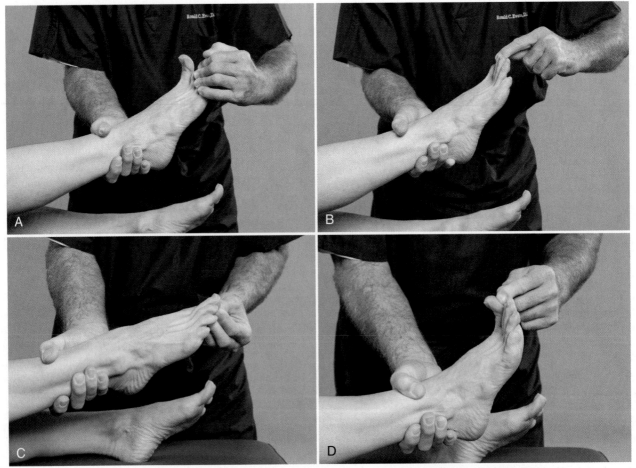

FIG. 12-20 The muscle power of the long toe extensors is tested by exerting a counter-force to the toes while the patient extends the metatarsophalangeal joints (A and B). The long toe flexors are tested by exerting a counter force to the tip of the toes while the patient flexes the interphalangeal joints (C and D).

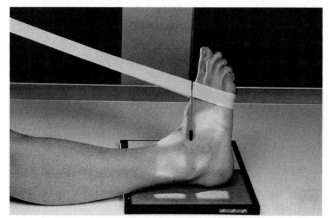

FIG. 12-21 Anteroposterior ankle in neutral position. (From Frank ED et al: *Merrill's atlas of radiographic positioning and procedures*, vol 1-3, ed 11, St Louis, 2007, Mosby.)

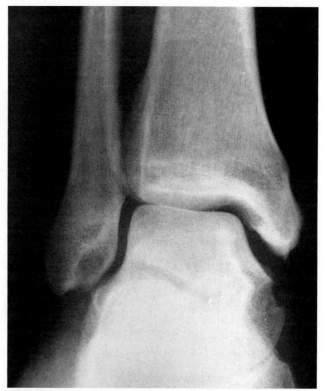

FIG. 12-22 Eversion stress. (From Frank ED et al: *Merrill's atlas of radiographic positioning and procedures,* vol 1-3, ed 11, St Louis, 2007, Mosby.)

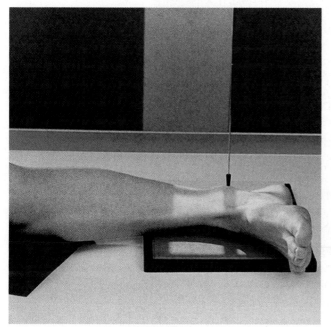

FIG. 12-23 Lateral ankle. (From Frank ED et al: *Merrill's atlas of radiographic positioning and procedures,* vol 1-3, ed 11, St Louis, 2007, Mosby.)

ORTHOPEDIC GAMUT 12-6

VIEWS OF THE FOOT

Three basic plain-film views of the foot are:
1. AP or dorsoplantar view (Figs. 12-26 and 12-27)
2. Oblique view (Figs. 12-28 and 12-29)
3. Lateral view

12

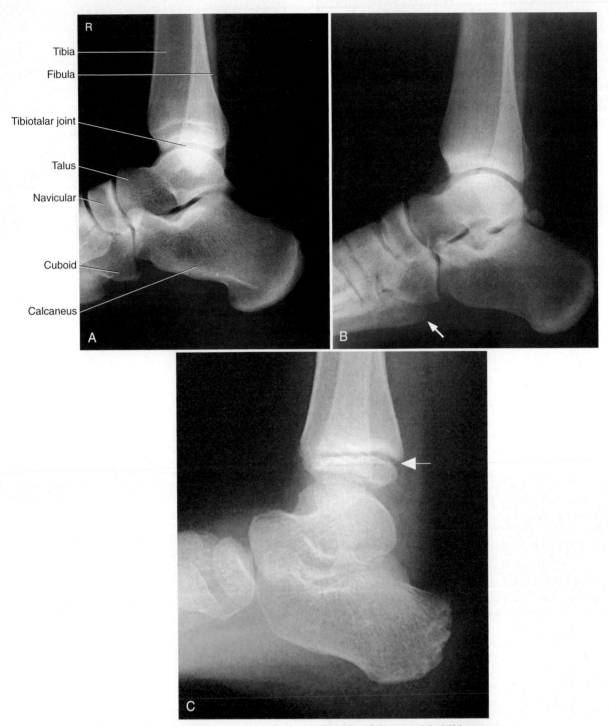

FIG. 12-24 **A** and **B,** Lateral ankle. **C,** Lateral ankle of 8-year-old child. (From Frank ED et al: *Merrill's atlas of radiographic positioning and procedures,* vol 1-3, ed 11, St Louis, 2007, Mosby.)

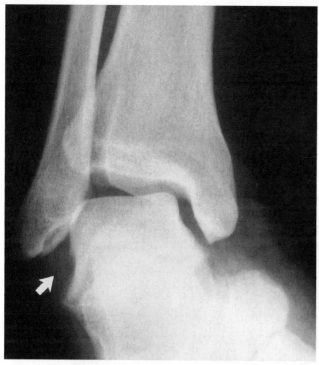

FIG. 12-25 Inversion stress. (From Frank ED et al: *Merrill's atlas of radiographic positioning and procedures,* vol 1-3, ed 11, St Louis, 2007, Mosby.)

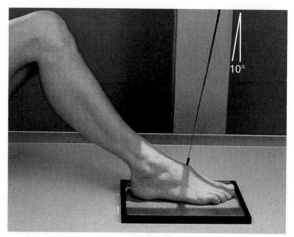

FIG. 12-26 Anteroposterior axial foot with posterior angulation of 10 degrees. (From Frank ED et al: *Merrill's atlas of radiographic positioning and procedures,* vol 1-3, ed 11, St Louis, 2007, Mosby.)

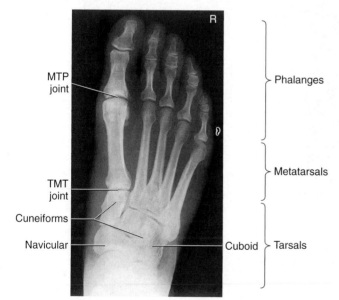

FIG. 12-27 Anteroposterior axial view of the foot with posterior angulation of 10 degrees. (From Frank ED et al: *Merrill's atlas of radiographic positioning and procedures,* vol 1-3, ed 11, St Louis, 2007, Mosby.)

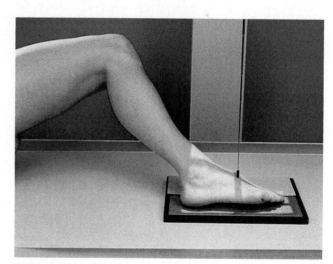

FIG. 12-28 Anteroposterior oblique view of the foot, medial rotation. (From Frank ED et al: *Merrill's atlas of radiographic positioning and procedures,* vol 1-3, ed 11, St Louis, 2007, Mosby.)

12

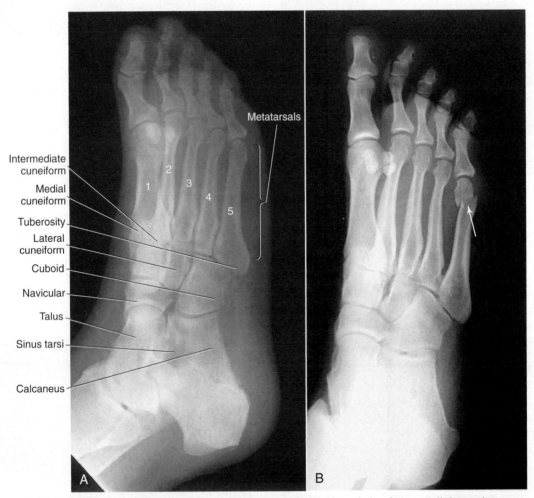

FIG. 12-29 **A** and **B,** Anteroposterior oblique projection of the foot, medial rotation. **B,** Fracture of the distal aspect of the fifth metatarsal *(arrow).* (From Frank ED et al: *Merrill's atlas of radiographic positioning and procedures,* vol 1-3, ed 11, St Louis, 2007, Mosby.)

ANTERIOR DRAWER SIGN OF THE ANKLE

Assessment for Anterior Talofibular Ligament Sprain

Comment

Ankle sprain is one of the most common diagnoses made in young active populations after low-energy traumatic events. This type of sprain is particularly prevalent in sports activities that involve jumping and cutting. The most common sprain is an inversion injury, with varying degrees of damage to the stabilizers of the lateral side of the ankle. Because of repetitive jumping, impact activities, athletic pursuits, and job requirements, ankle sprains are very common in active duty military populations. A study of United States Marine Corps recruits found an incidence of 0.53 ankle sprains per 1000 training days. The majority of patients (up to 80%) with lateral ankle instability return to function without requiring surgical intervention. Select patients with continued instability after 6 months are considered to have chronic lateral ankle instability (Bell et al, 2005).

Ankle sprain results from the stretching or tearing of ankle ligaments after inversion or eversion foot injuries. It is the most common injury in athletics but can occur in any age group with trauma not related to sports. Radiographs should be obtained when the ankle injury meets the Ottawa rules for ankle sprain (Fig. 12-30).

The most common fractures during ankle sprain are avulsions of the malleoli or tarsal bones. Other sites include the anterior process of the calcaneus, the base of the fifth metatarsal (insertion of the peroneus brevis tendon), the talar neck, the cuboid, and the bony epiphyses in children. The strength of the deltoid ligament makes it an uncommon site for injury. However, when injury occurs, malleolar fractures of concomitant sprains of the syndesmosis are more likely.

With injuries to the ankle, such a close association exists between sprain dislocation and fracture that placing them in separate categories is unwise, particularly because the same forces may cause a combination of injuries. Resultant pathologic conditions may be determined more by the strength and duration of the forces that cause the injury than by the exact type of stress. The injury is usually caused by stresses that may result in a sprain, a dislocation, a fracture, or all three.

Because the ankle is functionally a hinge joint that normally permits only dorsal and plantar flexion, injuries to the ankle are caused primarily by lateral stresses that force the ankle through an arc of motion that it does not normally possess. Less commonly, injuries are caused by hyperflexion or hyperextension (Fig. 12-31). The injuries that result from lateral stresses may be readily divided into two categories: inversion injuries and eversion injuries.

Inversion injuries to the ankle are usually not caused by pure inversion. The force consists of inversion, internal rota-

---

ORTHOPEDIC GAMUT 12-7

ANKLE SPRAIN CLASSIFICATIONS

Grade I: Localized tenderness, minimal swelling or ecchymoses, and normal range of motion without instability

Grade II: Moderate to severe pain, swelling or ecchymoses and restricted range of motion, potential mild instability, and painful weight bearing

Grade III: Severe pain, edema, hemorrhage, loss of motion, and inability to ambulate; ankle instability common, with complete functional loss

---

ORTHOPEDIC GAMUT 12-8

OTTAWA ANKLE RULES FOR FOOT AND ANKLE IMAGING IN ACUTE ANKLE INJURY

1. An ankle diagnostic image is required if the patient complains of any pain along the lateral malleolus or medial malleolus and any of these findings:
   - Bone tenderness at posterior edge or tip of lateral malleolus *or*
   - Bone tenderness at posterior edge or tip of medial malleolus *or*
   - Inability to bear weight both immediately and later
2. A foot diagnostic image is required if the patient has any pain in the mid foot tarsal area and any of these findings:
   - Bone tenderness at the base of the fifth metatarsal *or*
   - Bone tenderness at the navicular *or*
   - Inability to bear weight immediately or later

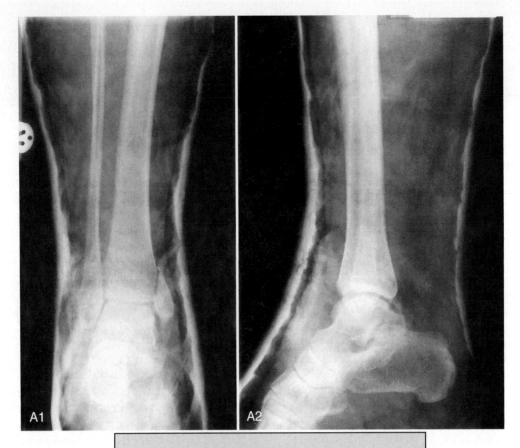

An ankle diagnostic image is required if there is any pain along the lateral malleolus or medial malleolus and any of these findings:

1. Bone tenderness at posterior edge or tip of lateral malleolus

               or

2. Bone tenderness at posterior edge or tip of medial malleolus

               or

3. Inability to bear weight both immediately and later

A foot diagnostic image is required if there is any pain in the midfoot tarsal area and any of these findings:

1. Bone tenderness at the base of the fifth metatarsal

               or

2. Bone tenderness at the navicular

               or

3. Inability to bear weight immediately or later

B

FIG. 12-30 **A,** A 45-year-old woman sustained an open injury to her right ankle, after an inversion injury. A clinical diagnosis of fracture dislocation of the ankle was made, and the dislocation was successfully reduced under sedation. AP and lateral radiographs were taken. They revealed an oblique fracture of the medial malleolus. The ankle mortice was well reduced. (From Shah K, Hakmi A: Unusual ankle injury–a case report, *Foot* 14(3):169-172, 2004.) **B,** The Ottawa ankle rules were prospectively derived, refined, and prospectively validated. They incorporate simple historical and physical findings that are well defined to determine if patients require radiography of their ankle and/or foot following a traumatic injury. Since their development, they have been further studied to determine their impact on clinical practice in a variety of settings and in multiple types of studies. (From Perry JJ, Stiell IG: Impact of clinical decision rules on clinical care of traumatic injuries to the foot and ankle, knee, cervical spine, and head, *Injury* 37[12]:1157-1165, 2006.)

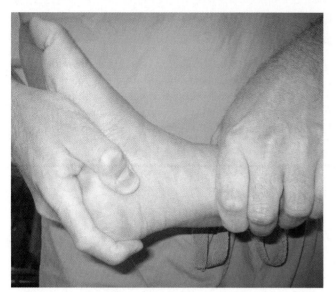

FIG. 12-31 Anterior drawer testing with ankle in slight plantar flexion. (From Bell SJ et al: Chronic lateral ankle instability: the Brostrom procedure, *Oper Tech Sports Med* 13[3]:176-182, 2005.)

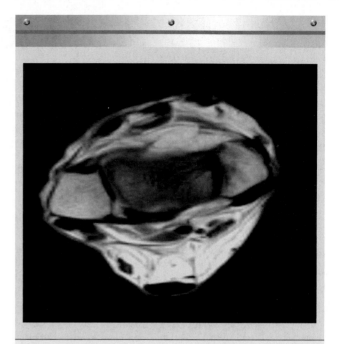

AT THE VIEWBOX

Axial MR image at the level of the ankle mortise demonstrates the normal low signal of the intact posterior talofibular ligament. Disruption of this ligament is seen with grade 2 or 3 ankle sprains, indicating increasingly unstable injuries that are associated with the anterior drawer sign of the ankle. (From the teaching file of Timothy Mick, DC, DACBR)

tion, and plantar flexion of the foot in relation to the leg so that the foot is inverted and the ankle and foot are thrown laterally. In this injury mechanism, the push is against the medial malleolus, and the pull is away from the lateral malleolus. As the foot inverts in relation to the leg, strain is placed on the lateral collateral ligament, the ligament primarily constructed to resist this motion. As a result of this overinversion, the ligament will tear slightly, partially, or completely according to the severity of the force. If the inverting force continues as the lateral ligament gives way, the ankle opens on the lateral side, and the talus is forcibly thrust against the medial malleolus. The medial malleolus acts as a fulcrum, and its tip impinges against the central portion of the medial face of the talus. The talus rotates over the malleolus rather than pushes off it. In such a case, the injury will probably be confined to the lateral side, and laceration of the lateral collateral ligaments will be complete. Breaking off the lateral malleolus is unusual for this type of force. In the geriatric patient in whom the bone is osteoporotic, the lateral malleolus may break before the ligament tears.

PROCEDURE

- The patient may be seated or supine.
- The examiner places one hand around the anterior aspect of the patient's lower tibia, just above the ankle, while gripping the calcaneus in the palm of the other hand.
- While the tibia is pushed posteriorly, the calcaneus and talus are drawn anteriorly (Figs. 12-32 and 12-33).
- Normally, no movement occurs from this action.
- The sign is present when the talus slides anteriorly under the ankle mortise.
- The test indicates anterior talofibular ligament instability, which is usually secondary to rupture.

Next Steps/Procedures
Keen sign, calf circumference test, and diagnostic imaging

12

CLINICAL PEARL

The drawer sign is a sensitive indicator of the amount of ligamentous damage in the ankle. Ankles with drawer sign will often require casting or rigid immobilization, at the least, in acute-stage management. Instability may sometimes follow tears of the anterior talofibular portion of the lateral ligament. This instability may be confirmed by radiographs after local anesthesia. The examiner supports the heel on a sandbag and presses firmly downward on the tibia for 30 seconds before exposure. A gap that is between the talus and the tibia and is greater than 6 mm is a pathologic condition.

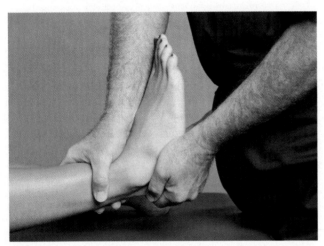

FIG. 12-32 The patient may be seated or supine. The examiner places one hand around the lower tibia, slightly above the ankle mortise. The calcaneus and talus are gripped in the palm of the other hand. The tibia is pushed posteriorly while the calcaneus and talus are drawn anteriorly. The sign is present if any movement of the talus is detected in the ankle mortise. The presence of this sign represents a talofibular ligament instability.

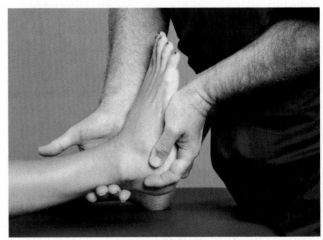

FIG. 12-33 In a reversal of this maneuver, the tibia is drawn anteriorly as the calcaneus and talus are pushed posteriorly. In this maneuver, a positive sign is indicated by a greater degree of mortise definition in the anterior. This positive sign may indicate insufficiency of the posterior talofibular portion of the lateral ligament.

Assessment for Vascular Compromise of the Lower Extremity

Comment

Peripheral arterial disease is mainly caused by impairment of the blood supply. This impairment may result from atheromatous narrowing of the artery, from thrombosis, or, much more rarely, from cardiac embolism (Fig 12-34).

Intermittent claudication (IC) is a cardinal symptom of lower-extremity peripheral arterial disease (PAD). With both asymptomatic and symptomatic PAD representing an independent risk factor for cardiovascular morbidity and mortality, a resurgence has taken place in epidemiologic and clinical interest in PAD. Approximately 12 million people in the United States alone have PAD, and, as the world population is aging, the incidence of PAD is expected to rise (Meru et al, 2006).

Chronic arterial insufficiency is much more common in the lower limb than other areas and usually produces IC. The patient is aware of pain in the leg, the thigh, or the buttock that comes on with walking and goes away when stopping to rest. The leg exhibits weak or absent foot, knee, and femoral pulses. The skin tends to become discolored and shiny, and hair is lost from the foot. Gangrene may affect the toes and foot (Fig. 12-35).

ORTHOPEDIC GAMUT 12-9

CATEGORIES OF PERIPHERAL VASCULAR DISEASE IN THE LOWER EXTREMITY

- Disease of the peripheral arterial system
- Disease of the peripheral venous system

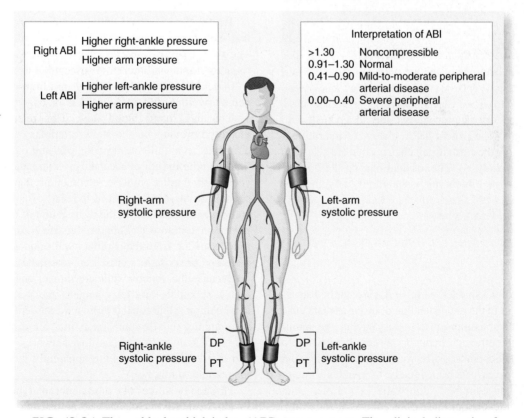

FIG. 12-34 The ankle–brachial index (ABI) measurement. The clinical diagnosis of atherosclerotic involvement of one or more arterial segments in the limb is usually detected as an ankle–brachial systolic blood pressure ratio (ABI) ≤ 0.90. Approximately 10% of individuals >55 years of age have asymptomatic PAD (ABI < 0.90), 5% have intermittent claudication, and 1% have critical leg ischemia. (From Braunwald E: *Primary cardiology*, ed 2, Philadelphia, 2003, Saunders.)

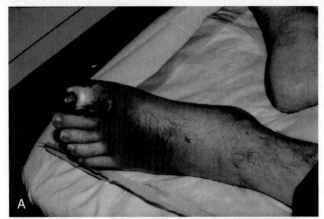

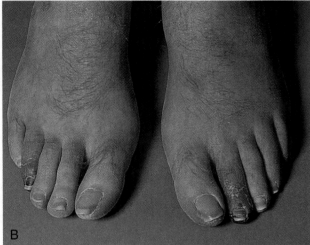

FIG. 12-35 **A,** Gangrene of the toe with cellulitis in a diabetic patient. (Courtesy of David Effron, MD.) (In Marx: *Rosen's emergency medicine: concepts and clinical practice,* ed 6, St Louis, 2006, Mosby.) **B,** Typical dry gangrene of two toes in a patient with diffuse atheroma. The patient had a history of intermittent claudication. Note the chronic nail changes that are also seen (resembling onycholysis). The residual hair on the dorsum of the feet is unusual in chronic ischemia; usually, the hair is lost. (From Forbes CD, Jackson WF: *Color atlas and text of clinical medicine,* ed 3, London, 2003, Mosby.)

Knowledge of the smaller, peripheral, vascular bed structures is important to the understanding of diseases that cause peripheral vascular compromise. After leaving the mainstream artery, the efferent circulatory system branches into smaller and smaller, muscularly walled precapillaries and arterioles. Arterioles can lead directly to venules through arteriovenous anastomoses (thin-walled arterioles that contain contractile smooth muscle for control of shunting). However, more often, arterioles channel into precapillaries, and then capillaries connect to the venules and larger venous

system. Fine-tuning of the systemic blood pressure can be controlled by the small, muscularly walled vessels and by shunting blood through collateral channels around the capillary bed. The pressures in capillaries of skeletal muscle range between 20 and 30 mm Hg. Therefore, external pressures that exceed this value may occlude these capillaries, which deliver oxygen and remove carbon dioxide during normal blood flow. This microvascular level is the point at which increased interstitial fluid pressure first affects compartmental contents and leads to a progressive pathologic condition.

Similar to the varying types of muscles, different patterns of blood supply within the muscles exist. Muscles in general have isolated vascular support systems with limited internal and external anastomoses, and therefore anatomic relationships may be inconsistent. In some muscles, abundant communications between arteriolar systems exist (longitudinal anastomotic chains, such as the soleus and peroneus longus). In other muscles, several mainstream arteries send arterial branches into the muscle; therefore, damage to a single vessel, such as the anterior tibialis and the flexor hallucis longus, may not be critical. However, some muscles, such as the extensor hallucis longus, have a single blood supply with few anastomoses. These latter systems are extremely susceptible to any circulatory compromise by virtue of their single vascular stem.

Tendons have a substantial and constant blood supply that may form an anastomosis with the muscular system. The vascularity of muscles may be isolated from the surrounding tissue and therefore susceptible to arterial injury.

In general, every major artery in a limb has one or two veins traveling with it. Any stasis or engorgement in this system may retard blood flow. This retardation causes increased pressure in the small arteriolar capillary system and leads to an alteration of the Starling equilibrium. The Starling equilibrium or mechanism is the alternation of the energy of cardiac muscle contraction that accompanies changes in the fiber length at the start of contraction. This component is essential in the dysfunction of cardiac decompensation syndromes. This circumstance might then cause fluid extrusion from the capillary walls and add to or create increased pressure in a closed compartment.

Because the venous walls are thinner and less muscular than comparable arterial channels, the venous walls are more compressible and therefore more susceptible to changes surrounding muscle and interstitial fluid pressure. The extremities have two venous flow networks: the superficial and the deep. Deep veins are apparently more efficient in maintaining blood flow.

Through the forces of external muscular pumping and the system of intimal valves and communicating branches, the blood is shunted to and transported through the deep vessels.

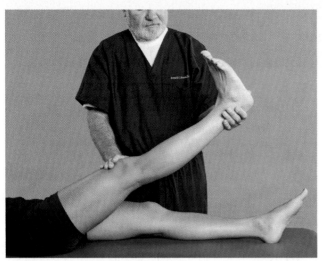

FIG. 12-36 The patient is lying supine. The examiner elevates the patient's leg to 45 degrees while the knee is fully extended. The patient actively dorsiflexes the foot.

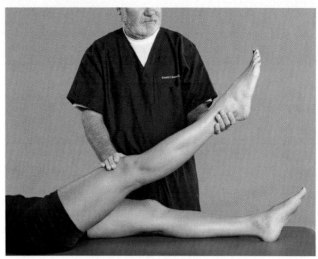

FIG. 12-37 After dorsiflexing the foot, as in Fig. 12-36, the patient plantar flexes the foot for at least 3 minutes. This maneuver diminishes the amount of blood in the distal vessels.

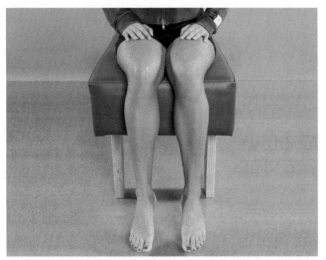

FIG. 12-38 After performing the maneuvers in Figs. 12-36 and 12-37, the patient sits at the edge of the examining table and dangles the legs. The test is positive for circulatory deficiency if the foot is blanched and the veins are collapsed. Also, the test is considered positive if more than 2 minutes is needed for the circulation to return to the dangling leg.

PROCEDURE

- While the patient is lying supine, the examiner elevates the patient's leg and extends the knee to a point of comfortable tolerance, approximately 45 degrees, for no less than 3 minutes (Figs. 12-36 and 12-37).
- The examiner lowers the limb, and the patient sits up, with both legs dangling side by side over the examining table (Fig. 12-38).
- The test measures arterial blood supply to the lower limbs.
- The blood supply is deficient if the dorsum of the foot blanches and the prominent veins collapse when the leg is initially raised.
- The test is also positive if, when the leg is lowered, 1 to 2 minutes is required for a ruddy (reddish) cyanosis to spread over the affected part and for the veins to fill and become prominent.

Next Steps/Procedures

Claudication test, foot tourniquet test, Homans sign, Moses test, Moszkowicz test, Perthes test, and vascular assessment

12

CLINICAL PEARL

Sciatic-like pain is not uncommon in lower extremity vascular disorders. This test allows a quick determination of neurogenic versus vascular pain. The test demonstrates loss of vascular integrity, but as circulation diminishes, the primary complaint is produced.

Assessment for Muscular Atrophy or Hypertrophy of the Lower Extremity

Comment

The efficiency of calf muscle pump relies on normally functioning venous valves, powerful contraction of calf muscle, full ankle joint movement, and normal muscular fasciae. Any malfunction in this system may contribute to calf pump dysfunction, influencing the venous hemodynamics and resulting in venous hypertension. Patients with chronic venous disease have venous reflux, weakness of calf muscle strength, and calf pump dysfunction (Qiao, Liu, Ran, 2005).

In the anterior compartment of the leg, the anterior tibial, the extensor hallucis, and the extensor digitorum longus muscles arise from the sides of the tibia, fibula, and interosseous membrane. These muscles completely fill the anterior compartment. This compartment is tightly roofed by the anterior fascia of the leg. With the anterior tibial syndrome, swelling of the muscle is rapid within its compartment. This swelling may come on after active exercise alone. In theory, this swelling occurs because muscles that have not been previously conditioned are overused, thus they respond with swelling and edema. The swelling also may come on after a direct injury in which swelling and hemorrhage into the space is excessive. The condition can also be caused by localized infection within the space. In fact, anything that causes intractable swelling may cause this syndrome (Fig. 12-39).

At the onset of anterior tibial syndrome, severe pain is felt over the involved area, and a loss of function occurs. Contraction of the muscles contained in the space rapidly becomes impossible, and foot drop can ensue. Even passive stretching of the muscles quickly becomes painful. However, this condition is not ordinarily preceded by the symptoms of tenosynovitis. The skin over the area becomes red, glossy, warm, and markedly tender. Woody tension is felt over the point of real hardness of the fascia over the space. The peroneal nerve may occasionally be involved, with sensory loss (Fig. 12-40). The loss of muscle function is not usually caused by nerve involvement but rather by pathologic changes within the muscle itself. The muscles develop ischemic necrosis, which is often called *Volkmann ischemia of the leg*.

The result is a firm, inelastic, and noncontractile muscle group. This condition can be extremely disabling and defies reconstructive treatment (Fig. 12-41).

ORTHOPEDIC GAMUT 12-10

THE FIVE LEG COMPARTMENTS

1. Anterior
2. Lateral
3. Posterior tibial
4. Deep posterior
5. Superficial posterior

ORTHOPEDIC GAMUT 12-11

CHARACTERISTICS OF VOLKMANN ISCHEMIA

1. Swelling
2. Edema
3. Extravasation of red blood cells
4. Destruction of blood cells
5. Replacement of muscle tissue by a fibrous scar

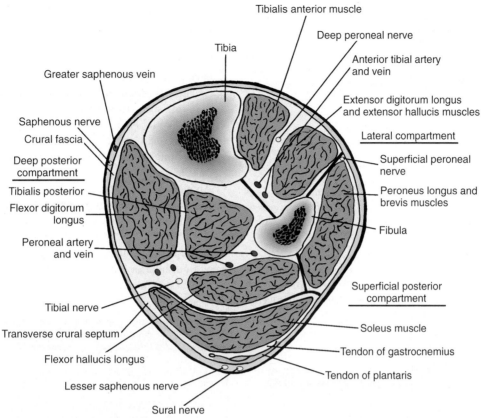

FIG. 12-39 Compartments of the leg. (From Nicholas JA, Hershman EB: *The lower extremity & spine in sports medicine,* vol 1-2, ed 2, St Louis, 1995, Mosby.)

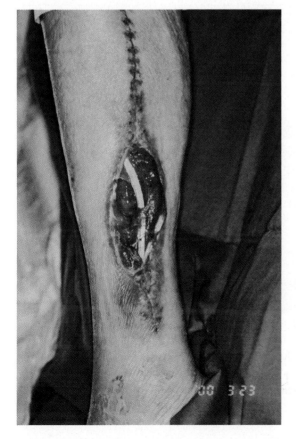

FIG. 12-40 In this patient an osteocutaneous fibular free flap was raised with a cuff of flexor hallucis longus and soleus. Direct closure of the leg wound was achieved (7 × 10 cm width skin paddle). Three weeks later wound dehiscence was observed with muscle necrosis including the middle-distal portion of the peroneus longus and brevis muscles and their tendons above the external maleolus. The peroneal muscles are vulnerable to compartment syndrome since they lie in a narrow and tight compartment limited by the deep fascia, the anterior and posterior intermuscular septa and the fibula. (From Villarreal PM, Monje F, Ganan Y et al: Vascularization of the peroneal muscles: critical evaluation in fibular free flap harvesting, *Int J Oral Maxillofac Surg* 33[8]:792-797, 2004.)

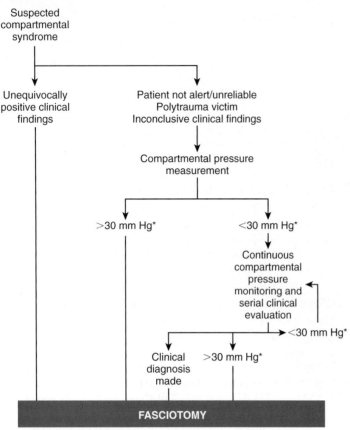

Suspected compartmental syndrome

Unequivocally positive clinical findings

Patient not alert/unreliable
Polytrauma victim
Inconclusive clinical findings

Compartmental pressure measurement

>30 mm Hg*   <30 mm Hg*

Continuous compartmental pressure monitoring and serial clinical evaluation

<30 mm Hg*

Clinical diagnosis made   >30 mm Hg*

FASCIOTOMY

*In patients with hypotension, compartmental syndromes may occur at pressures <30 mm Hg. Currently, we use 25 mm Hg as the critical pressure in these patients.

FIG. 12-41 Algorithm used in diagnosing and treating acute compartment syndromes of the lower leg. (From Bourne RB, Rorabeek CH: Compartment syndromes of the lower leg, *Clin Orthop* 240:97-104, 1989.)

PROCEDURE

- While the patient is lying supine, the circumference of the bellies of the gastrocnemius and soleus muscles are measured (Figs. 12-42 and 12-43).
- The measurement is compared with the calf circumference of the opposite leg.
- Because the dominance of a leg is not established, except in highly specialized sports or occupations, the measurements should be equal.
- A diminished calf circumference may represent simple loss of muscle tone, but it may also represent atrophy of muscle fibers.
- An increased calf circumference, corroborated with other pathologic findings, may indicate a fulminating compartment syndrome.

Next Steps/Procedures

Keen sign, anterior drawer sign of the ankle, vascular assessment, and diagnostic imaging

CLINICAL PEARL

In knee injuries, the first sign of internal joint derangement is loss of tone in the quadriceps. Internal derangement of the ankle joint produces the same phenomenon in its controlling musculature. The gastrocnemius-soleus mechanism weakens and loses tone to a degree sufficient to be quantified with a tape measure. This measuring can help differentiate the degree of ankle involvement.

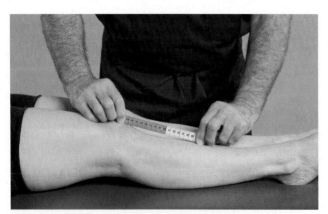

FIG. 12-42 The patient is lying supine with the knees extended. The examiner establishes a point in the leg approximately 15 cm below the midline of the patella.

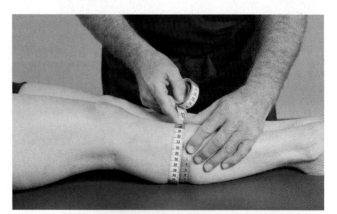

FIG. 12-43 The circumference of the leg is measured at the point selected in Fig. 12-42. The examiner should be cautious when drawing the tape measure tight. The tape should be snug, but skin depressions should be minimal. The measurement is recorded and compared with the circumference of the same point in the opposite leg.

Assessment for Chronic Arterial Occlusive Disease

Comment

PAD is a chronic arterial occlusive disease of the lower extremities caused by atherosclerosis. The most common presenting symptom of PAD is IC (PAD-IC), with exercise-induced pain experienced in the calves, thighs, or buttocks that is relieved with rest (Crowther et al, 2007).

Many patients with vascular diseases exhibit signs and symptoms evident at a site distal to the anatomic location of the abnormality. Because most of the vessels in the lower limb either terminate or originate in the foot, they are most often affected by circulatory problems.

Arterial diseases usually result in reduction of blood flow to the foot. Most commonly, this process is a type of occlusion involving the vessel itself or from mechanical obstruction of the vessel lumen by foreign material. The most common cause of occlusion is atherosclerosis and associated embolic atheromatous plaques.

Popliteal artery entrapment syndrome has a male predilection of 15:1 and typically occurs by the second or third decade of life. Symptoms are described as cramping in the calf and foot, often associated with paresthesias and numbness. Adventitial cystic disease of the popliteal artery generally affects men in their fourth or fifth decade. The patient experiences sudden claudication and absent pedal pulses in an otherwise healthy-appearing limb.

Frostbite occurs from freezing of the tissues and resultant vascular injury (Fig. 12-44). Long-term sensitivity to cold with vasospasm and Raynaud phenomenon is a common sequela of frostbite.

Erythromelalgia is a rare disorder, usually involving the feet, in which paroxysmal vasodilatation, erythema, and burning pain are brought on by exposure to heat. The cause may be primary or may be secondary to concomitant diseases such as diabetes, hypertension, venous insufficiency, or myeloproliferative disorders. Erythromelalgia should be suspected when the patient's subjective complaints of erythema and burning pain are associated with an objective elevation in skin temperature. It often begins as a mild discomfort mimicking neuropathy, but it may slowly progress to the point at which patients are severely disabled.

The most common causes of small-vessel diseases are arteriosclerosis and the collagen-vascular diseases. Micro-embolization will produce histologic changes in muscles that are comparable to those seen in myopathic diseases. An acute obstruction of small vessels is an example of such a change. The clinical conditions are chronic and usually progressive. The collagen-vascular diseases may have periods of acute exacerbation. During these periods, the diseases are rapidly progressive. In this case, the electromyographic (EMG) findings would be myopathic in nature and would resemble polymyositis. Nerve conduction studies would show normal or slightly slowed velocities, and the M wave would probably be reduced slightly. With slowly progressive arteriosclerosis, EMG studies are rarely performed. The changes would be very slow and would represent loss of individual muscle fibers from the motor units, as well as loss of small nerve fibers. The EMG findings would demonstrate myopathic and neuropathic, large-amplitude and small-amplitude motor units of brief duration. Fibrillation potentials would be a rare finding.

Symptomatic PAD, which affects 6% of the American population over 55 years of age, is a leading cause of morbidity. Patients experience lower extremity pain during ambulation because the impaired circulation cannot meet the energy needs of the active musculature. As a consequence, these patients have ambulatory dysfunction, decline in other domains of physical function—lower daily physical activity, impaired health-related quality of life—and difficulty in completing activities of daily living that require the use of the lower extremities. A widely recognized symptom of PAD

ORTHOPEDIC GAMUT 12-12

CONDITIONS AFFECTING THE POPLITEAL ARTERY

1. Popliteal artery entrapment syndrome
2. Adventitial cystic disease of the popliteal artery

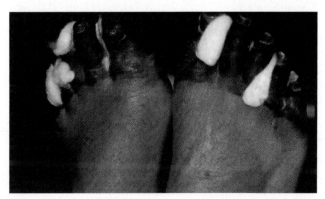

FIG. 12-44 Frostbitten toes demarcated at three weeks after injury. Note the cotton padding between the toes. Minimal tissue loss occurred. (Photo by Paul Auerbach, MD.) (In Auerbach: *Wilderness medicine*, ed 5, St Louis, 2007, Mosby.)

is IC, defined as ischemic calf pain that occurs during ambulation and resolves in 10 minutes or less of rest. However, patients with PAD are often asymptomatic or have symptoms that are atypical from the classic description of IC (Gardner, Montgomery, Afaq, in press).

PROCEDURE

- The patient walks at a rate of 120 steps per minute for 60 seconds (Fig. 12-45).
- This goal can be accomplished by having the patient walk on a treadmill.
- The time that elapses between the start of the test and the occurrence of leg cramping is the claudication time (Fig. 12-46).
- The site of the cramping and often the color change (pallor) in the tissues identifies the level of the lesion.
- A positive test indicates peripheral vascular disease of chronic arterial occlusion.

Next Steps/Procedures
Buerger test, foot tourniquet test, Homans sign, Moszkowicz test, Moses sign, Perthes test, and vascular assessment

CLINICAL PEARL

The claudication test may be an assumed finding in patients who complain of leg cramps during distance walking. The pain of neurogenic origin is differentiated from pain of arterial origin when the patient relates sitting with almost immediate cramp relief.

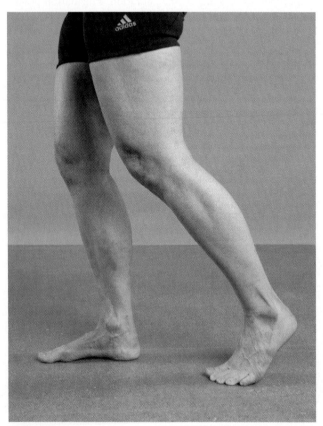

FIG. 12-45 The patient begins marching in place. The pace should be approximately 120 steps per minute and should be continued for 60 seconds. This maneuver also may be accomplished by using a treadmill.

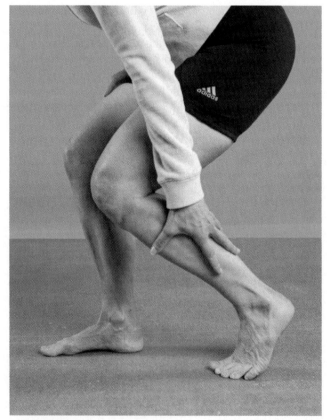

FIG. 12-46 The time elapsing between the start of the test and the onset of the leg cramping is the claudication time. The normal leg should not cramp. When positive, the test indicates chronic arterial occlusion.

DUCHENNE SIGN

Assessment for Lesions of the Superficial Peroneal Nerve

Comment

Compression or distortion of the superficial peroneal nerve may occur where the nerve exits the muscular layer of the leg and pierces the crural fascia at the level between the middle and the distal third of the leg. Chronic ankle sprains, a major underlying factor, subject the nerve to recurrent stretching (Fig. 12-47).

> Chronic ankle instability (CAI) is a subjectively reported phenomenon that has been defined as a tendency for the ankle to *give way* during normal activity and is comparable with the giving-way phenomenon that occurs in an unstable knee joint. Traditionally, CAI has been attributed to two potential causes: mechanical instability (MI) and functional instability (FI). MI has been defined as a 5-degree difference in the talar tilt test and a 4-mm side-to-side difference in the anterior drawer test, whereas FI is a subjective reported feeling of *giving way* during functional activity combined with negative talar tilt and anterior drawer objective tests (Monaghan, Delahunt, Caulfield, 2006).

At the entrance into the peroneal tunnel, near the head of the fibula, the common peroneal nerve divides into two terminal branches: the deep and the superficial peroneal nerve. This terminal branch point and the course of the superficial peroneal nerve may vary. The superficial branch continues distally between the fibula and the peroneus longus muscle, which lies on the intermuscular septum of the anterior compartment. The nerve also lies proximally between the peroneus longus and the extensor digitorum longus muscles and distally between the peroneus longus and the brevis muscles.

> Arthur William Meyer, a human anatomist, was the first to observe longitudinal peroneus brevis tears in both a Spanish sailor and an Irish dishwasher. Interestingly, Meyer noted that these tears, similar to other attritional tendon tears in the human body, lack a gross reparative process. Since this discovery, few studies have been conducted that explore the full clinical spectrum of peroneus brevis and longus tendon tears. Peroneal tendon tears are frequently overlooked because of the vague nature of pain along the lateral ankle region. These tears have been reported to occur after an acute traumatic event or without any identifiable traumatic episode. Warmth, edema, and tenderness along the course of the peroneal tendons in the fibular groove are the common physical findings. Manual muscle strength testing may show little or no weakness of the peroneal tendons, which further complicates the diagnosis (Dombek et al, 2003).

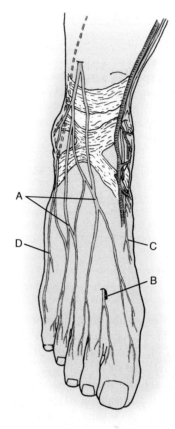

FIG. 12-47 Two main branches of superficial peroneal nerve: medial (intermediate) branch to medial side of hallux and second and third dorsal web spaces and lateral branch to third and fourth dorsal web spaces. **A,** Deep peroneal nerve courses between first and second metatarsals to innervate skin of first web space dorsally. **B,** Saphenous nerve courses anterior to medial malleolus and innervates skin over dorsomedial aspect of hindfoot and midfoot. **C,** Sural nerve passes posterior to lateral malleolus and divides near calcaneocuboid joint into dorsal branch (which innervates fourth web space dorsally) and main trunk (which continues distally to supply skin of lateral side of fifth toe). **D,** In practice, however, the branch of superficial peroneal nerve to dorsomedial aspect of hallux is most vulnerable to injury. (From: Canale ST: *Campbell's operative orthopaedics,* ed 11, St Louis, 2007, Mosby.)

At the level between the middle and the distal third of the leg, the nerve pierces the crural fascia and continues subcutaneously as the cutaneous dorsalis medialis and the cutaneous dorsalis intermedius nerves. Before piercing the fascia, the superficial peroneal nerve supplies the peroneus longus and brevis muscles. The cutaneous branches of the superficial nerves supply the skin of the anterolateral side of

959

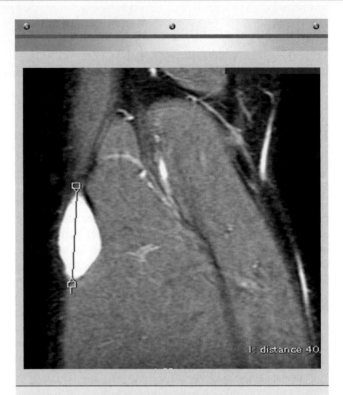

I: distance 40.

AT THE VIEWBOX

ORTHOPEDIC GAMUT 12-13

ADDITIONAL ANTEROLATERAL COMPARTMENT SYNDROME TEST PROCEDURES

1. Resisted dorsiflexion and eversion with pressure applied over the tunnel
2. Passive plantar flexion and inversion
3. Stretching of the nerve, as in the second test, with percussion over the tunnel

---

the leg; the dorsum of the foot; the dorsum of the first, second, and third toes; and the medial side of the fourth toe. The sural nerve, via the cutaneous dorsalis lateralis nerve, supplies the lateral sides of the fourth and fifth toes.

Trauma represents the most commonly proposed cause of this rarely diagnosed syndrome of the superficial peroneal nerve. Surgical trauma, lipomas, muscular hernias, tight boots, repetitive compression of the foot in sports, and dynamic compression of the narrow fascial tunnel have been offered as possible causes. Trauma in this area may lead to local inflammation, reactive swelling, and eventual compression of the fascial tunnel.

Dynamic compression, based on the functional anatomy of the leg, places the nerve at risk. The superficial peroneal nerve is fixed. Therefore forced inversion and extension of the foot further stretches the nerve over the fascial border. Although typically 1 cm long, surgical evidence shows that the tunnel may actually extend up 3 to 11 cm in length. Repetitive activities may cause scarring of the nerve or fascial borders, which narrows the tunnel even further.

Described as mononeuralgia, pain caused by compression or damage to the superficial peroneal nerve is felt on the dorsum of the foot and is occasionally accompanied by dysesthesia or complete anesthesia in the nerve's dermatome.

A positive result for these provocative tests is the production of pain or paresthesia over the nerve's dermatome. EMG studies of the peroneal and anterior tibial muscles and conduction velocities help in identifying the syndrome.

PROCEDURE

- The examiner pushes up the head of the patient's first metatarsal with the thumb, and the patient plantar flexes the foot (Fig. 12-48).
- The sign is present when the medial border of the foot dorsiflexes, with the lateral border plantar flexing (Fig. 12-49).
- The head of the first metatarsal offers no resistance to the pushing thumb.
- The plantar crease runs laterally from the medial side of the big toe to the heel, and the arch disappears.
- This result is caused by paralysis of the peroneus longus, which results from a lesion of the superficial peroneal nerve or a lesion at or above the L4, L5, and S1 roots.

Next Steps/Procedures
Tinel foot sign and electrodiagnosis

CLINICAL PEARL

Before diagnosing pes planus that is caused by structural problems, the examiner should attempt to elicit Duchenne sign. The presence of this sign indicates a pes planus phenomenon that is caused by neural lesions at a much higher level than the arch itself.

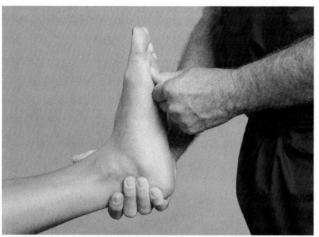

FIG. 12-48 The patient is lying supine, and the leg is extended. The examiner grasps the lower tibia with one hand slightly above the ankle mortise. With the thumb of the other hand, the examiner applies pressure to the head of the first metatarsal.

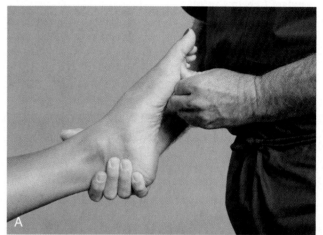

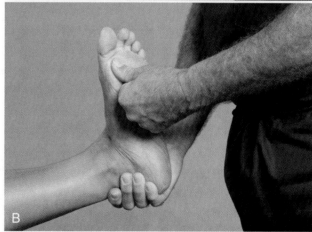

FIG. 12-49 The patient plantar flexes the foot as the examiner maintains pressure on the first metatarsal (A). The sign is present when the medial border of the foot dorsiflexes, the lateral border of the foot plantar flexes, and the arch of the foot disappears (B). The presence of this sign indicates paralysis of the peroneus longus muscle that is caused by a lesion of the superficial peroneal nerve.

12

Assessment for Arterial Insufficiency of the Lower Extremity

Comment

Chronic compartment syndrome is caused by high pressure within the noncompliant fascial boundaries of the leg, with resultant ischemia of muscles and nerves (Fig. 12-50). The elevated pressures are believed to arise from increased muscle volume and from increased intracellular and extracellular fluid accumulation with or without muscular microtears and hemorrhage. These increased pressures may cause venous and lymphatic compromise and further compound the situation (Fig. 12-51).

Compartment syndrome occurs when interstitial pressure within a limb muscle compartment is increased, reducing perfusion of the muscles and nerves below the level necessary for viability. Trauma is the most common cause of compartment syndrome. Untreated compartment syndrome results in irreversible nerve and muscle injury within 6 hours of onset. Treatment is an emergency surgery in which the fascial envelope around the muscle compartment is opened and the pressure within the compartment normalizes and blood flow is restored (Steinberg, 2005).

The diagnosis of chronic compartment syndrome can be made on clinical examination during or after exercise, but confirmation with compartmental pressures is warranted when considering surgical treatment (Fig. 12-52).

Pressures can be reproducibly obtained using the Stryker manometer or other handheld devices (Fig. 12-53).

Significant diminution of blood flow to individual toes or to an entire foot results in pale nail beds, slow capillary

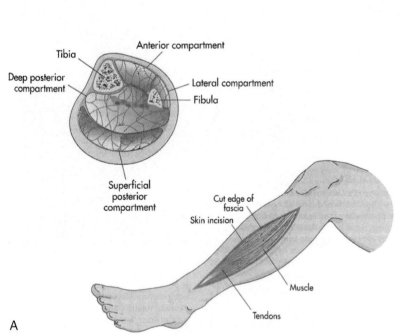

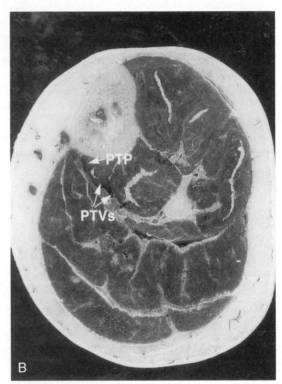

FIG. 12-50 **A,** Compartment syndrome. Often more than one compartment is involved, and anterior compartment is especially vulnerable. Causes include trauma, severe burn, or excessive exercise. A single incision may open more than one compartment. (From Beare PG, Myers JL: *Adult health nursing,* ed 3, St Louis, 1998, Mosby.) **B,** Cross-section of the upper third of the leg. Note a paratibial perforating vein (PTP) passing between the periosteum of the tibia and the fascia of the superficial posterior compartment. Veins were filled with blue Latex. PTVs, posterior tibial veins. (From Mozes G, Gloviczki P, Menawat SS, et al: A surgical anatomy for endoscopic subfascial division of perforating veins, *J Vasc Surg* 24:800–808, 1996.) (From Rutherford RB: *Vascular surgery,* ed 6, Philadelphia, 2005, Saunders.)

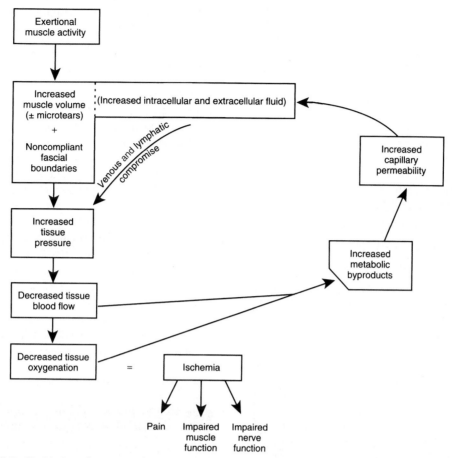

FIG. 12-51 Development of a compartment syndrome. (From Baxter DE: *The foot and ankle in sport*, St Louis, 1995, Mosby.)

ORTHOPEDIC GAMUT 12-14

DIAGNOSTIC CRITERIA OF COMPARTMENT SYNDROME

1. Pre-exercise compartment pressures of 15 mm Hg or greater
2. One-minute postexercise compartment pressures of 30 mm Hg or greater
3. Compartment pressure measured 5 to 10 minutes after cessation of exercise of 15 mm Hg or greater

recovery after skin compression, diminished bleeding after skin puncture, lowering of the skin temperature, and pain of varying intensity. Symptoms and signs of pain, pulselessness, pallor, paresthesia, and paralysis indicate arterial insufficiency or inadequate capillary perfusion. The coexistence of pallor with cyanosis and rubor (mottling) is consistent with vasoconstriction and, later, vasodilation.

The spectrum of causes for diminished blood flow is made apparent by observing the alterations that occur in the healthy extremity, which is affected temporarily by decreased blood flow as a result of environmental alterations, such as cooling of the feet, contact of a toe with ice, or sympathetic nervous stimulation from anxiety or fear. In each instance, the occurrence of pallor and a significant drop in skin temperature will cause pain that is moderately severe and is described as a deep, aching sensation. As the ischemic state persists, pain becomes more intense.

The term *Raynaud disease* is used to describe the occurrence of vasospasm within an underlying primary disease. If vasospasm is associated with a known connective-tissue disease, Raynaud phenomenon is implied. Recognition of Raynaud syndrome and the patient's response to this condition is important in explaining pain and cold tolerance associated with a known pathologic condition. When the symptoms of pain occur in a toe, the foot, or the entire lower extremity, the existence of adequate blood flow in the large and small vessels must be determined.

In patients known to have a nerve compression lesion, such as superficial peroneal nerve compression at the fascial tunnel, diminished blood flow will cause abnormal sensory changes to occur earlier than they would in the healthy patient. Motor weakness occurs more quickly when partial or complete ischemia occurs.

Various conditions—atherosclerotic stenosis, thromboembolism, or compression of major arteries in the lower abdomen—cause pain, claudication, paresthesia, and intermittent episodes of pallor. The lesions may be partial or complete, and the clinical symptoms may vary according to the degree of ischemia.

12

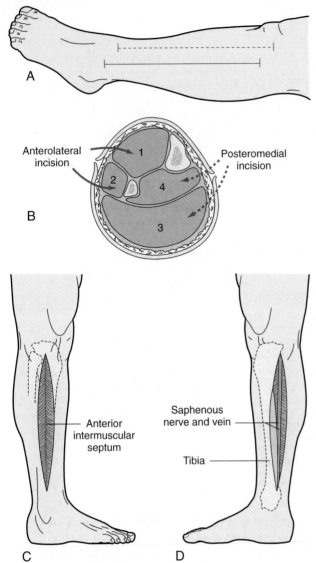

FIG. 12-52 **A,** The double-incision technique for performing fasciotomies of all four compartments of the lower extremity. **B,** Cross section of the lower extremity showing a position of anterolateral and posteromedial incisions that allows access to the anterior and lateral compartments (1 and 2) and the superficial and deep posterior compartments (3 and 4). **C,** A vertical anterior incision is centered midway between the tibia and fibula. The anterior intermuscular septum is identified, and two fasciotomy incisions are made: one anterior and one posterior to the septum. **D,** A vertical posteromedial incision is centered 2 cm to the rear of the tibia. Care is taken to avoid injury to the saphenous vein and nerve. (From Townsend CM: *Sabiston textbook of surgery,* ed 18, Philadelphia, 2007, Saunders.)

Acute occlusion of an artery is associated with unrelenting pain and pallor followed by rubor and cyanosis. Cold tolerance is diminished, and intrinsic muscle weakness occurs.

Obliteration of the artery results from trauma and the occurrence of an anterior compartment compression of the lower leg muscles, vessels, and nerves. This compression causes pallor of the foot, diminished pulse volume, and severe pain. The effect of diminished arterial inflow and lessened venous outflow during pain has been well calibrated by analyzing the effects of traumatic lesions at various levels of the extremity. Decompression of a tight compartment that is anterior to the leg will diminish pain almost immediately. Elimination of nerve compression syndromes at the ankle will provide measurable relief of pain.

Causalgia is considered a mixed nerve lesion with accompanying or secondary vascular insufficiency. The residual pain may require direct treatment of the peripheral nerve.

Sympathetic dystrophy is one condition that may occur, although a specific nerve injury cannot be demonstrated. However, a vasospastic element occurs secondary to a major or minor insult of the extremity or an adjacent organ.

Deep-venous thrombosis (DVT) is a common disorder affecting 250,000 people in the United States per year. Only a small percentage of individuals diagnosed with DVT progress to complications such as pulmonary embolism. However, the symptoms associated with critical venous occlusive and thrombotic disorders are severe, and patients may develop life- and limb-threatening complications such as phlegmasia cerulea dolens or the superior vena cava syndrome (SVC syndrome) (Dayal et al, 2005).

PROCEDURE

- Application of a pneumatic tourniquet, with pressure elevated to 20 mm Hg above the patient's resting diastolic blood pressure, to a normal extremity will obliterate arterial inflow and venous outflow, slow motor nerve conduction, decrease sensory conduction, and cause pain in the foot and at the site of tourniquet compression (Fig. 12-54).
- Anoxia and nerve compression occur simultaneously, and muscle weakness is evident within 3 to 5 minutes.
- Digital paresthesia occurs, and sensation diminishes gradually to anesthesia in approximately 30 minutes.
- These painful sensations are a combination of muscle and nerve ischemia and nerve compression.

Next Steps/Procedures

Buerger test, claudication test, Homans sign, Moszkowicz test, Moses test, Perthes test, and vascular assessment

CLINICAL PEARL

Tenderness at the front of the leg is characteristic in (1) Osgood-Schlatter disease, (2) Brodie abscess (or osteitis), (3) anterior tibial compartment syndrome, (4) stress fracture, and (5) shin splints. Tenderness at the back of the leg is characteristically situated (1) in the plantaris tendon in partial and complete ruptures, (2) over varicosities in superficial thrombophlebitis, and (3) over the tendocalcaneus in partial tears and complete ruptures.

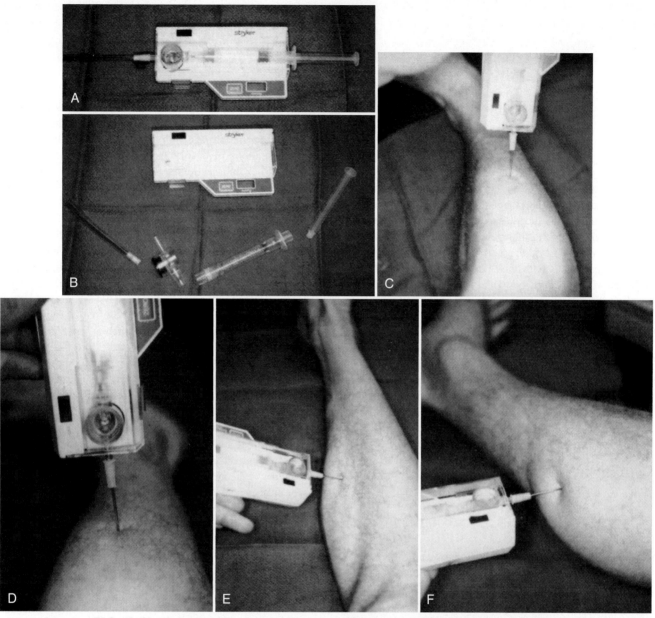

FIG. 12-53 Stryker handheld device for compartment pressure measurement **(A)**, disass-embled components **(B)**, measuring anterior **(C)**, lateral **(D)**, deep posterior **(E)**, and superficial posterior compartments **(F)**. (From Baxter DE: *The foot and ankle in sport*, St Louis 1995, Mosby.)

12

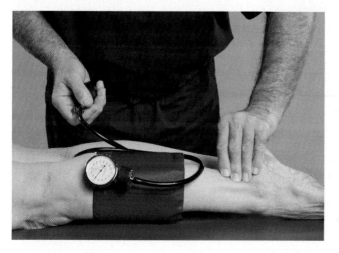

FIG. 12-54 The patient is lying prone on the examination table, and the leg is extended. The foot dangles over the end of the examining table. The calf musculature should be as relaxed as possible. A blood pressure cuff is applied to the leg, near the ankle, above the area of complaint. The cuff is inflated to 20 mm Hg above the patient's resting diastolic blood pressure. Pressure may need to be increased to reach blanching of the distal extremity. Foot pain, paresthesia, and muscle weak-ness appearing in less than 5 minutes indicate arterial insufficiency.

Assessment for Pes Planus

Comment

Flattening of the longitudinal arch, or flatfoot, is often asymptomatic but may result in muscle fatigue with aching and intolerance caused by long hours of standing or walking. Physical findings include loss of the medial longitudinal arch on weight bearing along with medial and plantar displacement of the navicular and the talar head. In severe cases, the calcaneus is everted (valgus), and the forefoot is abducted with *too many toes* when viewed from behind (Fig. 12-55).

Pes planus is attributed to deficiencies in the structure of the talus and calcaneus. Conversely, strong and well-shaped feet are attributed to tarsal bones so shaped and so integrated into one another that they cannot shift when weight is imposed on them. In symptomatic pes planus that does not involve osseous anomalies, the condition is often related to weak posterior tibial muscle function. This weakness permits an abnormal excursion of the talonavicular joint.

Rupture of the tendon of the posterior tibialis muscle is an etiologic factor in pes planus. These ruptures have occurred in middle-age individuals who have had one or more injections of a corticosteroid into the sheath of the tendon. Such an injection is used to relieve local discomfort or to alleviate an obvious synovitis. Rupture of the tendon occurs with prompt development of a markedly pronated foot. When the patient, attempting to rise on the toes, has difficulty doing so on the involved side, it is because the heel fails to invert and the longitudinal arch fails to rise during this maneuver. Rupture of the posterior tibial tendon should be suspected in any patient in which unilateral pes planus suddenly appears.

The symptomatic weak foot may be flat or may have a high longitudinal arch, especially when at rest. The flatfoot usually has a degree of abduction of the forefoot and eversion of the ankle. The Achilles tendon may be shortened and pulled at an angle instead of following a plumb line. The long, narrow, flaccid foot with a normal arch is likely to become symptomatic.

Injuries to the lateral column of the foot can involve the anterior aspect of the calcaneus, the cuboid, and the fourth and fifth metatarsals. These injuries are often associated with injuries of the medial column as well, many of which demonstrate operative indications. Isolated injuries of the lateral column, more specifically the cuboid, are rare but have been described. Missed fractures or nonoperative treatment of displaced cuboid injuries can lead to shortening of the lateral column with subsequent flatfoot deformity, which may be painful (Mihalich, Early, 2006).

Malunion of a cuboid fracture can cause poor outcomes, often resulting in a flatfoot deformity. This defect may be symptomatic and exhibit the attributes of the more commonly seen flatfoot associated with posterior tibial tendon insufficiency (Fig. 12-56).

PROCEDURE

- Medial curving of the Achilles tendon, when viewed posteriorly, indicates foot pronation (also known as "squinting of the toes") (Figs. 12-57 and 12-58).

Next Steps/Procedures
Hoffa test and Thompson test

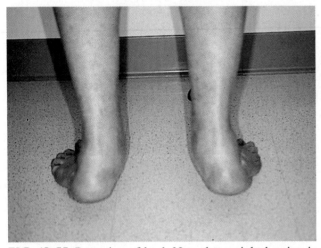

FIG. 12-55 Pronation of heel. Note that weight bearing is not through the midline of the foot. (From Seidel HM: *Mosby's guide to physical examination*, ed 4, St Louis, 1999, Mosby.)

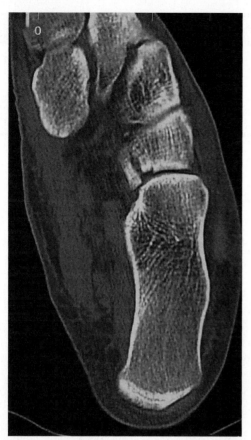

FIG. 12-56 CT scan of a stable cuboid fracture not requiring operative intervention. (From Mihalich RM, Early JS: Management of cuboid crush injuries, *Foot Ankle Clin North Am* 11[1]:121-126, 2006.)

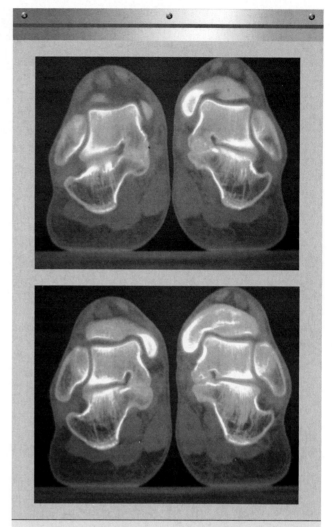

AT THE VIEWBOX

32-year-old male with right ankle sprain. Pain and swelling, slow to resolve. Long history of pes planus with foot pronation, rigid on clinical examination. CT scan demonstrates fibrous talocalcaneal coalition across the medial facet of the talus and the sustentaculum tali. Note associated degenerative changes of the subtalar joints, with reactive sclerosis. Tarsal coalition is associated with altered ankle and foot mechanics, often with chronic pain and dysfunction. Multiple ankle sprains, often associated with prolonged symptoms are frequently seen in patients with tarsal coalition. (From the teaching file of Timothy Mick, DC, DACBR)

12

CLINICAL PEARL

The arches of the foot do not become fully formed until a child has been walking for some years. The young child's foot is normally flat. If the arches fail to establish, an awkward gait and rapid, uneven wear and distortion of the shoes may occur, but it is rare for pain or other symptoms to develop. Persistent flatfoot may be associated with knock-knees, torsional deformities of the tibia, and valgus deformities of the heel.

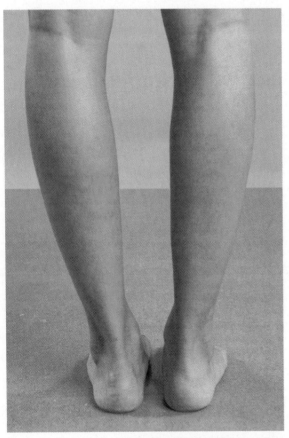

FIG. 12-57 The patient is standing, with the feet resting on a smooth, flat surface. From the posterior, the examiner observes the positions of the Achilles tendons. Normally, no curving of the tendons should be seen as the patient bears weight.

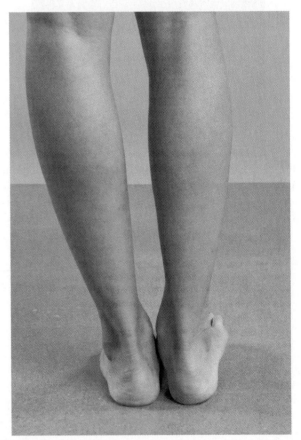

FIG. 12-58 The sign is present when a medial curving of the Achilles tendon is observed (as on the right). Also visible is the "squinting toes" sign, an effect of the pes planus. The sign indicates a pes planus condition.

HOFFA TEST

ALSO KNOWN AS HOFFA SIGN

Assessment for Fracture of the Calcaneus

Comment

The posterior portion of the foot is rarely fractured—if sprain-fractures are excluded. The ordinary fracture of the calcaneus is by direct compression, as in a fall from a height or from driving the foot into a hard surface. Approximately 2% of all fractures in adults are calcaneal fractures (Fig 12-59).

The calcaneus is the largest tarsal bone in the foot and plays an important role in walking and running. Motor-vehicle crashes and falls from elevation have been associated with calcaneal fractures. Although not life threatening, these injuries may result in permanent disability. This study used the Crash Injury Research and Engineering Network (CIREN) database to describe calcaneal fractures and concomitant lower-extremity skeletal injury patterns for occupants involved in motor-vehicle crashes (Benson et al, 2007).

Abnormal, forceful motion may cause avulsion or snubbing fractures of the talus. Also, the sustentaculum tali may be broken by forceful eversion of the foot. Restoring the contour of the calcaneus and particularly the integrity of the talocalcaneal joint is extremely important. Adduction or abduction of the foot may cause a snubbing or avulsion fracture of the superior portion of the calcaneus at the calcaneocuboid joint.

A fracture of the calcaneus usually results from a fall on the heel. It often is associated with a compression fracture of the lumbar spine. The os calcis is usually crushed, and the fragments are displaced in varying amounts (Fig. 12-60). The heel is often so painful that the spine injury may not be noticed initially.

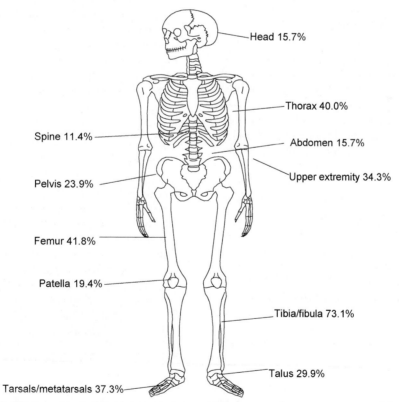

FIG. 12-59 Summary of the injury patterns and frequency for car occupants *with* calcaneal fractures. Overall, a large portion of occupants have injury to other body regions. Most occupants have other lower extremity injuries in addition to their calcaneal fracture.

(Adapted from Benson E, Conroy C, Hoyt DB, et al: Calcaneal fractures in occupants involved in severe frontal motor vehicle crashes, *Accident Analysis & Prevention* 39[4]:794-799, 2007.)

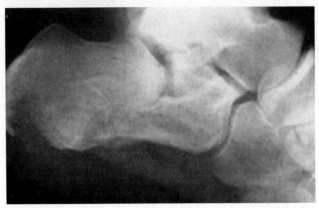

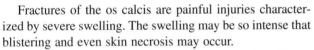

FIG. 12-60 Fracture of the calcaneus with moderate displacement. (From Mercier LR, Pettid FJ: *Practical orthopedics*, ed 4, St Louis, 1995, Mosby.)

Fractures of the os calcis are painful injuries characterized by severe swelling. The swelling may be so intense that blistering and even skin necrosis may occur.

Fracture of the calcaneus is the most common tarsal bone injury. A fracture involving the body of the calcaneus is the most common calcaneal fracture, and it often extends into the subtalar joint, with the posterior portion of the body displaced upward. This type of fracture is caused by a direct vertical force onto the calcaneus that usually occurs after a fall from a height. The spine should always be examined carefully because a compression fracture of the spine in the dorsolumbar area is often associated with calcaneal fractures.

The other types of calcaneal fractures such as an avulsion fracture of Achilles tendon insertion and fracture of the sustentaculum tali or anterior process are seen less frequently.

AP and lateral diagnostic imaging of the foot are necessary to evaluate the involvement of the subtalar joint. Fracture of the sustentaculum tali is demonstrable only in the axial views.

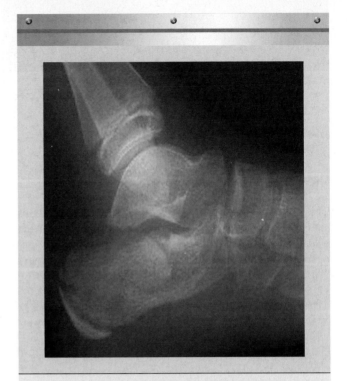

AT THE VIEWBOX

Adolescent male who fell from a second story balcony, landing on his feet. Resultant severe heel pain, with inability to bear weight. A lateral plain film of the ankle reveals depression of the mid-portion of the calcaneus. The angle created by intersection of lines drawn between the posterior and middle tubercles and the middle and anterior tubercles of the calcaneus (Boehler's angle) should be no less than 28 degrees. In this case, it is nearly zero. There are also mixed regions of lucency and sclerosis in the body of the calcaneus, further evidence of the impacted fracture. This type of impacted calcaneal fracture should prompt thorough evaluation to help exclude an associated vertebral body compression fracture or burst fracture in the thoracolumbar junction. Clinical focus on the more painful and debilitating calcaneal fracture could result in lack of attention to pain at the thoracolumbar junction, which would warrant imaging of the spine to further assess. Note the irregular, sclerotic appearance of the calcaneal tuberosity apophysis, which is seen as an age-related normal finding. (From the teaching file of Timothy Mick, DC, DACBR)

PROCEDURE

- While the patient is lying prone, the ankles hang well over the edge of the examining table in a symmetric position.
- Hoffa test is positive if the examiner, using movement and palpation, finds the patient's Achilles tendon on the injured side less taut than that on the contralateral side.
- Dorsiflexion of the foot in the relaxed position may also be increased on the affected side (Fig. 12-61).
- A loose fragment may be observed and felt behind either malleolus.
- The test is significant for fracture of the calcaneus.

Next Steps/Procedures

Helbings sign, Thompson test, and diagnostic imaging

CLINICAL PEARL

In geriatric patients, the Achilles tendon insufficiency that is caused by attrition also produces a positive Hoffa test. In this instance, the calcaneus remains intact.

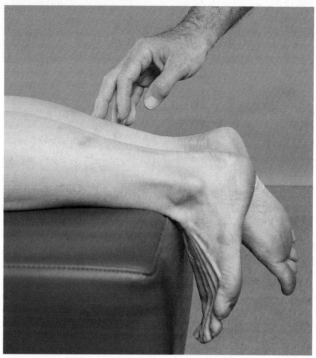

FIG. 12-61 The patient is prone on the examination table. The knees are extended, and the ankles hang well over the end of the table. The sign is present when the affected foot rests in a more dorsiflexed position (as noted on the left) than the opposite foot. The test is positive when the examiner determines by palpation the loss of Achilles tendon integrity. The sign implicates calcaneal fracture.

12

HOMANS SIGN

Assessment for Thrombophlebitis of the Lower Extremity

Comment

Superficial thrombophlebitis is inflammation and thrombosis of a superficial vein. This condition commonly results either from local trauma or from an intravenous infusion, but it may occur spontaneously. Thrombosis of the deep veins in the calf or pelvis usually occurs as a result of a combination of damage to the endothelial lining of the veins, with stasis of the blood within them as a consequence of physical inactivity.

In 1856, Virchow first described the constellation of stasis, hypercoagulability, and vascular injury as risk factors for development of DVT. In 1934, Homans further characterized clinical thromboembolic disease (TED). Today, despite multiple modalities for prevention, TED remains a significant source of morbidity and mortality. Trauma patients, especially those with advanced age, high severity of injury, prolonged immobilization, multiple blood transfusions, or elevated partial thromboplastin time, represent a group at particularly high risk for TED (Keller et al, 2000).

Intermittent claudication is the term applied to a condition that denotes an insufficient blood supply to the muscles of the lower extremities when they are called into activity during locomotion. IC occurs in atheroma, with or without thrombosis, and in embolism, Buerger disease, and rarely, syphilitic endarteritis. The condition is aggravated by anemia.

The patient complains of pain that occurs in one or both legs and in the calf muscles and comes on after walking a certain distance. The pain disappears during rest. The pain becomes so intolerable that the patient is obliged to stand or sit still until it passes. As time goes on, the distance that the patient can walk in comfort becomes progressively shorter.

Examination of the affected limb reveals nothing obvious. The legs are well nourished and normal in sensation and reflexes. The arteries at the ankle will be pulseless, and the popliteal pulsation behind the knee joint may not be felt. The femoral artery can usually be felt to pulsate in a normal manner.

After the patient walks, the foot may appear unduly pale. With rest, normal color returns and spreads gradually over the surface of the foot. The ankle jerk may be diminished or absent as a result of ischemia of the posterior tibial nerve. In later cases, paresthesia and objective sensory loss occur in the toes and foot. IC is not uncommon, and its diagnosis is not difficult.

The importance of recognizing the condition is paramount because of the tendency for the condition to develop into gangrene.

The postthrombotic syndrome (PTS) is a chronic, potentially debilitating complication of DVT of the lower extremity that is characterized by limb pain, heaviness, swelling, cramps, edema, varicosities, and, in severe cases, ulcers. PTS has been estimated to develop in 20% to 50% of patients after lower-extremity DVT and has adverse effects on quality of life and incurs high costs (Elman, Kahn, 2006).

PROCEDURE

- While the patient is lying in the supine position, the examiner dorsiflexes the patient's foot and squeezes the calf (Figs. 12-62 and 12-63).
- Deep-seated pain in the posterior leg or calf indicates thrombophlebitis.

Next Steps/Procedures

Buerger test, claudication test, foot tourniquet test, Moszkowicz test, Moses sign, Perthes test, and vascular assessment

CLINICAL PEARL

The use of Homans sign does not aid differentiation between a muscular lesion and thrombophlebitis. The differentiation occurs when the test is concluded. When the pain remits quickly, thrombophlebitis is suspected. When the pain persists or lags as an ache, calf strain is suspected.

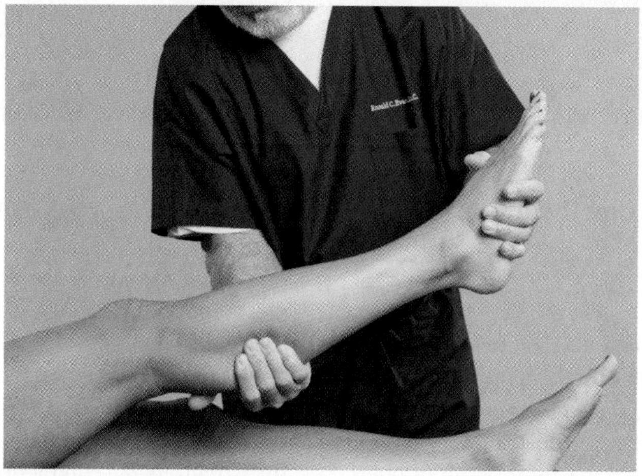

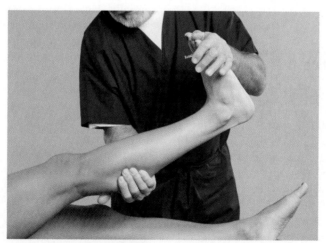

FIG. 12-62 The patient is lying supine with the knees extended and the legs resting on the examination table. The examiner elevates the affected leg to 45 degrees, and the calf is squeezed firmly.

FIG. 12-63 As the calf pressure is maintained, the examiner dorsiflexes the patient's foot. Deep calf or leg pain during this maneuver indicates thrombophlebitis.

12

Assessment for Distal Fibular Fracture

Comment

Fracture of the tibia is uncommon, but fracture of the fibula is common. In any fracture of the fibula, associated injury of the ankle must be investigated. Whenever complete fracture of the fibula occurs above the level of the tibiofibular syndesmosis, complete rupture of the inferior tibiofibular ligaments must be investigated. The possibility of rupture is the most serious and most important consideration in the fracture of the fibula. The actual fracture of the fibula is usually inconsequential, except that it does require a certain period of healing. If the fracture is accompanied by a rupture of the tibiofibular ligaments and results in instability or separation of the ankle mortise, a serious and permanent disability results (Fig. 12-64).

Fractures of the fibula result from direct blows that usually occur in the lower one third of the fibula. These blows may be caused by contact with a shoe or other hard object. Fracture of the fibula causes immediate pain but not severe disability. On examination, local tenderness will be present at the site of the injury. Local crepitus may or may not be present. Usually, prompt swelling occurs along with localized hematoma formation. The individual can usually walk quite well. In fact, the patient may be able to complete a walking task because, with a fracture of the fibula by direct blow, the integrity of the ankle is not involved, and disability is caused by contraction of the muscle attachments on the fibular shaft. Diagnosis is confirmed by diagnostic imaging, which should always be used in a case of localized tenderness over any bone.

Of all bones, the fibula is particularly prone to stress fracture and is second only to the metatarsals in this respect. This condition arises early in athletic or new job training requiring prolonged standing and first appears as an ache, with some soreness and distress during function. The ache is usually localized near the neck of the fibula. The patient has no history of injury.

Isolated, undisplaced fractures of either malleolus are usually stable (Fig. 12-68).

Fractures with significant displacement must be reduced, especially if any widening of the ankle joint is present (Fig. 12-69). Fractures with dislocation of the talus should be reduced as rapidly as possible (Fig. 12-70).

The incidence of nonunion in pediatric long bone lower extremity fractures is extremely low. Most uncomplicated

---

ORTHOPEDIC GAMUT 12-15

DISTAL TIBIAL AND FIBULAR FRACTURES

Types of distal tibial or fibular fractures include the following:

1. Bimalleolar fracture: fractures of the medial and lateral malleoli (Fig. 12-65)
2. Boot-top (skier's) fracture: spiral fracture of the distal diametaphyseal portions of the tibia and fibula
3. Maisonneuve fracture: fracture of the proximal fibula, as a result of severe inversion and external rotation of the ankle (often unobserved because of the severity of the ankle injury)
4. Pott fracture: fracture of the metadiaphyseal region of the distal fibula, with associated rupture of the distal tibiofibular ligament (Fig. 12-66) (Pott fracture that involves both the lateral and medial malleolus is highly likely to result in dislocation of the talus from the ankle mortise; isolated lateral [the more common] or medial malleolar fracture is less likely to destabilize the joint.) (Fig. 12-67)
5. Toddler's fracture: spiral fracture of the distal diametaphyseal region of the tibia in a toddler
6. Trimalleolar (Cotton) fracture: fracture of the medial and lateral malleoli, in addition to the posterior tibial lip, often with tibiotalar dislocation

---

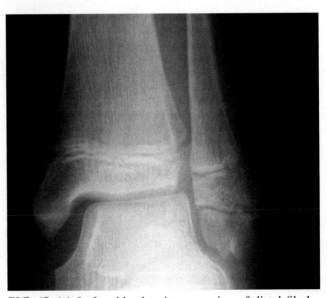

FIG. 12-64 Left ankle showing nonunion of distal fibular epiphyseal fracture and widened medial clear space. (From Mirmiran R, Schuberth JM: Non union of an epiphyseal fibular fracture in a pediatric patient, *J Foot Ankle Surg* 45[6]:410-412, 2006.)

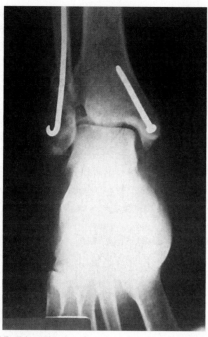

FIG. 12-65 Bimalleolar fracture. (From Deltoff MN, Kogon PL: *The portable skeletal x-ray library*, St Louis, 1998, Mosby.)

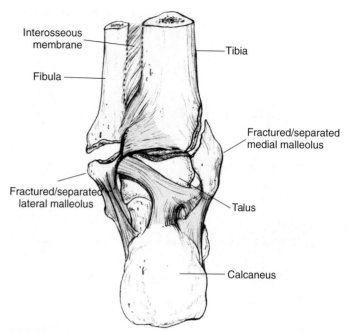

FIG. 12-67 Pott fracture. (From Mathers LH et al: *Clinical anatomy principles*, St Louis, 1996, Mosby.)

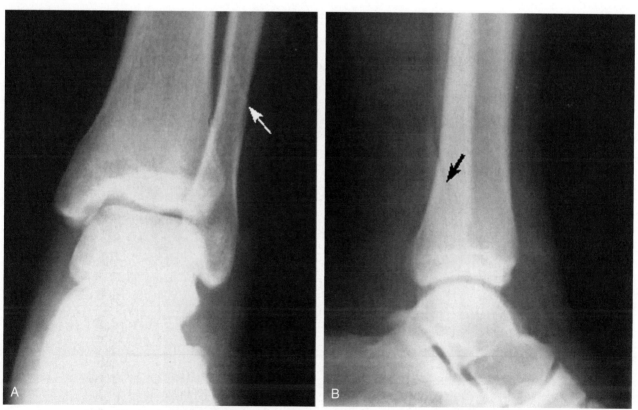

FIG. 12-66 **A** and **B,** Pott fracture *(arrows).* (From Deltoff MN, Kogon PL: *The portable skeletal x-ray library*, St Louis, 1998, Mosby.)

12

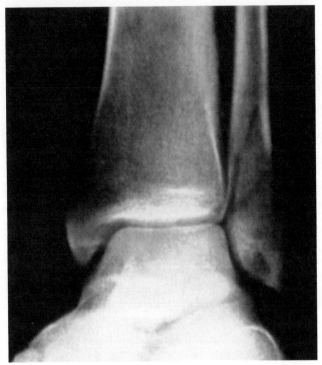

FIG. 12-68 Undisplaced fracture of the lateral malleolus. (From Mercier LR, Pettid FJ: *Practical orthopedics*, ed 4, St Louis, 1995, Mosby.)

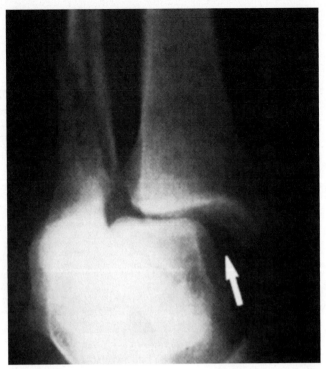

FIG. 12-69 Displaced fracture of the lateral malleolus with widening of the ankle mortise caused by lateral shift of the talus. (From Mercier LR, Pettid FJ: *Practical orthopedics*, ed 4, St Louis, 1995, Mosby.)

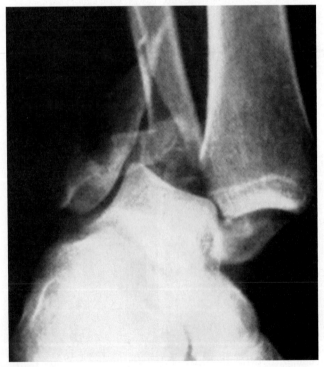

FIG. 12-70 Fracture-dislocation of the ankle. (From Mercier LR, Pettid FJ: *Practical orthopedics*, ed 4, St Louis, 1995, Mosby.)

pediatric fractures, if stable and not greatly displaced, heal with a short course of immobilization. Furthermore, the incidence of non-union seems to be increased if the fracture is open, has open reduction, or becomes infected. The rate of fracture non-union in long bones of pediatric patients has been reported in several relatively large series and ranges from 0% to 1.7% (Mirmiran, Schuberth, 2006).

PROCEDURE

- If a fracture of the distal fibula exists (as in Pott fracture), the diameter around the malleoli area of the affected ankle is increased (Fig. 12-71).

Next Steps/Procedures
Calf circumference test, anterior drawer sign of the ankle, and diagnostic imaging

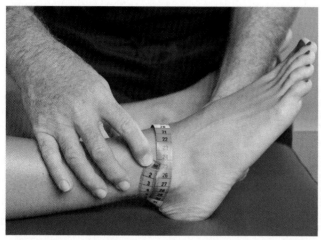

FIG. 12-71 The patient is lying supine on the examination table. The foot and ankle are in a resting position. A tape measure is placed around the ankle, passing over both malleoli. The diameter of the ankle is recorded and compared with the opposite ankle. An increased diameter, correlated with other pathologic findings, indicates a fracture of the distal fibula.

CLINICAL PEARL

Keen sign is an early indicator of ankle fracture. When it is present, the sign mandates diagnostic imaging of the joint.

12

Assessment for Metatarsalgia or Morton Neuroma

Comment

As the foot plantar flexes and the toes dorsiflex during push off, the interdigital nerves between the second and third, and third and fourth metatarsal (Fig. 12-72) may be compressed by the intermetatarsal ligament. This compression causes neuritic radiation of pain into the affected web space and toes. The pain often radiates proximally as well.

Morton neuroma is a common disorder in the adult. A fibroneuromatous reaction between the third and fourth metatarsal heads, over the deep transverse metatarsal ligaments, affects the lateral terminal branch of the median plantar nerve. The impinging effect on the nerve is accentuated during weight bearing, particularly during the push-off phase of walking or when the metatarsal heads are compressed or stretched (Fig. 12-73). Localized tenderness between the third and the fourth metatarsal heads on the plantar surface also occurs. Hypesthesia over the lateral and medial side of the third and fourth toes, respectively, may be present. Morton neuroma can occur in the web spaces that involve the corresponding terminal branch of either the medial or lateral plantar nerve, but this occurrence is uncommon.

Metatarsalgia, pain in the metatarsals, is very common in adults. This pain is caused by various foot deformities or arthritis of the metatarsophalangeal joints. This latter type of pain is most commonly caused by rheumatoid arthritis. The term *metatarsalgia* is used to refer to a pain syndrome and is not disease nomenclature per se (Table 12-4).

When clinically dealing with pain in the forefoot, the term *metatarsalgia* is often used. In reality, metatarsalgia is a descriptive but not a proper diagnostic term, and it incorporates a series of clinical situations of various etiologies—the exact identification of which, in any case—can be ascertained only in a minority of patients. In fact, the term metatarsalgia means *an acute or chronic pain in relation to one or more metatarsophalangeal joints caused by damage (whether or not of mechanical origin) to the anatomical structures that interact with the joint (bone, cartilage,*

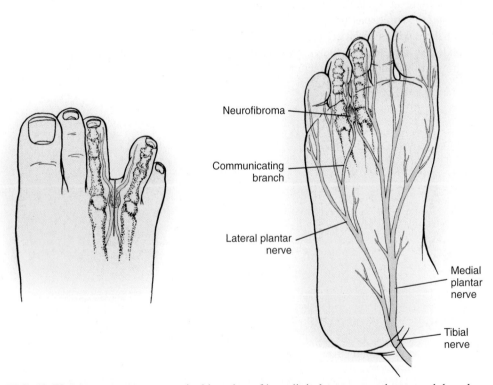

FIG. 12-72 Most common anatomical location of interdigital neuroma; plantar and dorsal views. (Modified from McElvenny RT: The etiology and surgical treatment of intractable pain about the fourth metatarsophalangeal joint (Morton's toe), *J Bone Joint Surg* 25:675, 1943.)

Labels on figure: Neurofibroma, Communicating branch, Lateral plantar nerve, Medial plantar nerve, Tibial nerve

TABLE 12-4

CLASSIFICATION OF METATARSALGIA

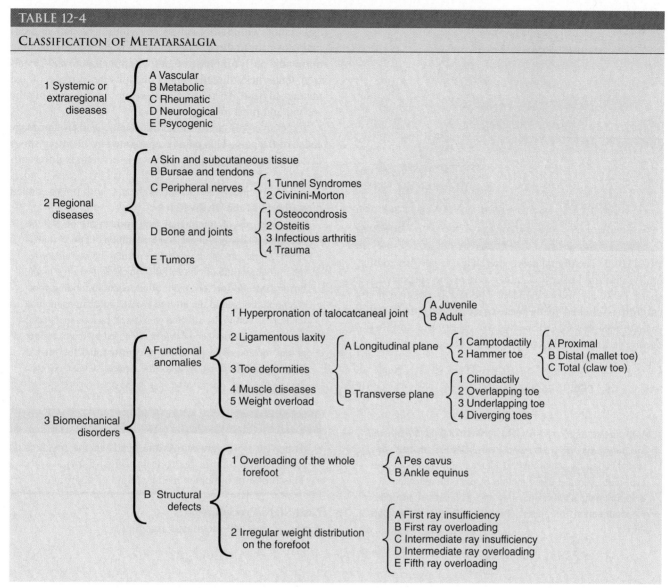

When clinically dealing with pain in the forefoot the term 'metatarsalgia' is often used. In reality, this is a descriptive, not a proper diagnostic term, and incorporates a series of clinical situations of various etiologies—the exact identification of which, in any case, can be ascertained only in a minority of patients. In fact, the term metatarsalgia "an acute or chronic pain in relation to one or more metatarsophalangeal joints caused by damage (whether or not of mechanical origin) to the anatomical structures that interact with the joint (bone, cartilage, capsule and ligaments, vessels, nerves, tendons, bursae and the subcutaneous tissue, and skin)" is meant. Defined in this way, metatarsalgia is not limited to plantar pain (as opposed to heel pain) because the symptom of pain, though more frequently on the plantar side, may be dorsal, lateral, medial, or a combination of these. (From Bardelli M, Turelli L, Scoccianti G: Definition and classification of metatarsalgia, *Foot Ankle Surg* 9[2]:79-85, 2003.)

12

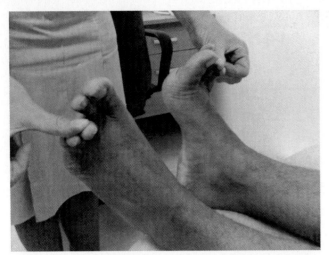

FIG. 12-73 The digital nerve stretch test is performed bilaterally with the lesser toes either side of the suspected web space passively fully extended. The test is positive if discomfort is elicited in the web space of the affected foot. (Adapted from Cloke DJ, Greiss ME: The digital nerve stretch test: A sensitive indicator of Morton's neuroma and neuritis, *Foot Ankle Surg* 12[4]:201-203, 2006.)

capsule and ligaments, vessels, nerves, tendons, bursae and the subcutaneous tissue, and skin). Defined in this way, metatarsalgia is not limited to plantar pain (as opposed to heel pain) because the symptom of pain, though more frequently on the plantar side, may be dorsal, lateral, medial or a combination of these (Bardelli, Turelli, Scoccianti, 2003).

The disease may occur as an isolated condition or in association with hallux valgus or rigidus. The patient complains of pain in the metatarsal heads or toes when standing during the push-off phase of gait. Examination reveals localized tenderness directly under the plantar surface of the metatarsal head. The most common sites for the pain are the second and third metatarsal heads.

Excessive pressure over the metatarsal heads is a primary cause of the pain. This pain is aggravated by ill-fitting shoes that squeeze the toes into a narrow toe-box and is differentiated from Morton neuroma by having its most severe tenderness directly under the metatarsal heads, with no associated hypesthesia of the involved toes.

The diagnosis of interdigital (intermetatarsal) or Morton neuroma is largely clinical. It is a condition of poorly understood origins but often coexists, and may be secondary to, other abnormalities in up to 80% of cases. Features in the history include forefoot pain, often worse in binding footwear and relieved in the unshod foot. Clinical signs include tenderness within the affected web space, pain on metatarsal head approximation, and ***Mulder click***, felt by the examiner as the metatarsal heads are approximated and the plantar tissues pushed dorsally into the space (Cloke, Greiss, 2006).

PROCEDURE

- Transverse pressure across the heads of the metatarsals causes sharp pain in the forefoot (Fig. 12-74).
- This pressure indicates metatarsalgia or neuroma.

Next Steps/Procedures
Strunsky sign and diagnostic imaging

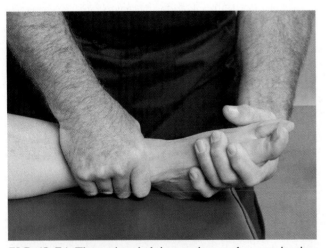

FIG. 12-74 The patient is lying supine on the examination table. The examiner grasps the affected forefoot with one hand and applies transverse pressure to the metatarsal heads. Sharp pain in the foot indicates a positive test and suggests metatarsalgia or neuroma.

CLINICAL PEARL

Anterior metatarsalgia is particularly common in the middle-age women and is often associated with some splaying of the forefoot. Symptoms may be triggered by periods of excessive standing or by an increase in weight, and the patient often has concurrent flattening of the medial longitudinal arch. Weakness of the intrinsic muscles is usually present; thus, a tendency exists for clawing of the toes.

MOSZKOWICZ TEST

ALSO KNOWN AS MOSCHCOWITZ TEST

Assessment for Inadequacy of the Collateral Circulation as in an Arteriovenous Fistula in the Lower Extremity

Comment

Most of the pathologic sequelae from venous diseases develop in the lower extremities.

DVT carries the threat of potentially fatal consequences and thus requires the immediate institution of bed rest and anticoagulation therapy. Such treatment reduces the likelihood of thrombus propagation and lessens the risk of emboli. Varicose veins are prominent, tortuous, abnormally distended veins that occur in approximately 20% of adults. They are five times more common in women than in men and are often associated with a family history of varicosities. Congenitally absent or defective valves are the usual underlying cause of varicose veins. Obstruction of outflow from venous thrombosis or pregnancy may also precipitate varicosities.

Patients with venous insufficiency complain of heaviness and tightness in the lower limbs with exercise. Exercise may greatly increase the degree of venous congestion and produce a deep-seated discomfort known as *venous claudication*. As the condition progresses, the deep and perforated system valves may fail, resulting in chronic stasis edema, dermatitis, and stasis ulcers.

Superficial thrombophlebitis is inflammation affecting a superficial vein with the presence of a blood clot. The underlying pathologic process can be explained by Virchow's triad of vascular stasis, endothelial injury, and hypercoagulability. Thrombophlebitis has been reported after air travel when in-flight stockings were worn. This report raises the suspicion that stockings are an etiologic factor in superficial thrombophlebitis in varicose veins by causing vascular stasis and trauma caused by a tourniquet effect at the top of the stockings (Ali, Riding, Tait, 2005).

Another source of edema in the lower extremities is dysfunction of the lymphatic system. The well-known but poorly understood problem of primary lymphedema is related to aberrant development or function of the lymphatic system. This condition is most common in women and is often unilateral. Manifestations may be evident at birth but usually appear no later than age 40. When suspected, the diagnosis may be confirmed with a radioisotope lymphogram and contrast lymphangiography. Chronic lymphedema predisposes patients to skin infections, which may, in turn, exacerbate fibrosis and obstruction of lymph flow.

Klippel-Trenaunay syndrome (KTS) is a complex congenital anomaly defined as a combination of (1) capillary malformations (port-wine stains) often located at the lateral aspect of the affected limb and, less often, at sites other than the hypertrophied limb; (2) soft tissue or bony hypertrophy (or both); and (3) varicose veins or venous malformations, frequently in the presence of persistent posterolateral embryologic veins. The presence of two or more of these criteria allows the diagnosis of KTS. Deep-venous abnormalities (hypoplasia, aplasia, and valvular incompetence) and lymphatic impairment also may occur (Delis et al, 2007).

Arteriovenous fistulas are abnormal communications, single or multiple, between arteries and veins, by which arterial blood enters the veins directly without traversing a capillary network.

Acquired arteriovenous fistulas, usually single and saccular, may develop after a bullet or stab wound involving an artery and a contiguous vein. Fistulas of the iliac vessels may occur after surgery for intervertebral disc disease. Con-

---

ORTHOPEDIC GAMUT 12-16
THROMBOPHLEBITIS

Thrombophlebitis, or intravascular coagulation, is usually related to three critical factors of the Virchow triad:
1. Venous stasis
2. Injury to the vein wall
3. Hypercoagulable state

ORTHOPEDIC GAMUT 12-17
COMMON CAUSES OF DEBILITATING PAIN IN PATIENTS WITH KLIPPEL TRENAUNAY SYNDROME

1. Chronic venous insufficiency
2. Cellulitis
3. Superficial thrombophlebitis
4. Deep-vein thrombosis
5. Calcification of vascular malformations
6. Intraosseous vascular malformation
7. Arthritis
8. Neuropathy
9. Unabated tissue growth

genital fistulas, which are present from birth, are usually multiple, and they result from defects in the differentiation of the common embryologic tissue into artery and vein. No special sex incidence has been found, and any part of the body may be involved.

Arterial blood, following the path of least resistance, flows directly into the vein and bypasses the corresponding capillary bed. The arterial blood pressure is transmitted to the venous side of the fistula. The distal vein pressure is increased, but the proximal vein pressure may actually be negative. The elevated venous pressure leads to the development of varicose veins and venous stasis changes in the leg. Increased blood flow makes the tissues near the fistula abnormally warm, and diminished flow distal to the fistula may produce peripheral coldness and trophic changes. Large fistulas impose a burden on the heart. The cardiac output must be increased above normal by an amount proportional to the size of the fistula to maintain the general circulation. Total blood volume may be increased. The low peripheral resistance of the involved area decreases diastolic and increases systolic and pulse pressure systemically. Large fistulas may lead to cardiac decompensation.

In the region of the fistula, the intima and the media of the involved veins become thickened, and newly developed elastic fibers appear. The arteries show a thinning of their walls, with a loss of elastic tissue and muscular fibers in the media.

Patients complain of ache, pain, edema, varicosities, or hypertrophied legs. Occasionally, cardiac symptoms—palpitations, substernal pain, and dyspnea on exertion—are present.

Examination reveals tortuous, dilated superficial veins in the leg. The venous pulsation can be felt unless the fistula is small and deeply placed. With congenital fistulas, the skin temperature is usually elevated locally but decreased distal to the fistulas, although in acquired lesions, the temperature of the toes may be greater than in the opposite normal foot. Bruits or thrills are common over acquired fistulas. The bruit lasts throughout systole and diastole and has a coarse, machinery-like quality. The tissues near the fistula may be tender, edematous, and either red or slightly cyanotic. The circumference of the leg is increased by edema or true hypertrophy, but bony structures are hypertrophied only if the fistula was present before epiphyseal closure. Temporary compression of the artery that supplies the large fistula diminishes the heart rate *(Branham sign)* and may be a helpful diagnostic sign.

PROCEDURE

- The patient's lower extremity is elevated, and an elastic bandage is wrapped firmly around the limb (Fig. 12-75).
- The elevated position is maintained for 5 minutes. Then the extremity is placed in a horizontal position, and the examiner quickly removes the applied bandage (Fig. 12-76).
- If the circulation is normal, a hyperemic blush occurs and rapidly flows into the area as the bandage is removed.
- The test is positive when the blush is absent or lags slowly behind the unbandaged area.
- The test demonstrates inadequacy of the collateral circulation as in an arteriovenous fistula.

Next Steps/Procedures

Buerger test, claudication test, foot tourniquet test, Homans sign, Moses test, Perthes test, and vascular assessment

CLINICAL PEARL

Thrombosis in the superficial veins of the calf and with local inflammatory changes is a common cause of recurrent calf pain, and the presence of tenderness and other inflammatory signs along the course of the calf vein makes diagnosis easy. Thrombosis in the deep veins is often silent, and its importance in the postoperative situation is well known.

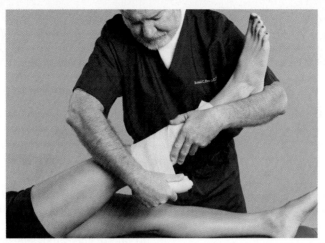

FIG. 12-75 The patient is lying supine on the examination table. The patient's legs are extended at the knees. The affected leg is elevated or flexed at the hip. While maintaining the leg in an elevated position, the examiner wraps the leg firmly with a 6-inch-wide elastic bandage and maintains the elevation of the leg for 5 minutes.

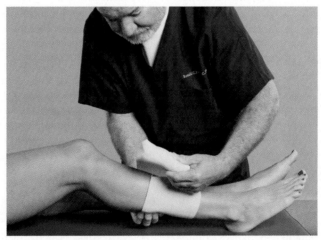

FIG. 12-76 At the end of 5 minutes, the leg is returned to the horizontal position, and the bandage is quickly removed. The test is positive if the area of the leg previously wrapped has no hyperemic blush. The lack of hyperemic blush indicates arteriovenous fistula formation.

12

MOSES TEST

Assessment for Arteriosclerosis Obliterans of the Lower Extremity

Comment

Arteriosclerosis obliterans is caused by arteriosclerotic narrowing or obstruction of large and small arteries that supply the extremities. Symptoms and signs are produced by ischemia.

Arteriosclerosis obliterans is the leading cause of obstructive arterial disease of the lower extremities after the age of 30. The superficial femoral artery is affected by stenosis or obstruction in approximately 90% of patients. The aortoiliac and popliteal arteries are the next most common sites. The greatest incidence of superficial femoral and more distal arterial disease occurs in the seventh decade, but aortoiliac disease has its peak a decade earlier. The disease is more common in men than in women, especially before menopause. Patients with diabetes mellitus develop arteriosclerosis obliterans more frequently and at an earlier age than nondiabetic patients.

> The majority of patients with arteriosclerosis obliterans are asymptomatic. According to the literature, only 22% of patients with arteriosclerosis obliterans have symptoms, such as pain in the legs or IC (Fujiwara et al, 2004).

Arteriosclerosis obliterans not only causes deterioration in activities of daily living and quality of life, but also worsens the life prognosis in elderly adults. Thus detection of asymptomatic arteriosclerosis obliterans should improve the prognosis of elderly people, 3.4% of whom have the disease.

The most common symptom of arteriosclerosis obliterans is IC (intermittent limping). The patient experiences cramping pain, tightness, numbness, or severe fatigue in the muscle group being exercised. The amount of exercise producing the pain is constant in each patient. The pain is relieved promptly by rest. In a few patients, pain may disappear after further walking because of an unconscious slowing of the gait. IC is typically seen in the calf muscles because femoral artery disease is so common. However, the calf is the most common site of claudication because these muscles do the most work during walking. Lower back, buttock, thigh, and foot claudication also may occur. The site of the symptom localizes the obstruction proximally.

Rest pain is the other important symptom of obstructive arterial disease. Rest pain is a grave sign that indicates that the blood supply is not sufficient even for the small nutritional requirements of the skin. Rest pain may be localized to one or more toes but often has a stocking distribution. The latter distribution means that ischemic neuritis is not usually the cause of rest pain. Rest pain is worse at night and is relieved somewhat by dependency and by cooling.

Other symptoms of arteriosclerosis obliterans include coldness, numbness, paresthesia, and color changes in the involved extremity.

Exercise-induced vascular claudication is unusual in young athletes. A rare cause of arterial occlusion has been reported in the adductor canal. An abnormal musculoskeletal band arising from the adductor magnus and lying adjacent and superior to the adductor tendon may lead to compression of the femoral artery at the adductor hiatus. The band may extend from the adductor magnus to the vastus medialis above and across the outlet of Hunter canal.

Symptoms in this syndrome are identical to those of other vascular occlusion problems. Exercise-induced claudication is present. On examination, the pulses distal to the occlusion are diminished or absent. The work-up of these patients consists of noninvasive vascular testing, such as Doppler studies and arteriography.

PROCEDURE

- Moses test is performed by grasping the patient's calf, which creates pain if phlebitis or vascular occlusion is present (Fig. 12-77).

Next Steps/Procedures

Buerger test, claudication test, foot tourniquet test, Homans sign, Moszkowicz test, Perthes test, and vascular assessment

CLINICAL PEARL

Pain in the calf is common for patients suffering from prolapsed intervertebral discs. Claudication pain is a feature of vascular insufficiency and spinal stenosis. Lesions of the foot and ankle that lead to protective muscle spasm during standing and walking often cause marked calf and leg pain.

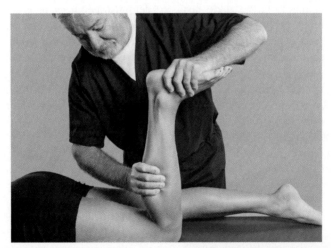

FIG. 12-77 The patient is lying prone on the examining table. The examiner flexes the patient's knee to 90 degrees. The examiner grasps and squeezes the calf of the affected leg. The sign is present if pain is elicited. The pain suggests phlebitis.

12

Assessment for Superficial Varicosities (Incompetency of the Valves of the Saphenous Vein) of the Lower Extremity

Comment

Thirty to fifty percent of patients with symptomatic chronic venous insufficiency (CVI) have a combination of superficial and perforator insufficiency without deep-venous disease (Mendes et al, 2003).

CVI results in a rise in tissue pressure in the skin and subcutaneous tissues. This increased pressure can interfere with adequate nutrient blood flow and may lead to skin necrosis and ulceration, most commonly at the ankle just above the malleoli. The skin is often dusky and indurated. Scarring as part of the healing process tends to impair the microcirculation further, and the condition may become self-perpetuating (Fig. 12-78).

Varicose veins are distended, tortuous veins with incompetent valves. The postphlebitic syndrome denotes the chronically swollen lower extremity with trophic changes secondary to chronic venous stasis. Despite the name, a history of thrombophlebitis is often not obtainable.

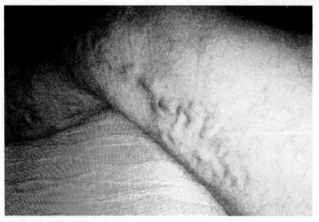

FIG. 12-78 Varicose veins. (From Barkauskas VH et al: *Health and physical assessment*, ed 2, St Louis, 1998, Mosby.)

Varicose veins are caused either by congenitally defective valves or by a condition that deforms valves or obstructs venous outflow over a long period. Varicosities that result from congenital defects are the most common and may develop early in life.

Primary lower limb **varicosities** classically arise from incompetence of the junction of the superficial and the deep-venous systems with retrograde flow into the saphenous veins. However, some patients with **superficial varicosities** have no demonstrable incompetence of the saphenofemoral or saphenopopliteal junctions (Olapade-Olaopa et al, 2000).

Because increased forearm vein distensibility has been demonstrated in patients with leg varicosities, a generalized abnormality of the veins has been suggested as the predisposing factor. Thrombophlebitis leads to deformation or destruction of venous valves and venous obstruction, and it is the second most common etiologic factor of venous problems. Pregnancy, ascites, abdominal tumor, excessive weight and height, or prolonged weight bearing may lead to increased venous pressure in the legs, distension of the veins, and, finally, incompetency of the valves.

Varicose veins are rather common. The condition appears in approximately 40% of all women, but the incidence is less in men. The saphenous veins in the lower extremity are the veins most commonly affected.

The dilated, tortuous, sacculated varices are easily visible. Some patients with extensive superficial varicosities have no other symptoms or signs, but some patients experience aching or easy fatigability of the calf muscles and edema after weight bearing. The edema usually disappears with bed rest overnight. When the communicating or deep veins are incompetent, symptoms and signs are more common. CVI is characterized by edema, which may later become fibrosed to produce brawny induration. Extravasation of blood locally may cause a brownish pigmentation. An itchy eczematoid rash may appear in the area. Finally, the skin may ulcerate, which produces an indolent, painless lesion that is usually above the medial malleolus, near a palpable, incompetent communicating vein. This picture of chronic swelling and stasis dermatitis is called postphlebitic syndrome. Arterial pulses are normal. When the deep-venous system is blocked, pain similar to intermittent claudication may rarely occur.

PROCEDURE

- While the patient is supine or standing, an elastic tourniquet is applied around the upper thigh to compress only the long saphenous vein (Fig. 12-79).
- The patient then exercises the limb briskly, by walking, kicking, or twisting, for up to 60 seconds.
- The examiner then notes the prominence of the varicosities.
- Normally, the muscular action of the exercise should empty the blood from the superficial system (long saphenous) through the communicating veins into the deep system.
- If superficial varicosities disappear, the valves of the communicating and deep veins are competent.
- If superficial varicosities remain the same, both the superficial and communicating valves are incompetent.
- If the varicosities become distended and more prominent and pain develops, the deep veins are obstructed, and the valves of the communicating veins are incompetent (Fig. 12-80).

Next Steps/Procedures

Buerger test, claudication test, foot tourniquet test, Homans sign, Moszkowicz test, Moses test, and vascular assessment

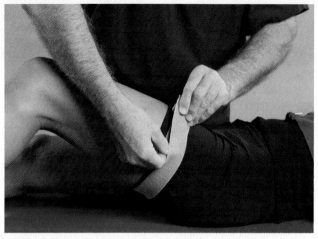

FIG. 12-79 The patient is lying supine on the examination table. A tourniquet is applied at the upper thigh of the affected leg. The tourniquet is only tight enough to compress the long saphenous vein.

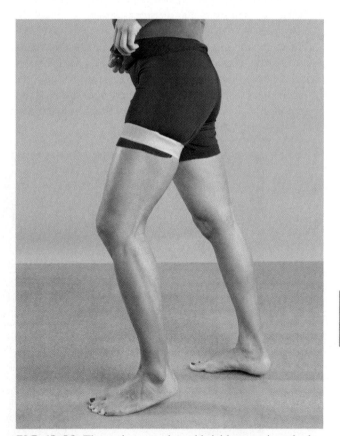

FIG. 12-80 The patient stands and briskly exercises the leg for up to 60 seconds. Prominent varicosities that do not disappear with exercise suggest that the valves of the communicating and deep veins are incompetent.

CLINICAL PEARL

Vascular damage may lead to gangrene of the foot and ankle. The circulation must always be observed if the vessels have likely been traumatized seriously by stretching or contusion, and the findings must be recorded. Neurologic damage often accompanies vascular injury.

12

STRUNSKY SIGN

Assessment for Metatarsalgia

Comment

Metatarsalgia in a patient can be a debilitating disorder leading to loss of athletic competitiveness or even loss of the ability to participate in a recreational fashion.

Forefoot pain cannot be assumed to be caused by biomechanical problems without a proper systems evaluation and until medical causes are ruled out. The examiner must distinguish between **primary** and **secondary metatarsalgia.** In primary metatarsalgia, the treatment will be directed primarily toward unloading the areas that are subjected to high pressure, whereas in metatarsalgia secondary to other causes the treatment should be directed to the systemic etiologic factors, as well as to the metatarsal symptoms (Fadel, Rowley, 2002).

The complaint of pain in the forefoot must be differentiated to make a correct diagnosis (Fig. 12-82). Most important is the exact location of pain.

The metatarsals are arranged in an arch both in an AP and in a transverse direction. The transverse arch, in which the

central three bones lie at a higher level than the peripheral bones, is pronounced proximally at the tarsometatarsal junctions and becomes shallower toward its distal extremity. The term *metatarsal arch* refers to the shallow concavity over the plantar aspect of the metatarsal heads. The central three

---

ORTHOPEDIC GAMUT 12-18

FOREFOOT DISORDERS

1. Lesser toe abnormalities
   a. Claw toes
   b. Mallet toes
   c. Hammertoes
   d. Hard and soft corns
2. More proximal problems
   a. Intractable plantar keratosis
   b. Bunionette (Fig. 12-81)
   c. Neuromas
   d. Metatarsophalangeal joint capsulitis and instability

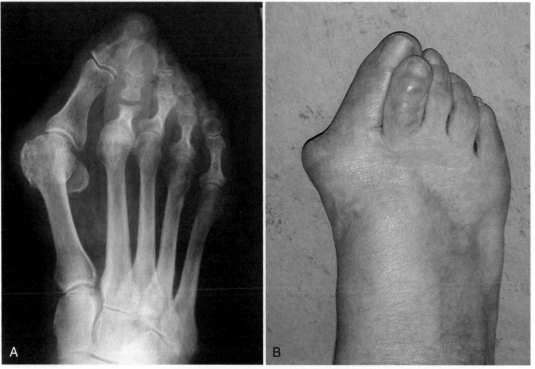

FIG. 12-81 An 82-year-old woman. **A,** Incongruent MTP joint, sesamoid position 3, intermetatarsal angle 15 degrees, hallux valgus angle 48 degrees. **B,** Preoperative photograph. (From Trnka H-J: Surgery of the hallux osteotomies for hallux valgus correction, *Food Ankle Clin North Am* 10[1]:15-33, 2005.)

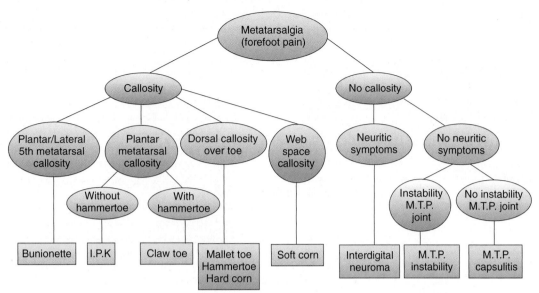

FIG. 12-82 Metatarsalgia algorithm. *I.P.K.*, Intractable plantar kelatosis; *M.T.P.*, metatar-sophalangeal. (From Baxter DE: *The foot and ankle in sport*, St Louis, 1995, Mosby.)

heads are elevated by the transverse metatarsal ligaments and the transverse head of the adductor hallucis muscle. The mechanism is ineffective during weight bearing, but it transfers pressure toward the medial and lateral tarsal heads when the arch is obliterated. During the push-off movement of a step, the intrinsic muscles flex the toes and help elevate the central metatarsal heads off the ground, thus relieving them of pressure. Paralysis of these muscles results in clawed toes, dropped metatarsal heads, and the inevitable plantar calluses.

> Patients with hallux valgus usually develop metatarsalgia as a result of splaying of the foot, with displacement of the first metatarsal in a medial and dorsal direction. The head of the first metatarsal moves to a different plane of weightbearing, dorsal to that of the metatarsal heads II through V (Saro et al, 2007).

Stretching of the transverse metatarsal ligaments is a major cause of pain in the forefoot. This pain is caused by congenital laxity, which typically results in flatfoot, in which the heel is everted, the longitudinal arch depressed, the metatarsals and the toes widely spread (splayfoot), and the forefoot supinated in relation to the hindfoot. An acquired stretching occurs as a result of obesity, prolonged standing, degenerative changes of aging, and acute illness.

The three central metatarsal heads drop and are prominent in the sole when palpated through the thinned subcutaneous fat.

Weakness of the intrinsics deprives the toes of strong flexor power, and the metatarsal heads drop. With poliomyelitis, paralysis of the foot dorsiflexors results in equinus that throws the weight forward on the foot. In addition, the common cavus deformity, which follows this disease, causes a downward tilting of the metatarsals, and added pressure is brought to bear distally.

Any form of arthritis can affect the metatarsophalangeal joints. In young and middle-age patients, rheumatoid arthritis is suspected. Severe degenerative arthritis favors the first metatarsophalangeal articulation. Degenerative changes in a single joint, other than the first, suggest an antecedent osteochondrosis.

An acute exacerbation of gout characteristically develops around the first metatarsophalangeal joint. Pain is severe and continuous and is aggravated by weight bearing and movement of the large toe.

Prolonged walking will cause a sprain of the transverse metatarsal ligament. Pain occurs throughout the distal metatarsal area during weight bearing and is intensified by spreading the toes passively.

12

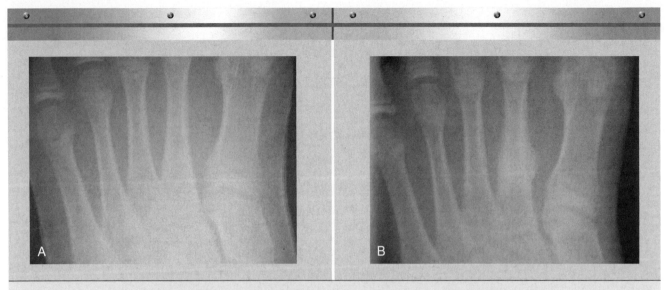

AT THE VIEWBOX

Adolescent male with ongoing metatarsal pain, increased with activity and relieved slightly with rest. Tenderness to palpation at the second metatarsal. Initial radiographs **(A)** were interpreted as normal and the patient diagnosed with likely Morton neuroma. Ongoing symptoms with conservative management prompted repeat plain films three weeks later **(B),** with obvious focal callus around the proximal diaphysis of the second metatarsal, indicative of a healing stress fracture. (From the teaching file of Timothy Mick, DC, DACBR)

Any deformity of the foot that changes the axis of the metatarsal to a more vertical direction throws forward the pressure of weight bearing.

PROCEDURE

• Sudden passive flexing of the toes is painless in a normal foot; however, if inflammation exists, pain is experienced in the anterior arch of the foot (Fig. 12-83).

Next Steps/Procedures
Morton test and diagnostic imaging

CLINICAL PEARL

Pain in the forefoot (called metatarsalgia) has many origins. A prominent metatarsal head is a common cause of pain and can follow any operation on the forefoot (including Keller operation) or dislocation of the second toe.

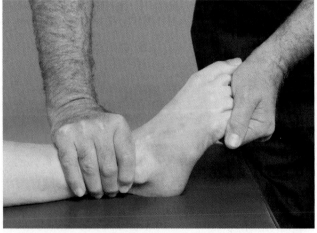

FIG. 12-83 The patient is lying supine, and the affected leg is extended on the examination table. The examiner grasps the toes of the affected foot. The examiner causes a sudden, passive flexion of the toes. The sign is present if the maneuver causes pain. The presence of this sign indicates inflammation of the anterior arch of the foot (metatarsalgia).

THOMPSON TEST

Assessment for Achilles Tendon Rupture

Comment

The history obtained in patients with a ruptured Achilles tendon is remarkably consistent. Typically, the individual is a middle-age, weekend, male athlete. A pop is often heard at the time of the rupture. The patient often thinks the heel was hit by an opponent's racquet. On turning, the patient realizes that no one is there. Most individuals are disabled enough to seek medical attention immediately but some are not. Only when the latter group fails to recover from this presumed *sprain* do they then seek help. As with epicondylitis of the elbow, the Achilles tendon is affected in exposure to fluoroquinolone antibiotics (Fig. 12-84).

The *Thompson-Doherty squeeze* test involves placing the patient prone with the knee at 90 degrees of flexion. A squeeze of the calf musculature normally results in passive plantar flexion. A positive Thompson-Doherty test is the absence of passive plantar flexion.

Calf pain with the Thompson-Doherty test indicates a probable medial gastrocnemius tear. A palpable gap is usually present in an Achilles rupture, particularly in an acute situation. This gap is best felt with the patient prone, the foot over the edge of the examination table, and the patient actively dorsiflexing the ankle.

O'Brien needle test involves placing a needle (acupuncture) 10 cm proximal to the superior border of the calcaneus into the tendon substance. If the needle is seen to swivel on passive motion of the foot, the Achilles tendon is intact. An absence of motion indicates a positive O'Brien test.

The final assessment is that of heel resistance strength. The examiner grasps the foot in a neutral position and instructs the patient to plantar flex. With an intact Achilles tendon, the grasp is easily broken. If the Achilles tendon is torn, the posterior tibial, peroneal, and flexor tendons will fail to break the grasp. In an acute case, usually palpation of a gap and a positive Thompson-Doherty test will suffice. However, with a delayed presentation, the other three techniques may be indicated.

Since the first report of the association of fluoroquinolone and tendon disorders in 1983, a causal relationship has emerged between these antibiotics and tendon ruptures from comparative studies, and a temporal relationship often exists between the intake of fluoroquinolone and the occurrence of tendon disorders in reported cases. The ratio of tendinitis to rupture is $3:1$, whereas another study reported revealed a rate of 2.4 and 1.2, respectively, per 10,000 patients. Although over 95% cases of tendinitis and rupture secondary to fluoroquinolone use involve the Achilles' tendon, other reported tendon involvement includes the quadriceps, peroneus brevis, and rotator cuff (Akali, Niranjan, in press).

The calf muscle may be partially or completely ruptured at any place, from its origin on the posterior part of the femoral condyles and back of the tibia to its attachment to the calcaneus. The tear may be in the muscle belly, but it occurs more often in the musculotendinous junction between the gastrocnemius and the conjoined tendon with the soleus. The muscle unit may rupture through the tendon or at the attachment to the heel, sometimes avulsing a fragment of bone. As with a muscle rupture anywhere, determination of the location and extent of injury is extremely important. The location is usually determined when the injury is examined early because the tenderness will be quite localized. After several hours, swelling, edema, and inflammation become diffuse, and the exact location may be in doubt. Both active and passive stretching will cause pain. If complete severance of the whole muscle-tendon unit from the head of the gastrocnemius or the entire gastrocnemius from the conjoined tendon or rupture of the tendon occurs, then loss of function will be noted, and the muscle will bunch up during contrac-

---

ORTHOPEDIC GAMUT 12-19

PHYSICAL EXAMINATION PROCEDURES FOR A RUPTURED ACHILLES TENDON

1. The Thompson-Doherty squeeze test
2. Palpation of the medial head of the gastrocnemius
3. Palpation of a gap in the tendon
4. O'Brien needle test
5. Assessment of heel resistance strength

ORTHOPEDIC GAMUT 12-20

FACTORS PREDISPOSING ACHILLES TENDON RUPTURE

1. *Mechanical:* The patient rapidly pushes off with the knee extended.
2. *Vascular:* The tendon that ruptures usually will do so in the zone of relatively diminished blood supply.
3. *Quality of the tissue substance:* Many studies have revealed that the ruptured Achilles tendon will have preexisting degenerative pathologic changes.

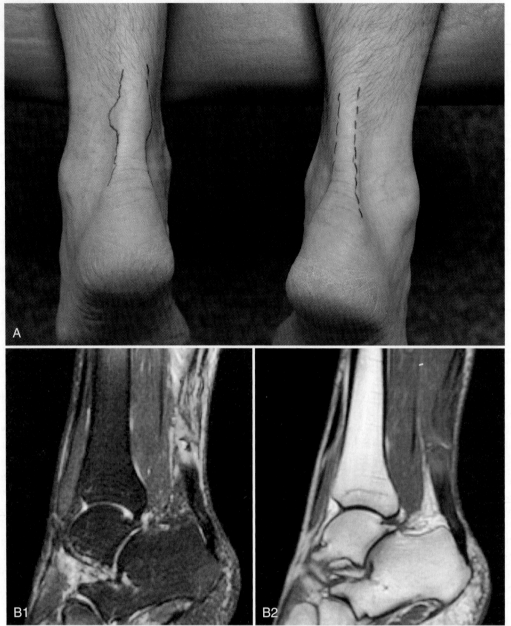

FIG. 12-84 **A,** 52-year old male elite-level body builder, runner, and athlete, with no known co-morbidities, was prescribed a five-day course of Levaquin (levofloxacin), 750 mg per day, for acute pneumonia. He had no other regular medication. Ten days after commencing the primary dosing, and in the absence of trauma, the patient developed an acute, persistent sharp pain in his left lower leg and at the Achilles tendon insertion on the heel. The patient developed a limp, as well as notable swelling of the Achilles tendon. Dorsiflexion of the foot was painful, worse on stairs or incline surfaces. Physical and orthopedic examination confirmed left Achilles tendinopathy of probable iatrogenic quinolone-therapy origin. The tendon remained intact, and advanced imaging was deferred. **B1** and **B2,** Complete rupture of the Achilles tendon. *(1)* T1- and *(2)* fat-saturated FSE T2-weighted MR images demonstrate swelling of the tendon, associated with hemorrhage (high signal on T1) and edema (high signal on T2). The tear itself is well demonstrated on both sequences. (**B** from From Adam: *Grainger & Allison's diagnostic radiology*, ed 5, Philadelphia, 2008, Churchill Livingstone.)

tion rather than flatten down, as it normally does. If the rupture is in the distal tendon or musculotendinous junction, a palpable defect can often be felt. The condition is disabling even with a minor degree of tearing, and it interdicts running or any activity that causes the patient to be on the toes. This loss of function may be caused by actual loss of continuity of the tendon, but it more commonly results from muscle spasm and pain.

- The patient is in a prone position with the feet hanging over the edge of the examination table.
- The examiner flexes the knee of the patient's affected leg to 90 degrees and squeezes the calf muscles just below the widest level of the posterior portion of the leg (Fig. 12-85).
- Normally, this maneuver causes a reflex plantar flexion motion of the foot (Fig. 12-86).
- The test is positive when the foot does not respond.
- The test indicates a complete rupture of the Achilles tendon.

Next Steps/Procedures
Helbings sign, Hoffa test, and diagnostic imaging

CLINICAL PEARL

The Achilles tendon can be torn by the same movements, such as a forward lunge on the sports field or a squash court, that tear the medial head of the gastrocnemius. The patient will feel as though someone has kicked the Achilles tendon. Legendary stories have been told in which the victim of such a tear turns around and punches the person behind in retribution.

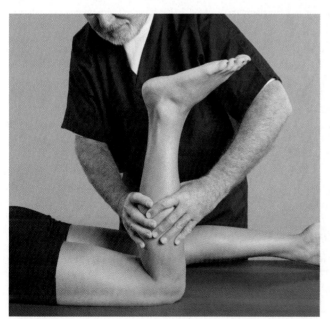

FIG. 12-85 The patient is lying prone on the examination table. The knee of the affected leg is flexed to 90 degrees by the examiner. The examiner grasps the patient's calf with both hands. The patient's musculature is relaxed.

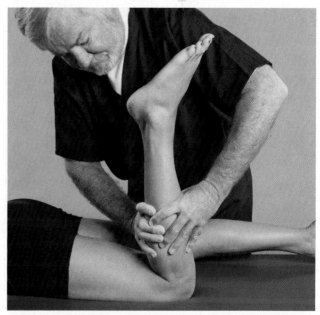

FIG. 12-86 The examiner squeezes the calf musculature at a point just distal to the widest level of the posterior portion of the leg. The test is positive if the foot does not plantar flex with this maneuver. A positive test indicates a rupture of the Achilles tendon.

12

Assessment for Tarsal Tunnel Syndrome

Comment

The tarsal tunnel is a fibroosseous tunnel formed by the flexor retinaculum or lacinate ligament, the medial wall of the calcaneus, the posterior portion of the talus, the distal tibia, and the medial malleolus.

The posterior tibial nerve may be compressed at several locations (Fig. 12-87). High tarsal tunnel syndrome exists when compression of the posterior tibial nerve occurs at the lower edge of the gastrocnemius muscle in the middle aspect of the posteromedial tibia. The traditional tarsal tunnel occurs behind the medial malleolus under the retinacular ligament. The compression may occur from a posterior bony preeminence of the talus (Fig. 12-88).

Accompanied by their corresponding arteries and veins, the tibial nerve's two terminal branches, the medial and the lateral plantar nerves, pass around the medial malleolus through a fibroosseous tunnel, which is the tarsal tunnel.

Although the causes of tarsal tunnel syndrome may be diverse, nerve compression or irritation is a common feature of them all. Mechanical pressure from changes in the tissue relationships within the tunnel remains the common denominator of the proposed causes. Therefore, trauma and congenital or acquired anomalies predispose these individuals to a higher risk of nerve compression because their tarsal tunnels are abnormally configured. Rather than change the bony components, autoimmune and inflammatory diseases affect the tunnel's soft tissues and decrease the tunnel's volume (Fig. 12-89). Because the tunnel's neural components remain most sensitive to increased pressure, changes in sensory and motor function are among the first symptoms of tunnel damage. The upper section of the tunnel, containing the medial plantar neurovascular structures, remains more sensitive to volume changes than the lower section, which contains the lateral plantar neurovascular structures.

Tarsal tunnel syndrome is a peripheral compression neuropathy of the tibial nerve and its branches, which results in a range of neuritic symptoms that affect the plantar aspect of the foot. Compression of the branches of the tibial nerve

---

ORTHOPEDIC GAMUT 12-21

TARSAL TUNNEL STRUCTURES

1. Posterior tibial nerve and its branches
2. Tendons of the posterior tibialis
3. Flexor digitorum longus
4. Flexor hallucis
5. Posterior tibial artery and vein

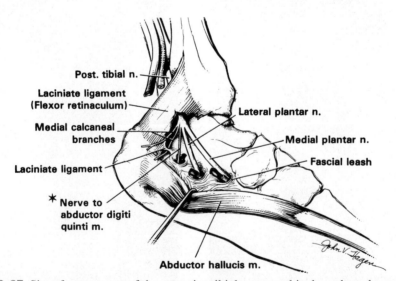

FIG. 12-87 Site of entrapment of the posterior tibial nerve and its branches, demonstrating possible entrapment beneath the laciniate ligament and at the point where the nerve passes through the fascia of the abductor hallucis muscle. (Redrawn from Baxter DE, Thigpen CM: Hell pain—operative results, *Foot Ankle* 5:16-25, 1984. Copyright American Orthopaedic Foot and Ankle Society, 1984.) (From DeLee: *DeLee and Drez's orthopaedic sports medicine*, ed 2, Philadelphia, 2003, Saunders.)

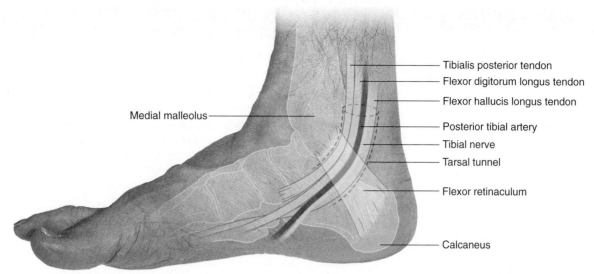

Medial malleolus

Tibialis posterior tendon
Flexor digitorum longus tendon
Flexor hallucis longus tendon
Posterior tibial artery
Tibial nerve
Tarsal tunnel
Flexor retinaculum

Calcaneus

FIG. 12-88 Testing for tarsal tunnel syndrome with EMG (electromyography) is often imprecise and misleading. The most reliable method of assessing tarsal tunnel syndrome is percussion of the nerve. This test is called a Tinel sign. Two fingers are used to briskly tap the medial ankle just behind the ankle bone (medial malleolus). An electrical shock sensation is called a positive Tinel sign and indicates the location of the entrapment. Two common areas of entrapment are found as the posterior tibial nerve passes beneath the flexor retinaculum and/or the upper margin of the abductor hallucis muscle. The posterior tibial nerve passes deep to the muscle at the dotted line. This is the most common location for entrapment of the posterior tibial nerve. (From Drake RL: *Gray's anatomy for students: with student consult online access,* New York, 2004, Churchill Livingstone.)

has been called *distal tarsal tunnel syndrome.* Patients often complain of sensory disturbances to portions of the foot, localized or radiating pain, burning pain, paresthesias, disturbances in the perception of temperature (feelings of coldness), or feeling as though a tight band is placed around the foot. However, in certain cases, no associated tingling is felt, and only a mild sensory loss or irritation of the pad and sole of the foot or heel is noted. Pain is often felt later in the development of chronic tarsal tunnel syndrome and is a less common complaint (Franson, Baravarian, 2006).

The tibial nerve, as with the median nerve, has a rich vascularity, but it is sensitive to ischemia. Compression of the vasa vasorum, which surrounds the nerve, will lead to ischemia and neurologic symptoms. Increased vascular compromise during standing and walking accounts for the crises that appreciate in patients with tarsal tunnel syndrome. In several idiopathic cases that have been relieved by surgery, the nerves were normal in appearance. These cases have been proposed to be vascular in nature.

Tarsal tunnel syndrome has historically been compared with, and even said to be analogous to, the well-known carpal tunnel syndrome. However, it has been more recently distinguished from carpal tunnel syndrome because of differences in anatomy, etiologic factors, treatment, and response to treatment. The tarsal tunnel is more analogous to the distal portion of the forearm than the carpal tunnel. Although synovium is present in the carpal tunnel, it is not present in the tarsal tunnel (Franson, Baravarian, 2006).

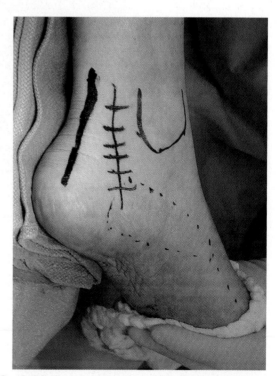

FIG. 12-89 Tarsal tunnel is centralized between the Achilles tendon and medial malleolus. (Adapted from Franson J, Baravarian B: Tarsal tunnel syndrome: A Compression neuropathy involving four distinct tunnels, *Clin Podiatr Med Surg* 23[3]:597-609, 2006.)

12

PROCEDURE

- Tapping the area over the posterior tibial nerve (medial plantar nerve) with a reflex hammer produces tingling distal to the percussion (Fig. 12-90).
- The paresthesia that radiates into the foot indicates tarsal tunnel syndrome.

Next Steps/Procedures
Duchenne sign and electrodiagnosis

CLINICAL PEARL

The medial plantar nerve enters the foot after passing beneath the medial ligament of the ankle, which it shares with the posterior tibial and flexor tendons. The structure of this feature is comparable to the carpal tunnel of the wrist. The medial plantar nerve is vulnerable to compression by swelling of the tendons or by space-occupying lesions, such as ganglia. Tarsal tunnel syndrome is not common, but it should be considered for patients who have neurologic symptoms in the hindfoot.

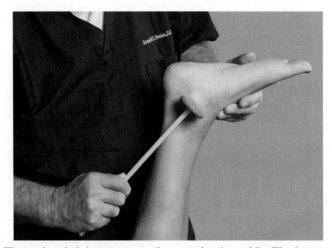

FIG. 12-90 The patient is lying prone on the examination table. The leg may be extended at the knee or flexed. The examiner percusses the posterior tibial nerve (medial plantar nerve) with a reflex hammer. Paresthesia elicited distal to the percussion indicates tarsal tunnel syndrome.

CRITICAL THINKING

1. What is medial tibial stress syndrome?
2. What is acute compartment syndrome?
3. What are the primary causes of acute compartment syndrome?
4. Who is most at risk for sustaining an Achilles tendon tear?
5. Describe the physical findings in an acute complete Achilles tendon rupture.
6. What is Thompson test?
7. What is the most common musculoskeletal injury?
8. What mechanism of injury most commonly produces an ankle sprain?
9. How is the anterior drawer test performed?
10. What indicates a positive anterior drawer test?
11. How are ankle sprains graded?
12. What is metatarsalgia?
13. What is Morton neuroma?
14. What is the tarsal tunnel?
15. What are the most common symptoms of tarsal tunnel syndrome?
16. Name four conditions that may cause swelling in the region of the Achilles tendon.
17. The anterior tibial compartment is one of the commonest sites affected by muscle herniation. Name the three muscles of the anterior compartment.
18. The muscles in the anterior and lateral compartments can be injured with a traumatic blow to the lateral leg. What nerve is damaged, and what is the most noticeable deficit the patient exhibits?
19. Inversion stress imaging views test which ligament for instability? Eversion tests which ligament?
20. The most common fractures during ankle sprain are of what type, and where are they located?
21. Describe the signs, symptoms, and potential complications that are exhibited in a patient with peripheral arterial disease in the lower extremities.
22. What structures are found within the tarsal tunnel?

12

BIBLIOGRAPHY

Abrams WB, Berkow R: *The Merck manual of geriatrics*, Rahway, NJ, 1990, Merck Sharp & Dohme Research Laboratories.

Adams JC, Hamblen DL: *Outline of orthopaedics*, ed 11, Edinburgh, 1990, Churchill Livingstone.

Agur A, editor: *Grant's atlas of anatomy*, Baltimore, 1991, Williams & Wilkins.

Alario AJ: *Practical guide to the care of the pediatric patient*, St Louis, 1997, Mosby.

Allison D, Strickland N: *Acronyms & synonyms in medical imaging*, Oxford, UK, 1996, ISIS Medical Media.

American Academy of Orthopaedic Surgeons: *Joint motion: method of measuring and recording*, Edinburgh, 1965, British Orthopaedic Association.

American Medical Association: *Guides to the evaluation of permanent impairment*, ed 4, Chicago, 1993, The Association.

American Medical Association: *How to use guides to the evaluation of permanent impairment*, ed 4, Falmouth, Conn, 1993, SEAK.

Anderson KN, Anderson LE: *Mosby's pocket dictionary of medicine, nursing, & allied health*, ed 2, St Louis, 1994, Mosby.

Andrish JT: The leg. In DeLee JD, Drez D editors: *Orthopaedic sports medicine, principles and practice*, vol 2, Philadelphia, 1994, WB Saunders.

Apley AG, Solomon L: *Concise system of orthopaedics and fractures*, London, 1988, Butterworth-Heinemann.

Barkauskas VH et al: *Health & physical assessment*, ed 2, St Louis, 1998, Mosby.

Barton NJ: Arthroplasty of the forefoot in rheumatoid arthritis, *J Bone Joint Surg* 55B:126, 1973.

Bassett FH III et al: Talar impingement by the anteroinferior tibiofibular ligament: a cause of chronic pain in the ankle after inversion sprain, *J Bone Joint Surg* 72A:55, 1990.

Baxter DE: *The foot and ankle in sport*, St Louis, 1995, Mosby.

Baxter DE, Pfeiffer GB: Treatment of chronic heel pain by surgical release of the first branch of the lateral plantar nerve, *Clin Orthop* 279:229, 1992.

Beeson PB, McDermott W: *Textbook of medicine*, ed 13, Philadelphia, 1971, WB Saunders.

Berkowitz JF, Kier R, Rudicel S: Plantar fasciitis: MR imaging, *Radiology* 179:665, 1991.

Binak K et al: Arteriovenous fistula: hemodynamic effect of occlusion and exercise, *Am Heart J* 60:495, 1960.

Boisen WR, Staples OS, Russell SW: Residual disability following acute ankle sprains, *J Bone Joint Surg* 37A:1237, 1955.

Bordelon RL: Heel pain. In DeLee JD, Drez D, editors: *Orthopaedic sports medicine: principles and practice*, vol 2, Philadelphia, 1994, WB Saunders.

Boytim MJ, Fischer DA, Neuman L: Syndesmotic ankle sprains, *Am J Sports Med* 19:294, 1991.

Bradley JP, Tibone JE: Percutaneous and open surgical repairs of Achilles tendon ruptures, *Am J Sports Med* 18:188, 1990.

Brahms MA: Common foot problems, *J Bone Joint Surg* 49A:1653, 1967.

Brook I: Superficial suppurative thrombophlebitis in children, caused by anaerobic bacteria, *J Pediatr Surg* 33(8):1279-1282, 1998.

Brooks M, Evans R, Fairclough J: *Sports injuries*, ed 2, London, 1992, Gower Medical.

Brotzman SB: *Clinical orthopaedic rehabilitation*, St Louis, 1996, Mosby.

Brown DE: Ankle and leg injuries. In Mellion MB, Walsh M, Shelton GL, editors: *The team physician's handbook*, Philadelphia, 1990, Hanley & Belfus.

Brown DE, Neumann RD: *Orthopedic secrets*, Philadelphia, 1995, Hanley & Belfus.

Bucholz RW: *Orthopaedic decision making*, ed 2, St Louis, 1996, Mosby.

Burns J, Crosbie J: Weight bearing ankle dorsiflexion range of motion in idiopathic pes cavus compared to normal and pes planus feet, *Foot* 15(2):91-94, 2005.

Cahill DR: The anatomy and function of the contents of the human tarsal sinus and canal, *Anat Rec* 153:1, 1965.

Calliet R: *Foot and ankle pain*, Philadelphia, 1979, FA Davis.

Campbell JB, Campbell JM: *Mosby's survival guide to medical abbreviations & acronyms prefixes & suffixes symbols Greek alphabet*, St Louis, 1995, Mosby.

Canale ST: *Campbell's operative orthopaedics*, vol 1-4, ed 9, St Louis, 1998, Mosby.

Carbayo JA et al: Using ankle-brachial index to detect peripheral arterial disease: prevalence and associated risk factors in a random population sample, *Nutr Metab Cardiovasc Dis* 17(1):41-49, 2007.

Chapman S, Nakielny R: *Aids to radiological differential diagnosis*, ed 3, London, 1995, Bailliere Tindall.

Cheetham DR et al: Is the Stresst'er a reliable stress test to detect mild to moderate peripheral arterial disease? *Eur J Vasc Endovasc Surg* 27(5):545-548, 2004.

Chiu M-C, Wang M-JJ: Professional footwear evaluation for clinical nurses, *Appl Ergon* 38(2):133-141, 2007.

Cipriano JJ: *Photographic manual of regional orthopaedic and neurological test*, ed 3, Baltimore, 1997, Williams & Wilkins.

Clain MR, Baxter DE: Achilles tendonitis, *Foot Ankle* 13:482, 1992.

Clanton TO, Schon LC: Athlete injuries to the soft tissues of the foot and ankle. In Mann RA, Coughlin MJ, editors: *Surgery of the foot and ankle*, ed 6, St Louis, 1993, Mosby.

Coffman JD, Mannick JA: An objective test to demonstrate the circulatory abnormality in intermittent claudication, *Circulation* 33:177, 1966.

Cohen HL, Brumlik J: *A manual of electroneuromyography*, New York, 1968, Harper and Row.

Cohen MS et al: Acute compartment syndrome: effect of dermotomy on fascial decompression in the leg, *J Bone Joint Surg* 73A:287, 1991.

Cohn RE: *Impairment rating examination and disability evaluation*, ed 3, Wilkesboro, NC, 1991, R Ernest Cohn.

Colter JM: Lateral ligamentous injuries of the ankle. In Hamilton WC, editor: *Traumatic disorder of the ankle*, New York, 1984, Springer-Verlag.

Cooke TDV, Lehmann PO: Intermittent claudication of neurogenic origin, *Can J Surg* 11:151, 1968.

Coughlin MJ: Conditions of the forefoot. In DeLee JD, Drez D, editors: *Orthopaedic sports medicine: principles and practice*, vol 2, Philadelphia, 1994, WB Saunders.

Craik RL, Oatis CA: *Gait analysis theory and application*, St Louis, 1995, Mosby.

Crenshaw AH, editor: *Campbell's operative orthopedics*, St Louis, 1992, Mosby.

Dambro MR, Griffith JA: *Griffith's 5 minute clinical consult*, Baltimore, 1997, Williams & Wilkins.

D'Ambrogio KJ, Roth GB: *Positional release therapy assessment & treatment of musculoskeletal dysfunction*, St Louis, 1997, Mosby.

D'Ambrosia RD: *Musculoskeletal disorders: regional examination and differential diagnosis*, Philadelphia, 1977, JB Lippincott.

Dandy DJ: *Essential orthopaedics and trauma*, Edinburgh, 1989, Churchill Livingstone.

Dejong RN: *The neurological examination incorporating the fundamentals of neuroanatomy and neurophysiology*, ed 3, New York, 1967, Harper & Row.

Delahunt E: Neuromuscular contributions to functional instability of the ankle joint, *J Bodywork Mov Ther* (in press, corrected proof).

Deltoff MN, Kogon PL: *The portable skeletal x-ray library*, St Louis, 1998, Mosby.

DeMaio M et al: Plantar fasciitis, *Orthopedics* 16:1153, 1993.

Demeter SL, Andersson GBJ, Smith GM: *Disability evaluation*, St Louis, 1996, Mosby.

Deshpande JK, Tobias JD: *The pediatric pain handbook*, St Louis, 1996, Mosby.

Dettenmeier PA: *Radiographic assessment for nurses*, St Louis, 1995, Mosby.

Di Marzo L et al: Diagnosis of popliteal artery entrapment syndrome: the role of duplex scanning, *J Vasc Surg* 13:434, 1991.

Doherty M: *Color atlas and text of osteoarthritis*, London, 1994, Wolfe.

Doherty M, Doherty J: *Clinical examination in rheumatology*, London, 1992, Wolfe.

Doherty M, George E: *Self-assessment picture tests in rheumatology*, London, 1995, Mosby-Wolfe.

DuVries HL: *Surgery of the foot*, ed 2, St Louis, 1965, Mosby.

DuVries HL: Five myths about your feet, *Today's Health* 45:49, 1967.

Eastwood DM, Gregg PJ, Atkins RM: Intra-articular fractures of the calcaneum, *J Bone Joint Surg* 75B:183, 1993.

Eisele SA, Sammarco GL: Fatigue fractures of the foot and ankle in the athlete, *J Bone Joint Surg* 75:290, 1993.

Elster AD: *Questions and answers in magnetic resonance imaging*, St Louis, 1994, Mosby.

Elstorm Pankovich A: Muscle and tendon surgery of the leg. In Evarts CM, editor: *Surgery of the musculoskeletal system*, ed 2, New York, 1990, Churchill Livingstone.

Epstein O et al: *Clinical examination*, ed 2, London, 1997, Mosby.

Espinola-Klein C et al: Inflammation, atherosclerotic burden and cardiovascular prognosis, *Atherosclerosis* (in press, corrected proof).

Farrar WE: *Atlas of infections of the nervous system*, London, 1993, Wolfe.

Fegan WG, Fitzgerald DE, Beesley WH: A modern approach to the injection treatment of varicose veins and its applications in pregnant patients, *Am Heart J* 68:757, 1964.

Feldmann E: *Current diagnosis in neurology*, St Louis, 1994, Mosby.

Ferezy JS: *The chiropractic neurological examination*, Gaithersburg, Md, 1992, Aspen.

Ferkel RD et al: Arthroscopic treatment of anterolateral impingement of the ankle, *Am J Sports Med* 19:440, 1991.

Fernandez-Palazzi F, Rivas S, Mujica P: Achilles tendinitis in ballet dancers, *Clin Orthop* 257:257, 1990.

Fornage B: *Musculoskeletal ultrasound*, New York, 1995, Churchill Livingstone.

Frank ED et al: *Merrill's atlas of radiographic positioning and procedures*, ed 11, St Louis, 2007, Mosby.

Frey C, Shereff M, Greenridge N: Vascularity of the posterior tibial tendon, *J Bone Joint Surg* 72A:884, 1990.

Friedman SA, Holling HE, Roberts B: Etiologic factors in aortoiliac and femoro-popliteal vascular disease, *N Engl J Med* 271:1382, 1964.

Gamstorp I: Normal conduction velocity of ulnar, median, and peroneal nerves in infancy, childhood and adolescence, *Acta Paediatra Suppl* 146:68, 1963.

Garcia JH: *Neuropathology: the diagnostic approach*, St Louis, 1997, Mosby.

Gardner E, Gray DJ, O'Rahilly R: *Anatomy: a regional study of human structure*, ed 4, Philadelphia, 1975, WB Saunders.

Gardner E, Gray DJ: The innervation of the joints of the foot, *Anat Rec* 161:141, 1968.

George VA et al: Morton's neuroma: the role of MR scanning in diagnostic assistance, *Foot* 15(1):14-16, 2005.

Gerard JA, Kleinfield SL: *Orthopaedic testing*, New York, 1993, Churchill Livingstone.

Gibbon WW, Cassar-Pullicino VN: Heel pain, *Ann Rheum Dis* 53:344, 1994.

Gilliatt RW: Normal conduction in human and experimental neuropathies, *Proc R Soc Lond B Biol Sci* 59:989, 1966.

Goldie BS: *Orthopaedic diagnosis and management: a guide to the care of orthopaedic patients*, ed 2, Oxford, UK, 1998, ISIS Medical Media.

Gomez D, Jha K, Jepson K: Ultrasound scan for the diagnosis of interdigital neuroma, *Foot Ankle Surg* 11(3):175-177, 2005.

Gray H: *Anatomy of the human body*, ed 28, Philadelphia, 1966, Lea & Febiger.

Greenspan A: *Orthopedic radiology*, ed 2, Philadelphia, 1992, JB Lippincott.

Greenstein GM: *Clinical assessment of neuromusculoskeletal disorders*, St Louis, 1997, Mosby.

Grossman ZD et al: *Cost-effective diagnostic imaging: the clinician's guide*, ed 3, St Louis, 1995, Mosby.

Hamilton WC: Anatomy. In Hamilton WC, editor: *Traumatic disorder of the ankle*, New York, 1984, Springer-Verlag.

Hammer WI: *Functional soft tissue examination and treatment by manual methods: the extremities*, Gaithersburg, Md, 1991, Aspen.

Harris J, Fallat L: Effects of isolated Weber B fibular fractures on the tibiotalar contact area, *J Foot Ankle Surg* 43(1):3-9, 2004.

Hart FD: *French's index of differential diagnosis*, ed 10, Baltimore, 1973, Williams & Wilkins.

Hartley A: *Practical joint assessment: lower quadrant*, ed 2, St Louis, 1995, Mosby.

Hassouna HZ, Singh D: The variation in the management of Morton's Metatarsalgia, *Foot* 15(3):149-153, 2005.

Hawkins RJ: *An organized approach to musculoskeletal examination and history taking*, St Louis, 1995, Mosby.

Hinkle CZ: *Fundamentals of anatomy & movement: a workbook and guide*, St Louis, 1997, Mosby.

Hopkinson WJ et al: Syndesmotic sprains of the ankle, *Foot Ankle* 10:325, 1990.

Hunt AE, Smith RM: Mechanics and control of the flat versus normal foot during the stance phase of walking, *Clin Biomech* 19(4):391-397, 2004.

Hunt GC: Injuries of peripheral nerves of the leg, foot and ankle: an often unrecognized consequence of ankle sprains, *Foot* 13(1):14-18, 2003.

Ibrahim T et al: Displaced intra-articular calcaneal fractures: 15-Year follow-up of a randomised controlled trial of conservative versus operative treatment, *Injury* (in press, corrected proof).

Inman VT: *The joints of the ankle*, Baltimore, 1976, Williams & Wilkins.

Jablonski S: *Dictionary of medical acronyms & abbreviations*, ed 3, Philadelphia, 1998, Hanley & Belfus.

Jackson BA, Schwane JA, Starcher BC: Effect of ultrasound therapy on the repair of Achilles tendon injuries in rats, *Med Sci Sports Exerc* 23:171, 1991.

Jahss MH: *Disorders of the foot*, Philadelphia, 1982, WB Saunders.

Jahss MH: Foot and ankle pain resulting from rheumatic conditions, *Curr Opin Rheumatol* 4:233, 1992.

Jehl J, Crummy P: *Essentials of radiologic surgery*, ed 6, Philadelphia, 1993, JB Lippincott.

Junqueira LC, Carneiro J, Kelly RO: *Basic histology*, ed 7, Norwalk, Conn, 1992, Appleton & Lange.

Kadel NJ, Teitz CC, Kronmal RA: Stress fractures in ballet dancers, *Am J Sports Med* 20:445, 1992.

Kainberger FM et al: Injury of the Achilles tendon: diagnosis with sonography, *Am J Roentgenol* 155:1031, 1990.

Kang PB et al: Atypical presentations of spinal muscular atrophy type III (Kugelberg-Welander disease), *Neuromusc Disord* 16(8):492-494, 2006.

Kanner R: *Pain management secrets*, Philadelphia, 1997, Hanley & Belfus.

Kannus P, Jozsa L: Histopathologic changes preceding spontaneous rupture of a tendon, *J Bone Joint Surg* 73A:1507, 1992.

Kannus P, Renstrom P: Current concepts review: treatment for acute tears of the lateral ligaments of the ankle, *J Bone Joint Surg* 73A:305, 1991.

Karasick D: Preoperative assessment of symptomatic bunionette deformity: radiologic findings, *Am J Roentgenol* 164:147, 1995.

Karasick D, Schweitzer ME: Tear of the posterior tibial tendon causing asymmetric flatfoot: radiographic findings, *Am J Roentgenol* 161:1237, 1993.

12

Karr SD: Subcalcaneal heel pain, *Orthop Clinic North Am* 25:161, 1994.

Katirji B: *Electromyography in clinical practice: a case study approach*, St Louis, 1998, Mosby.

Katz WA: *Rheumatic diseases diagnosis and management*, Philadelphia, 1977, JB Lippincott.

Keats TE: *Atlas of roentgenographic measurement*, ed 6, St Louis, 1990, Mosby.

Keene JA: Tendon injuries of the foot and ankle. In DeLee JD, Drez D, editors: *Orthopaedic sports medicine, principals and practice*, vol 2, Philadelphia, 1994, WB Saunders.

Kelikian H, Kelikian AS: *Disorders of the ankle*, Philadelphia, 1985, WB Saunders.

Kendall HP, Kendall RP, Wadsworth GE: *Muscles: testing and function*, ed 3, Baltimore, 1992, Williams & Wilkins.

Kerkhoffs GMMJ, Blankevoort L, van Dijk CN: A measurement device for anterior laxity of the ankle joint complex, *Clin Biomech* 20(2):218-222, 2005.

Kerkhoffs GMMJ et al: Anterior lateral ankle ligament damage and anterior talocrural-joint laxity: an overview of the in vitro reports in literature, *Clin Biomech* 16(8):635-643, 2001.

Kim JY et al: Non-traumatic peroneal nerve palsy: MRI findings, *Clin Radiol* 62(1):58-64, 2007.

Kleiger B: Mechanisms of ankle injury, *Orthop Clin North Am* 5:127, 1974.

Klenerman L: *The foot and its disorders*, ed 2, Boston, 1982, Blackwell Scientific.

Klippel JH, Dieppe PA: *Rheumatology*, vol 1-2, ed 2, London, 1998, Mosby.

Koenigsberg R: *Churchill's illustrated medical dictionary*, New York, 1989, Churchill Livingstone.

Konradsen L, Halmer P, Sondergard L: Early mobilizing treatment for grade III ankle ligament injuries, *Foot Ankle* 12:69, 1991.

Kontos HA: Vascular diseases of the limbs. In Wyngaarden JB, Smith LH, Bennett JC, editors: *Cecil textbook of medicine*, ed 19, Philadelphia, 1992, WB Saunders.

Kouchoukos NT et al: Operative therapy for femoral-popliteal arterial occlusive disease, *Circulation* 35(suppl 1):174, 1967.

Kuralay E et al: A quantitative approach to lower extremity vein repair, *J Vasc Surg* 36(6):1213-1218, 2002.

Larkin J, Brage M: Ankle, hindfoot, and midfoot injuries. In Reider B, editor: *Sports medicine: the school aged athlete*, Philadelphia, 1991, WB Saunders.

Larsen E, Angermann P: Association of ankle instability and foot deformity, *Acta Orthop Scand* 61:136, 1990.

Lavy CBD, Barrett DS: *Questions and answers on Apley's concise system of orthopaedics and fractures*, Oxford, UK, 1991, Butterworth-Heinemann.

Ledoux WR, Sangeorzan BJ: Clinical biomechanics of the peritalar joint, *Foot Ankle Clin North Am* 9(4):663-683, 2004.

Lee TH, Wapner KL, Hecht PJ: Plantar fibromatosis, current concepts review, *J Bone Joint Surg* 75A:1080, 1993.

Leppilahti J et al: Overuse injuries of the Achilles tendon, *Ann Chir Gynaecol* 80:202, 1991.

Lerner AJ: *The little black book of neurology*, ed 3, St Louis, 1995, Mosby.

Lewis CB, Knortz KA: *Orthopedic assessment and treatment of the geriatric patient*, St Louis, 1993, Mosby.

Lloyd-Roberts GC, Clark RC: Ball and socket ankle joint in metatarsus adductus varus (S-shaped or serpentine foot), *J Bone Joint Surg* 55B:193, 1973.

Lo YL et al: Superficial peroneal sensory and sural nerve conduction studies in peripheral neuropathy, *J Clin Neurosci* 13(5):547-579, 2006.

Loth TS: *Orthopedic boards review II: a case study approach*, St Louis, 1996, Mosby.

Lui TH: Arthroscopy and endoscopy of the foot and ankle: indications for new techniques, *Arthroscopy* (in press, corrected proof).

Lui TH, Ip K, Chow HT: Comparison of radiologic and arthroscopic diagnoses of distal tibiofibular syndesmosis disruption in acute ankle fracture, *Arthroscopy* 21(11):1370.e1-1370.e7, 2005.

Mabin D: Compressions nerveuses distales du membre inferieur. Etude clinique et electrophysiologique, *Clin Neurophysiol* 27(1):9-24, 1997.

Magee DJ: *Orthopedic physical assessment*, ed 3, Philadelphia, 1997, WB Saunders.

Malone TR, McPoil TG, Nitz AJ: *Orthopedic and sports physical therapy*, ed 3, St Louis, 1997, Mosby.

Mann RA et al: Chronic rupture of the Achilles tendon: a new technique of repair, *J Bone Joint Surg* 73A:214, 1991.

Mann RA: *Surgery of the foot*, St Louis, 1986, Mosby.

Marchiori DM: *Clinical imaging with skeletal, chest, and abdomen pattern differentials*, St Louis, 1999, Mosby.

Martens MA, Moeyersoons JP: Acute and recurrent effort-related compartment syndrome in sports, *Sports Med* 9:62, 1990.

Martin DJ, Gardner ER: Transfer metatarsalgia after hallux valgus correction alleviated by "auto-Helal" osteotomy of the second metatarsal, *Foot* 15(2):101-103, 2005.

Martin JH: *Neuroanatomy text and atlas*, ed 2, Stamford, Conn, 1996, Appleton & Lange.

Mathers LH et al: *Clinical anatomy principles*, St Louis, 1996, Mosby.

Maury AC, Southgate C, Owen T: Hypertrophic nonunion of the distal fibula after reduced triplane fracture of the distal tibia in a child, *Foot Ankle Surg* 9(4):229-232, 2003.

Mazion JM: *Illustrated manual of neurological reflexes/signs/tests, part I, orthopedic signs/tests/maneuvers for office procedure, part II*, Orlando, Fla, 1980, Daniels Publishing.

McBryde A: Disorders of ankle and foot. In Grana WA, Kalenak A, editors: *Clinical sports medicine*, Philadelphia, 1991, WB Saunders.

McBryde A: Stress fractures of the foot and ankle. In DeLee JD, Drez D, editors: *Orthopaedic sport medicine, principles and practice*, vol 2, Philadelphia, 1994, WB Saunders.

McRae R: *Clinical orthopaedic examination*, ed 3, Edinburgh, 1990, Churchill Livingstone.

McRae R: *Practical fracture treatment*, New York, 1994, Churchill Livingstone.

Medical Economics Books: *Patient care flow chart manual*, ed 3, Oradell, NJ, 1982, Medical Economics Books.

Mellion MB: *Sports medicine secrets*, Philadelphia, 1994, Hanley & Belfus.

Mellion MB: *Office sports medicine*, ed 2, St Louis, 1996, Mosby.

Mennell JM: *Foot pain*, Boston, 1969, Little, Brown.

Mennell JM: *The musculoskeletal system: differential diagnosis from symptoms and physical signs*, Gaithersburg, Md, 1992, Aspen.

Mercier LR, Pettid FJ: *Practical orthopedics*, ed 4, St Louis, 1995, Mosby.

Michelson JD et al: Examination of the pathologic anatomy of ankle fractures, *J Trauma* 32:65, 1992.

Milgram JE: Office measures for relief of painful foot, *J Bone Joint Surg* 46A:1095, 1964.

Miller M: *Review of orthopaedics*, Philadelphia, 1992, WB Saunders.

Moore KL: *Clinically oriented anatomy*, ed 3, Baltimore, 1992, Williams & Wilkins.

Morton DJ: *Biomechanics of the human foot, American Academy of Orthopaedic Surgeons Instructional Course Lectures*, vol 2, Ann Arbor, Mich, 1944, JW Edwards.

Mosby-Year Book, Inc: *Expert 10-minute physical examination*, St Louis, 1997, Mosby.

Mubarak SJ, Hargens AR: *Compartment syndromes and Volkmann's contracture*, vol 3, Philadelphia, 1981, WB Saunders.

Mubarak SJ et al: The medial tibial stress syndrome: a cause of shin splints, *Am J Sports Med* 10:201, 1992.

Mullark RE: *The anatomy of varicose veins*, Springfield, Ill, 1965, Charles C Thomas.

Musette P et al: Determinants of severity for superficial cellutitis (erysipelas) of the leg: a retrospective study, *Eur J Intern Med* 15(7):446-450, 2004.

Myerson MS, Quill GE: Late complications of fractures of the calcaneus, *J Bone Joint Surg* 75A:331, 1993.

Myerson MS: Injuries to the forefoot and toes. In Jahss MH, editor: *Disorders of the foot and ankle: medical and surgical management*, vol 2, ed 2, Philadelphia, 1991, WB Saunders.

Nettina SM: *The Lippincott manual of nursing practice*, ed 6, Philadelphia, 1996, JB Lippincott.

Newton RW: *Color atlas of pediatric neurology*, St Louis, 1995, Mosby-Wolfe.

Nicholas JA, Hershman EB: *The lower extremity & spine in sports medicine*, vol 1-2, ed 2, St Louis, 1995, Mosby.

Niranjan NS, Price RD, Govilkar P: Fascial feeder and perforator-based V-Y advancement flaps in the reconstruction of lower limb defects, *Br J Plast Surg* 53(8):679-689, 2000.

Nordin M, Andersson GBJ, Pope MH: *Musculoskeletal disorders in the workplace: principles and practice*, St Louis, 1997, Mosby.

O'Donoghue DH: *Treatment of injuries to athletes*, ed 3, Philadelphia, 1976, WB Saunders.

Olson WH et al: *Handbook of symptom-oriented neurology*, ed 2, St Louis, 1994, Mosby.

Omer GE, Spinner M: *Management of peripheral nerve problems*, Philadelphia, 1980, WB Saunders.

Orava S et al: Diagnosis and treatment of stress fractures located at the mid-tibial shaft in athletes, *Int J Sports Med* 12:419, 1991.

O'Reilly MAR, Massouh H: Pictorial review: the sonographic diagnosis of pathology in the Achilles tendon, *Clin Radiol* 48:202, 1993.

O'Young B, Young MA, Stiens SA: *PM&R secrets*, Philadelphia, 1997, Hanley & Belfus.

Pagana KD, Pagana TJ: *Mosby's manual of diagnostic and laboratory tests*, St Louis, 1998, Mosby.

Paley D, Hall H: Intra-articular fractures of the calcaneus, *J Bone Joint Surg* 75A:342, 1993.

Parmar HV, Triffitt PD, Gregg PJ: Intra-articular fractures of the calcaneum treated operatively or conservatively, *J Bone Joint Surg* 75B: 932, 1993.

Patten J: *Neurological differential diagnosis*, ed 2, London, 1996, Springer.

Pecina NM, Krmpotic-Nemanic J, Markiewitz AD: *Tunnel syndromes*, Boca Raton, Fla, 1991, CRC Press.

Pedowitz RA et al: Modified criteria for the objective diagnosis of chronic compartment syndrome of the leg, *Am J Sports Med* 18:35, 1990.

Pereira CE et al: Meta-analysis of femoropopliteal bypass grafts for lower extremity arterial insufficiency, *J Vasc Surg* 44(3):510, 2006.

Peters JW, Trevino SG, Renstrom PA: Chronic lateral ankle instability, *Foot Ankle* 12:182, 1991.

Pfeiffer WH, Cracchiolo A: Clinical results after tarsal tunnel decompression, *J Bone Joint Surg* 76A:1222, 1994.

Pheasant S: *Ergonomics, work and health*, Gaithersburg, Md, 1991, Aspen.

Post M: *Physical examination of the musculoskeletal system*, Chicago, 1987, Mosby.

Prichasuk S: The heel pad in plantar heel pain, *J Bone Joint Surg* 76B:140, 1994.

Prichasuk S, Subhadrabandhu T: The relationship of pes planus and calcaneal spur to plantar heel pain, *Clin Orthop* 306:192, 1994.

Prystowsky JB et al: Prospective analysis of the incidence of deep venous thrombosis in bariatric surgery patients, *Surgery* 138(4):759-765, 2005.

Puranen J: The medial tibial syndrome, *Ann Chir Gynaecol* 80:215, 1991.

Quirk R: Common foot and ankle injuries in dance, *Orthop Clin North Am* 25:123, 1994.

Raatikainen T, Mikko P, Puranen J: Arthrography, clinical examination, and stress radiograph in the diagnosis of acute injury to the lateral ligaments of the ankle, *Am J Sports Med* 20:2, 1992.

Raffetto JD et al: Differences in risk factors for lower extremity arterial occlusive disease, *J Am Coll Surg* 201(6):918-924, 2005.

Rao UB, Joseph B: The influence of footwear on the prevalence of flatfoot, *J Bone Joint Surg* 74B:525, 1992.

Rasmussen O, Tovberg-Jansen I: Anterolateral rotational instability in the ankle joint, *Acta Orthop Scand* 52:99, 1981.

Ravel R: *Clinical laboratory medicine clinical application of laboratory data*, ed 6, St Louis, 1995, Mosby.

Renstrom AFH: Persistently painful sprained ankle, *J Am Acad Orthop Surg* 2:270, 1994.

Renstrom AFH, Kannus P: Injuries of the foot and ankle. In DeLee JD, Drez D, editors: *Orthopaedic sports medicine, principles and practice*, vol 2, Philadelphia, 1994, WB Saunders.

Resnick D, Niwayama G: *Diagnosis of bone and joint disorders*, Philadelphia, 1995, WB Saunders.

Rich K: Effects of leg and body position on transcutaneous oxygen measurements in healthy subjects and subjects with peripheral artery disease after lower-extremity arterial revascularization: a pilot study, *J Vasc Nurs* 20(4):125-135, 2002.

Riddle DL: Foot and ankle. In Richardson JK, Iglarsh ZA, editors: *Clinical orthopaedic physical therapy*, Philadelphia, 1994, WB Saunders.

Riehl R: Rehabilitation of lower leg injuries. In Prentice WE, editor: *Rehabilitation techniques in sports medicine*, ed 2, St Louis, 1994, Mosby.

Robb CA et al: Comparison of non-operative and surgical treatment of displaced calcaneal fractures, *Foot* (in press, corrected proof).

Roberts DK, Pomeranz SJ: Current status of magnetic resonance in radiologic diagnosis of foot and ankle injuries, *Orthop Clin North Am* 25:61, 1994.

Roberts JM et al: Comparison of unrepaired, primarily repaired, and polygalactin mesh-reinforced Achilles tendon lacerations in rabbits, *Clin Orthop* 181:244, 1993.

Rolak LA: *Neurology secrets*, ed 2, Philadelphia, 1998, Hanley & Belfus.

Rooser B, Bengtson S, Hagglund G: Acute compartment syndrome from anterior thigh muscle contusion: a report of eight cases, *J Orthop Trauma* 5:57, 1991.

Rumack CM, Wilson SR, Charboneau JW: *Diagnostic ultrasound*, vol 1-2, ed 2, St Louis, 1998, Mosby.

Rust M: Achilles tendon injuries in athletes, *Ann Chir Gynaecol* 80:188, 1991.

Saidoff DC, McDonough AL: *Critical pathways in therapeutic intervention*, St Louis, 1997, Mosby.

Salter RB, Harris WR: Injuries involving the epiphyseal plate, *J Bone Joint Surg* 45A:587, 1963.

Sanada H et al: Vascular function in patients with lower extremity peripheral arterial disease: a comparison of functions in upper and lower extremities, *Atherosclerosis* 178(1):179-185, 2005.

Saro C et al: Plantar pressure distribution and pain after distal osteotomy for hallux valgus: a prospective study of 22 patients with 12-month follow-up, *Foot* 17(2):84-93, 2007.

Schadt DC et al: Chronic atherosclerotic occlusion of the femoral artery, *JAMA* 175:937, 1961.

Schepsis AA, Leach RE, Gorzyca J: Plantar fasciitis: etiology, treatment, surgical results and review of the literature, *Clin Orthop* 266:185, 1991.

Schneck CD: Mesgarzadeh M, Bonakdarpour A: MR imaging of the most commonly injured ankle ligaments, *Radiology* 184:507, 1992.

Schon LC: Nerve entrapment, neuropathy and nerve dysfunction in athletes, *Orthop Clin North Am* 25:47, 1994.

Schon LC, Glennon TP, Baxter DE: Heel pain syndrome, electrodiagnostic support for nerve entrapment, *Foot Ankle* 14:129, 1993.

Schumacher HR, Klippel JH, Koopman WJ: *Primer on the rheumatic diseases*, ed 10, Atlanta, 1993, Arthritis Foundation.

Scioli MW: Achilles tendinitis, *Orthop Clin North Am* 25:177, 1994.

Shankman GA: *Fundamental orthopedic management for the physical therapist assistant*, St Louis, 1997, Mosby.

Singh SK, Ioli JP, Chiodo CP: The surgical treatment of Morton's neuroma, *Curr Orthop* 19(5):379-384, 2005.

Smorto MP, Basmajian JV: *Clinical electroneurography: an introduction to nerve conduction tests*, Baltimore, 1972, William & Wilkins.

Specht NT, Russo RD: *Practical guide to diagnostic imaging*, St Louis, 1998, Mosby.

Spittell JA Jr et al: Arteriovenous fistula complicating lumbar disc surgery, *N Engl J Med* 268:1162, 1963.

12

Stanley K: Ankle sprains are always more than "just a sprain," *Postgrad Med* 89:251, 1991.

Stedman TL: *Stedman's medical dictionary*, ed 25, Baltimore, 1990, Williams & Wilkins.

Stephens MM: Haglund's deformity and retrocalcaneal bursitis, *Orthop Clinic North Am* 25:41, 1994.

Stevens A, Lowe J: *Histology*, New York, 1992, Gower Medical.

Stewart DL, Abeln SH: *Documenting functional outcomes in physical therapy*, St Louis, 1993, Mosby.

Stiell IG et al: Implementation of the Ottawa ankle rules, *JAMA* 271:827, 1994.

Stock G: *The book of questions*, New York, 1985, Workman Publishing.

Stoller DW: *Magnetic resonance imaging in orthopaedics & sports medicine*, Philadelphia, 1993, JB Lippincott.

Sutton D, Young JWR: *A concise textbook of clinical imaging*, ed 2, St Louis, 1995, Mosby.

Tachdjian MO: *The child's foot*, Philadelphia, 1985, WB Saunders.

Takao M et al: A case of superficial peroneal nerve injury during ankle arthroscopy, *Arthroscopy* 17(4):403-404, 2001.

Tan JC, Horn SE: *Practical manual of physical medicine and rehabilitation*, St Louis, 1998, Mosby.

Tavakkolizadeh A, Klinke M, Davies MS: Bilateral distal fibular stress fractures, *Foot Ankle Surg* 11(3):171-173, 2005.

Taybi H, Lachman RS: *Radiology of syndromes, metabolic disorders, and skeletal dysplasias*, ed 4, St Louis, 1996, Mosby.

Thibodeau GA, Patton KT: *Anatomy & physiology*, ed 3, St Louis, 1996, Mosby.

Thibodeau GA, Patton KT: *Pocket reference to accompany anatomy & physiology*, ed 3, St Louis, 1996, Mosby.

Thompson JM: *Clinical outlines for health assessment*, St Louis, 1997, Mosby.

Thompson TC: A test for rupture of the tendon of Achilles, *Acta Orthop Scand* 32:461, 1992.

Thompson TC, Doherty JH: Spontaneous rupture of the tendon of Achilles: a nonclinical diagnostic test, *J Trauma* 2:126, 1962.

Thompson TC, Doherty J: Spontaneous rupture of the tendon of Achilles: a new clinical diagnostic test, *Anat Rec* 158:126, 1967.

Toghill PJ: *Examining patients: an introduction to clinical medicine*, London, 1990, Edward Arnold.

Tollison CD, Satterthwaite JR, Tollison JW: *Handbook of pain management*, ed 2, Baltimore, 1994, Williams & Wilkins.

Torg JS, Shepard RJ: *Current therapy in sports medicine*, ed 3, St Louis, 1995, Mosby.

Tranier S et al: Value of somatosensory evoked potentials in saphenous entrapment neuropathy, *J Neurol Neurosurg Psychiatry* 55:461, 1992.

Turek SL: *Orthopaedics principles and their application*, ed 3, Philadelphia, 1977, JB Lippincott.

Turk N et al: Discriminatory ability of calcaneal quantitative ultrasound in the assessment of bone status in patients with inflammatory bowel disease, *Ultrasound Med Biol* 33(6):863-869, 2007.

Turnipseed WD, Pozniak M: Popliteal entrapment as a result of neurovascular compression by the soleus and plantaris muscles, *J Vasc Surg* 15:284, 1992.

Ubbink DT, Vermeulen H: Spinal cord stimulation for critical leg ischemia: a review of effectiveness and optimal patient selection, *J Pain Symptom Manage* 31(4, suppl 1):S30-S35, 2006.

Van Holsbeeck M, Introcaso JH: *Musculoskeletal ultrasound*, St Louis, 1991, Mosby.

Vasquez MA et al: The utility of the venous clinical severity score in 682 limbs treated by radiofrequency saphenous vein ablation, *J Vasc Surg* 45(5):1008.e2-1015.e2, 2007.

Verhaven EFC et al: The accuracy of three-dimensional magnetic resonance imaging in the diagnosis of ruptures of the lateral ligaments of the ankle, *Am J Sports Med* 19:583, 1991.

Wagner FW Jr: The dysvascular foot: a system for diagnosis and treatment, *Foot Ankle* 2:64, 1981.

Wakefield TS, Frank RG: *The clinician's guide to neuro musculoskeletal practice*, Abbotsford, Wis, 1995, Allied Health of Wisconsin, SC.

Weineck J: *Functional anatomy in sports*, ed 2, St Louis, 1990, Mosby.

Weinstein SL, Buckwalter JA: *Turek's orthopaedics principles and their application*, ed 5, Philadelphia, 1994, JB Lippincott.

Whitmore I, Willan PLT: *Multiple choice questions in human anatomy*, London, 1995, Mosby.

Wilkerson LA: Ankle injuries in athletes, *Primary Care* 19:337, 1992.

Wilkins RW, Coffman JD: Tests of peripheral vascular efficiency, *Practitioner* 188:346, 1962.

Windsor RE, Lox DM: *Soft tissue injuries: diagnosis and treatment*, Philadelphia, 1998, Hanley & Belfus.

Winter D: *Biomechanics and motor control of human movement*, ed 2, New York, 1990, Wiley-Interscience Publication.

Wood JE: *The veins*, Boston, 1965, Little, Brown.

Yao L et al: Plantar plate of the foot: findings on conventional arthrography and MR imaging, *Am J Roentgenol* 163:641, 1994.

Yochum T, Rowe L: *Essentials of skeletal radiology*, ed 2, Baltimore, 1996, Williams & Wilkins.

Zatouroff M: *Diagnosis in color physical signs in general medicine*, ed 2, London, 1996, Mosby-Wolfe.

Zitelli BJ, Davis HW: *Atlas of pediatric physical diagnosis*, ed 2, London, 1992, Wolfe.

Zsoter T, Cronin RFP: Venous distensibility in patients with varicose veins, *Can Med Assoc J* 94:1293, 1966.

Zwierska I et al: Upper- vs lower-limb aerobic exercise rehabilitation in patients with symptomatic peripheral arterial disease: a randomized controlled trial, *J Vasc Surg* 42(6):1122-1130, 2005.

CITATIONS

Akali AU, Niranjan NS: Management of bilateral Achilles tendon rupture associated with ciprofloxacin: a review and case presentation, *J Plast Reconstr Aesthetic Surg* (in press, corrected proof).

Ali M, Riding G, Tait WF: Superficial thrombophlebitis in varicose veins caused by inflight stockings, *EJVES Extra* 9(2):22-23, 2005.

Bardelli M, Turelli L, Scoccianti G: Definition and classification of metatarsalgia. *Foot Ankle Surg* 9(2):79-85, 2003.

Bell SJ et al: Chronic lateral ankle instability: the Broström procedure, *Oper Tech Sports Med* 13(3):176-182, 2005.

Benson E et al: Calcaneal fractures in occupants involved in severe frontal motor vehicle crashes, *Accid Anal Prev* 39(4):794-799, 2007.

Cloke DJ, Greiss ME: The digital nerve stretch test: a sensitive indicator of Morton's neuroma and neuritis, *Foot Ankle Surg* 12(4):201-203, 2006.

Crowther RG et al: Relationship between temporal-spatial gait parameters, gait kinematics, walking performance, exercise capacity, and physical activity level in peripheral arterial disease, *J Vasc Surg* 45(6):1172-1178, 2007.

Dayal R et al: Multimodal percutaneous intervention for critical venous occlusive disease, *Ann Vasc Surg* 19(2):235-240, 2005.

Delis KT et al: Hemodynamic impairment, venous segmental disease, and clinical severity scoring in limbs with Klippel-Trenaunay syndrome, *J Vasc Surg* 45(3):561-567, 2007.

Dombek MF et al: Peroneal tendon tears: a retrospective review, *J Foot Ankle Surg* 42(5):250-258, 2003.

Elman EE, Kahn SR: The post-thrombotic syndrome after upper extremity deep venous thrombosis in adults: a systematic review, *Thromb Res* 117(6):609-614, 2006.

Fadel GE, Rowley DI: Metatarsalgia, *Curr Orthop* 16(3):193-204, 2002.

Franson J, Baravarian B: Tarsal tunnel syndrome: a compression neuropathy involving four distinct tunnels, *Clin Podiatr Med Surg* 23(3):597-609, 2006.

Fujiwara T et al: Prevalence of asymptomatic arteriosclerosis obliterans and its relationship with risk factors in inhabitants of rural communities in Japan: Tanno-Sobetsu study, *Atherosclerosis* 177(1):83-88, 2004.

Gardner AW, Montgomery PS, Afaq A: Exercise performance in patients with peripheral arterial disease who have different types of exertional leg pain, *J Vasc Surg* (in press, corrected proof).

Keller ME et al: Evaluation of a disease management plan for prevention and diagnosis of thromboembolic disease in major trauma patients, *Curr Surg* 57(5):456-459, 2000.

Mendes RR et al: Treatment of superficial and perforator venous incompetence without deep venous insufficiency: is routine perforator ligation necessary? *J Vasc Surg* 38(5):891-895, 2003.

Meru AV et al: Intermittent claudication: an overview, *Atherosclerosis* 187(2):221-237, 2006.

Mihalich RM, Early JS: Management of cuboid crush injuries, *Foot Ankle Clin North Am* 11(1):121-126, 2006.

Mirmiran R, Schuberth JM: Non union of an epiphyseal fibular fracture in a pediatric patient, *J Foot Ankle Surg* 45(6):410-412, 2006.

Monaghan K, Delahunt E, Caulfield B: Ankle function during gait in patients with chronic ankle instability compared to controls, *Clin Biomech* 21(2):168-174, 2006.

Olapade-Olaopa EO et al: Primary lower limb varicosities arising directly from normal deep venous systems: a series report, *Ann Vasc Surg* 14(2):166-169, 2000.

Qiao T, Liu C, Ran F: The impact of gastrocnemius muscle cell changes in chronic venous insufficiency, *Eur J Vasc Endovasc Surg* 30(4):430-436, 2005.

Saro C et al: Plantar pressure distribution and pain after distal osteotomy for hallux valgus: a prospective study of 22 patients with 12-month follow-up, *Foot* 17(2):84-93, 2007.

Steinberg BD: Evaluation of limb compartments with increased interstitial pressure. An improved noninvasive method for determining quantitative hardness, *J Biomech* 38(8):1629-1635, 2005.

Williams DP, Hassan AI: Undiagnosed compartment syndrome following anterior tibialis muscle hernia repair, *Injury Extra* 38(2):59-60, 2007.

12

MALINGERING

INTRODUCTION

In a framework for disability, examining physicians need to understand the interaction between the disability and the factors affecting a return to work (Fig. 13-2). In this model of interaction, *pathology* is the disturbance of normal bodily processes at the cellular level. *Impairment* is a specific loss of function. *Functional limitation* is the lack of ability to perform an action or activity. *Disability* is the inability to perform socially defined activities. *Quality of life* refers to the patient's concept of total well-being. *Risk* or *cofactors* include biologic, environmental, lifestyle, and behavioral characteristics that are associated with musculoskeletal conditions (Fig. 13-3). Whether people with specific physical limitations are disabled depends on their expectations, resources, and the demands of their physical environment.

Feigned illness, or malingering, is a sensitive medicolegal issue. Illness or injury that cannot be supported by medical fact confounds the physician's diagnostic procedures and health care delivery; it also serves as an element of fraud in the third-party payer system. Patients participating in this behavior are a bane.

Forensic neuropsychology has experienced enormous growth over recent years. Thus the percentage of articles on neuropsychology in the most widely read neuropsychologic journals (*Archives of Clinical Neuropsychology, Journal of Clinical and Experimental Neuropsychology,* and *Clinical Neuropsychology*) increased from 4% in 1990 to 14% in 2000. The predominant issue in these studies is malingering, addressed by 86% of the forensic papers. The upsurge of interest in this issue results from the increasingly frequent demand for neuropsychologists to give expert opinion in personal injury litigation, especially in cases of mild or moderate brain damage. Thus a large proportion of individuals undergoing neuropsychologic assessment in the United States are implicated in legal cases that would afford them considerable economic benefits if cognitive damage were demonstrated, whether genuine or not. In many cases, neuropsychologic test data are the only objective source of evidence of deficits, especially in cases of mild brain damage in which neuroimaging techniques generally give negative results and neurologic signs are usually absent (Vilar-Lopez et al, 2007).

Not all patients who feign an illness are completely aware of their actions. Some patients embellish symptoms and physical signs as learned responses or traits, whereas others describe physical problems with hysterical emotional overlays. The latter group is influenced mostly by fear of the unknown. Depression bears a significant relationship to pain (Fig. 13-4 and Box 13-1).

Text continued on p. 1013

TABLE 13-1

MALINGERING CROSS-REFERENCE TABLE BY ASSESSMENT PROCEDURE

Malingering, Hysterotia, and Embellishment	DISEASE PORTRAYED													
Test/Sign	Lower Back	Sciatica	General Pain	Facial Pain	Olfactory Nerve	Trigeminal Nerve	Cerebellar Lesions	Blindness	Facial Anesthesia	Deafness	Anesthesia	Consciousness	Stoicism	Paresis
Pain														
Axial trunk-loading test	•													
Burn bench test	•													
Flexed-hip test		•												
Flip sign		•												
Libman sign			•											
Magnuson test	•													
Mannkopf sign			•											
Marked part pain-suggestibility test			•											
Plantar flexion test	•	•												
Related joint motion test			•											
Seeligmuller sign				•										
Trunk rotational test	•													
Sensory														
Anosmia testing					•	•								
Coordination-disturbance testing							•							
Cuignet test								•						
Facial anesthesia testing									•					
Gault test										•				
Janet test											•			
Limb-dropping test (upper extremities)												•		
Lombard test										•				
Marcus Gunn sign								•						
Midline tuning-fork test											•			
Optokinetic nystagmus test								•						
Position-sense testing							•							
Regional anesthesia testing									•		•			
Romberg sign							•							
Snellen test								•						
Stoicism indexing												•	•	
Motor														
Bilateral limb-dropping test (lower extremities)														•
Hemiplegic posturing							•							•
Hoover sign														•
Simulated foot-drop testing							•							•
Simulated forearm-and-wrist-weakness testing														•
Simulated grip-strength-loss test														•
Tripod test (bilateral leg-fluttering test)	•													

13

TABLE 13-2

MALINGERING, HYSTERIA, AND EMBELLISHMENT CROSS-REFERENCE TABLE BY SUSPECTED SYNDROME

Anesthesia	Janet test	Lower back	Axial trunk-loading test
	Midline tuning-fork test		Burn bench test
	Regional anesthesia testing		Flexed-hip test
Blindness	Cuignet test		Magnuson test
	Marcus Gunn sign		Plantar flexion test
	Midline tuning-fork test		Trunk rotational test
	Snellen test		Tripod test (bilateral leg-fluttering test)
Cerebellar lesions	Coordination-disturbance testing	Olfactory nerve	Anosmia testing
	Position-sense testing	Paresis	Bilateral limb-dropping test (lower extremities)
	Romberg sign		
	Hemiplegic posturing		Hemiplegic posturing
	Simulated foot-drop testing		Hoover sign
Consciousness	Limb-dropping test (upper extremities)		Simulated foot-drop testing
	Stoicism indexing		Simulated forearm-and-wrist-weakness testing
Deafness	Gault test		Simulated grip-strength-loss testing
	Limb-dropping test (lower extremities)	Sciatica	Flip sign
Facial anesthesia	Facial anesthesia testing		Plantar flexion test
	Lombard test	Stoicism	Stoicism indexing
Facial pain	Seeligmuller sign	Trigeminal nerve	Anosmia testing
General pain	Libman sign		
	Mannkopf sign		
	Marked part pain-suggestibility test		
	Related joint motion test		

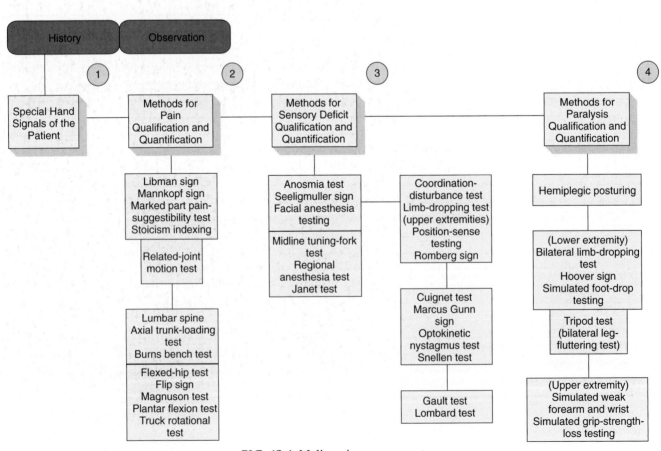

FIG. 13-1 Malingering assessment.

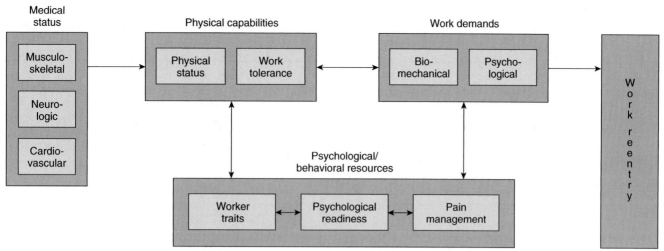

FIG. 13-2 Multiple factors potentially affecting return to work following occupational musculoskeletal injury/illness. Conceptual Model of Work Disability. (From Demeter SL, Andersson GBJ, Smith GM: *Disability evaluation,* St Louis, 1996, Mosby.)

ORTHOPEDIC GAMUT 13-1

COMMONLY USED PROCEDURES IN DETERMINING EXISTENCE OF COGNITIVE MALINGERING

- *Victoria Symptom Validity Test (VSVT):* The VSVT is a computer-administered and computer-scored test. It includes a total of 48 items, presented in three blocks of 16 items each. During the study trial, a single five-digit study number is presented for 5 seconds in the center of the computer screen. This presentation is followed by the retention interval and then by the recognition trial, in which the target and a five-digit distractor are displayed. The respondents are asked to choose the number they saw in the study trial. The retention interval is 5 seconds in the first block, 10 seconds in the second, and 15 seconds in the third.

- *Test of memory malingering (TOMM):* The TOMM is an instrument designed to provide an assessment whether an individual is falsifying symptoms of memory impairment. It consists of 50 pictures of common objects that the subject must remember. After the presentation of the 50 pictures, the individual has to recognize which one is the correct picture between two alternatives. The TOMM consists of two learning trials and an optional retention trial and has good face validity as a test of learning and memory.

- *The b test:* The b test is a measure to identify malingering requiring recognition of overlearned information. This test is a letter recognition and discrimination task that consists of a 15-page *stimulus booklet.* The examinee is asked to circle all occurrences of the letter *b* that appear on each page, working as quickly as possible.

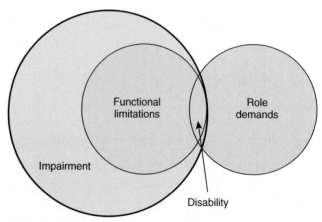

FIG. 13-3 Disability lies at the interface between functional limitations and role demands. (From Demeter SL, Andersson GBJ, Smith GM: *Disability evaluation*, St Louis, 1996, Mosby.)

BOX 13-1

SYMPTOMS OF DEPRESSION

1. Depressed or irritable mood
2. Markedly diminished interest or pleasure in activities
3. Significant weight loss or weight gain when not dieting
4. Insomnia or hypersomnia nearly every day
5. Psychomotor agitation or retardation—observable by others
6. Fatigue or loss of energy
7. Feelings of worthlessness or excessive or inappropriate guilt, which may be delusional
8. Diminished ability to think or concentrate; indecisiveness
9. Recurrent thoughts of death, recurrent suicidal ideation without a plan, a suicide attempt, or a specific plan for committing suicide
10. Lack of reactivity to usually pleasurable stimuli
11. Depression worse in the morning
12. Early morning awakening

From White AH, Schofferman JA: *Spine care,* vol 1-2, St Louis, 1995, Mosby.

13

**Psychiatric History
and Mental Status Examination**

(To be completed by attending psychiatrist or psychiatric resident under direct supervision of the attending psychiatrist)

Psychiatric History

Chief Complaint(s)

_____
_____
_____

Present Illness(es) (Presenting symptoms, precipitating events, details of outpatient therapy, medications and pt.'s response)

_____
_____
_____
_____
_____
_____
_____
_____
_____
_____

Past Psychiatric History (Include previous mental illnesses, suicide attempts, hospitalizations, treatments, medications)

_____
_____
_____
_____
_____

Habits (Include use of tobacco, caffeine, laxatives, alcohol and non-prescription drugs)

_____
_____
_____

Personal History (Education, occupational functioning, military, legal, marital, history of childhood abuse, etc.)

_____
_____
_____
_____

Family History (Include all information relevant to this admission)

_____
_____
_____

FIG. 13-4 Psychiatric history and mental status examination (From Akron Medical Center, 1995.)

Mental Status Examination

General Observations
General Appearance
General Demeanor

(Behavior/Activity
Check all that apply)

○ Neat/well-groomed	○ Casually groomed and dressed	○ Dishevelled/unkempt
○ Spontaneous	○ Overtly negativistic and hostile	○ Mistrustful and suspicious
○ Preoccupied	○ Regressed	○ Demanding and manipulative

○ Hyperactive	○ Hypoactive	○ Stuporous	○ Agitated	○ Silly
○ Grimaces	○ Mannerisms	○ Tics	○ Compulsions	○ Hypervigilant
○ Bored	○ Stooped	○ Tearful	○ Elated	

○ Facial expression and body posture appropriate to interview   ○ Other (specify)

Eye Contact:

○ Avoids direct gaze	○ Most of the time	○ Often	○ Occasionally
○ Stares into space	○ Most of the time	○ Often	○ Occasionally
○ Glances furtively	○ Most of the time	○ Often	○ Occasionally

Motor Behavior
  Psychomotor Retardation
  Psychomotor Excitement
  Specific Observations

○ None	○ Mild	○ Moderate	○ Marked
○ None	○ Mild	○ Moderate	○ Marked
○ Posturing	○ Waxy Flexibility	○ Catatonic Rigidity	○ Catatonic Stupor
○ Pacing	○ Fidgeting	○ Tremors Gait: ○ Rigid	○ Unsteady

Comments on Behavior:

_____

_____

Mood and Affect

Depression	○ None	○ Mild	○ Moderate	○ Severe
Anxiety	○ None	○ Mild	○ Moderate	○ Severe
Anger	○ None	○ Mild	○ Moderate	○ Severe
Anhedonia	○ None	○ Mild	○ Moderate	○ Severe
Loneliness	○ None	○ Mild	○ Moderate	○ Severe
Euphoria	○ None	○ Mild	○ Moderate	○ Severe
Diurnal mood variation	○ None	○ Worse in a.m.	○ Worse in p.m.	

Affect

Range	○ Full	○ Restricted		
Inappropriate	○ None	○ Mild	○ Moderate	○ Severe
Flat	○ None	○ Mild	○ Moderate	○ Severe
Labile	○ None	○ Mild	○ Moderate	○ Severe

Comments on Mood and Affect:

_____

_____

Thought Processes

Ability of speech

○ Clear, comprehensible	○ Blocking	○ Slow	○ Slurred
○ Rapid	○ Pressured	○ Flight of Ideas	○ Talkative

Incoherence	○ None	○ Mild	○ Moderate	○ Severe
Irrelevance	○ None	○ Mild	○ Moderate	○ Severe
Evasiveness	○ None	○ Mild	○ Moderate	○ Severe
Circumstantiality	○ None	○ Mild	○ Moderate	○ Severe
Loose associations	○ None	○ Mild	○ Moderate	○ Severe
Concrete thinking	○ None	○ Mild	○ Moderate	○ Severe
Other finding:	○ None	○ Mild	○ Moderate	○ Severe

○ None	○ Clang Associations	○ Neologisms	○ Flight of Ideas
○ Echolalia	○ Perseverations	○ Word play	○ Excessive profanity

Comments on Thought Processes: ○ Unintelligible muttering

_____

_____

FIG. 13-4, cont'd

Mental Status Examination—cont'd

Thought Content

Delusions   ○ Absent   ○ Present
                 ○ Grandiose   ○ Persecutory   ○ Somatic ○ Bizarre   ○ Religious   ○ Nihilistic
Other Findings   ○ Phobic Ideas ○ Ambivalence   ○ Obsessive Ideas   ○ Autistic Thinking
                 ○ Guilt   ○ Self Reproach   ○ Ideas of Reference   ○ Suicidal ideation
                 ○ Suspicious   ○ Self-derogatory ○ Resentful of Others   ○ Preoccupation with death
                 ○ Preoccupied w/ self-harm

Comments on Thought Content:
_____
_____

Somatic Functioning and Concern

Appetite Disturbance: ○ None   ○ Poor   ○ Excessive
Energy Disturbance: ○ None   ○ Easily Fatigued   ○ Excessively Energetic
Libido Disturbance   ○ None   ○ Decreased   ○ Markedly increased
Insomnia   ○ None   ○ Diff. falling asleep ○ Early a.m. awakening   ○ Awakening at night
Incontinence   ○ None   ○ Occasional   ○ Often   ○ Very often
Seizures (past week)   ○ None   ○ One   ○ Several   ○ Daily   ○ Several/day
Sensory impairment (organic)   ○ None   ○ Visual   ○ Hearing
Preoccup. with physical health ○ None   ○ Mild   ○ Moderate   ○ Marked

Somatic concerns (e.g., constipation, diarrhea, GI disturbance, short of breath, headaches, backaches, sweating, itching, etc):
_____
_____

Perception

Hallucinations   ○ Unknown   ○ None   ○ Suspected   ○ Definite
   Auditory   ○ Slight   ○ Mild   ○ Moderate   ○ Marked
   Visual   ○ Slight   ○ Mild   ○ Moderate   ○ Marked
   Olfactory   ○ Slight   ○ Mild   ○ Moderate   ○ Marked
   Gustatory   ○ Slight   ○ Mild   ○ Moderate   ○ Marked
   Tactile   ○ Slight   ○ Mild   ○ Moderate   ○ Marked
   Visceral   ○ Slight   ○ Mild   ○ Moderate   ○ Marked
   Belief that hallucinations are real   ○ Knows unreal   ○ Unsure   ○ Convinced they are real

Hallucinatory content (threatening, accusatory, self-derogatory, grandiose, flattering, reassuring, sexual, religious):
_____
_____

Illusions   ○ None   ○ Mild   ○ Moderate   ○ Marked
Depersonalization ○ None   ○ Mild   ○ Moderate   ○ Marked
Derealization   ○ None   ○ Mild   ○ Moderate   ○ Marked
Misperceptions of Role and Meaning:
_____
_____

Sensorium

Orientation Disturbances   ○ Tested   ○ Too disturbed to test
   Time   ○ None   ○ Mild   ○ Moderate   ○ Marked
   Place   ○ None   ○ Mild   ○ Moderate   ○ Marked
   Person   ○ None   ○ Mild   ○ Moderate   ○ Marked
Clouded Consciousness   ○ None   ○ Mild   ○ Moderate   ○ Marked
                           ○ Fluctuating   ○ Continuous
Dissociation   ○ None   ○ Mild   ○ Moderate   ○ Marked
Comments on Sensorium:
_____
_____

FIG. 13-4, cont'd

Mental Status Examination—cont'd

Cognitive Functions

Memory Disturbances	○ Tested	○ Too disturbed to test		○ Confabulations	
Immediate	○ Unknown	○ None	○ Mild	○ Moderate	○ Marked
Recent	○ Unknown	○ None	○ Mild	○ Moderate	○ Marked
Remote	○ Unknown	○ None	○ Mild	○ Moderate	○ Marked

Attention Disturbances	○ None	○ Mild	○ Moderate	○ Marked	
Distractibility	○ None	○ Mild	○ Moderate	○ Marked	
Intelligence (estimated)	○ Unknown	○ Retarded	○ Borderline	○ Average	○ Bright

Comments on Cognitive Functions:

_____

_____

Judgment

Family Relations	○ Poor	○ Fair	○ Healthy	
Other social relations	○ Poor	○ Fair	○ Healthy	
Employment	○ Poor	○ Fair	○ Healthy	
Future Plans	○ No Plans	○ Poor	○ Fair	○ Realistic

Comments on Judgment:

_____

_____

Insight and Attitude Toward Illness

Recognition of one's illness
  ○ Unknown   ○ Too sick to be tested   ○ Physically ill only
  ○ None   ○ Little   ○ Fair   ○ Full recognition

Awareness of one's contribution to problem
  ○ Unknown   ○ Too sick to be tested   ○ Not applicable
  ○ None   ○ Little   ○ Fair   ○ Full awareness
  ○ Blames others   ○ Blames circumstances

Motivation for getting well
  ○ Unknown   ○ Too sick to be tested
  ○ None   ○ Little   ○ Fair   ○ Highly motivated
  ○ Accepts offered treatment   ○ Refuses offered treatment

Comments on Insight:

_____

_____

Potential for Self-Injury, Suicide and Violence

Self-Injury	○ Unknown	○ Absent	○ Minimal	○ Potentially present	○ Marked (specify precautions)
Suicide Risk	○ Unknown	○ Absent	○ Minimal	○ Potentially present	○ Marked (specify precautions)
Assaultiveness	○ Unknown	○ Absent	○ Minimal	○ Potentially present	○ Active (specify interventions)

Comments on self-injury, suicide/violence potential (e.g., plan, history, behavior):

_____

_____

_____

Reliability and Completeness of Information:
  ○ Very good   ○ Good   ○ Only Fair   ○ Poor   ○ Very Poor

13

FIG. 13-4, cont'd

Mental Status Examination—cont'd

Barriers to Communication/reliability due to (Complete only if reliability rated poor/very poor):

○ Dialect/Foreign language   ○ Quality of speech   ○ Deafness   ○ Physical illness

○ Refuses to give information   ○ Massive Denial   ○ Conscious falsification

○ Pt. psychopathology   Other (explain) _____

_____

_____

Attitude Toward Examiner:

○ Positive   ○ Neutral   ○ Ambivalent   ○ Negative   ○ Unknown

Overall Severity of Illness:

○ Mild   ○ Moderate   ○ Marked   ○ Severe   ○ Extremely Severe

Discussion and Formulation (include description of patient's strengths/assets)

_____

_____

_____

_____

_____

_____

Diagnoses (DSM-IV)

Axis I _____

Axis II _____

Axis III _____

Axis IV (assessment of psychosocial/environmental problems) _____

Axis V (Global Assessment of Functioning score) Current _____ Past year _____

Recommendations:

_____

_____

_____

_____

_____

_____

_____

Examiner's Name, Title   Date

_____

Examining Psychiatrist Signature   Date

FIG. 13-4, cont'd

In many areas of human suffering, patients often exhibit symptoms that are in excess of objective physical evidence. A clear illustration of this phenomenon is the individual who, while being monitored with video-electroencephalographic telemetry, appears to exhibit a generalized seizure. The individual's convulsions may ostensibly be indistinguishable from those of patients with genuine epilepsy in every respect, including postictal confusion, with the exception of normal brain electrical activity concomitant to the symptom presentation. Many patients with nonepileptic seizures are unwavering in their beliefs of the authenticity of their disorder, thereby suggesting a conversion (unconscious) mechanism of their presentation, whereas others may have a more intentional component to their symptom

amplification. Nonepileptic seizures are one of a myriad of conditions with excessive symptom presentation, but the clear dissociation between the pronounced motor symptoms and normal brain substrates provides such a poignant lesson on the potential of human nature to manufacture illness behavior unconsciously or consciously (Delis, Wetter, 2007).

No specific guideline has been offered with regard to the maximal number of malingering tests that should be given or the appropriateness of a battery of tests exclusively designed to detect malingering. Greve and Bianchini (2006) report the standard practice of their clinic of always administering the TOMM [test of memory malingering] Retention Trial regardless of outcome on trial 2 in addition to at least one other symptom validity test, usually the Portland Digit Recognition Test. The authors also report using the malingering indices on the Minnesota Multiphasic Personality Inventory-2 (MMPI-2) and stated that some subjects were also given the *word memory test*. Administering several malingering measures (especially in their longest forms, despite good early performance) might increase the likelihood of diagnosing malingering or probable malingering based on statistical chance alone, or it may even elicit suboptimal performance. The point made by Rogers and Cavanaugh (1983) that malingering may, in some cases, represent a unique response to unusual and often trying circumstances, rather than sociopathic tendencies, may apply in this instance (Booksh, Aubert, Andrews, 2007).

Two major categories of hysterical disorders are identified: patients with a fictitious illness, such as in malingering, and patients with Munchausen syndrome. Both types of patients are those with signs and symptoms that have no organic basis but who are not deliberately attempting to mislead the examiner.

Trivial physical trauma or disease is often at the root of a portrayed illness or injury. In many instances, by the time

---

ORTHOPEDIC GAMUT 13-2

DSM-IV SYMPTOM-SPECIFIC CATEGORIES IN EXCESSIVE COGNITIVE SYMPTOMS

A. Somatization disorder requires:
   a. At least four pain symptoms
   b. Two gastrointestinal symptoms
   c. One sexual symptom
   d. One pseudoneurologic symptom
B. *Undifferentiated somatoform disorder*—requires one or more physical complaints, with no reference made to cognitive difficulties
C. *Conversion disorder*—requires one or more symptoms or deficits affecting voluntary motor or sensory function without mention of cognitive or memory difficulties
D. *Pain disorder*—requires only excessive pain symptoms
E. *Somatoform disorder NOS*—includes individuals with predominantly excessive cognitive symptoms
F. *Dissociative amnesia*—requires one specific type of cognitive problem, such as the inability to recall important personal information, usually of a traumatic or stressful nature
G. *Dissociative fugue* requires:
   a. One specific cognitive difficulty, such as the inability to recall some or all of one's past
   b. This difficulty must surface in the context of a sudden, unexpected travel away from home or one's customary place of daily activities
H. *Dissociative identity disorder*—occurs in individuals with multiple personalities in which they exhibit an inability to recall important information about one or more personality states when they are in a different personality state
I. *Dissociative disorder NOS*—encompasses individuals with excessive cognitive complaints

---

ORTHOPEDIC GAMUT 13-3

PREDICTORS OF WORK INCAPACITY AND WORK LOSS BECAUSE OF DEPRESSION

1. Incoherent presentation of pain localization and stable symptoms
2. Inability to influence pain and function by movement or change of position
3. Relapse of a preexisting condition and lack of response in previous episodes
4. Work dissatisfaction
5. Problems of communicating realistic treatment goals
6. Poor self-perceived prognoses with unrealistically high perception of impairment

13

symptom embellishment is clinically recognized, the complaints are of such a magnitude that they are completely incongruous with the original illness or injury. A patient who originally experienced a minor, clinically documented upper respiratory infection now describes symptoms and subjective complaints that resemble those for histoplasmosis or black lung disease. Yet another patient may complain of total leg disability after a minor thigh contusion. Both patients have in common the total lack of clinical findings to support the complaints, and some type of secondary gain serves as a driving force behind the medical charade.

Individuals may feign physical symptoms to continue in a less strenuous job at work, or they may receive a parking space closer to their place of employment. These individuals may also fake symptoms to gain control over family members or fellow workers. The injured party may also allow others to do work the patient would ordinarily do.

The diagnosis of hysteria should be established based only on positive evidence. Even if the patient has an obvious hysterical disorder, a serious organic illness may still be present.

Conversion symptoms have a physiologic or pathologic substrate. A conversion disorder denotes a process in which a patient's emotions become transformed into physical (motor or sensory) manifestations. These patients are asking for help but in an inappropriate way. Conversion symptoms often occur in mentally defective individuals or in adolescents as a way of coping (albeit inadequately) with the environment. Common presentations include blindness, deafness, paresis, sensory disturbances, ataxia, seizures, and unconsciousness.

Posttraumatic stress disorder (PTSD) arises after exposure to a traumatic stressor. That is, after exposure to a situation or event that is, or is perceived to be, threatening to the safety or physical integrity of oneself or others. PTSD symptoms include reexperiencing of the trauma (e.g., recurrent and intrusive thoughts, distressing dreams), avoidance and emotional numbing (e.g., avoidance of reminders of the traumatic event, restricted range of affect), and hyperarousal (e.g., exaggerated startle response). In other words, to diagnose PTSD, these symptoms must persist for at least 1 month and must be associated with significant distress or impairment in functioning. Traumatic events are common, yet PTSD is comparatively rare. Estimates indicate that 40% to 60% of community adults have been exposed to trauma, whereas the lifetime prevalence of PTSD is 8%. Vulnerability factors, such as particular learning experiences, or genetic factors likely influence the person's risk of meeting criteria for PTSD after exposure to a trauma. To diagnose PTSD according to the *Diagnostic and Statistical Manual of Mental Disorders,* fourth edition, text revision (DSM-IV-TR), malingering needs to be ruled out (Taylor, Frueh, Asmundson, 2007).

Malingering is the conscious misrepresentation of thoughts, feelings, and facts, and it is a condition in which symptoms and signs associated with pain or dysfunction are either partially or entirely feigned for secondary gain. Most commonly, malingering occurs in the setting of the workplace, where workers' compensation is an issue.

Labeling patients as hysterics, frauds, or malingerers is difficult. This task is rarely accomplished without reaping the wrath of the patient or substantial legal repercussions.

The actual percentage of patients who are malingerers is undetermined. However, estimates indicate that 2% of all patients seeking health care are malingering. Obviously, the ascertainment of the inaccuracy of a patient's report of pain and disability is a difficult process, but the possibility of malingering should be raised in the mind of the treating physician when major discrepancies or inconsistencies

---

ORTHOPEDIC GAMUT 13-4

THE FIVE Ds OF GLOBAL HEALTH STATUS

1. Death
2. Disability—upper or lower limb functional problems
3. Discomfort—physical or psychologic
4. Drug reactions—or other medical or surgical iatrogenic problems
5. Dollars—both direct and indirect costs

ORTHOPEDIC GAMUT 13-5

IMPORTANCE OF MALINGERING ASSESSMENT

Examiners should be concerned about whether treatment-seeking patients are malingering for several important reasons:

- Diagnosis and treatment planning
  - Malingering needs to be ruled out before establishing a diagnosis.
  - If the diagnosis is incorrect, the resulting treatment may be misguided.
- Threat to the therapeutic alliance with clinicians: Clinicians routinely working with traumatized populations that have high rates of suspected but undetected malingering often become suspicious of the motives of all patients.
- Economic impact
  - In 1995 the total cost of insurance fraud in the United States was estimated to be $85.3 billion.
  - Most of the cost was the result of health insurance fraud, including (but not limited to) the malingering of posttraumatic stress disorder.
- Threat to research databases: Researchers commonly recruit people studies from treatment-seeking populations.

appear in the patient's medical situation. In this effort, outcome measures for the assessment of work capacity, work tolerance, dependable ability, and task demand are useful tools (Table 13-3).

OUTCOMES ASSESSMENTS

The *health assessment questionnaire* (HAQ) is a self-administered instrument that assesses discomfort and disability. It is used to measure outcomes in many different neuromusculoskeletal diseases (Fig. 13-5). Disease-specific instruments have been produced to help follow outcomes in several other neuromusculoskeletal diseases. This group includes a Fibromyalgia Impact Questionnaire (Fig. 13-6). The activity of inflammatory neuromusculoskeletal diseases can be assessed through serologic measures. Separate measures of both tender and swollen joints can be charted on a homunculus (Fig. 13-7). A generic measure of anxiety and depression, such as the *hospital anxiety and depression (HAD) scale* (Fig. 13-8), allows psychologic variables to be assessed independently from orthopedic disease-related outcomes. The EuroQuol Thermometer is one of the instruments that uses a simple visual technique to allow people to assess their own health status (Fig. 13-9); the *disease repercussion profile* is another such resource (Box 13-2).

Armed with Borg Pain Scales, Oswestry Disability Indices, symptom magnification indexing, Dallas Pain Questionnaire (Fig. 13-10), Waddell Indexing (Table 13-4), and neuroorthopedic malingering tests, the physician is able to substantiate or refute the existence of malingering in any given case. These tests and indices are usually used in combination with the more traditional neuroorthopedic physical examinations. A singular positive finding or test does not indicate that the patient is magnifying or faking symptoms. Rather, the malingering diagnosis is based on the preponderance of positive malingering test findings and the absence of findings from traditional neuroorthopedic tests. Any positive findings must be further correlated with the medical history of the patient. The constellation of positive malingering tests, normal findings in traditional tests, and medical history discrepancies form the malingering diagnosis. Malingering and psychogenic rheumatism patients complain primarily of pain, sensory losses, or paralysis in any combination.

Text continued on p. 1025

TABLE 13-3

DISTINCTIONS AMONG WORK CAPACITY, WORK TOLERANCE, DEPENDABLE ABILITY, AND TASK DEMAND

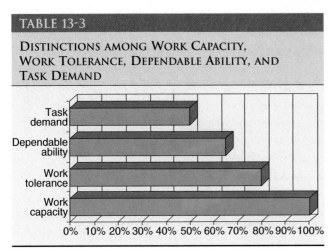

From Demeter SL, Andersson GBJ, Smith GM: *Disability evaluation,* St Louis, 1996, Mosby.

BOX 13-2

DISEASE IMPACT INDEX

Patients report severity of problems on a 0-to-10 scale in six dimensions:
- Functional activities
- Social activities
- Relationships
- Emotions
- Socioeconomic factors
- Body image

From Carr AJ, Thompson PW: Towards a measure of patient-perceived handicap in rheumatoid arthritis, *Br J Rheumatol* 33:378, 1994.

CLINICAL PEARL

Standardized instruments are often used in survey research. Many of these instruments are devised in clinic settings in which trained health care professionals complete health assessments. However, prohibitive cost and relative ease make participant-assessed outcome measures a more feasible approach to obtain constructs describing functional and mental health outcomes. With these more-convenient measures of health increasingly used as primary outcomes in epidemiologic studies, selecting an appropriate assessment tool involves thorough review of the many standard survey instruments available. The Millennium Cohort, the largest cohort study ever undertaken by the U.S. Department of Defense, was launched in 2001 to gather health outcome information along with occupational and environmental exposures employing a longitudinal approach. In the first panel of enrollment, more than 77,000 participants joined the 22-year-long study, filling out either a mailed survey or an identical Web-based survey.

13

Name [   ]   Date [   ]

In this section we are interested in learning how your illness affects your ability to function in daily life. Please feel free to add any comments on the back of this page.

Please check the response which best describes your usual abilities

over the past week:

Dressing & grooming Are you able to:	Without any difficulty	With some difficulty	With much difficulty	Unable to do
Dress yourself, including tying shoelaces and doing buttons?	☐	☐	☐	☐
Shampoo your hair:	☐	☐	☐	☐

Arising Are you able to:				
Stand up from a straight chair?	☐	☐	☐	☐
Get in and out of bed?	☐	☐	☐	☐

Eating Are you able to:				
Cut your meat?	☐	☐	☐	☐
Lift a full cup or glass to your mouth?	☐	☐	☐	☐
Open a new milk carton?	☐	☐	☐	☐

Walking Are you able to:				
Walk outdoors on flat ground?	☐	☐	☐	☐
Climb up five steps?	☐	☐	☐	☐

Please check any **aids or devices** that you usually use for any of these activities:

☐ Cane   ☐ Devices used for dressing (button hook, zipper pull, long-handled shoe horn, etc.)
☐ Walker   ☐ Built up or special utensils
☐ Crutches   ☐ Special or built up chair
☐ Wheelchair   ☐ Other (specify . . . .)

Please check (x) the response which best describes your usual abilities

Over the past week:

Hygiene Are you able to:	Without any difficulty	With some difficulty	With much difficulty	Unable to do
Wash and dry your body?	☐	☐	☐	☐
Take a tub bath?	☐	☐	☐	☐
Get on and off the toilet?	☐	☐	☐	☐ ☐ Hygiene

Reach Are you able to:				
Reach and get down a 5 pound object (such as bag of sugar) from just above your head?	☐	☐	☐	☐
Bend down to pick up clothing from the floor?	☐	☐	☐	☐ Reach

Grip Are you able to:				
Open car doors?	☐	☐	☐	☐
Open jars which have been previously opened?	☐	☐	☐	☐
Turn faucets on and off?	☐	☐	☐	☐ Grip ARA

Activities Are you able to:				
Run errands and shop?	☐	☐	☐	☐
Get in and out of a car?	☐	☐	☐	☐
Do chores such as vacuuming or yardwork?	☐	☐	☐	☐ Activity

Please check (x) any **aids or devices** that you usually use for any of these activities:

☐ Raised toilet seat   ☐ Bathtub bar
☐ Bathtub seat   ☐ Long-handled appliances for reach
☐ Jar opener   ☐ Long-handled appliances in bathroom
☐ (for jars previously opened)   ☐ Other (specify. . . . .)

Please check (x) any categories for which you usually need **help from another person:**

☐ Hygiene   ☐ Gripping and opening things
☐ Reach   ☐ Errands and chores

We are also interested in learning whether or not you are affected by pain because of your illness. How much pain have you had because of your illness **In the past week:**

Place a vertical (I) mark on the line to indicate the severity of the pain

No pain [=====================================] Severe pain
0   100

FIG. 13-5 The Health Assessment Questionnaire (HAQ): disability and discomfort scales.
(From Fries JF et al: Measurement of patient outcomes in arthritis, *Arthritis Rheum* 23:137, 1980.)

Fibromyalgia Impact Questionnaire

1. Were you able to:

	Always	Most times	Occasionally	Never
a. Do shopping	0	1	2	3
b. Do laundry with a washer and dryer	0	1	2	3
c. Prepare meals	0	1	2	3
d. Wash dishes/cooking utensils by hand	0	1	2	3
e. Vacuum a rug	0	1	2	3
f. Make beds	0	1	2	3
g. Walk several blocks	0	1	2	3
h. Visit friends/relatives	0	1	2	3
i. Do yard work	0	1	2	3
j. Drive a car	0	1	2	3

2. Of the 7 days in the past week, how many days did you feel good?

1	2	3	4	5	6	7

3. How many days in the past week did you miss work because of your fibromyalgia?
(If you don't have a job outside the home leave this item blank.)

1	2	3	4	5

4. When you did go to work, how much did pain or other symptoms of your fibromyalgia interfere with your ability to do your job?

No problem |————————————————| Great difficulty

5. How bad has your pain been?

No pain |————————————————| Very severe pain

6. How tired have you been?

No tiredness |————————————————| Very tired

7. How have you felt when you got up in the morning?

Awoke well rested |————————————————| Awoke very tired

8. How bad has your stiffness been?

No stiffness |————————————————| Very stiff

9. How tense, nervous or anxious have you felt?

Not tense |————————————————| Very tense

10. How depressed or blue have you felt?

Not depressed |————————————————| Very depressed

FIG. 13-6 Fibromyalgia Impact Questionnaire (FIQ). (From Burkhardt CS, Clark SR, Bennett RM: The Fibromyalgia Impact Questionnaire: development and validation, *J Rheumatol* 18:728, 1991.)

13

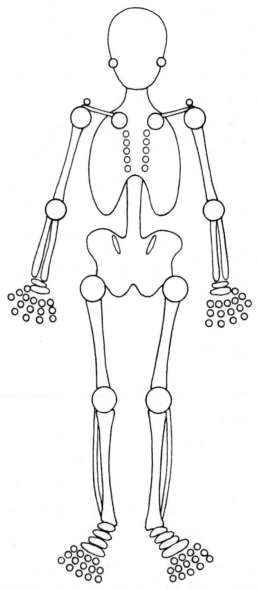

FIG. 13-7 Skeletal diagram for recording joint examination findings. (From Polley HF, Hunder GG: *Rheumatologic interviewing and physical examination of the joints*, ed 2, Philadelphia, 1978, WB Saunders.)

1. Are you basically satisfied with your life?		Yes	No
2. Have you dropped many of your activities and interests?		Yes	No
3. Do you feel that your life is empty?		Yes	No
4. Do you often get bored?		Yes	No
5. Are you hopeful about the future?		Yes	No
6. Are you bothered by thoughts you can't get out of your head?		Yes	No
7. Are you in good spirits most of the time?		Yes	No
8. Are you afraid that something bad is going to happen to you?		Yes	No
9. Do you feel happy most of the time?		Yes	No
10. Do you often feel helpless?		Yes	No
11. Do you often get restless and fidgety?		Yes	No
12. Do you prefer staying at home rather than going out and doing new things?		Yes	No
13. Do you frequently worry about the future?		Yes	No
14. Do you feel that you have more problems with memory than most?		Yes	No
15. Do you think it is wonderful to be alive now?		Yes	No
16. Do you often feel downhearted and blue?		Yes	No
17. Do you feel pretty worthless the way you are now?		Yes	No
18. Do you worry a lot about the past?		Yes	No
19. Do you find life very exciting?		Yes	No
20. Is it hard for you to get started on new projects?		Yes	No
21. Do you feel full of energy?		Yes	No
22. Do you feel that your situation is hopeless?		Yes	No
23. Do you think that most individuals are better off than you are?		Yes	No
24. Do you frequently get upset over little things?		Yes	No
25. Do you frequently feel like crying?		Yes	No
26. Do you have trouble concentrating?		Yes	No
27. Do you enjoy getting up in the morning?		Yes	No
28. Do you prefer to avoid social gatherings?		Yes	No
29. Is it easy for you to make decisions?		Yes	No
30. Is your mind as clear as it used to be?		Yes	No

FIG. 13-8 Geriatric depression screening form. (Modified from Yesavage JA et al: Development and validation of a geriatric depression screening scale: a preliminary report, *J Psych Res* 17:37, 1983.)

13

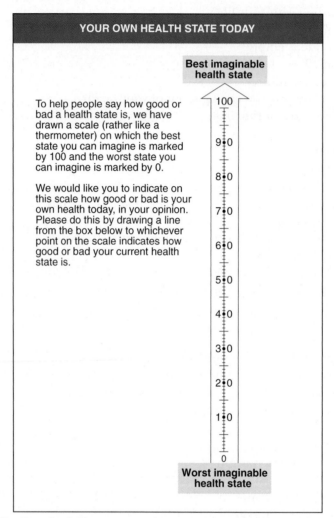

FIG. 13-9 The EuroQuol Thermometer for assessing health status. (From Euroquol Group: Euroquol: a new facility for the measurement of health-related quality of life, *Health Policy* 16:199, 1990.)

DALLAS PAIN QUESTIONNAIRE

Name:_____   Date of Birth:_____

Today's Date:_____   Occupation:_____

PLEASE READ: *Mark an "X" along the line from 0 to 100 for each question that tells your doctor how your pain has affected your life. Be sure to mark your own answers. Do not ask someone else to answer the questions for you.*

For example: I feel bad.

Never		Some		Mostly all the time
0%	0 1 X 2 3 4 5			100%

SECTION I: DAILY ACTIVITIES

1. PAIN AND INTENSITY - to what degree do you rely on pain medications or pain relieving substances for you to be comfortable?

None		Some		All the time
0%	0 1 2 3 4 5			100%

2. PERSONAL CARE - how much does pain interfere with your personal care (getting out of bed, teeth brushing, dressing, etc.)?

None (no pain)		Some		Cannot get out of bed
0%	0 1 2 3 4			100%

3. LIFTING - how much limitation do you notice lifting?

Can lift as I did		Some		Cannot lift anything
0%	0 1 2 3 4 5			100%

4. WALKING - compared to how far you could walk before your injury or back trouble, how much does pain restrict your walking now?

None (can walk the same)		Some		Cannot walk
0%	0 1 2 3 4 5			100%

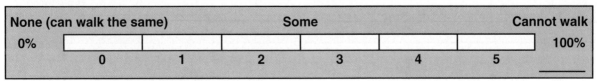

FIG. 13-10 **A,** Dallas Pain Questionnaire. (From White AH, Schofferman JA: *Spine care,* vol 1-2, St Louis, 1995, Mosby.)

13

5.   SITTING - back pain limits my sitting in a chair to:

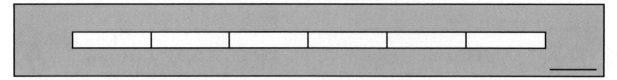

6.   STANDING - how much does your pain interfere with your tolerance to stand for long periods of time?

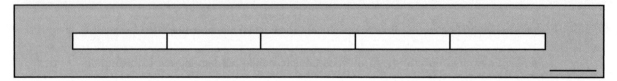

7. SLEEPING - how much does your pain interfere with your sleeping?

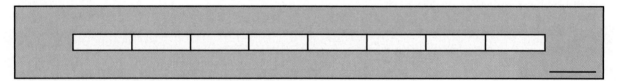

$$D = \underline{\hspace{1cm}} \times 3 = \underline{\hspace{1cm}}\%$$

SECTION II: WORK AND LEISURE

8.   SOCIAL LIFE - how much does pain interfere with your social life (dancing, games, going out, eating with friends, etc.)?

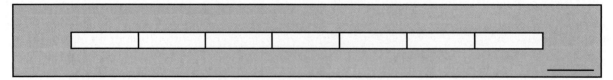

9.   TRAVELING - how much does pain interfere with traveling in a car?

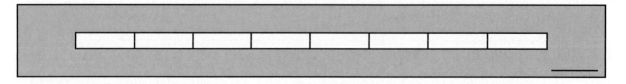

10.   VOCATIONAL - how much does pain interfere with your job?

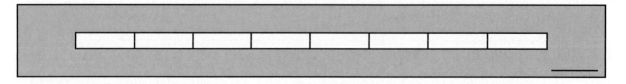

$$W = \underline{\hspace{1cm}} \times 5 = \underline{\hspace{1cm}}\%$$

FIG. 13-10, cont'd

SECTION III: ANXIETY/DEPRESSION

11. ANXIETY/MOOD - how much control do you feel that you have over the demands made on you?

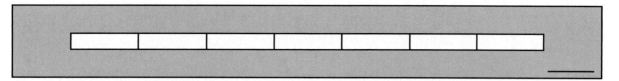

12. EMOTIONAL CONTROL - how much control do you feel you have over your emotions?

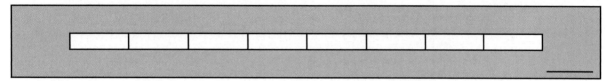

13. DEPRESSION - how depressed have you been since the onset of pain?

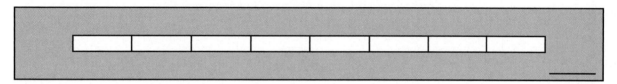

SECTION IV: SOCIAL INTERESTS

A = ____ × 5 = ____%

14. INTERPERSONAL RELATIONSHIPS - how much do you think your pain changed your relationship with others?

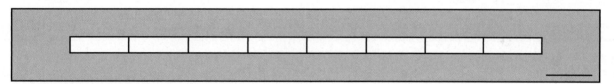

15. SOCIAL SUPPORT - how much support do you need from others to help you during this onset of pain (taking over chores, fixing meals, etc.)?

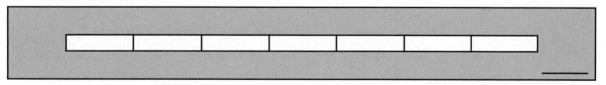

16. PUNISHING RESPONSE - how much do you think others express irritation, frustration, or anger toward you because of your pain?

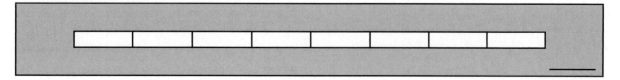

S = ____ × 5 = ____%

FIG. 13-10, cont'd

13

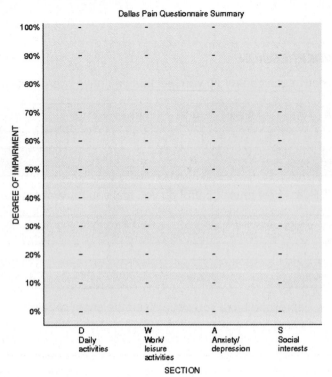

FIG. 13-10, cont'd

TABLE 13-4

NONORGANIC PHYSICAL SIGNS INDICATING ILLNESS BEHAVIOR

	Physical Disease/Normal Illness Behavior	Abnormal Illness Behavior
Symptoms		
Pain	Anatomic distribution	Whole leg pain
		Tailbone pain
Numbness	Dermatomal	Whole leg numbness
Weakness	Myotomal	Whole leg giving way
Time pattern	Varies with time and activity	Never free of pain
Response to treatment	Variable benefit	Intolerance of treatments
		Emergency admissions to hospital
Signs		
Tenderness	Anatomic distribution	Superficial
		Widespread nonanatomic
Axial loading	No lumbar pain	Lumbar pain
Simulated rotation	No lumbar pain	Lumbar pain
Straight leg raising	Limited on distraction	Improves with distraction
Sensory	Dermatomal	Regional
Motor	Myotomal	Regional, jerky, giving way

From Waddell G et al: Symptoms & signs: physical disease or illness behavior? *Br Med J* 289:739, 1984, British Medical Association.

GENERAL PROCEDURES

General Patient Observation

Consensus among physicians asserts that malingering is readily detected with appropriate medical and psychologic tests. Most patients who have remained conscious during an injury can give an adequate description of what happened. A malingerer is vague and on guard while describing the incidents of an injury or accident. However, some patients who also remain conscious at the time of injury are not as observant as others are, and these patients will be somewhat vague.

A malingerer often appears quarrelsome, nervous, and ill at ease. General observation of the patient before and after the physical examination may reveal that the patient is fully capable of movements or activities that were claimed to be impossible in the physical examination. The examiner should note how the patient enters and behaves in the reception room. It is helpful if a nonprofessional staff person takes the patient's history and engages the claimant in conversation.

When hearing loss is the complaint, the examiner should speak to the patient calmly and in a very low tone of voice to test the patient's response. With visual-disturbance complaints, the examiner should give the patient a magazine with fine print to read while waiting and later ask something about the subject matter.

The patient should be asked to describe the accident in detail. The examiner should encourage the patient to go through as many of the painful motions as possible. In many instances, the extreme interest of the examiner in the patient's story will cause the patient to move the arms, legs, or back in a normal manner.

The examiner should try to observe the patient tying the shoes, walking down a hallway, bending at the waist, drinking at a fountain, pulling or pushing a door, or many other unguarded activities of daily living.

> What distinguishes malingering from conditions such as factitious disorder is the conscious motivation to deceive (lie) for a secondary gain. In factitious disorder, the intentional production of symptoms is undertaken to assume the patient role. Unlike factitious disorder, in which patients are most often encountered in hospitals and clinics, malingerers are more often seen in outpatient settings and are usually involved in legal proceedings (civil or criminal). They are often uncooperative with examinations and are unwilling to undergo painful procedures or medication trials with potential side effects. Malingerers commonly display axis II traits, if not frank disorders. They often have histories of (1) previous lawsuits, (2) run-ins with the law, (3) acting-out behavior in school, workplace, or the military, (4) sporadic employment and attendance at work, (5) substance use, (6) turning down jobs that accommodate or accept their professed *partial* disability, and (7) few, if any, longstanding financial responsibilities (Hall, Hall, 2006).

Detailed History

Occasionally, the physician is compelled to distinguish fraud or exaggeration from organic injury. As should be apparent by now, this task is not easy. An examination, when deception or exaggeration is suspected, should be completed with a strictly impartial attitude on the part of the examiner. The patient must be accorded all the tact and courtesy that is ordinarily extended to any other patient. If the physician-patient rapport is compromised, confidence is destroyed, and questions and tests, which are constructed to evoke sincerity on the part of the patient, become unreliable.

In many instances, the patient grudgingly gives the history. The malingering patient may remark, "I've told this to the last doctor, and I don't see any reason to repeat it."

The patient may also deny permission to review previous X-ray findings or case histories, stating that only the attorney can grant such permission. The genuine patient will not usually hesitate to furnish all patient information or permissions in this regard.

Malingerers will give an involved and long history, most of which is often discovered to be false. When the patient's history, actions, and examination findings suggest that symptoms are exaggerated, one of the duties of the physician is to make the examination so complete that no question exists as to the actual extent of any organic disease or injury.

The physician's next duty is to decide whether the patient is a malingerer attempting to defraud and deceive or whether hysteria or neurasthenia exists, in which case the patient benignly imagines the disability. Many patients become convinced that a certain type of disability is caused by a specific injury. If the physician can establish sufficient confidence with the patient to explain and treat the condition effectively, the exaggerated symptoms will often disappear. However, with malingering, any attempt on the part of the physician to confront the patient results in further exaggeration.

To achieve a secondary gain, the malingerer must use subterfuge. Exaggeration is usually obvious no matter how cleverly it is performed. The malingerer exhibits slyness of expression and watches the examiner carefully during the various procedures. The patient may try to impress the examiner with the importance of the case and often reiterates a great degree of personal honesty.

The patient appears to be constantly suspicious that detection is likely and attempts to avoid disclosure.

A detailed history is the first essential, and many times the answers to questions must be requested repeatedly (Fig. 13-11). The patient may give strange stories about the exact nature of an accident or the treatment that was previously administered for the condition (Figs. 13-12 to 13-14).

Psychogenic Rheumatism Profile

Patients with psychiatric disorders may develop pain as part of the symptoms associated with mental illness. Patients

Text continued on p. 1043

13

Patient History

Please take time to fill out the appropriate spaces

Name _____ Date _____

Age _____ Medication allergies _____ Current Rx'd medicine _____

Present job _____

Type of work done _____

When did your back or neck pain originally start? _____

When did your arm or leg pain originally start? _____

When did your current episode begin? _____

Did your pain start gradually? _____ Suddenly? _____ Injury _____

What type of injury? _____

What time of day is your pain worse?   Morning _____ Later in the day _____

                     Middle of the night _____

Do you have numbness or tingling in an arm or leg? Please describe.

_____

Are there any recent changes in bowel or bladder habits? Please describe.

_____

Do you feel stiffness in the morning? _____

My pain is: check the appropriate column:	Better	Worse	No different
With cough or sneeze	_____	_____	_____
With straining	_____	_____	_____
Sitting in straight chair	_____	_____	_____
Sitting in soft, easy chair	_____	_____	_____
Bending forward to brush teeth	_____	_____	_____
Walking up stairs	_____	_____	_____
Walking down stairs	_____	_____	_____
Lying flat on stomach	_____	_____	_____
On side with knees bent	_____	_____	_____
When bending	_____	_____	_____
When lifting	_____	_____	_____
When working overhead	_____	_____	_____
Lying on back	_____	_____	_____
Standing	_____	_____	_____

	Yes	No
My back sometimes gets stuck when I bend forward.	_____	_____
After walking, bending forward relieves my pain.	_____	_____
My back feels like giving way when I bend forward.	_____	_____
Do you have headaches?	_____	_____

FIG. 13-11 Patient history and examination forms. (From Watkins RG: *The spine in sports*, St Louis, 1996, Mosby.)

Patient History—cont'd

	Yes	No
Have you had a change in hearing, vision?	_____	_____
Have you had dizzy spells?	_____	_____
My pain stops me when I walk a certain distance.	_____	_____
Have you been in a hospital for back, leg, or neck pain?	_____	_____

Number of times hospitalized _____ Please give dates. _____

How long can you sit? _____

How long can you walk? _____

If you have to stop walking, how long does the pain last? _____

Have you had myelograms? _____

Number of times _____

Have you had neck or back surgery? _____

Number of times _____ Please give dates and types. _____

Have you been in the hospital with other medical problems? _____

Number of times _____ Please describe. _____

What treatments have made your pain better? _____

What treatments have made your pain worse? _____

Who referred you to this office? _____

Do you have an attorney helping you? _____

Do other members of your family have significant back trouble? _____

Who? _____

Did you have to change jobs? _____ To what? _____

Are you under any pressure at home? _____ At work? _____

Mild _____ Moderate _____ Severe _____

What can you not do because of your pain that you want to do? _____

_____

What was the date of your last physical exam and the name of the doctor? _____

Who did it? _____

Pelvic done? _____ Rectal done? _____

FIG. 13-11, cont'd

13

Patient Pain/Sensation Chart

Date _____

Please give this paper to the doctor at the time of examination

Mark the areas on your body where you feel the described sensations. Use the appropriate symbol. Mark areas of radiation. Include all affected areas. Just to complete the picture, please draw in your face.

	—		oooo		XXXX		////
NUMBNESS	—	PINS AND NEEDLES	oooo	BURNING	XXXX	STABBING	////
	—		oooo		XXXX		////

Have you had prior back or neck surgery? ( )Yes   ( )No

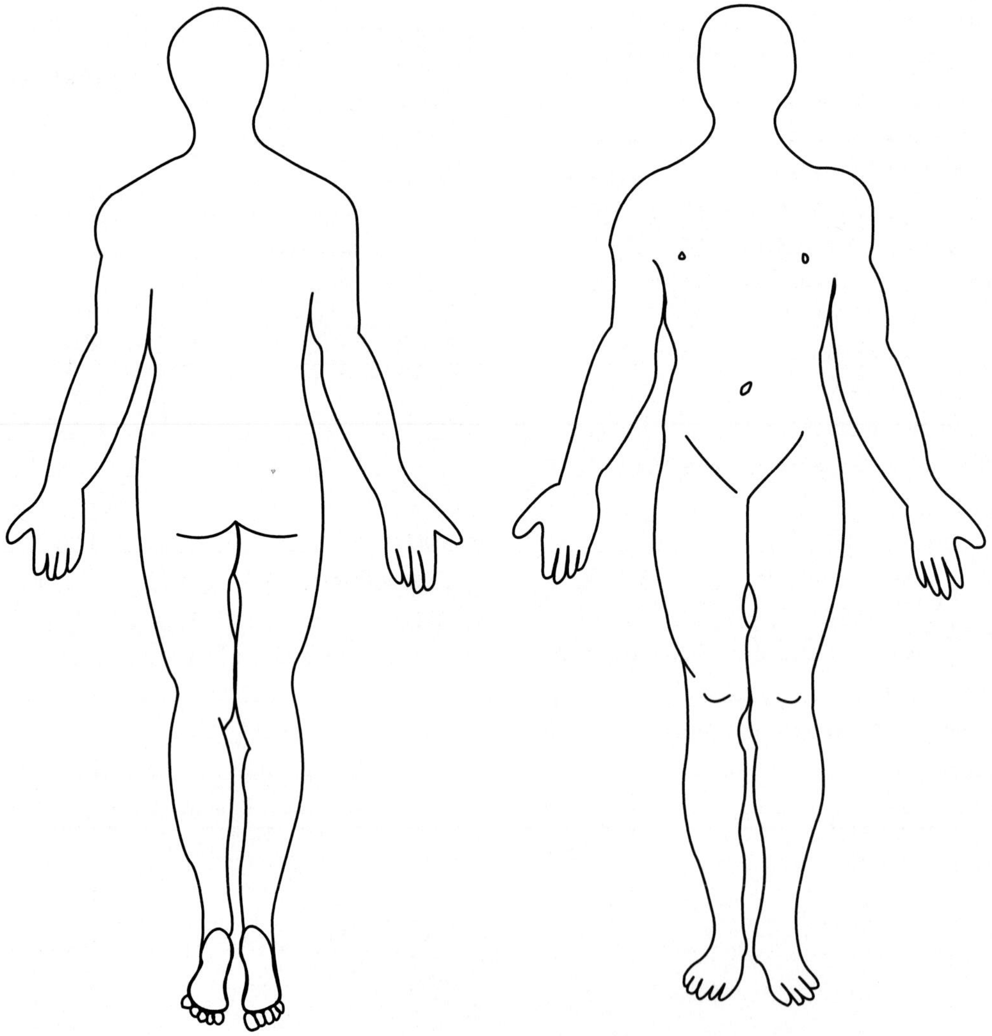

FIG. 13-11, cont'd

Oswestry Function Test

Please choose one answer only per section

Pain Intensity

1. I can tolerate my pain without having to use pain killers.
2. My pain is bad, but I manage without taking pain killers.
3. Pain killers give me complete relief from my pain.
4. Pain killers give me moderate relief from my pain.
5. Pain killers give me very little relief from my pain.
6. Pain killers have no effect on my pain, and I do not use them.

Personal Care

1. I can look after myself normally without causing extra pain.
2. I can look after myself normally, but it causes extra pain.
3. It is painful to look after myself, and I am slow and careful.
4. I need some help, but I manage most of my personal care.
5. I need help every day in most aspects of self-care.
6. I do not get dressed, wash with difficulty, and stay in bed.

Lifting

1. I can lift heavy objects without causing extra pain.
2. I can left heavy objects, but it gives me extra pain.
3. Pain prevents me from lifting heavy objects off the floor, but I can manage light to medium objects if they are conveniently positioned.
4. I can lift only very light objects.
5. I cannot lift anything at all.

Walking

1. Pain does not prevent me from walking any distance.
2. Pain prevents me from walking more than 1 mile.
3. Pain prevents me from walking more than ½ mile.
4. Pain prevents me from walking more than ¼ mile.
5. I can only walk using a cane or crutches.
6. I am in bed most of the time and have to crawl to the toilet.

Sitting

1. I can sit in any chair as long as I like.
2. I can sit only in my favorite chair as long as I like.
3. Pain prevents me from sitting more than 1 hour.
4. Pain prevents me from sitting more than ½ hour.
5. Pain prevents me from sitting more than 10 minutes.
6. Pain prevents me from sitting at all.

Standing

1. I can stand as long as I want without extra pain.
2. I can stand as long as I want, but it gives me extra pain.
3. Pain prevents me from standing more than 1 hour.
4. Pain prevents me from standing more than ½ hour.
5. Pain prevents me from standing more than 10 minutes.
6. Pain prevents me from standing at all.

Sleeping

1. Pain does not prevent me from sleeping well.
2. I can sleep well only by taking medication for sleep.
3. Even when I take medication, I have less than 6 hours' sleep.
4. Even when I take medication, I have less than 4 hours' sleep.
5. Even when I take medication, I have less than 2 hours' sleep.
6. Pain prevents me from sleeping at all.

Sex Life

1. My sex life is normal and gives me no extra pain.
2. My sex life is normal but causes some extra pain.
3. My sex life is nearly normal but is very painful.
4. My sex life is severely restricted by pain.
5. My sex life is nearly absent because of pain.
6. Pain prevents any sex life at all.

Social Life

1. My social life is normal and gives me no extra pain.
2. My social life is normal but increases the degree of pain.
3. Pain has no significant effect on my social life apart from limiting my more energetic interests, like dancing, etc.
4. Pain has restricted my social life, and I do not go out as often.
5. Pain has restricted my social life to my home.
6. I have no social life because of pain.

Traveling

1. I can travel anywhere without extra pain.
2. I can travel anywhere, but it gives me extra pain.
3. Pain is bad, but I manage journeys over 2 hours.
4. Pain restricts me to journeys of less than 1 hour.
5. Pain restricts me to short necessary journeys of less than ½ hour
6. Pain prevents me from traveling except to the doctor or hospital.

FIG. 13-11, cont'd

History and Present Status of the Back/Neck Problem

Patient's name _____ Date _____

CHIEF COMPLAINT (Major items only) _____

_____

_____

ONSET: Time—sudden or gradual—Date and time of day _____

*Cause—injury, sickness, etc. _____

_____

†Immediate symptoms _____

_____

_____

_____

COURSE: Detailed chronologic study of symptoms and medical care and reaction to each procedure

_____

_____

_____

_____

_____

_____

_____

_____

PAST RELEVANT HISTORY: Previous and recent attacks, etc. _____

_____

Pain	1	2	3	4
Function	1	2	3	4
Occupation	1	2	3	4

PROGRESS: Better, worse, stationary _____

Relation to Activity

Lying down—position of greatest comfort: _____

Does rest or activity relieve? _____

Awakened often and why? _____

Sitting—one side, or shifts _____ How most comfortable? _____

Getting up from sitting—need assist? _____ Hard or soft _____ Driving _____

Standing—one side or shifts _____ Time, and what happens? _____

Walking—distance _____ What happens? _____

Stairs, inclines, irregular ground _____

Bending—degree _____ Pain and assist returning to erect position _____

Lifting: Wt. _____ lbs. _____ Fatigue _____

Working _____ Type _____ Date discontinued _____ Returned _____

Effect of manipulation _____ Support: type and effect _____

Effect of exercise _____

*Describe carefully just how forces of the accident affected the patient, how he or she was thrown, fell, landed: twists to back or limbs. Just mechanical factors. (Don't include extraneous material, such as who was to blame.)
†How patient felt immediately: unconscious—how long, ache, severe pain, gradual increase, inability to walk or use certain joints, numbness, and/or paralysis.

FIG. 13-11, cont'd

History and Present Status of the Back/Neck Problem—cont'd

Neurologic Effects

Ratio of neck/arm pain: _____ / _____

Radiation of pain: Where? _____ When? _____

Effects of coughing, sneezing, and straining during bowel movements: On back, where? _____

On referred pain, how far? _____

Areas of skin tingling, numbness, coldness _____ Muscle weakness? _____

Chronic Inflammatory Factors

Stiffness after rest: Getting out of bed _____ After sitting _____

Effect of change of weather _____ Cold, damp weather _____ Hot _____

Effect of heat to part _____ Type of heat _____

(Women) Relation to menstrual periods _____

Remarks: _____

Physical Examination

Review of Systems
HEENT

Chest
Cardiovascular
Abdomen
Rectal
Fundi
Prostate

Pulses	Right	Left
Femoral		
Popliteal		
Pedal		
Bruits		

Back and Lower Extremity Examination

Range of motion	Right	Left
Flexion		
Extension		
Left lateral flexion		
Right lateral flexion		

Muscle strength	Right	Left
Hip abduction		
Hip adduction		
Hip flexion		
Hip extension		
Knee flexion		
Knee extension		
Ankle dorsiflexion		
Ankle plantar flexion		
Ankle inversion		
Ankle eversion		

FIG. 13-11, cont'd

13

Physical Examination—cont'd

Muscle strength—cont'd	Right	Left
Toes dorsiflexion		
Toes plantar flexion		
Big toe dorsiflexion		

Reflex grades	Right	Left
Patella		
Achilles		
Posterior tibia		

Pain radiation	Right	Left
Thighs		
Calves		
Feet		
Foot top		
Foot bottom		
Heel		
Big toe		
Little toe		

Sensory function	Right	Left
Light touch		
Pinprick		
Vibratory		

Tests	Right	Left
Leg lengths		
Thighs		
Calves		
Muscle spasm		
Convexity scoliosis		
Kyphosis		
Lordosis		

Tests	Right	Left
Babinski		
Clonus		
Laségue		
Flip		
Bowstring		
Cram		
Foot dorsiflexion		
Neck flexion		
Faber		
Hip range of motion		
Femoral stretch		

Point tenderness

Thoracic spine
L1
L2
L3
L4
L5
S1
S2 to S5
Coccyx
Anterior spine

FIG. 13-11, cont'd

Physical Examination—cont'd

Point tenderness—cont'd	Right	Left
Sacroiliac joint		
Sciatic notch		
Greater trochanter		
Ischial tuberosity		
Paraspinous		

Straight leg raising	Right	Left
Supine—leg pain		
Sitting—leg pain		
Contralateral—leg pain		
Sitting—low back pain		
Contralateral—low back pain		

Neck and Upper Extremity Examination

Muscle strength	Right	Left
Trapezius		
Cuff		
Deltoid		
Rhomboid		
Serrant		
Pectoralis		
Biceps		
Triceps		
Forearm supination		
Forearm pronation		
Wrist extension		
Wrist flexion		
Thumb		
Grip		
Intrinsics		

Sensory function

Light touch
Pinprick
Vibratory

PERRLA

Gag
Tongue
Smile
Hearing
Sight
Thyroid
Neck mass
Bruits:
   Carotids
   Subclavicular
   Axillary
Torticollis

Range of motion	Right	Left
Flexion		
Extension		
Left flexion		
Right flexion		
Left rotation		
Right rotation		

FIG. 13-11, cont'd

North American Spine Society Back Pain Questionnaire-Baseline Medical History, Expectations and Outcomes*

1. HOW LONG AGO did your current episode begin?

    1   Less than 2 weeks ago

    2   2 weeks to less than 8 weeks ago

    3   8 weeks to less than 3 months ago

    4   3 months to less than 6 months ago

    5   6 to 12 months ago

    6   More than 12 months ago

2. HOW did your current episode begin?

    0   Suddenly

    1   Gradually

3. Have you had back symptoms before your current episode?

    0   No (IF NO, GO TO QUESTION 6)

    1   Yes, one episode

    2   Yes, two or more episodes

    Answer #4–5 about your PAST back symptoms.

    ---

    4.   Did you receive Worker's Compensation for your PAST back symptoms?

         1   No   0   Yes

    5.   How much work did you miss because of your worst prior episode?

         0   None

         1   1 day to 2 weeks

         2   More than 2 weeks to 4 weeks

         3   More than 4 weeks to 12 weeks

         4   More than 12 weeks to 24 weeks

         5   More than 24 weeks

    ---

6. Have you had previous back surgery?

    0   No (If NO, go to question 9)

    1   Yes: How many surgeries? # _____

FIG. 13-12 North American Spine Society Back Pain Questionnaire—Baseline Medical History, Expectations, and Outcomes. (Courtesy: North American Spine Society, 1993.)

North American Spine Society Back Pain Questionnaire-Baseline Medical History, Expectations and Outcomes—cont'd
Answer #7–8 about your PAST back surgeries.

7. After your most recent surgery, did you return to work?
    0 No
    1 Yes, with limitations
    2 Yes, with no limitations
    3 Never stopped working
    4 Did not work: _____ Homemaker
                      _____ Student
                      _____ Retired
                      _____ Other
8. After your most recent surgery, did you return to full function?
    0 No   1 Yes

There will be several questions about leg and back pain in this questionnaire. When we say LEG, we mean your thigh, calf, ankle, and foot. When we say BACK, we mean your low back and buttocks.

9. Which hurts you more, your legs or back?
    1 Legs hurt much more
    2 Legs hurt somewhat more
    3 Legs and back hurt about the same
    4 Back hurts somewhat more
    5 Back hurts much more

Please answer every question in the box below.

In the PAST WEEK, how often have you suffered:	None of the time	A little of the time	Some of the time	A good bit of the time	Most of the time	All the time
10. low back and/or buttock pain	1	2	3	4	5	6
11. leg pain	1	2	3	4	5	6
12. numbness or tingling in leg and/or foot	1	2	3	4	5	6
13. weakness in leg and/or foot (such as difficulty lifting foot)	1	2	3	4	5	6

Please answer every question in the box below.

In the PAST WEEK, how bothersome have these symptoms been?	Not at all bothersome	Slightly bothersome	Somewhat bothersome	Moderately bothersome	Very bothersome	Extremely bothersome
14. low back and/or buttock pain	1	2	3	4	5	6
15. leg pain	1	2	3	4	5	6
16. numbness/tingling in leg and/or foot	1	2	3	4	5	6
17. weakness in leg and/or foot (such as difficulty lifting foot)	1	2	3	4	5	6

FIG. 13-12, cont'd

North American Spine Society Back Pain Questionnaire-Baseline Medical History, Expectations and Outcomes—cont'd

In the LAST WEEK, please tell us HOW PAIN HAS AFFECTED YOUR ABILITY TO PERFORM the following daily activities.
Mark the ONE statement that best describes your average ability.

18. Getting Dressed (in the LAST WEEK)
    1 I can dress myself without pain.
    2 I can dress myself without increasing pain.
    3 I can dress myself but pain increases.
    4 I can dress myself but with significant pain.
    5 I can dress myself but with very severe pain.
    6 I cannot dress myself.

19. Lifting (in the LAST WEEK)
    1 I can lift heavy objects without pain.
    2 I can lift heavy objects but it is painful.
    3 Pain prevents me from lifting heavy objects off the floor but I can manage if they are on a table.
    4 Pain prevents me from lifting heavy objects but I can manage light to medium objects if they are on a table.
    5 I can lift only light objects.
    6 I cannot lift anything.

20. Walking (in the LAST WEEK)
    1 Pain does not prevent me from walking.
    2 Pain prevents me from walking more than 1 hour.
    3 Pain prevents me from walking more than 30 minutes.
    4 Pain prevents me from walking more than 10 minutes.
    5 I can only walk a few steps at a time.
    6 I am unable to walk.

21. Sitting (in the LAST WEEK)
    1 I can sit in any chair as long as I like.
    2 I can only sit in a special chair for as long as I like.
    3 Pain prevents me from sitting more than 1 hour.
    4 Pain prevents me from sitting more than 30 minutes.
    5 Pain prevents me from sitting more than a few minutes.
    6 Pain prevents me from sitting at all.

22. Standing (in the LAST WEEK)
    1 I can stand as long as I want.
    2 I can stand as long as I want but it gives me pain.
    3 Pain prevents me from standing for more than 1 hour.
    4 Pain prevents me from standing for more than 30 minutes.
    5 Pain prevents me from standing for more than 10 minutes.
    6 Pain prevents me from standing at all.

23. Sleeping (in the LAST WEEK)
    1 I sleep well.
    2 Pain occasionally interrupts my sleep.
    3 Pain interrupts my sleep half of the time.
    4 Pain often interrupts my sleep.
    5 Pain always interrupts my sleep.
    6 I never sleep well.

24. Social and Recreational Life (in the LAST WEEK)
    1 My social and recreational life is unchanged.
    2 My social and recreational life is unchanged but it increases pain.
    3 My social and recreational life is unchanged but it severely increases pain.
    4 Pain has restricted my social and recreational life.

FIG. 13-12, cont'd

North American Spine Society Back Pain Questionnaire-Baseline Medical History, Expectations and Outcomes—cont'd

 5 Pain has severely restricted my social and recreational life.

 6 I have essentially no social and recreational life because of pain.

26. Traveling (in the LAST WEEK)

 1 I can travel anywhere.

 2. I can travel anywhere but it gives me pain.

 3 Pain is bad but I can manage to travel over 2 hours.

 4 Pain restricts me to trips of less than 1 hour.

 5 Pain restricts me to trips of less than 30 minutes.

 6 Pain prevents me from traveling.

26. Sex Life (in the LAST WEEK)

 1 My sex life is unchanged.

 2 My sex life is unchanged but causes some extra pain.

 3 My sex life is nearly unchanged but is very painful.

 4 My sex life is severely restricted by pain.

 5 My sex life is nearly absent because of pain.

 6 Pain prevents any sex life at all.

Please answer every question in the box below.

HOW OFTEN do you need to use the following assistive devices?	Never	Sometimes	About half the time	Often	All the time
27. One or two canes	1	2	3	4	5
28. One or two crutches	1	2	3	4	5
29. Walker	1	2	3	4	5
30. Wheelchair	1	2	3	4	5

31. Which health care providers have you used for your current back condition? (CIRCLE ALL THAT APPLY)

 A Acupuncturist

 B Chiropractor

 C Emergency room

 D General practitioner

 E Immediate care clinic

 F Internist

 G Massage Therapist

 H Neurosurgeon

 I Osteopath

 J Orthopaedic Surgeon

 K Pain Clinic

 L Physical Therapist

 M Rheumatologist

 N Work Hardening Clinic

 O Other: _____

 P None of the above

32. During the LAST WEEK, how often have you taken narcotic medication such as codeine, Demerol, Percodan, or Vicodin for your back and/or leg pain?

 1 3 or more times a day

 2 Once or twice a day

 3 Once every couple of days

 4 Once a week

 5 Not at all

33. During the LAST WEEK, how often have you taken non-narcotic medication such as aspirin, Motrin, or Tylenol for your back and/or leg pain?

 1 3 or more times a day

 2 Once or twice a day

 3 Once every couple of days

 4 Once a week

 5 Not at all

FIG. 13-12, cont'd

13

North American Spine Society Back Pain Questionnaire-Baseline Medical History, Expectations and Outcomes—cont'd

34. Have you used alcoholic beverages (beer, wine, liquor) to relieve your current back or leg pain?

    0 No

    1 Yes, once in a while

    2 Yes, often

35. If you had to spend the rest of your life with your back condition as it is right now, how would you feel about it?

    1 Extremely dissatisfied

    2 Very dissatisfied

    3 Somewhat dissatisfied

    4 Neutral

    5 Somewhat satisfied

    6 Very satisfied

    7 Extremely satisfied

What expectations do you have for your treatment at this office?

As a result of my treatment, I expect	not likely	slightly likely	somewhat likely	very likely	extremely likely
36. Complete pain relief	1	2	3	4	5
37. Moderate pain relief	1	2	3	4	5
38. To be able to do more everyday household or yard activities	1	2	3	4	5
39. To be able to sleep more comfortably	1	2	3	4	5
40. To be able to go back to my usual job	1	2	3	4	5
41. To be able to do more sports, go biking, or go for long walks	1	2	3	4	5

42. What other results do you expect from your treatment? Please describe:

    _____

    _____

    _____

How important are the following treatment outcomes for you?

How important is...	not important	slightly important	somewhat important	very important	extremely important
43. Pain relief	1	2	3	4	5
44. To be able to do more everyday household or yard activities	1	2	3	4	5
45. To be able to sleep more comfortably	1	2	3	4	5
46. To be able to go back to my usual job	1	2	3	4	5
47. To be able to do more sports, go biking, or go for long walks	1	2	3	4	5
48. Other (see your answer to #42 above): _____	1	2	3	4	5

FIG. 13-12, cont'd

North American Spine Society Back Pain Questionnaire-Baseline Medical History, Expectations and Outcomes—cont'd

Following are some questions about your general health.

49. In general would you say your health is:

    1 Excellent

    2 Very Good

    3 Good

    4 Fair

    5 Poor

    6 Terrible

50. Have you ever had any of the following conditions?
    (CIRCLE ALL THAT APPLY)

    A Diabetes

    B Heart Disease

    C Stroke

    D Arthritis other than in your back

    E Asthma or other lung disease

    F Depression

    G High Blood Pressure (hypertension)

    H Colitis

    I Psoriasis

    J None of the above

51. Do you currently smoke cigarettes?

    0 I have never smoked

    1 Yes

    2 No, I quit in the last 6 months

    3 No, I quit more than 6 months ago

52. Has the treatment for your back condition met your expectations so far?

    1 Yes, totally

    2 Yes, almost totally

    3 Yes, quite a bit

    4 More or less

    5 No, not quite

    6 No, far from it

    7 No, not at all

53. Would you have the same treatment again if you had the same condition?

    1 Definitely not

    2 Probably not

    3 Not sure

    4 Probably yes

    5 Definitely yes

54. If you had back pain, how has your back pain been affected by the treatment?

    (CHECK ONLY ONE STATEMENT)

    1 I did not have back pain to start with.

    2 The pain is totally gone.

    3 The pain is much better than before treatment.

    4 The pain is somewhat better than before treatment.

    5 The pain is about the same as before treatment.

    6 The pain is somewhat worse than before treatment.

    7 The pain is much worse than before treatment.

55. If you had leg pain, how has your leg pain been affected by the treatment?

    (CHECK ONLY ONE STATEMENT)

    1 I did not have leg pain to start with.

    2 The pain is totally gone.

    3 The pain is much better than before treatment.

    4 The pain is somewhat better than before treatment.

FIG. 13-12, cont'd

13

North American Spine Society Back Pain Questionnaire-Baseline Medical History, Expectations and Outcomes—cont'd

   5 The pain is about the same as before treatment.

   6 The pain is somewhat worse than before treatment.

   7 The pain is much worse than before treatment.

The following questions are about how you feel and how things have been with you during the last week. For each question, please indicate the one answer that comes closest to the way you have been feeling. Please, CIRCLE ONE ANSWER ON EACH LINE.

How much of the time during the LAST WEEK	All of the time	Most of the time	A good bit of the time	Some of the time	Little of the time	None of the time
56. Have you been a very nervous person?	1	2	3	4	5	6
57. Have you felt so down in the dumps nothing could cheer you up?	1	2	3	4	5	6
58. Have you felt calm and peaceful?	1	2	3	4	5	6
59. Have you felt downhearted and blue?	1	2	3	4	5	6
60. Have you been a happy person?	1	2	3	4	5	6

North American Spine Society Back Pain Questionnaire-Baseline Medical Employment History, and Work Status.*

1.   How many jobs have you had in the last 3 years?

   0 None

   1 1 or 2

   2 3 or more

2.   Which statements describe your current employment situation?   CIRCLE ALL THAT APPLY

   A Currently working

   B On paid leave

   C On unpaid leave

   D Unemployed

   E Homemaker

   F Student

   G Retired (not due to health)

   H Disabled and/or retired because of my back problems

   I   Disabled due to a health problem not related to my back

   J Other, please specify: _____

3.   Are you self-employed?

   0 No   1 Yes

4.   If NOT WORKING now, how long has it been since you stopped?

   1 Less than 1 week ago

   2 1 week to less than 3 months ago

   3 3 months to less than 6 months ago

   4 6 months to less than 12 months ago

   5 1 to 2 years ago

   6 More than 2 years ago

   8 Currently working

   9 Never employed

FIG. 13-12, cont'd

North American Spine Society Back Pain Questionnaire-Baseline Medical Employment History, and Work Status—cont'd

5. What is your primary occupation? If you are not working now, what was your primary occupation? (Please be as specific as possible)

   Occupation: _____

6. Is your current job the same one you had when your current back symptoms started?

   1 Yes, exact same job

   2 Yes, but job was modified or hours reduced because of my back

   3 No, I have changed jobs because of my back symptoms

   4 No, I have changed jobs but for reasons unrelated to my back

   5 Not working now

7. How long have you worked at your current job?

   0 less than 6 months

   1 6 to 12 months

   2 more than 12 months

   3 not working now

Please answer each of the following questions about your current job (or the one you plan to go back to if on leave).
CIRCLE ONE ANSWER ON EACH LINE.

	All of the time	Most of the time	A good bit of the time	Some of the time	Little of the time	None of the time
8. How much sitting does your work involve?	1	2	3	4	5	6
9. How much standing or walking does your work involve?	1	2	3	4	5	6
10. How often do you lift 25 lbs. on the job?	1	2	3	4	5	6
11. How often do you lift 50 lbs. on the job?	1	2	3	4	5	6

Please answer each of the following questions about your current job (or the one you plan to go back to if on leave):

	Extremely	Very much	Quite a bit	Somewhat	A little	Not at all
12. Is your current work physically demanding?	1	2	3	4	5	6
13. Is your work stressful to you?	1	2	3	4	5	6
14. How much do you like your job?	1	2	3	4	5	6
15. How much do you like your co-workers?	1	2	3	4	5	6
16. How much do you like your supervisor?	1	2	3	4	5	6

FIG. 13-12, cont'd

North American Spine Society Back Pain Questionnaire-Baseline Medical Employment History, and Work Status—cont'd

17. Other than your salary, what other sources of income does your household receive?
CIRCLE ALL THAT APPLY:

   A   Another person's salary

   B   State Support

   C   Social Security

   D   Disability

   E   Other (Investments, Retirement Plan, etc.)

   F   No other source of income

18. Are you experiencing financial difficulties because of your back condition?

   0   None at all

   1   Only a little

   2   Some

   3   A lot

Please answer the questions in the box, or check below if none applies.

Are you on or planning to apply for any of the following programs?	Already on it	Applied for it	Planning to apply for it
19. Social Security	1	2	3
20. Disability	1	2	3
21. Workers Compensation	1	2	3
22. Other (please specify): _____	1	2	3

[ ]   Check here if none of the above applies.

23. Do you think the fault for your current back condition is: (CIRCLE ALL THAT APPLY)

   A   Yours?

   B   Your employer's?

   C   A co-worker's?

   D   Another person's?

   E   Nobody's?

24. Have you hired a lawyer because of your back condition?

   0   No, I have not hired a lawyer.

   1   Yes, I have and the case is in litigation.

   2   Yes, I have and the case has been settled.

Thank you for your help. Please take a moment to go over the questionnaire to make sure you have not missed any pages or questions. Then return it to the person who gave it to you or in the envelope provided.

FIG. 13-12, cont'd

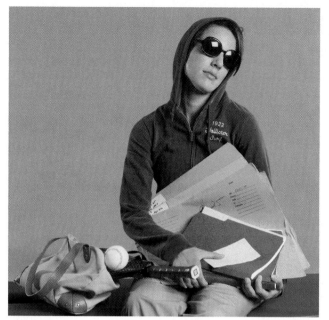

FIG. 13-13 When observing a malingering patient, the examiner may note that the patient (1) often fails to make consistent eye contact and may obscure eye contact with sunglasses, (2) may dress in clothing suitable for activities inappropriate for the injury complaint or disability, (3) may make the record voluminous, with an aggregation of notations and images (plain and advanced) from numerous sources, often containing minimal and disjointed evidence to support the complaint, (4) may be impatient, and (5) may be unwilling to participate in a full or complete examination. Other subtle signs include activities—a sport or other physical activity scheduled immediately after the examination of the disabled lower back—that are inappropriate for the disability.

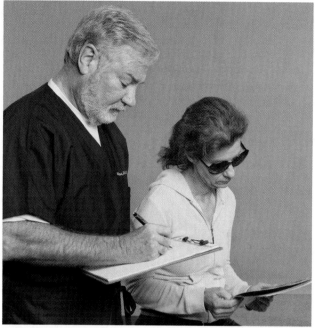

FIG. 13-14 Furthermore, a detailed history from a malingering patient is difficult to acquire and assess. The patient may act disinterested and distant in the history interview, avoiding eye contact and relating odd and exaggerated stories concerning the injurious event.

ORTHOPEDIC GAMUT 13-6

REASONS FOR PSYCHOLOGIC ILLNESS THAT CAUSE THE APPEARANCE OR EXACERBATION OF PAIN

1. Anxiety
2. Psychiatric hallucination
3. Increased tension in the muscles, with associated inadequate circulation and the accumulation of metabolic byproducts (lactic acid)
4. Hysteria with conversion reactions

---

with pain may also develop psychiatric disorders as part of the symptoms associated with the physical illness. Pain associated with neurosis is more common than pain associated with schizophrenia or endogenous depression.

Psychogenic rheumatism is a term used to describe patients who have musculoskeletal psychiatric disorders. An example of psychogenic rheumatism that is associated with back pain is camptocormia, which is a special form of conversion hysteria that occurs mainly in military service personnel and industrial workers. The disease is characterized by the patient's assumption of a posture in which the back is flexed acutely, the arms hang loosely, and the patient's eyes are directed downward. The posture disappears when the patient assumes a recumbent position. The short-form McGill Pain Questionnaire, a pain scale, and pain drawings represent a few of the many methods to document psychogenic rheumatism (Figs. 13-15 to 13-17).

Many of the afflicted individuals are men whose parents have had back disorders. Therapy for the condition involves separation of the individual from the source of stress.

The malingerer exaggerates or fakes a condition or injury. Believing the history the patient relates, even though malingering is suspected, is important.

In many instances, a malingerer can be extremely convincing during the examination. The malingering patient usually complains of sensory loss, paralysis, pain, or a combination of these symptoms. A hysterical patient will claim similar problems. Unlike the hysterical patient, the malingerer consciously attempts to deceive the physician.

Two separate sets of criteria have been developed to document the likelihood of malingering: the Emory Pain Control Center Inconsistency Profile and Ellard's Profile of Inconsistency.

13

ORTHOPEDIC GAMUT 13-7

PSYCHOGENIC RHEUMATISM

Symptoms and signs of psychogenic rheumatism are:

1. Dramatic urgency for an appointment that is not justified by the severity of the disease
2. A list (in writing) of complaints so long and detailed that no fact is left out
3. Multiple test results, including electrocardiogram, electromyelogram, electroencephalogram, barium enema, upper gastrointestinal series, computed tomography scans, myelograms, and magnetic resonance imaging, with no positive findings
4. Patient demands to review the laboratory data first to determine the cause of the symptoms; patient highlights any minor abnormalities
5. Preoccupation with future disability from minor physical changes
6. Persons who accompany the patient may be entirely separated from the patient's condition or intensely supportive; the companion may be highlighting every abnormality, often using the pronoun *we* during the description of tests or treatments
7. Inability of the patient to relax during the examination (Boxes 13-3 and 13-4)
8. Marked theatrical responses to questions concerning pain
9. The patient often holds onto the physician during the examination, as a gesture of seeking support

From Rotes-Querol J: The syndrome of psychogenic rheumatism, *Clin Rheum Dis* 5:797, 1979.

ORTHOPEDIC GAMUT 13-8

COMBINED EMORY AND ELLARD INCONSISTENCY PROFILES

1. Discrepancies become apparent between a patient's complaints of terrible pain and an attitude of calmness and well being.
2. A complete work-up for organic disease by two or more physicians is negative.
3. The patient makes dramatized complaints that are vague or have global implications. "It just hurts," or "I hurt bad." This statement may be further attested by malingering hand signals.
4. The patient exaggerates a trivial pathologic condition (e.g., a mild strain, muscular cramp, contusion) and embellishes it with medical terms learned from previous contact with physicians. "My back spasms paralyze my legs."
5. The patient overemphasizes gait or posture abnormalities that develop suddenly, persist, and cannot be substantiated objectively. For example, the patient complains of a limp that is not confirmed by a specific pattern of wear on old shoes; or the patient reports daily use of a cane or back brace, but these items show little wear.
6. The patient resists evaluation or rehabilitation when the stated goal of therapy is a return to gainful employment.
7. The patient exhibits a lack of motivation to learn new coping skills, despite verbal reports of compliance with treatment. (For instance, the patient will show no increase in back motion despite claims of completing range-of-motion exercise daily.)
8. The patient misses appointments for objective studies that measure function, motion, or vocational capabilities.
9. The patient has an unconventional response to treatment, such as reports of increased symptoms after therapy that follows no anatomic or physiologic pattern. For example, the patient may respond to tranquilizers as if they are stimulants and vice versa.
10. The patient shows resistance to treatment procedures, especially in the presence of intense complaints of pain.
11. Psychologic or emotional disturbances are absent (Box 13-5).
12. Psychologic tests are inconsistent and without clinical presentations. For example, the Minnesota Multiphasic Personality Index profile indicates a psychotic disorder, but no clinical signs of psychosis are present (Box 13-6).
13. Discrepancies arise between reports by the patient and spouse or other close relatives.
14. Personal and occupational history appears unstable.
15. The patient's personal history reflects a character disorder that might include drug or alcohol abuse, criminal or compulsive behavior, erratic personal relationships, and violence.

From Evans RC: Malingering/symptoms exaggeration. In Sweere JJ, editor: *Chiropractic family practice*, Gaithersburg, Md, 1992, Aspen.

SHORT-FORM McGILL PAIN QUESTIONNAIRE

Please tick which of these words describes your pain. Put the tick in the box which gives the intensity of that particular quality of your pain.

	None	Mild	Moderate	Severe
Throbbing	0) _____	1) _____	2) _____	3) _____
Shooting	0) _____	1) _____	2) _____	3) _____
Stabbing	0) _____	1) _____	2) _____	3) _____
Sharp	0) _____	1) _____	2) _____	3) _____
Cramping	0) _____	1) _____	2) _____	3) _____
Gnawing	0) _____	1) _____	2) _____	3) _____
Hot-burning	0) _____	1) _____	2) _____	3) _____
Aching	0) _____	1) _____	2) _____	3) _____
Heavy	0) _____	1) _____	2) _____	3) _____
Tender	0) _____	1) _____	2) _____	3) _____
Splitting	0) _____	1) _____	2) _____	3) _____
Tiring-exhausting	0) _____	1) _____	2) _____	3) _____
Sickening	0) _____	1) _____	2) _____	3) _____
Fearful	0) _____	1) _____	2) _____	3) _____
Punishing-cruel	0) _____	1) _____	2) _____	3) _____

Please put a mark on the scale to show how bad your   usual pain has been these days.

```
No                                                          Worst
pain   _____            possible
                                                            pain
```

How bad is your pain now?

0	No pain	_____
1	Mild	_____
2	Discomforting	_____
3	Distressing	_____
4	Horrible	_____
5	Excruciating	_____

FIG. 13-15 The Short-Form McGill Pain Questionnaire. *(From Melzack R: The short-form McGill Pain Questionnaire,* Pain *30:191, 1987.)*

13

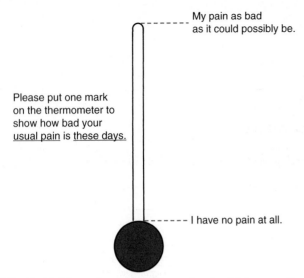

FIG. 13-16 The pain scale. The scale should be exactly 100 mm long, and the level marked by the patient is scored as a percentage. *(From Pope MH et al: Occupational low back pain assessment, treatment and prevention, St Louis, 1991, Mosby.)*

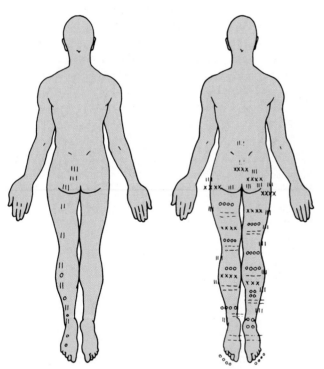

FIG. 13-17 The pain drawing provides information about the physical and emotional aspects of the patient's pain. *(From Pope MH et al: Occupational low back pain assessment, treatment and prevention, St Louis, 1991, Mosby.)*

BOX 13-3

CLINICAL SYMPTOMS OF ANXIETY

Motor Tension
- Trembling, twitching, or feeling shaky
- Muscle tension, aches, or soreness
- Restlessness
- Easy fatigability

Autonomic Hyperactivity
- Shortness of breath or smothering sensation
- Palpitations or accelerated heart rate
- Sweating or cold clammy hands
- Dry mouth
- Dizziness or light-headedness
- Nausea, diarrhea, or other abdominal distress
- Flushes (hot flashes) or chills
- Frequent urination
- Trouble swallowing or lump in throat

Vigilance and Scanning
- Feeling keyed up or on edge
- Exaggerated startle response
- Difficulty concentrating or *mind going blank* because of anxiety
- Trouble falling or staying asleep
- Irritability

From White AH, Schofferman JA: *Spine care,* vol 1-2, St Louis, 1995, Mosby.

BOX 13-4

DSM-III-R* CRITERION FOR ANXIETY

300.02 Generalized anxiety disorder—unrealistic or excessive anxiety and worry more days than not.
Other anxiety disorders
Panic disorder
300.21 with agoraphobia or
300.01 without agoraphobia
300.22 Agoraphobia without history of panic disorder
300.23 Social phobia
300.29 Obsessive-compulsive disorder
300.89 Posttraumatic stress disorder
300.00 Anxiety disorder not otherwise specified

Diagnostic and Statistical Manual of Mental Disorders, third edition, revised.
From White AH, Schofferman JA: *Spine care,* vol 1-2, St Louis, 1995, Mosby.

Special Hand Signals by the Patient

Chronic pain is revealed to be widespread by community epidemiologic studies. Nonspecific chronic low back pain is a common variant of this problem and presents both physician and patient with difficulties in explanation and treatment because of the frequently poor *fit* between expressed symptoms (and consequent perceived disability) and observable spinal disease. Indeed, one authority has noted that approximately 80% of such cases resist definitive diagnosis. For this reason, chronic low back pain is frequently characterized as a product of somatization that is as a problem of mind rather than of biomechanical dysfunction. This cir-

CLINICAL PEARL

In distinguishing psychogenic rheumatism from primary fibromyalgia, the patients with primary fibromyalgia are usually women, 25 to 40 years of age, who complain of diffuse musculoskeletal aches, pains or stiffness associated with tiredness, anxiety, poor sleep, headaches, irritable bowel syndrome, subjective swelling in the articular and peri-articular areas, and numbness. Physical examination reveals the presence of multiple tender points at specific sites and absence of joint swelling. Symptoms are influenced by weather and activities, as well as by time of day (worse in the morning and the evening). In contrast, symptoms of patients with psychogenic rheumatism have little fluctuation, if any, and are modulated by emotional rather than physical factors. In psychogenic rheumatism, diffuse tenderness is felt rather than tender points at specific sites.

BOX 13-5

MOOD DISORDERS—DSM-III-R* CLASSIFICATIONS

Bipolar Disorders
296.6x Mixed—both manic and depressed features
296.4x Manic
296.5x Depressed
301.13 Cyclothymia
296.70 Bipolar disorder not otherwise specified

Depressive Disorders—Major Depression
296.6x Single episode
296.3x Recurrent
300.40 Dysthymia

Diagnostic and Statistical Manual of Mental Disorders, ed 3, revised. Fifth digit (x) allows coding of current state of disorder: 1 = mild; 2 = moderate; 3 = severe, without psychotic features; 4 = with psychotic features; 5 = in partial remission; 6 = in full remission; 0 = unspecified. From White AH, Schofferman JA: *Spine care,* vol 1-2, St Louis, 1995, Mosby.

---

cumstance leads to conflicts and resentments in the consulting room, when clinicians and patients contest the *reality* of expressed symptoms—the former, regarding it as a function of psychosocial distress, and the latter, experiencing symptoms and disability that are understood as a product of injury or degeneration. This problem has a long history, but it has become increasingly pressing, given that the prevalence of chronic low back pain appears to have grown and given that it has become a disproportionate drain on the resources of health care systems. Although uncertainty about the *real* nature of this pain may be dispiriting for the clinician, it also poses important difficulties for the patient. Without evidence of an organic pathologic condition, it demands that the patient effects an account of pain that is convincing to the *skeptical* clinician (May, Rose, Johnstone, 2000).

How a patient uses the hands to describe the area of pain is useful in determining the validity of the complaints. At first, malingering patients take care to avoid touching the area they claim experiences pain. Because the complaint is a sham, touching of the part abets the lie. The examiner often inadvertently aids this process by physically touching the area of complaint before the patient has. The patient now only has to agree with the frustrated examiner concerning the exact location of the pain (Fig. 13-18).

The psychogenic rheumatic patient uses the whole hand to *paint* the area of involvement with pain. Because this type of patient perceives the lesion abnormally, the distribution is painted to cover a whole body part. This pain crosses more than one dermatome boundary, and this patient's discomfort is real. The discomfort may have origin in an organic lesion, but because of learned responses or fear, the patient rubs the whole part with the hand to indicate its extent. Careful questioning and guidance will help this patient better define the most focal trigger areas (Fig. 13-19).

Patients with organic, pain-producing lesions are concerned that the source of the pain might be missed. When directed to point to the pain, this type of patient will touch the part with one or two fingers, which is representative of a more focal appreciation of the discomfort. In severe expression of the symptoms, this patient also may place the examiner's hand on the exact location of the pain. These patients do not want to risk having the source missed and not treated (Fig. 13-20).

PAIN QUALIFICATION AND QUANTIFICATION

Overview

The description of individuals with congenital insensitivity and indifference to pain provided one of the bases for Melzack and Casey's (1968) seminal distinction between the sensory and affective components of pain. In addition, the observation that these people often die in childhood because they fail to notice injuries and illnesses has been viewed as compelling evidence that the ability to perceive pain has great survival value. That is, the sensation of pain protects humans (and other species) from the tissue-damaging effects of dangerous stimuli and appears to be critical for survival of the organism (Nagasako, Oaklander, Dworkin, 2003).

13

BOX 13-6

DESCRIPTION OF MMPI-2*

L, F, and K are validity scales.

L is called the *lie scale* and measures willingness to admit minor social faults. It gives information about social conformity, self-image and self-insight, and denial.

F refers to infrequency and consists of items that are socially unacceptable or have disturbing content. Persons scoring on the low end of this scale are usually conventional and unassuming. Those with elevations are admitting to severe emotional distress or psychopathologic condition or both. Very high scores suggest an invalid profile.

K refers to correction, and the items measure personal resources required to cope with life. Low scores suggest exaggeration of problems or severe emotional distress. Higher scores can result when patients are very confident and in charge or when they are being defensive in their efforts to present themselves as adequate and in control when in fact their lives are in disarray.

Scales 1 through 10 are the basic clinical scales of the MMPI-2. The information is presented using T scores. A T score of 50 is average; T scores over 65 are in the abnormal range.

Scale 1 is also known as the *Hypochondriasis (HS) scale*. This scale consists of items that concern bodily functioning. Many of the items are vague in their content. Persons scoring low on this scale do not have or are denying that they have any physical complaints. Those whose scores are elevated have many physical complaints and concerns. If scores are above 65, physical complaints are often the major focus of the person's life.

Scale 2 is known as the *Depression (D) scale*. It consists of items that measure subjective depression, psychomotor slowing and immobilization, physical complaints, mental dullness, and brooding. High scores indicate the presence of depression, and low scores indicate persons whose affective functioning is within normal limits.

Scale 3 is referred to as *Hysteria (Hy)*. It consists of items that indicate whether the individual tends to avoid emotional and social unpleasantness. Those that do may then experience their emotions and stress as somatic complaints. High scorers will often deny psychologic problems and look for concrete solutions to their problems.

Scale 4 is known as *Psychopathic Deviate (PD)*. Eight items refer to authority conflicts, and the rest of the items deal with family conflicts, denial of social and dependency needs, social alienation, and self-integration. High scorers are often angry, impulsive, in conflict with authority figures in their lives, and are feeling isolated and despondent. High scorers who are not psy-

chopathic are often undergoing stressful transitions in their lives.

Scale 5 is known as *Masculinity-Femininity (MF)*. Scores on this reflect traditional versus nontraditional masculine or feminine interests and beliefs, conflicts about sexuality, and interests in aesthetics. Low scores for women suggest feelings of helplessness and dependency, whereas low scores for men suggest an action-oriented *macho* approach to life. High-scoring men often hold interests in activities usually considered as feminine and may be experiencing insecurity, helplessness, and conflicts of sexuality. High-scoring women report interest in traditional male patterns and are often seen as unfriendly, dominating, and aggressive.

Scale 6 is known as *Paranoia (Pa)*. In addition to paranoia and externalization of blame, this scale contains items related to hypersensitivity, subjectivity, naiveté, righteousness, and denial of hostility and distrust. Very high scorers are outright paranoid and may have a thought disorder, whereas low scorers may be insensitive to others and unaware of others' motives. They may also be denying the presence of paranoid thoughts.

Scale 7 is known as *Psychasthenia (Pt)*. Items center around the presence of worries, brooding, and rumination. High scorers are seen as anxious and insecure, and may be indecisive. If scores are very high, the individual may be compulsive and agitated with feelings of guilt and fear disrupting everyday functioning.

Scale 8 is known as *Schizophrenia (Sc)*. High scorers are having difficulty with their thinking and feelings. They often feel out of control and unable to take positive action in their own behalf. Extremely high scores are suggestive of severe situational stress. More moderate elevations are seen in those with thought disorders, with difficulties in logic concentration and judgment common.

Scale 9 is known as *Hypomania (Ma)*. This scale provides information about motivation, physical and emotional activity levels, confidence in social situations, and feelings of self-importance. High scorers are restless, agitated, emotionally labile and may have racing thoughts. They may also have difficulty delaying gratification and can be impulsive. Manic features appear as scores elevate.

Scale 10 is known as *Social Introversion (SI)*. This scale provides information about social interests, interpersonal skills, self-consciousness, and feelings of alienation from self or others. High scorers are often depressed. They withdraw from social interactions and feel shy and insecure. Low scorers are usually socially extroverted and outgoing.

MMPI-2, Minnesota Multiphasic Personality Inventory-2.
From White AH, Schofferman JA: *Spine care,* vol 1-2, St Louis, 1995, Mosby.

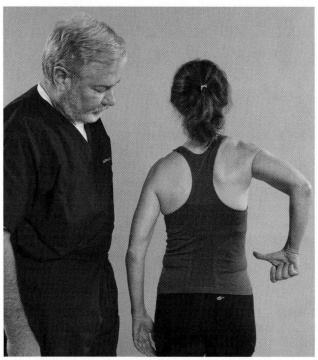

FIG. 13-18 At first in the physical examination, the malingering patient takes care to avoid touching the area of concern. The complaint is a sham; thus, the patient allows the examiner to touch the part or area of supposed complaint first. Then the patient simply agrees with the suggested origin of pain.

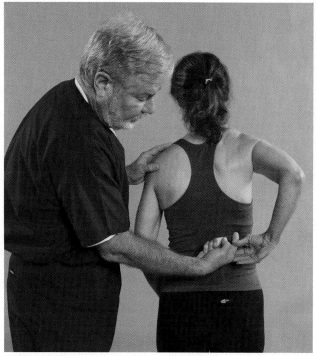

FIG. 13-20 Patients experiencing organic pain for the first time are concerned that the lesion may be missed. This patient touches the part or tissue, precisely locating it with one or two fingers. The patient may also hold the examiner's finger on the spot of worst complaint.

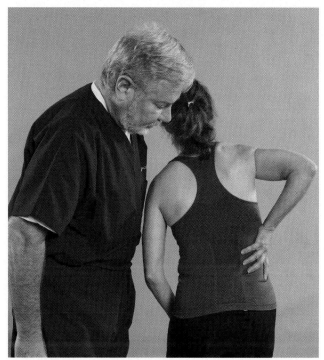

FIG. 13-19 The hysterical patient, or the patient with psychogenic rheumatism, *paints* the area of complaint with the whole hand. The discomfort is real, but the borders of the complaint exceed the known anatomic distributions. Thorough investigation will define the focal triggers.

Pain disrupts the life of the individual in terms of relationships with others, self-esteem, ability to complete tasks of daily living and to work, and ability to function as a member of the community. Disability is strongly correlated with attitude to illness; these considerations underlie the importance of assessing patients' beliefs regarding the nature and prognosis of their pain (Box 13-7).

Low back pain (LBP) is one of the least understood painful conditions. Such is the case despite evidence that it is among the most frequently occurring conditions, affecting over 80% of people at some point in their lifetime. LBP is believed to be the most frequent cause of morbidity, disability, and perceived threat to health in middle-age men and women. The cost of LBP, however, is not the same for all individuals. Marked variability exists in how individuals respond to the condition. A significant number of individuals experience much larger personal costs in terms of psychologic distress and disability and who also inflict substantial cost to industry (e.g., in compensation, work days lost) and the medical system as a result of a slower rate of recovery, if any at all. Preliminary research suggests anxiety might be important in understanding the variability in adjustment to LBP. An association between anxiety and chronic pain has been recognized for years. Findings in this area have revealed that persons with chronic pain are more anxious and fearful and that the incidence of anxiety disorders is elevated in patients with chronic pain relative to the general population.

13

BOX 13-7

ACTIVITIES OF DAILY LIVING AND VISUAL ANALOG QUESTIONNAIRE

A. How often is it painful for you to:

	Never	Sometimes	Most of the Time	Always
Dress yourself?	_____	_____	_____	_____
Get in and out of bed?	_____	_____	_____	_____
Lift a cup or glass to your lips?	_____	_____	_____	_____
Walk outdoors on flat ground?	_____	_____	_____	_____
Wash and dry your entire body?	_____	_____	_____	_____
Bend down to pick up clothing from the floor?	_____	_____	_____	_____
Turn faucets on or off?	_____	_____	_____	_____
Get in and out of a car?	_____	_____	_____	_____

B. How much pain have you had in the past week (mark the scale):

No pain _____ **Pain as bad as it could be**
    0   100

From Callahan LF et al: Quantitative pain assessment for routine care of rheumatoid arthritis patients, using a pain scale on activities of daily living and a visual analog pain scale, *Arthritis Rheum* 30:630, 1987.

The majority of studies in this area have shown that higher levels of anxiety are associated with increased pain reports and prolonged pain experiences (Hadjistavropoulos, LaChapelle, 2000).

Pain is an image that becomes perfected in the sensorium of the cerebral cortex. This pain image is created by stimuli that have passed through a chain of lower centers in which they are modified and refined. Even at the cortical level, the pain image is subject to changes by associated constitutional and emotional factors. Stimuli coming from the same source and passing through the same modifications by the lower centers will produce, in one patient, a pain image of bright and burning colors and, in another, a faded out, unimpressive design. The patient's constitution is mirrored in this difference (Fig. 13-21).

In general, the closer to the axis of the body, the more scant is the distribution of sensory end organs in the tissues and the less precise the allocation of the pain source. Some exceptions exist. Some deep-lying structures are intensely sensitive because of their rich endowment with pain-conducting terminal fibers, in contrast to other structures occupying the same anatomic plane. Sensory nerves are obvious exceptions to the rule because they are the conductors of pain.

The differential diagnosis and evaluation of pain depend on a description of the intensity of the unpleasant sensation, a comparison by the patient to other known sensations, and an attempted designation of the severity of the pain based on a number system.

The spectrum of pain awareness and severity varies from a minimal pain response that is tolerated and easily overlooked to an unbearable sensation that interferes with the individual's productive activities.

ORTHOPEDIC GAMUT 13-9

RELAY STATIONS

Three main relay stations for sensory stimuli from the periphery to the sensory cortex include:
1. The peripheral sensory nervous system, with its cell station in the spinal ganglia
2. The pathways and centers in the spinal cord and medulla
3. The sensory centers of the diencephalon, especially the thalamus

---

Patients with chronic nonmalignant pain often have medical symptoms, including loss of physical function that cannot be explained by organic disease. Waddell (1987) and colleagues have argued that disease alone cannot account for the prevalence of disability or the frequency of health care utilization among many of these patients. One of the more compelling explanations for nonorganic symptom reporting in this population is the somatization hypothesis. Somatization occurs when affective or other benign impulses associated with psychologic distress or with normal physiologic function are misconstrued as symptoms of physical disease. For many people, the process of somatization is adaptive rather than pathologic and can be viewed as a normative response to psychologic stress (Ciccone, Just, Bandilla, 1996).

Physiologic variations of the pain threshold can be found from one person to another. An inherent, definable differ-

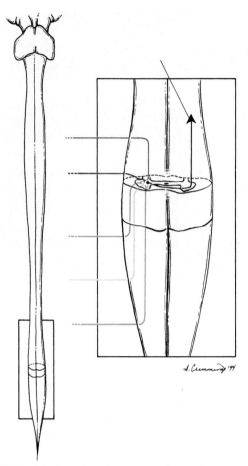

FIG. 13-21 Nociception from a variety of sources may influence the same pool of tract neurons. *(From Cramer CD, Darby SA: Basic and clinical anatomy of the spine, spinal cord, and ANS, St Louis, 1995, Mosby.)*

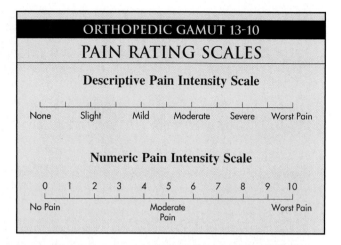

ORTHOPEDIC GAMUT 13-10

PAIN RATING SCALES

Descriptive Pain Intensity Scale

None | Slight | Mild | Moderate | Severe | Worst Pain

Numeric Pain Intensity Scale

0 1 2 3 4 5 6 7 8 9 10

No Pain .... Moderate Pain .... Worst Pain

ence in the pain level exists that varies from congenital insensitivity to pain to a state of hypersensitivity to almost any external stimulus.

Changes in pain produced by psychologic factors (e.g., placebo analgesia) are thought to result from the activity of specific cortical regions. However, subcortical nuclei, including the periaqueductal gray and the rostroventral medulla, also show selective activation when subjects expect pain relief. These brainstem regions send inhibitory projections to the spine and produce diffuse analgesic responses. Regrettably, the precise contribution of spinal mechanisms in predicting the strength of placebo analgesia is unknown (Goffaux et al, 2007).

Congenital insensitivity to pain is recognized as a true syndrome in which the person does not respond to epicritic stimuli, or even fractures of the extremities, by anything other than a descriptive comment concerning the injury (Fig. 13-22). These patients do not complain of pain.

Charcot originally described the progressive, destructive process that bears his name in the setting of tabes dorsalis. This process can occur in any joint of the body; however, it

is less common in the spine. Although seen in complex spine practices secondary to quadriplegia and paraplegia, treatment of Charcot spine is lacking in the spine literature. Indeed, no discussion has been found of congenital insensitivity to pain in the adult spine patient. Any disease process that affects the nervous system can cause the characteristic changes of neuropathic arthropathy. Some of the more common causes reported for spinal arthropathy are tertiary syphilis and post–spinal cord injury. A much less common cause of neuropathic arthropathy is congenital insensitivity to pain (Cassidy, Shaffer, in press).

A high threshold of pain is recognized in many individuals who tolerate painful stimuli—such as heat, cold, sharp prick, or heavy pressure—and who recognize the abnormal sensation and the kind of sensation but are able to accept the stimulus with minimal response.

Experience with the many scales that exist to document pain intensity in children is limited in the context of an emergency department. The visual analog scale is commonly used as a mechanical slide rule or on paper for the quantification of pain and usually consists of a 100-mm scale from 0 to 100. It has been validated in children ages 5 to 6 years and older for acute, recurrent, and chronic pain. The visual analog scale is considered to have excellent reliability, validity, and responsiveness. The standardized color analog scale uses a mechanical slide rule and provides gradations of pain in color (usually from white to red to black) and sometimes width (narrow to wide). It has been validated in children ages 4 to 5 years and older for acute, recurrent, and chronic pain, as well as in a pediatric emergency department. The color analog scale is also considered to have excellent reliability and validity and adequate responsiveness. The Wong-Baker FACES Pain Rating Scale is a 6-point *faces* scale ranging from a smiley to a crying child face; the child points to the level of pain. It has been validated in children ages 3 to 6 years and older for acute pain and is considered to have adequate reliability and validity but poor responsiveness. Finally, the verbal numeric scale is a verbal scale that asks

13

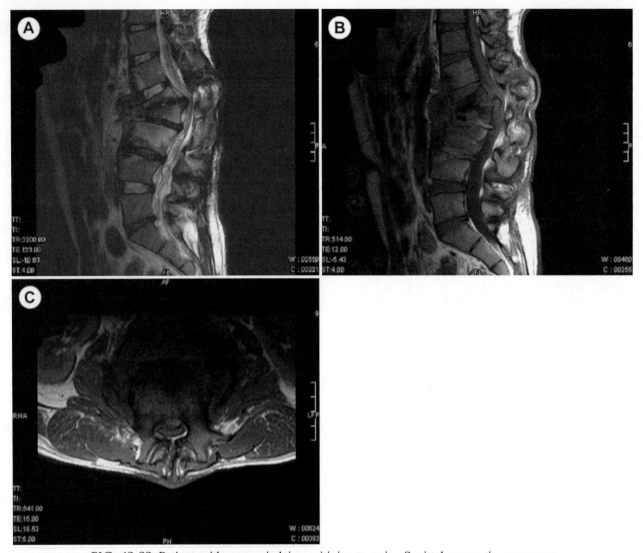

FIG. 13-22 Patient with congenital insensitivity to pain. Sagittal magnetic resonance image showing focal kyphosis at L1–L2. Compression of the thecal sac is significant. The patient was myelopathic because of severe spinal cord compression from postinfectious kyphosis. (Adapted from Cassidy RC, Shaffer WO: Charcot arthropathy because of congenital insensitivity to pain in an adult, *Spine J* 8(4):691-695, 2008.)

the child to grade his or her pain from 0 to 10, representing no pain to the worst pain (Bailey et al, 2007).

A temporary, limited awareness of pain occurs immediately after certain severe injuries, such as a tear of major ligaments around the knee during a football game or a severe inversion injury to the ankle resulting in massive ligamentous tear. The individual experiences sudden, exquisite pain at the time of the injury and may become hypotensive, nauseated, and faint. During the recovery phase, the injured part may be manipulated with little or no discomfort in certain instances. However, within several minutes after injury, the pain pattern associated with periosteal injury, distended synovium and capsule, and pressure from hematoma becomes severe.

An average reaction to pain stimuli is the one that most individuals have to a sudden sharp point, to excessive heat, or to a severe rotary injury to a joint. The individual with an average pain tolerance will describe pain in the shoulder as dull and aching but compatible with moderate limitation of the activities of daily living. If the pain is more severe, the condition will be described as sharp, lancinating, and intermittently severe. The circadian cycle affects the intensity of the pain. Complaints of pain are usually greater at night and may increase as barometric pressure increases. External modalities—excessive heat or cold or an unusual degree of compression or forcible rotation—cause pain to increase.

The individual's personality affects the average reaction to pain. Those with hysterical personalities or with a tendency for hypochondriasis or those who are anxious and depressed respond with more frequent and intense complaints concerning pain, and they overreact to the severity

CLINICAL PEARL (ASSESSMENT OF PAIN)

Feigning or pretense of nonexistent symptoms by word, gesture, action, or behavior is simulation (*positive malingering*) or dissimulation (*negative malingering*). The deliberate and designed feigning of disease or disability or the intentional concealment of disease, if it exists, is *pure malingering*. The magnification or intensification of symptoms that already exist is partial malingering or exaggeration. Ascribing morbid phenomena or symptoms to a definite cause, although the cause may be recognized or ascertained to have no relationship to the symptoms, is false imputation. The six areas of psychologic forensic practice are (1) mental state at the offense, (2) risk for violence, (3) risk for sexual violence, (4) competency to stand trial, (5) competency to waive *Miranda* rights, and (6) *malingering*.

of the stimulus. Sleep deprivation and an unnaturally high anxiety level affect pain. Individuals with a labile personality who have acute pain may overreact to painful stimulus. The same individuals may become dependent and passive and accept chronic pain, although they often complain about the effect of the pain on their personality. For example, they state that the pain lessens their sex drive and performance and alters their disposition. The emotional aspects of pain cannot be separated from the physical aspects. A severe toothache that interferes with sleeping, eating, and working is represented by a much higher degree of pain and responds less readily to medications and external applications than does the acute form of pain that is present for only a short period and does not affect rest and nutrition.

> Measurements of reported pain intensity are of great importance in clinical practice and are often used to determine the need and dosage of analgesics. Unidimensional scales are often used to assess pain intensity, for example, numerical rating scales and visual analogue scales anchored by pain descriptors at each extreme (e.g., from *no pain* to *pain as bad as it could be*). However, overwhelming experimental and clinical evidence has been found that pain has at least two dimensions, a sensory and an affective one. Thus unidimensional pain intensity scales might be inadequate because there is no way to know which dimension or dimensions of pain the patient is rating and how he or she is *weighting* the different dimensions to arrive at a unidimensional rating result. The *multidimensional affect and pain survey* (MAPS) questionnaire consists of three scales (super clusters) measuring somatosensory pain sensations and negative and positive emotions related to the pain experience (Huber et al, 2007).

A patient who actually is in pain demonstrates a definite pallor or change in the facial features. Pain often will produce positive evidence, through involuntary muscle spasm and contractures, leading to postural attitudes for relief. The patient who is in genuine pain will perspire freely and flinch consistently. In addition, the pulse will increase suddenly, the blood pressure may rise, and the pupils will dilate. In a malingerer, the pulse does not change, the pupils do not dilate abnormally, and the complaints of pain will usually be greater than the clinical findings can support.

Anesthesia denotes a state in which a patient gives no demonstrable recognition of eternal stimuli except for stimuli

ORTHOPEDIC GAMUT 13-11

CLINICAL FEATURES OF BURNING MOUTH SYNDROME*

Pain
Descriptors: burning
Intensity: variable, weak to intense
Pattern: continuous, not paroxysmal
Localization:
- Independent of a nervous pathway
- Often bilateral and symmetrical

Paroxysmal: not
Pain during sleep: infrequent
Associated signs and symptoms:
Dysgeusia
Xerostomia
Thirst
Sensory:
Chemosensory anomalies
Psychologic changes

*Adapted from Patton LL et al: Management of burning mouth syndrome: systematic review and management recommendations, *Oral Surg Oral Med Oral Pathol Oral Radiol Endod* 103(suppl 1):S39.e1-S39.e13, 2007.

that involve movement of the part with extreme pressure that causes tendon or bone stimulation.

Hypesthesia (hypoesthesia) is the diminution of the ability to recognize cutaneous stimulation caused by pressure made with a sharp point or a dull object. This description usually designates alteration of a dermatome.

Dysesthesia is an uncomfortable, unpleasant sensation that results from stimulation of a cutaneous region caused or affected by peripheral nerve trauma or regeneration. Stimulation of one side of a digit may actually be felt in an adjacent digit.

> Primary burning mouth syndrome (BMS) is a chronic, idiopathic intraoral mucosal pain condition that is not accompanied by clinical lesions or systemic disease. Some uncertainty exists whether this condition should be labeled as a disease, a disorder, or a syndrome, but data are insuf-

13

ficient to justify any change in taxonomy at present. BMS occurs most often among women and is often accompanied by xerostomia and taste disturbances. More recently, a neuropathologic basis has been proposed so that BMS may be regarded as an *oral dysesthesia* or painful neuropathy (Patton et al, 2007).

Paresthesia is painful tingling, aching, or burning along the course of a peripheral nerve that results from percussion of the involved nerve or stimulation of the skin in the autonomous zone of the involved nerve.

Hyperesthesia is the unpleasant feeling of excessive sensation that results from cutaneous stimulation. When a finger or toe is affected, hair follicles in the geographic dermatome are excessively sensitive to touch, as are the skin and cuticle of that digit.

Cold intolerance is the dull, deep, aching sensation in a segment of the extremity that occurs as the environmental temperature is lowered. The more rapidly the temperature drops, the greater the pain will be. The pain distribution is not well localized and is not relieved immediately by warming the part. The pain associated with cold intolerance may be minimal if the temperature is dropped slowly but may be severe if warm-up is accomplished too rapidly.

Burning, searing, cutting, and *hot* are terms commonly used by individuals with peripheral dysfunction lesions that result from complete or partial nerve trauma.

Determining the most relevant factors, whether biologic or psychologic, should be incorporated into a prospective assessment of each patient. The goal is the identification of individuals who will and will not benefit from medical and surgical management of pain.

A multitude of procedures have been used to evaluate the outcome of therapeutic interventions in LBP. They range from the single overall rating scale traditionally used to

---

ORTHOPEDIC GAMUT 13-12

CATEGORIES OF PAIN

1. Pure nerve pain
2. Pain associated with nerve and vascular insufficiency
3. Pain related to numerous local alterations, such as inadequate skin coverage, fibrosis, bone pressure, tendon irritation, and collagen fibrosis

---

assess surgical outcome (excellent, good, fair, poor) to the more complex, multiitem, multidimensional questionnaires most commonly used in psychosocial studies. Some instruments evaluate treatments in terms of their effects on pain severity; others assess treatments in terms of their effects on functional status, return to work, symptoms other than pain, psychologic status, health care utilization, or some combination of these variables. None of the studies cover all the constructs that are now considered relevant in evaluating treatments for LBP. As a result, outcome studies often require use of multiple questionnaires to evaluate treatment outcomes adequately. Disease-specific questionnaires are generally considered superior to their generic counterparts for clinical applications. Generic questionnaires are more appropriate when comparing different disease conditions or when evaluating types of care across disease categories. No single questionnaire is available that was specifically designed to measure clinical outcomes after site-specific surgical therapy in patients with LBP as the presenting complaint (BenDebba, diZerega, Long, 2007).

ORTHOPEDIC GAMUT 13-13

OSWESTRY-TYPE PAIN-DISABILITY QUESTIONNAIRE*

This questionnaire has been designed to give the examiner information about pain and how it affects your ability to manage in everyday life. Please circle, in each section, only one statement that most closely applies to you.

Section 1: Pain Intensity

1. I can tolerate the pain I have without having to use painkillers.
2. The pain is bad, but I manage without taking painkillers.
3. Painkillers give complete relief from pain.
4. Painkillers give moderate relief from pain.
5. Painkillers give very little relief from pain.
6. Painkillers have no affect on the pain, and I do not use them.

Section 2: Personal Care (e.g., Washing, Dressing)

1. I can look after myself normally, without causing extra pain.
2. I can look after myself normally, but it causes extra pain.
3. Looking after myself is painful, and I am slow and careful.
4. I need some help, but I manage most of my personal care.
5. I need help every day in most aspects of self-care.
6. I do not get dressed. I wash with difficulty and stay in bed.

Section 3: Lifting

1. I can lift heavy weights without increased pain.
2. I can lift heavy weights, but it gives added pain.
3. Pain prevents me from lifting heavy weights off the floor, but I can manage if they are conveniently positioned, such as on a table.
4. Pain prevents me from lifting heavy weights, but I can manage light to medium weights if they are conveniently positioned.
5. I can lift only very light weights.
6. I cannot lift or carry anything at all.

Section 4: Walking

1. Pain does not prevent me from walking any distance.
2. Pain prevents me from walking more than 1 mile.
3. Pain prevents me from walking more than 1/2 mile.
4. Pain prevents me from walking more than 1/4 mile.
5. I can walk only using a cane or crutches.
6. I am in bed most of the time and have to crawl to the toilet.

Section 5: Sitting

1. I can sit in any chair as long as I like.
2. I can sit only in my favorite chair as long as I like.
3. Pain prevents me from sitting more than 1 hour.
4. Pain prevents me from sitting for more than 30 minutes.
5. Pain prevents me from sitting more than 10 minutes.
6. Pain prevents me from sitting at all.

Section 6: Standing

1. I can stand as long as I want without added pain.
2. I can stand as long as I want, but it gives me added pain.
3. Pain prevents me from standing for more than 1 hour.
4. Pain prevents me from standing for more than 30 minutes.
5. Pain prevents me from standing for more than 10 minutes.
6. Pain prevents me from standing at all.

Section 7: Sleeping

1. Pain does not prevent me from sleeping well.
2. I can sleep well only by using sleeping tablets.
3. Even when I take sleeping tablets, I have less than 6 hours of sleep.
4. Even when I take sleeping tablets, I have less than 4 hours of sleep.
5. Even when I take sleeping tablets, I have less than 2 hours of sleep.
6. Pain prevents me from sleeping at all.

Section 8: Sexual Activity

1. My sexual activity is normal and causes no extra pain.
2. My sexual activity is normal but causes some extra pain.
3. My sexual activity is nearly normal but is very painful.
4. My sexual activity is severely restricted by pain.
5. My sexual activity is nearly absent because of pain.
6. Pain prevents any sexual activity at all.

Section 9: Social Life

1. My social life is normal and gives me no extra pain.
2. My social life is normal but increases the degree of pain.
3. Pain has no significant effect on my social life other than limiting my more energetic interests, such as dancing.
4. Pain restricts my social life, and I do not go out often.
5. Pain has restricted my social life to my home.
6. I have no social life because of pain.

continued

13

ORTHOPEDIC GAMUT 13-13—CONT'D

OSWESTRY-TYPE PAIN-DISABILITY QUESTIONNAIRE*

Section 10: Traveling
1. I can travel anywhere without added pain.
2. I can travel anywhere, but it gives me added pain.
3. Pain is bad, but I manage journeys of more than 2 hours.
4. Pain restricts me to a journey of less than 1 hour.
5. Pain restricts me to short, necessary journeys that take no longer than 30 minutes.
6. Pain prevents me from traveling, except to the physician or hospital.

Scoring
Each item is given a point value ranging from 0 to 5, from top to bottom, for a potential total score of 0 to 50. The score is doubled for a total percentage score. If an item is not answered or the patient makes up an answer, it is dropped from the total potential score, and the total percentage is calculated using the remaining answers. The percentages are interpreted as follows: 0% to 20% indicates minimal disability in the activities of daily living (ADL), 20% to 40% represents moderate ADL disability, 40% to 60% is severe ADL disability, 60% to 80% is crippled ADL disability, and 80% to 100% represents symptom magnification or bed bound.

*From Fairbank JTC: The Oswestry low back disability questionnaire, *Physiotherapy* 66:271, 1980, Chartered Society of Physiotherapy.

ORTHOPEDIC GAMUT 13-14

CHARACTERISTICS OF PURE MALINGERING

- The simulation of a nonexistent illness or injury
- The voluntary provocation, aggravation, and protraction of disease by artificial means
- False allegations about the existence of some malady, such as epilepsy

Assessment for Lumbar Spine Malingering

Comment

In the valid patient, any antalgic position can be taken as a sign that pain can be alleviated or abolished. The Quebec Task Force Classification System for categorizing spinal disorders lends in the differentiation of spinal pain validity (Table 13-5).

> Simulation in LBP is often suspected but difficult to prove. No known variables exist that correlate with motivation to deceive. Recent work suggests that people who simulate pain employ pain language differently than patients with clinical pain (Leavitt, 1987).

An antalgic position, which is assumed automatically, cannot easily be simulated, and it is a protective measure. With uncomplicated lumbosacral strain, the typical antalgic position when standing is slight forward flexion. When maintaining this position, it is not only the abdominal muscles, as forward flexors of the trunk, that are under tension, but also the long back muscles, even though they are extensors. The antalgic position does not merely block extension; it also prevents an excess of forward flexion.

Axial back pain with underlying degenerative lumbar disc disease affects a large percentage of the population. It encompasses a myriad of pathologic features, including degenerative change, annular tears, nucleus pulposus protrusion, and internal disc derangement. With progressive age and pathologic change, the discs can deform to a greater degree and are less able to provide stability and the appropriate distribution of the loads. Tears may develop within the annulus. Efforts by the body to heal these defects can result in neurovascular invasion of the disc material, making the disc nociceptive under weight-bearing conditions. The disc is a composite structure, with the nucleus serving to minimize vertebral end plate stress concentration and the annulus acting as a restraining ligament. Magnetic resonance imaging findings show dehydration of the nucleus pulposus in the majority of people over the age of 40 and in discs that have undergone significant trauma. These changes affect the behavior of the intervertebral disc and its response to loading by altering the hydrophilic and viscoelastic properties. The hydrostatic properties in the nucleus pulposus and integrity of the annulus fibrosis together are necessary for normal attenuation and transmission of spinal loads during activity. Both the subchondral bone of the vertebral end plates and

TABLE 13-5			
THE QUEBEC CLASSIFICATION SYSTEM			
Classification	**Symptoms**	**Duration of Symptoms from Onset**	**Working Status at Time of Evaluation**
1	Pain without radiation	a (<7 days)	W (working)
2	Pain radiation to extremity, proximally	b (7 days-7 weeks)	I (idle)
3	Pain radiation to extremity, distally	c (>7 weeks)	
4	Pain radiation to upper or lower limb neurologic signs		
5	Presumptive compression of a spinal nerve root on a simple roentgenogram (i.e., spinal instability or fracture)		
6	Compression of a spinal nerve root confirmed by (1) specific imaging techniques (i.e., computed axial tomography, myelography, or magnetic resonance imaging) or (2) other diagnostic techniques (e.g., electromyography, venography)		
7	Spinal stenosis		
8	Postsurgical status, 1-6 mos after intervention		
9	Postsurgical status, >6 mos after intervention 9.1 Asymptomatic 9.2 Symptomatic		
10	Chronic pain syndrome		
11	Other diagnoses		W (working) I (idle)

From Spitzer WO et al: Scientific approach to the assessment & management of activity related spinal disorders: a monograph for clinicians. Report of the Quebec Task Force on Spinal Disorders, *Spine* 12(suppl 7):S1, 1987.

the fibers of the annulus fibrosus are innervated and may be a source of pain. A microinstability environment may be created that promotes increased discal strain under loading even from normal activity (Ferrara et al, 2005).

PROCEDURE

- The examiner presses the patient's cranium in a downward direction (Fig. 13-23).
- The existing antalgic positioning must not be disturbed during the axial loading.
- The axial loading may elicit pain in the neck,* but it should not elicit pain in the lower back.
- Malingering should be suspected if the patient indicates that pain is felt in the lower back.

Next Steps/Procedures
Burns bench test, flexed-hip test, flip sign, Magnuson test, plantar flexion test, and trunk rotational test

---

*Whiplash syndrome (WS) is characterized by a cluster of symptoms such as neck pain, headache, restricted head movement and cognitive impairments that are the consequence of sudden extension-acceleration forces to the neck, often as a result of a motor-vehicle accident. WS has a high incidence of approximately 1 per 1000 per year and is the reason for 80% of all insurance litigations. However, legislation-related elimination of compensation for pain and suffering greatly reduced the incidence of and improved the prognosis for WS, thus suggesting that simulation and exaggeration of symptoms may be important, especially in insurance cases. Given that the symptoms of WS are exclusively subjective and cannot be properly quantified, determining if the symptoms are invented, prolonged, exaggerated or if previously present symptoms are attributed to the accident is difficult (Sartori et al, 2003).

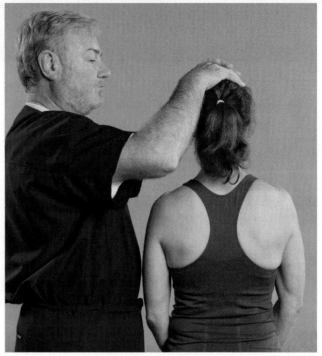

FIG. 13-23 The patient is in the standing position. The examiner presses downward on the patient's head with both hands carefully and not disturbing the existing antalgic posture. The axial loading may elicit pain in the neck but should not elicit pain in the lower back. Lower back pain is a positive finding and indicates a lack of organic basis for the lower back complaint.

CLINICAL PEARL

Back pain sufferers express a fear that the reality of their pain is being questioned. Many of these individuals strive and frequently fail to achieve clinical and social characteristics that make up appropriate sickness behavior. A lack of proof that they are sick, including a lack of medical diagnosis, appropriate health care treatment, and visible disabilities, often leads to accusations, both felt and enacted, of malingering, hypochondria, mental illness, or any combination.

BURNS BENCH TEST

Assessment for Lumbar Spine Malingering

Comment

The yearly incidence of LBP in the United States is between 15% and 20%, and the lifetime prevalence of LBP is approximately 70% to 80%. It is the most frequent cause of physical limitations in patients younger than age 45, the second most common reason for physicians' visits, and the third ranking reason for surgical procedures. Approximately 1% to 2% of the population of the United States is either chronically or temporarily disabled secondary to back pain. These disorders have a significant impact on patients in terms of loss of activities and lifestyle, lost wages and productivity, and disability (Pahl et al, 2006).

A herniated disc can be defined as the herniation of the nucleus pulposus through the fibers of the annulus fibrosus.

The patient's major complaint is a sharp lancinating pain. The patient often has a history of intermittent episodes of localized back pain. The pain also radiates down the leg in the anatomic distribution of the affected nerve root, and it is usually described as deep and sharp, progressing from above downward. The onset of pain may be insidious or sudden and may be associated with a tearing or snapping sensation in the spine. Occasionally, when sciatica develops, the back pain resolves. Once the annulus is ruptured, it may no longer be under tension. Disc herniation occurs with sudden physical effort when the trunk is flexed or rotated. The sciatica may vary in intensity, and it may be so severe that a patient is unable to ambulate and feels as if the back is locked.

ORTHOPEDIC GAMUT 13-15

COMMON LUMBAR SPINE DISORDERS

- Herniated lumbar discs
  - Younger patients
  - Causes radicular type symptoms in the lower extremities
- Spinal stenosis
  - Elderly patients
  - Most common diagnoses in Medicare patients undergoing lumbar spine surgery
  - Back pain
  - Radicular type symptoms
  - Problems walking secondary to neurogenic claudication
- Degenerative spondylolisthesis
  - Segmental instability
  - Occurs in conjunction with spinal stenosis
  - Affects patients in their fifth and sixth decades of life
  - May cause symptoms of neurogenic claudication and radiculopathy
- Lumbar disc degeneration or collapse
  - Observed at one or more levels in the vast majority of all patients by the age of 50
  - May begin as early as age 20

PROCEDURE

- The patient is instructed to kneel on a stool (Fig. 13-24) and bend the trunk forward (Fig. 13-25) far enough to allow touching of the floor with fingertips or hands (Fig. 13-26).
- Patients who may be expected to perform this test successfully include those afflicted with sciatica, sacralization, spondylolisthesis, compression fractures of vertebra, and so on.
- A malingerer will fail to perform the maneuver and usually states, "I can't do it," or words to this effect, even before attempting the move.

Next Steps/Procedures

Axial trunk-loading test, flexed-hip test, flip sign, Magnuson test, plantar flexion test, and trunk rotational test

---

CLINICAL PEARL

Patients with lumbar disc degeneration can have back pain without associated radiculopathy or neurologic dysfunction in the lower extremities and represent a much greater challenge in terms of presentation, clinical imaging, and management than the other three diagnoses.

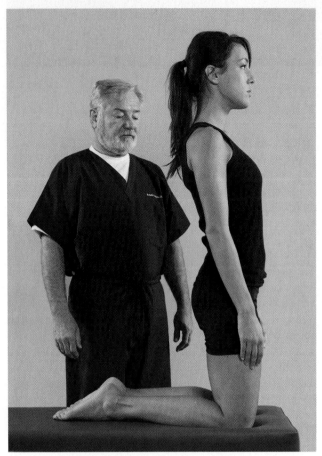

FIG. 13-24 The patient is instructed to kneel on a table or stool, approximately 18 inches from the floor.

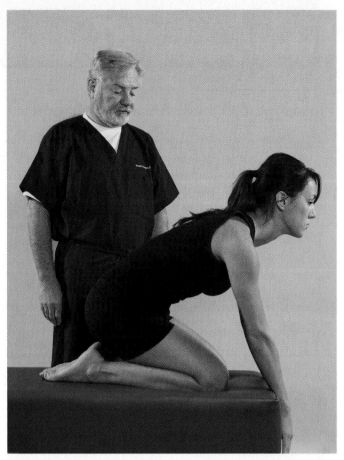

FIG. 13-25 The patient is then instructed to flex the trunk forward.

FIG. 13-26 This flexion should be far enough to allow the patient to touch the floor. This maneuver does not affect the lumbar tissues to any significant degree. A malingering patient will fail to perform the maneuver, stating, "I can't do it," or words to this effect.

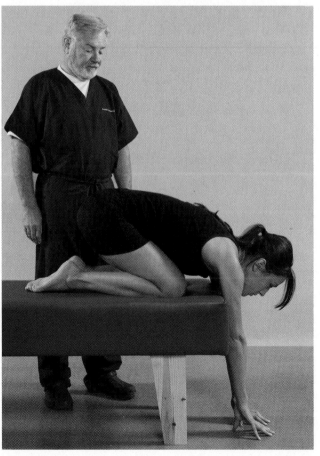

FLEXED-HIP TEST

Assessment for Lumbar Spine Malingering

Comment

Acute pain in the back that radiates down to the knee but will not radiate beyond this point without neurologic abnormality is usually caused by an acute muscle or ligament injury in the lumbar spine. The symptoms can be precipitated by a sudden violent movement or by a comparatively trivial movement after a period of hard work.

Although classically considered a rheumatic and nontraumatic condition, LBP episodes are commonly ascribed today to minor traumatic injuries to the spine. Clinical and population studies of subjects developing serious LBP illness demonstrate significant genetic, psychologic, and social predisposing factors and a high degree of non–spinal chronic pain comorbidity (60% to 70%) and mental disorders (35%). Despite such evidence, many LBP episodes are described as *spinal injury,* apparently occurring in the absence of bone or ligament injury. Experts have often postulated that minor trauma, though unlikely to injure a normal spinal segment, does cause serious structural injury to already degenerative components. The degenerative intervertebral disc is most commonly implicated as the *injured* structure, and many findings seen on imaging studies have been attributed to these *injuries.* On the other hand, studies of asymptomatic subjects have shown that loss of disc signal, annular bulging, and facet arthrosis are frequently seen in subjects with no traumatic history or serious back pain problems. Similarly, these findings appear to be most clearly associated with aging. Annular fissures, disc herniation, and end-plate fractures have been more commonly attributed to acute events (Carragee et al, 2006).

The sacroiliac joints are also subject to acute strains. Although the joints have a large surface area, they have poor mechanical cohesion, and violent twisting strains can cause severe pain around the joints.

PROCEDURE

- The examiner places one hand under the patient's lumbar spine and the other hand under the patient's knee.
- The examiner lifts the knee while flexing the hip (Fig. 13-27).
- If the patient indicates LBP, or if leg pain is felt in the lower back before the lumbar spine moves, malingering should be suspected.

Next Steps/Procedures

Axial trunk-loading test, Burns bench test, flip sign, Magnuson test, plantar flexion test, and trunk rotational test

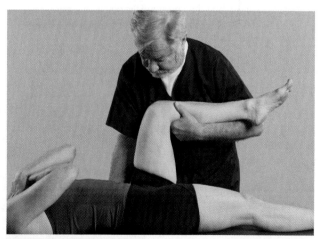

FIG. 13-27 The patient is supine on the examination table. The examiner places one hand under the patient's lumbar spine, palpating the bony landmarks of the L5 and S1 spinous processes. The examiner maintains contact with these landmarks. While the patient's knee is passively held in 90 degrees of flexion, the examiner flexes the patient's hip to 90 degrees. If lower back or leg pain is experienced before the L5 and S1 spinosus separate, malingering is suspected.

CLINICAL PEARL

The causes of low back pain in most people are unclear. Serious structural lesions such as tumors, infection, fractures, and severe deformities are frequently painful and are diagnosed with modern imaging studies. Such patients with serious structural problems are uncommon in outpatient clinical settings. Much more often, people have back pain episodes of varying degrees and either do not seek care or are treated symptomatically without a diagnosis.

Assessment for Feigned Low Back Pain

Comment

With the patient who has a valid lower back injury, a full neurologic examination is warranted if continued root symptoms exist. Enhanced imaging (computed tomography [CT], magnetic resonance imaging [MRI]) is indicated if disabling pain continues, despite a period of absolute rest, and if the distribution of the pain does not give a clear indication of which root is involved. Enhanced studies are required in the setting of paralysis of any muscle that does not recover within a few days. Further investigation is required if any disturbance of micturition exists. If the pain is clearly in the distribution of a lumbar root but is not accompanied by any stiffness of the back, enhanced studies are warranted. This situation may be observed in spinal neurofibromata.

Documentation of both subjective and objective findings is key to the diagnosis and treatment of lumbar disk injury with and without radiculopathy. Subjects in the personal injury protection (PIP) group were significantly more likely to have abnormal straight leg raising (SLR) compared with subjects in the Workers' Compensation (WC) group. A significant proportion of subjects with positive bilateral SLR (89%) had attorney involvement. These findings may reflect several provocative issues in health care today, including physicians erroneously documenting physical examination findings to support their requests for further testing or treatment, the influence of pending litigation, and the potential for improper interpretation of physical examination findings by treating providers in the PIP system (Nadler, Malanga, Ciccone, 2004).

Nadler and colleagues (2004) found that a positive (unilateral, bilateral) SLR in women was 7.4 times more likely if they were covered by PIP than by WC. For men, a positive SLR was 23.5 times more likely if they were covered by a PIP. The odds of bilateral SLR (radicular pain on both sides) were even more strongly associated with type of reimbursement. For women, bilateral SLR was 105.1 times more likely if covered by a PIP than by WC. For men, bilateral SLR was 38.9 times more likely if covered by a PIP.

PROCEDURE

- While the patient is lying in a supine position on the examining table, the examiner raises the patient's affected leg, keeping the patient's knee straight (Fig. 13-28).
- If this movement is limited by pain or muscle resistance, the examiner then directs the patient to sit up, making sure the legs are kept flat on the table.
- If the patient can sit in this manner without pain, the test is positive.
- Sitting with the legs straight out reproduces the same maneuver as a straight-leg-raising test (Fig. 13-29).

Next Steps/Procedures

Axial trunk-loading test, Burns bench test, flexed-hip test, Magnuson test, plantar flexion test, and trunk rotational test

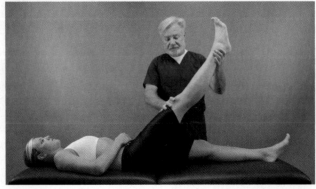

FIG. 13-28 The patient is lying supine on the examination table. The examiner performs a straight-leg-raising test on the affected side, noting the limitation of movement because of pain or muscle spasm.

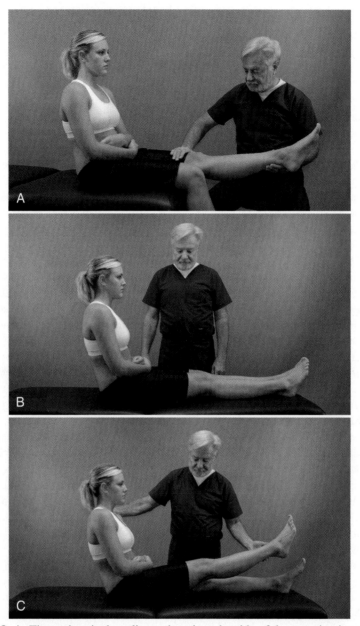

FIG. 13-29 **A,** The patient is then directed to sit at the side of the examination table, with the legs dangling over the edge. On pretext of examining an uninvolved joint of the leg, the examiner fully extends the knee of the affected leg, effecting a straight-leg-raising sciatic stretch maneuver. If the maneuver does not elicit pain, the test is positive, and malingering should be suspected. **B,** In a modification of this test, the patient is directed to sit up from the position shown in Fig. 13-28, with the legs extended and flat on the examination table. If the patient can sit up in this manner, the test is positive. **C,** The examiner can further elevate the leg to increased tissue traction effect. If the maneuver does not elicit pain, the test is positive, and malingering should be suspected.

Assessment for Hypersensitivity of Mastoid Process

Comment

Management of patients with chronic whiplash-associated disorders (WAD) remains a challenge. Even though many individuals recover within a few weeks of injury, a significant proportion (14% to 42%) has persistent ongoing pain, with 10% reporting constant severe pain. Berglund and colleagues (2000) estimated that a relative risk of 2.7 (95% confidence interval [CI] 2.1, 3.5) exists of developing chronic neck pain if acute neck pain began soon after the motor-vehicle crash. Persons with persistent symptoms are the ones who contribute substantially to the significant economic and personal costs related to this condition internationally. Currently, many patients seek ongoing physical therapies from a variety of practitioners for their persistent neck pain, months after their injury. Decisions as to who should receive physical therapies at this stage appear to be largely indiscriminate (Jull et al, 2007).

Spontaneous pain, hyperpathia, and hyperalgesia usually characterize central pain. The term *spontaneous pain* is used to denote the absence of extrinsic stimuli, which ordinarily produce pain. Spontaneous pain is often differentiated from evoked pain in which the stimuli are obvious. Hyperpathia designates a painful overreaction to different stimuli and is associated with diminished sensibility to the form of stimulation that excites such a reaction. Hyperalgesia is an overreaction without diminished sensibility or sensory loss. In the last two instances, regardless of the threshold value, the sensation evoked is abnormal. These painful sensations always develop in an explosive manner; are of an excessive, compelling, diffuse, and complex nature; and continue unduly after stimulation has ceased.

Tenderness and pain thresholds in pericranial muscles were studied in a general population. A random sample of 1000 adults ages 25 to 64 years was drawn as part of the Glostrup Population Studies, and 740 adults were examined. This study was part of a multifacetted, epidemiologic study of different headache disorders according to the new headache classification. Manual palpation and pressure pain threshold with an electronic pressure algometer were performed by observers blinded to other information such as the person's history of headache, previous illness, and mental state. The muscles most commonly tender to manual palpation were the lateral pterygoid (55%), the trapezius (52%), and the sternocleidomastoid muscles (51%). Women were more tender than men in all the muscles examined by manual palpation. In total, the young age group was more tender than the old age group ($p = .03$). Pressure pain thresholds on temporal muscles showed lower thresholds in women than in men ($p < 10-3$), and in the total population thresholds increased with age ($p < .05$). No side-to-side difference in tenderness by manual palpation was found, whereas the right side showed increased pain thresholds in right-handed individuals ($p < 10-4$). No side-to-side difference was found in left-handed persons. This study provides data about the normal population and forms the necessary basis for evaluating the importance of muscle tenderness in headache subjects and other selected groups (Jensen et al, 1992).

PROCEDURE

- The examiner applies finger pressure to the mastoid process (Fig. 13-30).
- The pressure is gradually increased until the patient states that it is becoming noticeably uncomfortable.
- This point is an indication of that patient's pain threshold, which varies from patient to patient.
- The threshold gives the examiner an idea if this patient has a low, high, or moderate pain threshold.
- The threshold is not to be used specifically as a criterion for malingering.
- Identifying a patient's pain threshold will quantify discomfort in this patient and applies to this patient only.
- This testing procedure will be useful during interpretation of palpation findings or subjective statements concerning pain or discomfort.

Next Steps/Procedures

Mannkopf sign, marked part pain-suggestibility test, and related joint motion test

CLINICAL PEARL

Chronic pain patients are typically more impaired on more complex attention-demanding tasks. However, tasks that require fewer attentional resources are unaffected even when pain levels were high. Nonetheless, the relationship between pain and cognitive impairment is complex.

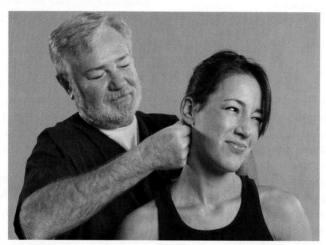

FIG. 13-30 The patient is seated, and the examiner is positioned behind the patient. The examiner applies thumb pressure to the mastoid process and gradually increases the pressure until the patient states that it is becoming noticeably uncomfortable. The test may be repeated for comparison on the opposite mastoid process. This test provides an indication of the patient's pain threshold and is a useful index for interpretation of palpation finding in later examination procedures.

13

MAGNUSON TEST

Assessment for Feigned Low Back Pain

Comment

Identifying any single musculoskeletal factor that adequately explains why some patients with LBP experience rapid and uncomplicated remission while others continuously develops chronic LBP and disability is difficult. Several psychosocial factors, such as job dissatisfaction, secondary gain, and anxiety, are positively associated with a poorer prognosis for patients with LBP; but whether this relationship is causal or associative is controversial (O'Neill et al, 2007).

Cutaneous tenderness is present when pain and discomfort are elicited by a normally innocuous amount of pressure. This tenderness may be related to, but is slightly different from, hyperalgesia. Pain may or may not be concomitantly present. The tenderness may be caused by a direct, underlying pathologic condition, such as occurs with inflammatory lesions or after trauma to the skin, subcutaneous, and muscular tissue. The tenderness may occur as a result of peripheral nerve lesions, or it may occur as a result of a visceral or deep, somatic pathologic condition at some distance from the tenderness. The tenderness may be present over the area where pain is felt, or it may be absent entirely from that area and found at some distant point. The latter condition exists in visceral disease, for example, in cholecystitis, in which the pain is felt in the back at the angle of the scapula, and the tenderness is felt in the skin of the upper right quadrant. Cutaneous tenderness may be elicited by pinching the skin or pressing on it, and it should always be compared with a symmetrically identical area on the opposite side.

PROCEDURE

- The patient with lower back pain is directed to point to the site of the pain.
- The examiner marks that site (Fig. 13-31).
- The examiner then distracts the patient by performing an examination away from the marked site of pain and later resumes the examination of the lower back.
- The test is positive with any change in the location of the pain of greater than 1 to 2 cm (Fig. 13-32).
- The test is significant as evidence of simulated pain, hysteria, or malingering.

Next Steps/Procedures

Axial trunk-loading test, Burns bench test, flexed-hip test, flip sign, plantar flexion test, and trunk rotational test

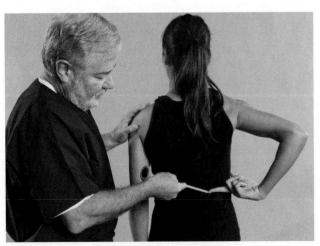

FIG. 13-31 The patient may be standing or seated for this test. The patient is directed to point to the site of lower back pain. The examiner marks the site.

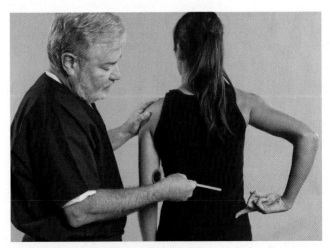

FIG. 13-32 After distraction by other examination procedures, the patient is instructed once again to point to the location of the lower back pain. The test is positive when the patient identifies any site other than the original. The test is significant for simulated lower back pain, hysteria, or malingering.

MANNKOPF SIGN

Assessment for Simulated Pain

Comment

Pain intensity and associated distress in patients with non-malignant pain is at least as high as in patients with cancer pain. A recent World Health Organization survey of primary care patients in 15 countries reported that 22% of patients had pain for at least 6 months that required medical attention or medication or that interfered significantly with daily activities. This statistic is consistent with a previous meta-analysis and subsequent surveys. The majority of these patients have pain that is not proportional to objective disease, such as back pain and headache. Nonetheless, 13% of patients with headache and 18% of those with back pain in the United States report that they have been unable to work full time because of their pain. In a 1999 nationwide telephone survey, 9% of Americans reported moderate to severe chronic nonmalignant pain (CNMP) (≥ 5 on 10-point scale), with one third of them (3%) rating the pain as 10 (worst they could imagine). This pain had been present an average of 6 days per week for more than 5 years. Approximately one half of these participants thought their pain was "pretty much under control." The social burden of CNMP is large because, in contrast to cancer pain, it occurs in the midst of life (Sullivan, Ferrell, 2005).

The autonomic nervous system is a division of the peripheral nervous system that distributes to smooth muscle and glands throughout the body. By definition, the autonomic nervous system is entirely a motor (efferent) system and is automatic in the sense that most of its functions are carried out below the conscious level.

The sympathetic division of the autonomic nervous system is thrown into activity in preparing the organism for fight or flight, and it causes a mass response because of the existence of sympathetic ganglion chains or plexuses where the preganglionic synapse occurs. In action, the sympathetic nervous system produces vasoconstriction of the skin and viscera, shifting more blood to the brain, skeletal muscles, and heart.

Further hindering a clear understanding of the impact of pain on cognitive function is the fact that the presence of financial incentive influences symptom report and test performance. For example, pain patients without head injury who were involved in worker's compensation claims reported more cognitive symptoms than nonlitigating patients with head injury. Furthermore, chronic pain patients involved in disability litigation fail cognitive symptom validity indicators at much higher rates than nonlitigating pain patients and even patients with nonlitigating traumatic brain injury, indicating that some litigating pain patients exaggerate impairment on tasks that appear to measure cognitive ability. A reasonable assumption is that a substantial portion of this exaggeration is intentional, given that the base rate of malingering in pain may be as high as 30%. Thus a clear understanding of the cognitive impact of pain requires consideration of variables other than pain, including intentional exaggeration (Etherton et al, 2006).

PROCEDURE

- The examiner establishes the patient's resting pulse rate, and the patient is made as comfortable as possible (Fig. 13-33).
- Then, without changing the patient's position, the examiner applies mechanical pressure or electrical stimulation over the painful area while monitoring the pulse rate (Fig. 13-34).
- An increase in pulse rate of 10 or more beats per minute constitutes a positive sign.
- The sign is absent in simulated pain.

Next Steps/Procedures
Libman sign, marked part pain-suggestibility test, and related joint motion test

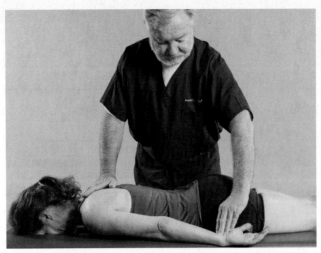

FIG. 13-33 The test may be applied for any area of musculoskeletal pain. The examiner palpates the patient's resting radial pulse and establishes a baseline index.

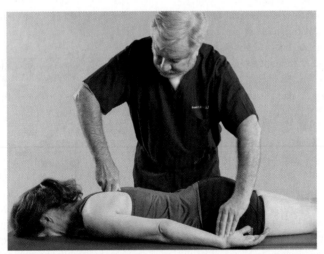

FIG. 13-34 The examiner applies firm pressure, or any form of noxious stimulation, over the area of the pain. The examiner again palpates the patient's radial pulse. An increase of 10 or more beats per minute in the pulse rate is a positive sign. The sign is absent in simulated pain.

MARKED PART
PAIN-SUGGESTIBILITY TEST

PAIN-SUGGESTIBILITY TEST

Assessment for Pain Exaggeration

Comment

Hypochondriacal neurosis denotes a preoccupation with bodily processes, in which the individual becomes unduly concerned about possible dysfunctions that are largely imagined or exaggerated. Health issues occupy the patient's thoughts, and concern exists that one or more illnesses exist. Contrary facts are not reassuring. The symptoms chosen for expression are often those experienced by close associates. In psychodynamic terms, the hypochondriacal person is immature and never achieved an external object relationship, focusing instead on the body for the major and often sole means of communicating with others.

Hypochondriasis has been theorized to relate to self-assessed health (SAH) both through differences in symptom perception and through processes related to medical excuse making (MEM). In symptom-perception views of hypochondriasis, the tendency to experience benign physical symptoms as painful and distressing has been argued to be a perceptual bias common to hypochondriac individuals. Alternatively, hypochondriasis is theorized to relate to SAH through more motivated psychologic influences. Smith and colleagues (1983) found that hypochondriacal college students reported poorer health in an evaluative setting in which poor performance *could* versus *could not* be attributed to poor health. Additionally, in an interpersonal model of hypochondriasis, Noyes and colleagues suggest that hypochondriacal patients elicit emotional support from friends, family, and physicians through attachment-driven care-seeking behaviors. In support of their model, the researchers found that hypochondriacal patients attending a general medical clinic were insecurely attached. Hypochondriasis therefore may relate to SAH through both MEM and anxious attachment (Fortenberry, Wiebe, 2007).

Underlying these complaints is the need for continual reassurance that an illness does not exist and that someone cares and is willing to listen.

Because physical well being is essential to our survival, not surprisingly, most people experience health-focused thoughts and concerns from time to time. Among persons suffering from serious medical illnesses (and those at risk), health concerns serve an adaptive function in that they motivate the person to attend closely to bodily sensations to ensure that serious signs and symptoms are dealt with in a timely fashion. In fact, as part of their self-care, at-risk patients are often instructed to monitor their bodies for possible symptoms. In other instances, intense health concerns (or health anxiety) develop in the absence of organic disease, such as when individuals perceive themselves as seriously ill based on a misinterpretation of benign bodily sensations (e.g., "This headache means I have a brain tumor," "My stomach pain is caused by a rare gastrointestinal disorder"). Hypochondriasis involves a pattern of intense health anxiety that is based on these sorts of misattributions. In hypochondriasis, catastrophic overestimates of the probability and seriousness of medical conditions give rise to preoccupation with the suspected illness, selective attention to illness-related stimuli, and irresistible urges to seek medical advice and reassurance to the extent that it impairs psychosocial functioning (Abramowitz, Olatunji, Deacon, 2007).

PROCEDURE

- The examiner applies pressure to the described painful point and marks it (Figs. 13-35 and 13-36).
- The patient is distracted by examination of some other part of the body and pressing on new, tender areas.
- The examiner returns to the area of original complaint and asks the patient to close the eyes and then locate the tender points (Figs. 13-37 to 13-39).
- If the patient cannot place the points of pain or tenderness closer than 2 inches from the marked area, exaggeration is suspected (Fig. 13-40).

Next Steps/Procedures
Libman sign, Mannkopf sign, and related joint motion test

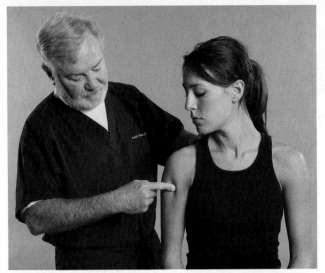

FIG. 13-35 The patient is seated. The examiner instructs the patient to identify the area of pain. The examiner applies pressure to the site, confirming the pain reaction. The site is marked or noted by some non-stimulating method. The patient is distracted with other examination procedures.

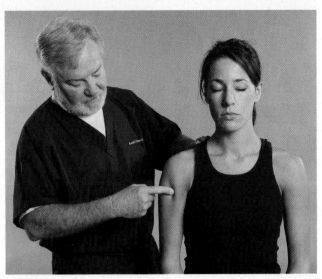

FIG. 13-36 The patient is instructed to close the eyes.

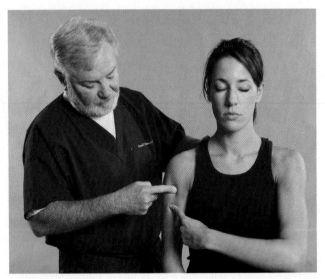

FIG. 13-37 With the eyes closed, the patient is asked to, once again, identify the site of pain. If the patient cannot place the point of pain within 2 inches of the original site, exaggeration is suspected. *The examiner must not remind the patient of the original location, especially by touch.* (In these photographs, the examiner reminds the reader of the original point of pain.)

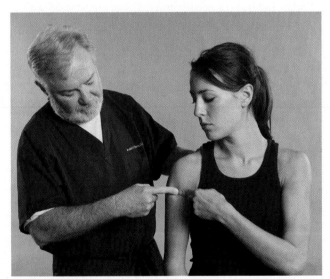

FIG. 13-38 In an alternative method of determining pain suggestibility, the examiner first suggests a certain point as the source of pain and marks it.

CLINICAL PEARL

Human babesiosis was first recognized in Europe in 1957. In 1999, the southern-most range of human babesiosis on America's Atlantic coast was reported to be northwestern New Jersey. Other agents such as *Borrelia burgdorferi*, the Lyme disease (LYD) spirochete, the rickettsiae of ehrlichiosis, and bacterial rods of *Bartonella* spp. within tick saliva often accompany *Babesia* spp.; increasingly, patients are coinfected with LYD and babesiosis. If the disease is misdiagnosed as influenza, for example, and therefore goes untreated, infected humans tend to decompensate, often being mislabeled as depressed, *hypochondriacal*, and so forth, rarely receiving optimum treatment for smoldering but active babesiosis—a sometimes fatal disease, especially if the patient is older or becomes immunocompromised.

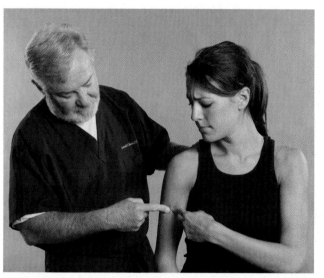

FIG. 13-39 By distracting the patient with different testing procedures, the examiner suggests a nearby but new point of discomfort and notes whether the pain shifts with the suggestion.

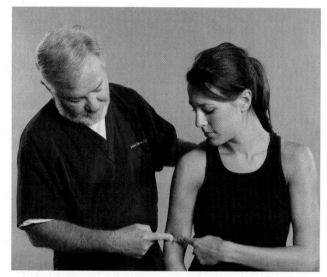

FIG. 13-40 If the site of pain does shift, this suggests exaggeration of pain. It is important that the examiner not remind the patient of the original location, especially by touch.

13

PLANTAR FLEXION TEST

Assessment for Feigned Low Back Pain

Comment

Several maneuvers can be used to tighten the sciatic nerve and, in doing so, further compress an inflamed nerve root against a herniated disc. With the straight-leg-raising maneuver, the L5 and S1 nerve roots move 2 to 6 mm at the level of the foramen. The L4 nerve root moves a shorter distance, and the more proximal nerve roots show little motion. Thus, the straight-leg-raising test is important and has value in detecting lesions of the L5 and S1 nerve root.

ORTHOPEDIC GAMUT 13-16

ACTIVE PLANTAR FLEXION

Active plantar flexion stresses the calf muscles similarly to the treadmill test but with less effect on the cardiovascular system. The procedure is as follows:

- Both feet are placed in an adjustable brace, stabilizing the isolating the lower limbs.
- The patient pushes with both feet against pedals simultaneously until the pedals stop and holds the position for 2 seconds.
- The patient releases the pedals gently over 2 seconds.
- The patient presses the pedals in time to an audible signal set at 30 beats per minute; one signal to push is followed by a signal to release the pedals.
- The time in which the patient feels pain in the calf muscles is recorded (pain-free exercise time).
- The time at which the patient claims to reach their limit of exercise is recorded (maximal exercise time).
- The patient is allowed to stop for other symptoms; as in the treadmill test, symptoms, as well as blood pressure and heart rate before and after exercise, are recorded.

In the vascular laboratory, stress tests are used to evaluate the severity of the peripheral arterial disease (PAD). Stress tests can also be used to confirm PAD in patients who appear normal at rest. The most commonly used stress test is to walk on a treadmill. Treadmill stress testing produces maximal flow demands to the most symptomatic leg, its parameters correlate well with calf blood flow measurements, and it is readily available for assessing the severity of PAD. However, one problem with treadmill tests is that they induce stress on the whole body, including the cardiovascular system. Patients with PAD have a high risk for ischemic heart disease, and performing treadmill tests on these patients can lead to angina. Another problem is that not all patients with PAD can walk sufficiently. For example, patients with PAD may also have arthritic hip or knee joints, and some may have had their other leg amputated. Active plantar flexion is a type of exercise known to use mainly the calf muscles, the location of symptoms in most patients with PAD. Plantar flexion is widely used as a stress test in physiology and sports medicine but is not commonly used for to assess patients with limb ischemia (Yamamoto et al, 2007).

PROCEDURE

- The patient is instructed to raise the legs, one at a time, until pain is felt in the lower back or the leg (Fig. 13-41).
- The angle at which the pain occurs is noted, and the patient lowers the leg.
- The examiner places one hand under the patient's knee and one hand under the patient's foot and raises the lower extremity, keeping the patient's knee slightly flexed (Fig. 13-42).
- The leg is raised to half of the height at which the pain was originally elicited.
- The foot is passively plantar flexed at this point (Fig. 13-43).
- If the patient indicates that this move causes LBP, malingering should be suspected.

Next Steps/Procedures
Axial trunk-loading test, Burns bench test, flexed-hip test, flip sign, Magnuson test, and trunk rotational test

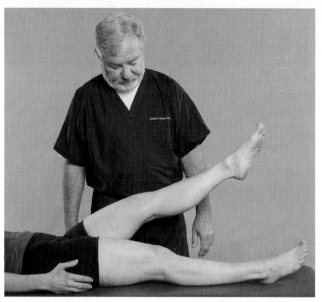

FIG. 13-41 The patient is lying supine on the examination table. The patient is instructed to raise the extended, affected leg until pain is felt in the lower back or in the leg. The examiner notes the angle at which pain occurs. The patient lowers the leg to the table.

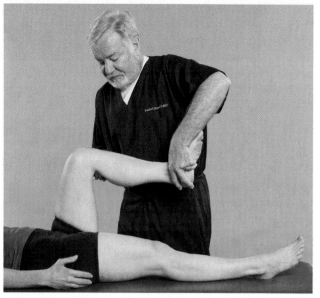

FIG. 13-42 The examiner places one hand under the patient's knee and one hand under the ankle and elevates the leg, keeping the knee slightly flexed. The leg is elevated to a point below the production of the original pain.

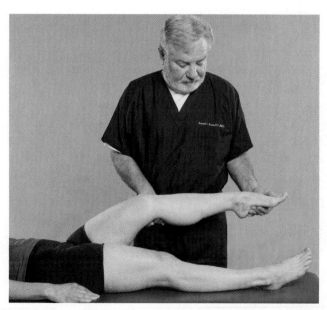

FIG. 13-43 The examiner plantar flexes the foot. If the patient indicates that the final maneuver caused lower back pain, malingering is suspected.

13

Assessment for Feigned Pain

Comment

Most orthopedic conditions are associated with some restriction of movement in the related joint. Complete loss of movement follows surgical ablation of a joint (arthrodesis) or may occur during some pathologic process, such as infection, in which fibrous or bony tissue binds the articular surfaces together. The joint then cannot be moved, either actively or passively. In many conditions, loss occurs of that part of the range of motion that allows the joint to be brought into its neutral position. The common loss of movement usually prevents the joint from being fully extended. This condition is known as a *fixed flexion deformity*.

Although individuals do have some voluntary control over the duration of imagined goal-directed movements, they cannot exert voluntary control over speed and accuracy relationships in imagined motor task performance. When performing the motor sequencing task and imagining performance on the same task under normal conditions, healthy subjects showed the expected speed-accuracy trade-off, described by Fitts' law, for both real and imagined movements (provided that they were instructed to make the movements as fast and as accurate as possible). Furthermore, the general duration of real and imagined motor task performance was equivalent. When required to feign an injury, the duration of performance on the motor sequencing task increased dramatically, although more so for real movements than for imagined movements (Maruff, Velakoulis, 2000).

PROCEDURE

- The painful part is either actively or passively moved.
- This move is performed with isometric resistance of a muscle group that is nearby but is in no way associated with the pain (Fig. 13-44).
- If the patient complains of pain, the examiner moves the muscle group or related joint later, judging the inaccuracy of the statements and the correlated reactions (Fig. 13-45).
- This assessment is accomplished by using a flexor group in which an extensor group may produce pain in the joint.
- Where the same muscle serves more than one movement, all movements should be tested.

Next Steps/Procedures

Libman sign, Mannkopf sign, and marked part pain-suggestibility test

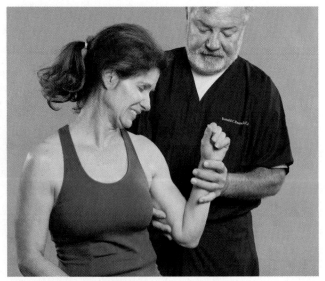

FIG. 13-45 The examiner places the painful joint or part into isometric testing of a muscle group that is nearby but unrelated to the primary injury group. For example, the examiner isometrically tests the triceps muscle group. If the patient complains of the original pain, the examiner moves the primary muscle group later in the examination, noting the accuracy of statements and reactions to the original findings. Discrepancies suggest exaggeration of symptoms or malingering.

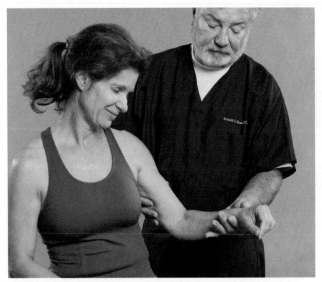

FIG. 13-44 The patient identifies the area of musculoskeletal complaint, especially the point at which motion of the affected joint is uncomfortable. The examiner confirms this reported site of pain with the patient. For example, the patient identifies that flexion of the elbow hurts the biceps musculature.

SEELIGMULLER SIGN

Assessment for Hysterical Face Pain

Comment

Trigeminal neuralgia is characterized by a sudden attack of excruciating pain of short duration along the distribution of the fifth cranial nerve. The attack is normally precipitated by mild stimulation of a trigger zone in the area of the pain and is characterized by recurrent paroxysms of sharp, stabbing pains in the distribution of one or more branches of the nerve. The onset is usually in middle or late life, and the incidence is higher in women than in men. The pain may be described as a burning or searing pain that occurs in lightning-like jabs, lasting only 1 to 2 minutes or as long as 15 minutes. The frequency of attacks varies from many times a day to several times a month or year. The patient often tries to immobilize the face during conversation or attempts to swallow food without chewing to prevent irritating the trigger zone.

Neurologic conversion symptoms include muscular weakness or paralysis, affecting one, two, or all four limbs, or resulting in loss of speech, convulsions simulating epilepsy, or a loss of sensation (commonly blindness or tunnel vision, deafness, or a circumscribed loss of cutaneous sensation) assumed to depend on the psychoanalytic mechanism of conversion. As the extent of the paralysis or sensory loss reflects the patient's ideas rather than anatomic facts, and because it can often be demonstrated neurologically that the relevant motor or sensory pathways are undamaged, the diagnosis of hysteria can usually be made with some confidence. Hysterical pain and other psychophysiologic reactions include visceral symptoms such vomiting or otherwise unexplained pain assumed to be produced by the same conversion mechanism. Unlike neurologic conversion symptoms, usually, no easy way exists of demonstrating that such symptoms must be psychogenic, and, as a result, the diagnosis of hysteria remains uncertain (Kendell, Neil, Paul, 2001).

Research has isolated *core* pain-related facial actions common to acute pain, exacerbations of chronic pain, and various types of experimentally induced pain. These facial actions are a lowered brow, raised cheeks, tightened eye lids, a raised upper lip or opened mouth, and closed eyes. Research has less consistently identified horizontal or vertical stretching of the lips, a wrinkled nose, deepening of the nasolabial fold, and drooping eyelids as pain-related actions. These discrepancies may reflect methodologic variations such as the type of pain experienced, pain severity, and situational and individual difference variables. Various predictive correlates of facial expression contribute to its clinical utility. The magnitude of facial activity increases with the intensity of noxious stimulation, correlates with self-reports of pain severity and unpleasantness, and is discriminable by naive observers, suggesting that facial expressions of pain can communicate quantitatively graded pain information. The pain expression also seems relatively specific to pain, given that it can be differentiated from other negative subjective states, such as disgust, fear, anger, and sadness. In addition, research has not found a relationship among anxiety, depression, and the facial expression of pain, despite consistent findings of a correlation among anxiety, depression, and verbal pain reports (Hill, Craig, 2002).

PROCEDURE

- Mydriasis (dilated pupil) is present on the side of the face that is afflicted with neuralgia.
- The sign is present as long as pain is present.
- The sign is absent in cases of hysteria and malingering (Fig. 13-46).

Next Steps/Procedures
Anosmia testing and facial anesthesia testing

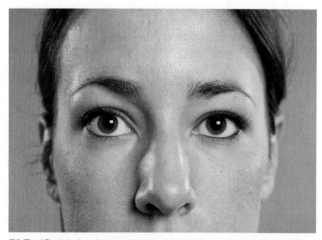

FIG. 13-46 In the patient complaining of facial neuralgia, the examiner observes the pupils for mydriasis. A dilated pupil is a usual finding with facial neuralgia and is absent, **as in this photograph,** in cases of hysteria or malingering.

Assessment for Nonorganic Low Back Pain

Comment

During flexion of the trunk, the strain falls first on the iliolumbar ligament. Next, strain is transmitted to the interspinous ligaments, from the L5 vertebra upward, and then to the dorsolumbar fascia, particularly to the sacral triangle. During extension, the impingement signs prevail over the tension effects. The articulation comes first, and the interspinous ligaments follow. The ligamentum flavum escapes impingement. During axial rotation, the iliolumbar ligament becomes strained first and then the intertransverse.

> The response of an individual experiencing acute pain has been hypothesized to fall along a continuum between two extremes: confrontation or avoidance. Where on this continuum an individual patient will fall is determined by his or her fear of pain. Confrontation is generally considered to be an adaptive response in which the individual views pain as a nuisance and has strong motivation to return to normal levels of activity. This response is seen as gradually leading to a reduction in fear and a return to normal activity. Avoidance is a maladaptive response, causing the patient to avoid certain activities that are anticipated to cause an increase in pain and suffering. An avoidance response may lead to a reduction in physical and social activities, an exacerbation of the fear and avoidance behaviors, prolonged disability, and adverse physical and psychologic consequences (Fritz, George, Delitto, 2001).

The legs transmit their effects through the pelvis. Single leg raising causes no pelvic movement, although it does cause contraction of the contralateral gluteus maximus. Double leg raising tilts the pelvis into extension. The ischial tuberosities serve as fulcrums.

- The patient rotates the trunk.
- The examiner ensures that the patient's pelvis rotates as well (Fig. 13-47).
- If the patient indicates that this rotation causes LBP, malingering should be suspected.
- The lumbar spine is not moving.
- Instead, the whole spine is rotated from the hips and thighs.

Next Steps/Procedures

Axial trunk-loading test, Burns bench test, flexed-hip test, flip sign, Magnuson test, and plantar flexion test

SENSORY DEFICIT QUALIFICATION AND QUANTIFICATION

Overview

The nervous system does not perceive external events directly. Instead, the brain receives an abstract picture that is a composite of nerve impulses that originate at the periphery. The transformation of external stimuli into conductible impulses is called *transduction*. *Sensibility* is the reception or encoding of external stimuli and the transmission of impulses along nerve fibers.

> Pain is caused by the activation of A-δ (1- to 4-μ thinly myelinated fibers) or C-fibers (1-μ unmyelinated nociceptor units). A-δ fibers entrain sharp, lancinating, well-localized first pain, whereas C-fibers encode slow, poorly localized, diffuse, burning second pain. Natural and tissue-destructive stimuli coactivate different pain and somatosensory tissue receptors, the summated activity of which results in a

CLINICAL PEARL

Although episodes of acute low back pain (LBP) are nearly universal human experiences, the subsequent development of chronic disability and diminished work capacity occurs in only a limited percentage of individuals. In 1987, the Quebec Task Force on Spinal Disorders reported that 7% of individuals with work-related LBP accounted for 76% of compensation costs and work absence as a result of LBP.

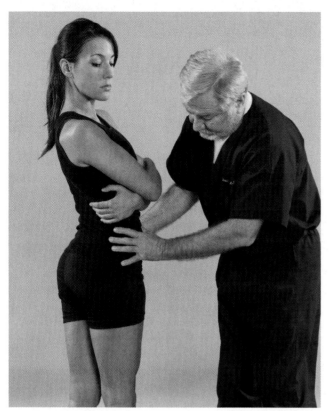

FIG. 13-47 The patient is in the standing position with the arms folded across the chest. The examiner instructs the patient to rotate the trunk, while making sure that the pelvis is rotated siumltaneously. If the patient indicates that this move causes pain in the lower back, the test is positive and indicates malingering.

blended sensation. Thus burning or cold pain is a combination of activation of specific A-δ cold receptors and C-fiber nociceptors. At the site of nerve injury is the production and release of algesiogenic substances, cytokines, inflammatory mediators, and products of wallerian degeneration that produce inhomogeneous receptor sensitization and activation of polymodal C-nociceptors (Schwartzman, Maleki, 1999).

Sensibility is the modality of prime importance. Touch pressure is the ability to recognize touch, whether moving across the surface or continually applied to a single spot.

In contrast to sensibility, which is primarily a peripheral phenomenon, sensation is the central reception and conscious recognition of external stimuli. Sensation involves several facets of central nervous system function. Some of these facets are voluntary, and some are involuntary. Among these facets are the orderly reception and integration of impulses from several sources, association with other information (either current or from memory storage), assimilation and interpretation of such data, and, finally, elevation to the conscious level. All of these facets may result, at the patient's discretion, in an appropriate response.

ORTHOPEDIC GAMUT 13-18

SPECIFIC ASPECTS OF POSTINJURY NEUROPATHIC PAIN SYNDROMES

1. Mechanoallodynia and thermal allodynia
   a. Allodynia refers to pain provoked by an innocuous mechanical or thermal stimulus.
   b. Dynamic mechanoallodynia and hyperalgesia refers to a gentle moving stimulus over the skin surface that elicits pain, whereas static mechanoallodynia and hyperalgesia is pain produced by a stationary pressure stimulus.
2. Mechanohyperalgesia and thermal hyperalgesia—hyperalgesia signifies a lowered threshold to a normally painful stimulus and enhanced pain perception.
3. Hyperpathia—hyperpathia is a reflection of disordered central pain processing in which the pain threshold is increased, but once exceeded pain reaches maximal intensity too rapidly, is more severe than expected and is not stimulus bound.

ORTHOPEDIC GAMUT 13-19

NEURAL SENSIBILITY

Neural sensibility encompasses :
1. Sight
2. Smell
3. Sound
4. Taste
5. Temperature change
6. Pain
7. Touch-pressure
8. Movement or change in position

The transmission of impulses from skin surface to the cerebral cortex requires a chain of three afferent neurons. The cell body of the first-order afferent neuron lies in the dorsal ganglion, and the other two are in the spinal cord and brain. From a practical standpoint, the examiner has access only to the axon of the first-order afferent neuron, its receptors, and the skin that contains them.

Superficial sensation is concerned with touch, pain, temperature, and two-point discrimination; deep sensation is concerned with muscle and joint position sense (proprioception) and deep muscle pain and vibration sense (pallesthesia). The combination of superficial and deep sensory mechanisms is involved in stereognosis, the recognition and naming of familiar objects placed in the hand, and topognosis, the ability to localize cutaneous stimuli. Stereognosis depends on the integrity of the cerebral cortex.

13

ORTHOPEDIC GAMUT 13-20
SENSATION

Sensation is divided into three groups:
1. Superficial
2. Deep
3. Combined

ORTHOPEDIC GAMUT 13-21
TWO GROUPS OF CUTANEOUS SENSIBILITY

1. Epicritic
2. Protopathic

Each is served by a different neuron. Epicritic senses are involved in perception of light touch, two-point discrimination, and small differences in temperature; the protopathic senses are involved with pain and more marked changes of temperature.

Phantom limbs are a seemingly curious phenomenon, nevertheless perceived by up to 98% of amputees after amputation, nerve avulsion, or spinal cord injury and by approximately 20% of children with congenital limb aplasia. Phantom pain is experienced by up to 80% of amputees, with pain usually characterized as (a) burning, tingling, or throbbing; (b) cramping or squeezing; or (c) shocking or shooting. Phantom sensations are perceived immediately after limb loss by most amputees; however, for some, they may emerge years or even decades after limb loss. The dura-tion of phantom limb perception also varies between individuals, and phantom sensations may be perceived for anything from a few days to weeks, months, years, or even decades after limb loss before they fade completely, if at all. Phantom sensations are reported most commonly after the amputation of an arm or leg, or some part thereof, although they have also been reported after removal of the breast, penis, eye, teeth, bladder, and rectum. Phantom sensations after removal of visceral organs may be painful in nature (e.g., menstrual pain after hysterectomy or phantom pain that resembles presurgical pain) and tend to be characterized by functional sensations—for example, sensations of urina-tion or erection following penis removal (Giummarra et al, 2007).

CLINICAL PEARL (SENSORY DEFICIT ASSESSMENT)

In the evaluation of what appears to be psychogenic changes in sensation, the fact that some variation in the nerve supply exists in normal individuals must always be remembered. Furthermore, hysterical or malingered changes may be superimposed on organic anesthesia in peripheral nerve lesions and other neurologic disorders. An ipsilateral decrease or loss of the senses of vision, hearing, smell, and taste may occasionally accompany hysterical (or malingered) hemianesthesia, which almost invariably occurs on the left side.

ANOSMIA TESTING

Assessment for Feigned Anosmia

Comment

The central connections of the olfactory nerve are complex. Association fibers to the tegmentum and pons pass directly as third-order neurons from the anterior perforated substance and indirectly from the hippocampus via the fornix and olfactory projection tracts through the mammillary bodies and anterior nuclei of the thalamus. Reflex connections, thus established within the nuclei of the other cranial and spinal nerves, may be functionally significant during swallowing and digestion.

> Most odorous compounds stimulate not only the olfactory, but also the intranasal trigeminal system, at least when presented at higher concentrations whereby they produce sensations such as irritation, pain, or tickling. Olfactory activation is transmitted from the olfactory epithelium via the olfactory bulb to the brain, including the piriform, orbitofrontal, and insular cortices. Trigeminal activation is generated at free nerve endings located within both the respiratory and the olfactory epithelium of the nasal cavity. This information receives significant processing in the spinal cord, the thalamus, and the primary and secondary somatosensory cortex, SI and SII (Iannilli et al, 2007)

The olfactory nerve may serve as a portal of entry for cryptogenic infections of the brain and meninges (poliomyelitis, epidemic meningitis, and encephalitis).

Anosmia may be of significance. Bilateral anosmia commonly occurs with colds, rhinitis, and so on. Unilateral anosmia may be of diagnostic significance in locating brain lesions, such as tumors, at the base of the frontal lobe.

The presence of olfactory dysfunction in individuals with different types of dementia is well documented. For example, Alzheimer disease (AD) produces deficits in one's ability to detect, identify, and remember odors. In addition, individuals with Huntington disease (HD) and a subset of those with Parkinson disease (PD) also display olfactory deficits. Cognitively intact persons who are at risk for AD via the presence of the apolipoprotein E (ApoE) 4 allele and individuals with Down syndrome also demonstrate deficiencies in olfactory functioning. Given the presence of dementia in all of these disorders, a need exists for assessment tools that involve minimal cognitive demands. One such tool is the *olfactory event-related potential* (OERP). The OERP can be evoked in a single-stimulus paradigm by presenting an odor and requiring the patient to press a button when it has occurred. Delayed OERP latencies have been reported in individuals with AD and PD compared with normal controls. These findings suggest that the OERP may be useful for detecting deficits in olfactory functioning in these individuals in a clinical setting. In addition, the OERP would be a useful tool to detect malingering in nasal dysfunction clinics, where patients may feign olfactory deficits on standard psychophysical measures (Wetter, Murphy, 2003).

The classical presentation of Refsum disease includes progressive retinitis pigmentosa, cerebellar ataxia, and chronic symmetrical sensory-motor neuropathy. Additional features include cataract, ichthyosis, sensory neural deafness, anosmia, cardiac involvement (abnormalities of conduction and cardiomyopathy), aminoaciduria, and epiphyseal dysplasia. The diagnosis of the disease is confirmed by the detection of elevated plasma levels of phytanic acid. In addition, the cerebral spinal fluid protein level is usually elevated. Refsum disease follows a generally progressive course, with alternating episodes of remission and relapse. The three most frequent triggers for relapse include (1) weight loss (possibly at the beginning of the diet low in phytanic acid), (2) pregnancy and (3) severe infections.

ORTHOPEDIC GAMUT 13-22

CAUSE OF DISORDERS OF THE SENSE OF SMELL

1. Inflammatory and other lesions of the nasal cavity
2. Fracture of the anterior fossa of the skull
3. Tumors of the frontal lobe and pituitary region
4. Meningitis
5. Hydrocephalus
6. Posttraumatic cerebral syndrome
7. Arteriosclerosis
8. Cerebrovascular accidents
9. Certain drug intoxications
10. Psychoses
11. Neuroses
12. Congenital defects

ORTHOPEDIC GAMUT 13-23

SPECIAL SYNDROMES INVOLVING THE OLFACTORY NERVE

1. Foster-Kennedy syndrome (unilateral optic atrophy, with or without anosmia and contralateral papilledema)
2. Aura of epilepsy

These conditions have been associated with acute and sub-acute presentations that may mimic the Guillain-Barré syndrome and chronic inflammatory demyelinating polyneuropathy (Verny et al, 2006).

PROCEDURE

- With complaints involving the loss of the sense of smell, the patient is directed to index various odors by smelling aromatics such as peppermint, clove, vanilla, coffee grounds (uncooked), and then, finally, spirit of ammonia (Fig. 13-48).
- An individual with psychogenic loss of smell often claims the inability to smell any of these substances.
- Ammonia is extremely pungent and actually irritates the trigeminal nerve endings in the nose rather than being smelled by the olfactory nerve proper.
- Hence a damaged olfactory nerve does not impair a patient's ability to notice (smell) the pungent ammonia fumes.

Next Steps/Procedures
Seeligmuller sign and facial anesthesia testing

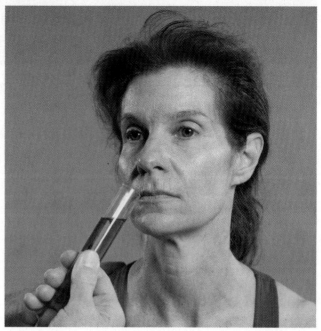

FIG. 13-48 In complaints of loss of smell, the patient is instructed to index various odors by smelling aromatics, such as peppermint, clove, vanilla, coffee grounds, and finally, spirit of ammonia. An individual with feigned anosmia will claim the inability to smell any of the substances. Using spirit of ammonia directly irritates the trigeminal nerve endings in the nose. A damaged olfactory nerve does not impair the patient's ability to notice (smell) pungent ammonia. Anosmia to ammonia suggests a psychogenic or manufactured complaint.

CLINICAL PEARL

One challenge to the implementation of the olfactory event-related potential in a clinical setting is the need for measurement of habituation-free brain potentials. The neuronal recovery time for the olfactory system is significantly longer than that of both the auditory and the visual systems. Specifically, the presentation of two olfactory stimuli 45 seconds apart results in habituation to the second presentation, which does not completely recover even after 90 seconds. This phenomenon is the result, in part, of adaptation of olfactory receptor cells and, in part, of habituation to the original presentation of the stimulus.

COORDINATION-DISTURBANCE TESTING

Assessment for Nonorganic Loss of Coordination

Comment

Symptomatic or secondary myoclonus constitutes one symptom of an identifiable underlying disorder, which can be neurologic or nonneurologic. Symptomatic myoclonus (72%) is the most common type of myoclonus, followed by epileptic (17%) and essential myoclonus (11%). Myoclonus may be present in a huge number of neurologic diseases (Borg, 2006).

Tremors are involuntary movements in one or more parts of the body produced by rhythmical alternate contractions of opposing muscle groups. Tremors are symptoms of constitutional diseases or disorders rather than clinical entities.

In differentiating tremors, the examiner should note their rate, rhythm, and distribution and the effect of movement or rest. A rapid tremor oscillates 8 to 10 times per second, a slow tremor 3 to 5 times per second. Tremors may be fine or coarse. Intention tremor appears during, or is accentuated by, volitional movements of the affected part. Resting tremors are present when the involved part is at rest, but they diminish or disappear during active movements.

Transient tremors, without particular significance, may occur in healthy individuals during hunger, chilling, or excitement or after physical exertion.

Tremor is an involuntary movement characterized by regular or irregular oscillations of one or several body segments. It can be classified according to its anatomic allocation, the circumstances under which it occurs, its frequency and amplitude, and whether it is physiologic or pathologic. Physiologic and pathologic tremor in motor control can be defined as roughly sinusoidal movements with particular amplitude and frequency profiles. For example, patients with Parkinson disease exhibit a resting tremor of increased amplitude and a modal frequency between 4 and 6 Hz, whereas the postural tremor is between 5 and 12 Hz. Among the pathologic cases, Parkinsonian and essential tremor are the most often observed types. PD is a growing problem with 120 to 180 victims in every 100,000 people. Most patients are over 40 years of age, although the disease can appear in younger subjects. Essential tremor affect up to 5000 people in every 100,000. The mean age at onset is 45

years, but the disorder may start in adolescence or early adulthood (Engin et al, 2007).

PROCEDURE

- The patient with coordination disturbances is instructed to touch the tip of the nose while the eyes are open.
- The patient is then instructed to close the eyes and again touch the tip of the nose (Fig. 13-49).
- With organic cerebellar lesions, an intention crescendo tremor occurs as the finger approaches the nose.
- The malingerer will move the finger in a guided but devious course toward the nose without exhibiting the intention tremor (Fig. 13-50).

Next Steps/Procedures

Limb-dropping test (upper extremities), position-sense testing, and Romberg test

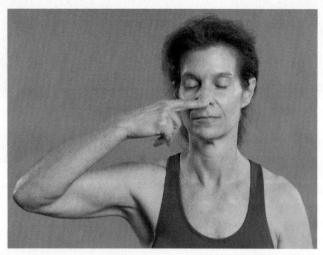

FIG. 13-49 The seated patient is instructed to touch the tip of the nose while the eyes are open. The patient is then instructed to close the eyes and again touch the tip of the nose. With organic cerebellar lesions, an intention crescendo tremor occurs as the finger approaches the nose.

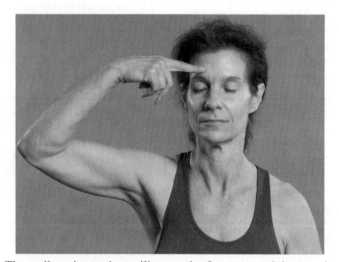

FIG. 13-50 The malingering patient will move the finger toward the nose in a guided but devious course, without the intention tremor.

Assessment for Simulated Blindness

Comment

Optic atrophy is commonly divided into primary and secondary (or postneuritic) categories. Primary optic atrophy results from a degeneration of the nerve fibers after retrobulbar neuritis that results from syphilis, central retinal artery occlusion, glaucoma, trauma, or any condition or drug that causes injury to the optic nerve along its intracanalicular or intracranial course. With secondary optic atrophy, degeneration of the nerve fibers is accompanied by glial formation on the nerve head and is caused by optic neuritis or severe and prolonged papilledema.

Visual loss is directly proportional to the degree of nerve atrophy. This appreciation of light is demonstrated by the Marcus Gunn phenomenon. With the Marcus Gunn phenomenon, the examiner is able to recognize the quantitative difference in the pupillary light reflex between the two eyes by means of alternately illuminating the pupils of the two eyes and observing the difference in pupillary constriction. In optic atrophy, total blindness and a dilated, fixed pupil may result (Figs. 13-51 and 13-52). In primary optic atrophy, the disc is white or grayish with sharp edges and a saucer-shaped excavation. The lamina cribrosa is clearly visible. The retina is usually normal.

In secondary optic atrophy, the disc is dirty white with irregular and indistinct margins and is covered by glial tissue that conceals the lamina cribrosa. Evidence of previous inflammation, such as sheathed vessels, may be seen in the retina.

Periorbital cellulitis, largely seen in pediatric patients, affects visual activity, if only from visual obstruction of the swollen eyelid. However, periorbital cellulitis is associated with collagen-vascular disease, systemic disease, or neoplasms (Fig 13-53).

Functional visual loss (FVL) refers to subnormal vision or altered visual fields in which no underlying disease of the visual system can be found. It is a clinical diagnosis that is made when the physician demonstrates that visual acuity is better than subjectively alleged. FVL may be seen in a continuum of clinical settings, from frank malingering with the aim of secondary gain to a factitious disorder that is symptom focused or is hysteria based, with subconscious expression of visual symptoms. FVL may be seen in any age group but is seen in 1% to 5% of referrals to ophthalmologists. The total incidence may be greater, given that patients may also visit their general practitioners, internal medicine physicians, psychiatrists, or neurologists. The financial impact of FVL is estimated at an average of greater than $500 per patient spent on diagnosis and a potential of millions of dollars in claims for disability benefits, workers' compensations, or insurance claims. A thorough ophthalmologic and neuroophthalmologic examination should be undertaken before entertaining a diagnosis of FVL and a high level of suspicion is important for early diagnosis of FVL to prevent unnecessary investigations and false claims (Chen et al, 2007).

ORTHOPEDIC GAMUT 13-25

SUMMARY OF CLINICAL TESTS FOR FUNCTIONAL VISUAL LOSS

Clinical tests	Principle
Total binocular blindness	
Observation	Clue to true or simulated difficulties in visual tasks
Finger tip test	Proprioceptive tasks and does
Signature test	not require vision
Mirror test	Convergence, miosis and accommodation reflex
Optokinetic test	Optokinetic reflex of smooth pursuit
Pupil response	Detection of afferent and efferent pathway
Menace reflex	Shock value
Tearing reflex	Tearing with bright light
Monocular blindness	
Pupil response	Direct afferent visual pathway light testing
Fogging test	Elicit better vision than claimed
Stereopsis testing	Require binocular vision
Prism shift test	Demonstrates binocular vision
Reduced visual acuity	
Fogging test and stereoacuity	As above
Reduced visual field	
Visual field to confrontation, kinetic and static perimetry	Physiologic visual field characteristics

Adapted from Chen CS et al: Practical clinical approaches to functional visual loss, *J Clin Neurosci* 14(1):1-7, 2007.

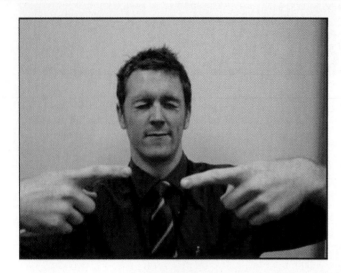

FIG. 13-51 The fingertip touching test is performed by asking the patient to bring the index fingers together. A truly blind patient can easily touch the tips of the fingers together. Those who are functionally blind tend not to. Similarly, the signature test is also a nonvisual task. A patient with organic visual loss can easily sign his or her name without difficulty, but a patient with functional visual loss may produce a bizarre signature. (Adapted from Chen CS et al: Practical clinical approaches to functional visual loss, *J Clin Neurosci* 14[1]:1-7, 2007.)

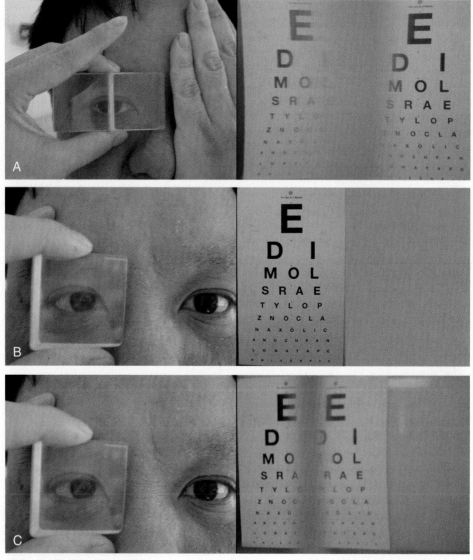

FIG. 13-52 The Prism Shift test or The diplopia test. **A,** The "blind eye" is occluded and a strong prism is placed over the "good eye" to produce monocular diplopia. **B,** The prism is then placed over the good eye. If only the good eye is seeing, it will see a single displaced image. **C,** If both eyes are seeing, there will be two images, one from the displaced image of the "good eye", the second image from the "blind eye". Hence if the patient admits to diplopia, he/she is seeing out of both eyes. (From Chen CS, Lee AW, Karagiannis A et al. Practical clinical approaches to functional visual loss, *J Clin Neurosci* 14[1]:1-7, 2007.)

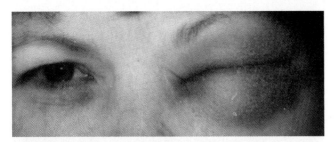

FIG. 13-53 Periorbital cellulitis (POC) presents as unilateral or bilateral periorbital inflammation and is seen most commonly in the pediatric age group. Common causes include paranasal sinusitis, upper respiratory tract infections, local cutaneous trauma, conjunctivitis, dacryocystitis and other causes. POC may also herald more grave underlying conditions, such as collagen-vascular disorders, systemic diseases, intraorbital or paranasal neoplasms. This 40-year-old female nurse had a history of 4 episodes of left POC. The POC appeared as a well-demarcated erythema limited to the left eyelid region with minimal edema. A CT scan revealed no evidence of sinus opacification or osteo meatal complex obstruction. The patient was suspected of self-injecting with an unknown irritant as a likely cause of POC. (Adapted from Sorin A, April MM, Ward RF: Recurrent periorbital cellulitis: an unusual clinical entity, *Otolaryngol Head Neck Surg* 134[1]:153-156, 2006.)

PROCEDURE

- The examination starts from the moment the patient walks into the consulting room, and much information can be gained by careful observation. A truly blind patient will move cautiously and bump into objects naturally. A functionally blind patient will deliberately bump into objects or exaggerate movements. Observe hand-shaking. Furthermore, observe the accompanying person and their behavior toward the patient. It provides a very strong clue to the *overall picture*.
- Without a positive Marcus Gunn phenomenon but with continued complaint of unilateral blindness, the examiner places a refractive lens over the *good* eye, ostensibly to test it (Fig. 13-54).
- The lens actually deprives the eye of any effective vision.
- The malingering patient is directed to read a Snellen chart (Fig. 13-55).
- This task is accomplished perfectly with the blind eye.

Next Steps/Procedures
Marcus Gunn sign, optokinetic nystagmus test, and Snellen test

13

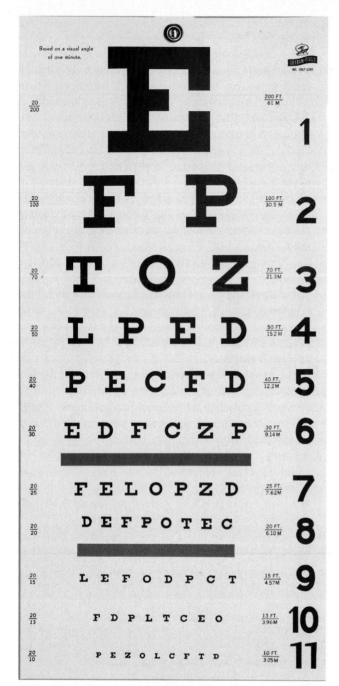

FIG. 13-54 The seated patient is placed at an appropriate distance from a Snellen eye chart. The patient is instructed to read the chart with one eye at a time. With simulated unilateral blindness, the patient will claim that the blind eye cannot read the chart.

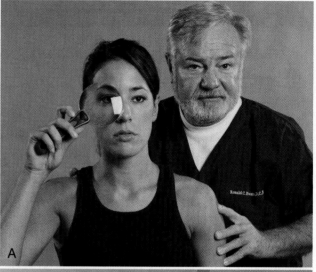

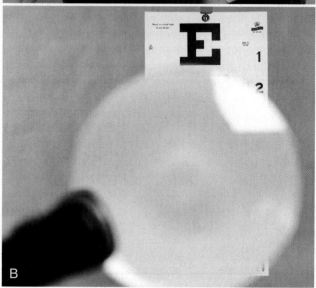

FIG. 13-55 The examiner places a refractive, but myopic lens over the *good eye,* ostensibly to aid its vision and test it (**A**). The patient is again instructed to read the Snellen chart. The lens deprives the eye of any effective vision. If the chart is read, *it was done so with the blind eye* (**B**). If the chart can be read, the test is positive and indicates simulated unilateral blindness.

Assessment for Hysterical or Simulated Face Anesthesia

Comment

The trigeminal nerve is one of the largest cranial nerves, sending fibers to innervate all muscles controlling jaw movements and the skin of virtually the whole face and skull. The trigeminal nerve and nuclei (the trigeminal

---

Adapted from Valls-Sole J: Neurophysiological assessment of trigeminal nerve reflexes in disorders of central and peripheral nervous system, *Clin Neurophysiol* 116(10):2255-2265, 2005.

---

complex) have interesting anatomic and physiologic peculiarities. No Renshaw cells have been identified in the trigeminal motor nucleus, and therefore trigeminal motoneurons have no recurrent inhibition. The trigeminal sensory nucleus is a complex structure, divided into many subnuclei extending from the mesencephalon to the spinal cord. One of the most striking anatomic peculiarities of the trigeminal complex is that the first-order sensory neurons for proprioceptive information are located inside the central nervous system, in the mesencephalic nucleus, when comparable sensory neurons from other muscles in the body are located in the dorsal root ganglia, one half covered only by the blood-brain barrier. *Vibration, which causes a decrease of the H reflex in limb muscles, induces potentiation in trigeminal motoneurons* [emphasis added] (Valls-Sole, 2005).

Neuritis is a disease of a nerve. As an affectation of a single nerve, it is called mononeuritis. As an affectation of two or more nerves in separate areas, the disease is called mononeuritis multiplex, and if it affects many nerves simultaneously, it is called polyneuritis. The term implies a syndrome of sensory, motor, reflex, and vasomotor symptoms, singly or in combination, produced by lesions of the nerve roots or peripheral nerves.

Sensory symptoms may be prominent. Descriptive terms—tingling, pins-and-needles sensation, burning, boring, and stabbing—are used by the patient. Pain, often worse at night, may be aggravated by touching the affected area or by temperature changes. Numbness and objective loss of sensation occur, in severe cases, in stocking-and-glove distributions. The nerve trunks may be tender. When sensory loss is profound, painless ulcers may appear on the digits or joints may be painlessly enlarged (Charcot joints).

Pain initiated by a primary lesion or dysfunction of the nervous system is defined as neuropathic pain. Neuropathic pain (NP) may be primary (no recognized pathologic process) or secondary, as in painful posttraumatic neuropathies. When affecting the orofacial region, NP is conveniently termed neuropathic orofacial pain (NOP) and includes a heterogeneous group of entities. Based on symptoms, NOP may be divided into two broad categories: paroxysmal and continuous. Paroxysmal neuropathies such as trigeminal neuralgia are characterized by short electrical or sharp pain. Continuous pain, sometimes of a burning quality, is characteristic of posttraumatic neuropathy and is a common feature in postherpetic neuralgia. Signs and symptoms highly associated with NP also include thermal and mechanical allodynia (Lewis et al, 2007).

ORTHOPEDIC GAMUT 13-26
LESIONS INVOLVING THE TRIGEMINAL COMPLEX

- Trigeminal nerve branches
- Isolated idiopathic trigeminal neuropathy
- Vasculitis
- Traumatism
- Lymphoma, bone tumors, metastasis
- Trigeminal tumors
- Trigeminal ganglion
- Herpes zoster
- Immunologic aggressions to Gasserian ganglia neurons
- Trigeminal neuralgia surgery
- Trigeminal nerve roots
- Meningioma, acoustic neurinoma, trigeminal neurinoma
- Aneurysms, vascular malformations
- Polyradiculoneuritis
- Vascular compression
- Trigeminal nuclei
- Infarcts, other vascular lesions in the brainstem
- Encephalitis and intraaxial tumors
- Demyelinating diseases of the central nervous system
- Syringobulbia
- Changes in excitability in trigeminal nerve mediated reflexes
- Parkinson disease and other parkinsonisms
- Cranial and cervical dystonia
- Huntington disease
- Various movement disorders (tics, head tremor; hemifacial spasm)

ORTHOPEDIC GAMUT 13-27

CLINICALLY APPLICABLE BRAINSTEM REFLEXES MEDIATED BY THE TRIGEMINAL NERVE

- Blink Reflex
- Corneal Reflex
- Masseteric Inhibitory Reflex
- Mandibular Reflex

PROCEDURE

- In a patient with symptoms of facial anesthesia, the examiner applies a vibrating tuning fork to the numb side of the patient's forehead near the midline (Fig. 13-56).
- The malingerer or hysteric will state that no sensation is felt.
- When the examiner moves the application of the tuning fork just across the midline, the patient now reports sensing the vibrations immediately.
- The **lack of vibration sense on the *numb* side is impossible** because the bone tissue conducts the vibration that is applied to the area of claimed anesthesia to the normal side.
- This test is valid even for a pathologic bone condition or an organic bone disease.

Next Steps/Procedures
Seeligmuller sign and anosmia testing

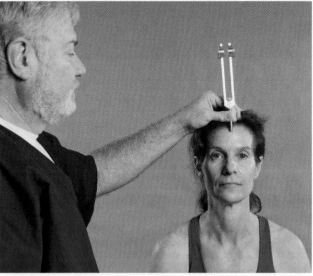

FIG. 13-56 The patient is seated. The examiner applies a vibrating tuning fork to the numb side of the forehead, near the midline of the forehead. The patient is asked to identify sensations of vibration across the forehead. If the patient denies feeling the vibration on the numb side of the forehead, the test is repeated just across the midline on the normal side of the forehead. If the patient feels the vibration only on the normal side, hysteria or malingering is suspected.

Assessment for Simulated Deafness

Comment

Perceptive deafness is impaired hearing caused by disorders of the inner ear, the eighth (auditory) nerve, cerebral pathways, or the auditory center.

Excessive noise is a common cause of hearing loss. The loss is more pronounced in the high frequencies and has traditionally been caused by industrial noise and exposure to heavy gunfire. Recently, the condition has appeared in adolescents, caused by excessive electronic amplification of music.

> Children with deafness are at risk of vestibular dysfunction because in some forms of inner ear deafness the damage extends to the vestibular receptor as well. Reports have been published of peripheral vestibular dysfunction and delayed postural control in some types of congenital or early-acquired deafness such as in inner ear malformations, meningitis, viral labyrinthitis, and some forms of hereditary deafness. Children with bilateral vestibular loss since birth or early life exhibit delayed gross motor development. These children stand and walk later than healthy children. However, the postural disturbances that result from isolated peripheral dysfunction are usually corrected by the time these children grow to be adolescents (Suarez et al, 2007).

Deafness is a form of sensory deprivation easily feigned and as easily tested. Although the complaint is the inability to hear any sound, the patient with such a conversion reaction may startle to a loud noise and can be awakened from a sound sleep by the same. A startled response to sound is an important finding when an examiner is testing a noncooperative, hysterical, or malingering patient. This phenomenon is based on the acoustic reflex. The reflex occurs with contraction of the stapedius and tensor tympani muscles in the middle ear in response to a loud sound. The muscle contractions pull the stapes out of the oval window and thus protect the inner ear from damage caused by a loud noise. The acoustic reflex threshold is the lowest level of sound that will elicit an acoustic reflex and is in the range of the 85- to 90-dB hearing level in individuals with normal hearing. Acoustic reflexes are usually elevated or absent in cases of conductive or neural hearing loss and present at normal or lower levels in the case of cochlear (inner ear) hearing loss.

> Given that neural changes take place following the early loss of hearing, investigation of visual perceptual processes from a lateralized perspective may be useful in understanding perceptual specialization. For instance, deaf individuals have demonstrated a right visual field-left hemisphere advantage for visual motion perception when compared with controls and left visual field-right hemisphere presentations. However, more recently, research revealed that lateralization effects for visual motion perception may be more influenced by experience with sign language relative to hearing loss per se. Finally, a left hemisphere advantage for motion processing has been supported by neuroimaging findings and by findings of studies employing evoked response potentials (Heming, Brown, 2005).

The eyelid movements are mediated mainly by the orbicularis oculi (OO) and the levator palpebrae superioris (LPS) muscles. Dissociated upper lid functions exhibit different counterbalanced action of these muscles, and in blinking they show a strictly reciprocal innervation. The disturbance of this close LPS-OO relationship likely leads to many of the central lid-movement disorders. Three groups of supranuclear motor impairment of lid movements are considered: (1) the disorders of the lid-eye movements' coordination, (2) the disturbances of blinking and lid *postural* maintenance, and (3) the alteration of voluntary lid movements (Esteban, Traba, Prieto, 2004).

ORTHOPEDIC GAMUT 13-28

CAUSES OF IMPAIRED HEARING

1. Involvement of the auditory structures in infectious diseases such as meningitis, syphilis, typhoid, mumps, measles, and hemolytic streptococcal infection
2. Tumors of the cerebellopontine angle, temporal lobe, eighth nerve, or cochlea
3. Trauma, such as from skull fracture
4. Injury by such toxic substances as quinine, arsenic, alcohol, salicylates, mercury, or aminoglycoside antibiotics (kanamycin)
5. Psychogenic disturbances
6. Physiologic dysfunction that may occur in senility and from excessive noise

---

ORTHOPEDIC GAMUT 13-29

COMPONENTS OF REFLEX BLINKING

- The inhibition of the basal tonic levator palpebrae superioris muscles, which keeps the eyes open
- The concurrent activation of the orbicularis oculi muscles

ORTHOPEDIC GAMUT 13-30
CONSIDERATIONS IN BLINKING

- Levator palpebrae superioris inhibition precedes and outlasts the orbicularis oculi activation.
- This normal configuration is impaired in parkinsonism and blepharospasm.
- Spontaneous blinking demonstrates a highly interindividual rate variation (among 10 to 20 per minute in adults).
- Abnormal blink rates occur in neurologic diseases related to dopaminergic transmission impairments.

PROCEDURE

- The examiner can gain a crude estimate of the patient's hearing ability by using the auditory-palpebral reflex.
- When a patient hears a loud sound, an involuntary blink is the response.
- With the patient's normal ear covered, an assistant standing behind the patient (out of the patient's line of sight) can clap the hands or pop a bag (Fig. 13-57).
- The examiner observes the patient for blinking or a startled response (Fig. 13-58).
- If the patient has a response, the examiner can be certain that the patient heard something.
- If the patient does not respond, the significance of the test is doubtful.

Next Steps/Procedure
Lombard test

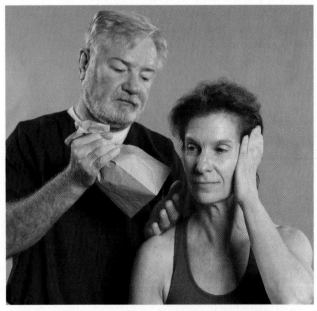

FIG. 13-57 The patient is seated and is instructed to cover the normal ear. The examiner or an assistant is positioned behind the patient, out of the patient's peripheral vision.

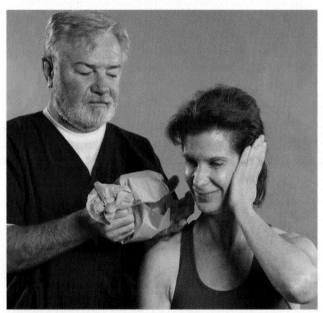

FIG. 13-58 The examiner or an assistant claps hands loudly or pops a bag. The examiner observes the patient for involuntary blinking or a startle response (auditory-palpebral reflex). If the response is present, the test is positive and indicates that the deaf ear heard something. This result suggests malingering.

JANET TEST

Assessment for Simulated Anesthesia

Comment

Hysterical paralysis of one limb usually provides little difficulty during diagnosis. The affected limb may be either rigid or flaccid, and there is no true muscular atrophy and no alteration in the muscular response to electrical stimulation. The reflexes provide the most information. With hysterical paralysis, the reflexes may be exaggerated, but they are never lost.

More often than not, a limb that is the seat of hysterical paralysis also presents complete insensibility to all forms of stimulation, and the upper limit of such anesthesia may end abruptly at a level for which no anatomic basis is found (Fig 13-59).

> Functional neuroimaging has revealed selective decreases in the activity of frontal and subcortical circuits involved in motor control during hysterical paralysis, decreases in somatosensory cortices during hysterical anesthesia, or decreases in visual cortex during hysterical blindness. Such changes are usually not accompanied by any significant changes in elementary stages of sensory or motor processing as measured by evoked potentials, although some changes in later stages of integration (such as P300 responses) have been reported (Vuilleumier, Steven, 2005).

PROCEDURE

- If anesthesia is the complaint, the patient is instructed to close the eyes (Fig. 13-60).
- The patient is then directed to answer *yes* if a pinprick is felt on the skin or *no* if not (Fig. 13-61).
- Obviously, the only appropriate answer is silence when the supposedly anesthetic area is touched.

Next Steps/Procedures
Facial anesthesia testing, midline tuning-fork test, and regional anesthesia testing

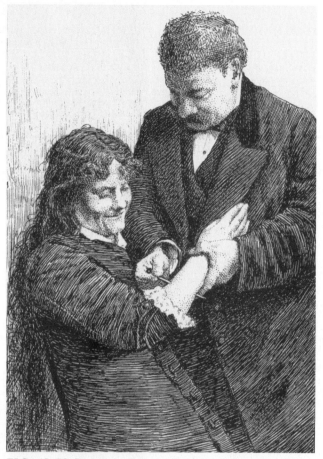

FIG. 13-59 In some respects, the most important change since classical descriptions of hysteria by Charcot and others at the end of the nineteenth century is related to the fact that the term *hysteria* was recently eliminated from the official psychiatric terminology. *L'anesthésie hystérique,* a cruel demonstration of anesthesia in a patient at La Salpêtrière, while in a state of hysteria (etched from photograph by P. Régnard, 1887, Les maladies épidémiques de l'esprit—Sorcellerie, magnétisme, morphinisme, délire des grandeurs, Plon-Nourrit, Paris). (From Uilleumier P, Steven L: *Hysterical conversion and brain function.* In: Progress in brain research, vol 150, Amsterdam, 2005, Elsevier.)

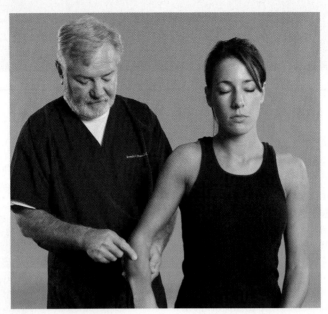

FIG. 13-60　In this test for anesthesia, the patient may be seated or recumbent. The patient is instructed to close the eyes.

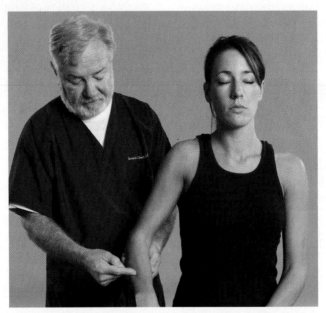

FIG. 13-61　As the examiner touches the involved part, either with a finger or sharp object, the patient is directed to **indicate feeling the touch by saying "yes" and not feeling the touch by saying "no."** The only appropriate answer, when the anesthetic area is touched, is silence. The test is positive when the patient identifies with the answer *no*. The test indicates hysteria or malingering.

LIMB-DROPPING TEST (UPPER EXTREMITIES)

Assessment for Feigned Unconsciousness

Comment

"Impaired consciousness is an expression of dysfunction in the brain as a whole," wrote Teasdale and Jennett in 1974, that "may be due to agents acting diffusely . . . or to the combination of remote and local effects produced by brain damage which was initially focal." The authors were from the Glasgow University Department of Neurosurgery Institute of Neurologic Sciences. In their view, the clinical assessment of unconsciousness suffered from the practice by many physicians to "retreat from any formal scheme in favor of a general description of the patient's state, without clear guidelines as to what to describe and how to describe it." This tendency, in turn, led to "ambiguities and misunderstandings when information about patients is exchanged and when groups of patients treated by alternative methods are compared" (Sternbach, 2000).

Level of consciousness is a term that refers to certain processes that provide awareness of one's self and the environment. Terms used to describe pathologic alterations in the level of consciousness are determined, largely by the degree of patient arousal. These alterations range from confusion to somnolence, stupor, and coma.

The examiner should be familiar with conditions that, in some respects, resemble stupor or coma. Akinetic mutism is a state of wakeful unresponsiveness in which the patient has no meaningful mental content or purposeful movement but seems to be awake. This condition may follow bilateral cerebral damage (the apallic state), lesions of the upper midbrain or diencephalon, and, rarely, hydrocephalus. The locked-in syndrome is a condition in which the patient is conscious and aware but paralyzed and anarthric. Eye movements are preserved and may be of use for communication. The condition is caused by a lesion of the ventral portion of the pons. Disease processes involving two general areas of the central nervous system can alter consciousness. These disease processes are lesions, either in both cerebral hemispheres or in the deep midline structures, in the upper brainstem near the central core of the gray matter.

The best known example use of the Glasgow Coma Scale (GCS) is the well-known recommendation that a patient with a GCS score of 8 or less is unable to protect the airway and requires endotracheal intubation. Another use is the categorical division of severity of head injury by GCS score of mild (13 to 15), moderate (9 to 12), and severe (8 or less).

Reduced awareness or faked stoicism is attempted to portray a reduced level of consciousness. In a conversion reaction or malingering, the pupillary and corneal reflexes and plantar responses will be normal, although reduced awareness or increased pain tolerance is exhibited.

ORTHOPEDIC GAMUT 13-31

THREE COMPONENTS OF THE GLASGOW COMA SCALE

- *Motor response:* The ease with which motor responses can be elicited in the limbs, together with the wide range of different patterns that can occur, makes motor activity a suitable guide to the functioning state of the central nervous system.
- *Verbal response:* Probably the commonest definition of the end of a coma, or the recovery of consciousness, is the patient's first understandable utterance.
- *Eye opening:* Spontaneous eye opening indicates that the arousal mechanisms in the brainstem are active.

ORTHOPEDIC GAMUT 13-32

GLASGOW COMA SCALE

Eye Opening	
Spontaneous	4
To speech	3
To pain	2
None	1
Best verbal response	
Oriented	5
Confused conversation	4
Inappropriate words	3
Incomprehensible sounds	2
None	1
Best motor response	
Obeys commands	6
Localizes pain	5
Withdrawal (normal flexion)	4
Abnormal flexion (decorticate)	3
Extension (decerebrate)	2
None	1

ORTHOPEDIC GAMUT 13-33

LEVEL OF CONSCIOUSNESS

Diseases producing disturbances of the level of consciousness fall into the following four main categories:

1. Supratentorial mass lesions that secondarily compress deep midline structures
2. Infratentorial lesions that directly damage the central brainstem core
3. Metabolic disorders that widely depress or interrupt cortical function
4. Psychiatric disorders resembling coma

ORTHOPEDIC GAMUT 13-34

GLASGOW-LIEGE SCALE

The five brainstem reflexes selected disappear in descending order during rostral-caudal deterioration. The disappearance of the last, the oculocardiac, coincides with brain death.

Brainstem Reflex	Points
Frontoorbicular	5
Vertical oculovestibular	4
Pupillary light	3
Horizontal oculovestibular	2
Oculocardiac	1
No response	0

PROCEDURE

- In many instances, when the examiner holds up the hand of a patient who is feigning reduced consciousness and lets the hand drop over the patient's face, the arms will consciously swerve to keep the hand from striking the face.
- A patient with an organically reduced level of consciousness will not make this movement of avoidance and will usually have pupillary abnormalities and other positive neurologic signs (Figs. 13-62 to 13-65).

Next Steps/Procedures

Coordination-disturbance testing, position-sense testing, and Romberg test

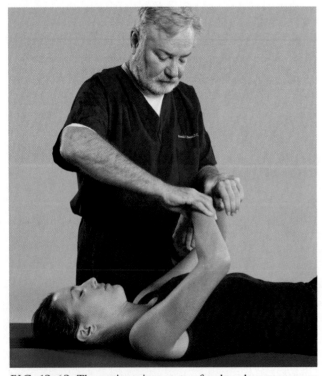

FIG. 13-62 The patient, in a state of reduced awareness or consciousness, is recumbent on the examination table. The examiner elevates the patient's arms by the wrists.

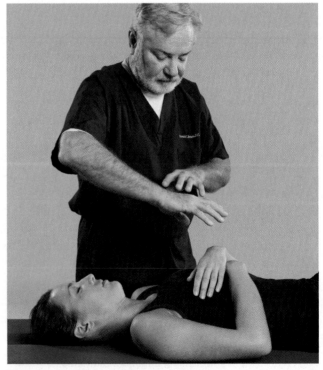

FIG. 13-63 The arms are allowed to drop over the patient's chest.

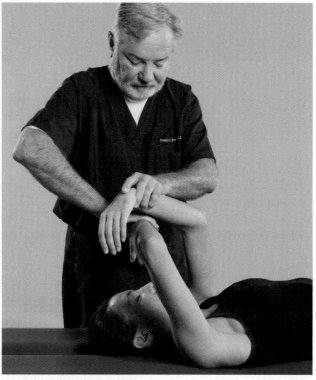

FIG. 13-64 The test is repeated, this time with the examiner holding the arms over the patient's head and face.

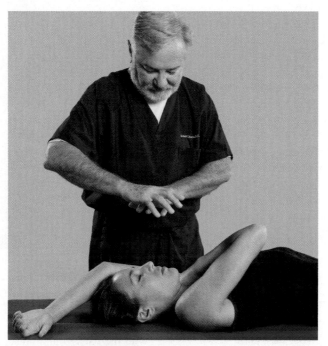

FIG. 13-65 The arms are allowed to drop. The test is positive when the arms are swerved to avoid striking the face. A positive test indicates a lack of organic basis for the reduced level of awareness or consciousness.

13

LOMBARD TEST

Assessment for Simulated Deafness

Comment

Anomalies of the external auditory canal, eardrum, middle ear, or eustachian tube that interfere with the conduction of sound waves to the inner ear may be responsible for conductive deafness. In this category are mechanical obstructions of the external auditory canal from a foreign object, cerumen, furuncle, osteoma, or stenosis. Perforation, scarring, or inflammation of the tympanic membrane also restrict sound-wave movement in the ear. Ankylosis of the ossicles, middle-ear inflammation (acute or chronic), tumor, or osteosclerotic involvement of the oval window margin restricts the vibration of the footplate of the stapes. Obstruction of the eustachian tube by inflammation, stenosis, tumor, or lymphoid hypertrophy at the ostium also diminishes conductive hearing.

Sudden deafness is defined as sensineural hearing loss with a deficit over 30 dB in at least three consecutive frequency areas during a 3-day period.

Psychologic factors or psychogenic stresses can be the cause of sudden hearing loss. Functional hearing loss or psychogenic hearing loss is used to describe any hearing loss that cannot be explained by an organic cause. Psychogenic hearing loss is classified as part of a conversion disorder in the field of psychiatry. The features include neurologic symptoms that cannot be explained by known neurologic or medical diseases, psychologic stress that is coexistent with symptoms, and confirmation that the symptoms are not purposeful or consciously motivated. The diagnosis of psychogenic hearing loss must be differentiated from malingering. Both can have a discrepancy in pure tone audiometry (PTA) and speech audiometry, but, in malingering, some distinctive features exist. When PTA and auditory brainstem response (ABR) tests are repeated, more than a 15-dB difference is found at the time of testing. In addition, the history given reveals inconsistencies that may be uncovered by psychiatric consultation (Ban, Jin, 2006).

- Lombard auditory test is a test of hearing that relies on the effect of induced noise on a subject's hearing responses (ABR).
- The test is used in the investigation of nonorganic hearing loss.
- The patient with hearing loss is seated for this examination.
- The examiner engages the patient in conversation or has the patient read aloud from a page.
- As the reading progresses or the conversation continues, background noise is induced and amplified (Fig. 13-66).
- If the patient's voice grows louder with the background noise, the testing is positive and indicates nonorganic hearing loss.

Next Steps/Procedure
Gault test

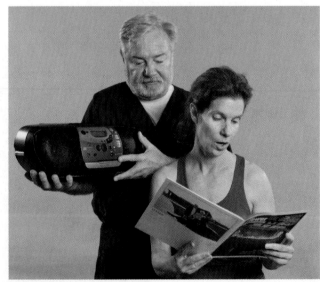

FIG. 13-66 The patient with hearing loss is seated for this examination. The examiner engages the patient in conversation or has the patient read aloud from a page. As the reading progresses or the conversation continues, background noise is induced and amplified. If the patient's voice grows louder with the background noise, the testing is positive and indicates nonorganic hearing loss.

Assessment for Normal Optic Neural Function

Comment

Fibrous dysplasia is an uncommon disease characterized by replacement of normal cancellous bone by fibrous tissue and immature woven bone.

The most notable ocular complication of fibrous dysplasia involving the sphenoid bone is visual loss secondary to optic nerve compression. Because the optic nerve lacks the potential to regenerate, damage to the nerve may be permanent, and the progressive nature of this disease can lead to irreversible blindness. Loss of vision may occur rapidly because of hemorrhage or mucocele within the dysplastic tissue. When constriction of the optic canal has occurred, decompression is technically more difficult, with a greater risk of optic nerve injury. In addition, once radiologic evidence of optic canal involvement is found, a 33% incidence of severe visual loss occurs (Edelstein, Goldberg, Rubino, 1998).

Optic neuritis is inflammation of that portion of the optic nerve that is ophthalmoscopically visible (Fig 13-67). This inflammation occurs with meningitis, encephalitis, syphilis, and acute febrile diseases; with foci of infection and multiple sclerosis; and with poisoning by methyl alcohol, carbon tetrachloride, lead, and thallium. Optic neuritis is almost always unilateral. Disturbances of vision are the only symptoms, which vary from minimal contraction of the visual field to enlargement of the blind spot to complete blindness and pain during motion of the globe.

Although the clinical presentation of optic neuritis (ON) has been documented for well over 100 years, only recently has organized clinical efforts codified the relevant clinical symptoms. ON is typically characterized by acute painful vision loss. It is typically monocular but may be bilateral in 15% of cases. Sixty-five percent of cases, however, are subclinically bilateral, as evidenced by visual field analysis. Vision loss ensues over a few hours to days but rarely extends beyond 2 weeks. Pain occurs in 90% of affected individuals, and the discomfort typically increases with eye movement. Overall, the clinical signs and symptoms of ON are identical to any other optic neuropathy: reduced central acuity, diminished color vision, visual field loss, and a relative afferent pupillary defect. In two thirds of cases, the optic nerve appears normal; however, one third of the time, optic disc swelling occurs. Typically, the swelling is mild, but in 5% of cases, severe swelling with hemorrhages occurs. The presence of disc edema in patients with monosymptomatic ON may modify the risk of developing multiple sclerosis (MS); therefore every patient should receive a careful funduscopic examination (Kaur, Bennett, Alireza, 2007).

Marcus Gunn sign represents an afferent pupillary defect caused by a lesion of the optic nerve. Resting pupil sizes are normal. Both direct and consensual pupillary responses are decreased (reduced constriction) with bright illumination of the involved side. Both responses are normal with illumination of the normal side. When moving the light back to the involved eye, both pupils dilate and both constrict with stimulation on the normal side. When applied monocularly, high-intensity stimulation normally results in a sustained contraction; when alternated between the two eyes, it is found to produce small transient responses similar to those obtained with low-intensity monocular stimulation.

Autonomic nervous system disturbances have been studied in several neurodegenerative disorders, such as multiple-system atrophy, but have also been reported in MS. Many patients with MS develop disturbances of sexual functions or urinary bladder and bowel functions. In addition, simple bedside tests have demonstrated abnormalities of sweating and cardiovascular tone. Furthermore, pupillary impairment, irrespective of the presence of ON, seems to be underestimated in MS. Both afferent and efferent pupillary defects have been reported in MS. The latter disturbances are clearly less frequent than visual-evoked potential abnormalities and appear to be caused by a different mechanism, which still remains unclear (de Seze et al, 2001).

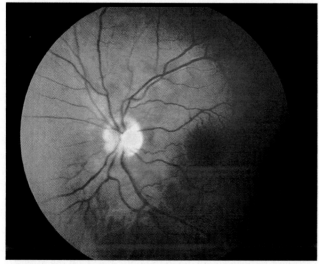

FIG. 13-67 Optic nerve head edema in optic neuritis, evidenced by peripapillary nerve fiber layer edema. (Adapted from Kaur P, Bennett JL, Alireza M: *Optic neuritis and the neuro ophthalmology of multiple sclerosis. In: International review of neurobiology,* vol 79, New York, 2007, Academic Press.)

PROCEDURE

- If an organic basis exists for unilateral blindness, the lesion must be situated anteriorly to the optic chiasm, and the pupillary reaction is usually abnormal.
- Marcus Gunn sign is especially useful for evaluating the existence of unilateral blindness.
- To elicit Marcus Gunn sign, the patient's eyes are fixed at a distant point and a strong light shone on the intact eye (Fig. 13-68).
- A crisp, bilateral contraction of the pupils is noted.
- On moving the light to the affected eye, both pupils dilate for a brief period (Fig. 13-69).
- When the light is returned to the intact eye, both pupils contract promptly and remain contracted (Fig. 13-70).
- This response indicates damage to the optic nerve on the affected side.

Next Steps/Procedures
Cuignet test, optokinetic nystagmus testing, and Snellen test

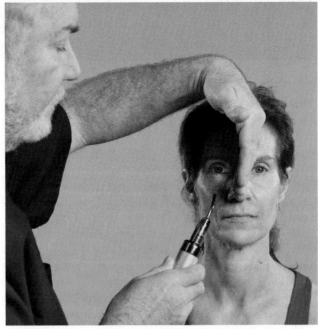

FIG. 13-68 To elicit the Marcus Gunn sign, the seated patient's eyes are fixed at a distant point. The examination room is dimmed, and a strong light is shone on the normal eye. The examiner notes a crisp bilateral contraction of the pupils.

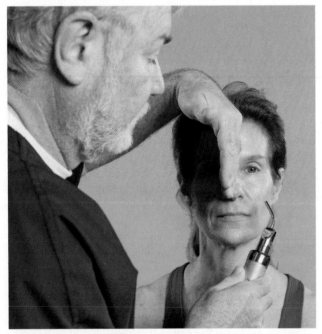

FIG. 13-69 On moving the light to the affected eye, both pupils dilate for a brief period.

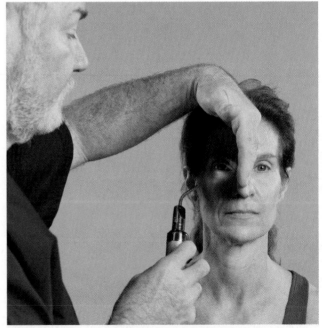

FIG. 13-70 On return of the light to the intact eye, both pupils contract promptly and remain contracted. This response indicates damage to the optic nerve on the affected side. The absence of Marcus Gunn sign in unilateral blindness indicates a nonorganic basis for the complaint.

MIDLINE TUNING-FORK TEST

Assessment for Simulated Anesthesia

Comment

Fibers conveying touch, superficial pain, and temperature pass via cutaneous nerves to mixed nerves, where they are joined by fibers carrying impulses from joints, ligaments, and muscles. Lesions of cutaneous nerves will not cause proprioceptive sensory loss, but interruption of mixed nerves and pure motor nerves will. All sensory fibers have their cell station in the ganglia of the cranial nerves or the posterior spinal roots. The spinal roots enter the posterolateral aspect of the cord in the root entry zone. Fibers conveying touch and postural sensibility pass upward in the posterior columns to the nuclei gracilis and cuneatus in the medulla. Those from the lower half of the body lie medially, and those from the upper half of the body occupy the lateral portion of the posterior column. These fibers cross the midline of the central nervous system as sensory decussation, form the medial lemniscus, and then pass upward through the brainstem to the thalamus.

> Radiating back pain is usually divided into pseudoradicular and radicular syndromes. The rationale behind this distinction stems from the assumption that neuropathic versus nociceptive pain types differ concerning their underlying pain generating mechanism. In pseudoradicular LBP, a proximal nociceptive event–like mechanical factor, musculoskeletal dysfunctions, degenerative changes in connective tissues, and local or even systemic inflammation are regarded to lead to a referred sensation in proximal dermatomes of the leg (nociceptive component). A convergent afferent input from deep somatic and cutaneous domains to spinothalamic tract neurons may explain this phenomenon (convergence-projection theory). In contrast, compression or damage to a nerve root by a protruded intervertebral disc or an inflammatory cause (e.g. leakage of inflammatory substances from the ruptured nucleus pulposus) are suspected to be the main causes of radicular pain that is therefore categorized as pain with a neuropathic component (Freynhagen et al, 2008).

Many feigned complaints fall in the category of sensory loss. Complaints of this kind are usually associated with numbness or anesthesia of a body part. The major distinguishing factor between feigned numbness and organic anesthesia is the disregard of the former for anatomic continuity. Indeed, feigned numbness includes all levels of sense (e.g., light touch, heat, cold, position, deep pressure). However, such instances of sensory loss are physically impossible without

spinal cord transection. Conversion reactions that involve only the sensory systems are difficult to prove. Organic sensory losses follow known anatomic distributions, but conversion reaction sensory disturbances follow the patient's perception of human anatomy.

PROCEDURE

- Patients with organic sensory disturbances are able to perceive a vibrating tuning fork placed on either side of the head or on either side of the sternum because the conduction vibrates through the bone (Fig. 13-71).
- In a conversion reaction, the sternum or head is split.
- For example, vibration is perceived on one side of the midline of the forehead or sternum but not on the other.

Next Steps/Procedures
Janet test and regional anesthesia testing

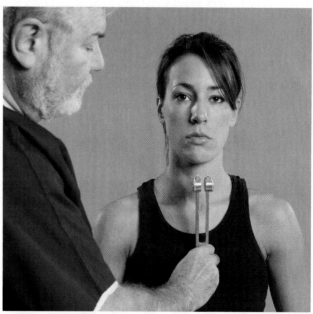

FIG. 13-71 The patient may be seated or recumbent. The examiner places a vibrating tuning fork on the affected side of the sternum near the midline. The patient is instructed to identify areas of perceived vibration. If the patient does not feel the vibration, the tuning fork is moved across the midline to the normal side. The test is positive if the patient identifies that vibration is felt only on the normal half of the body and not on the affected side. The positive test indicates hysteria, conversion reaction, or malingering.

Assessment for Feigned Blindness

Comment

Objective measurement of visual acuity by optokinetic nystagmus (OKN) can be used to differentiate FVL; to estimate visual acuity in children, in patients with developmental delay, mental retardation, or psychiatric disorders, and in animals; and to judge visual disturbance or to evaluate disease courses. The validity of visual acuity measurement by OKN suppression and OKN induction has been established (Shin et al, 2006).

Nystagmus is a rhythmic horizontal or vertical oscillation of the eyeballs. This oscillation is more pronounced when the patient is looking in certain directions (Bard sign) (Fig 13-72). Nystagmus is often a sign of cerebellar, vestibular, or labyrinthine disease, and it is a common sign in certain systemic diseases, such as MS. Prolonged use of the eyes with insufficient illumination and in strained positions, such as that maintained by miners, and fatigue of the eye muscles, especially when caused by errors of refraction, also may be causative. Vestibular stimulation causes nystagmus. Bard's sign is demonstrated by the increased oscillations of the eyeball in organic nystagmus when the patient tries to follow visually a target moved from side to side across the line of

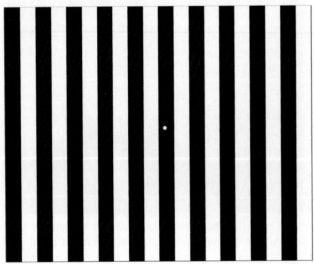

FIG. 13-72 Optokinetic nystagmus is elicited with alternating white and black vertical stripes. Induction of OKN response is a sign that patients recognize the stimuli. The superimposition of a stationary white dot detection stimulus is used to suppress OKN response. Suppression of OKN response is a sign that the stimuli is recognized by patients. (Adapted from Shin YJ, Park KH, Hwang J-M et al: Objective measurement of visual acuity by optokinetic response determination in patients with ocular diseases, *Am J Ophthalmol* 141[2]:327-332, 2006.)

sight. Such oscillations usually cease during the same test if the patient has congenital nystagmus.

The control of gaze can be considered as the coordination of eye movements around three rotational axes (horizontal, vertical, and torsional eye movements) in harmony with the coordination of head movements. The coordination of eye and head movements presents a challenging scenario to the brain, given that the head rotates around three rotational axes, which are not equivalent to the axes of eye rotations, and the head can also move in three translational directions. With respect to oculomotor control in humans, a sophisticated array of eye movements are available to optimize the acquisition of visual information falling on the retina. Saccades serve to bring a target of interest onto the fovea rapidly. Fixational eye movements keep a static target on the fovea, and smooth pursuit tracks a moving target. If the whole visual field is moving, the vestibulo-ocular reflex, driven by vestibular input, and OKN, driven by visual input, act to reduce movement of retinal images (Proudlock, Gottlob, 2007).

PROCEDURE

- With faked blindness, the patient will often avoid personal injury when walking and will blink to unexpected physical threats.
- Pupillary reactions are normal, and OKN is normal.
- To demonstrate optokinetic nystagmus, the examiner instructs the patient to keep the eyes open.
- The examiner holds a ruler or a tape measure 10 inches in front of the patient's face, ostensibly to measure pupillary distances (Fig. 13-73).
- As the pupils constrict, which demonstrates attempted focusing, the ruler is moved from left to right across the patient's field of vision (Fig. 13-74).
- A patient who can see the ruler will fix the vision on the vertical markings and develop an involuntary eye movement, which is known as OKN.
- This phenomenon is a similar to the one a person exhibits while riding in a vehicle and looking out the window and watching telephone poles go by.
- This test is used when routine eye examination reveals a normal fundus and intact pupillary reactions to light.
- With organic blindness, pupillary reflexes are abnormal, and OKN is absent.
- Hysterical field defects, when plotted out on a tangent screen, will not change with the varying distance between the patient and the screen.

Next Steps/Procedures

Cuignet test, Marcus Gunn sign, and Snellen test

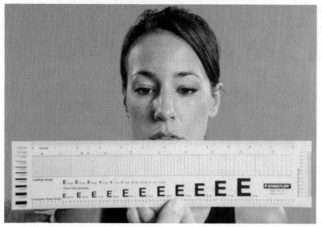

FIG. 13-73 The patient is seated. The examiner instructs the patient to keep the eyes open. A ruler or a tape measure is held approximately 10 inches in front of the patient's face. The examiner holds the ruler still and observes the patient's eyes for slight pupil constriction, indicating the attempt of the eyes to focus on the ruler markings.

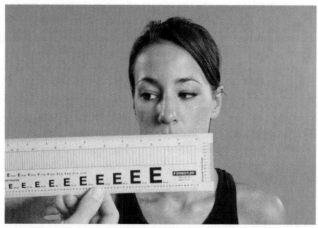

FIG. 13-74 The ruler is moved from left to right, across the patient's field of vision. A patient who can see the ruler will fix the vision on the vertical markings and develop an involuntary eye movement, called *optokinetic nystagmus*. This test is used when routine eye examination reveals a normal fundus and intact pupillary reactions to light. Optokinetic nystagmus OKN suggests a lack of organic basis for the blindness.

13

Assessment for Feigned Loss of Position Sense

Comment

Hereditary spastic paraplegia is characterized by a gradual onset of progressive lower-extremity weakness and spasticity. This condition is genetically heterogeneous, and, thus far, more than 30 genes have been implicated. Autosomal-dominant hereditary spastic paraplegia is the most common mode of inheritance, accounting for almost 80% of all familial cases. The diagnosis is typically straightforward in patients with a clear family history but can be more challenging if this history is unknown or is absent (Blair et al, 2007).

Hereditary spastic paraplegia is familiar, but it may be present without a history of cases in previous generations because sporadic cases do occur. The symptoms are those of a slowly progressive degeneration of the pyramidal tracts, starting between 3 and 15 years of age but rarely at older ages. For a time, only a spastic paraplegia is present, but gradually spastic weakness spreads to the upper limbs and ultimately to the bulbar muscles. No sensory loss occurs, but optic atrophy may occur. The disease takes many years to run its course and is one of the heredofamilial groups, of which Friedreich's ataxia is the best known. With Friedreich's ataxia, symptoms usually come on in childhood or adolescence, and the earliest complaints are of weakness and clumsiness of the legs. Ataxia of gait is apt to obscure the presence of weakness because of pyramidal degeneration, more so because tendon reflexes are diminished or absent, and tone is reduced. The ataxia is caused partly by degeneration of the spinocerebellar tracts and partly by loss of position sense.

Discriminative sensory loss is common after stroke but may not be adequately detected by routine neurologic measures. Loss of body sensations, such as touch and proprioceptive discrimination, occur in 50% to 85% of people who experience a stroke. This loss is important in its own right and impairs effective exploration of the environment and performance of everyday tasks such as grasp and manipulation of objects. This loss adversely affects quality of life, personal safety, and motor recovery and has been found to be a factor contributing to poor functional outcome and longer rehabilitation in several studies. Clinicians in acute and rehabilitation hospitals are frequently required to assess and monitor the presence of tactile and proprioceptive discrimination impairment. Because the decision to treat a patient is dependent on this detection, accurate identification of sensory loss is clinically important. If incorrect decisions are made, a patient who requires treatment may not receive it, or valuable treatment time may be used inappropriately (Carey, Matyas, Oke, 2002).

PROCEDURE

- If a patient claims that the position of a body part cannot be differentiated, the patient is directed to close the eyes, and the examiner bends the patient's fingers or toes up or down (Fig. 13-75).
- The patient is instructed to state what direction the examiner is bending the digit.
- A patient may report contrary findings by saying "up" when the examiner is bringing the digit down, and vice versa (Fig. 13-76).
- With organic sensory loss, the patient has a 50% chance of correctly guessing the digit position.
- The malingerer's reporting average is always contrary to the actual digit position and therefore incorrect a majority of the time.

Next Steps/Procedures
Coordination-disturbance testing, limb-dropping test (upper extremities), and Romberg test

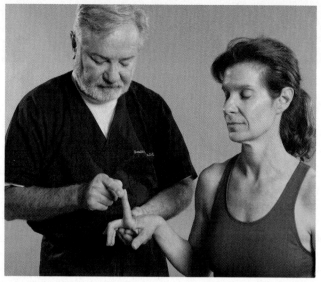

FIG. 13-75 The patient may be seated or recumbent. The patient is instructed to close the eyes. The examiner bends the patient's finger (or toe) up.

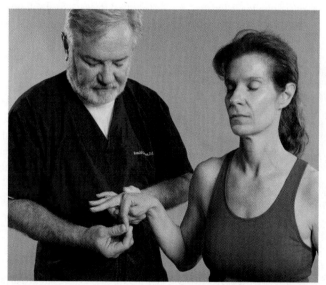

FIG. 13-76 The finger or toe is then bent down. The patient is instructed to identify the direction of the digit movement. The patient may report contrary findings to the actual position of the digit. In organic sensory loss, the patient has a 50% chance of success rate at guessing the digit position. The test is positive when the patient is consistently wrong. This result suggests malingering.

13

Assessment for Feigned Anesthesia

Comment

Physical findings of Dejerine-Roussy syndrome are largely sensory phenomena, although impairment of proprioception, hemiplegia, hemiparesis, or other motor abnormalities may be present. Additionally, no pathognomonic or universal pain features exist describing pain of thalamic origin or any form of central poststroke pain. It may affect the entire ipsilateral body, or it may be concentrated in only the upper or lower quadrants. The crucial factor for development of central *thalamic-type* pain is the presence of a spinothalamic pathway lesion. This tract is significant for transmitting temperature and pain sensibility, converging with sensation pathways in the ventral posterior lateral nucleus of the thalamus. Specifically, the spinoreticular fibers are thought to play a role in the nonspecific discomfort and pain of Dejerine-Roussy syndrome. Of note, the level of the lesion along the central neuraxis is not critical for the development of pain sensation; the location, however, is important for the characterization of associated neurologic symptoms (i.e., sensory and emotional reactions) (Ferrante, Rana, Ferrante, 2004).

Conversion of anxiety into symptoms of dysfunction of various organs or parts of the body is a common characteristic of conversion hysteria. The emotional conflict, instead of being experienced consciously, is converted into physical symptoms involving voluntary muscles or special sense organs. The patient often appears unconcerned about the sensory or motor paralysis (la belle indifference). The reaction not only serves to allay anxiety but may also provide some secondary gain. The conversion symptom does not always follow the anatomic distribution of the sensorimotor nerves, but it is determined symbolically (glove or stocking anesthesia, tunnel vision). These reactions help in understanding the nature of the unconscious conflict.

PROCEDURE

- To define a regional complaint of numbness, the examiner uses a straight pin or a Wartenberg pinwheel and delineates the areas where the claimed numbness ceases.
- The usual organic cause of anesthesia or paresthesia is peripheral neuritis.
- With peripheral neuritis, the upper border of the anesthesia is blurry and usually different for each different sensation tested, such as pain, touch, heat, and vibration.
- In the hysterical or malingering patient, the border of anesthesia is extremely abrupt, stopping at a wrist crease or some other external anatomic area that is unrelated to the dermatome pattern (Fig. 13-77).
- This numbness landmark may even vary from examination to examination.
- Most malingerers claim a simultaneous loss of all forms of sensation, including touch, pain, temperature, and vibratory sensation.
- All losses are identical as to extent and accurate neural distribution or dermatome patterns are not present.

ORTHOPEDIC GAMUT 13-35
THALAMIC PAIN

Patients with thalamic pain exhibit the following characteristics:

- Ipsilateral, constant, severe pain, described as "crushing, aching, or burning"
- Paroxysmal episodes of hypersensitivity to stimulation, making sensory examinations difficult if not impossible
- Increased sensory threshold and referred pain over a wide area
- A distinct lag between the time of application and the subsequent recognition of a stimulus also noted
- Coupled with this delayed appreciation, stimulus-induced pain described as having a more prolonged duration than that of the stimulus duration itself

Next Steps/Procedures
Janet test and midline tuning-fork test

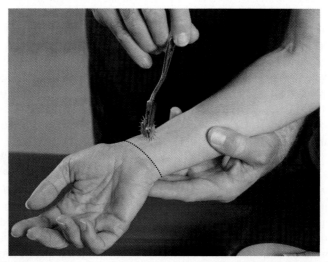

FIG. 13-77 The patient may be seated or recumbent for this test. The patient identifies the area of numbness. The examiner, using a pin or Wartenberg pinwheel, delineates the boundaries of the numbness. The test is positive when the borders of the anesthesia are extremely abrupt, stopping at some anatomic landmark unrelated to the dermatome involved. Such a sensory deficit distribution suggests malingering or hysteria.

13

ROMBERG SIGN

ALSO KNOWN AS STATION TEST

Assessment for Nonorganic Ataxia

Comment

Vestibular neuritis is the second most common cause of peripheral vestibular vertigo; its incidence in the population is 3.5 in 100,000. The most distinctive clinical features of the disease are sudden onset of rotatory vertigo, spontaneous horizontal or horizonto-rotatory nystagmus, nausea, and vomiting. This disease is also termed *neuronitis* because both the labyrinth and the vestibular nerve can be affected. The cause of the disease is multifactorial. Preceding respiratory infection may have a role in the cause of pediatric cases. Only in 7% of vertigo cases, viral pathogens were demonstrated, especially mumps, rubella, herpes simplex virus type 1, cytomegalovirus, and Epstein-Barr virus. Enteroviruses are among the other rare viral causes (Ergul et al, 2006).

These patients may also exhibit a positive Romberg sign and a positive head-thrust test.

Tabetic or ataxic gait is characteristic of posterior column disease and results from the loss of proprioceptive sense in the extremities. The patient walks on a wide base, slapping the feet, and usually watches the legs to know where they are. When the eyes are closed or the patient is in the dark, the ataxia is much worse. Clumsiness and uncertainty are characteristic. The feet are placed too widely apart, and in taking a step, the patient lifts the advancing leg abruptly and too high and then stamps or slaps the foot solidly to the ground. Uneven spacing of steps, tottering, and swaying occur, usually with deviation to one side or the other. Gait disturbance may be the result of obturator nerve compression, with pressing of the *Howship-Romberg* sign.

Romberg sign is no longer thought to be pathognomonic of tabes, but it may occur with a significant loss of position sense in the lower extremities as a result of any cause. Some authors use the term if imbalance occurs only with the eyes closed. Gowers thought that *in tabes* (locomotor ataxia) imbalance occurred with the eyes closed early in the disease, but as the disease progressed, unsteadiness would occur, although to a lesser degree with the eyes open. Finally, Adams and colleagues state that the term Romberg sign should be used if only discrepancy in balance is marked with the eyes open and closed. Some worsening of imbalance occurs with the eyes closed in cerebellar disease, but usually the discrepancy is not as marked as it is when position sense is significantly impaired (Cole, Michael, Robert, 2003).

The *Howship-Romberg* sign is the term used to describe pain along the distribution of the obturator nerve caused by compression of the nerve and is thought to be a specific symptom of an obturator hernia (Fig 13-78).

PROCEDURE

- With this disorder of balance loss, the patient is instructed to stand with the feet together, first with the eyes open, then with the eyes closed (Fig. 13-79).
- With organic sensory ataxia, the patient will sway the body from the ankles (Fig. 13-80).
- Swaying from the hips toward a wall to catch one's self in the nick of time suggests malingering (Fig. 13-81).

Next Steps/Procedures

Coordination-disturbance testing, limb-dropping test (upper extremities), and position-sense testing

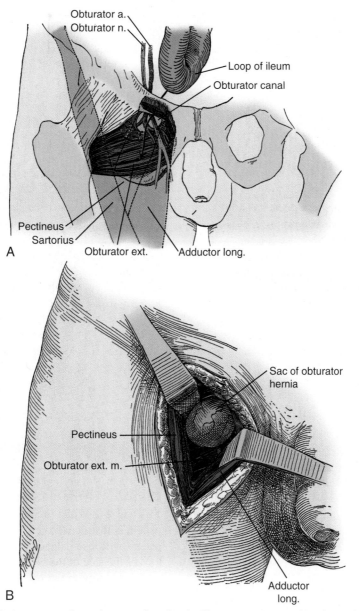

FIG. 13-78 Anatomy of an obturator hernia. **A,** The structures passing through the obturator canal, in order of their superposition behind the hernial sac, are the obturator nerve, artery, and vein. **B,** Hernia in the obturator canal, the most common type of obturator hernia. The sac lies on the obturator externus muscle and is covered by the pectineus. The obturator nerve is seen directly behind the sac. Three clinical signs are specific to incarceration of an obturator hernia. Obturator neuralgia is manifested as cramping or as hypoesthesia or hyperesthesia extending from the inguinal crease to the anteromedial aspect of the thigh. The Howship-Romberg sign is characterized by pain radiating down the medial aspect of the thigh to the knee and less often to the hip. The pain is a result of compression of the obturator nerve (anterior division) by the hernia sac within the canal and is relieved by flexion and external rotation of the thigh and exacerbated by extension, adduction, and medial rotation of the leg. The Howship-Romberg sign is considered pathognomonic for an incarcerated obturator hernia and is present in 25% to 50% of patients. The Hannington-Kiff sign is absence of the obturator reflex in the thigh, which is caused by compression on the obturator nerve. This reflex can usually be elicited by placing an extended index finger across the adductor muscle approximately 5 cm above the knee and percussing over the finger. Muscle contraction should be seen or felt with an intact reflex. If the patellar reflex of the ipsilateral side is present in the absence of an obturator reflex, it is highly likely that the obturator nerve is compressed. (From Watson LF: *Hernia,* ed 3, St Louis, 1948, CV Mosby.)

13

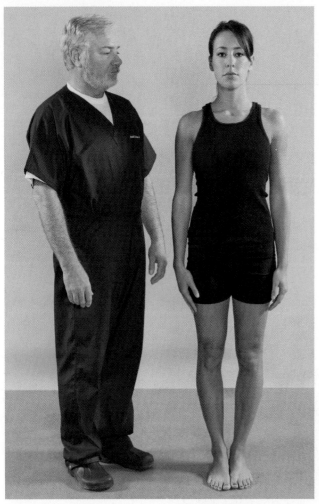

FIG. 13-79 The patient is standing and instructed to place the feet close together. The patient's eyes are open.

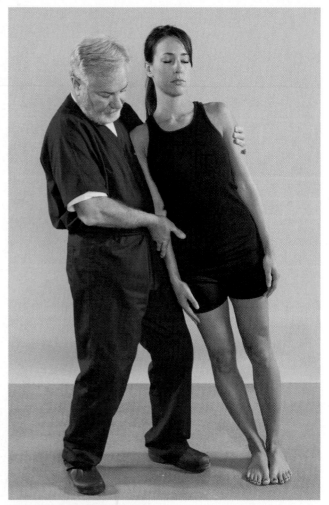

FIG. 13-80 While maintaining this narrowed base, the patient is instructed to close the eyes. In organic ataxia, the patient will lose balance usually by falling from the ankles toward the side of the cerebellar lesion. The examiner maintains proximity to the patient for safety.

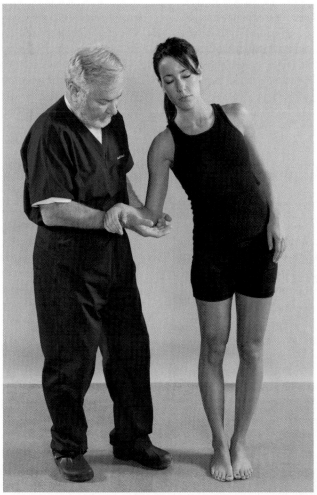

FIG. 13-81 The malingering patient will sway from the pelvis, usually toward a wall, catching the fall in the nick of time. In this instance, the sign is absent and indicates a lack of organic basis for the patient's loss of balance.

13

SNELLEN TEST

Assessment for Feigned Color Blindness

Comment

Defective color vision can be acquired by any kind of agent with the capacity to disturb the normal functioning of the visual system—the result of ocular disease, intracranial injury, the use of therapeutic drugs, aging, and so on. Frequently, color disturbances are initial symptoms of diseases and can be used for early detection, indicating when therapeutic measures should begin or when they should be discontinued (Lillo, Moreira, Charles, 2004).

ORTHOPEDIC GAMUT 13-36

COLOR BLINDNESS

Color blindness may be hereditary or acquired. Hereditary types are transmitted as recessive characteristics, sometimes X-linked. These characteristics include the following:
1. Achromatopsia (total color blindness)
2. Monochromatism (partial color blindness, with ability to recognize one of the three basic colors remaining)
3. Dichromatism (ability to recognize two of the three basic colors)

In normal (trichromatic) vision, the eye can perceive three light primaries (red, blue, and green) and can mix these in suitable portions; thus, white or any color of the spectrum can be matched. Color blindness can result from a lessened capacity to match three primary colors. It can be dichromatic vision, in which only one pair of the primary colors is perceived, the two colors being complementary to each other. Most dichromats are red-green blind and confuse red, yellow, and green (Table 13-6).

The mechanism of color vision depends critically on a comparison of the photon catch of different types of cone photoreceptors that are maximally sensitive at different wavelengths. This is the process of *opponency* whereby different photoreceptors are stimulated to different extents by light of differing spectral content. Comparison of these signals by the brain provides the sensation of color. From this process, it follows that color vision requires a minimum of two different types of cone photoreceptors to be present (Hunt, Sydney, Jeffrey, 2001).

Clinical characteristics of achromatopsia include reduced visual acuity, pendular nystagmus, increased sensitivity to light, a small central scotoma, normal peripheral visual fields, eccentric fixation, significant refractive error, and reduced or complete loss of color discrimination. Electrodiagnostic testing shows an extinguished or markedly reduced photopic response in combination with normal scotopic function. Paradoxical pupillary constriction in darkness has been reported in patients with achromatopsia. Fundus appearance is usually normal, although subtle macular changes and vessel narrowing may be present in some patients. Unlike conditions that cause progressive cone degeneration, achromatopsia results in relatively stable

---

TABLE 13-6

COMPARISON OF ACQUIRED AND CONGENITAL COLOR VISION DEFICIENCIES

Acquired Color Vision Defect	Congenital Color Vision Defect
Onset after birth	Onset at birth
Monocular differences in the type and severity of the defect occur frequently	Both eyes are equally affected
Color alterations are frequently associated with other visual problems such as low acuity and reductions in the useful visual (except in rod monochromatism) or visual field	The visual problems are specific to color perception; there are no problems with acuity field
The type and severity of the deficiency fluctuate throughout life	The type and severity of the defect are the same
The type of defect might not be easy to classify; combined or nonspecific defects occur frequently	The type of defect can be classified precisely
Predominantly either protan or deutan	Predominantly tritan
Higher incidence in men	Same incidence in both sexes

Adapted from Lillo JA, Moreira H, Charles S: Color blindness. In *Encyclopedia of applied psychology,* New York, 2004, Elsevier.

visual acuity throughout the patient's lifetime. The most debilitating symptom of achromatopsia has repeatedly been identified as severe photophobia. The absence of normal cone inhibition of rod function leads to a significant degradation of image quality in bright illumination (Schornack, Brown, Siemsen, 2007).

PROCEDURE

- For pretended color blindness in one eye, the patient is requested to look at alternate red and green letters (Fig. 13-82).
- The admittedly good eye is covered with a red glass (Fig. 13-83).
- If the green letters are read, evidence of fraud is present.

Next Steps/Procedures
Cuignet test, Marcus Gunn sign, and OKN testing

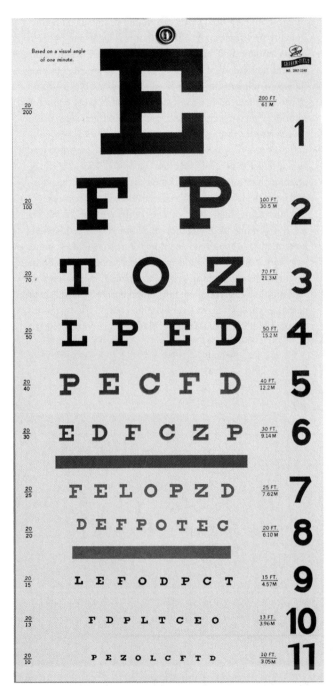

FIG. 13-82 The seated patient is placed an appropriate distance from a Snellen eye chart. The patient is instructed to read the red and green letters, using one eye at a time. The patient will state that the color blind eye cannot read the chart.

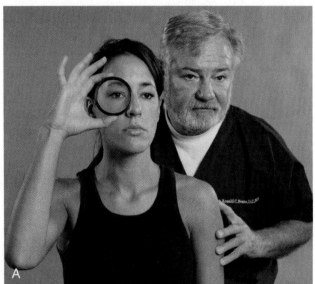

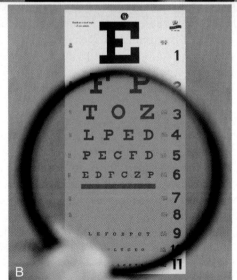

FIG. 13-83 The *vision of the good eye is obscured with a red lens,* and the patient is instructed to reread the chart (**A**). If the *green letters are read,* the test is positive (**B**). A positive test indicates that the vision of the alleged colorblind eye is preserved, suggesting malingering.

Assessment for Congenital Insensitivity to Pain

Comment

Although it is rare, some patients are born with a lack of any pain appreciation. This condition is a congenital indifference to pain or an inability to perceive it at all. Whether the patient feels the pain but is indifferent to it or whether the patient lacks any pain sensation is difficult to determine. The patient does not suffer. The cause of this congenital absence of pain perception is unknown. As children, these patients undergo falls and bumps but never cry. The defect is central rather than peripheral because the child recognizes the stimulus without exhibiting signs of pain. Normal nerve endings, which subserve pain sensibilities, are found in the skin and periosteum. Free nerve endings are also found in the glandular tissue. Progressive degenerative changes of the Charcot type are observed in the adult joints of these patients.

Individuals vary widely in their sensitivity to painful stimuli. Some exhibit heightened reactions to pain (hyperpathia), whereas others show relative indifference. This variability can be attributed, in part, to the cultural context and to individual psychologic factors. However, varying sensitivities to pain also can be caused by underlying differences in nociceptive neurophysiologic responses. For example, peripheral inflammation or central sensitization can produce heightened sensitivity. Conversely, insensitivity to pain can represent a blunted or absent response of the sensory nervous system, either on a congenital basis or secondary to disease or injury. Studying cases of insensitivity or apparent indifference to pain is useful because these *experiments of nature* may provide insights into the structure and function of nociceptive systems. Furthermore, cases of insensitivity to noxious stimuli in the presence of preserved function of other sensory modalities may provide clues to therapeutic targets for patients who suffer from painful illnesses and injuries. Congenital disorders of the sensory nervous system that reduce sensitivity to noxious stimuli include the hereditary sensory and autonomic neuropathies. Acquired diseases that decrease pain sensation include small fiber neuropathies, such as can be seen in diabetes or leprosy. Underlying disorders of the nervous system have been identified in all reported instances of decreased sensitivity to pain. A unifying observation is the disruption of small-fiber function. This fact is evident in test results that demonstrate, among other findings, decreased sweating and decreased small-fiber counts on nerve biopsy (Sandroni et al, 2006).

Intact corneal sensation plays a vital role in maintaining the integrity of the corneal epithelium. Not only is it an important mechanism in preventing injury through the blink reflex and reflex tearing, it also aids healing of epithelial defects by promoting epithelial cell proliferation. Enhanced epithelial-cell proliferation is thought to be mediated by neurotransmitters and nerve growth factors released from corneal nerve ending. Reduced or absent corneal sensation therefore renders the corneal surface vulnerable to occult injury and delayed healing of established corneal epithelial injuries. Punctate keratitis and epithelial loss may also occur spontaneously in the presence of reduced corneal sensation and may progress to corneal perforation. They may also lead to the development of infectious keratitis. The lack of the afferent limb of corneal sensation causes the mucous component of the tear film to increase, causing it to become more viscous. More than 24% of eyes with corneal anesthesia after trigeminal root alcohol injection developed serious keratopathy, although the potential for neurotrophic keratitis can vary. Absent or reduced corneal sensation may be acquired or congenital in origin. Congenital lack of corneal sensation may be complete congenital corneal anesthesia or partial to varying degrees (congenital corneal hypoesthesia) (Ramaesh et al, 2007). (Fig. 13-84)

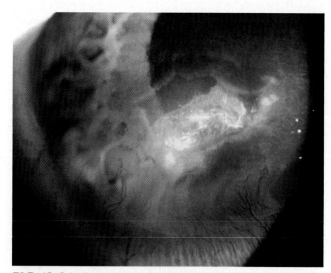

FIG. 13-84 Corneal opacity observed in a patient with congenital insensitivity to pain with anhidrosis. (Adapted from Ramaesh K et al: Congenital corneal anesthesia, *Surv Ophthalmol* 52[1]:50-60, 2007.)

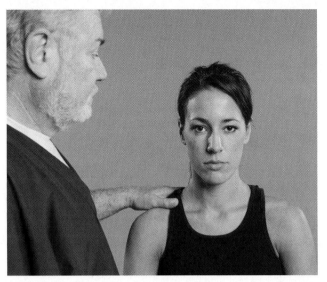

FIG. 13-85 The patient is seated, and the examiner observes the interval between blinks as the patient stares straight ahead.

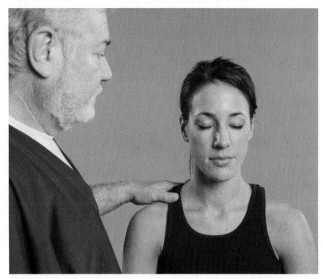

FIG. 13-86 A lapse of 60 seconds or more between blinks indicates decreased sensitivity to pain. A lapse of less than 20 seconds indicates a patient hypersensitive to pain.

- The interval between eye blinks in the average patient is 25 to 30 seconds (Fig. 13-85).
- A 60-second lapse between blinks while staring straight ahead indicates a patient who is stoic (Fig. 13-86).
- A stoic patient can be described as impassive and calm in the face of pain and discomfort.
- Stoic patients may also be cool and indifferent to the sensations elicited in testing.

Next Steps/Procedures
Libman sign, Mannkopf sign, marked part pain-suggestibility test, and related joint motion test

PARALYSIS QUALIFICATION AND QUANTIFICATION

Overview

Motion is a fundamental property of most animal life. The lowest multicellular animals possess rudimentary neuromuscular mechanisms. In higher forms, motion is based on the transmission of impulses from a receptor through an afferent neuron and ganglion cell to muscle. This same principle is found in the reflex arc of higher animals, including humans, in whom the anterior spinal cord has developed into a central regulating mechanism. This central regulating mechanism is involved in initiating and integrating movements.

Motor disturbances include weakness and paralysis, which may result from lesions of the voluntary motor path-

ways or of the muscles themselves. Impaired motor functioning may result from involvement of muscle, myoneural junction, peripheral nerve, or the central nervous system.

The types of paralysis or paresis are based on the location. Hemiplegia is a spastic or flaccid paralysis of one side of the body and extremities, limited by the median line sagittally. Monoplegia is a paralysis of one extremity only. Diplegia is a paralysis of any two corresponding extremities, both of which are usually lower extremities but may be upper extremities. Paraplegia is a symmetric paralysis of both lower extremities. Quadriplegia, or tetraplegia, is a paralysis of all four extremities. Hemiplegia alternans (crossed paralysis) is a paralysis of one or more ipsilateral cranial nerves and contralateral paralysis of the arm and leg.

Psychogenic movement disorders are substantial diagnostic and management challenges for both neurologists and psychiatrists. The term *psychogenic* is traditionally used to describe disorders that cannot be attributed to any known structural or neurochemical disease but that result from an underlying psychiatric illness or malingering. The disorders are commonly associated with various complex movements. Symptoms can mimic the full range of organic abnormal involuntary movements, affect gait and speech, or exhibit as unusual undifferentiated movements that do not fit into a known category. The disorders most commonly fulfill psychiatric criteria for a conversion disorder, a form of somatoform disorder, along with somatization disorder, hypochondriasis, body dysmorphic disorder, and pain disorder. Psychogenic movement disorders can be disabling and the health care cost associated with somatoform disorders in

13

ORTHOPEDIC GAMUT 13-37

MOVEMENT DISORDERS OF ORGANIC ORIGIN

- Tremor
- Dystonia
- Chorea
- Bradykinesia
- Myoclonus
- Tics
- Athetosis
- Ballism
- Incoordination

ORTHOPEDIC GAMUT 13-38

PSYCHOGENIC MOVEMENT DISORDERS

Psychogenic movement disorders in order of clinical frequency:
- Action tremor
- Resting tremor
- Dystonia
- Bradykinesia
- Myoclonus
- Incoordination resembling cerebellar dysfunction
- Tics
- Chorea
- Athetosis
- Ballism

TABLE 13-7

CLINICAL CHARACTERISTICS OF PSYCHOGENIC MOVEMENT DISORDERS

Mode of onset	• Abrupt • Precipitating event • Fast progression to maximal symptom severity and disability
Clinical signs	• Signs incongruent with organic disease • Distractibility and variability • Multiple abnormal movements • Increased movement with attention to the affected body part • Deliberate slowness of movement • Entrainment, coactivation • Association with false weakness, sensory loss, and pain • Unresponsiveness to drugs for organic movement disorders, response to placebo drugs and suggestion

Adapted from Hinson VK, Haren WB: Psychogenic movement disorders, *Lancet Neurol* 5(8):695-700, 2006.

---

general is substantial, amounting to an estimated cost of $20 billion per year. Many physicians are reluctant to make the diagnosis of psychogenic movement disorder for fear of missing an underlying organic and potentially treatable disorder or because of the general reluctance of the patient to accept the diagnosis (Hinson, Haren, 2006).

Typically, 60% of psychogenic movement disorders patients will have a gait disorder and 28% will have a speech dysfunction. Most patients (74%) will exhibit two or more signs. The upper hands and arms are most frequently affected, followed by the legs and feet, the neck, trunk, head, face, and shoulders.

The mode of onset typifies the clinical presentation of psychogenic movement disorders; symptoms begin abruptly, sometimes in the context of a minor injury or another precipitating event, and maximal symptom severity and disability are reached quickly.

Disabilities might be selective and affect only specific functions, such as walking, whereas movement of the extremities is normal when engaged in other motor tasks (rapid alternating movements, strength testing).

Other signs that implicate psychogenicity are abnormal movements incongruent with an organic movement disorder, deliberate slowness of movement, distractibility, variability, and simultaneous occurrence of various abnormal movements and dysfunctions (e.g., tremor associated with myoclonus and gait dysfunction).

Movements may resolve when a patient is unaware of being observed and increase when the affected body part is being examined.

Distractibility and variability are especially common in psychogenic tremor (80% of cases) and commonly coexist with entrainment and coactivation signs (Table 13-7).

Paralyses occur in many patients with hysteria, and they may be spastic or flaccid. With hysterical contracture, the affected muscles are not atrophied, except in severe cases of long duration. The deep-tendon reflexes are increased, and a spurious ankle-clonus may be present, but the Babinski sign is not observed. The limbs are most affected, as is the case with hemiplegia, monoplegia, or paraplegia. Less often, the muscles of the face are affected. Certain attitudes are characteristic of hysterical paralyses. The elbows, wrists, and fingers are kept flexed, and the arms are adducted. The hip and knee are extended, and the foot is held in a position of talipes equinovarus. Ptosis of the face may be simulated by spasm of the orbicularis palpebrarum, torticollis by contracture of the sternomastoid. In the less severe cases, the stiffness and paresis are neither complete nor marked enough for the condition to be called a contracture. The deformity produced is the result of active muscular spasm. In severe and longstanding cases, a true contracture results and the limb cannot be straightened by ordinary mechanical means. Highly characteristic of hysterical contracture is the patient's use of antagonistic muscles to prevent passive or active correction of the deformity exhibited.

CLINICAL PEARL (PARALYSIS ASSESSMENT)

Abnormalities of the motor system, which may be manifestations of both hysteria and malingering, include disturbances of muscle strength and power, disorders of tone. dyskinesia, and abnormalities of coordination, station, and gait. Rarely do changes in volume or contour occur (except for wasting from disuse), and no abnormalities are found on electromyographic examination. These motor changes of psychic origin may resemble almost any type of motor disturbance that is brought about by organic disease of the nervous system.

In both hysterical and malingered paralyses, the patient makes little effort to contract the muscles necessary for executing the desired movement. The patient may remain calm and indifferent while demonstrating the lack of strength. The patient may also show little sign of alarm at the presence of complete paralysis and may smile cheerfully during the examination. Reliable evidence that the patient is not exerting all available power in an attempt to carry out a voluntary movement can be elicited by watching and palpating the contraction of the antagonists, as well as the agonists.

13

BILATERAL LIMB-DROPPING TEST (LOWER EXTREMITIES)

Assessment for Feigned Paresis of Lower Extremity

Comment

Muscle imbalance at the hip encourages subluxation and dislocation. When the equilibrium between the flexor-adductor group and the abductor-extensor group is altered, as the former overpowers the latter, the femoral neck is pulled medially to a more vertical position.

Disproportionate muscle forces necessary for producing subluxation and dislocation occur most often in children with myelomeningocele. Paralysis or paresis in one or both lower extremities is present at birth in more than 90% of the infants with thoracolumbar or lumbar myelomeningocele and in more than 50% with lumbosacral or sacral myelomeningocele. The peculiar muscle imbalance is also found—but this is uncommon—in cerebral palsy, poliomyelitis, and diseases and injuries of the cauda equina.

After a stroke, people develop multiple impairments and disabilities (e.g., motor deficits, difficulties in activities of daily living, sphincter muscle control, perceptive faculties, communication and cognitive capacities, mobility, walking problems), all of which must be considered to assess rehabilitation outcomes adequately. Thus clinicians tend to use an overall functional index that provides a comprehensive view of a patient's status. The Barthel Index and the FIM™ instrument are examples of such an index, although many more exist. However, one of the most valued and important aspects for patients and relatives is the patient's recovery of walking function, probably because changes in walking function are among the most frequent causes for physical dependency in these patients (Viosca et al, 2005).

ORTHOPEDIC GAMUT 13-39
FUNCTIONAL AMBULATION CLASSIFICATION

Level 0: Nonambulation
Level 1: Nonfunctional or dependent ambulation
Level 2: Household ambulation
Level 3: Surroundings of the house ambulation (neighborhood)
Level 4: Community ambulation
Level 5: Normal ambulation

PROCEDURE

- Lower extremities are usually portrayed to be either weak or completely paralyzed.
- To determine whether the patient has a weak hip or leg, the patient is placed on the examination table in a supine position.
- The examiner flexes the patient's legs at the hip, keeping the knees straight.
- The examiner holds the legs in an elevated position by cradling the patient's feet in a hand and instructs the patient to push the legs downward and hard against the examiner's hand (Fig. 13-87).
- The examiner suddenly pulls the hand away (Fig. 13-88).
- If leg weakness is of an organic origin, the affected leg will fall to the examination table.
- If the weakness is faked, the leg may move up or hang in midair for a moment before falling because of hip muscle flexor actuation.

Next Steps/Procedures
Hoover sign, simulated foot-drop testing, and tripod test (bilateral leg-fluttering test)

ORTHOPEDIC GAMUT 13-40

THE BARTHEL INDEX

Patient Name: _____

Rater Name: _____

Date: _____

Activity	Score
Feeding	
0 = unable	_____
5 = needs help cutting, spreading butter, etc. or requires modified diet	
10 = independent	
Bathing	
0 = dependent	_____
5 = independent (or in shower)	
Grooming	
0 = needs to help with personal care	_____
5 = independent face/hair/teeth/shaving (implements provided)	
Dressing	
0 = dependent	_____
5 = needs help but can do about half unaided	
10 = independent (including buttons, zips, laces, etc.)	
Bowels	
0 = incontinent (or needs to be given enemas)	_____
5 = occasional accident	
10 = continent	
Bladder	
0 = incontinent, or catheterized and unable to manage alone	_____
5 = occasional accident	
10 = continent	
Toilet Use	
0 = dependent	_____
5 = needs some help, but can do something alone	
10 = independent (on and off, dressing, wiping)	
Transfers (bed to chair and back)	
0 = unable, no sitting balance	_____
5 = major help (one or two people, physical), can sit	
10 = minor help (verbal or physical)	
15 = independent	
Mobility (on level surfaces)	
0 = immobile or < 50 yards	_____
5 = wheelchair independent, including corners, >50 yards	
10 = walks with help of one person (verbal or physical) >50 yards	
15 = independent (but may use any aid; for example, stick) >50 yards	

Activity	Score
Stairs	
0 = unable	_____
5 = needs help (verbal, physical, carrying aid)	
10 = independent	
Total (0-100)	_____

1. The index should be used as a record of what a patient does, not as a record of what a patient could do.
2. The main aim is to establish degree of independence from any help, physical or verbal, however minor and for whatever reason.
3. The need for supervision renders the patient not independent.
4. A patient's performance should be established using the best available evidence. Asking the patient, friends or relatives, and nurses are the usual sources, but direct observation and common sense are also important. However, direct testing is not needed.
5. Usually the patient's performance over the preceding 24 to 48 hours is important, but occasionally longer periods will be relevant.
6. Middle categories imply that the patient supplies over 50% of the effort.
7. Use of aids to be independent is allowed.

Full credit is not given for an activity if the patient needs even minimal help or supervision. A score of 0 is given when patient cannot meet criteria as defined. (Maximum score: 100.)

The advantage of the BI is its simplicity. It is useful in evaluating a patient's state of independence before treatment, patient progress undergoing treatment, and patient status when reaching maximum benefit. The total score is not as significant or meaningful as the breakdown into individual items, because these indicate where the deficiencies are.

13

From Mahoney FI, Barthel D: Functional evaluation: the Barthel Index, *Maryland State Med J* 14:56-61, 1965. Used with permission.

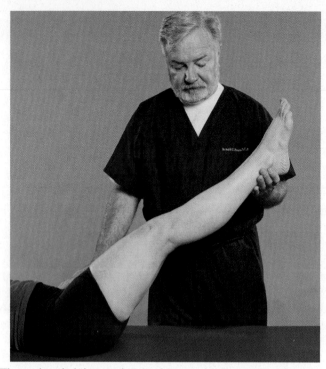

FIG. 13-87 The patient is lying supine on the examination table. The examiner performs a bilateral straight-leg-raising test. As the legs are in the elevated position, the examiner instructs the patient to push the heels of the legs downward, against the examiner's resistance.

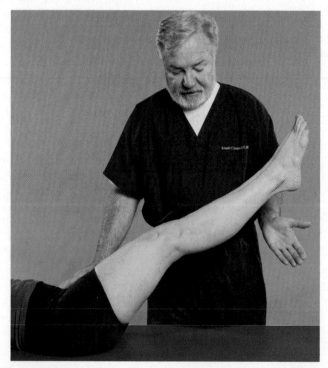

FIG. 13-88 The examiner unexpectedly pulls the supporting hand away from the legs. The leg affected with simulated paralysis will hang in the air momentarily before falling to the table. This result represents a positive test and indicates hysteria or malingering.

Assessment for Nonorganic Hemiplegia

Comment

Postural unsteadiness represents a very common impairment in patients who experienced a hemiplegic stroke and is the major source of falls and limitation in functional independence. Recovery of a stable standing position is a crucial step in the rehabilitation process of the hemiplegic subject (Paillex, So, 2005).

Hemiplegic cerebral palsy is mostly characterized by unilateral paresis and spasticity. Although children with hemiplegic cerebral palsy often acquire motor milestones within the late-normal range, their patterns of motor development differ from that of unimpaired children. Because of

---

ORTHOPEDIC GAMUT 13-41

HEMIPLEGIC MOVEMENT PATTERNS IN CHILDREN WITH CEREBRAL PALSY

Movement Patterns for the Task of Rising from a Supine Position to a Standing Position	Segmental Score
I. Upper Limb Categories	
a. Push and reach to bilateral push	1
b. Push and reach to asymmetric push	2
c. Symmetric push	3
d. Symmetric reach	4
e. Push and reach followed by pushing on one leg	5
f. Push and reach to bilateral push followed by pushing on leg	6
II. Axial Categories	
a. Full rotation with abdomen down	1
b. Full rotation with abdomen up	2
c. Partial rotation	3
d. Forward with rotation	4
e. Symmetric	5
III. Lower limb categories	
a. Pike	1
b. Pike jump to squat	2
c. Kneel	3
d. Jump to squat	4
e. Half-kneel	5
f. Asymmetric wide based squat	6
g. Narrow based symmetric squat	7

---

unilateral weakness and variable pelvic stability, they often favor side-sitting and asymmetric prone shuffling. Whole-body motor tasks such as standing up and walking are achieved at greater physiologic cost, primarily supported by the unaffected leg that bears more of the body weight in the upright position. Quality of movements and efficiency is impaired in these children who display less selective and more global whole-body movements. Whole-body movements have been used to identify specific strategies of motor control involving changes in posture in children with cerebral palsy (Mewasingh et al, 2004).

Intracerebral hemorrhage destroys the parenchyma. Cerebral thrombosis or embolism causes necrosis of the parenchyma (infarction, encephalomalacia) in the area supplied by the occluded vessel. If the embolus is septic and infection spreads beyond the vessel wall, encephalitis, brain abscess, or meningitis may result.

The site of the lesion determines specific symptoms. Cerebral hemorrhage is most common in the region of the thalamus and internal capsule and is usually accompanied by severe hemiplegia, hemianesthesia, speech disturbance, and sometimes hemianopsia. Because the middle cerebral artery or its branches are often the site of thrombosis or embolism, common symptoms are hemiplegia (affecting the arm more than the leg) and cortical sensory loss in the affected limbs. Various disturbances (aphasia and apraxia) may follow damage to the dominant hemisphere.

After stroke, patients may develop hemiparesis, which can have a profound effect on walking ability. A common gait deviation, often occurring unilaterally after a stroke, is an equinus deformity of the foot, which is caused by total or partial central paralysis of the muscles innervated by the common peroneal nerve or spasticity of the plantar flexors or both. The incidence of equinus deformity of the foot in adult stroke patients has been reported to vary between 10% and 20% (Kinsella, Moran, in press).

PROCEDURE

- Paralysis is yet another symptom presentation from the repertoire of the hysteric, psychogenic, rheumatic, or malingering patient.
- A patient with a feigned paralyzed leg and arm may incorrectly assume the existence of difficulty in turning the head toward the paralyzed side (Fig. 13-89).
- Pronation drift (the inability to hold the pronated arms still) is absent on station and gait.

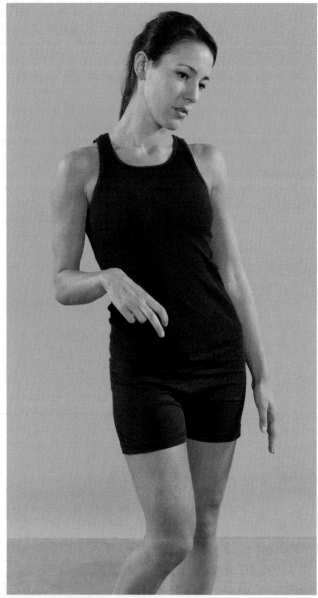

FIG. 13-89 The patient is standing, and the examiner assesses the patient's posture. In feigned paralysis, the paralyzed arm and leg are held in typical flexion contractures. The patient incorrectly assumes that the **head cannot be turned toward the paralyzed side**. Pronation drift is absent. This behavior indicates malingering or hysteria.

HOOVER SIGN

Assessment for Feigned Leg Paresis

Comment

Charcot (1889) conjectured that hysterical paralysis implicated what he called "dynamic or functional lesions" in the cortical motor zone opposite the paralysis. These functional lesions were regarded as akin to localized edema, anemia or active hyperemia "of which no trace is found after death" (Freud, 1893) (Marshall et al, 1997).

Neurologic loss is usually described as a sensory or motor deficit. The sensory loss may produce hypoesthesia, paresthesia, or hyperesthesia and may produce pain or numbness over a specific area. The motor deficits may be described as a weakness, as stiffness, or, more commonly, as difficulty in walking far, running, or jumping. If outright paralysis exists, the onset may have been sudden or insidious (Table 13-8). The paralysis may be flaccid or spastic. Flaccidity is associated with lower motor neuron disorders and spasticity with upper motor neuron disorders. The examiner must determine whether the symptoms have increased or decreased and to what degree the patient is disabled. The examiner must also determine whether a loss of sphincter control of the bladder and rectum has occurred.

Cerebral palsy (CP) is a neuromotor disorder caused by damage to the brain before, during, or shortly after birth. Common clinical manifestations of CP include muscle hypertonicity and joint malposition during gait in cases of lower-limb involvement in ambulant patients. The musculoskeletal system adaptations associated with these movement and posture impairments are not fully understood. At the ankle joint, for example, CP is often associated with hyperextension during gait (equinus gait), indicative of shortening in one or more of the following structures: (1) the gastrocnemius and the other ankle plantar flexor muscles, (2) the tendons of these muscles, and (3) soft-tissue structures in the joints of the foot (e.g., joint capsules and ligaments) (Mohagheghi et al, 2007).

Acute muscle hypoasthenia has various causes and is sometimes of multifactorial origin. If extreme weakness is

---

TABLE 13-8

COMMON CAUSES OF HYPOKALEMIC PARALYSIS

Potassium deficit

Group 1
Hypochloremic metabolic alkalosis

- Excessive vomiting
- Diuretics
- Licorice ingestion
- Mineralocorticoid syndromes
- Bartter or Gitelman syndrome
- Liddle syndrome

Group 2
Hyperchloremic metabolic acidosis and low NH_4^+ excretion

- Distal renal tubular acidosis (medullary-sponge kidney, Sjögren syndrome)
- Proximal renal tubular acidosis, Fanconi syndrome

Group 3
Hyperchloremic metabolic acidosis and high NH_4^+ excretion

- Toluene abuse
- Diarrheal state
- Urethral diversion

Intracellular potassium shift
Normal acid-base balance

- Thyrotoxic periodic paralysis
- Familial periodic paralysis
- Sporadic periodic paralysis
- Hypernatremic hypokalemic paralysis
- Barium poisoning

NH_4^+, Ammonium.
From Pompeo A et al: Thyrotoxic hypokalemic periodic paralysis: an overlooked pathology in western countries, *Eur J Intern Med* 18(5):380-390, 2007.

associated with hypokalemia, the differential diagnosis is of hypokalemic paralysis, which can be further classified as either a deficiency, caused by loss or decreased intake of potassium, or a periodic form (hypokalemic periodic paralysis [HPP]) that is caused by a critical intracellular movement of this electrolyte. For the latter instance, the most frequent in western countries is familial HPP (FHPP), while the thyrotoxic form (THPP) and the subgroup of sporadic periodic paralysis (without hyperthyroidism and without a family history of periodic paralysis) are more frequent in Asian populations. The migration of peoples has resulted in the loss of this geographical confinement for these diseases. At the same time, THPP is not limited to populations of Asian origin but can also be found on rare occasions in other ethnic groups (Pompeo et al, in press).

PROCEDURE

• Hoover sign is helpful in differentiating between organic and hysterical paralysis.
• When a supine patient is directed to lift the paralyzed or affected one leg, normally the patient unconsciously presses the heel of the unaffected leg against the examination table.
• In organic hemiplegia, this downward pressure is accentuated on the healthy side as the patient attempts to raise the paretic leg.
• If the examiner places a hand under the patient's heel, this pressure can be felt (Fig. 13-90).
• In malingering, the patient will feel no, or very little, pressure on the opposite side of the affection as the patient attempts to raise the involved extremity.

Next Steps/Procedures
Bilateral limb-dropping test (lower extremities), simulated foot-drop testing, and tripod test (bilateral leg-fluttering test)

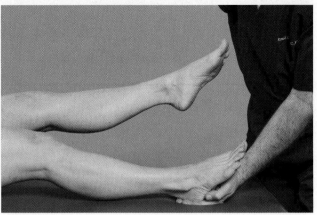

FIG. 13-90 The patient is lying supine on the examination table. The examiner places one hand under the heel of the unaffected leg. The patient attempts to lift the paralyzed leg off the table. The organically paralyzed patient presses the unaffected leg firmly downward, when attempting to flex the paralyzed hip. Because the malingerer is not trying, this synergistic action does not occur. The sign is present when the counterpressure is absent on the unaffected side. The sign indicates malingering or hysteria.

SIMULATED FOOT-DROP TESTING

Assessment for Feigned Steppage Gait or Foot Drop

Comment

Foot drop is defined as severe weakness of ankle dorsiflexion (extension) with intact plantar flexion. It should be distinguished from a flail foot in which ankle or foot movement is minimal or nonexistent in all directions, including severe weakness of ankle dorsiflexion, plantar flexion, and intrinsic foot muscles. In contrast to a flail foot, voluntary movement at or distal to the ankle occurs in foot drop caused by intact plantar flexion and intrinsic foot muscles. Many patients with peripheral polyneuropathy, such as Charcot-Marie-Tooth disease, are often mislabeled as having bilateral foot drop, whereas thorough examination reveals foot and ankle weakness in all directions, compatible a bilateral flail foot. Foot drop is a direct effect of tibialis anterior muscle weakness. It is often associated with weakness of toe extension caused by weakness of the extensor hallucis and extensor digitorum longus and brevis. Unilateral foot drop is caused by disorders distinct from those leading to bilateral foot drop, with very little overlap. In general, most cases of bilateral foot drop are caused by generalized disorders such as motor neuron disease, neuropathy, or myopathy, whereas unilateral foot drop is often caused by focal disorders such as a mononeuropathy or radiculopathy. Common causes of unilateral foot drop include peroneal neuropathy, L5 radiculopathy, sciatic nerve lesion, and lumbosacral plexopathy (Katirji, Michael, Robert, 2003).

Complicated, coordinated movements are examined by observing the patient's manner of walking (Table 13-9).

TABLE 13-9

CAUSES OF UNILATERAL FOOT DROP AND BILATERAL FOOT DROP

I. Unilateral foot drop	a. Deep peroneal mononeuropathy
	b. Common peroneal mononeuropathy
	c. Anterior compartmental syndrome of the leg
	d. Sciatic mononeuropathy
	e. Lumbosacral plexopathy (lumbosacral trunk)
	f. L5 radiculopathy
	g. L4 radiculopathy
	h. Multifocal motor neuropathy
	i. Hereditary neuropathy with liability to pressure palsy
	j. Amyotrophic lateral sclerosis
	k. Poliomyelitis and postpoliomyelitis syndrome
	l. Cortical or subcortical parasagittal cerebral lesion
II. Bilateral foot drop	a. Myopathies
	b. Distal myopathies
	c. Scapuloperoneal muscular dystrophy
	d. Facioscapulohumeral muscular dystrophy
	e. Myotonic dystrophy
	f. Neuropathies
	g. Multifocal motor neuropathy with conduction block
	h. Chronic inflammatory demyelinating polyneuropathy
	i. Bilateral peroneal neuropathies
	j. Bilateral sciatic neuropathies
	k. Bilateral lumbosacral plexopathies
	l. Radiculopathies
	m. Bilateral L5 radiculopathies
	n. Conus medullaris lesion
	o. Anterior horn cell disorders
	p. Amyotrophic lateral sclerosis
	q. Poliomyelitis and the postpoliomyelitis syndrome
	r. Cerebral lesions
	s. Bilateral cortical or subcortical parasagittal lesions

Adapted from Katirji B, Michael JA, Robert BD: Foot drop. In: *Encyclopedia of the neurological sciences,* New York, 2003, Academic Press.

Paresis will produce a slow, guarded, short-stepped, and shuffling gait. Paralysis of the anterior tibial muscles, especially by anterior horn or peripheral nerve lesion, causes a drop foot and produces a steppage gait. To prevent tripping over the plantar-flexed foot, the extremity is advanced with the knee and hip flexed. With spasticity, the legs are advanced slowly with shortened steps, and the toes scrape the ground. Adductor tightness produces a scissors gait, by which the legs are alternately crossed. With the ataxic, or tabetic, gait, the patient must constantly observe the placement of the feet because of the absence of deep position sense. The hip is flexed and externally rotated, and the forefoot is strongly dorsiflexed before being thrown down with the heel striking first. The patient is unable to stand with the eyes closed. In contrast, cerebellar ataxia is not aided by visual assistance. The gait appears stumbling and drunken because the patient sways from side to side, and a tendency to fall toward the side of the lesion is present.

Charcot-Marie-Tooth disease (CMT) describes a group of inherited polyneuropathies with both motor and sensory manifestations. A tendency exists to supersede this term with the synonymous descriptive term *hereditary motor sensory neuropathy*. However, CMT remains in common use and historically attached to the three physicians who first identified it in 1886: Jean-Martin Charcot and Pierre Marie in Paris, France, and Howard Henry Tooth in Cambridge, England. Inherited polyneuropathies are the most frequent inherited peripheral neuropathies, with a prevalence ranging between 10 and 28 per 100,000. In most cases, weakness, wasting, and sensory dysfunction progress centripetally, affecting first the intrinsic foot muscles and then spreading to the leg muscles. As a consequence, foot deformities develop, as well as abnormalities in gait pattern. The lower extremities are usually more affected than the upper limbs, but most patients will exhibit a certain degree of associated hand weakness. In the majority of cases, patients either deteriorate very slowly or remain clinically stable for relatively long periods, in most cases decades (Newman et al, 2007).

PROCEDURE

- With feigned total leg weakness or paralysis, a patient may pretend to be unable to raise the forefoot while walking.
- This complaint must be separated from organic foot drop.
- The patient is standing, and the examiner is positioned behind the patient (Fig. 13-91).
- The patient is instructed to maintain a rigid and narrow-based posture, with the feet close together.
- In a surprise move, the examiner grasps the shoulders of the patient and pulls the patient's body backward (Fig. 13-92).
- The examiner notes the movement of the patient's toes and forefoot.
- If the forefoot rises, the test is positive.
- A positive test indicates feigned foot drop.

Next Steps/Procedures
Bilateral limb-dropping test (lower extremities), Hoover sign, and tripod test (bilateral leg-fluttering test)

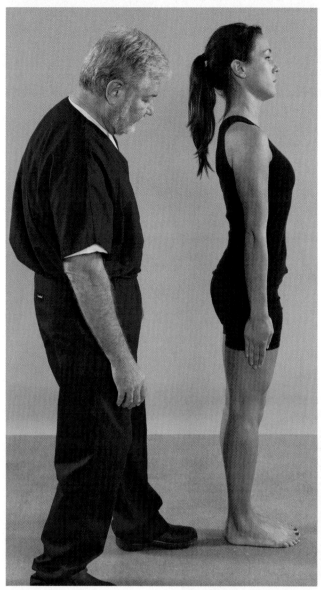

FIG. 13-91 The patient is standing, and the examiner is positioned behind the patient. The patient is instructed to maintain a rigid and narrow-based posture with the feet close together.

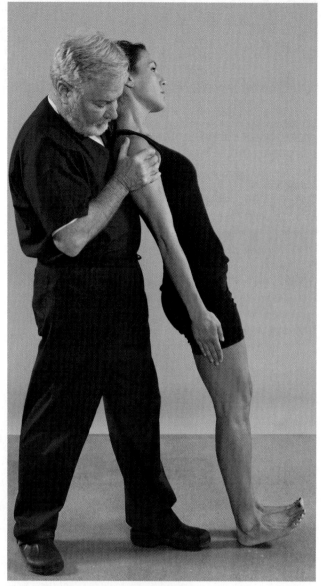

FIG. 13-92 In a surprise move, the examiner grasps the shoulders of the patient and pulls the patient's body backward. The examiner notes the movement of the toes and forefoot. If the forefoot rises, the test is positive. The positive test indicates feigned foot drop.

13

SIMULATED FOREARM-AND-WRIST-WEAKNESS TESTING

Assessment for Simulated Weakness of Forearm and Wrist

Comment

Pinch and grip strength have been shown as the most important factors related to hand function. Fowler and Nicols (2001) noted that pinch and grip strength along with range-of-motion measurements were able to provide a robust alternative to detailed biomechanical measures with the additional benefit of being efficient in terms of cost and time. Goniometric measurements of joint range of motion have undergone exponential development, from simple clinical tools to more complex systems such as the Sheffield Instru-

mented Glove. As with the questionnaire-based assessments, these too have their benefits and limitations, often with accuracy being sacrificed in response to clinical practicality and time constraints. Thus the clinical assessment of hand function and disability remains complex and controversial (Goodson et al, 2007).

Although the function of one hand may be assessed (Fig 13-93), the impairment of function in one hand may clearly affect many activities that normally involve both hands performing together. The degree of overall functional impairment may be investigated by inquiring about or testing the patient's ability to perform certain tasks. This ability can be assessed efficiently with the Lamb Bilateral Hand Activity Index.

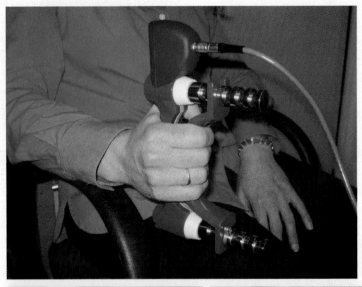

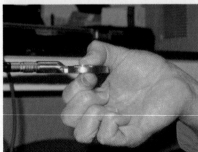 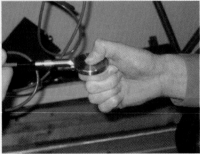

FIG. 13-93 The three prehensile patterns are the key grip, the pinch grip, and the power grip. Pinch-grip strength (opposition of thumb tip with ipsilateral fingertips) is assessed in each finger separately. Key grip and pinch grip are measured using the pinch dynamometer. Power grip is assessed using the grip dynamometer. (From Goodson A et al: Direct, quantitative clinical assessment of hand function: usefulness and reproducibility, *Man Ther* 12[2]:144-152, 2007.)

ORTHOPEDIC GAMUT 13-42

LAMB BILATERAL HAND ACTIVITY INDEX OF ACTIVITIES PERFORMED WITH BOTH HANDS ACTING SIMULTANEOUSLY AND TOGETHER*

- Unscrew the top from a bottle.
- Fill a cup or glass and drink.
- Open a can with a manual can opener.
- Remove a match from a box or book and light it.
- Use a knife and fork for eating.
- Apply toothpaste to a toothbrush and clean teeth.
- Put on a jacket.
- Close buttons on clothing.
- Fasten a belt around the waist.
- Tie shoelaces.
- Sharpen a pencil in a manual sharpener.
- Write messages.
- Use a dial telephone.
- Staple papers together.
- Wrap string around a package.
- Use playing cards.

When progress is being measured, each of these items listed in may be scored on a scale of 0 to 5, or 0 to 10, and added. A total score of 80 or 160, respectively, represents a return to normal bilateral hand functions.

*Modified from McRae R: *Clinical orthopaedic examination,* ed 3, Edinburgh, 1990, Churchill Livingstone.

Clinically, stroke survivors commonly have a flexed wrist at the affected side, mainly caused by the muscular contractures in the upper limb after the upper motor neuron lesion. Therefore subjects would usually have lengthening wrist extensors and shortening wrist flexors. Researchers had found that skeletal muscles adapt to a shortened (lengthened) position by reducing (increasing) the number of sarcomeres. Spastic muscles with shortening fiber length result in a shortening resting fiber length. These changes can bring shifts in the muscle length-force curve of each active muscle during affected wrist contractions. As compared with the unaffected wrist contraction over the wrist range of motion, the peak values of the affected normalized torque during wrist flexion and extension shifted to more flexed positions (Hu et al, 2006).

PROCEDURE

- If the complaint is persisting forearm or wrist weakness that is not associated with grip-strength loss, the patient is directed to dorsiflex the wrist, usually by making a fist.
- If this action cannot be performed, the patient is then asked to squeeze a dynamometer while the examiner palpates the patient's forearm (Fig. 13-94).
- In functional or feigned weakness, the examiner will feel the patient's forearm extensors contract synergistically and will see the wrist extend when the patient squeezes.

Next Steps/Procedure
Simulated grip-strength-loss testing

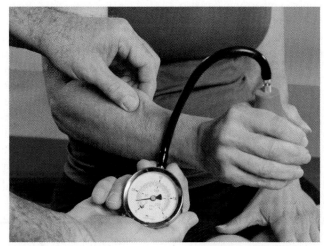

FIG. 13-94 The patient is seated and is directed to dorsiflex the wrist. If this move cannot be accomplished, the examiner instructs the patient to grip and squeeze a dynamometer. As the patient squeezes, the examiner palpates the forearm musculature. The test is positive when the examiner notes synergistic contraction of the forearm extensors and observes slight wrist dorsiflexion. The test is significant for feigned muscular weakness.

13

SIMULATED GRIP-STRENGTH-LOSS TESTING

Assessment for Simulated Grip Strength Loss

Comment

The two basic approaches to assessing muscle imbalance are the measurement of muscle strength and of muscle fatigability in agonist and antagonist groups for a specific movement, and this study uses both. Muscle fatigue (defined as exercise-induced reduction in the maximal capability to produce force or power output) can be measured indirectly by electromyelogram (EMG), notably by median frequency, which falls alongside the force, and has been shown to provide a reliable, sensitive, and relatively unbiased means to detect fatigue, especially during sustained voluntary contractions. By contrast, changes in EMG amplitude with fatigue are often too inconsistent for this purpose. Very few direct wrist-strength studies are found in the literature; in these few, the focus has been mainly on wrist extension. Probably because of lack of proper instrument for directly measuring wrist strength, grip-strength measurement has been generally used for assessing outcomes of tennis elbow and hand and wrist function. However, this measurement depends both on wrist flexor and on extensor muscles; it cannot differentiate between them (Alizadehkhaiyat et al, 2007).

When a patient complains of weakness, the physician must consider many possible causes. Because of the wide range of differential diagnosis, evaluation for all the possible causes of weakness would be not only cumbersome but also costly for the patient and time-consuming for the examiner. Perhaps even more important, the patient is exposed to potentially hazardous and painful tests that might be unnecessary. Therefore, ascertaining the anatomic locus of the patient's weakness is desirable.

When a weak patient shows evidence of motor unit disease and the cause is not myopathic, the patient probably has a neuropathy.

In the evaluation of peripheral nerve function, grip- and pinch-strength measurements with dynamometers have often been recommended as a measure of outcome. An

> ### ORTHOPEDIC GAMUT 13-43
> # NEUROPATHY
>
> **The differential diagnosis of neuropathy includes many diseases that present with similar symptoms (symmetric distal sensory losses). However, patients with neuropathy occasionally may complain of the following symptoms:**
> 1. Thickened nerves (hypertrophic neuropathy)
> 2. Mononeuritis
> 3. Radiculopathy
> 4. Cranial nerve involvement
> 5. Autonomic disturbances
> 6. Ascending neuritis
> 7. Weakness without sensory findings

important caution in using these dynamometers was made by Strickland and colleagues, who argued that grip- and pinch-strength data may be used only as an indirect measurement of nerve recovery. A commonly overlooked point is that grip-strength measurements provide information on the combined function of all the intrinsic and extrinsic muscles of the hand. Researchers have observed frequently that patients with weak intrinsic muscles of the hand after ulnar or median nerve lesion have a considerably strong grip. The strength of the intrinsic muscles of the hand affect the grip strength only to a certain level. Improvement in grip strength can merely be a reflection of compensatory strengthening of the uninvolved extrinsic musculature. Therefore grip-strength measurements do not provide decisive information about the motor function of the ulnar and median nerves in the lower arm. Hand surgery literature, however, is replete with grip-strength data used to measure the outcome after nerve repair (Schreuders et al, 2004).

PROCEDURE

- When grip strength loss is the complaint, the patient is directed to squeeze the examiner's fingers with the paralyzed hand as hard as possible (Fig. 13-95).
- While the patient performs this task, the examiner suddenly tears the fingers away.
- If grip weakness is caused by organic disease, a sudden tug will break the grasp easily.
- If the weakness is being faked, strong resistance is likely to be encountered before the malingerer realizes the error or contradiction and releases the grip (Fig. 13-96).

Next Steps/Procedure
Simulated forearm-and-wrist-weakness testing

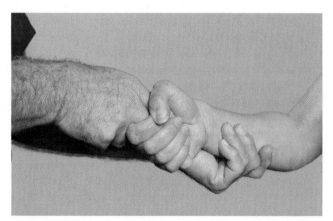

FIG. 13-95 The seated patient is instructed to grip and squeeze the examiner's fingers with the paralyzed hand as hard as possible.

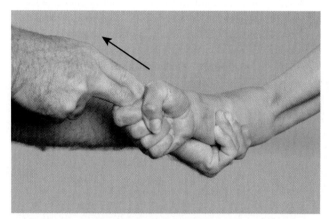

FIG. 13-96 As the patient continues the grip, the examiner unexpectedly tears the fingers from the grip. Strong resistance is likely to be encountered before the patient realizes the error and releases the grip. In organic disease, the sudden tug will break the grasp easily. The test is positive for feigned loss of grip.

13

TRIPOD TEST (BILATERAL LEG-FLUTTERING TEST)

Assessment for Simulated Lumbar Pain

Comment

In Western industrialized countries, the incidence of LBP varies between 60% and 90%, and its prevalence is estimated to be 5%, but pain and disability disappear within 3 months in 85% to 95% of patients. However, the costs of chronic LBP are considerable and continue to grow. Chronic LBP has become the second cause of disability after cardiovascular diseases. In industrialized countries, LBP has become the most common cause of work loss and absenteeism. Only 10% of patients are still on sick leave after 6 months, but this minority is responsible for more than 80% of LBP costs. Functional prognosis is rather poor, with only 50% of patients on sick leave for 6 months returning to their previous job and almost none after 2 years. Usual treatments have failed to reduce the burden of chronic LBP, and physicians who fail to follow guidelines may have contributed to this problem. Therefore, in a search for new solutions, functional restoration programs were developed. The ideas of a deconditioning syndrome and of functional restoration programs for patients with disabling chronic LBP were proposed by Mayer and colleagues in 1985. This deconditioning syndrome appears after 4 to 6 months of limited activities because of LBP and is associated with decreased lumbar spine mobility and back muscle strength and endurance, with psychosocial implications such as increased anxiety and depression (Poiraudeau, Rannou, Revel, 2007).

Lesions of the lower motor neurons may be located in the ventral gray column of the spinal cord or brainstem or in their axons, which constitute the ventral roots of the spinal nerves or the cranial nerves. Lesions may result from trauma, toxins, infections, vascular disorders, congenital malformations, degenerative processes, or neoplasms. Signs of lower motor neuron lesions include flaccid paralysis of the involved muscles, muscle atrophy, and a degeneration reaction. Reflexes of the involved muscle are diminished or absent, and no pathologic reflexes are obtainable.

In many cases, patients do not complain of loss of muscle power in itself but have noted difficulty in walking or in using a limb for a particular activity. The hand is an integrated motor sensory organ, and early symptoms of manipulatory difficulty are similar in pure motor and pure sensory disorders. Furthermore, some patients who complain of weakness may be suffering from numbness, inhibition from using a painful limb, or incoordination. Weakness of particular muscle groups can lead to distinctive symptoms. Proximal arm muscle weakness impairs lifting objects from high shelves or combing hair. Isolated weakness of small hand muscles is frequently not noted, although loss of grip for unscrewing tight bottle tops will be revealed by direct questioning. Posterior interosseous nerve lesions impairing finger extension may lead to difficulties in sliding the hand into a pocket. Focal triceps weakness may account for difficulty in pushing the motor-vehicle gear shift lever forward. Proximal leg muscle weakness affecting quadriceps causes difficulty on stairs or rising from sitting. Distal leg muscle weakness produces foot drop or loss of the normal bounce from gait. The pattern of weakness produced by lower motor neuron lesions directly reflects the topography of damage to anterior horn cells, spinal nerve roots, or individual peripheral nerves (Donaghy, Michael, Robert, 2003).

PROCEDURE

- A patient may attempt to fake a leg paralysis as the result of a further faked lumbar intervertebral disc syndrome.
- In this instance, the patient is instructed to sit on the examination table with the knees flexed at 90 degrees and the legs hanging dependent (Fig. 13-97).
- The patient is directed to extend and relax, or flex, the legs rapidly and repeatedly (Fig. 13-98).
- If lumbar disc involvement exists, the patient will need to lean back to perform this maneuver, if able to do it at all (Fig. 13-99).
- The patient feigning disc involvement can accomplish the maneuver without assuming such a tripod posture (Fig. 13-100).

Next Steps/Procedures

Bilateral limb-dropping test (lower extremities), Hoover sign, and simulated foot-drop testing

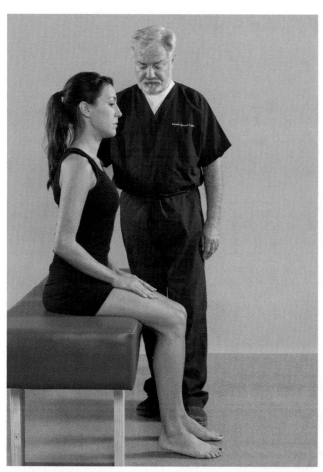

FIG. 13-97 The patient is instructed to sit on the examining table with the knees flexed at 90 degrees and the legs hanging dependent.

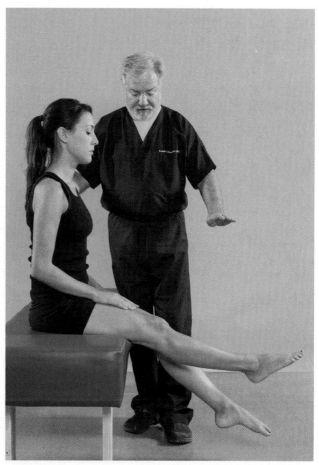

FIG. 13-98 The patient is directed to rapidly and repeatedly extend the legs, in a flutter maneuver.

13

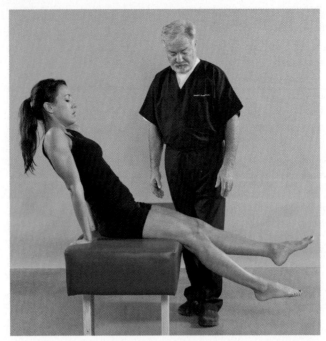

FIG. 13-99 If a lumbar disc involvement exists, the patient will need to lean back to perform this maneuver, if the patient is even able to perform the maneuver at all.

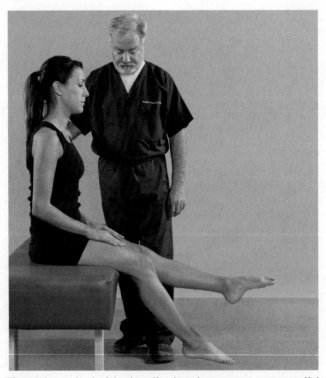

FIG. 13-100 The patient who is feigning disc involvement can accomplish the maneuver without assuming such a tripod posture.

CRITICAL THINKING

1. What are the predictors of work incapacity and work loss caused by depression?
2. To consider posttraumatic stress disorder, what are the signs and symptoms that have to be present?
3. What is the definition of malingering?
4. What criteria are needed in the examination process for the clinician to suspect malingering?
5. Psychogenic rheumatism is a term used to describe patients who have musculoskeletal psychiatric disorders. What are the reasons for psychologic illness that cause the appearance or exacerbation of pain?
6. Describe the symptoms and signs of psychogenic rheumatism.
7. Pure malingering is suggested by what characteristics?
8. How is Libman sign performed? What information does the clinician extract from this test?
9. The examiner establishes the patient's resting pulse rate, and the patient is made as comfortable as possible. Then, without changing the patient's position, the examiner applies mechanical pressure or electrical stimulation over the painful area. While monitoring the pulse rate, an increase of a pulse rate of 10 or more beats per minute is noted, which constitutes a positive sign. The sign is absent in simulated pain. What test was just performed?
10. How should the *trunk rotational twist* test be performed?
11. How is Janet test for simulated anesthesia performed?
12. What sign is useful to evaluate the possibility of organic unilateral blindness?
13. What is the Howship-Romberg sign?
14. What is the mode of onset and clinical characteristics of psychogenic movement disorders?
15. Hoover sign is helpful in what conditions? How is the test performed?

13

BIBLIOGRAPHY

Abenhaim L et al: The prognostic consequences in the making of the initial medical diagnosis of work-related back injuries, *Spine* 20:791, 1994.

Abramowitz JS, Moore EL: An experimental analysis of hypochondriasis, *Behav Res Ther* 45(3):413-424, 2007.

Abrams WB, Berkow R: *The Merck manual of geriatrics,* Rahway, NJ, 1990, Merck Sharp & Dohme Research Laboratories.

Adams JC, Hamblen DL: *Outline of orthopaedics,* ed 11, Edinburgh, 1990, Churchill Livingstone.

Agnew LRC, editor: *Dorland's illustrated medical dictionary,* ed 27, Philadelphia, 1988, WB Saunders.

Alario AJ: *Practical guide to the care of the pediatric patient,* St Louis, 1997, Mosby.

Allaire SH et al: Management of work disability, resources for vocational rehabilitation, *Arthritis Rheum* 36:1663, 1993.

Allison D, Strickland N: *Acronyms & synonyms in medical imaging,* Oxford, UK, 1996, ISIS Medical Media.

American College of Sports Medicine: *Guidelines for exercise testing and prescription,* ed 4, Philadelphia, 1991, Lea & Febiger.

American Medical Association: *Guides to the evaluation of permanent impairment,* ed 4, Chicago, 1993, The Association.

American Medical Association: *How to use guides to the evaluation of permanent impairment,* ed 4, Falmouth, Conn, 1993, SEAK.

American Psychiatric Association: *Diagnostic and statistical manual of mental disorders,* ed 3, Washington, 1980, The Association.

Anderson KN, Anderson LE: *Mosby's pocket dictionary of medicine, nursing, & allied health,* ed 2, St Louis, 1994, Mosby.

Apley AG, Solomon L: *Concise system of orthopaedics and fractures,* London, 1988, Butterworth-Heinemann.

Arbisi PA, Butcher JN: Failure of the FBS to predict malingering of somatic symptoms: response to critiques by Greve and Bianchini and Lees Haley and Fox, *Arch Clin Neuropsychol* 19(3):341-345, 2004.

Aronoff GM et al: Pain treatment programs: do they run workers to the workplace? *Spine* 2:123, 1987.

Aronoff GM: *Evaluation and treatment of chronic pain,* Baltimore, 1985, Urban and Schwartzenberg.

Auvin S et al: Neuropathological and MRI findings in an acute presentation of hemiconvulsion-hemiplegia: a report with pathophysiological implications, *Seizure* 16(4):371-376, 2007.

Barkauskas VH et al: *Health & physical assessment,* ed 2, St Louis, 1998, Mosby.

Battie MC et al: Managing low back pain: attitudes and treatment preferences of physical therapist, *Phys Ther* 74:219, 1994.

Benito MB, Gorricho BP: Acute mastoiditis: Increase in the incidence and complications, *Int J Pediatr Otorhinolaryngol* 71(7):1007-1011, 2007.

Benson DF, Blumer D: *Psychiatric aspect of neurologic disease,* New York, 1975, Grune & Stratton.

Bianchini K et al: Detection and diagnosis of malingering in electrical injury, *Arch Clin Neuropsychol* 20(3):365-373, 2005.

Bianchini KJ, Greve KW, Glynn G: On the diagnosis of malingered pain-related disability: lessons from cognitive malingering research, *Spine J* 5(4):404-417, 2005.

Black HC: *Black's law dictionary,* St Paul, 1990, West Publishing.

Bongers PM et al: Psychosocial factors at work and musculoskeletal disease, *Scand J Work Environ Health* 19:297, 1993.

Borenstein DG, Wiesel SW: *Low back pain, medical diagnosis and comprehensive management,* Philadelphia, 1987, WB Saunders.

Borg G: Psychophysical bases of perceived exertion, *Med Sci Sport Exercise* 14:377, 1982.

Bradley LA: Multivariate analysis of the MMPI profiles of low back pain patients, *J Behav Med* 1:253, 1978.

Brena SF, Chapman SL: *Pain and litigation, textbook of pain,* Edinburgh, 1984, Churchill Livingstone.

Brooks M, Evans R, Fairclough J: *Sports injuries,* ed 2, London, 1992, Gower Medical.

Brotzman SB: *Clinical orthopaedic rehabilitation,* St Louis, 1996, Mosby.

Brown DE, Neumann RD: *Orthopedic secrets,* Philadelphia, 1995, Hanley & Belfus.

Bucholz RW: *Orthopaedic decision making,* ed 2, St Louis, 1996, Mosby.

Buschbacher RM: *Musculoskeletal disorders, a practical guide for diagnosis and rehabilitation,* Boston, 1994, Andover Medical Publishers.

Bush SS et al: Symptom validity assessment: practice issues and medical necessity: NAN Policy & Planning Committee, *Arch Clin Neuropsychol* 20(4):419-426, 2005.

Campbell JB, Campbell JM: *Mosby's survival guide to medical abbreviations & acronyms prefixes & suffixes symbols Greek alphabet,* St Louis, 1995, Mosby.

Canale ST: *Campbell's operative orthopaedics,* vol 1-4, ed 9, St Louis, 1998, Mosby.

Cassidy JD et al: Quebec task force on whiplash-associated disorders, redefining "whiplash" and its management (abridged), *Spine* 20(suppl):S1, 1995.

Chan CK et al: Ocular features of West Nile virus infection in North America: a study of 14 eyes, *Ophthalmology* 113(9):1539-1546, 2006.

Chen Y-L: Effectiveness of a new back belt in the maintenance of lumbar lordosis while sitting: a pilot study, *Int J Industr Ergon* 32(4):299-303, 2003.

Cho K-J et al: A case of an inflammatory myofibroblastic tumor of the mastoid presenting with chronic suppurative otitis media, *Auris Nasus Larynx* (in press, corrected proof).

Cipriano JJ: *Photographic manual of regional orthopaedic and neurological test,* ed 3, Baltimore, 1997, Williams & Wilkins.

Cohn RE: *Impairment rating examination and disability evaluation,* ed 3, Wilkesboro, NC, 1994, R Ernest Cohn.

Cole AJ, Herring SA: *The low back pain handbook: a practical guide for the primary care clinician,* Philadelphia, 1997, Hanley & Belfus.

Conwell TD: *Documenting patient progress "daily office charting seminar" thorough accurate quick procedures,* ed 11, Lakewood, Colo, 1990, Clinical Advancement Plus Seminars.

Cousins MJ, Phillips GD: *Acute pain management,* New York, 1986, Churchill Livingstone.

Cramer GD, Darby SA: *Basic and clinical anatomy of the spine, spinal cord, and ANS,* St Louis, 1995, Mosby.

Dambro MR, Griffith JA: *Griffith's 5 minute clinical consult,* Baltimore, 1997, Williams & Wilkins.

D'Ambrosia RD: *Musculoskeletal disorders regional examination and differential diagnosis,* Philadelphia, 1977, JB Lippincott.

Dandy DJ: *Essential orthopaedics and trauma,* Edinburgh, 1989, Churchill Livingstone.

Dawes HN et al: Borg's Rating of Perceived Exertion Scales: do the verbal anchors mean the same for different clinical groups? *Arch Phys Med Rehabil* 86(5):912-916, 2005.

Demeter SL, Andersson GBJ, Smith GM: *Disability evaluation,* St Louis, 1996, Mosby.

DeMeyer W: *Technique of the neurologic examination: a programmed text,* New York, 1969, McGraw-Hill.

Deshpande JK, Tobias JD: *The pediatric pain handbook,* St Louis, 1996, Mosby.

DeVellis B: The psychological impact of arthritis: prevalence of depression, *Arthritis Care Res* 8:284, 1995.

Doherty M, Doherty J: *Clinical examination in rheumatology,* London, 1992, Wolfe.

Doherty M, George E: *Self-assessment picture tests in rheumatology,* London, 1995, Mosby-Wolfe.

Doherty M: *Color atlas and text of osteoarthritis,* London, 1994, Wolfe.

Duhamel P: Criterion, construct and concurrent validity of a norm-referenced measure of malingering in pain patients, *J Pain* 6(3, suppl 1): S70-S426, 2005.

Dupoux E et al: Persistent stress "deafness": the case of French learners of Spanish, *Cognition* (in press, corrected proof).

Ellard J: Psychological reactions to compensable injury, *Med J Aust* 8:349, 1970.

Epstein O et al: *Clinical examination,* ed 2, London, 1997, Mosby.

Etherton JL et al: Pain, malingering and the WAIS-III Working Memory Index, *Spine J* 6(1):61-71, 2006.

Evans RC: Malingering/symptoms exaggeration. In Sweere JJ, editor: *Chiropractic family practice, a clinical manual,* Gaithersburg, Md, 1992, Aspen.

Evans RC: Overview of orthopedic malingering, CAPIT Homecoming and Educational Symposium, Rotorura, New Zealand, 1986, Phillip Institute of Science and Technology.

Eyler VA, Diehl KW, Kirkhart M: Validation of the Lees-Haley Fake Bad Scale for the MMPI-2 to detect somatic malingering among personal injury litigants, *Arch Clin Neuropsych* 15(8):834-835, 2000.

Fairbank JTC: The Oswestry low back pain disability questionnaire, *Physiotherapy* 8:66, 1980.

Farrar WE: *Atlas of infections of the nervous system,* London, 1993, Wolfe.

Feldmann E: *Current diagnosis in neurology,* St Louis, 1994, Mosby.

Ferezy JS: *The chiropractic neurological examination,* Gaithersburg, Md, 1992, Aspen.

Ferraz MB et al: EPM-ROM scale: an evaluative instrument to be used in rheumatoid arthritis trials, *Clin Exp Rheumatol* 8:491, 1990.

Finneson BE: *Low back pain,* ed 2, Philadelphia, 1981, JB Lippincott.

Foreman SM, Stahl MJ, Sportelli L: *Medical-legal issues in chiropractic,* Palmerton, Pa, 1993, PracticeMakers Products.

Forestier R et al: French version of the Copenhagen neck functional disability scale, *Joint Bone Spine* 74(2):155-159, 2007.

Frank ED et al: *Merrill's atlas of radiographic positioning and procedures,* ed 11, St. Louis, 2007, Mosby.

Fries JF: *Arthritis, a take care of yourself health guide for understanding your arthritis,* ed 4, 1995, Addison-Wesley.

Garcia JH: *Neuropathology: the diagnostic approach,* St Louis, 1997, Mosby.

Gips H, Yannai U, Hiss J: Self-inflicted gunshot wound mimicking assault: a rare variant of factitious disorder, *J Forensic Leg Med* 14(5):293-296, 2007.

Glenton C: Chronic back pain sufferers—striving for the sick role, *Soc Sci Med* 57(11):2243-2252, 2003.

Goldie BS: *Orthopaedic diagnosis and management: a guide to the care of orthopaedic patients,* ed 2, Oxford, UK, 1998, ISIS Medical Media.

Goldner JL, Bright DS: The effect of extremity blood flow on pain and cold tolerance. In Omer G, Spinner M, editors: *Peripheral nerve injuries,* Philadelphia, 1979, WB Saunders.

Goldner JL: Musculoskeletal aspects of emotional problems [editorial], *South Med J* 69:1, 1976.

Goldner JL: Volkmann's ischemia contracture. In Flynn JE, editor: *Hand surgery,* ed 2, Baltimore, 1975, Williams & Wilkins.

Gondipalli P, Tobias JD: Anesthetic implications of Möbius syndrome, *J Clin Anesth* 18(1):55-59, 2006.

Grassi L et al: Psychosomatic characterization of adjustment disorders in the medical setting: some suggestions for DSM-V, *J Affect Disord* 101(1-3):251-254, 2007.

Greenstein GM: *Clinical assessment of neuromusculoskeletal disorders,* St Louis, 1997, Mosby.

Greve KW, Bianchini KJ, Ameduri CJ: Use of a forced-choice test of tactile discrimination in the evaluation of functional sensory loss: a report of 3 cases, *Arch Phys Med Rehabil* 84(8):1233-1236, 2003.

Grilo RM et al: Clinically relevant VAS pain score change in patients with acute rheumatic conditions, *Joint Bone Spine* (in press, uncorrected proof).

Gunn CC, Bilbrandt WE: Early and subtle signs in low back sprain, *Spine* 3:267, 1978.

Guyton AC: *Structure and function of the nervous system,* Philadelphia, 1972, WB Saunders.

Hale BS, Raglin JS, Koceja DM: Effect of mental imagery of a motor task on the Hoffmann reflex, *Behav Brain Res* 142(1-2):81-87, 2003.

Hart FD: *French's index of differential diagnosis,* ed 10, Baltimore, 1973, Williams & Wilkins.

Hartley A: *Practical joint assessment lower quadrant,* ed 2, St Louis, 1995, Mosby.

Hashiba Y et al: A comparison of lower lip hypoesthesia measured by trigeminal somatosensory-evoked potential between different types of mandibular osteotomies and fixation, *Oral Surg Oral Med Oral Pathol Oral Radiol Endod* (in press, corrected proof).

Haustgen T, Bourgeois ML: L'evolution du concept de mythomanie dans l'histoire de la psychiatrie, *Ann Med Psychol Rev Psychiatr* 165(5):334-344, 2007.

Hawkins RJ: *An organized approach to musculoskeletal examination and history taking,* St Louis, 1995, Mosby.

Heilman KM, Watson RT, Greer M: *Handbook for differential diagnosis of neurologic signs and symptoms,* New York, 1977, Appleton-Century-Crofts.

Heroux ME et al: Upper-extremity disability in essential tremor, *Arch Phys Med Rehabil* 87(5):661-670, 2006.

Holmquist LA, Wanlass RL: A multidimensional approach towards malingering detection, *Arch Clin Neuropsychol* 17(2):143-156, 2002.

Holvey DN, Talbott JH: *The Merck manual of diagnosis and therapy,* ed 12, New Jersey, 1972, Merck.

Iowa Trial Lawyers Association: *Medical damages,* Des Moines, Iowa, 1995, The Association.

Jabaley ME et al: Comparison of histologic and functional recovery after peripheral nerve repair, *J Hand Surg (Am)*1:119, 1976.

Jablonski S: *Dictionary of medical acronyms & abbreviations,* ed 3, Philadelphia, 1998, Hanley & Belfus.

Jacobs JW: Screening for organic mental syndromes in the medically ill, *Ann Intern Med* 86:40, 1977.

Kanner R: *Pain management secrets,* Philadelphia, 1997, Hanley & Belfus.

Kasdan ML: *Occupational hand & upper extremity injuries & diseases,* ed 2, Philadelphia, 1998, Hanley & Belfus.

Katirji B: *Electromyography in clinical practice: a case study approach,* St Louis, 1998, Mosby.

Katz JN et al: Stability and responsiveness of utility measures, *Med Care* 32:183, 1994.

Katz WA: *Rheumatic diseases diagnosis and management,* Philadelphia, 1977, JB Lippincott.

Keefe FJ: Behavioral assessment and treatment of chronic pain: current status and future directions, *J Consult Clin Psychol* 50:896, 1982.

Kelsey JL: An epidemiological study of acute herniated lumbar intervertebral disc, *Rheum Rehab* 14:144, 1975.

Kendall HO, Kendall FP, Wadsworth GE: *Muscles testing and function,* ed 2, Baltimore, 1971, Williams & Wilkins.

Kirby RL et al: Wheelchair-skill performance: controlled comparison between people with hemiplegia and able-bodied people simulating hemiplegia, *Arch Phys Med Rehabil* 86(3):387-393, 2005.

Klippel JH, Dieppe PA: *Rheumatology,* vol 1-2, ed 2, London, 1998, Mosby.

Knutsson E, Martensson A: Isokinetic measurements of muscle strength in hysterical paresis, *Electroencephalogr Clin Neurophysiol* 61(5):370-374, 1985.

Koenigsberg R: *Churchill's illustrated medical dictionary,* New York, 1989, Churchill Livingstone.

Lally SJ: What tests are acceptable for use in forensic evaluations?: a survey of experts, *Professional Psychology: Res Pract* 34(5):491-498, 2003.

Lavy CBD, Barrett DS: *Questions and answers on Apley's concise system of orthopaedics and fractures,* Oxford, UK, 1991, Butterworth-Heinemann.

13

Leavitt F, Sweet JJ: Characteristics and frequency of malingering among patients with low back pain, *Pain* 25(3):357-364, 1986.

Leavitt F: Pain and deception: use of verbal pain measurement as a diagnostic aid in differentiating between clinical and simulated low-back pain, *J Psychosom Res* 29(5):495-505, 1985.

Lee TMC et al: Neural correlates of feigned memory impairment, *NeuroImage* 28(2):305-313, 2005.

Lephart SM, Henry TJ: Functional rehabilitation for the upper and lower extremity, *Orthop Clin North Am* 26:579, 1995.

Lerner AJ: *The little black book of neurology,* ed 3, St Louis, 1995, Mosby.

Lewis CB, Knortz KA: *Orthopedic assessment and treatment of the geriatric patient,* St Louis, 1993, Mosby.

Lorish DK et al: Disease and psychosocial factors related to physical functioning in rheumatoid arthritis, *J Rheumatol* 18:1150, 1991.

Loth TS: *Orthopedic boards review II: a case study approach,* St Louis, 1996, Mosby.

Lucas CE, Vlahos AL, Ledgerwood AM: Kindness kills: the negative impact of pain as the fifth vital sign, *J Am Coll Surg* (in press, corrected proof).

Magee DJ: *Orthopedic physical assessment,* ed 3, Philadelphia, 1997, WB Saunders.

Magerl W, Treede R-D: Secondary tactile hypoesthesia: a novel type of pain-induced somatosensory plasticity in human subjects, *Neurosci Lett* 361(1-3):136-139, 2004.

Maihofner C, DeCol R: Decreased perceptual learning ability in complex regional pain syndrome, *Eur J Pain* (in press, corrected proof).

Malone TR, McPoil TG, Nitz AJ: *Orthopedic and sports physical therapy,* ed 3, St Louis, 1997, Mosby.

Martinez MA et al: Facial nerve neuropathy in congenital vascular and lymphatic malformations of the face, *Clin Neurophysiol* 117(suppl 1):1-2, 2006.

Mayer TG: A prospective two year study of functional restoration in industrial low back injury: an objective assessment procedure, *JAMA* 258:1763, 1987.

Mayo Clinic and Mayo Foundation: *Clinical examinations in neurology,* ed 5, Philadelphia, 1981, WB Saunders.

Mazion JM: *Illustrated manual of neurological/reflexes/signs/tests, part I, orthopedic signs/tests/maneuvers for office procedure, part II,* Orlando, Fla, 1980, Daniels Publishing.

McBride ED: *Disability evaluation and principles of treatment of compensable injuries,* ed 6, Philadelphia, 1963, JB Lippincott.

McKechnie B: Low back pain in the 1990's. In McKechnie B, McRae R, editors: *Clinical orthopaedic examination,* ed 3, Edinburgh, 1990, Churchill Livingstone.

McNair PJ et al: Acute neck pain: cervical spine range of motion and position sense prior to and after joint mobilization, *Man Ther* (in press, corrected proof).

Medical Economics Books: *Patient care flow chart manual,* ed 3, Oradell, NJ, 1982, Medical Economics Books.

Mellion MB: *Office sports medicine,* ed 2, St Louis, 1996, Mosby.

Mellion MB: *Sports medicine secrets,* Philadelphia, 1994, Hanley & Belfus.

Melzack R: *The McGill pain questionnaire: pain measurement and assessment,* New York, 1983, Raven.

Mengel MB, Schwiebert LP: *Ambulatory medicine the primary care of families,* ed 2, Stamford, Conn, 1996, Appleton & Lange.

Mennell JM: *The musculoskeletal system differential diagnosis from symptoms and physical signs,* Gaithersburg, Md, 1992, Aspen.

Mercier LR, Pettid FJ: *Practical orthopedics,* ed 4, St Louis, 1995, Mosby.

Merle H et al: Natural history of the visual impairment of relapsing neuromyelitis optica, *Ophthalmology* 114(4):810.e2-815.e2, 2007.

Merskey H: *Pain and psychological medicine, textbook of pain,* Edinburgh, 1984, Churchill Livingstone.

Meyers JE, Millis SR, Volkert K: A validity index for the MMPI-2, *Arch Clin Neuropsychol* 17(2):157-169, 2002.

Meyers JE, Volbrecht ME: A validation of multiple malingering detection methods in a large clinical sample, *Arch Clin Neuropsychol* 18(3):261-276, 2003.

Million T, Green CJ, Meagher RB: *Million behavioral health inventory,* ed 3, Minneapolis, 1982, Interpretive Scoring System.

Momeni M, Baele P, Lavand'Homme P: Postoperative mapping of sensitive dysesthesia and residual pain after sternotomy for cardiac surgery, *J Pain* 8(4, suppl 1):S30, 2007.

Mosby-Year Book, Inc: *Expert 10-minute physical examination,* St Louis, 1997, Mosby.

Mountcastle VB: The view from within: pathways to the study of perception, *Johns Hopkins Med J* 136:109, 1975.

Nachemson AL: The lumbar spine: an orthopaedic challenge, *Spine* 1:59, 1976.

Neblett R et al: Quantifying lumbar flexion-relaxation phenomenon: theory and clinical applications, *Spine J* 2(5, suppl 1):97, 2002.

Nelson EC: Using outcome measures to improve care delivered by physicians and hospitals. In Heithoff KA, Lohr KN, editors: *Effectiveness and outcomes in healthcare,* Washington DC, 1990, Institute of Medicine, National Academy Press.

Nettina SM: *The Lippincott manual of nursing practice,* ed 6, Philadelphia, 1996, JB Lippincott.

Newton RW: *Color atlas of pediatric neurology,* St Louis, 1995, Mosby-Wolfe.

Nicholas JA, Hershman EB: *The lower extremity & spine in sports medicine,* vol 1-2, ed 2, St Louis, 1995, Mosby.

Nicholas JA, Hershman EB: *The upper extremity in sports medicine,* ed 2, St Louis, 1995, Mosby.

Nordin M, Andersson GBJ, Pope MH: *Musculoskeletal disorders in the workplace: principles and practice,* St Louis, 1997, Mosby.

O'Donoghue DH: *Treatment of injuries to athletes,* ed 3, Philadelphia, 1976, WB Saunders.

Olden KW, Drossman DA: Psychologic and psychiatric aspects of gastrointestinal disease, *Med Clin North Am* 84(5):1313-1327, 2000.

Olson WH, Brumback RA: *Handbook of symptom-oriented neurology,* Chicago, 1989, Mosby.

Omer GE, Spinner M: *Management of peripheral nerve problems,* Philadelphia, 1980, WB Saunders.

Osterweis M, Kleinman A, Mechanic D: *Pain and disability: clinical, behavioral and public policy perspectives, report of the Institute of Medicine Committee on Pain, Disability and Chronic Illness Behavior,* Washington, DC, 1987, National Academy Press.

O'Young B, Young MA, Stiens SA: *PM&R secrets,* Philadelphia, 1997, Hanley & Belfus.

Parker JC, Wright GE: The implications of depression for pain and disability in rheumatoid arthritis, *Arthritis Care Res* 8:279, 1995.

Patten J: *Neurological differential diagnosis,* ed 2, London, 1996, Springer.

Pilling LF, Brannick TL, Swenson WM: Psychological characteristics of patients having pain as a presenting symptom, *Can Med Assoc J* 97:287, 1967.

Pope AM, Tarlov AR: *Disability in America: toward a national agenda for prevention,* Washington, DC, 1991, National Academy Press.

Pope MH et al: *Occupational low back pain assessment, treatment and prevention,* St Louis, 1991, Mosby.

Powell MR et al: Detecting symptom- and test-coached simulators with the test of memory malingering, *Arch Clin Neuropsychol* 19(5):693-702, 2004.

Raphael BA et al: Validation and test characteristics of a 10-item neuro-ophthalmic supplement to the NEI-VFQ-25, *Am J Ophthalmol* 142(6):1026.e2-1035.e2, 2006.

Reed R: *Malingering, symposium papers,* Los Angeles, 1986, American College of Chiropractic Orthopedists.

Ridehalgh C, Greening J, Petty NJ: Effect of straight leg raise examination and treatment on vibration thresholds in the lower limb: a pilot study in asymptomatic subjects, *Man Ther* 10(2):136-143, 2005.

Rockwood CA Jr, Eilbert RE: Camptocormia, *J Bone Joint Surg* 51A:533, 1969.

Rode S et al: Health anxiety levels in chronic pain clinic attenders, *J Psychosom Res* 60(2):155-161, 2006.

Rolak LA: *Neurology secrets,* ed 2, Philadelphia, 1998, Hanley & Belfus.

Rotes-Querol J: The syndrome of psychogenic rheumatism, *Clin Rheum Dis* 5:797, 1979.

Saidoff DC, McDonough AL: *Critical pathways in therapeutic intervention,* St Louis, 1997, Mosby.

Sasai K et al: Two-level disc herniation in the cervical and thoracic spine presenting with spastic paresis in the lower extremities without clinical symptoms or signs in the upper extremities, *Spine J* 6(4):464-467, 2006.

Schram S, Taylor T: Tension signs in lumber disc prolapse, *Clin Orthop* 75:195, 1971.

Schumacher HR, Klippel JH, Koopman WJ: *Primer on the rheumatic diseases,* ed 10, Atlanta, 1993, Arthritis Foundation.

Schurch B: The predictive value of plantar flexion of the toes in the assessment of neuropathic voiding disorders in patients with spine lesions at the thoracolumbar level, *Arch Phys Med Rehabil* 80(6):681-686, 1999.

Scrivani SJ et al: Taste perception after lingual nerve repair, *J Oral Maxillofac Surg* 58(1):3-5, 2000.

Shankman GA: *Fundamental orthopedic management for the physical therapist assistant,* St Louis, 1997, Mosby.

Sherman MS: The nerves of bones, *J Bone Joint Surg* 45A:522, 1963.

Sherr VT: Human babesiosis—an unrecorded reality: absence of formal registry undermines its detection, diagnosis and treatment, suggesting need for immediate mandatory reporting, *Med Hypotheses* 63(4):609-615, 2004.

Simon D et al: Recognition and discrimination of prototypical dynamic expressions of pain and emotions, *Pain* (in press, corrected proof).

Sledge CB, Poss R: *The year book of orthopedics 1997,* St Louis, 1997, Mosby.

Slick DJ et al: Detecting malingering: a survey of experts' practices, *Arch Clin Neuropsychol* 19(4):465-473, 2004.

Smith TC et al: Reliability of standard health assessment instruments in a large, population-based cohort study, *Ann Epidemiol* 17(7):525-532, 2007.

Stedman TL: *Stedman's medical dictionary,* ed 25, Baltimore, 1990, Williams & Wilkins.

Stewart DL, Abeln SH: *Documenting functional outcomes in physical therapy,* St Louis, 1993, Mosby,

Strauss E et al: Intraindividual variability as an indicator of malingering in head injury, *Arch Clin Neuropsychol* 17(5):423-444, 2002.

Sun F, Tauchi P, Stark L: Binocular alternating pulse stimuli: experimental and modeling studies of the pupil reflex to light, *Math Biosci* 67(2):225-245, 1983.

Sweere JJ: *Chiropractic family practice: a clinical manual,* Gaithersburg, Md, 1992, Aspen.

Teichner G, Wagner MT: The test of memory malingering (TOMM): normative data from cognitively intact, cognitively impaired, and elderly patients with dementia, *Arch Clin Neuropsychol* 19(3):455-464, 2004.

Thompson JM: *Clinical outlines for health assessment,* St Louis, 1997, Mosby.

Toghill PJ: *Examining patients: an introduction to clinical medicine,* London, 1990, Edward Arnold.

Tollison CD, Satterthwaite JR, Tollison JW: *Handbook of pain management,* ed 2, Baltimore, 1994, Williams & Wilkins.

Torg JS, Shepard RJ: *Current therapy in sports medicine,* ed 3, St Louis, 1995, Mosby.

Truex RC, Carpenter MB: *Human neuroanatomy,* ed 6, Baltimore, 1969, Williams & Wilkins.

Turek SL: *Orthopaedics principles and their application,* ed 3, Philadelphia, 1977, JB Lippincott.

Waddell G: A new clinical model for the treatment of low back pain, *Spine* 12:632, 1987.

Waddell G: An approach to backache, *Br J Hosp Med* 28:187, 1982.

Wakefield TS, Frank RG: *The clinician's guide to neuro musculoskeletal practice,* Abbotsford, Wis, 1995, Allied Health of Wisconsin, SC.

Wall JR, Millis SR: Can motor measures tell us if someone is trying? An assessment of sincerity of effort in simulated malingering, *Arch Clin Neuropsychol* 14(1):40-41, 1999.

Walshe FMR: *Diseases of the nervous system,* ed 11, Baltimore, 1970, Williams & Wilkins.

Walters A: Psychogenic regional pain alias-hysterical pain, *Brain* 84:1, 1961.

Watkins RG: *The spine in sports,* St Louis, 1996, Mosby.

Weineck J: *Functional anatomy in sports,* ed 2, St Louis, 1990, Mosby.

Weinstein SL, Buckwalter JA: *Turek's orthopaedics principles and their application,* ed 5, Philadelphia, 1994, JB Lippincott.

White AH, Schofferman JA: *Spine care,* vol 1-2, St Louis, 1995, Mosby.

Whitmore I, Willan PLT: *Multiple choice questions in human anatomy,* London, 1995, Mosby.

Windsor RE, Lox DM: *Soft tissue injuries: diagnosis and treatment,* Philadelphia, 1998, Hanley & Belfus.

Wing PC, Wilfling FJ, Kokan PJ: *Comprehensive analysis of disability following lumbar intervertebral fusion: medical diagnosis and management,* Philadelphia, 1987, WB Saunders.

Yamamoto M et al: Psychological aspects of psychogenic deafness in children, *Int J Pediatr Otorhinolaryngol* 21(2):113-120, 1991.

Yelin E: Musculoskeletal conditions and employment, *Arthritis Care Res* 8:311, 1995.

Yunus M et al: Primary fibromyalgia (fibrositis): clinical study of 50 patients with matched normal controls, *Semin Arthritis Rheum* 11(1):151-171, 1981.

Zamir E, Read RW, Rao NA: Self-inflicted anterior scleritis, *Ophthalmology* 108(1):192-195, 2001.

Zatouroff M: *Diagnosis in color physical signs in general medicine,* ed 2, London, 1996, Mosby-Wolfe.

Zitelli BJ, Davis HW: *Atlas of pediatric physical diagnosis,* ed 2, London, 1992, Wolfe.

13

CITATIONS

Abramowitz JS, Olatunji BO, Deacon BJ: Health anxiety, hypochondriasis, and the anxiety disorders, *Behav Ther* 38(1):86-94, 2007.

Alizadehkhaiyat O et al: Strength and fatigability of selected muscles in upper limb: assessing muscle imbalance relevant to tennis elbow, *J Electromyogr Kinesiol* 17(4):428-436, 2007.

Bailey B et al: Comparison of four pain scales in children with acute abdominal pain in a pediatric emergency department, *Ann Emerg Med* 50(4):379-382, 2007.

Ban J-H, Jin SM: A clinical analysis of psychogenic sudden deafness, *Otolaryngol Head Neck Surg* 134(6):970-974, 2006.

BenDebba M, diZerega GS, Long DM: The lumbar spine outcomes questionnaire: its development and psychometric properties, *Spine J* 7(1):118-132, 2007.

Blair MA et al: Infantile onset of hereditary spastic paraplegia poorly predicts the genotype, *Pediatr Neurol* 36(6):382-386, 2007.

Booksh RL, Aubert MJ, Andrews SR: Should the retention trial of the test of memory malingering be optional?: a reply, *Arch Clin Neuropsychol* 22(1):87-89, 2007.

Borg M: Symptomatic myoclonus, *Clin Neurophysiol* 36(5-6):309-318, 2006.

Carey LM, Matyas TA, Oke LE: Evaluation of impaired fingertip texture discrimination and wrist position sense in patients affected by stroke: comparison of clinical and new quantitative measures, *J Hand Ther* 15(1):71-82, 2002.

Carragee E et al: Are first-time episodes of serious LBP associated with new MRI findings? *Spine J* 6(6):624-635, 2006.

Cassidy RC, Shaffer WO: Charcot arthropathy because of congenital insensitivity to pain in an adult, *Spine J* (in press, uncorrected proof).

Chen CS et al: Practical clinical approaches to functional visual loss, *J Clin Neurosci* 14(1):1-7, 2007.

Ciccone DS, Just N, Bandilla EB: Non-organic symptom reporting in patients with chronic non-malignant pain, *Pain* 68(2-3):329-341, 1996.

Cole M, Michael JA, Robert BD: Romberg's sign. In: *Encyclopedia of the neurological sciences,* New York, 2003 Academic Press.

de Seze J et al: Pupillary disturbances in multiple sclerosis: correlation with MRI findings, *J Neurol Sci* 188(1-2):37-41, 2001.

Delis DC, Wetter SR: Cogniform disorder and cogniform condition: proposed diagnoses for excessive cognitive symptoms, *Arch Clin Neuropsychol* 22(5):589-604, 2007.

Donaghy M, Michael JA, Robert BD: Lower motor neuron lesions. In: *Encyclopedia of the Neurological Sciences,* New York, 2003, Academic Press.

Edelstein C, Goldberg RA, Rubino G: Unilateral blindness after ipsilateral prophylactic transcranial optic canal decompression for fibrous dysplasia, *Am J Ophthalmol* 126(3):469-471, 1998.

Engin M et al: The classification of human tremor signals using artificial neural network, *Expert Syst Appl* 33(3):754-761, 2007.

Ergul Y et al: Vestibular neuritis caused by enteroviral infection, *Pediatr Neurol* 34(1):45-46, 2006.

Esteban A, Traba A, Prieto J: Eyelid movements in health and disease. The supranuclear impairment of the palpebral motility, *Clin Neurophysiol* 34(1):3-15, 2004.

Etherton JL et al: Pain, malingering and the WAIS-III Working Memory Index, *Spine J* 6(1):61-71, 2006.

Ferrante FM, Rana MV, Ferrante MA: Conversion disorder mimicking Dejerine-Roussy syndrome (thalamic stroke) after spinal cord stimulation, *Reg Anesth Pain Med* 29(2):164-167, 2004.

Ferrara L et al: A biomechanical assessment of disc pressures in the lumbosacral spine in response to external unloading forces, *Spine J* 5(5):548-553, 2005.

Fortenberry KT, Wiebe DJ: Medical excuse making and individual differences in self-assessed health: the unique effects of anxious attachment, trait anxiety, and hypochondriasis, *Person Individ Dif* 43(1):83-94, 2007.

Freynhagen R et al: Pseudoradicular and radicular low-back pain—a disease continuum rather than different entities? Answers from quantitative sensory testing, *Pain* 135(1-2):65-74, 2008.

Fritz JM, George SZ, Delitto A: The role of fear-avoidance beliefs in acute low back pain: relationships with current and future disability and work status, *Pain* 94(1):7-15, 2001.

Giummarra MJ et al: Central mechanisms in phantom limb perception: the past, present and future, *Brain Res Rev* 54(1):219-232, 2007.

Goffaux P et al: Descending analgesia—when the spine echoes what the brain expects, *Pain* 130(1-2):137-143, 2007.

Goodson A et al: Direct, quantitative clinical assessment of hand function: usefulness and reproducibility, *Man Ther* 12(2):144-152, 2007.

Hadjistavropoulos HD, LaChapelle DL: Extent and nature of anxiety experienced during physical examination of chronic low back pain, *Behav Res Ther* 38(1):13-29, 2000.

Hall RCW, Hall RCW: Malingering of PTSD: forensic and diagnostic considerations, characteristics of malingerers and clinical presentations, *Gen Hosp Psychiatry* 28(6):525-535, 2006.

Heming JE, Brown LN: Sensory temporal processing in adults with early hearing loss, *Brain Cogn* 59(2):173-182, 2005.

Hill ML, Craig KD: Detecting deception in pain expressions: the structure of genuine and deceptive facial displays, *Pain* 98(1-2):135-144, 2002.

Hinson VK, Haren WB: Psychogenic movement disorders, *Lancet Neurol* 5(8):695-700, 2006.

Hu X et al: Joint-angle-dependent neuromuscular dysfunctions at the wrist in persons after stroke, *Arch Phys Med Rehabil* 87(5):671-679, 2006.

Huber A et al: Dimensions of "unidimensional" ratings of pain and emotions in patients with chronic musculoskeletal pain, *Pain* 130(3):216-224, 2007.

Hunt DM, Sydney B, Jeffrey HM: Color blindness. In: *Encyclopedia of genetics,* New York, 2003, Academic Press.

Iannilli E et al: Intranasal trigeminal function in subjects with and without an intact sense of smell, *Brain Res* 113:235-244, 2007.

Jensen R et al: Cephalic muscle tenderness and pressure pain threshold in a general population, *Pain* 48(2):197-203, 1992.

Jull G et al: Does the presence of sensory hypersensitivity influence outcomes of physical rehabilitation for chronic whiplash?—a preliminary RCT, *Pain* 129(1-2):28-34, 2007.

Katirji B, Michael JA, Robert BD: Foot drop. In: *Encyclopedia of the neurological sciences,* New York, 2003, Academic Press.

Kaur P, Bennett JL, Alireza M: Optic neuritis and the neuro[hyphen (true graphic)]ophthalmology of multiple sclerosis. In: *International review of neurobiology.* vol 79, New York, 2007, Academic Press.

Kendell RE, Neil JS, Paul BB: Hysteria. In: *International encyclopedia of the social & behavioral sciences,* New York, 2001, Pergamon.

Kinsella S, Moran K: Gait pattern categorization of stroke participants with equinus deformity of the foot, *Gait Posture* (in press, corrected proof).

Leavitt F: A linguistic pain signature in simulated low back pain, *J Pain Sympt Manage* 2(2):83-88, 1987.

Lewis MAO et al: Management of neuropathic orofacial pain, *Oral Surg Oral Med Oral Pathol Oral Radiol Endod* 103(suppl 1):S32.e1-S32.e24, 2007.

Lillo JA, Moreira H, Charles S: Color Blindness. In: *Encyclopedia of applied psychology,* New York, 2004, Elsevier.

Marshall JC et al: The functional anatomy of a hysterical paralysis, *Cognition* 64(1):B1-B8, 1997.

Maruff P, Velakoulis D: The voluntary control of motor imagery. Imagined movements in individuals with feigned motor impairment and conversion disorder, *Neuropsychologia* 38(9):1251-1260, 2000.

May CR, Rose MJ, Johnstone FCW: Dealing with doubt: how patients account for non-specific chronic low back pain, *J Psychosom Res* 49(4):223-225, 2000.

Mewasingh LD et al: Motor strategies in standing up in children with hemiplegia, *Pediatr Neurol* 30(4):257-261, 2004.

Mohagheghi AA et al: Differences in gastrocnemius muscle architecture between the paretic and non-paretic legs in children with hemiplegic cerebral palsy, *Clin Biomech* 22(6):718-724, 2007.

Nadler SF, Malanga GA, Ciccone DS: Positive straight-leg raising in lumbar radiculopathy: is documentation affected by insurance coverage? *Arch Phys Med Rehabil* 85(8):1336-1338, 2004.

Nagasako EM, Oaklander AL, Dworkin RH: Congenital insensitivity to pain: an update, *Pain* 101(3):213-219, 2003.

Newman CJ et al: The characteristics of gait in Charcot-Marie-Tooth disease types I and II, *Gait Posture* 26(1):120-127, 2007.

O'Neill S et al: Generalized deep-tissue hyperalgesia in patients with chronic low-back pain, *Eur J Pain* 11(4):415-420, 2007.

Pahl MA et al: The impact of four common lumbar spine diagnoses upon overall health status, *Spine J* 6(2):125-130, 2006.

Paillex R, So A: Changes in the standing posture of stroke patients during rehabilitation, *Gait Posture* 21(4):403-409, 2005.

Patton LL et al: Management of burning mouth syndrome: systematic review and management recommendations, *Oral Surg Oral Med Oral Pathol Oral Radiol Endod* 103(suppl 1):S39.e1-S39.e13, 2007.

Poiraudeau S, Rannou F, Revel M: Functional restoration programs for low back pain: a systematic review, *Ann Readapt Med Phys* 50(6):425-429, 2007.

Pompeo A et al: Thyrotoxic hypokalemic periodic paralysis: an overlooked pathology in western countries, *Eur J Intern Med* (in press, corrected proof).

Proudlock FA, Gottlob I: Physiology and pathology of eye-head coordination, *Prog Retin Eye Res* 26(5):486-515, 2007.

Ramaesh K et al: Congenital corneal anesthesia, *Surv Ophthalmol* 52(1):50-60, 2007.

Sandroni P et al: Congenital idiopathic inability to perceive pain: a new syndrome of insensitivity to pain and itch with preserved small fibers, *Pain* 122(1-2):210-215, 2006.

Sartori G et al: A brief and unobtrusive instrument to detect simulation and exaggeration in patients with whiplash syndrome, *Neurosci Lett* 342(1-2):53-56, 2003.

Schornack MM, Brown WL, Siemsen DW: The use of tinted contact lenses in the management of achromatopsia, *Optometry* 78(1):17-22, 2007.

Schreuders TAR et al: Measuring the strength of the intrinsic muscles of the hand in patients with ulnar and median nerve injuries: reliability of the Rotterdam Intrinsic Hand Myometer, *J Hand Surg* 29(2):318-324, 2004.

Schwartzman RJ, Maleki J: Postinjury neuropathic pain syndromes, *Med Clin North Am* 83(3):597-626, 1999.

Shin YJ et al: Objective measurement of visual acuity by optokinetic response determination in patients with ocular diseases, *Am J Ophthalmol* 141(2):327-332, 2006.

Sternbach GL: The Glasgow Coma Scale, *J Emerg Med* 19(1):67-71, 2000.

Suarez H et al: Balance sensory organization in children with profound hearing loss and cochlear implants, *Int J Pediatr Otorhinolaryngol* 71(4):629-637, 2007.

Sullivan M, Ferrell B: Ethical challenges in the management of chronic nonmalignant pain: negotiating through the cloud of doubt, *J Pain* 6(1):2-9, 2005.

Taylor S, Frueh BC, Asmundson GJG: Detection and management of malingering in people presenting for treatment of posttraumatic stress disorder: methods, obstacles, and recommendations, *J Anxiety Disord* 21(1):22-41, 2007.

Valls-Sole J: Neurophysiological assessment of trigeminal nerve reflexes in disorders of central and peripheral nervous system, *Clin Neurophysiol* 116(10):2255-2265, 2005.

Verny C et al: Refsum's disease may mimic familial Guillain-Barré syndrome, *Neuromusc Disord* 16(11):805-808, 2006.

Vilar-Lopez R et al: Detection of malingering in a Spanish population using three specific malingering tests, *Arch Clin Neuropsychol* 22(3):379-388, 2007.

Viosca E et al: Walking recovery after an acute stroke: assessment with a new functional classification and the Barthel Index, *Arch Phys Med Rehabil* 86(6):1239-1244, 2005.

Vuilleumier P, Steven L: Hysterical conversion and brain function. In Laureys S, editor: *Progress in brain research,* vol 150, Amsterdam, 2005, Elsevier.

Wetter S, Murphy C: A paradigm for measuring the olfactory event-related potential in the clinic, *Int J Psychophysiol* 49(1):57-65, 2003.

Yamamoto K et al: Plantar flexion as an alternative to treadmill exercise for evaluating patients with intermittent claudication, *Eur J Vasc Endovasc Surg* 33(3):325-329, 2007.

13

GLOSSARY OF ABBREVIATIONS

A

a artery, before

aa equal part of each

AA affected area

AAA abdominal aortic aneurysm

A2 aortic second sound

AAL acute lymphoblastic, leukemia, anterior axillary line

ab antibody

abd abdomen

ABG arterial blood gasses

ABN abnormal

ABP arterial blood pressure

abs absent

a/c. before meals (ante sebum)

Ac acute

AC anterior chamber

acc accident

accom accommodation

acid phos acid phosphate

ACL anterior cruciate ligament

ACTH adrenocorticotrophic hormone

AD right ear

add. abductor or abduction

ADH antidiuretic hormone

ADL activates of daily living

ad lib as desired

adm. admission

AE above elbow

AEA above elbow amputation

AF atrial fibrillation, afebrile

AFB acid-fast bacilli

AFO ankle–foot orthosis

A/G albumin globulin ratio (blood)

AI aortic insufficiency

AIDS acquired immunodeficiency syndrome

AJ ankle jerk

a.k. above knee

aka alcoholic ketoacidosis

AKA above knee amputation

alb. albumin

alc. alcohol

alk. phos. alkaline phosphate

ALL acute lymphocytic leukemia

ALS amyotrophic lateral sclerosis

ALT alternating with, alanine aminotransferase (formerly serum glutamate pyruvate transaminase [SGPT])

AMA against medical advice

amb. ambulating, ambulatory

AMI acute myocardial infarction

AML acute myeloid leukemia

amp. amputation, ampule

ANA antinuclear antibody

anes. anesthesia

ann. fib. annulus fibrosis

ANS autonomic nervous system

ant. anterior

ante before

Anxty anxiety

A/O alert and oriented

AOB alcohol on breath

AODM adult-onset diabetes mellitus

A&P auscultation and percussion

AP anteroposterior

APC atrial premature contractions

aph aphasia

AP & lat anteroposterior and lateral

aq. water

AR aortic regurgitation

ARD acute respiratory distress

ARDS adult respiratory distress syndrome

ARF acute respiratory failure, acute rheumatic fever

art arterial

AS left ear, aortic stenosis

ASA acetylsalicylic acid, aspirin

A.S.A. 1 normal healthy patient

A.S.A. 2 patient with mild systemic disease

A.S.A. 3 patient with severe systemic disease

A.S.A. 4 patient with incapacitating systemic disease that is a constant threat to life

ASAP as soon as possible

ASCVD atherosclerotic cardiovascular disease

ASD atrial septal defect

ASHD arteriosclerotic heart disease

ATNR asymmetrical tonic neck reflex

AU both ears

aud. auditory

Aur. Fib auricular fibrillation

A-V arteriovenous

AVF arteriovenous fistula

AVR aortic valve replacement

Ax. axilla, axillary

B

B. bath

BA barium

Bab. Babinski sign

Ba.E barium enema
Bas. basal, basilar
baso basophile
BBB bundle branch block
BBT basal body temperature
BCA basal cell atypia
BCD basal cell dysplasia
BCE basal cell epithelioma
BDC burn dressing change
BE below elbow, barium enema
BEA below-elbow amputation
BFP biological false-positive
Bic. biceps
b.i.d. twice daily
BIH bilateral inguinal hernia
bilat. bilateral, bilaterally
bili bilirubin
b.i.n. twice per night
BiW twice weekly
BJ biceps reflex
bk. back
BK below knee
BKA below-knee amputation
bl cult blood culture
bld. blood
Bl.T bleeding time
BM black male, bone marrow, bowel movement
BMR basal metabolic rate
body wt. body weight
BOMA otitis media, both ears, acute
BP blood pressure
BPD bronchopulmonary dysplasia
BPH benign prostatic hypertrophy
BPM beats per minute
BR bedrest, bathroom
brach. brachial
broncho bronchoscopy
BS blood sugar, bowel sounds
B.S. breath sounds
BSA body surface area
BST blood serologic test
BT bleeding time
BUN blood urea nitrogen
Bx. biopsy

C
c. with
C cervical, Caucasian
C. centigrade, Celsius complement
CI–XII First to twelfth cranial nerve
C–1 to C–7 cervical vertebrae
Ca calcium
CA carcinoma, cancer
CABG coronary artery bypass graft
CAD coronary artery disease
CAHD coronary atherosclerotic heart disease
Cal calorie, calories

CAPD continuous ambulatory peritoneal dialysis
Caps capsules
car. carotid
card. cardiac
Card Cath cardiac catheterization
CAT computerized axial tomography
cath catheterization, catheter
CBC complete blood count
CBD common bile duct
CBF cerebral blood flow
CBG capillary blood gas
CBR complete bed rest
cc. cubic centimeter
CC chief complaint
CCU coronary care unit
CD cardiac disease, contagious disease
CEA carcinoembryonic antigen
Cerv. cervix, cervical
CF cardiac failure, cystic fibrosis
CHD congenital heart disease, coronary heart disease
Chem. chemotherapy
CHF congestive heart failure
CHO carbohydrate
Chol cholesterol
Chr chronic
C.I color index
CI cardiac insufficiency, cardiac index
CIS carcinoma *in situ*
CK creatinine kinase
Cl chlorine, chloride
Clav. clavicle
cldy cloudy
CLL chronic lymphocytic leukemia
Cl.T clotting time
cm. centimeter
CML chronic myeloid leukemia
CMV cytomegalovirus
CN cranial nerve
CNS central nervous system
cnst. constipation
c/o complains of, complaints
CO₂ carbon dioxide
comb. combine, combination
comm. communicable
comp. compound, compress
conc. concentrated
cons. consultation
cont. contractions, continued
COPD chronic obstructive pulmonary disease
Cor heart
CPAP continuous positive airway pressure
CPC clinicopathological conference
CPK creatinine phosphokinase
CPPB continuous positive pressure breathing
CPR cardiopulmonary resuscitation
CPT chest physical therapy
CR closed reduction

cran. cranial
CRD chronic respiratory disease
creat. creatinine
CRF chronic renal failure
C/S, CS cesarean section
C&S culture and sensitivity
CSF cerebrospinal fluid
C-spine cervical spine
CT computed tomography
CV cardiovascular
CVA cerebrovascular accident, costovertebral angle
CVL central venous line
CVP central venous pressure
CVS cardiovascular system
Cx cervix, culture
CxR chest X-ray
Cysto cystoscopy

D
DAP distal airway pressure
dB decibel
DBE deep-breathing exercise
d/c discontinue
DC discharges, discontinue
DD discharge diagnosis
DDx differential diagnosis
decr. decreased
dehyd. dehydrated
Derm. dermatology
DES diethylstilbestrol
DI diabetes insipidus, diagnostic imaging
DIAG. diagnosis
diam. diameter
DIC disseminated intravascular coagulation, disseminated coagulopathy
diff. differential
dil. dilute
dim. diminished
DIP distal interphalangeal (joint)
dis. disease
disch. discharge
disp. disposition
dist. distilled, distal
div. divorced
DJD degenerative joint disease
DKA diabetic ketoacidosis
DLE disseminated lupus erythematosus
D/L, dL deciliter
DM diabetes mellitus, diastolic murmur
DNA deoxyribonucleic acid
DNKA did not keep appointment
DOB date of birth
DOE dyspnea on exertion
Dors dorsal
D.P. dorsal pedia
DPT diphtheria, pertussis, tetanus vaccine
drsg. dressing

D/S discharge summary
DTR deep tendon reflexes
DTs delirium tremens
DUI driving under influence
Dx diagnosis

E
e without
EBV Epstein-Barr virus
ECG electrocardiogram
ECHO enterocytopathogenic human orphan virus
E. coli *Escherichia coli*
ED emergency department
EEG electroencephalogram
EENT eyes, ears, nose, throat
EEX electrodiagnosis
EKG electrocardiogram
elev. elevated
EMG electromyogram
ENT ears, nose, throat
Eos. eosinophiles
EOM extraocular movement
ESR erythrocyte sedimentation rate
ETIOL. etiology
ETOH ethanol
EVAL evaluation
ex. exercise, example
ext. extremities, external

F
F finger, female, Fahrenheit
FA fluorescent antibody
F.A. first aid
F.B. foreign body
FBS fasting blood sugar
FDP flexor digitorum profundus
Fe def. iron deficiency
FEF forced expiratory flow
fem. femoral
fem. pop. femoral popliteal
FEV forced expiratory volume
f.f. force fluid
FH family history, fetal heart
Fio$_2$ faction of inspired oxygen concentration
fl. fluids
flac. flaccid
flex. flexor, flexion
fl. oz. fluid ounce
FM finger movement
fract. fractional
FRC functional residual capacity
FS finger stick
FSH follicle-stimulating hormone
F/U, F-U, F.U. follow-up
FUO fever of unknown origin
FVC forced vital capacity
Fx fracture

G

G

G globulin
G.A. general anesthesia
GB gallbladder
GBS gallbladder series
G.C. gonococcus
GCS Glasgow Coma Scale
GE gastroenterology
G/E gastroenteritis
gen, genl. general
GFR glomerular filtration rate
GI gastrointestinal
gluc glucose
gm gram
Gm+ gram positive
Gm− gram negative
gm.% grams per 100 cc
GMA grand mal attack
Gt.tr. gait training
GSW gunshot wound
GTT glucose tolerance test
GU genitourinary
G/W glucose and water

H

h hour
H hydrogen, history, hour, hypodermic
H/A headache
HASCVD hypertensive arteriosclerotic cardiovascular disease
Hb., Hgb hemoglobin
HB heart block
HBP high blood pressure
H&C hot and cold
HCO₃ bicarbonate
Hct. hematocrit
HCVD hypertensive cardiovascular disease
h.d. at bedtime
Hd head, Hodgkin disease
HDL high-density lipids
HEENT head, eyes, ears, nose, throat
hern. hernia
Hem hematology
Hem Pro hematology profile
HH hard of hearing
hist. history, histology
HIV human immunodeficiency virus
HKAFO hip knee ankle foot orthosis
HLA human leukocyte group A, histocompatibility leukocyte focus
HM hand movement
HNP herniated nucleus pulposus
h/o history of
HOB head of bed
horiz. horizontal
H&P history and physical
HPI history of present illness

HR heart rate
H.R.S.T. heat, reddening, swelling, tenderness
HS bedtime
H₂O water
H₂O₂ hydrogen peroxide
Ht height, heart
HVD hypertensive vascular disease
Hx history
Hz hertz (cycles/second)

I

I radioactive iodine
IA intra-arterially
IABP intra-aortic balloon pump
i.c. intracutaneous(ly)
ICCU intensive coronary care unit
ICF intracellular fluid
ICS intercostal space
ICU intensive care unit
i.d. during the day
ID intradermal, identification, infectious disease
IDDM insulin-dependent diabetes mellitus
I/E inspiratory, expiratory
Ig immunoglobulin
IgA immunoglobulin A
IgE immunoglobulin E
IgG immunoglobulin gamma (G)
IgM immunoglobulin M
IH infectious hepatitis
IHD ischemic heart disease
IM intramuscular, intramedullary
imp. impression
In. inches
incr. increased(ing)
inf infusion, inferior
inj injured, injection
inspir inspiration, inspiratory
int. internal
INTHC intrathecally
IO inferior oblique
IPJ interphalangeal joint
irreg. irregular
IS intercostal space
IST insulin shock therapy
ITP idiopathic thrombocytopenic purpura
I.U., IU International Unit
IV intravenous(ly)
IVD intervertebral disc

J

J joint
JRA juvenile rheumatoid arthritis
jt. joint
JVP jugular venous pulse

K

K potassium, kidney
KC1 potassium chloride

Kcal. kilocalorie, calorie
kg kilogram
KJ, K-J knee jerk
KK knee kick
17 KS 17 ketosteroids
KUB kidney, ureter, bladder (X-rays)

L
L left, liver, liter, lower, light, lumbar
L2, L3 second, third lumbar vertebrae
LA left antrum
lab. laboratory
lac. laceration
LAD left anterior descending coronary artery
lam. laminectomy
lat. lateral
lb. pound
LBP lower back pain
LCA left coronary artery
L.D. lethal dose
LDH lactic dehydrogenase
LDL low-density lipids
LE lupus erythematosus
L.E. lower extremities
leuc. leukocytes
lg large, leg
LICS left intercostal space
lig. ligament
LIH left inguinal hernia
liq. liquid
LKS liver, kidneys, spleen
LLE left lower extremity
LLG left lateral gaze
LLL left lower lobe
LLQ left lower quadrant
LMA left mentoanterior
L/min liter per minute
LML left mediolateral
LMP left mentoposterior, last menstrual period
LMT left mentotransverse
L.N. lymph node
LNMP last normal menstrual period
L.O.C. loss of consciousness, level of consciousness, laxative of choice
LOM left otitis media
LOP left occipital posterior
LOS length of stay
LP lumbar puncture, light perception
LRQ lower right quadrant
L.S. lumbosacral
LSA lateral sacrum anterior
LSK liver, spleen, kidneys
LSP left sacrum posterior
LST left sacrum transverse
Lt. left, light
LUE left upper extremity
LUL left upper lobe

LUQ left upper quadrant
Lymphs lymphocytes
lytes electrolytes

M
m. minimum
m, M married, male, mother murmur, meter, mass, molar
MA mental age
macro. macrocytic, macroscopic
MAP mean arterial pressure
max. maximum, maxillary
mcg. microgram
MCH mean corpuscular hemoglobin
MCHC mean corpuscular hemoglobin concentration
MCL midclavicular line
MCP metacarpophalangeal joint
MCV mean corpuscular volume
MD muscular dystrophy
Mdnt. midnight
ME middle ear, medical examiner
Med. medicine
MEq/L milliequivalents per liter
Mets. metastasis
mg. milligram
Mg. magnesium
MG myasthenia gravis
mg/dL milligrams per deciliter
mg.% milligrams per 100 cc (mL)
MI myocardial infarction, mitral insufficiency
micro microcytic, microscopic
Min minute
mL. milliliter
mm millimeter
mm. muscles
MMPI Minnesota Multiphasic Personality Inventory
mod moderate
mono. monocyte
MP metacarpophalangeal
MRI magnetic resonance imaging
mss massage
MT metacarpophalangeal (joint)
M.T. muscles and tendons
MVA motor vehicle accident

N
n. nerve
N₂ nitrogen
N₂O nitrous oxide (anesthetic)
Na sodium
NaCl sodium chloride
NED no evidence of disease
neg. negative
NER no evidence of recurrence
NERD no evidence of recurrent disease
Neur. neurology
NKA no known allergies
NM neuromuscular

G

NMR nuclear magnetic resonance
noct. nocturnal
NOS not otherwise specified
Ns. nerves
N.S. nervous system
NSA no significant abnormality
NSAID nonsteroidal anti-inflammatory drug
N&V nausea and vomiting
NS neurosurgery
NTP normal temperature and pressure
NVD nausea, vomiting, diarrhea
NWB non–weight–bearing
NYD not yet diagnosed

O
o none, without
O oral
O2 oxygen
O$_2$ cap. oxygen capacity
O$_2$ sat. oxygen saturation
OA osteoarthritis
Obs observation
OCC. occipital, occasional
O/E on examination
OH occupational history
OOB out of bed
Op. operation
OR operating room, open reduction
OR-IF open reduction with internal fixation
Ortho. orthopedic surgery
os opening, mouth, bone
OTC over-the-counter (pharmaceuticals)
O.T. occupational therapy, old tuberculin
oz. ounce

P
P after, phosphorus, pulse
PA posteroanterior
p&a percussion and auscultation
palp. palpate, palpated, palpable
Path. pathology
PA view posterior-anterior view on X-ray
Pb lead
PBI protein bound iodine
p/c., p.c. after meals
PCL posterior cruciate ligament
PCO$_2$ carbon dioxide concentration
PCV packed cell volume (of blood)
PE physical examination, pulmonary embolism
PERRLA pupils equal, round, reactive to light and accommodation (normal)
PET positron emission tomography
PH past history
PID pelvic inflammatory disease
PIP proximal interphalangeal
plts. platelets
P.M. afternoon, post-mortem

PMH past medical history
PMN polymorphonuclear (leukocytes)
PM&R physical medicine and rehabilitation
PNI peripheral nerve injury
POMR problem-oriented medical record
poplit. popliteal
pos. positive
post. posterior
PRE progressive resistive exercise
p.r.m. according to circumstances
p.r.n. PRN, as often as necessary
prod. productive
Prog. prognosis
PROM passive range of motion, premature rupture of membranes
pron. pronator, pronation
pros. prostate, prostatic
prosth. prosthesis
prot., Prot protein, Protestant
pro.time prothrombin time
PSH past surgical history
psi pounds per square inch
PSMA progressive spinal muscular atrophy
pt., Pt. patient
PT physical therapy
P.T. physical therapy, posterior tibial artery pulse
PTB patellar tendon bearing
PTCA percutaneous transvenous coronary angioplasty (balloon angioplasty)
PVD peripheral vascular disease
PVT previous trouble
PWB% partial weight-bearing with percent
Px, PX physical examination

Q
q every
q.d. every day
q.h. every hour
q2h every two hours
q4h every four hours
q.i.d. four times per day
q.i.w. four times per week
q.l. as much as desired
qn, q.n. every night
q.n.s., QNS quantity not sufficient
q.o.d. every other day
q.o.n. every other night
q.p. as much as you please
q.q., Q.Q. each, every
q.q.h. every four hours
q.s. quantity, sufficient
qt. quart
qts. drops
quad. quadriplegic
quant. quantitative or quantity
q.v. as much as you wish
q.w. every week

R

r., R right, rectal, roentgen, X-ray
RA rheumatoid arthritis, right atrium
rad. radial
r.a.m. rapid alternating movements
R.A.S. right arm sitting
rbc, RBC red blood count, red blood cell
RE reconditioning exercise
reg. regular
rehab. rehabilitation
resp. respiratory, respirations
RF rheumatic fever
R to L&A react to light and accommodation
RLE right lower extremity
RMSF Rocky Mountain spotted fever
RNA ribonucleic acid
RO, R/O rule out
ROM range of motion, rupture of membranes,
ROS review of systems
RRE, RR&E round, regular, and equal
RSD reflex sympathetic dystrophy
Rt. right
RUE right upper extremity
Rx therapy, prescription

S

s without
S sensation, sensitive, serum
sec second
sed. rate erythrocyte sedimentation rate
Sens. sensory, sensation
Serol. serology, serological test
SGOT, SGO-T serum glutamic oxalacetic transaminase
SH social history, serum hepatitis
SI sacroiliac joint, stroke index
SIDS sudden infant death syndrome
skel. skeletal
SLE systemic lupus erythematosus
SLR straight leg raising
sm small
SMA-14 routine admission chemistry
SNS sympathetic nervous system
S.O.A.P. subjective, objective assessment plan
SOB shortness of breath
sp. spine, spinal
sp.cd. spinal cord
stat., STAT immediately
STD sexually transmitted disease
sup. superior
supin. supination
SWD short wave diathermy
Sx symptoms
sys. system

T

T3 triiodothyronine
T4 total serum thyroxine

TA tendon Achilles
T&A tonsils and adenoids, tonsillectomy and adenoidectomy
tab. tablet
TB tuberculosis
tbsp. tablespoon
TCDB turn, cough, deep breath
temp temperature
TENS transient electric nerve stimulation
T.F. tuning fork
THERAP. therapy, therapeutic
thor. thorax, thoracic
THR total hip replacement
TIA transient ischemic attack, transient ischemic shock
t.i.d. three times per day
TIP terminal interphalangeal (joint)
t.i.w. three times per week
TJ triceps reflex
TKR total knee replacement
TMJ temporomandibular joint
TPR temperature, pulse, respiration
tr trace
TSH thyroid-stimulating hormone
tsp. teaspoon
TSS toxic shock syndrome
Tx treatment, traction

U

U. unit
U/A urinalysis
UCD usual childhood diseases
UCHD usual childhood diseases
uln ulnar
ULQ upper left quadrant
unilat. unilateral
Ur. urine
URD upper respiratory disease
URI upper respiratory infection
Urol. urology
URQ upper right quadrant
u/s, US ultrasound
UTI urinary tract infection
UVL ultraviolet light

V

V vein
VA visual acuity
VC, (vit.cap) vital capacity
VD venereal disease
VDRL venereal disease research laboratory test; blood test for syphilis
vert. vertical
Via by way of
vit. vitamin
VLDL very-low-density lipoproteins
vol volume
VS, V.S. vital signs

G

W

W widowed, white

wbc, WBC white blood count, white blood cell

WBT weight bearing to tolerance

WF white female

wk week

WM white male

w/n within

WN well–nourished

WNL within normal limits

WP whirlpool

wt. weight

w/u workup

X

x times

Y

y.o. years old

yrs. years

APPENDIX A
LISTING OF TESTS, ALPHABETICALLY AND ANATOMICALLY

APPENDIX B
LISTING OF TESTS ACCORDING TO THE POSITION OF THE PATIENT

Side-Lying Examination

Prone Examination

ANSWERS TO CRITICAL THINKING QUESTIONS

Chapter 1

1. The essential points of the complaint history include trying to establish the physical issues that are of greatest importance to the patient. Try to differentiate the anatomic and pathologic aspects of any disease or injury that might be present. A history of trauma may help differentiate between inherent laxity and past instability. An accurate description of the injury event, including the exact position of the injured part at the time of injury, is essential. Observe and examine the movements and mannerisms of the patient as well as listen to the patient. An experienced examiner can form an idea of the extent and magnitude simply from the patient's history.

2. The five essential steps in formulating a working diagnosis are history taking, observation, palpation, orthopedic testing, and clinical laboratory and diagnostic imaging procedures.

3. The 5 critical questions in orthopedics are:
   - Are any joints abnormal?
   - What is the nature of the abnormality?
   - What is the extent of the involvement?
   - Are other features of diagnostic importance present?
   - Do the answers to questions 1 to 4 provide sufficient clues?

4. Jendrassik maneuver is a distraction technique used if less-than-normal reactivity is encountered in the upper or lower extremities. The patient is instructed to perform an isometric contraction in the opposite upper or lower extremity.

5. The patient exhibits the possibility of viscerosomatic pain or psychosocial causes. These conclusions mandate further examination, diagnostic testing, or other appropriate tests.

6. The five-rung test involves performing one repetition (trial) with the handle of the Jamar dynamometer on each of the five handle settings, whereas the maximal static grip test involves performing three repetitions with the handle on either the second or third setting.

7. During the static grip test, the duration of muscular contraction of each hand grip is 3 to 5 seconds, whereas during the rapid exchange grip maneuver, the hands alternate rapidly, resulting in a shorter duration of each grip (less than 1.5 seconds per grip).

8. A "positive REG test" is obtained when REG scores are greater than static grip scores, which indicates a submaximal or a feigned effort. A "negative REG test" is obtained when static grip scores are greater than REG scores, indicating a maximal or a sincere effort. Remember, grip strength is another tool to evaluate the myoneural function *versus* sincerity of effort.

9. Scleratogenous pain is from somatic structures such as cartilage, ligament, joint capsule, or bone. It *does not* follow a dermatome pattern. The pain is described as dull, achy, diffuse, and difficult to pinpoint. Scleratogenous pain is one of the more common spinal pain patterns.

10. It is very useful in measuring structural damage and features such as erosions, joint space narrowing and disease-specific findings.

11. In rheumatoid arthritis, this can help gauge the response or lack of response to therapy. The areas to monitor would include PA view of the hands, wrists, and feet.

12. This should be done at 6-month intervals for a minimum of 2 years.

13. In early AS, studies are reasonable at 6 months from the baseline study.

14. The areas monitored include pelvis, sacroiliac joints, and axial spine annually or every other year. Plain films (PA) views of the hands and feet at baseline, to be followed up based on clinical features of the area.

15. Bone scanning has become common in the evaluation of child abuse. Very young children typically do not develop stress fractures of multiple fracture sites in normal living situations.

16. This test is helpful in evaluation of variations from the peripheral nerve through the spinal cord to the somatosensory region of the brain. This includes diseases of the spinal cord, trauma to the spine, neuromuscular diseases, and demyelinating conditions.

Chapter 2

1. Inflammatory disease, mechanical articular or periarticular disorder, systemic disease presenting with musculoskeletal symptoms or signs, functional disorder and idiopathic.

2. Such referred pain is a perceptual error occurring at the sensory cortex and reflects shared innervations by structures derived from the same embryonic segment.

3. Nerve entrapment—electric shock
   Vascular—throbbing
   Articular—joint ache

4. Pain with use suggests a mechanical problem
   Pain at rest or at the beginning of use rather than the end implies inflammatory component
   Pain at night suggests a serious problem, avascular necrosis, bone neoplasm, or bone collapse around a joint
5. Falls, 185,000 hip fractures happen yearly. Fat embolism is the danger.
6. Working age adults with subacute lower back pain (duration of more than 4 weeks and less than 12 weeks).
7. 1. **P** Preventable course of disability (e.g., falls, direct trauma)
   2. **I** Independence (e.g., self-care)
   3. **L** Lifestyle (roles, goals)
   4. **S** Social factors (e.g., family, friends, shelter)
8. Attention must be directed to possible extrinsic disorders. Determination of extrinsic disorders requires the examination of the regions of the body that might be responsible, such as cervical spine pathology may be causing pain anywhere in the upper extremity.
9. Localized pigmented villonodular synovitis and giant cell tumor.
10. Dermatomyositis
11. The papules are frequently found on the hands, elbows, or feet. They can be in any combination.
12. Chronic pain, fibromyalgia or neuropathic syndromes
13. • Comprehensive history and physical examination
    • Laboratory to evaluate electrolytes
    • Urinalysis for blood and/or myoglobin
14. Spasticity
15. Ataxia

Chapter 3

1. The vertebral artery is the major source of blood for the cervical cord and cervical spine.
2. The atlantoaxial joints are unstable because of their opposed convexity with a small contact area between the joint surfaces.
3. The mechanism of injury is hyperflexion.
4. The initial radiograph is a lateral radiograph of the cervical spine, preferably made with the patient still on the transportation stretcher.
5. Because swelling is noted in the prevertebral soft tissue after cervical spine fractures, the mid-position of C3–C7, where most fractures occur, should be evaluated. At C3, 3.5 mm is standard; at C4, 5.0 mm; and at C5, C6, and C7, approximately 15 mm, with up to 20 mm at the distal portion. If abnormal widening is noted at any area along the anterior cervical spine, fracture should be suspected.
6. The most common congenital abnormality is stenosis of the cervical spine canal, with the quadriplegia occurring at the stenotic level.

7. 1. Compressive flexion
   2. Vertical compression
   3. Distractive flexion
   4. Compressive extension
   5. Distractive extension
   6. Lateral flexion
8. The most common anatomic finding is a unilateral vertebral arch fracture that involves the articular process.
9. The patient often feels marked apprehension and fear with a sense of subjective instability. Pain radiating along the course of the greater occipital nerve (C2), so-called occipital neuralgia, is frequent and leads to marked guarding of neck motion.
10. The most common occur from the occiput to C3. Lesions at the atlantoaxial joint are noted in 70% of children under 15 years of age but in only 16% of adults.
11. In C4 quadriplegia, the patient is expected to breathe spontaneously because C4 innervates the diaphragm. The patient is able to shrug the shoulders independently but lacks functional abdominal muscles. Sensation is present in the upper anterior chest wall but not in the upper extremities. All reflexes are absent.
12. In quadriplegia, the deltoid muscle and a portion of the biceps muscle are functioning. The patient is able to perform shoulder abduction and flexion/extension as well as some elbow flexion. However, all these functions are weak. Sensation is normal over the upper portion of the anterior chest wall and the lateral aspect of the arm from the shoulder to the elbow crease. The biceps reflex may be normal or slightly decreased.
13. Both the biceps and rotator cuff muscles continue to function. The extensor carpi radialis longus and brevis and extensor carpi ulnaris may not be functioning. The patient has almost full function of the shoulder, full flexion of the elbow, full supination and partial pronation of the forearm, and partial extension of the wrist. The strength of wrist extension is normal, because some power for the extension is supplied predominantly by the extensor carpi radialis longus and brevis. The lateral side of the entire upper extremity as well as the thumb, index, and half of the middle finger have normal sensory power. Both the biceps and the brachioradialis reflexes are normal.
14. C7 quadriplegia involves the vertebral level of C7, T1. With the C7 nerve root intact, the triceps, wrist flexors, and long-finger extensors are functional. The patient can hold objects, but the grasp is extremely weak. Although still confined to a wheelchair, the patient may be able to attempt parallel bar and brace function for general exercise.
15. The most common pain pattern for the cervical disc is radiation into the scapular area and down the lateral aspect of the arm into the forearm and hand.
16. The tests designed for cervical spine complaints test for dural tension, foraminal, central canal and vertebral canal patency, muscle, tendon, and ligamentous injuries.

17. At-level pain, which occurs in dermatomes near the spinal injury, develops shortly after spinal cord injury, and is often characterized as either stabbing pain or a stimulus-independent type that is accompanied by allodynia.

18. Children often have lax ligaments, which increases spinal motion. This most commonly occurs in the cervical region. Increased motion seen during physical or X-ray examination should be differentiated from pathologic subluxation.

19. On imaging of the cervical spine, the predental space (atlantodental–ADI) should not exceed 3 mm. A predental space greater than 3 mm has been found in 20% of normal patients younger than 8 years of age and can be followed on patients into early adulthood.

20. Pathologic subluxation of the atlas on the axis that compromises the spinal cord (compressive myelopathy) is associated with rheumatoid arthritis and ankylosing spondylitis. The common characteristic of these disorders is the destructive weakening of the atlantooccipital ligament system, with resultant translation of the structures.

21. In addition to the basic cervical study (APOM, APLC, and LCN) flexion and extension views will allow measurement of the ADI.

22. Cranial nerve (CN) XI supplies the sternocleidomastoid (SCM) muscle.

23. The patient pushes their cheek against the examiner's hand, pushes the back of the head against the examiner's hand and pushes the forehead against the examiner's hand testing the strength of the SCM.

24. The symptoms of nerve root compression include proximal (root) pain and neck pain, distal paresthesia in dermatome patterns, muscle weakness in one or several muscles supplied by a single root, loss of deep tendon reflexes, muscle fasciculation, and radiating pains that are further aggravated by movements of the neck. With CRPS, there is burning pain, skin sensitivity, changes in skin temperature (warmer or cooler compared to opposite extremity), change in skin color (often blotchy purple, pale or red), change in skin texture (shinny and thin), and changes in nail and hair growth patterns. Neurovascular compression (thoracic outlet) can result in swelling or puffiness in the arm and hand, bluish discoloration of the hand, feeling of heaviness in arm and hand, deep boring tooth ache like pain in the neck and shoulder that increases at night, easily fatigued arm and hand.

25. Bakody sign is used to define the difference between the two.

26. The brachial plexus is made up of the anterior primary rami of the four lower cervical nerves, C5 through C8, and the greater part of T1. The C5 and C6 rami form the upper trunk, the C7 ramus forms the middle trunk, and the C8 and T1 rami form the lower trunk. The C5 nerve root is assessed with this orthopedic test. It is the most common level involved. The fifth cervical nerve root is the root irritated most often, and the sixth, fourth, third, second, and seventh roots become irritated in that order of frequency.

27. The subclavian "steal" is caused by basilar artery insufficiency. With the subclavian steal syndrome, occlusion occurs at the portion of the subclavian artery that is proximal to the origin of the vertebral artery. Because of this occlusion, blood flow is diverted from the opposite vertebral artery into the artery on the obstructed side, which results in perfusion of the distal subclavian bed with blood that was intended for cerebral circulation.

28. Muscle cramping due to ischemia with vigorous work activity, dizziness and vertigo can occur. TIA-like symptoms can occur.

29. 1. Widened retropharyngeal space (in excess of 7 mm)
    2. Widened retrotracheal space (in excess of 21 mm)
    3. Displacement of the prevertebral fat stripe
    4. Tracheal deviation and laryngeal dislocation

30. From C3 through C7, the average AP measurement of the cervical canal is 17 mm.

31. Spinal cord compression will occur only if the canal is reduced to 11 mm or less. Myelopathy is a significant result of central cervical stenosis.

32. The sleep cycle is characterized by waking the patient after several hours of sleep and then relieved after approximately 15 to 30 minutes with the patient sitting up. This occurs because when the patient lies down the spinal cord lengthens and shortens when sitting up.

33. A sharp pain radiating down the spine and into the upper or lower limbs is a positive finding.

34. Multiple sclerosis, intra-and extra-axial tumor, huge central disc herniation, and hydro-syringomyelia are four conditions that can contribute to a positive finding.

35. Other IVD or space occupying tests are recommended in place of this test. Naffziger test is not good for a geriatric or atheromatous patient to endure. The resulting increase in cerebrospinal fluid pressure is uncomfortable, and the momentary circulatory obstruction may result in significant syncope.

36. In all varieties of strain, contraction of the muscle against resistance will increase pain. This response is a characteristic finding of strains and differentiates the injury from sprains. A sprain is an injury to a ligamentous tissue that results in some degree of damage to the fibers of the ligament or its attachments.

37. Strains are divided into three categories according to the degree of muscle tissue damage:
    1. A *mild* strain is a low-grade inflammatory reaction accompanied by no appreciable hemorrhage, minimal amounts of swelling and edema, and some disruption of adjacent fibers.
    2. A *moderate* strain involves laceration of fibers and appreciable hemorrhaging into the surrounding tissue (hematoma), followed by an inflammatory reaction

A

with swelling and edema.

3. A *severe* strain is the consequence of a single, violent incident that results in complete disruption of the muscle unit. These strains occur when a tendon is torn from the bone or pulled apart, when the musculotendinous junction ruptures, or when the muscle ruptures through its belly.

38. Sprains are divided into four categories according to the severity of the ligamentous injury: A *mild* sprain describes an injury in which only a few of the ligamentous fibers are severed. A *moderate* sprain is a more severe tearing but less than a complete separation of the ligament. A *severe* sprain is a complete tearing of a ligament from its attachments or a complete separation within its substance. A *sprain-fracture* has occurred when the ligamentous attachment pulls loose with a fragment of bone (avulsion). The examination of a sprain initially will reveal discomfort when an attempt is made to stretch the ligament or the mechanism of injury is repeated. This one maneuver, when positive, will differentiate a sprain from a strain.

39. Rust sign suggests severe upper cervical (atlantoaxial) instability.

40. The patient spontaneously grasps the head with both hands when lying down or when arising from a recumbent position; this is a positive sign that indicates severe sprain, rheumatoid arthritis, fracture, or severe cervical subluxation. No other physical finding is as important or as revealing as Rust sign. The presence of this sign mandates that (1) no further passive or active testing be undertaken, (2) imaging be performed immediately, and (3) the neck be adequately supported by using a cervical collar. Rust sign has never been observed in conditions of minor consequence.

41. The febrile patient may be suffering from meningeal irritation and nuchal rigidity. Confirmation should be performed with Kernig or Brudzinski sign. This patient is a high-risk candidate for meningitis.

Chapter 4

1. The process is secondary to repetitive microtrauma, degeneration, or impingement.

2. The supraspinatus is tested with the shoulder abducted to 90 degrees, flexed 30 degrees, and then maximally internally rotated. Downward pressure exerted by the examiner is resisted primarily by the supraspinatus. The infraspinatus is tested with the shoulder abducted at the side while the elbows are flexed 90 degrees. The examiner resists active external rotation.

3. The tendon has an important contribution as a humeral head depressor.

4. The inferior glenohumeral ligament complex is the most important because it resists anteroinferior shoulder translation when the arm is placed in abduction, external rotation, and extension.

5. The Bankart lesion is a detachment of the anteroinferior glenoid labrum from the bony glenoid rim.

6. A Hill-Sachs lesion is an osteochondral depression in the posterior humeral head.

7. Most dislocations occur through an indirect force applied to the arm. Anterior dislocations are produced by an external rotation and/or hyperextension force applied to the shoulder that is already in about 90 degrees of abduction. Posterior dislocations are caused by indirectly applied force to the arm when the shoulder is variably flexed, adducted, and internally rotated.

8. External rotation and elevation are limited. The anterior shoulder is flattened and the coracoid process may be prominent.

9. The sulcus test demonstrates the degree of inferior laxity; it is thought to be a test of the superior glenohumeral ligament and the coracohumeral ligament.

10. As a whole, the rotator cuff functions center the humeral head in the glenoid, thus adding stability and maximum leverage to shoulder motions.

11. *Impingement* is a general term used to describe pain originating from compression of inflamed tissue between the humeral head and the coracoacromial arch. Any condition that causes a narrowing of this "subacromial space" (structural abnormalities, physiologic abnormalities, or both) can lead to impingement.

12. Rotator cuff tears are associated with impingement in 95% of cases. Impingement lesions have three progressive stages:
    1. Edema and hemorrhage
    2. Fibrosis and tendinopathy
    3. Rotator cuff tears, biceps tendon ruptures, and bony changes

13. Inflammation of the tendon of the long head of the biceps occurs by the same mechanisms responsible for impingement. With elevation and rotation of the arm, the biceps tendon can be compressed between the head of the humerus, the acromion, and the coracoacromial ligament.

14. The four primary articulations of the shoulder include the glenohumeral, acromioclavicular, sternoclavicular, and scapulothoracic.

15. • Rotator cuff tendonopathy/impingement syndrome
    • Calcific tendinopathy
    • Rotator cuff tear
    • Bicipital tendonopathy
    • Acromioclavicular arthritis

16. • Gallbladder disease
    • Splenic trauma
    • Subphrenic abscess
    • Myocardial infarction
    • Thyroid disease
    • Diabetes mellitus
    • Kidney disease

17. It arises mainly from the fifth through the seventh cervical nerve roots via its formation into the brachial plexus.

18. The number one predisposing factor is age degeneration. This is more than likely accelerated from repeated friction and angulation at the point where the tendon enters the bicipital groove.

19. The subclavian artery can be compressed as it passes between the anterior and medial scalene muscles and the first rib.

20. The lower roots of the brachial plexus (C8–T1) are at higher risk that more superior roots because of their location in the plexus.

21. The supraspinatus tendon is most commonly involved in the upper limb.

22. This condition occurs most often in athletes that do repeated overhead movements. This would include sports such as swimming and tennis.

23. This describes the traumatic injury of rotator cuff tear, anterior glenohumeral dislocation and neurologic injury.

24. This injury occurs when the arm is in abduction, extension, and external rotation. This results in an anterior dislocation.

25. The axillary artery is vulnerable to traumatic incidents much like the popliteal in the knee.

26. The cardinal sign of rotator cuff rupture is persistent weakness.

27. The patient may be able to lift the arm, but placing any downward pressure on the arm is unable to be supported by the patient. An incomplete tear is one cause of the painful arc syndrome, and a complete tear seriously impairs the patient's ability to abduct the shoulder.

28. Codman drop arm test is described.

29. The etiology of rotator cuff tears have been described from a number of causes. Decreased tensile strength of the tendon and trauma may be the most important factor. This includes degenerative changes of the tendon in association with microtrauma.

30. 1. Cervical rib syndrome
    2. Scalenus-anticus syndrome
    3. Wright hyperabduction syndrome
    4. Pectoralis minor syndrome
    5. Costoclavicular syndrome

31. Castagna test is helpful in determining minor chronic shoulder instability. Patients often describe snapping, popping, or transient locking.

32. The test is performed with the patient on their back with the arm positioned with a 45 degrees glenohumeral abduction. The arm is maximally externally rotated. If the pain is relieved with relocation is a positive Castagna test.

33. The difference from Jobe test is the arm is abducted to 90 degrees.

34. Patients usually experience sensory symptoms as the first manifestation of thoracic outlet syndrome. Paresthesias are common, which follow the ulnar nerve distribution along the medial aspect of the arm and forearm and then to the fourth and fifth fingers.

35. Wasting of the thenar, hypothenar, and intrinsic muscles of the hand may be the earliest involved. This distribution of atrophy, following a definite peripheral nerve pattern, is in contrast to progressive muscular atrophy, in which there is generalized involvement that does not follow a specific pattern.

36. With calcific tendinopathy there is severe pain, but full range of motion on passive movement. Calcific deposits are evident on the radiographs. With osteoarthritis, there is loss of passive shoulder movement and classic OA radiographic findings.

37. Adhesive capsulitis, nerve compression (C5–C6 disc), suprascapular neuropathy or other brachial plexus lesions, and shoulder instability has to be considered.

38. Speed test is performed to determine bicipital tendinopathy. Conditions involving the bicipital tendon and the bicipital groove are particularly pertinent to athletes because many sports involve the throwing motion of the arm. These athletes include baseball pitchers, football quarterbacks, batters, and tennis players. The throwing motion is especially inhibited by bicipital tendon problems. It is especially pertinent to recognize if the defect is an adhesive tenosynovitis, fraying of the tendon, or subluxation or dislocation of the tendon.

Chapter 5

1. Humeroulnar joint, humeroradial joint, and proximal radioulnar joint

2. The elbow positions the hand in space, effectively lengthens and shortens the upper extremity, stabilizes the upper extremity for power and detailed work activities, and provides power to the arm for lifting.

3. The carrying angle of the elbow is the normal anatomic valgus angulation between the upper arm and forearm when the elbow is fully extended. The normal angle is 5 to 10 degrees in males and 10 to 15 degrees in females.

4. A gunstock deformity refers to a cubitus varus deformity of the elbow.

5. Flexor carpi radialis, flexor carpi ulnaris, palmaris longus, flexor digitorum superficialis, flexor digitorum profundus, and pronator teres

6. Extensor carpi radialis, extensor carpi radialis longus, palmaris longus, extensor digitorum communis, supinator, and anconeus

7. Medially, the ulnar collateral ligament; laterally, the radial collateral ligament and annular ligament

8. 90 degrees flexion with the forearm midway between supination and pronation

9. Radial head dislocation

10. Panner disease is osteochondrosis of the capitellum. It is seen most often in young males.

11. Osteochondritis dissecans is an idiopathic disorder affecting the capitellum of the humerus, with avascular necrosis.

A

12. This term has traditionally been used to describe numerous symptoms of the elbow. It most commonly refers to lateral epicondylitis, in which the extensor carpi radialis brevis is affected by repetitive strain injury.

13. The examiner stabilizes the elbow. The patient makes a fist, pronates the forearm, and extends the wrist against resistance. This can cause pain in the lateral epicondyle.

14. Repetitive strain injury of the flexor-pronator musculature at or near its insertion on the medial epicondyle.

15. The examiner resists wrist flexion and forearm pronation, causing medial epicondyle pain.

16. Boxer elbow is a hyperextension overload syndrome or olecranon impingement syndrome caused by repetitive valgus extension of the elbow.

17. Little leaguer elbow is an injury occurring in children and adolescents in which the medial epicondyle is inflamed and there is partial separation of the apophysis.

18. The cubital tunnel, which is a passageway, formed by the two heads of the ulnar collateral ligament and the tendon of the flexor carpi ulnaris

19. Draftsman elbow is inflammation of the olecranon bursa. It is also known as *student elbow* and *miner elbow.*

20. Pushed elbow is subluxation of the radial head in proximal direction, which often occurs after a person falls on an outstretched hand. Pulled elbow is subluxation of the radial head in a distal direction, which may follow a forceful traction to the forearm.

21. Pain, location of the swelling, presence of point tenderness, specific examination procedures, and the results of range-of-motion studies gives the clinician diagnostic information.

22. Serious problems such as posterior dislocation of the elbow, fracture of the epicondyle, intracondylar fracture and fracture of the olecranon.

23. This is a combination of posterior dislocation of the elbow, fracture of the radial head and coronoid process. This is a serious entity as it may lead to instability, arthrosis and stiffness.

24. The most common ages are 11 to 21 years.

25. This is a potentially sport-ending injury for an athlete, with long-term sequelae of degenerative arthritis.

26. The flexion motion is 130 degrees or less.

27. Extension is 10 degrees or more.

28. A gunstock deformity is a cubitus varus deformity of the elbow

29. Gunstock deformities are usually secondary to fractures or epiphyseal injury to the distal humerus.

30. The muscles are the biceps brachii, brachialis, and brachioradialis.

31. The innervation is from C5 and C6.

32. The triceps brachii muscle is the prime mover.

33. The anconeus muscle is an accessory

34. Innervation comes from C7 and C8.

35. The sites include the arcade of Struthers, the proximal edge of the cubital tunnel retinaculum, cubital tunnel, and the deep flexor pronator aponeurosis.

36. If the grip improves, the brace is helping the musculature and epicondylar tissue. If not, the support is not adequate or the condition may be so severe the brace is not helpful.

37. The presentation of the radial tunnel syndrome is with pain and the posterior interosseous nerve syndrome presents in painless paralysis.

Chapter 6

1. The extensor pollicis brevis and the adductor pollicis longus.

2. The second dorsal tunnel in on the radial side of the radial tubercle. The third tunnel is on the ulnar side of the radial tubercle and defines the ulnar border of the anatomic snuff box. The fourth tunnel lies just to the ulnar side of the tunnel three and contains the extensors digitorum communis and extensor indicis to the hand.

3. The structure is a ganglion cyst, which is usually in the radial scaphoid joint where a collection of mucopolysaccharide fluid forms a cystic mass.

4. The median nerve, the median artery, and obviously the median vein; the tendons of the flexor digitorum profundus and flexor digitorum superficialis, as well the flexor palmaris longus.

5. 1. Tinel sign: percussion over the carpal ligament causes pain and/or radiation of pain distally or occasionally distally and proximally
   2. Phalen test: the wrist are palmar flexed and symptoms of numbness, tingling, or pain occur in the thumb or middle fingers.

6. The flexor pollicis longus, the pronator quadratus, and the flexor digitorum profundus.

7. The examiner holds the elbow flexed and palpates over the medial epicondyle with one hand and with the opposite hand pronates the patient's wrist and extends the patient's elbow, which will cause compression of the median nerve in the pronator mass. The second provocative test in this instance is caused by having the patient resist flexion of the superficialis flexor tendon of the middle finger. This will cause pain along the margin of the pronator teres and the muscle belly of the flexor digitorum superficialis. The third provocative maneuver is to have the patient try to contact the biceps tendon with the examiner supinating the forearm. This will cause pain at the biceps tendon aponeurosis.

8. It is a longitudinal tear in the extensor digitorum communis tendon or the sagittal bands that overlie the metacarpal heads. It most commonly occurs in the third metacarpophalangeal joint.

9. The normal carpal tunnel contains the median nerve and nine flexor tendons: the four sublimis tendons, the four profundus tendons, and the flexor pollicis longus.

10. Guyon canal is the triangular canal immediately ulnar to the carpal tunnel in the wrist. The ulnar nerve and ulnar artery traverse the canal.

11. The snuff box lies just distal to the radial styloid process. The radial border is composed of the abductor pollicis longus and extensor pollicis brevis. The ulnar border is the extensor pollicis longus. The floor of the snuff box is the scaphoid bone.

12. Allen test evaluates the circulation of the radial and ulnar arteries in the hand. The patient opens and closes the fist several times, then the examiner occludes the radial and ulnar arteries at the wrist with the fist closed. Next the patient opens the fist and the examiner releases one of the arteries. The hand should flush immediately. The procedure is repeated, with release of the other artery. Failure to flush or slow return of color to the hand suggests occlusion of one of the arteries.

13. Bunnell first described no man's land, the area in which both the flexor tendons of the fingers pass through a tight fibrous tunnel. Designated as zone II, it is the area between the distal palmar crease and the insertion of the flexor superficialis at the midportion of the middle phalanx.

14. Dupuytren contracture is a progressive contracture of the fingers into the palm caused by cords of palmar fascia. It commonly begins with the fourth and fifth fingers and may involve the entire palm.

15. The most common ganglion is the dorsal wrist ganglion, which originates from the scapholunate ligament and accounts for approximately 60 to 70% of all hand ganglia. The second most common is the volar ganglion (18-20%). Ganglia of the flexor tendon sheath at the A-1 pulley are the third most common (10 to 12%).

16. A boxer fracture is a fracture of the fifth metacarpal neck. It is one of the most common hand fractures and is usually seen in brawlers or persons who strike a wall or other unyielding object in anger.

17. To evaluate rotational alignment, have the patient flex the metacarpophalangeal (MCP) and PIP joints, and look at the alignment of the fingers. They should point toward the scaphoid bone. Subtle differences sometimes can be seen by looking at the semiflexed fingers end-on and comparing the planes of the fingernails to those of the unaffected side.

18. A Bennett fracture is actually a fracture-dislocation of the base of the thumb metacarpal joint. The shaft is displaced radially and dorsally at the base by the abductor pollicis longus.

19. The term *gamekeeper thumb* has come to mean almost any injury of the ulnar collateral ligament of the thumb MCP. Specifically it refers to an occupational deformity in the hands of British gamekeepers due to their methods of killing rabbits.

20. The scaphoid (carpal navicular) is the most commonly fractured bone in the carpus. After distal radius fractures, it is the most common fracture of the wrist.

21. Fractures of the proximal third of the scaphoid have nonunion or avascular necrosis rates around 30%. Fractures of the tuberosity or distal third have healing rates approaching 100%, and waist fractures heal in 80 to 90% of cases.

22. The forearm and hand have a classic dinner-fork deformity after a fall onto the outstretched hand. Radiographs demonstrate dorsal angulation and displacement as well as radial shortening and angulation. A fracture of the ulnar styloid also may be present.

23. Plantar fibromatosis
    Knuckle pads
    Peyronie disease

24. Heberden nodes are bone spurs that form on the dorsal aspect of the DIP joints of the fingers.

25. Caput ulna syndrome refers to the destructive process initiated by synovitis of the distal radioulnar joint. Characteristic findings include loss of wrist rotation (pronation/supination) and dorsiflexion, weakness, dorsal prominence and instability of the distal ulna, soft-tissue swelling over the distal ulna secondary to synovitis, loss of normal action of the extensor carpi ulnaris tendon, and occasionally loss of extension of the small, ring, and long fingers as a result of extensor tendon ruptures.

26. Trauma or acute fracture is implicated as a cause of the avascular necrosis (AVN).

27. Kienbock disease is a radiographic diagnosis based on characteristic density changes that in later stages are accompanied by fracture lines, fragmentation, and collapse.

28. The most common compressive neuropathy of the upper extremity is carpal tunnel syndrome or median nerve compression at the wrist.

29. Median nerve compression may occur with decreased canal size or increased volume of the contents in the carpal canal. Nonspecific tenosynovial proliferation in otherwise healthy individuals is the most common cause of increased canal contents. The mnemonic PRAGMATIC can be used to remember the other common causes of carpal tunnel syndrome:

    P = Pregnancy
    R = Rheumatoid arthritis
    A = Arthritis (degenerative)
    G = Growth hormone abnormalities (acromegaly)
    M = Metabolic (hypothyroidism, gout, diabetes mellitus)
    A = Alcoholism
    T = Tumors
    I = Idiopathic
    C = Connective tissue disorders (amyloidosis, hemochromatosis)

30. A median nerve percussion test is performed by percussion with a finger or reflex hammer over the median nerve in the wrist or palm. A positive test produces paresthesias in the median nerve distribution (Tinel sign).

A

31. De Quervain disease is stenosing tenosynovitis of the first dorsal compartment at the wrist.

32. The diagnosis is made by patient history and physical exam. In addition to pain and tenderness, patients occasionally have swelling over the compartment.

A provocative test for de Quervain disease is the Finkelstein test.

33.
- The type of three-dimensional loading
- The magnitude and direction of the forces involved
- The position of the hand at the time of impact
- The biomechanical properties of the bones and ligaments

34. The roof is formed by the flexor retinaculum or the transverse carpal ligament.

35. The median nerve is contained in the tunnel along with nine tendons.

36. The bones are the scaphoid, trapezium, pisiform, and the hamate.

37. The ulnar nerve, artery, and vein occupy the tunnel.

38. The scaphoid

39. Disruption of arterial blood supply to the bone results in avascular necrosis.

40. A tear of the scapholunate interosseous ligament, it is between the scaphoid and lunate carpal bones.

41. A gap of 3 mm is considered normal.

42. A supinated, clenched-fist anteroposterior view is the best study.

43. The most common cause is wrist rotary subluxations of the scaphoid.

44. Other causes may include Preiser disease, Kienböck disease, midcarpal instability or post traumatic, following injuries involving the radioscaphoid or capitolunate joints

45. Complex regional pain syndrome (CRPS), this also has been called reflex sympathetic dystrophy (RSD). The clinician must be alert to what may seem as a trivial injury and the patient's severe pain complaints.

46. The patient would exhibit a "touch me not" reaction to palpation; they are averse to touch and pressure to the area.

47. On observation, shiny, dry skin is noted, as well as loss of use and a stiffness of the soft tissue. Joint motion is lost, strength and function diminish. The warmth of hypervascularity turns to a sense of coldness.

48. Significant osteoporosis of the distal radius is present on imaging.

49. Heberden nodes are located in the distal interphalangeal (DIP) and Bouchard are in the proximal interphalangeal joints of the hand.

50.
- Symmetric swelling of the PIP joints
- Boutonniere or swan-neck deformities of several pip joints
- Swelling or tenderness of the MCP joints
- Ulnar deviation or subluxation of these MCP and PIP joints

- Synovitis of the wrist (especially at the distal ulna)
- Tenderness of the distal ulna
- Swelling of the extensor carpi ulnaris tendon

51. Scaphoid

52. Opponens

53. Stenosing tenosynovitis of the tendon sheath of the abductor pollicis longus and the extensor pollicis brevis is examined with Finkelstein test.

54. The abductor pollicis longus and the extensor pollicis brevis.

55. Repetition or over use is the most common cause. Lymphedema factors in to the cause, but it is a minor factor. In this process, an additional etiologic agent may be the presence of accessory tendons in the sheath.

56. It is more common in females between the ages of 30 to 60 years of age.

57. Tingling sensations that radiate into the thumb, the index finger, and the middle and lateral half of the ring finger constitute a positive sign.

58. 60 seconds.

59. The carpal compression test is preferred as the most accurate provocative sign in CTS. The patient opposes the thumb to the small finger and flexes the wrist. The examiner's thumb firmly compresses the area between the two tendons, indenting the skin 4 to 5 mm. In CTS, paresthesias in the median nerve distribution occur within 60 seconds. Paresthesias within 15 seconds or less indicate more advanced disease.

60. Anterior interosseous nerve syndrome, in this syndrome, the pronator quadratus is nonfunctioning. Compression of the anterior interosseous branch of the median nerve in the forearm, usually secondary to anomalous muscle and tendon origins, produces the anterior interosseous syndrome. The ligament of Struthers is a fibrous band in the elbow that may compress the nerve. This may be the least common of the causes.

61. Vasospasm is present without an underlying primary disease, and the patient complaint of pain with an intolerance to cold.

62. The ulnar nerve is the most commonly injured. Open wounds at the wrist are the most common cause. Compression or irritations of the nerve at the elbow or wrist can occur. Loss of all the interossei and adductor pollicis interferes with the strength and effectiveness of hand grasp.

63. The most common causes are old fractures of the elbow and arthritis. This can cause weakness of the intrinsic muscles of the hand. Tinel sign at the epicondylar groove will produce a tingling or paresthesias along the course of the nerve.

64. Front of the thumb, index finger, middle finger, and the radial half of the ring finger. The palm of the hand is not involved. The symptoms are worse at night, and the patient will wake and fling the hand up and down to try and relieve the symptoms. In time, the paresthesia is replaced by pain, which can be felt as far up as the

elbow, and eventually by numbness in the median distribution. The differential diagnosis includes peripheral neuropathy, mononeuritis, cervical spondylosis, and tumors of the thoracic outlet that involve the brachial plexus, but these are often forgotten because CTS is such a common condition. If there is any doubt, the diagnosis can be confirmed by nerve conduction studies.

Chapter 7

1. (1) Ankylosing spondylitis, (2) psoriatic arthritis, (3) reactive arthritis (Reiter syndrome), and (4) juvenile ankylosing spondylitis
2. 1. Predilection for inflammatory lesions of axial skeleton
   2. Oligoarticular peripheral joint arthritis
   3. Enthesitis-inflammation at bony insertion of tendons, ligaments, and articular capsules
   4. Frequent extraarticular inflammation of eye (uveitis), heart (aortitis), skin, and mucous membranes
   5. Tendency to afflict young adults (mostly men)
   6. Strong association with HLA-B27
   7. Negative rheumatoid factor
3. Scoliosis, kyphosis, and lordosis
4. • Congenital scoliosis
   • Adolescent idiopathic scoliosis
   • Infantile and juvenile idiopathic scoliosis
   • Neuromuscular scoliosis
5. • Neurofibromatosis
   • Spinal cord injuries
   • Metabolic disorders
   • Marfan syndrome
   • Infections
   • Tumors
   • Dwarfism
6. Curves of more than 10 degrees occur in approximately 3% of the population in North America, whereas curves greater than 20 degrees occur in 0.2 to 0.3% of the population. Curves greater than 20 degrees have a female: male ratio of 9:1.
7. Asymmetries in the shoulder, scapula, waistline, or pelvic regions are identified. Adams positions are performed.
8. The patient stands with feet together and knees straight and bends forward at the waist. The arms are held dependent with the hands together, palms and fingers opposed. The examiner compares the sides of the back for asymmetry. Prominence of the scapula or rib (called *rib hump*) is observed.
9. Infantile scoliosis occurs from 0 through 3 years of age. Juvenile scoliosis occurs between ages 4 and 10 years.
10. Kyphosis is a change in the alignment of a segment of the spine in the sagittal plane that increases the posterior convex angulation.

11. Scheuermann disease is found in approximately 1% of the general population, with a slight female dominance (female: male ratio is 1.4:1).
12. The *anterior* column includes the anterior longitudinal ligament, the anterior portion of the annulus, and the anterior half of the vertebral body. The *middle* column consists of the posterior longitudinal ligament, the posterior portion of the annulus, and the posterior portion of the vertebral body. The *posterior* column is made up of the pedicles, facets, lamina, and posterior ligamentous complex, including the interspinal ligaments, ligamentum flavum, and facet joint capsule.
13. A compression fracture results in a typical anterior wedging of the vertebral body in the anterior column. The middle and posterior columns generally are not involved.
14. A burst fracture is a fracture of the anterior and middle columns; varying degrees of the fracture fragments are displaced into the neural canal.
15. A flexion-distraction injury, also known as a *Chance fracture,* is common in motor vehicle accidents when the victim is wearing only a lap seatbelt. The fracture involves the anterior, middle, and posterior columns or the posterior ligaments.
16. 1. The first element is the vertebral articular process. The interlocking arrangement of the thoracic facets prevents anterior displacement of the vertebra and forms the imbrication of the thoracic spine.
    2. The second primary stabilizing influence of the thoracic spine is the vertebral body. At the posterior of the vertebral bodies, the height of the body is greater than in the anterior. This contributes to the thoracic spine kyphosis.
    3. The third stabilizing influence is the structure of the ribs and their attachments to the spine. The ribs help stiffen the thoracic spine.
    4. The fourth primary stabilizing influence for the thoracic spine is the structure of the intervertebral disc. The thoracic spine intervertebral discs are more narrow and thin than in the cervical or lumbar spines. They are also less elastic than all the other disc tissues of the spine.
17. The Lenke Classification System is simple, accurate, and easy to reproduce and communicate between different surgeons. It relies on measurements taken from standard radiographs (X-rays). In this method, the surgeon evaluates X-rays of the patient from the front, the side, and in bending positions. The Lenke system helps surgeons to get a more complete picture of the patient's condition by understanding the scoliosis as multidimensional and considering it from more than one view. This allows the surgeon to focus treatment where it is needed and to optimize the patient's balance and curve correction from the treatment.
18. 1. Curves less than 20 degrees will improve spontaneously more than 50% of the time.

A

2. There is no accurate method of predicting which curves will improve or worsen.

3. In curves of less than 30 degrees, 20% will progress.

4. Progression is more common in young children, at the beginning of their growth spurt.

5. The larger the curve at detection, the greater the chance of progression.

6. Curves in females and double curves in males or females are more likely to progress.

7. Scoliosis is more common in females (idiopathic), 9:1 ratio.

19. • Clinical criteria
   • Low back pain and stiffness for more than 3 months improves with exercise, but is not relieved by rest
   • Limitation of motion of the lumbar spine both the sagittal and frontal planes
   • Limitation of chest expansion relative to normal values corrected for age and sex
   • Radiological criterion
   • Sacroiliitis grade 2 bilaterally or sacroiliitis grade 3 to 4 unilaterally

20. Reiter disease and psoriatic arthritis will exhibit a close relationship with ankylosing spondylitis.

21. The clinician has to be aware of chest wall pain and the distribution of the thoracic nerve roots, thoracic myelopathy involving the lowers extremities (weakness and numbness), cardiopulmonary, gastrointestinal, demyelinating disease, neoplasm, genitourinary disorders, and psychiatric disease.

22. Chest expansion is restricted because of disease of the costovertebral joints. The chest measurement is taken at the fourth intercostal space. When the chest expansion is less than 0.75 inches in the female and 1 inch in the male, this indicates, ankylosing spondylitis.

23. Injury to the long thoracic nerve is the most common cause of scapular winging. The nerve root level is C5–C6–C7; this nerve is easily injured because it is superficial.

24. Schepelmann sign is used to differentiate intercostal neuritis from myofascitis. The patient is seated with arms extended about the head. They are asked to bend to one side and then the other. If the pain is on the convex side of the ribs, the diagnosis of intercostal myofascitis is probable. If the pain is on the concave side of the ribs, it is caused by intercostal neuritis.

25. The second through fifth costal cartilage areas are most commonly involved.

Chapter 8

1. Cauda equina syndrome is a large midline disc herniation that compresses several roots of the cauda equina.

2. Herniation at L3–L4 compresses the L4 nerve root. There are sensory deficits in the posterolateral thigh, anterior knee, and medial leg. Motor weakness is in the quadriceps and hip adductors. Patellar reflex is diminished or absent.

3. The L5 nerve root is compressed with herniation at L4–L5. Sensory deficit noted in the anterolateral leg, dorsum of the foot, and great toe. Motor weakness is of the extensor hallucis longus, gluteus medius, and extensor digitorum longus and brevis. No reflex changes are present.

4. Herniation at L5–S1 compresses the S1 nerve root. Sensory deficits are in the lateral malleolus, lateral foot, heel, and web of the fourth and fifth toes. Motor weakness involves the peroneus longus and brevis, gastrocnemius–soleus complex, and gluteus maximus. The Achilles reflex is usually diminished.

5. 1. Lasègue test
   2. Forestier bowstring sign
   3. Lasègue sitting test
   4. Fajersztajn test
   5. Femoral nerve traction

6. Herniation of a disc lateral to the nerve root produces antalgia posture away from the side of the irritated nerve root. Herniation of the disc medial to the nerve root produces a list toward the side of the irritated nerve root.

7. 1. Plain film radiography
   2. Magnetic resonance imaging
   3. Computed axial tomography
   4. Myelography

8. Lumbar spinal stenosis is an abnormal narrowing of the osseoligamentous vertebral canal or vertebral foramina.

9. Spinal stenosis

10. Pain that increases with walking or standing and that is relieved by sitting and leaning forward or lying down

11. Spondylolisthesis is the forward slippage of one vertebral body on another.

12. Spondylolysis is the clinical entity in which the pars interarticularis is not intact or is separated.

13. 1. Congenital
   2. Isthmic
   3. Traumatic
   4. Pathologic
   5. Degenerative

14. The most common level of the cyst is the L4–5 level.

15. The patient usually presents with a history of slowly progressive or intermittent radicular pain that is commonly neuroclaudicatory in nature.

16. Symptoms that correlate with Z-joint arthrography, computed tomography, magnetic resonance imaging can be used to correlate the findings and complaints. Myelography has also been used.

17. • With the patient in the supine position, the examiner moves the patient's leg until it is above the examiner's shoulder.
   • At this point, firm pressure should be exerted on the hamstring muscles.

- If pain is not elicited, pressure is applied to the popliteal fossa.
- Pain in the lumbar region or radiculopathy is a positive sign for nerve root compression.

18. Suspicion of a single nerve root compression syndrome should be prompted by the combination of a history of pain and the presence of paresthesia in the appropriate distribution of one nerve root only. Findings necessary to confirm the diagnosis are those that relate spinal movement to the radiating pain, those that demonstrate muscular weakness and tenderness in the myotome, and those that localize sensory and reflex deficits to the dermatome and myotome.

19. The degree of slip in patients with lytic spondylolisthesis is greater at L4/5 above an L5 transition than at L5/S1 above an S1 transition. This is postulated to be due to the restraining action of the iliolumbar ligament, which stabilizes the L5 vertebra.

20. • Cox sign occurs during straight leg raising when the *pelvis rises* from the table instead of the hip flexing.
    • Cox sign is positive when there is a prolapse of the nucleus into the intervertebral foramen.

21. 1. Symmetric destruction of adjacent end-plate surfaces of two vertebrae
    2. Loss of disc height
    3. Reactive new bone formation
    4. Sclerosis of bone end-plates, with or without evidence of bone destruction or bone formation
    5. Soft-tissue abscesses
    6. Kyphosis or subluxation after there has been significant bone destruction

22. The patients inability to walk on the toes indicates a L5–S1 disc problem based on weakness of the calf muscles supplied by the tibial nerve. Their inability to walk on the heels would indicate a L4–L5 disc problem based on weakness of the anterior leg muscles supplied by the common peroneal nerve.

23. The test is positive when pain radiating down the leg aggravates a pattern of radicular pain the patient has described.

24. If the pain is localized, it should be noted as it may connote strain-sprain of the facet joints or pericapsular inflammation. It is not a positive Kemp test.

25. When the patient is seated, it increases the intradiscal pressure. Standing maximizes the stress to the facets.

26. Patients with neurogenic claudication primarily complain of pain radiating down the legs as well as weakness, numbness, and tingling in the lower extremities. Vascular claudication differs from neurogenic claudication in several ways. Neurogenic claudication occurs with little or no exercise and, in some cases, with just standing. In contrast, vascular claudication typically requires some exertion on the part of the patient to stress the blood supply to the musculature of the lower extremities. One of the key differences between the conditions is that standing and resting fail to relieve leg pain in neurogenic, whereas cessation of activity, regardless of posture or position, relieves the pain in the vascular group. Because of poor circulation in the lower extremities associated with vascular claudication, the feet are cool to the touch and pedal pulses are weak or absent. Other findings include smooth skin and a paucity of hair on the lower legs. Venous stasis and atrophic skin may also be associated with vascular claudication. Furthermore, the character of the pain may be described differently, with vascular claudication manifesting as a dull ache in a calf muscle, for example, whereas neurogenic claudication may describe more of a radicular pain radiating from the back or buttocks down the leg and into the calf or foot.

27. This test is helpful in determining that pain in the sacroiliac is caused by strained superior sacroiliac ligaments.

28. It is an entrapment of the lateral femoral cutaneous nerve, which is initiated by obesity and local trauma such as a tight belt or waist band. This occurs when it passes under the inguinal ligament medial to the anterior superior iliac spine.

29. This entrapment results in dysesthesia and pain along the lateral thigh. Some loss of sensitivity to pain and touch is often typical in a small area. The skin may become sensitive to touch and pinching. There is no atrophy and no motor or reflex change.

30. This may occur in diabetic patients or patients with thyroid disease as a mononeuropathy.

31. Quick test is accomplished with the patient standing and then asked to squat down and stand up.

32. If the patient has lower extremity pain, this test assesses the integrity of the ankles, knees, and hips.

33. If the patient can fully squat without any symptoms, these joints are free of pathology related to the pain complaint.

34. The spinous process of S2 is marked, and then .5 cm below S2 and 10 cm above the S2 mark.

35. Lumbar rigidity from ankylosing spondylitis would be your concern.

36. Normally, the S2 reference points should separate at least 5 to 8 cm.

37. Evidence of localized pain indicates a possible ver-tebra fracture. Osteoporotic compression fractures typically present as acute, excruciating back pain, the onset of which does not usually occur as a result of obvious trauma but is precipitated by minor stress such as bending forward. Loss of vertebral body height and kyphotic deformity following osteoporotic compression fractures may cause muscle spasm, stress on ligaments, and/or nerve-root irritation, which, in turn, produce chronic back pain. Severe neurolo-gical deficits following osteoporotic fractures are unusual but may develop in the late stages. Fractures, which are frequently multiple, occur most commonly at the thoracolumbar junctions, followed in order of frequency by the middle thoracic and lower lumbar vertebrae.

A

38. Dural movement begins at 30 degrees.

39. Sciatica that is in the leg and produced from 0 to 30 degrees is caused by nerve root compression. Sciatica that is in the leg and produced from 30 to 60 degrees is probably caused by sacroiliac joint disease. Sciatica that is in the leg and produced above 60 degrees is probably caused by lumbosacral disease.

40. A midline herniation may not cause sciatica during straight-leg-raising, and the test will be negative. In a classically positive test, sciatica is produced at 30 degrees or less on one side, while the other side has full range.

41. In hamstring tightness, leg pain occurs at about the same angle on each leg, and pain is confined to the posterior thigh and does not go below the knee.

42. 1. Viscerogenic pain: Pain that originates from the kidneys, sacroiliac, pelvic lesions, and retroperitoneal tumors. This type of pain is neither aggravated by activity nor relieved by rest.

    2. Neurogenic pain: Pain commonly caused by neurofibromas, cysts, and tumors of the nerve roots in the lumbar spine.

    3. Vascular pain: Pain characterized by intermittent claudication from aneurysms and peripheral vascular disease.

    4. Spondylogenic pain: Pain directly related to the pain originating from soft tissues of the spine and sacroiliac joint.

    5. Psychogenic pain: Pain that is uncommon and ascribed to nonorganic causes.

Chapter 9

1. Ankylosing spondylitis, psoriatic arthritis, reactive arthritis (Reiter syndrome), juvenile ankylosing spondylitis, and arthropathies that complicate inflammatory bowel diseases (regional enteritis and ulcerative colitis)

2. An anteroposterior radiograph of the pelvis usually suffices to demonstrate the bilateral sacroiliitis of ankylosing spondylitis.

3. OCI is characterized by a triangular area of dense sclerotic bone limited to iliac bones of the pelvis adjacent to the lower half of normal sacroiliac joints.

4. Malgaigne fractures usually refer to unstable fracture–dislocations of the pelvis, of both the superior and inferior pubic rami.

5. Transfer weight from the single axis of the upper body to the bipolar weight-bearing of the lower extremity, and secondarily it provides protection to the viscera.

6. This is a common fatty nodule in the sacroiliac area. The fatty tissue herniates through the normal deep fascia and becomes a source of pain. Clinically, the patient complains of pain in the nodules. They are often bilateral. It has been called a "back mouse" or ESIL nodes.

7. The most common areas are the groin, hamstrings, knee, back of the thigh, and possibly into the lower abdomen. Many provocative tests used to evaluate for intervertebral disc, sciatic neuritis, and lumbosacral sprain can cause pain in the sacroiliac joint, if it is also involved with the patients' complaints.

8. Extraspinal compression of the sciatic nerve is cause of "sciatica." With any patient having leg pain, evaluation of extraspinal causes is an essential part of the differential diagnosis. The clinician needs to evaluate for the presence of myofascial trigger points in the piriformis.

9. This type of collision is the number one cause of pelvic injuries. Pelvic fracture is associated with high mortality and morbidity rates, as well as economic costs.

10. Osteitis pubis is a painful inflammation of the pubic symphysis. This can develop after childbirth, urologic infection and certain athletic activities. Things such as coughing aggravate the pain. This can be a serious problem and full recovery may take months to resolve. It is thought to be an overuse injury and is a bony stress reaction. Degenerative and rheumatic causes must be considered.

11. Pain is elicited in the sacroiliac joint before lumbar spine movement.

12. Ankylosing spondylitis (AS) is most often confused with osteitis condensans ilii. The difference is striking, however; in AS, both sides of the joint are involved. In OCI, the increased bone density is in the ilium and is almost always bilateral.

13. The elderly are generally osteoporotic and any fall is capable of resulting in possible fracture. Fracture of the pelvis in the elderly will usually occur in pairs. It is usually the pubic rami and the ischial rami. This can be confirmed with diagnostic imaging of the pelvis.

Chapter 10

1. In the groin area, with possible radiation into the anterior portion of the thigh

2. The patient holds one leg to the abdomen and lowers the other leg until it is flat on the examination table. Failure of the hip to extend fully indicates a fixed flexion contracture.

3. The patient stands on one leg. As the patient stands erect, the gluteus medius muscle on the supported side should contract to keep the pelvis level. If the pelvis remains unsupported and the opposite side drops, the gluteus medius muscle is either weak or nonfunctioning, and the test is positive.

4. 1. Galeazzi sign is a check for apparent thigh length. Galeazzi sign indicates apparent shortening of one femur in comparison with the normal contralateral femur.

   2. Barlow test assesses the potential for dislocation of the hip.

3. Ortolani maneuver usually is combined with Barlow test. If abducting the hip with a little pressure over the trochanter produces a clunk that is felt rather than heard, Ortolani test is positive.

5. The femoral capital epiphysis of the hip displaces or "slips" on the femoral neck.

6. LCP disease is necrosis of the bony nucleus of the proximal femoral epiphysis and impairment of the growth of the physis, with subsequent remodeling of regenerated bone in the pediatric patient.

7. Hip dislocation occurs when the femoral head is forcibly dislocated from the acetabulum.

8. A sudden, violent muscle contraction (eccentric or concentric) or an increased muscular stretch causes an avulsion fracture across an open epiphysis.

9. Iliotibial band friction syndrome and iliotibial band tendinopathy

10. It should be considered when a young athlete (9 to 15 years old) presents with medial thigh pain, hip or knee pain, or a positive Trendelenburg gait.

11. They occur secondary to repetitive microtrauma and often are seen in runners with persistent groin pain.

12. Excessive anteversion causes a "toe-in" gait. This leads to tight hip internal rotator muscles, internal rotation of the tibia, and flexion at the knee and hip, thus altering normal biomechanics.

13. Craig test will give an approximation of the degree of anteversion.

14. This finding would be consistent with adhesive capsulitis of the hip joint. Pain in the posterior aspect of the hip is most often referred from the lumbar spine.

15. Thoracic/lumbar junction (T12–L1)

16. Trochanteric bursa
    1. Iliopsoas bursa
    2. Ischiogluteal bursa

17. Nerves from the femoral, sciatic, obturator, superior, and inferior gluteal nerves all send fibers to the hip joint. L3 is the sclerotome.

18. 1. Intertrochanteric fracture
    2. Slipped capital femoral epiphysis
    3. Legg-Calvé-Perthes disease
    4. Congenital hip dislocation
    5. Rickets
    6. Paget disease

19. Congenital dislocation of the hips or developmental dysplasia of the hip joint is the likely cause. Congenital dislocation of the hip is a condition in which one or both hips are dislocated at birth or are dislocated in the first few weeks of life. There is a familial tendency and a well-established geographic distribution for the disorder. The disorder may occur with other congenital defects.

20. Nonunion of the femoral neck

21. 1. Steroid use
    2. Alcohol use
    3. Trauma
    4. Gout

5. Metabolic problems
6. Genetic problems

22. The iliotibial band is a thickened portion of the tensor fascia latae along its lateral aspect. The tensor fascia latae arises from the coccyx, the sacrum, the iliac crest, Poupart ligament, and the pubic ramus.

23. The patient is supine with the legs extended on the examination table. Using a cloth tape measure, the examiner measures the circumference of the thigh, passing the tape over the level of the greater trochanter. The distance is recorded and compared to that of the opposite leg. An increased diameter indicates that the trochanter has rolled laterally. Fracture of the neck of the femur occurs mainly among elderly females whose bones are osteoporotic.

Chapter 11

1. Grade I: mild sprain—microscopic disruption of the ligamentous structure but no loss of integrity
   Grade II: moderate sprain—partial disruption of ligamentous fibers with structures still intact
   Grade III: severe sprain—complete disruption of ligamentous integrity

2. Medial meniscus tear, rupture of the anterior cruciate ligament, rupture of the medial collateral ligament

3. The quadriceps angle is formed by two lines, one projecting from the anterosuperior iliac spine to the mid-patella and the second from the mid-patella to the tibial tubercle.

4. A posterior drawer test is performed in a similar fashion to the anterior drawer test, except that a posterior force is applied on the proximal tibia.

5. Rotational force as the flexed knee moves toward an extended position

6. Longitudinal tear of the posterior horn of the medial meniscus

7. With the knee completely flexed, the leg is externally rotated as far as possible; then the knee is slowly extended. As the femur passes over a tear in the medial meniscus, a painful click or pop is felt or heard if the test is positive. The lateral meniscus is checked by palpating the posterolateral margin of the joint, internally rotating the leg as far as possible, and slowly extending the knee while listening and feeling for a click.

8. A discoid lateral meniscus

9. Lachman test is performed in approximately 15 to 30 degrees of flexion. The femur is stabilized with the examiner's hand. The opposite hand is used to apply an anteriorly directed force to the posterior tibia while stabilizing the femur. The examiner senses any tibial displacement and compares it with the uninvolved knee.

10. The posterior sag test detects the amount of posterior displacement caused by gravity when the knee and hip are flexed to 90 degrees.

A

11. The clinical appearance is bow-leggedness, which causes the mechanical axis to go through or inside the medial compartment of the knee.
12. The weight-bearing axis falls outside the lateral compartment of the knee. The patient appears knock-kneed.
13. Osteochondritis dissecans is a disorder of one or more ossification centers with sequential degeneration and/or aseptic necrosis and recalcification.
14. Medial femoral condyle of the knee
    Capitellum of the distal humerus
    Talus
15. The fracture usually results from a direct blow to the knee sustained in a fall or a motor vehicle or pedestrian accident.
16. Age groups as age pain tends to be age-related. Further classified by intraarticular, periarticular, or referred.
17. Anterior and posterior cruciate, tibial and fibular collateral ligaments are the major stabilizers. The quadriceps muscle and its tendinous expansion contribute to the stability of the knee. The earliest clinical indication of internal knee derangement is atrophy of the quadriceps.
18. The fabella. It may act as a source of atypical knee pain. It may be confused with an intraarticular loose body or osteophytes. Without considering this as a potential problem, unnecessary arthroscopy may be ordered.
19. Gracilis—obturator nerve
    Sartorius—femoral nerve
    Semitendinosus—tibial nerve
20. • Lateral view—is most sensitive for evaluating effusion of the joint
    • Tangential view—provides an axial depiction of the patella and its relationship
    • Tunnel view—allows excellent visualization of the intercondylar region of the femoral–tibial articulation.
    • AP and lateral is the typical study, but to further evaluate the patella, a PA view would be useful.
21. The medial collateral ligament
22. It is a combined injury to the medial collateral ligament (MCL), anterior cruciate ligament (ACL), and the medial meniscus.
23. Grade I: 0 to 5 mm of joint opening with no instability
    Grade II: 5 to 10 mm of joint opening with some degree of instability
    Grade III: 10 to 15 mm of joint opening with moderate instability
    Grade IV: Greater than 15 mm of joint opening with gross ligament instability
24. Apley and McMurray test are the most common.
    1. Pain or tenderness on the lateral surfaces of the knee joint
    2. Popping, snapping, or grating sounds with movement
    3. Inability to fully extend the knee ("locking")

25. A high riding patella, or patella Alta, is a predisposing factor. Recurrent dislocation is also common in females with a genu valgum deformity.
26. The entrapped meniscus often splits longitudinally, and its free edge may displace inward, toward the center of the joint. The handle remains attached to the body of the meniscus. This can occur when the affected knee is involved in a twisting strain that is applied to the flexed weight bearing leg.
27. Group I—Trauma related repeated or acutely induced. Changes include fissuring, absorption and fragmentation of the cartilage.
    Group II—This is a disturbance of the rhythm of patellar function. This group is commonly called tracking disorders.
    Group III—Primary malacia that is usually a bilateral condition without any demonstrable etiologic factor. These cases can be perplexing and the clinician needs to search for other causes other than simple contusion.
28. • ACL, especially the anteromedial bundle
    • Posterolateral capsule
    • MCL, especially the deep fibers
    • Iliotibial band
    • Posterior oblique ligament
    • Arcuate–popliteus complex
29. • PCL
    • Arcuate–popliteus complex
    • Posterior oblique ligament
    • ACL
30. ITB is widely recognized as an overuse injury. Exercise-related tenderness over the lateral femoral epicondyle and location of the pain excluding other pathology. Ober test may result in a sharp burning pain over the lateral epicondyle when the knee is flexed at 30 degrees.
31. There is skeletal alignment differences between sexes, such as a greater hip width to femoral length ratio, and a larger quadriceps angle (Q-angle) are thought to contribute to excessive amounts of knee valgus (lateral angulation or abduction of the tibia with respect to the femur). The combination of knee valgus (tibial abduction) and external rotation positions contribute to ACL impingement and injury.
32. • Diabetes mellitus
    • Gout
    • Repetitive microtrauma
    • Endocrine disorders

Chapter 12

1. Medial tibial stress syndrome is an inflammatory condition involving the periosteal attachment of the deep posterior compartment.
2. An acute increase in tissue pressure within the enclosed anatomic space (the muscle compartment that is surrounded by semirigid fascia) results in increased local

venous pressure, leading to a decrease in the arteriovenous gradient and thus a decrease in arterial inflow.

3. Eighty-five percent of cases of acute compartment syndrome are caused by overuse of the musculature (strain).

4. Tears are most commonly seen in males between the ages of 30 and 50.

5. There will be palpable defect in the tendon as the proximal tendon retracts following rupture. The gap is usually 2 to 3 cm long. Within 24 to 48 hours, marked swelling and ecchymosis usually occur. The patient is able to weakly plantar flex the foot. Thompson's test is positive.

6. With the patient supine and the affected foot hanging over the end of the table, the examiner squeezes the calf and observes for ankle motion. A positive Thompson test occurs when there is no plantar flexion of the ankle when the calf is squeezed.

7. Sprain of the lateral ankle ligaments

8. Inversion of the supinated, plantar flexed foot produces 85% of ankle sprains.

9. The examiner stabilizes the distal tibia with one hand and then grasps the posterior heel with the opposite hand. The examiner applies anterior force in an attempt to displace the talus anteriorly.

10. A "clunk" and increased laxity of the ankle are noted when the examiner attempts to displace the talus anteriorly.

11. Grade I: no laxity, minimal pain with range of motion, and mild swelling.

Grade II: mild to moderate laxity, soft-tissue swelling, and slight laxity on anterior drawer and talar tilt tests.

Grade III: moderate to severe swelling and pain. The patient is usually unable to bear weight.

12. It is pain in the region of the metatarsophalangeal joints.

13. Morton neuroma is a perineural thickening of the common digital nerves of the second or third interspace of the foot.

14. The tarsal is a fibro-osseous tunnel formed by the flexor retinaculum or laciniate ligament, the medial wall of the calcaneus and talus, and the medial malleolus.

15. Patients with tarsal tunnel syndrome complain of plantar numbness, diffuse plantar burning sensations, and tingling pain that increases with activity and decreases with rest.

16. The four conditions include the following: tendon rupture, calcaneal bursitis, rheumatoid nodules, and urate tophi.

17. The three muscles of the anterior compartment include the tibialis anterior, extensor hallucis longus, and extensor digitorum longus.

18. This damages the common peroneal nerve. The most noticeable deficits to result from such an injury are weakness in extension (dorsiflexion) of the ankle and a dragging of the toes ("foot drop") in walking.

19. Inversion stress tests the lateral collateral ligament and eversion tests the medial collateral or deltoid ligament.

20. The mechanism of the ankle sprain leads to avulsions of the malleoli or tarsal bones.

21. There is an impairment of the blood supply to the lower extremities. It may be from atheromatous narrowing of the artery, from thrombosis, or much more rarely, from cardiac embolism. It presents as intermittent claudication in either or both legs. The pain could be in the buttocks, thighs, or legs. The pain goes away when the patient rests and resumes after a short distance walking. The cycle repeats. The pulse is absent or very weak in the foot, knee, or femoral pulse locations. The skin is shiny and discolored with loss of hair from the foot. Nail bed may be bluish and the patient may complain of coldness in the foot. This has a 15:1 male predilection.

22. • Posterior tibial nerve and its branches
   • Tendons of the posterior tibialis
   • Flexor digitorum longus
   • Flexor hallucis
   • Posterior tibial artery and vein

Chapter 13

1. • Incoherent presentation of pain localization and stable symptoms.
   • Inability to influence pain and function by movement or change of position.
   • Relapse of a preexisting condition and lack of response in previous episodes.
   • Work dissatisfaction.
   • Problems of communicating realistic treatment goals.
   • Poor self-perceived prognoses with unrealistically high perception of impairment.

2. • Re-experiencing the trauma (recurrent and intrusive thoughts and dreams)
   • Avoidance and emotional numbing (avoiding reminders of traumatic event)
   • Hyperarousal (exaggerated startle response)
   • Symptoms persist at least one month and associated with significant distress or impairment in function.
   • To make a conclusive diagnosis, malingering needs to be ruled out.

3. *Malingering* is the conscious misrepresentation of thoughts, feelings, and facts and is a condition in which symptoms and signs associated with pain or dysfunction are either partially or entirely feigned for secondary gain.

4. The malingering diagnosis is based on the preponderance of positive malingering test findings and the absence of findings from traditional neuro orthopedic tests. Any positive findings must be further correlated

with the medical history of the patient. It is the constellation of positive malingering tests, normal findings in traditional tests, and medical history discrepancies that form the malingering diagnosis.

5. 1. Anxiety
   2. Psychiatric hallucination
   3. Increased tension in the muscles, with associated inadequate circulation and the accumulation of metabolic byproducts (lactic acid)
   4. Hysteria with conversion reactions
6. 1. Dramatic urgency for an appointment that is not justified by the severity of the disease
   2. A list (in writing) of complaints so long and detailed that no fact is left out
   3. Multiple test results, including electrocardiogram (ECG), electromyelogram (EMG), electroencephalogram (EEG), barium enema, upper gastrointestinal (GI) series, computed tomography (CT) scans, myelograms, and magnetic resonance imaging (MRI), with no positive findings
   4. Patient demands to review the laboratory data first to determine the cause of the symptoms; patient highlights any minor abnormalities
   5. Preoccupation with future disability from minor physical changes
   6. Those who accompany the patient may be entirely separated from the patient's condition or intensely supportive; the companion may be highlighting every abnormality, often using the pronoun *we* during the description of tests or treatments
   7. Inability of the patient to relax during the examination
   8. Marked theatrical responses to questions concerning pain
   9. The patient often holds onto the physician during the examination, as a gesture of seeking support.
7. 1. The simulation of a nonexistent illness or injury
   2. The voluntary provocation, aggravation, and protraction of disease by artificial means
   3. False allegations about the existence of some malady or injury.
8. The examiner applies finger pressure to the mastoid process. The pressure is gradually increased until the patient states that it is becoming noticeably uncomfortable. This point is an indication of that patient's pain threshold, which varies from patient to patient. The threshold gives the examiner an idea if this patient has

a low, high, or moderate pain threshold. The threshold is not to be used specifically as a criterion for malingering. Identifying a patient's pain threshold will quantify discomfort in this patient and applies to this patient only.

9. Mannkopf sign
10. The patient rotates the trunk. The examiner ensures that the pelvis rotates as well. If the patient indicates that this causes lower back pain, malingering should be suspected. *The lumbar spine is not moving.* Instead, the whole spine is rotated from the hips and thighs.
11. The patient is instructed to close their eyes. The clinician then uses a sharp instrument. The limb that has the possible anesthesia is pricked with the sharp object. The patient is then directed to answer "yes" if a pinprick is felt on the skin or "no" if not. If the patient remains silent, that is the correct response.
12. The Marcus Gunn sign
13. It is the term used to describe pain along the distribution of the obturator nerve caused by compression of the nerve, and is thought to be a specific symptom of an obturator hernia.
14. **Mode of onset:**

    Abrupt, precipitating event and fast progression to maximum symptom severity and disability.

    Clinical signs:

    Signs incongruent with organic disease, distractibility and variability, multiple abnormal movements, increased movement with attention to the affected body part, deliberate slowness of movement, entrainment, co-activation, association with false weakness, sensory loss, and pain and unresponsiveness to drugs for organic movement disorders, response to placebo drugs and suggestion.
15. Hoover sign is helpful in differentiating between organic and hysterical paralysis. When a supine patient is directed to lift the paralyzed or affected one leg, it is normal for the patient to unconsciously press the heel of the unaffected leg against the examination table. In organic hemiplegia, this downward pressure is accentuated on the healthy side as the patient attempts to raise the paretic leg. If the examiner places a hand under the heel, this pressure can be felt. In malingering, there will be no, or very little, pressure on the opposite side of the affection as the patient attempts to raise the involved extremity.

INDEX

I

I

I

Perfect your testing and assessment skills with the companion DVD!

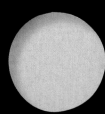

COMPANION DVD

ILLUSTRATED
Orthopedic Physical Assessment
Third Edition

MOSBY
ELSEVIER

RONALD C. EVANS

WIN/MAC

999604632X

Copyright © 2009, 2005, 2001 by Mosby, Inc.,
an affiliate of Elsevier Inc.
All rights reserved.
Produced in the United States of America.

TRY IT NOW!

Use the enclosed DVD to see how to perform each assessment test in the book to achieve accurate diagnoses.

Simply insert the DVD into your computer or DVD player to get started!

- Watch videos of all 237 orthopedic tests in the book.
- Listen to voiceover instructions and commentary from the book's author, Ron Evans, DC, FACO, FICC.
- Gain a depth of understanding that isn't possible with still photos or drawings.
- See the many subtleties and nuances of assessment — giving you more confidence in testing!

MOSBY
ELSEVIER